Modules for
Basic
Nursing
Skills

Seventh Edition

Janice Rider Ellis, PhD, RN
Professor Emeritus and Nursing Education Consultant
Shoreline Community College
Seattle, WA

Patricia M. Bentz, EdD, RN
Professor Emeritus
Shoreline Community College
Seattle, WA

. Lippincott Williams & Wilkins
a Wolters Kluwer business
Philadelphia · Baltimore · New York · London
Buenos Aires · Hong Kong · Sydney · Tokyo

Senior Acquisitions Editor: Elizabeth Nieginski
Managing Editor: Michelle Clarke
Development Editor: Deedie McMahon
Senior Project Editor: Debra Schiff
Director of Nursing Production: Helen Ewan
Senior Managing Editor/Production: Erika Kors
Art Director: Joan Wendt
Manufacturing Manager: Karin Duffield
Indexer: Angie Wiley
Compositor: Circle Graphics
Printer: RRD-Willard

7th Edition

9 8 7 6 5 4 3 2 1

Library of Congress Cataloging-in-Publication Data
Ellis, Janice Rider.
  Modules for basic nursing skills / Janice Rider Ellis, Patricia M. Bentz.
—7th ed.
    p. ; cm.
  Includes bibliographical references and index.
  ISBN-10: 0-7817-5380-5
  1. Nursing—Outlines, syllabi, etc. 2. Nursing—Problems, exercises, etc.
I. Bentz, Patricia M. II. Title.
  [DNLM: 1. Nursing Care—Programmed Instruction. 2. Nursing
—methods—Programmed Instruction. 3. Nursing Process—Programmed
Instruction. WY 18.2 E47m 2006]
RT52.E44 2006
610.73'076—dc22

                                                                    2005029796

LWW.com

Our special dedication of this work goes to
our longtime friend and colleague
Elizabeth A. Nowlis, EdD, RN,
who wrote with us through six prior editions.
Her joyful approach to nursing, teaching, and all of life
enriched those who knew her and is a lasting legacy
of a life well-lived.
This one's for you, Betsy!

Contributors

Andrea S. Breedlove, MSN, RN, FNP
Nursing Instructor
University of Arkansas at Little Rock
Little Rock, Arkansas

Michelle Byrne, PhD, CNOR, RN
Associate Professor
North Georgia College and State University
Dahlonega, Georgia

Virginia Dare Domico, DSN, RN
Associate Professor
Georgia Baptist College of Nursing
Atlanta, Georgia

Marie Kerr Emery, MSN, APRN, BC, RN
Nurse Practitioner, Family Practice
Toccoa Clinic
Toccoa, Georgia

Valerie S. Eschiti, MSN, CHTP, AHN, BC, RN
Assistant Professor
Wilson School of Nursing
Midwestern State University
Wichita Falls, Texas

Cynthia Kay Gilbert, MS, RN
Associate Professor
University of Arkansas at Little Rock
Little Rock, Arkansas

Mary Grabowski, BSN, RN
Clinical Associate
Puget Sound Blood Center
Seattle, Washington

Nancy Johnson Stahl, MSN, RN
Assistant Professor, Assistant Department Head
  of Nursing
North Georgia College and State University
Dahlonega, Georgia

Dee Townsend-McCall, BSN, RN
Transfusion Nurse Specialist
Children's Hospital and Regional Medical Center
Seattle, Washington

Trish Wittig, MSN, RN
Nursing Instructor
Department of Health Service Occupations
Waukesha County Technical College
Pewaukee, Wisconsin

Reviewers

We would like to thank the following individuals for their reviews of the manuscript at various stages and for their many useful suggestions.

Teresa Aprigliano, EdD, RN
Director RN/Dual Degree/LPN-BS Program
Molloy College
Rockville Centre, New York

Linda Berry, PhD, MN, BN, RN
Associate Professor
Eastern Michigan University
Ypsilanti, Michigan

Teresa Britt, MSN, RN
Assistant Clinical Professor
University of Memphis, Loewenberg School
of Nursing
Memphis, Tennessee

Lou Ann Boose, MSN, BSN
Associate Professor of Nursing
Harrisburg Area Community College
Harrisburg, Pennsylvania

Betty L. Hanrahan, MSN, CNS, CWCN, RN, BC, ARNP
Regional Director Wound Programs
Kindred Hospitals West Region
Westminster, California
Co-Director Wound Management Education
Program
Department of Continuing Nursing Education
University of Washington
Seattle, Washington

Nicole Harder, MPA, RN
Coordinator, Learning Laboratories
University of Manitoba, Helen Glass Centre
for Nursing
Winnipeg, Manitoba, Canada

Catherine Hasson
Nursing Professor
Drexel University, College of Nursing and
Health Professions
Philadelphia, Pennsylvania

Dorothy G. Herron, PhD, RN, CS
Assistant Professor
University of Maryland, School of Nursing
Baltimore, Maryland

Janet T. Ihlenfeld, PhD, RN
Nursing Professor
D'Youville College
Buffalo, New York

Barbara A. Ihrke, PhD, RN
Associate Professor of Nursing
Indiana Wesleyan University
Marion, Indiana

Rosie Jackson, MSN, BSN, RN
Nursing Instructor
Hinds Community College
Jackson, Mississippi

Patricia T. Ketcham, MSN, RN
Adjunct Assistant Professor, Nursing Laboratory
Manager
Oakland University, School of Nursing
Rochester, Michigan

Trudy L. Klein, MS, BS, RN
Associate Dean
Walla Walla College, School of Nursing
College Place, Washington

Jeanie Krause-Bachand, EdD, MSN, RN, BC
Associate Professor
York College of Pennsylvania
York, Pennsylvania

Eloise Lewis, MSN, RN
Assistant Professor
Ivy Tech State College
Columbus, Indiana

Denise Marshall, MEd, BSN, RN
Department Head of Nursing
Worwic Community College
Salisbury, Maryland

Acknowledgments

would like to acknowledge the nursing faculty and staff with whom we have worked throughout our careers for their commitment to the development of new nursing professionals. Their willingness to be teachers and learners together with us and with students has created a climate for excellence in nursing education.

We appreciate all the efforts of the staff at Lippincott Williams & Wilkins: This has been a prodigious effort and it would not have been possible without the help of many different individuals but a few deserve special mention. We owe special thanks to Deedie McMahon, who continued editing for us when she was ready to relax into retirement; Michelle Clark, who coordinated photographers, artists, and the multitude of details needed to create a text this varied; and Debra Schiff, who labored with us through getting everything together in final printed pages.

But perhaps most importantly, we want to acknowledge those who provided the personal support needed for so great a project. Patricia Bentz especially acknowledges her family and those special friends who provided support, patience, and a listening ear throughout the development and writing of this text. Janice Ellis acknowledges her husband Ivan, whose support has been a constant river keeping her boat afloat.

Using the Modules

The seventh edition of *Modules for Basic Nursing Skills* continues to provide a resource for nursing students to learn basic skills and procedures. We have used a nursing-process–oriented, self-instructional approach that has proven valuable in previous editions, while improving visual appeal through the use of full-color photos and illustrations.

In preparing this edition, we have examined our instructions and directions from a student's standpoint. We have added definitions and clarifications for the new language of healthcare that students are learning at the same time they are mastering skills. We recognize that the formal, official terms used for equipment and skills are not always the same as the "shorthand" that students will hear in a clinical setting. Therefore, in many instances we have provided both sets of terms.

As more students enter the university setting with varied educational backgrounds, language and reading levels become ever more important. In a skills text, perhaps more than anywhere else, the focus must be on clear, straightforward language. We are grateful for the responses of our students in helping us with this task.

COMPREHENSIVE SKILLS COVERAGE

There are now 53 modules, each containing multiple skills that are related. Because programs vary considerably from state to state and from institution to institution, we have tried to make it possible to use them in whatever order meets the curricular needs of the program.

ORGANIZATION

The modules are organized into nine units that reflect broad concepts of nursing care. This structured presentation will help students understand how individual skills relate to their own practice of nursing. The first two units focus on concepts and skills that students must master in order to provide basic care. In Unit 3, the modules move through assessment skills, and then on to more complex skills. As in the previous edition, each module is self-contained so that skills can be omitted or reordered according to the needs of particular programs.

SELF-INSTRUCTIONAL FORMAT

By consistently emphasizing the nursing process and appropriately highlighting rationales (with the symbol "**R:**" throughout the text, and in a second column in the Implementation sections), the format of the modules focuses on the student's practice and mastery of skills and procedures. The elaborate program of features is designed to encourage understanding, independent learning, and self-instruction.

Module 1, An Approach to Nursing Skills, provides the foundation for all that follows. It places technical skills in the broader context of nursing competence and the patient's needs and rights. The goal is that students see the common thread of a problem-solving, nursing-process approach to each skill. The authors challenge students to formulate their own approach as they encounter the need for skills not included in the modules. The framework can be the student's own building block for an evolving practice of nursing.

Throughout the modules we have referred to the recipient of nursing care as a patient. The term *patient* is used by all hospitals and most ambulatory care facilities and by the regulatory agencies, both governmental and voluntary, that oversee them. Our experience is that the recipients of care refer to themselves as patients and prefer to use that term. We made our choice for very practical reasons. Most students learn their skills in hospitals and care settings that use the term patient. We also prefer to call recipients of care by the term they themselves use. While the term *resident* is used in long-term care facilities and by their regulatory bodies, it is only pertinent to a setting where the person is making his or her home. Throughout the home health arena and in mental health settings, the term *client* is commonly used. We acknowledge that many individuals prefer to use the term client in all settings for a variety of reasons. Students can easily adapt to use other terminology that is in use where they are practicing or which is used by their nursing program.

SKILL MODULE CONTENTS

Each module includes the following features, designed to assist students to approach each module in a logical and organized fashion.

LIST OF SKILLS

Each module begins with a list of skills that are found within the module. This facilitates the student's self-directed study.

PREREQUISITES

The list of prerequisites lets the student know what other modules and significant material are essential to successful completion of the particular module. This information is especially helpful when the order of modules is adjusted to meet the needs of individual nursing programs. It can also be used advantageously by the student who wishes to prepare for a particular patient-care situation.

OVERALL OBJECTIVE(S) AND LEARNING OUTCOMES

A general statement of the overall objective(s) concisely describes what the student can expect to learn in the module.

The list of learning outcomes previews the important steps and concepts in the skill and indicates what basic knowledge and application of knowledge are required in addition to psychomotor skills.

KEY TERMS

A list of key terms for each skill is provided. These terms are defined in the glossary at the back of the text and are discussed within each module, as well.

NURSING DIAGNOSES

Nursing diagnoses relevant to the particular skill are presented in a separate display. These are provided in standardized NANDA-I terminology. This reinforces for beginning students the importance of understanding nursing language.

DELEGATION

Today's healthcare environment requires that nurses appropriately delegate care to families and to assistive personnel. Module 1 introduces the concept of delegation for the nurse. The concept is defined and the student helped to understand the essential elements in determining whether a particular patient care task can be delegated. In each module, the student will find a discussion of this important concept and of the factors that must be considered when determining whether to delegate the skills addressed within the context of the module.

MODULE CORE

The discussion of each procedure includes necessary background information and step-by-step instructions, with carefully chosen photographs and technically precise illustrations. The illustrations are designed to help the students as they work through the module independently.

Skills are presented in a **nursing process format** when the skill is one that is used with patients and when the nursing process is appropriate to the skill. The steps in the process—**Assessment, Analysis, Planning, Implementation,** and **Evaluation**—are explained in Module 1 and clearly delineated by headings in subsequent modules. This emphasis reinforces for students the fact that nursing process is relevant to practice. New to this edition is an emphasis on developing patient-centered outcomes during planning. Clearly identified outcomes help the student to focus and provide the basis for effective evaluation.

Documentation is included with every skill. The increasing emphasis on documentation for both evaluative and legal reasons makes the learning of correct documentation essential. Our premise is that although systems differ in how documentation is done, what needs to be documented is fairly standard. We have indicated what needs to be included in documentation as well as some specific examples of flow sheets to help students make the transition to the record system they will be asked to use.

Rationale for the specific actions that are part of the procedure is introduced throughout the discussion by the use of the symbol "**R:**" in the assessment, analysis, planning, evaluation, and documentation sections and a *two-column format* in the implementation section, with the left-hand column describing the nursing actions and the right-hand column explaining the rationale.

Because the approach to many skills is the same, whenever possible a general procedure for a group of specific procedures has been identified. The purpose of this is to facilitate the student's ability to transfer basic principles from one situation to another. We have tried to do this in a way that does not create confusion and that can be followed when practicing the skill.

SPECIAL FEATURES

Throughout the modules an icon provides emphasis for actions that require attention to hand hygiene. Detailed information on infection control is found in several different modules. Module 4 presents the basic requirements for infection control with an emphasis on Standard Precautions and effective hand hygiene. Isolation precautions are presented in Module 23. Actions required for sterile technique are presented in Modules 24 and 25.

A second major emphasis is safety. An ▲ icon emphasizes actions taken to further safety goals. Both the Joint Commission on the Accreditation of Healthcare Organizations (JCAHO) and the Institute of Medicine have provided the impetus for the development of programs supporting safe practice in all care settings. Some of these include the JCAHO standard of using two iden-

tifiers before performing any treatment or invasive procedure. The foundations of safety are provided in Module 3, where basic body mechanics that protect the nurse are discussed and in Module 5, where overall safety in the healthcare environment is presented. Safe practice in the context of every skill is emphasized.

REFERENCES

The references cited are to research data regarding the skill or the recommendations of an authoritative agency such as the Centers for Disease Control and Prevention (CDC). The most recent research is cited. In the case of skills, this research may be older than expected. For example, the information on infection control processes are based on the Guidelines originally published in 1994 and still in use throughout the United States. The CDC changes recommendations only when their decision-making bodies determine that the new data warrant a change.

Unfortunately, there is little research data to support many of the nursing techniques used. Therefore, you will also note an emphasis within the modules on consulting policies and procedures in place in specific institutions. These are generally established by groups of nurses working together with legal as well as healthcare goals in mind. Learning to use the official policy and procedure manual will be an asset both to the student and to the practicing nurse.

LEARNING ACTIVITIES

The learning activities provide additional guidance to the student about what steps to take in order to accomplish the desired outcomes. Note that each module directs the student to prepare as if planning to teach the skill to others. Because teaching is so integral to the nursing role, we believe students should consider that from the start. They must be prepared to teach other nurses, families, and assistive personnel.

LEARNING TOOLS AND CRITICAL THINKING EXERCISES

Skill development for the nurse must constantly be framed within the context of the individual patient. In order to focus on this [...] critical thinking [...] cises assist the stud[...] text of providing nu[...] Students are asked to [...] has problematic aspects [...] ities, or approaches that w[...] particular patient. There are [...] situations. They might form t[...] for a written paper, or for person[...]

SELF-QUIZ

A self-test is provided at the end of each [...] students to test their mastery of the m[...] module. The quizzes may also be used by in[...] evaluation purposes. Answers to quizzes are p[...] the end of the text.

GLOSSARY

The key terms in the vocabulary lists are defined in th[...] glossary at the back of the text. The glossary is a convenient reference source for students.

The glossary defines terms within the context in which they are used in nursing and healthcare. This is particularly useful for the beginning student who often finds that words have special connotations in nursing and healthcare that are not included in the traditional dictionary definition.

INDEX

An index is provided at the back of the text.

CD-ROM PERFORMANCE CHECKLISTS

A new feature of this edition is the CD-ROM accompa[...] nying the text. It contains Performance Checklists f[...] each skill that match the skills instructions. They ca[...] used for a quick review or be printed out and use[...] tool for self or instructor evaluation. To facilitate [...] and evaluation, all steps of each procedure, i[...] those that are first presented as part of a gen[...] dure, are outlined in the Performance Chec[...]

Using the Modules

The seventh edition of *Modules for Basic Nursing Skills* continues to provide a resource for nursing students to learn basic skills and procedures. We have used a nursing-process–oriented, self-instructional approach that has proven valuable in previous editions, while improving visual appeal through the use of full-color photos and illustrations.

In preparing this edition, we have examined our instructions and directions from a student's standpoint. We have added definitions and clarifications for the new language of healthcare that students are learning at the same time they are mastering skills. We recognize that the formal, official terms used for equipment and skills are not always the same as the "shorthand" that students will hear in a clinical setting. Therefore, in many instances we have provided both sets of terms.

As more students enter the university setting with varied educational backgrounds, language and reading levels become ever more important. In a skills text, perhaps more than anywhere else, the focus must be on clear, straightforward language. We are grateful for the responses of our students in helping us with this task.

COMPREHENSIVE SKILLS COVERAGE

There are now 53 modules, each containing multiple skills that are related. Because programs vary considerably from state to state and from institution to institution, we have tried to make it possible to use them in whatever order meets the curricular needs of the program.

ORGANIZATION

The modules are organized into nine units that reflect broad concepts of nursing care. This structured presentation will help students understand how individual skills relate to their own practice of nursing. The first two units focus on concepts and skills that students must master in order to provide basic care. In Unit 3, the modules move through assessment skills, and then on to more complex skills. As in the previous edition, each module is self-contained so that skills can be omitted or reordered according to the needs of particular programs.

SELF-INSTRUCTIONAL FORMAT

By consistently emphasizing the nursing process and appropriately highlighting rationales (with the symbol "**R:**" throughout the text, and in a second column in the Implementation sections), the format of the modules focuses on the student's practice and mastery of skills and procedures. The elaborate program of features is designed to encourage understanding, independent learning, and self-instruction.

Module 1, An Approach to Nursing Skills, provides the foundation for all that follows. It places technical skills in the broader context of nursing competence and the patient's needs and rights. The goal is that students see the common thread of a problem-solving, nursing-process approach to each skill. The authors challenge students to formulate their own approach as they encounter the need for skills not included in the modules. The framework can be the student's own building block for an evolving practice of nursing.

Throughout the modules we have referred to the recipient of nursing care as a patient. The term *patient* is used by all hospitals and most ambulatory care facilities and by the regulatory agencies, both governmental and voluntary, that oversee them. Our experience is that the recipients of care refer to themselves as patients and prefer to use that term. We made our choice for very practical reasons. Most students learn their skills in hospitals and care settings that use the term patient. We also prefer to call recipients of care by the term they themselves use. While the term *resident* is used in long-term care facilities and by their regulatory bodies, it is only pertinent to a setting where the person is making his or her home. Throughout the home health arena and in mental health settings, the term *client* is commonly used. We acknowledge that many individuals prefer to use the term client in all settings for a variety of reasons. Students can easily adapt to use other terminology that is in use where they are practicing or which is used by their nursing program.

SKILL MODULE CONTENTS

Each module includes the following features, designed to assist students to approach each module in a logical and organized fashion.

LIST OF SKILLS

Each module begins with a list of skills that are found within the module. This facilitates the student's self-directed study.

PREREQUISITES

The list of prerequisites lets the student know what other modules and significant material are essential to successful completion of the particular module. This information is especially helpful when the order of modules is adjusted to meet the needs of individual nursing programs. It can also be used advantageously by the student who wishes to prepare for a particular patient-care situation.

OVERALL OBJECTIVE(S) AND LEARNING OUTCOMES

A general statement of the overall objective(s) concisely describes what the student can expect to learn in the module.

The list of learning outcomes previews the important steps and concepts in the skill and indicates what basic knowledge and application of knowledge are required in addition to psychomotor skills.

KEY TERMS

A list of key terms for each skill is provided. These terms are defined in the glossary at the back of the text and are discussed within each module, as well.

NURSING DIAGNOSES

Nursing diagnoses relevant to the particular skill are presented in a separate display. These are provided in standardized NANDA-I terminology. This reinforces for beginning students the importance of understanding nursing language.

DELEGATION

Today's healthcare environment requires that nurses appropriately delegate care to families and to assistive personnel. Module 1 introduces the concept of delegation for the nurse. The concept is defined and the student helped to understand the essential elements in determining whether a particular patient care task can be delegated. In each module, the student will find a discussion of this important concept and of the factors that must be considered when determining whether to delegate the skills addressed within the context of the module.

MODULE CORE

The discussion of each procedure includes necessary background information and step-by-step instructions, with carefully chosen photographs and technically precise illustrations. The illustrations are designed to help the students as they work through the module independently.

Skills are presented in a **nursing process format** when the skill is one that is used with patients and when the nursing process is appropriate to the skill. The steps in the process—**Assessment, Analysis, Planning, Implementation,** and **Evaluation**—are explained in Module 1 and clearly delineated by headings in subsequent modules. This emphasis reinforces for students the fact that nursing process is relevant to practice. New to this edition is an emphasis on developing patient-centered outcomes during planning. Clearly identified outcomes help the student to focus and provide the basis for effective evaluation.

Documentation is included with every skill. The increasing emphasis on documentation for both evaluative and legal reasons makes the learning of correct documentation essential. Our premise is that although systems differ in how documentation is done, what needs to be documented is fairly standard. We have indicated what needs to be included in documentation as well as some specific examples of flow sheets to help students make the transition to the record system they will be asked to use.

Rationale for the specific actions that are part of the procedure is introduced throughout the discussion by the use of the symbol "**R:**" in the assessment, analysis, planning, evaluation, and documentation sections and a *two-column format* in the implementation section, with the left-hand column describing the nursing actions and the right-hand column explaining the rationale.

Because the approach to many skills is the same, whenever possible a general procedure for a group of specific procedures has been identified. The purpose of this is to facilitate the student's ability to transfer basic principles from one situation to another. We have tried to do this in a way that does not create confusion and that can be followed when practicing the skill.

SPECIAL FEATURES

Throughout the modules an icon provides emphasis for actions that require attention to hand hygiene. Detailed information on infection control is found in several different modules. Module 4 presents the basic requirements for infection control with an emphasis on Standard Precautions and effective hand hygiene. Isolation precautions are presented in Module 23. Actions required for sterile technique are presented in Modules 24 and 25.

A second major emphasis is safety. An icon emphasizes actions taken to further safety goals. Both the Joint Commission on the Accreditation of Healthcare Organizations (JCAHO) and the Institute of Medicine have provided the impetus for the development of programs supporting safe practice in all care settings. Some of these include the JCAHO standard of using two identifiers before performing any treatment or invasive procedure. The foundations of safety are provided in Module 3, where basic body mechanics that protect the nurse are discussed and in Module 5, where overall safety in the healthcare environment is presented. Safe practice in the context of every skill is emphasized.

REFERENCES

The references cited are to research data regarding the skill or the recommendations of an authoritative agency such as the Centers for Disease Control and Prevention (CDC). The most recent research is cited. In the case of skills, this research may be older than expected. For example, the information on infection control processes are based on the Guidelines originally published in 1994 and still in use throughout the United States. The CDC changes recommendations only when their decision-making bodies determine that the new data warrant a change.

Unfortunately, there is little research data to support many of the nursing techniques used. Therefore, you will also note an emphasis within the modules on consulting policies and procedures in place in specific institutions. These are generally established by groups of nurses working together with legal as well as healthcare goals in mind. Learning to use the official policy and procedure manual will be an asset both to the student and to the practicing nurse.

LEARNING ACTIVITIES

The learning activities provide additional guidance to the student about what steps to take in order to accomplish the desired outcomes. Note that each module directs the student to prepare as if planning to teach the skill to others. Because teaching is so integral to the nursing role, we believe students should consider that from the start. They must be prepared to teach other nurses, families, and assistive personnel.

LEARNING TOOLS AND CRITICAL THINKING EXERCISES

Skill development for the nurse must constantly be framed within the context of the individual patient. In order to focus on this important concept, we have added critical thinking exercises to each module. These exercises assist the student in placing the skills into the context of providing nursing care for each unique patient. Students are asked to consider a patient situation that has problematic aspects and to determine needs, priorities, or approaches that would be appropriate for the particular patient. There are no "right" answers to these situations. They might form the basis for a discussion, for a written paper, or for personal thoughtful study.

SELF-QUIZ

A self-test is provided at the end of each module to allow students to test their mastery of the material in the module. The quizzes may also be used by instructors for evaluation purposes. Answers to quizzes are provided at the end of the text.

GLOSSARY

The key terms in the vocabulary lists are defined in the glossary at the back of the text. The glossary is a convenient reference source for students.

The glossary defines terms within the context in which they are used in nursing and healthcare. This is particularly useful for the beginning student who often finds that words have special connotations in nursing and healthcare that are not included in the traditional dictionary definition.

INDEX

An index is provided at the back of the text.

CD-ROM PERFORMANCE CHECKLISTS

A new feature of this edition is the CD-ROM accompanying the text. It contains Performance Checklists for each skill that match the skills instructions. They can be used for a quick review or be printed out and used as a tool for self or instructor evaluation. To facilitate review and evaluation, all steps of each procedure, including those that are first presented as part of a general procedure, are outlined in the Performance Checklist.

Acknowledgments

We would like to acknowledge the nursing faculty and staff with whom we have worked throughout our careers for their commitment to the development of new nursing professionals. Their willingness to be teachers and learners together with us and with students has created a climate for excellence in nursing education.

We appreciate all the efforts of the staff at Lippincott Williams & Wilkins: This has been a prodigious effort and it would not have been possible without the help of many different individuals but a few deserve special mention. We owe special thanks to Deedie McMahon, who continued editing for us when she was ready to relax into retirement; Michelle Clark, who coordinated photographers, artists, and the multitude of details needed to create a text this varied; and Debra Schiff, who labored with us through getting everything together in final printed pages.

But perhaps most importantly, we want to acknowledge those who provided the personal support needed for so great a project. Patricia Bentz especially acknowledges her family and those special friends who provided support, patience, and a listening ear throughout the development and writing of this text. Janice Ellis acknowledges her husband Ivan, whose support has been a constant river keeping her boat afloat.

Contents

UNIT 7

Supporting Oxygenation and Circulation, 587

UNIT 8

Performing Special Therapeutic and Supportive Procedures, 693

UNIT 9

Administering Medications and Intravenous Therapy, 819

U N I T 1

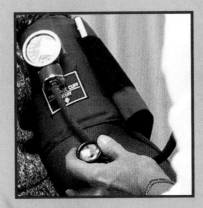

Foundations for Nursing Skills

MODULES

1 An Approach to Nursing Skills

2 Documentation

3 Basic Body Mechanics

4 Basic Infection Control

5 Safety in the Healthcare Environment

MODULE
1

An Approach to Nursing Skills

CONCEPTS INCLUDED IN THIS MODULE

Patients' Rights
Evidence-Based Nursing Practice
Delegation
The Nursing Process
Critical Thinking
Technical Competence
Methods for Developing Technical Competence
Using a Psychomotor Taxonomy for Self-Assessment

KEY TERMS

advocate
analysis
assessment
communication
confidentiality
consent
critical thinking
dexterity
dignity
documentation
ethical rights
evaluation
health status
Health Insurance
    Portability and
    Accountability
    Act (HIPAA)
implementation

implied consent
informed consent
legal rights
mental practice
nursing diagnosis
nursing process
ombudsman
organization
physical practice
planning
privacy
respect
sanctions
self-care
self-determination
technical
    competence

OVERALL OBJECTIVE

▸ To understand how patients' rights, the nursing process, and critical thinking relate to performing nursing skills with technical competence and safety.

LEARNING OUTCOMES

The student will be able to
1. Support and maintain patients' rights when implementing nursing skills.
2. Use the nursing process as a framework for approaching skills.
3. Incorporate critical thinking into each step of the nursing process in the performance of nursing skills.
4. Establish mechanisms to develop technical competence in learning each skill, including the development of correct technique, organization, dexterity, and speed.

Nursing is more than just performing skills. The nursing process provides a framework for the total role of the nurse and for all nursing activities. Concerns for patients' rights, **communication,** and the nursing process should be part of your approach to any nursing skill or intervention. Technical competence is important, but it must be situated within the broad context of the nursing role.

Although each nursing skill is presented separately for learning purposes, no single nursing skill exists outside the context of the individual patient and the specific situation. Nursing skills are most valuable when the rights of the patient, communication, the framework of the nursing process, and the value of technical competence are kept in mind.

PATIENTS' RIGHTS

The patient in the healthcare system has both ethical and **legal rights.** Legal rights include rights that are supported by law and would be upheld in court. **Ethical rights** are those that the healthcare community recognizes as important to the patient's well-being but may not be included in actual laws. Various groups, such as the American Hospital Association, individual healthcare agencies, and state nurses' associations, have adopted statements related to their view of patients' rights. These statements differ slightly because each focuses on the healthcare services provided by a particular agency or group. This module presents some general concepts usually included in discussions of patients' rights and focuses on how you can support these in your nursing practice.

The nursing student must approach every patient with both ethical and legal rights in mind. Failure to provide ethical rights can result in ethical **sanctions** (penalties), such as reprimand or even termination. Failure to provide legal rights can result in legal action against the care provider and the institution, resulting in major fines and payment of monetary damages to the patient.

RIGHTS SUPPORTED BY LAW

Patients' rights either are specifically stated in the laws of a particular state or jurisdiction or have consistently been supported in court.

RIGHT TO SELF-DETERMINATION/CONSENT

The patient has the right to make personal decisions regarding health care. This is often called the right to **consent.** All adults older than 18 years (21 years in some states) have the right to make their own decisions about health care. Only those who have been declared incompetent by a court (and who therefore have a court-appointed guardian) and those who are unconscious do not have this personal right. Advanced age is never a valid reason for ignoring the right to **self-determination.** For children, parents or guardians exercise these rights. Even young children, however, are often included in the decision-making process. This enhances their ability to participate in care, even though final authority rests with the parents or guardians.

Some minors (those under the legal age of consent) do have the right to self-determination. Examples include those who are considered to be emancipated because they are married and those who are living independently of parents as prescribed by law. In most states, minors can give consent for care related to reproduction, such as birth control, abortion, and treatment for sexually transmitted diseases. The facility where you practice should have specific policies that are based on applicable state law and court decisions to guide you in knowing who can legally give consent for care. One of your responsibilities is to review these policies.

Self-determination means that the patient has the right to accept or refuse any aspect of care and the right to decide whether to use the healthcare system at all, to use any part of the system, to ask for adaptations of the system, or to totally refuse the care available. It is the care provider's responsibility to give sufficient information to enable the patient to make an informed decision with an adequate understanding of related consequences. This is called **informed consent.** For example, if you ask the patient to consent to having a procedure such as an enema, you are responsible for making sure the patient understands the purpose of the enema and the possible consequences of not having it at that time. The patient's choice is then truly informed.

Sometimes consent is implied by the patient's previous actions or statements. When a patient consents to have surgery, there is **implied consent** to procedures and routines that are necessary for successful preparation for and recovery from the surgery. Although a patient is free at any time to change his or her mind with regard to the original procedure or to refuse any aspect of care, care proceeds on the basis of the implied consent. Another factor to be considered in such a situation is the patient's current **health status.** The individual who has just had surgery and is weakened and in pain is not in a position to make the best decisions about care. Thus, immediately after surgery, do not ask a patient if he or she is willing to turn. You say, "It is time to turn now." When you believe that pain medication is needed, you say, "It is time for your pain medication. It will help you to rest more comfortably and move as you need to." The patient does have the right to refuse the pain medication, but this seldom happens; the patient is interested in recovery and willing to accept the care provider's judgment as to the best action.

Consent is also implied by the patient's behavior in response to your statements. If you say, "It is time for your injection," and the patient rolls over to receive the injection, this is considered implied consent. If you offer a patient an oral medication, and he or she reaches for it, implied consent is present.

Decision making is shared between the care provider and the patient in some situations. The nurse instructs a new diabetic how to self-administer an insulin injection. At some point, the patient will need to perform the procedure independently. The nurse and patient will consider the progress the patient has made in learning, and together, they will agree on when the patient is ready to take on this responsibility. The nurse must agree that the patient has the necessary knowledge and skills, and the patient must agree that he or she is ready to undertake the task. For many situations in nursing, joint decision making is the most appropriate course of action.

Nurses and other care providers do make all the decisions for certain patients in certain situations. The patient who is disoriented as to time and place is sometimes unable to make decisions about safety and care. In such cases, the nurse and physician may consult and decide that, for example, raised side rails or other safety devices are necessary to prevent falls. For a newborn, nurses must decide on the amount of covering needed to maintain proper body temperature, the optimum position for safety, and other details of the infant's daily routine. If the patient is unconscious, all aspects of daily life must be controlled by those responsible for care. Decisions, such as the amount of a feeding, the length of time to lie in one position, and more technical aspects of care, must all be made by caregivers.

Correctly assessing the patient's ability to make decisions is an important responsibility for the nurse. Consult with your instructor and more experienced staff nurses to make sure you are providing maximum self-determination consistent with the patient's health status.

RIGHT TO INFORMATION ON WHICH TO BASE DECISIONS

The patient has the right to information on which to base decisions. This means that the nurse has an obligation to provide information related to the care that he or she is giving. When you measure blood pressure, you have an obligation to provide that reading if the patient asks. You do not, however, speak for others. Thus, when the patient asks what the medical diagnosis is, explain that this question should be directed to the physician who has made the diagnosis. It is then the physician's responsibility to discuss the diagnosis with the patient.

Care providers are sometimes reluctant to give information to patients for fear that it will upset them and increase their anxiety. This fear is usually groundless. Not knowing what is happening usually produces much more anxiety than knowing the truth. Fear of the unknown can be paralyzing to the patient. However, some people prefer not to have information about their health status because it would make them anxious. These people will simply avoid asking for information with which they are not ready to cope. Explaining what you are doing and why you are doing it can be an effective way to initiate a discussion with an individual who might otherwise not ask any questions.

In some instances, it is essential that patients have information regarding their current health status. A patient who is on a special diet, for example, must have sufficient information to manage **self-care.** In these instances, the nurse does not wait for the patient to ask questions but initiates discussion and specifically plans for health teaching based on the nurse's understanding of the knowledge needed by the patient.

RIGHT TO PRIVACY/CONFIDENTIALITY

The patient has the right to **confidentiality,** which means that personal and private information is carefully protected and held in confidence. In today's complex society, it is too easy for confidential information to reach those who have no need for it. Keep in mind that people can be harmed when information spreads unnecessarily. The information might change someone's attitude toward the patient, adversely affect the patient's employment opportunities, or result in financial loss, to name only a few possibilities. Even when no objective harm is demonstrated, the individual may feel exposed and vulnerable.

The **Health Insurance Portability and Accountability Act (HIPAA)** provides federal protection for individual health information under the privacy rule. This Act requires that institutions develop many safeguards for patient health information and that they provide instruction to all employees and others providing care about these safeguards. In addition, the act imposes penalties for healthcare agencies that fail in their responsibilities. You will need to know how this rule affects handling of patient information and records in the institution for which you work.

To maintain patient **privacy,** you should discuss information about a patient only with those who have a need for that information, such as nurses or the healthcare team. Discussions should take place only where others will not overhear you. An appropriate place might be a conference room, a patient's room, or the nurses' station. Even these places, however, may be inappropriate. For example, a nurses' station with several visitors at the desk might be too public. The cafeteria or elevator are never appropriate, and anywhere outside of the facility is inappropriate.

Written communication must also be safeguarded. Watch your patient care notes carefully, and do not leave them in patient's rooms or in the cafeteria. When you no longer need informal notes, shred them or discard them in the designated receptacle; do not leave them around on desks or counters. Patient's records, whether written or electronic, should be read only by those involved in care, those who have the patient's permission, and those involved in healthcare education. This means that you should not read a patient's chart or access a computer record if you do not have a valid need to know about that patient.

The use of patient information for learning experiences is valid but requires you to take special care. Do not identify patients by name when you choose them as subjects for a paper. Doing so would be a breach of confidentiality. When using a patient as an example in a class discussion, share only information pertinent to the topic. In most cases, information of a personal or private nature should not be shared.

When gathering information from a patient, explain that you will be sharing information you receive with the nurse assigned to the patient's care or with your instructor or both. You should not accept the responsibility of receiving confidences that cannot be shared in these ways. Doing so might put you in a situation that would be difficult to manage. If the patient asks you to promise to tell no one what is said, explain that you cannot make that promise. State that to plan appropriate care, you need to be free to discuss concerns with your instructor or the staff nurse. Then if the patient does not want the information shared in this way, per-

haps he or she should not share it with you. This does not indicate rejection of the patient but clearly outlines your obligations. The patient is then free to choose what to share, and you are free to consult with others as necessary.

RIGHT TO SAFE CARE

The patient has the right to expect that those who are providing care are knowledgeable and competent and will provide safe care. This means that the patient will receive safe care no matter who is providing it. Therefore, as a nursing student, you are held to the same standard of safety in care as a registered nurse. The patient cannot be expected to accept poor-quality care because you are learning. It is your responsibility to learn skills before you perform them, to know the necessary safety precautions, and to seek supervision. These actions safeguard the patient and protect you from legal action. To function safely at all times requires constant self-evaluation and a willingness to accept help and strive toward excellence.

RIGHTS SUPPORTED BY ETHICS

These rights are based on ethical beliefs as to what constitutes high-quality care. They are concerned with supporting optimum health for the patient, not merely with ensuring the absence of harm. In most cases, these rights would not be upheld by a court. If they were violated, recourse would come only from within the healthcare system or from community pressure.

RIGHT TO PERSONAL DIGNITY

The patient has the right to care that respects personal **dignity** and worth, unrestricted by considerations of nationality, race, creed, color, status, age, or gender. **Respect** for a person's dignity means that you treat each person as if he or she has intrinsic value at all times. Although this attitude is an internal characteristic, you give it meaning through your behavior.

One behavior that reflects this attitude is addressing the patient by the name he or she chooses. Therefore, the older person who prefers to be addressed as Mr. or Mrs. is so addressed, and the person who asks to be called by his or her first name or a nickname is addressed in that way. You also can show respect for the patient's dignity by displaying concern for privacy and modesty, for example, by knocking on closed doors, pulling curtains, and providing appropriate garments and draping. You show respect for individual dignity when you help a person have the best possible appearance through careful attention to hygiene and personal care. By doing so, you reflect your view of the patient as a human being who is valuable to you and to others.

The attitude you convey to patients by the manner in which you communicate with them is very important.

Listening to the thoughts and concerns of the patient conveys respect. By his or her attitude, an attentive, concerned listener says, "What you have to say is important." Explaining expectations and new situations so that the individual is more able to cope reflects your belief that the patient is capable of coping when given the opportunity and the necessary information.

Accepting the individual's feelings without judging them as right or wrong is another way of showing respect. Feelings are personal and arise from internal and external circumstances. Even though you may not understand a patient's feelings, you can accept them.

RIGHT TO INDIVIDUALIZED CARE

The patient has the right to individualized care related to his or her unique needs and lifestyle. Each of us is unique, with a different combination of physical attributes, thoughts, feelings, values, and beliefs. Care that is precisely uniform will fit no one precisely. Adaptations in care plans are made to provide for each patient's special needs and attributes. You might adapt a bathing method to respect a patient's attitude about modesty. You might alter visiting hours to help maintain an important family bond. You might request a special dietary consultation to fit the patient's cultural background. The patient has the right to expect this kind of individualized approach to **planning** care.

RIGHT TO ASSISTANCE TOWARD INDEPENDENCE

Being able to care for oneself is important in building self-esteem and is critical to being able to function as an independent person. Patients have the right to expect that care will have the goal of returning them to maximum independence. Nurses can support this right in many ways. Put simply, this means that you will encourage the patient to perform self-care whenever possible. When bathing a patient, you might encourage the patient to wash his or her own face. When helping the patient move in bed, take the extra time to give directions carefully so that the patient can move independently without strain. To function independently at home, the person with a health problem may need considerable knowledge and skill. The nurse is typically the person who plans and carries out the teaching program.

RIGHT TO EVALUATE AND OBTAIN CHANGES IN CARE

The patient has the right to evaluate care, criticize when care has not been of high quality, and obtain changes to improve the quality of care.

Most hospitals now provide patients with a form that lists evaluation criteria and asks the patient to respond. In a less formal way, patients may be given information on admission as to what they can expect with regard to care. Some facilities provide patients with a list of their rights, so they can knowledgeably exercise them. Legal recourse is always available when care has been so poor as to cause harm; however, this is a complex process that is not suited to lesser issues that are nevertheless important to the patient.

Some facilities now employ a "patient **advocate**" or "**ombudsman.**" It is this person's responsibility to discuss problems with the patient and then work with the healthcare system to improve the patient's care. In many facilities, however, no one is officially designated to do this job, and the role of patient advocate falls to the nurse. It is logical for the nurse to fulfill this role, because nurses are the only care providers who are in contact with the patient 24 hours a day, 7 days a week. Nurses also understand the institutional structure and can interface with that structure on behalf of the patient. This role is not an easy one. It demands a great deal of understanding of human behavior, understanding of the institution, and excellent communication skills.

You can support this right by listening carefully to patients' concerns and complaints and then discussing them with your instructor or a knowledgeable nurse on the unit. There may be simple remedies that you can implement, or you may begin the process by which others will resolve the patient's concerns. When you are criticized or when the care of another healthcare provider is mentioned in a negative way, do not become defensive, but carefully consider how this information might help you and other staff to provide better care to this individual as well as to other patients.

EVIDENCE-BASED NURSING PRACTICE

Although nursing is moving toward a research base for practice, it does not yet exist for many nursing procedures and skills. Evidence-based practice is defined as "the application of the best, most cost-effective and clinically meaningful evidence to nursing practice" (Lee, 2003, p. 618). The definition by Goode & Piedalue (1999, p.15) identifies all the types of evidence that are commonly used: "Evidence-based clinical practice involves the synthesis of knowledge from research; retrospective or concurrent chart review; quality improvement and risk data; international, national, and local standards; infection control data; pathophysiology; cost effectiveness analysis; benchmarking data; patient preferences; and clinical expertise."

References to the research that is available to support certain methods or approaches to a skill are presented in the modules. Future research may further refine what nurses do or significantly alter how they proceed. For some nursing skills, there is little or no research base. In these instances, the skills should be based on past practice and sound deductive reasoning from known facts. Future research may support traditional methods, or it may not, even though the reasoning behind the methods may seem logically correct.

Because nursing is an applied science, nurses' knowledge is incomplete. Given this reality, it is the responsibility of all nurses to be aware of the reasoning, or rationale, underlying what they do, to evaluate this rationale, and to be willing to alter their practice when research brings more specific information.

DELEGATION

Delegation in nursing is the transfer of authority to a competent individual to accomplish a specific nursing skill or task in a selected situation. The nurse who delegates remains accountable. That is, the nurse must assess the patient, the circumstances, and the ability of the delegatee to perform the task before delegating it.

Box 1-1 lists the Five Rights of Delegation as identified by the National Council of State Boards of Nursing (NCSBN, 1995). When you delegate a task to assistive personnel, your knowledge of the patient, the situation, the task itself, the competence of the proposed delegatee, and the direction and supervision you provide are critical to the success of the delegatee and the safe care of the patient.

THE NURSING PROCESS

The **nursing process** is a thoughtful, deliberate use of a problem-solving approach to nursing. This process forms a structure within which you can function. Most skills included in this text will be presented in a nursing process format, to assist you in establishing a pattern by which to approach nursing interventions. You will need to consult a nursing theory text for a complete understanding of the nursing process in the broader scope of nursing practice. Each step is defined here, followed by a discussion of how that step is used in performing nursing skills.

ASSESSMENT

Assessment is the process of gathering information. The basic purpose of some skills is to gather information. These skills are grouped together in Unit 3. For every skill that you use, however, you must gather the necessary information to implement it appropriately and safely. In each module, directions for carrying out the skill begin by indicating the assessment data you must gather before you proceed.

In addition to carrying out the specific assessment listed, you should always be observant while carrying out the procedure. It is an excellent time to gain further information about the patient. You may extend your knowledge of existing problems or gain insight that will lead you to identify new ones.

ANALYSIS/NURSING DIAGNOSIS

Analysis includes the intellectual processes of sorting and classifying the data collected, recognizing patterns and discrepancies, comparing these with norms, and identifying patient responses to health problems that are amenable to nursing intervention. This process is referred to as analysis because you are analyzing the data obtained. In many instances, analysis results in a statement of a patient concern or problem called a **nursing diagnosis.** The problem-solving processes involved in assessment, planning, implementation, and evaluation are always appropriate, but in the context of specific skills, a nursing diagnosis may not be appropriate. The purpose of analysis is to enable you to individualize the procedure to the patient and ensure safety. Although you may identify concerns, these may not fall into the classifications currently accepted by NANDA–International (formerly North American Nursing Diagnosis Association). During the process, you may uncover data that contribute significantly to the development of nursing diagnoses for the patient. In many instances, a skill is used to help resolve a patient problem or nursing diagnosis that has already been identified.

Two nursing diagnoses that are commonly identified in patients receiving treatment are Deficient Knowledge related to the specific procedure and Anxiety related to the specific procedure.

PLANNING

Planning is the phase during which you identify specific desired outcomes and plan for nursing actions. For each skill, specific desired outcomes are listed. You will

---

box 1-1 *Five Rights of Delegation*

1. The right **task** (the task must be within the purview of delegatee).
2. The right **circumstances** (the situation must be one in which the delegatee would reasonably be expected to complete the task successfully).
3. The right **person** (the person must have the education and skills necessary to perform the task).
4. The right **direction/communication** (it must be clear to the delegatee exactly what is expected in the situation).
5. The right **supervision/evaluation** (monitoring and evaluation appropriate to the situation and to the delegatee) must be provided.

need to adapt those outcomes to the specifics of individual situations. For example, if one of the desired outcomes is stable vital signs, it is essential to identify what the specific desired vital signs are for this particular patient.

Within the planning phase, you also must plan for carrying out the skill. Equipment must be identified and obtained. The need for additional personnel must be considered. Timing must be determined. Careful planning is the main factor in organization.

IMPLEMENTATION

Implementation is the phase of the nursing process during which you carry out the actions you planned. The specific nursing skills you use are only part of the implementation for a given problem. Nursing implementation includes your task, along with your attitude toward and communication with the patient. Because implementation is the most visible part of nursing, some people make the mistake of thinking that it is the most important. It is important, but it can never be more important than the careful data gathering and planning that goes before it or the communication that accompanies it.

For each technical skill presented, step-by-step instructions are given to guide you in your implementation of the skill. The implementation phase is the "hands-on" segment of any procedure.

EVALUATION

Evaluation is the process by which you measure the patient outcomes set forth in the planning phase. Another focus of evaluation is the patient's response. Finally, you also will want to evaluate your own nursing ability and whether you functioned well.

You must also be alert for adverse outcomes. Some adverse outcomes are directly related to the procedure and are known hazards. You should be planning to observe specifically for these. Other adverse effects are unusual and totally unexpected. When these occur, you must be alert to respond appropriately.

DOCUMENTATION

Documentation is establishing a written or electronic record of the assessment, the care provided, and the patient's responses. It usually is not considered an independent step in the nursing process, but rather an extension of each of the other steps. That is, you assess, and then you record your assessment; you plan, and then you record your plan; and so forth. For the beginner, it is often much easier to consider all documentation at the same time. Therefore, we have grouped all information about documentation as a sixth section in each skill. You will find more complete information about documentation in Module 2, Documentation.

CRITICAL THINKING

Critical thinking is organized, purposeful, disciplined thinking focused on deciding what to believe or do (Ennis, 1985). It is seen as both an attitude and an approach to ideas and decisions (Bucher & Melander, 1999). The nursing process provides a framework for critical thinking and is at its best when critical thinking is incorporated into it. If nursing process is conceptualized as cyclical in nature, with every component interacting with every other component, and with critical thinking at the center, you can approach care in a thoughtful, questioning, analytical way.

Use of critical thinking in *assessment* includes deciding what data to collect and differentiating which data are relevant and which irrelevant. You will identify what more you need to know and figure out where to find the needed information.

During *analysis, or the statement of a nursing diagnosis,* critical thinking is employed to sort and cluster information, to identify contributing factors, and to recognize the need to refer some problems to others on the healthcare team. Analysis leads you to the identification of individual problems that will affect how you should proceed with a skill.

Critical thinking is infused into the *planning* phase when you reflect on the desired outcomes for the individual patient and the context, set priorities among the problems, consider alternatives among the interventions, and identify rationale for the selected interventions. During the *planning* phase, critical thinking prompts the nurse to ask the following questions:

- Am I prepared to carry out the action and to answer client questions? If not, what do I need to do to prepare?
- Will I need additional equipment or personnel to carry out the action(s) safely?
- Have I considered the strengths of the individual or group as well as the context of *this* situation?

Critical thinking in the *implementation phase* involves being alert to what is happening as you proceed, responding to unexpected results in the patient and recognizing whether your technique is effective. Critical thinking leads you to adapt as you proceed in order to perform the skill more effectively.

Finally, critical thinking in *evaluation* includes asking whether the intervention was effective in achieving the desired outcomes (or whether it should be changed), whether more information is needed, and whether one of the alternatives *not* chosen should be considered.

Documentation is examined critically to ensure that it includes the reason for the action (nursing intervention), a description of the action taken, and a description of the response of the individual or group receiving the care.

As Figure 1-1 illustrates, critical thinking may result in your returning to the assessment phase from the implementation phase. It shows that the planning phase relates to the evaluation phase and all other phases. Thus, critical thinking makes the nursing process an evolving and adaptive approach. If critical thinking is integrated into every phase of the nursing process, you can approach nursing care in a thoughtful, questioning, analytical way.

TECHNICAL COMPETENCE

When people reflect on being skillful at any task, they most often are referring to **technical competence.** Technical competence has four components: the technique itself, the organization of the skill, the dexterity with which the task is accomplished, and the speed with which you implement nursing skills (see Box 1-2).

APPROPRIATE TECHNIQUE

Appropriate technique is always the most important component of technical competence because it maintains safety and is most likely to achieve the optimum outcome for the patient. In each module, appropriate technique is outlined and discussed in detail in the implementation phase. Some elements of each procedure may be different, depending on the circumstances and the policy in your facility. These elements are carefully pointed out. When practicing a skill, the most important element is to make sure that you always use

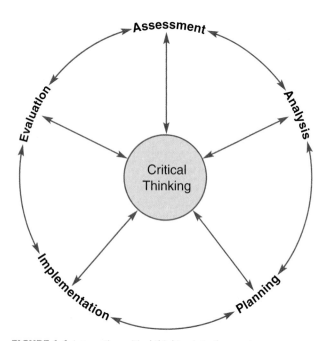

FIGURE 1-1 Integrating critical thinking into the nursing process.

box 1-2   *Components of Technical Competence*

1. Technique
2. Organization
3. Dexterity
4. Speed

appropriate technique, regardless of how slow or awkward it may be at first.

ORGANIZATION

Organization, having a systematic approach to technical skills, has many advantages. First, if you are well organized, you do not waste your time or others' time. Second, being well organized makes you appear competent and enhances the patient's trust in your skill. Third, you are less likely to make errors in technique when you are well organized; therefore, you will give safe care.

During the planning of any procedure, you will be organizing your work. One part of this is carefully identifying all the equipment you will need so that you can obtain it all at once. Nothing makes one look more disorganized than repeated trips to get forgotten items. Trips of this kind also take time and energy that can be better spent in other ways. The equipment needed for each skill is listed in the planning phase of the directions. You will often find a list of equipment specific to your facility when you consult the procedures or policies there.

At the same time, it is important to identify the need for additional personnel to carry out a given procedure. Whether the personnel are needed to assist with moving and positioning the patient, assisting the patient to remain in a certain position throughout the procedure, or simply to make the procedure go more quickly when the patient is in pain, the need for people to assist you adds additional complexity to the planning process.

Another part of organization is determining at what point in your schedule it is most appropriate to carry out a task. For example, an irrigation that is likely to result in a wet bed should be done before the bed linen is changed so that you do not end up changing the bed twice. The patient's schedule and needs must also be considered when deciding when to perform a procedure. The patient may wish to have a bath after a procedure to feel fresher. In other instances, the patient should have the bath before the procedure so that after the procedure, the patient can rest without interruptions. Because planning for the timing of any procedure is a highly individual matter, it is not included in the directions for each skill. You will need to keep it in mind, however, in each situation.

DEXTERITY

Dexterity refers to your skill or adroitness in the use of your hands. When you are dexterous, your movements are deliberate, coordinated, and purposeful. You do not use awkward or inappropriate movements. Dexterity requires practice. To increase your dexterity, you must work with the equipment enough to develop the neural pathways that coordinate your movements. You develop your sense of touch to provide accurate feedback about the position of your hands and the equipment. Although some people are naturally more dexterous than others, everyone needs practice to develop dexterity with a new skill. Going slowly and thinking carefully about your movements at first will help you to develop dexterity.

SPEED

The speed with which you carry out a nursing skill can be important. When you perform a procedure quickly, you help yourself in terms of overall time management, and more important, you help the patient. If a procedure is uncomfortable, and you perform it in 5 minutes instead of 15, the patient is only uncomfortable for 5 minutes. If a procedure creates anxiety, the anxiety decreases if you are quick and dexterous. The value to you in terms of time management is a serious consideration. Nurses often find that the many demands on their time present challenges to the completion of quality patient care. When you perform an individual skill more quickly, you are freer to plan for all patients' needs. Be cautious, however, in your quest for speed. Never sacrifice appropriate technique or neglect patients' rights. Developing your organizational ability and your dexterity are the first steps in gaining speed in performance. After you have mastered the appropriate technique, developed your organizational ability, and achieved some dexterity, you can work on speed alone.

METHODS FOR DEVELOPING TECHNICAL COMPETENCE

Developing technical competence in routine nursing skills is an important part of your education as a nurse. Various techniques will help you in this endeavor.

READING THE MODULE

Before attempting any skill, you should first read through the entire module. This provides you with the background information to understand the procedure and an overview of what you will be doing. Read as though you will be expected to teach the procedure to someone else, which in many cases will be true. You may be required to teach or assist patients, their families, and other caregivers. Look carefully at photos and drawings to help you identify new equipment and relate these to the steps of the procedure. You may also wish to point out the photos and drawings if you are teaching the skill.

MENTAL PRACTICE

Mental practice is a technique to help you establish the mental patterns that govern your actions when performing the procedure. In mental practice, you imagine yourself performing the actions in the procedure. You should attempt to "feel" and "see" yourself doing the movements and skills as they are described and illustrated as you go through each step. Bucher (1993) found that students who had used mental and **physical practice** increased their competence slightly more than those who used all of their time for physical practice. Because mental practice may be done at home or in a study room, it is an efficient use of your time and resources. "Techniques such as watching a demonstration, while sound, are not always available or possible. In contrast, mental practice is not context-dependent; it can be used at any time" (Doheny, 1993, p. 263).

PHYSICAL PRACTICE

When you go to your practice setting to perform physical practice skills, the most important aspect is the time you spend doing the task. Focus your attention so that you do not waste this valuable time. Repeat the procedure following the module directions, being careful to practice the skill correctly. When you believe you have learned the skill, try doing it with just the checklist to remind you of the steps. When you can do this satisfactorily, you are ready to ask a partner to check your performance, using the checklist. Repeating a particular skill correctly five to six times is usually necessary to be able to do it without reference to directions. It is also important to be aware of the value of spaced practice to maintenance of a given skill. Spaced practice implies that one to several days have passed between practice sessions. If you are not able to complete the entire procedure and check off in one practice session, use mental practice before you go to the practice setting again. This will maximize your ability to perform the skill.

USING A PSYCHOMOTOR TAXONOMY FOR SELF-ASSESSMENT

Dave (1970) proposed a taxonomy for psychomotor skill performance that Reilly and Oermann (1992) applied to nursing. The taxonomy includes five levels of performance: imitation, manipulation, precision, articulation, and naturalization. Expected behaviors for each level

table 1-1. Dave's Taxonomy of Skill Acquisition Applied to Nursing

Category	Behavior
Imitation—Performance of a skill following a demonstration	Observed actions copied; errors present; coordination poor; time and speed based on learner need
Manipulation—Able to perform skill following written instructions and/or verbal cues	Practice stage; improved coordination; accuracy improved; time and speed variable
Precision—Refining; becoming more exact	Accurate; able to perform skill without cues; logical sequence of actions; good coordination; minimal errors—do not involve critical decisions; time and speed variable
Articulation—Performance coordinated; able to combine more than one skill in a sequence	Logical sequence; good coordination; limited errors; skillful; efficient; improved speed
Naturalization—High level of proficiency; efficient; meets criteria for professional competence	Sequence of actions automatic; coordination consistently at high level; timely

Adapted from Reilly, D., & Oermann, M. (1992).

were developed by Reilly and Oermann to develop performance criteria for nursing skills (see Table 1-1).

The first two levels, *imitation* and *manipulation,* may be achieved in a practice laboratory setting, a non-threatening and predictable environment, where you may use printed directions and where speed and time are not important. At the *precision* level, you will be able to perform the skill without cues in the laboratory setting, but may need some help in the nonpredictable and distracting clinical setting. At the *articulation* level, you will be accurate and able to perform the skill in a timely manner. A synthesis of cognitive, affective, and psychomotor domains will have occurred when you reach the *naturalization* level. At this level, skill performance reflects professional competence. You will reach this level only when you have performed a skill frequently in the clinical setting. Therefore, you will not reach this level for skills that you perform only occasionally. You may find it helpful to use this model to evaluate your own progress (Morris & Harr, 2004).

LEARNING TOOLS

DEVELOP YOUR BACKGROUND KNOWLEDGE

1. Review the Learning Outcomes.

2. Read the material on patient rights, the nursing process, the nursing role, and direct care skills in your assigned text.

3. Look up the Key Terms in the glossary.

4. Review the module as though you were preparing to teach the content to another person.

DEVELOP YOUR SKILLS

1. Check the policy manual of the facility where you will practice for information on
   - confidentiality/privacy
   - patients' rights
   - consent
   - patient evaluation of care.

2. Arrange to go to a nursing unit as an observer. Make observations in the following four categories:
   Patients' rights—identify any behaviors that interfere with patients' rights. Identify and record staff actions that support any of the patients' rights emphasized in the module.
   Communication—notice communication between staff members, between staff and patients, and between staff and visitors. Identify and write down communication that you see as positive or negative. Be ready to state the rationale for your opinions.
   Nursing process—write down examples of nurses carrying out various steps of the nursing process.
   Technical competence—observe two different staff members perform an uncomplicated procedure (such as bed making).
   - Obtain their consent before observing.
   - Time each person doing the task.
   - Identify the factors that contributed to or interfered with timely completion of the task.
   - Compare the dexterity of the two staff members.
   - Compare the organization of the two staff members.

3. In a discussion with other students, share your observations.

CRITICAL THINKING EXERCISES

1. You have been caring for Mrs. B. for 3 sequential days. On the third day of care, Mrs. B. begins to share personal information with you as you are bathing her. You believe this information should be shared with others on the healthcare team because it has implications for approaches to her care. Mrs. B. has not said that you must keep the information confidential. Describe how you should proceed.

2. You will be learning to measure blood pressures in your skills lab. Review your personal schedule, and identify how you can include mental practice and spaced practice in your schedule.

SELF-QUIZ
SHORT-ANSWER QUESTIONS

1. List patients' rights in eight major areas that are of special concern to nurses.

   a. _____

   b. _____

   c. _____

   d. _____

   e. _____

   f. _____

   g. _____

   h. _____

2. Give an example of a behavior that demonstrates respect for the individual.

   _____

   _____

3. List the five rights of delegation.

   a. _____

   b. _____

   c. _____

   d. _____

   e. _____

4. List the steps of the nursing process.

   a. _____

   b. _____

   c. _____

   d. _____

   e. _____

5. Define assessment.

   _____

   _____

6. Define critical thinking.

   _____

   _____

7. How is critical thinking incorporated into assessment?

   _____

   _____

8. List four components of technical competence.

   a. _____

   b. _____

   c. _____

   d. _____

9. If research data are not available, how is the decision made as to what nursing action is correct?

   _____

   _____

   _____

10. What is the purpose of evaluation in nursing practice?

    _____

    _____

    _____

11. Describe the process of mental practice.

    _____

    _____

    _____

Answers to Self-Quiz questions appear in the back of this book.

MODULE 2

Documentation

SKILLS INCLUDED IN THIS MODULE

General Procedure for Documentation

PREREQUISITE MODULES

Module 1   An Approach to Nursing Skills

KEY TERMS

APIE	legibility
assessment	military time
charting by exception	minimum data set
	narrative charting
computerized records	objective
	password
DARP	problem-oriented medical record
data	
flow sheet	problem-oriented record
focus charting	
graphic record	protected health information (PHI)
HIPAA	
infused	SOAP
ingested	subjective

OVERALL OBJECTIVE

▸ To provide effectively structured and written records that document the various aspects of the nursing process to facilitate care by the entire healthcare team and maintain a legal record.

LEARNING OUTCOMES

The student will be able to

1. Assess what needs to be documented in the patient record to meet legal requirements and professional standards.
2. Maintain privacy and confidentiality of patient health information.
3. Use healthcare vocabulary accurately and effectively when documenting care.
4. Use flow sheets and checklists according to the policies of the agency.
5. Write clear, effective progress notes in narrative, **SOAP** (abbreviation for **s**ubjective, **o**bjective **a**ssessment analysis, **p**lan narrative format), and focus formats.
   a. Record assessment using objective and subjective terminology accurately.
   b. State problems correctly.
   c. Document nursing plan of care.
   d. Describe nursing actions taken.
   e. Record patient response.
6. Evaluate completed documentation.

The patient's healthcare record is used by all members of the healthcare team to communicate the patient's progress and the current treatment. Therefore, entries in the record must be clear, accurate, and comprehensive. The chart also serves as a legal record of care and the patient's progress. It is used to determine the appropriateness and quality of care being given; therefore, accuracy, **legibility** (decipherable writing), clarity, and completeness are very important. Finally, each healthcare facility establishes its own format for patients' records. This format must be used for all documentation in the facility.

TYPES OF RECORDS

TEMPORARY RECORDS

A nursing unit will almost always have a variety of temporary records that are used to facilitate communication or to maintain information for easy accessibility. These are valuable, but they must be recognized as temporary and should not be the only record of important information about the patient. Although they are temporary, these records must be accurate.

A vital signs list is typically maintained. This form may include **data** on the temperature, pulse, respiration, and blood pressure of every patient on the unit. If one person is assigned to take all these measurements, a one-page form is a convenient way to record the data as they are obtained. This list also is a quick reference for a nurse in charge of the unit. The list may be used for immediate access; the information is later transferred to the patient's permanent record by the nurse responsible for care or by a unit secretary.

The front of the chart may have a page on which the nurses make brief notations to remind the physicians of pertinent timelines such as "The narcotic order is due for renewal within the next 24 hours." These are to facilitate communication, but the official record of these matters is elsewhere in the chart.

Many nursing units maintain a whiteboard or other display for noting patients, rooms, physicians, and the caregivers assigned. What other special needs are noted often depends upon whether the whiteboard is in a location that cannot be viewed by the public or whether it is in public. A board that is private might, for example, indicate patients who are not allowed to take oral food and fluids, are to be weighed daily, have intravenous infusions, or are going for special tests or surgery. This allows staff members to obtain information quickly and conveniently. The display needs to be updated whenever a change in the patient's plan of care occurs so that care can be appropriately adjusted.

Temporary records may also be placed at the bedside to facilitate carrying out specific measures. An example would be a "turning record" that specifies when the patient is to be turned and which position is to be used. Having the information at the bedside makes it easier for the staff person to check what needs to be done and when.

Another common temporary record is a fluid intake and output worksheet. This is used to document all fluids **ingested** and lost by a patient. This might be kept on the bathroom door for easy accessibility. The information may be transcribed onto the permanent record once each shift (see Module 13, Monitoring Intake and Output, for further instructions).

Temporary bedside records that are designed to be discarded must be differentiated from actual chart forms that are kept at the bedside in some facilities. For example, a neurologic assessment flow sheet might be placed at the patient's bedside to facilitate documentation. When the flow sheet has been filled out, it is then placed in the permanent chart.

In some facilities, the nursing care plan is kept on a card file (such as a Kardex), and some parts may be changed as the patient's needs change. In most settings, this nursing plan of care is considered a permanent part of the record and is written in ink and retained along with the other permanent parts of the chart. In some facilities, a Kardex care plan may be written in pencil and considered temporary. This is used for quick reference by direct care providers. A permanent plan of care resides in the chart in these settings.

THE PERMANENT RECORD

A permanent paper record of the patient's healthcare may be referred to either as the "chart" or the "record." When it is contained in a computerized system, it is usually referred to as the "record." Whether on paper or in a computer (or sometimes both), this record is the legal record of care; it is the proof of the patient's condition and care in legal proceedings. It is also proof of care rendered for reimbursement purposes. During the patient's stay in a healthcare facility, the record is a means of communication among members of the healthcare team in regard to the patient's condition and care. It also is used to evaluate the quality of care given. In addition, data from the record are used for teaching and research.

RECORD CONTENT

An overview of the content of the patient's record is shown in Table 2-1. All patients' records provide personal data. This includes home address and telephone number, next of kin, insurance coverage, and attending physician. The admitting diagnosis and the date of admission to the agency or facility also are included.

Every type of care given is documented in the record. The physician documents the history and physical examination and then continues with medical progress notes and medical orders for care. All diagnostic and laboratory data are permanently documented in the record. Other healthcare disciplines, such as physical therapy, occupational therapy, or respiratory therapy, are responsible for documenting their contributions to the patient's healthcare.

Nursing personnel are responsible for documenting all nursing care. Each step of the nursing process is included. *Assessments* are documented on a routine schedule as well as at more frequent intervals when the patient's condition is changing. The *analysis of data* that reveals problems or nursing diagnoses is noted. *Plans* of care are documented to provide continuity of care. *Actions implemented* to support the patient or return the

table 2-1. Elements of the Patient's Record	
Element	**Description**
Database	■ Patient identifying information with social and financial data
	■ Initial physician's history and physical examination
	■ Laboratory and diagnostic test results
	■ Nursing admission interview and examination
Flow sheets	Forms arranged in columns or graphs that allow information to be recorded quickly and progress to be monitored with ease. Commonly used flow sheets include vital signs record, intake and output, medications given, and routine personal care.
Progress notes	■ Documentation of the patient's status on an ongoing basis
	■ Source-oriented records: progress identified by discipline, each on separate forms; most are in narrative form
	■ Problem-oriented records (POR), all progress notes (from all sources) use the same form. The notes have a formal, specific structure that makes them easier to use.
Problem list	This list is a combination table of contents and index to the patient's condition and progress. Each problem is numbered and titled for easy reference. Titles may refer to medical diagnoses, patient problems, or nursing diagnoses, depending on the setting. The date when the problem was initially identified is included, and when the problem is resolved, that fact and the date of resolution are added.

patient to health are documented. This includes both nursing-determined actions and those actions that are carried out as part of the medical plan of care (such as administering medications). *Evaluation* of the patient's overall status as well as response to the various treatments is also essential.

Each facility has its own approach to where and how all these aspects of nursing care are recorded. It will be your responsibility to understand what you need to document and then learn the appropriate place to document in that facility's records.

SYSTEMS FOR ORGANIZING CONTENT

The two major systems for organizing the information in a patient's record are the source-oriented system and the problem-oriented record (POR) or problem-oriented medical record (POMR) system. A facility may use one system or a combination of these two systems to meet its needs and staff preferences.

In the source-oriented method, the majority of the information is organized according to the source of that information. Progress notes written by the physician are found in the medical progress notes. Nursing progress notes are in another section of the record. Notes written by other disciplines, for example, by the respiratory therapist or the dietitian, are found on other forms in the patient's record. Some facilities combine certain of these records to facilitate effective use.

The POR in its purest form is organized according to the identified problems of the patient. The patient's problem list serves as a table of contents. All members of the healthcare team write progress notes about the same problem on the same form in the chart. This allows an individual problem to be followed clearly. It may lead to fragmentation and a failure to recognize the interdependence of problems.

COMPUTERIZED RECORDS

Computerized information systems are used in many healthcare facilities, and the use of **computerized records** is increasing. Scheduling, diagnostic and laboratory results, and information related to billing is computerized in almost all agencies. In some facilities or agencies, comprehensive patient care information systems provide a complete "paperless" record and include all aspects of nursing assessment, care planning, documentation of actions taken, and evaluation of the patient's response. There are acute care hospitals with computer terminals at each patient's bedside to facilitate immediate entry and retrieval of data.

The hardware components of these computerized systems vary, but they generally include a keyboard and a monitor/terminal and possibly a light pen and a printer. Information is input using the keyboard, although some systems use hospital-defined menus to reduce typing to a minimum. The monitor screen displays information and, in many cases, questions (Fig. 2-1).

In most healthcare facilities, staff members must use a special **password** to gain access to patient information. Other types of safeguards to access include identification cards that are "swiped" through an access indicator and nametags that contain a microchip that will enable computer access when you are close to the machine.

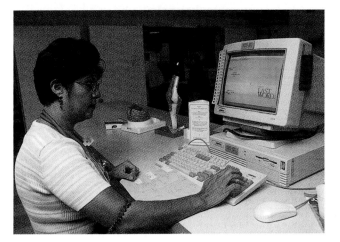

FIGURE 2-1 A nurse working on a computer.

Access to system functions may be limited by job category, level of authorization, and location of the terminal being used. For example, some data may be available only on the unit where the patient is located. Limiting by occupation may permit only registered nurses to change the nursing care plan but other nursing personnel (such as nursing assistants or students) to read it. Level of authorization may limit access to certain information to a limited number of people.

MECHANICS OF CHARTING

Mechanics include all of the standards relating to legal requirements and also those that are policies of the institution.

MEETING LEGAL STANDARDS

As a legal record, a patient record must conform to certain legal standards of legibility, clarity, and accuracy. Legibility and clarity are hallmarks of computerized documents. All entries in a printed chart must be in ink so that changes are noticeable, and the record is permanent. Your facility may specify a particular color of ink to be used. If the facility has no such policy, remember that black and dark blue ink reproduce especially well on microfilm and on photocopiers. Legibility is critical; obviously, statements that are not legible are not usable either for care or for the various other purposes of records, such as quality review or legal proceedings.

Computerized patient records maintain this legal standard by not permitting changes once the information has been entered into the record. The healthcare worker can usually edit the note being composed, but after permanently entering the information in the record, the computer program blocks any changes. Errors in documentation, blank spaces, legal signatures, time frames, and privacy are all major legal concerns in documentation.

ERRORS

An error in a computerized record requires a specific type of amendment to the notation. Each system differs somewhat, but you must learn what to do in your system if you enter information erroneously (for example, making an entry on the wrong patient's record).

For printed paper charts, if you make an error, draw a single line through the incorrect entry so that it remains legible. Traditionally the word "error" followed by initials (or first initial, last name, and title) was written above the lined-out entry. Recently, some attorneys have suggested that entering the word "error" may give an uninformed layperson the idea that this means an error was made in care. To avoid this, include a note as

Date/Time	Nurses Progress Notes
3-20-06 0700	~~Refused breakfast due to nausea.~~ Wrong chart. JE Ate all breakfast with no nausea. States feels much better this a.m. J. Ellis, RN

FIGURE 2-2 Error correction: Draw a line through the error and indicate the reasons for the change. Initial the change.

to the nature of the error. This is helpful if the chart is needed in a legal proceeding. Such a note might read "charted on wrong chart" or "mistaken entry" and your initials. This notation and the traditional "error" are both legally correct, so follow the policy of your facility. If it has no policy, the more descriptive notation is preferable (Fig. 2-2).

Documentation errors should never be corrected by erasing, using correction fluid, or obliterating the first entry. This may create the impression that the information recorded was damaging to the care provider or is being hidden for other reasons. When the mistake can be clearly read, the situation can be evaluated more readily.

If you have omitted information that should have been included in earlier charting, it may be essential to record that information. For example, you may have noted a series of assessments on a pocket note pad and failed to record them on the patient's chart in a timely manner. This information may help to identify an ongoing pattern in the patient. It is legally acceptable to add a notation as long as it is clear when the notation was made. Your facility may have a policy on how to note this. If there is no policy, a heading that indicates "delayed entry" with a date and time will clearly indicate that these data were collected in a timely manner but not recorded at the appropriate time.

A delayed entry for the purpose of protecting oneself or the agency from legal liability is more problematic. This may arouse suspicion as to whether the entry is accurate. If this situation arises, consult with an instructor or supervisor before making an entry.

BLANK SPACES

When blank spaces are left in charting, there is potential for an individual to enter information at a later time, above someone else's signature. Because of this, if you are using the narrative form of charting, chart on consecutive lines, and do not leave any blank spaces. Draw a single line through any empty spaces to prevent subsequent entries from being made above your signature (Fig. 2-3). Some facilities specify that you place your signature at the end of the note, and follow it with a line to the margin.

In some PORs, the standard is to start each segment of the note on a separate line. You would then draw a straight line through any unused space on a line before starting the next segment. *Note:* Computerized, or electronic, charting omits this problem. Each entry is recorded independently, and the computer maintains separation. It is not possible for anyone to insert information into a note that has been entered.

SIGNATURE

Computerized records base the origin of the information by the password or other confidential entry code. This clearly identifies the entry as yours. This makes it very important that you not use another person's entry code nor share yours.

When you sign a notation on a paper record, use your first initial and full last name followed by the abbreviation of your position. If you were a nursing student named Jane Smith, you would sign the record "J. Smith, NS." In large facilities where there is more chance of two individuals having the same initials, the facility may require that you sign your full name.

Traditionally, nursing students used the abbreviation SN (student nurse) to designate their position; however, most now use the abbreviation NS (nursing student). If

Date/Time	Nurses Progress Notes
12-26-06	Ambulated to bathroom c̄ one person assist. Urinated 250 mL clear urine. Up in chair until after dinner.
1815	Completed all activities c̄ no complaint of breathing difficulty or fatigue. Stated "I'm so glad I can get
	around some now. I was so short of breath when I came in." Returned to bed after dinner. Resting quietly.
	——————————————————————————— S. Chin, NS
1900	Husband in to visit. ——————————————————— S. Chin, NS

FIGURE 2-3 Filling blank spaces with lines.

more than one nursing program uses the facility or agency, you may also need to add initials designating your educational institution, for example, "Jane Smith NS, SCC." Your instructor will indicate the notation your facility prefers. In some cases, the facility may require your instructor to co-sign your progress notes, flow sheets, or medication records. There has been considerable discussion about what this co-signature means. Many facilities expect that it means the instructor has verified the accuracy of the information in the notation. If this is the case in your facility, you must ask that the instructor verify the accuracy of your information before entering it into the record.

You must use the designation appropriate to your position at the time you are giving care. For instance, a licensed practical nurse (LPN) who is enrolled in a program preparing registered nurses would use the SN or NS designation while working as a student. The nurse would use the LPN designation only when employed by and working for a facility as an LPN.

Flow sheets are often signed once per shift in a designated signature section where the signature and the initials are documented together. All data entries are then identified by the initials of the person collecting the data. You may be asked to use two initials or, in some facilities, three initials. This often depends on the size of the facility and the likelihood of multiple people with the same first and last initial.

ABBREVIATIONS AND SPECIALIZED TERMINOLOGY

Abbreviations are used throughout healthcare records to save the time of providers and reduce the size of the chart. However, abbreviations sometimes make it more difficult to understand the meaning of the document. That is why abbreviations are standardized. Each facil-

ity is required by the national accreditation standards to have a list of approved abbreviations. The use of nonstandard abbreviations increases the potential for error because different people may interpret them differently. For example, a set of initials may be interpreted as two different diseases. There are also abbreviations that should be prohibited because of their frequent involvement in safety errors. These abbreviations are easily mistaken for different terms and may be used incorrectly. Handwriting may further confuse these abbreviations. The Joint Commission on the Accreditation of Healthcare Organizations (JCAHO) has identified a list of abbreviations that must be prohibited as part of their national safety goals. Any facility is free to add additional abbreviations to this list of prohibited abbreviations as they determine it is appropriate (Table 2-2).

In addition to avoiding easy-to-misinterpret abbreviations, your charting should be descriptive and precise. Charting that the patient ate chicken soup, a cheese sandwich, fruit, and tea for lunch tells caregivers more than stating that the patient ate a good lunch (see Table 2-3 for a list of descriptive charting terms).

ESTABLISHING A TIME FRAME

Computers have internal clocks and calendars that allow times and dates to be automatically appended to any entry. You will have to specify the time of the event within your note if you are charting after the fact.

You can note time in conventional notation or according to **military time,** a 24-hour time clock. The 24-hour clock works as follows: When the time reaches 12:00 noon (or 1200), instead of returning to 1:00 p.m., the time goes on to 1300, continuing until 2400 is reached at midnight. The hours before noon are recorded

---

table 2-2. Prohibited Abbreviations: Safeguarding Patient Care

Set	Item	Abbreviation	Potential Problem	Preferred Term
1	1	U (for unit)	Mistaken as zero, four, or cc	Write "unit."
2	2	IU (for international unit)	Mistaken as IV (intravenous) or 10 (ten)	Write "international unit."
3	3	Q.D.	Mistaken for each other. The period after the Q can be mistaken for an "I" and the "O" can be mistaken for "I."	Write "daily" and "every other day."
	4	Q.O.D. (Latin abbreviation for once daily and every other day)		
4	5	Trailing zero (X.0 mg) [*Note: Prohibited only for medication-related notations*]; lack of leading zero (.X mg)	Decimal point is missed.	Never write a zero by itself after a decimal point (X mg), and always use a zero before a decimal point (0.X mg).
	6			
5	7	MS	Confused for one another	Write "morphine sulfate" or "magnesium sulfate."
	8	MSO_4	Can mean morphine sulfate or magnesium sulfate	
	9	$MgSO_4$		

Source: Joint Commission for the Accreditation of Healthcare Organizations. (2005). *National safety goals.* (Online.) Available at http://www.jcaho.org.

table 2-3. Descriptive Charting Terms

Descriptive Category	Observations
Physical Attributes	
Body location (use specific anatomic terms)	Right upper quadrant Left upper quadrant Right lower quadrant Left lower quadrant Distal/proximal
Body functions	Urination—void Have a bowel movement—defecate Profuse sweating—diaphoresis Walk—ambulate
Skin characteristics	Intact—not open, broken, or blemished Moist or dry Smooth, roughed, cracked Warm, brown (light, medium, dark): describes healthy color of the black- or brown-skinned person Warm, pink: describes healthy color of what is usually termed white skin Warm, tan: healthy color of most Asians and those termed dark-complected Dull, ash brown: African-American person's skin without adequate blood supply Dull, gray-brown: African-American or dark-complected person's skin with unoxygenated blood apparent Pale, pallor: white person's skin without adequate blood supply Cyanotic: blue-gray color in skin of white person and in conjunctiva, mucous membranes, and nail beds of all people with unoxygenated blood apparent
Nutrition	List percent of meal eaten, not poor or good. Specify types of foods eaten and amounts when more specific information is needed
Urine Description	Color: pale, yellow, amber, dark amber Clarity: clear, cloudy, smoky Contents: mucus, clots, sediment
Stool description	Color: black, brown, clay-colored (gray) Consistency: liquid, watery, semiformed, soft, formed, hard Tarry: indicates black, sticky Mucoid: indicates contains mucus
Drainage or secretions	Quantity, specify exact measurement as possible Estimate milliliters if you have a standard to compare Specify number of dressings saturated slight, scanty, small, moderate, large, copious, profuse Other terms: Watery, thin Thick, tenacious Stringy Mucoid (like mucus) Serous (like serum) Sanguineous (with blood) Serosanguineous (serum and blood mixed) Purulent (containing pus)

Mental Attitude or Mood
When you observe behavior, ask patients for an appraisal of their own feelings.
Chart both the patient's statement of feelings (left column) and your description of a patient's behavior (right column).

"I feel depressed." "I feel sad."	Does not smile Avoids eye contact Drooping posture Cries when alone
"I am glad to go home." "I am happy."	Speaks with animation Smiles and jokes Moves about room briskly
"I am worried." "I feel anxious."	Asks many questions Paces the floor In constant movement Short attention span Worried look on face
"I am mad." "I feel angry."	Loud and belligerent language Frown on face Vigorous movements

as 0100, 0200, 0300, and so on (Table 2-4). The 24-hour clock eliminates confusion as to whether something took place before noon (a.m.) or after noon (p.m.). In the past, confusion was decreased by using different ink colors for different shifts or different times of day. This method is quite effective in the original, but when records are photocopied or microfilmed as they are in most facilities, the color distinction is lost, and certain colors do not reproduce (on photocopies) as well as others. Therefore, most facilities use black ink.

On flow sheets, the times that events occurred or actions were taken are noted with initials in the "Time" column. This is clear on most records. Notations of time and date are important for healthcare reasons and legal reasons. Time sequences can be crucial in certain problems.

Policies differ regarding time notations on narrative or SOAP progress notes. The policy in most facilities is to note in the "Time" column the time you write on the nursing progress notes, rather than the time the event occurred. The time of the event can be reflected in the body of the note if that is appropriate to the charting. Often the charting reflects a process or series of events rather than one event. For particularly important events such as a sudden change in a patient's condition, your documentation may be done immediately.

Some facilities, however, have a policy of noting the time of the events in the "Time" column on the narrative or SOAP progress notes even if they are documented

later. It is critical that you understand the policy of the facility in regard to this time notation so that your notes conform to the policy.

RIGHT TO PRIVACY

A federal law titled Health Insurance Portability and Accountability Act (**HIPAA**) has an extensive section of requirements for protection of the patient's health information. HIPAA refers to this as **PHI (protected health information)**. Each facility is obligated to provide training for employees and volunteers on the specific ways that it carries out the mandate of maintaining confidentiality of PHI. All institutions are required to institute certain strategies such as having a compliance officer to whom breaches of patient confidentiality can be reported.

Access to a patient record is restricted to those in the facility using it for care and, in some instances, for research or teaching. The patient may also give permission for others such as health insurance plan, an attorney, or family members to have access to PHI.

Copying a patient chart presents many potential problems for protecting privacy, and therefore, special procedures are required. A chart may not be photocopied except for specific allowed purposes, and then you must follow careful procedures designed to protect the patient's privacy. Faxing of records and using the Internet to exchange patient information requires that the institution put in place specific procedures to guard privacy. If you, as a student, are using a chart as a learning tool, it is your responsibility to protect the patient's privacy by not using the patient's name or any identifying statements in any notations you make for your own use. Papers or case studies based on a patient's care should likewise protect the anonymity of the patient.

The medical record is the property of the hospital, but a patient has a right to the information contained in that record (state laws differ as to whether or not a patient has the legal right to review the chart itself). Usually, however, the patient must follow a procedure to obtain this information, and you must know what that procedure is. This should be found in the facility's policy and procedure manual. If there is no such procedure, you should consult with your supervisor for assistance. Clear and timely explanations and progress reports to patients and families may result in fewer requests to see the chart.

The same policies cover computerized charting. Privacy is maintained by limiting access to those with an appropriate password. Even those with a password, however, do not have a right to access the computerized record unless they are participating in care in some way. For example, a nurse on a medical-surgical unit may not access the record to determine whether her friend had a

table 2-4. What Time Is It?	
Conventional 12-Hour Time (U.S.A.)	**24-Hour (Military) Time**
1 a.m.	0100
2 a.m.	0200
3 a.m.	0300
4 a.m.	0400
5 a.m.	0500
6 a.m.	0600
7 a.m.	0700
8 a.m.	0800
9 a.m.	0900
10 a.m.	1000
11 a.m.	1100
12 p.m. (noon)	1200
1 p.m.	1300
2 p.m.	1400
3 p.m.	1500
4 p.m.	1600
5 p.m.	1700
6 p.m.	1800
7 p.m.	1900
8 p.m.	2000
9 p.m.	2100
10 p.m.	2200
11 p.m.	2300
12 a.m. (midnight)	2400

baby boy or baby girl. While this might appear innocent, it is a breach of the patient's privacy and will result in disciplinary action against the person violating privacy. Many computer systems have a program that traces all computer access to any record. Therefore, it is possible to identify any inappropriate or unauthorized use.

USING FORMS CORRECTLY

Many different forms are in use. You must become familiar with all the forms used in your facility so that you know where to look for information and where to record your own data. Initially, concentrate on forms that nurses are responsible for maintaining.

FLOW SHEETS

Flow sheets allow information to be recorded in tables or graphs. These may be referred to as the **graphic record.** This facilitates charting in that it takes less time to record information on a table than to write it in a paragraph. In most instances, it also is easier to review data or to recognize relationships among data when they appear in a table or graph. All systems of charting use some standard flow sheets, such as a graph for temperature, pulse, and respirations and a table for intake and output.

Some facilities have more flow sheets than others. The **charting by exception** assessment flow sheet shows how the normal assessment is described at the bottom of the page and is indicated by a "√" in the box on the flow sheet. The functional independence measures (FIM) key is printed at the top of the form so that a single digit can be entered on the flow sheet for those areas (Fig. 2-4).

In the **problem-oriented record** (POR) system, you are encouraged to initiate flow sheets whenever you will be collecting data or performing actions on a regular basis. Blank forms are usually available for this purpose. Thus, it will be your responsibility to figure out how best to represent the information in a table. Be sure you provide a place to note the date and time of each item in your table. Some computer programs do this for you. In the source-oriented system (SOS) of charting, anything that does not fit onto one of the existing forms is written into the appropriate progress notes of the specific discipline (see below).

NARRATIVE PROGRESS NOTES

Narrative charting, known also as narrative progress notes, is simple narration, or telling, of information. Narrative progress notes are usually differentiated by professional discipline. Most narrative charting is done in chronological order. You begin your statement with the data that were observed or that occurred first and move forward in time (Fig. 2-5). This type of narration is easy to follow, and most people find that it traces thought patterns well.

Finding relevant data regarding a single problem can be difficult, however, because a great deal of material must be read to gather specific data. Thus, many healthcare agencies have made some modifications to narrative charting. The narration itself may be organized according to functional assessment categories, body systems, or a focus of concern (**focus charting**). In this case, you would chart in chronological order all the information appropriate to one category before going on to another category.

All types of narrative notes should be characterized by brevity and clarity. Brevity is important because it is respectful of the time of those who must review notes, lessens the bulk of the chart, and conserves your own time. Brevity is accomplished by using the minimum number of words and by not necessarily using complete sentences (such as omitting the subject of the sentence when the patient is the subject). Clarity means that people can clearly understand what you mean. See Figures 2-6, 2-7, and 2-8 for more information.

PROBLEM-ORIENTED MEDICAL RECORDS

In the **problem-oriented medical record** (POMR) style of patient record, progress notes are written for significant data regarding any problem. Detailed data may be entered by any member of the healthcare team. The following format is frequently used (sometimes not all components are included).

Problem—identified by number and title

Subjective *data*—the patient's perception or statements regarding the problem

Objective *data*—your observations regarding the problem. Sometimes, it is appropriate to summarize or refer to specific information found on flow sheets, for example, the pattern of an elevated temperature or the progression of a falling blood pressure.

Assessment/*analysis*—the conclusions you reach based on the data gathered. (This use of the term assessment is slightly different from the common meaning of assessment within the nursing process, which is why the term analysis also is used for this section.) The analysis may consist of a newly identified nursing diagnosis, a general problem area, or a summary of the evaluation of the patient's progress.

Plan—your plan of action to deal with the problem. This format is commonly called SOAP notation, and the process has been called "SOAPing" (Fig. 2-9), from the terms subjective, objective,

SHIFT	23–07	07–15	15–23	23–07	07–15	15–23	23–07	07–15	15–23	23–07	07–15	15–23
PERSONAL HYGIENE:		bedbath c̄ assist	back rub	∅								
ACTIVITY: (Bedrest, Amb c̄ help, Dangle, Chair c̄/s̄ help, Up Ad Lib.		up in chair 15"	amb c̄ help 50 ft.	up to bath room								
ELIMINATION: BM (Number & Description)		∅	1̄ med soft brown	∅								
SLEEP PATTERNS: (Naps, 1 hour intervals, etc).		nap 90"	slept 2130–23	slept 23–03 04–07								
DIET 2 gm. Na	Breakfast	Lunch	Dinner	Breakfast	Lunch	Dinner	Breakfast	Lunch	Dinner	Breakfast	Lunch	Dinner
Type	soft	soft	reg.									
Amount taken (All, none, fraction)	All	3/4	3/4									

ADDITIONAL NURSING ACTIONS & TREATMENTS: I.E. (Restraints, Decubitus Care, T.C.D.B., Wound Care, Dressing Changes, Traction Anti-Embolic Stockings, ROM, Suctioning, Positioning, Cath. Care, O₂, etc.

O₂ @ 2 liters per nasal prong prn		11–13	18–21	∅								
ONE TIME ONLY NURSING ACTIONS & TREATMENTS:												

SIGNATURES:	23–07		A. Carlson RN				
	07–15	R. Gomez NS					
	15–23	K. Jones RN					
DATE:		3–17–06	3–18–06				

HOSPITAL MEDICAL CENTER
Seattle, Washington 98104

FIGURE 2-4 Flow sheet for routine care.

assessment, and plan. Although the SOAP format was developed for use with POR, it may be used for progress notes even when the record is not entirely problem-oriented. The actual implementation of the plan is documented on flow sheets. When a one-time action has been taken, some facilities suggest adding an "I" to the format of the note for the purpose of recording "intervention."

On occasion, facilities modify the POMR. Some of these modifications include the use of PIE (problem, intervention, and evaluation); **APIE** (assessment,

Date/Time	Nurses Progress Notes
1-22-06	Pt. states he has abd discomfort and feels bloated. No flatus
3:30 PM	passed. Abd hard and tense. Encouraged Pt. to ambulate and
	consume fluids.
	———————————————————— J. Jones, RN

FIGURE 2-5 Example of chronological narrative charting.

Date/Time	Nurses Progress Notes
1-1-06	Hygiene: AM care ā bkft. Complete bedbath.
10:30 AM	Activity: Up in chair c̄ assistance for bkft. No c/o fatigue or
	weakness. ROM p̄ bath.
	Nutrition: Ate all of soft diet.
	Elimination: Voided 250 ml clear amber urine @ 8:00. Moderate amt
	soft, dark brown BM @ 8:00.
	Pain: c/o abd incisional pain, 3 on scale of 1–5, @ 8:00. Demerol
	75 mg 1M given. Stated relief in 20 min. No further pain in AM.
	Fluids and Elec: IV running at 22 gtt/min into R forearm. Site s̄
	redness, pain, swelling. ———————— J. Jones, RN

FIGURE 2-6 Example of narrative charting organized by functional assessment.

Date/Time	Nurses Progress Notes
1-1-06	Circ: IV running at 22 gtt/min into R forearm. Abd drg dry and
10:30 AM	intact.
	GI: Ate all of soft diet. Mod amt soft, dark brown BM @ 8:00.
	GU: Voided 250 ml clear amber urine @ 8:00.
	Musc-Skel: Up in chair c̄ assistance for 30 minutes. No c/o
	weakness or fatigue. ROM to lower extremities p̄ bath. Rested p̄
	ROM. Near: c/o abd incisional pain, 3 on scale of 1–5, @ 8:00.
	Demerol 75 mg IM given. Stated relief in 20 min. No further
	pain in AM.
	———————————————————— J. Jones, RN

FIGURE 2-7 Example of narrative charting organized by body systems.

Date/Time	Nurses Progress Notes
1-28-06	Shortness of breath: Data: Able to walk to bathroom with O_2 @
2200	2l without shortness of breath. Became S.O.B. with R 32 and
	labored after shower without O_2. Action: O_2 restarted at 2l.
	Response: Respirations became less labored and rate @ 22 in 10 min.
	———————————————————— J. Jones, RN

FIGURE 2-8 Example of narrative charting organized by a focus of concern.

Date/Time		Nurses Progress Notes
12-28-06	3.	Pain related to developing wound infection.
11:30 PM	S	Has c/o of "increased pain" in incisional area changed from
		3 to 4.
	O	Had pain med q4h yesterday and q3h today (see Med Record).
		Temp increasing steadily to 101.6 (see graphic). Wound
		drainage has increased from scant serosanguineous to moderate
		and odorous (see Drsg Flow Sheet).
	A	Wound infection developing.
	P	Notify Dr. Jones immediately. Culture wound drainage.
		Increase fluid intake to a minimum of 3000 ml/24 h. Change drsg
		q 2 h. Establish dressing isolation.
		J. Stuart, RN

FIGURE 2-9 A SOAP format nursing progress note.

problem, intervention, and evaluation); and DARP (data, action, client response, and plan). See Figures 2-10, 2-11, and 2-12, respectively. Because it is common for facilities to make individual modifications in documentation style, you should consult the procedure book in your clinical setting for specific policies and procedures related to documentation.

SPECIAL NOTES

At times, information must be recorded that does not seem to fit within the scope of a single problem, and therefore SOAPing or its variations may not be appropriate. Information of this kind is placed in the progress notes and identified as a special note. Some types of

special notes used are temporary problems, discharge planning, family involvement, and interim notes.

Temporary problems are concerns that could be SOAPed but that are so quickly resolved that it is inappropriate to place them on the problem list. An example might be a misplaced valuable that is found or urinary retention that is resolved through nursing action (Fig. 2-13).

Discharge planning is important for a patient, but it often encompasses many problems and cannot be SOAPed in the conventional manner. A section of the progress notes is titled Discharge Planning, and the relevant information is recorded (Fig. 2-14).

Recognition of the family's role in the patient's life has led to an increased emphasis on including the

Date/Time		Nurses Progress Notes
3-20-06	P	Nausea and vomiting after breakfast
0800	I	Antiemetic given (see MAR).
		Clear fluids. Will hold regular diet and provide fluids until more
		stable.
0900	E	States nausea relieved — T. Williams, RN

FIGURE 2-10 PIE (problem, intervention, evaluation) format progress note.

Date/Time		Nurses Progress Notes
3-20-06	A	Pt. states that she is feeling dizzy and weak when getting up.
1400		BP lying of 132/90 drops down to 102/60 when standing.
	P	Postural hypotension related new antihypertensive medications.
	I	Pt. taught to get up slowly and sit on the edge of the bed
		until balance restored. Pt. directed to seek assistance when
		ambulating.
	E	If pt. changes position slowly, states dizziness is less. Pt. is
		following Instructions to seek help when ambulating.
		W. Stevenson, RN

FIGURE 2-11 APIE (assessment, problem, implementation, evaluation) format progress note.

Date/Time	Nurses Progress Notes
3-20-06 1630	D States pain is 8 on a scale of 1–10. Holds self still and does not move.
	A Pain med as indicated on MAR. Taught to splint when moving.
	R In 30 min. pain 4 of 10. Able to turn, cough and deep breathe.
	P Provide pain med. q4h for 24 hr and encourage moving. — N. Doe, RN

FIGURE 2-12 DARP (data, action, response, plan) format progress note.

Date/Time	Nurses Progress Notes
3-10-06 1600	Temporary problem: Missing hearing aid.
	S Wife thought it was with patient when he entered through Emergency Room.
	O Hearing aid not listed in initial personal effects list and not found in belongings.
	A
	P 1. Emergency Room to be contacted.
	2. Wife to search at home for hearing aid.
	3. Recheck tomorrow evening when wife visits. — J. Jones, RN
3-11-06 1700	Temporary problem: missing hearing aid, resolved: Wife brought in hearing aid this evening. — J. Jones, RN
3-11-06 2000	3. Urinary incontinence
	S States: "I think I'm doing better. I was only wet once today."
	O Voiding when offered urinal on q2h schedule. See flow sheet.
	A Current program successful.
	P Continue bladder rehab. program without change. — J. Jones, RN

FIGURE 2-13 Temporary problem note.

Date/Time	Nurses Progress Notes
12-30-06 3:30 PM	Discharge Planning
	S Mrs. E. wishes to go to her own home for convalescence.
	O Resources for home care equipment and assistance with care discussed. Expected activity limitations reviewed.
	A Pt will be able to manage home care only with some outside assistance.
	P Contact social services. —— M. Rosen, RN

FIGURE 2-14 Discharge planning note.

Date/Time	Nurses Progress Notes
1-15-06	Family involvement
2200	Growth and development information regarding common 2-yr-old behavior discussed with mother. Mother encouraged to let nurse know when she must leave and to be direct with Robbie and not to sneak out. Reassured mother that nurses understand why he cries when she leaves, and this is Ok. ——— R. Filipi, SN

FIGURE 2-15 Family involvement note.

family in care. This may be accomplished by teaching family members and discussing the patient's care needs with them. When *family involvement* occurs, it is appropriate to make a legal record of it. This is done by writing a note titled *Family Involvement* in the progress notes (Fig. 2-15).

Another special note is the *interim note*. This note is most often used to provide a legal record of nursing action that is not directly related to observations of the patient. For example, if a patient's condition is becoming worse, and you cannot locate the physician, your interim note might be a series of entries recording your attempts to contact the physician, your conferences with the nursing supervisor, and your contact with another physician. This provides the necessary legal record that appropriate nursing action was taken (Fig. 2-16). Your observations of the patient would be recorded in a conventional SOAP note. An interim note might also be used to record the time of departure and return of a patient leaving a facility on a temporary pass.

INCIDENT OR QUALITY ASSURANCE REPORTS

An important issue in healthcare today is that of quality assurance (QA), which means measurement and ongoing monitoring of the quality of patient care. Most healthcare facilities have an active QA committee composed of a variety of staff members, including nurses. The incident or quality assurance report is used to document any unusual occurrence, accident, or error in the facility. Some facilities use different forms for different kinds of events (for example, medication errors and falls), whereas others use one standard form for all incidents. The incident report is useful for determining the quality of the care provided and can facilitate improvements.

Incident reports serve several purposes. First, they objectively document the event. Second, they are a record for insurance and legal reference. Last, they help identify the need to modify or correct procedures, policies, or situations within the healthcare facility.

The incident report is completed by the staff person who discovers or is involved in the incident. Because the report may become a legal document, it should contain proper language, pertinent facts, and the exact times and proper sequence of events. Only facts—not opinions or conclusions—are documented. If a report concerns a patient, the report is not incorporated into the patient's chart but is sent to the immediate supervisor and finally to administration. A notation about the incident is made in the chart. The report does not constitute an admission of liability, and the fact that one was filed is not documented in the patient's chart. Complete and file an

Date/Time	Nurses Progress Notes
1-23-06	Interim Note
11:30 PM	Phone call to Dr. Johnson regarding patient's condition. His answering service was notified that immediate contact is needed. ——— C. Chang, RN
11:45 PM	Call to Dr. Johnson has not been returned. Nursing Supervisor notified of pt's condition and of call placed to physician. ——— C. Chang, RN
12:00 midnight	Supervisor here. Dr. Johnson's answering service contacted again. Unable to reach him. ER doctor contacted and arrived at 12:10 PM. ——— C. Chang, RN

FIGURE 2-16 Interim note.

incident report in a timely fashion, because recall is more difficult once time has elapsed.

GENERAL PROCEDURE FOR DOCUMENTATION

When you are responsible for documenting care, you will find it easier to be sure that your documentation is complete if you develop a systematic approach. Use your nursing process framework to assist you.

ASSESSMENT

1. Identify the assessment data you have obtained:
   a. presence or absence of abnormal findings
   b. changes in status
   c. information significant to the patient's diagnosis and problems, such as drainage and excretions; condition of devices, tubes, and dressings; feelings and concerns expressed

ANALYSIS

2. Note the new nursing diagnoses or problems identified and their etiology as thoroughly as you can.

PLANNING

3. Note new plans that you have developed for care.

IMPLEMENTATION

4. Review the nursing interventions completed:
   a. routine care activities and safety measures
   b. special procedures and interventions, such as prn medications, treatments, dressing changes, fluids instilled or **infused**
   c. patient or family teaching
   d. psychosocial interventions

EVALUATION

5. Identify how you evaluated the patient's status and progress.

DOCUMENTATION

6. Identify where to document data in the system you are using.
7. Complete each flow sheet with information, date, times, signatures.
8. Write progress notes related to information not on flow sheets.
   a. Use correct format for facility.
   b. Use only approved abbreviations.
   c. Write legibly.
   d. Make sure your wording is brief and clear for others to understand.
   e. Include date, time, and signature.
9. Do a final self-check.
   a. Correct format
   b. Correct use of abbreviations
   c. Legibility
   d. Clarity
   e. Date, time, and signature

Acute Care

Patients are in acute care because of the seriousness of their conditions or the fact that there is a potential for adverse events. Therefore, acute care patients require frequent assessment and evaluation of their response to care. Documentation of the assessment and evaluation are also completed frequently. These are usually required at least every 8 hours and often more frequently. Documentation is also used as a basis for overall system evaluation through audits of charts. When audits are conducted, assessments and actions not documented are considered to not have been done. Thus there are multiple demands for careful documentation.

Long-Term Care

The regulations for documenting nursing care in long-term care facilities are federally mandated and interpreted at both federal and state levels. Specifically, these regulations state that the director of nursing services ensures that all nurses' notes are informative and descriptive of the nursing care provided and of the patient's response to care. With regard to the patient care plan, the surveyor is charged to verify that the record indicates that the plan of care is followed, and the goal of care is being met (Centers for Medicare & Medicaid Services, 2004).

In long-term care facilities, admitting assessments and monthly assessments must be recorded on a form known as the **minimum data set** (MDS). This form is required by the federal regulations regarding reimbursement by Medicare and Medicaid. The MDS standardizes the collection of data on long-term care residents and thus facilitates policymaking and research. Based on the MDS data, ongoing assessment is specified by resident assessment protocols (RAPs). These protocols help to standardize follow-up on actual or potential problems frequently seen in long-term care residents. Most facilities have a specific form on which to record the data required by the RAP.

In long-term care facilities, summary narrative notes are often written monthly. These notes may address each problem that appears on a resident's nursing care plan, providing an evaluation of that problem. Many nursing homes use computerized systems that integrate all of the required data.

Home Care

The federal government and third-party payers require specific types of documentation to justify paying for home care. In home healthcare, documentation is directed toward nursing activities that are reimbursable. Reimbursement for home care is usually available only when a person is homebound and continues to need acute or skilled (not chronic) care. Because specific terminology is used in reimbursement policies, the documentation of visits must use correct terminology. To facilitate this type of documentation, many home care agencies have special forms with headings that guide documentation.

Some home care agencies have developed computerized systems that allow home care nurses to document care using a laptop computer and then communicate that information to the main agency computer through a modem or by transferring files at the office location. Whatever the system used, each visit must be correctly documented for the agency to receive reimbursement.

Ambulatory Care

In ambulatory care settings, keeping records has often been challenging. In large clinics, charts move from office to office. When a patient has many appointments, it is sometimes hard for the chart to be completed from one appointment and then forwarded to the next. Computerized patient records have facilitated continuity of care and assure that each provider has access to all the information about the patient's health status.

LEARNING TOOLS

DEVELOP YOUR BACKGROUND KNOWLEDGE

1. Review the Learning Outcomes.
2. Read the section on documentation in your assigned text.
3. Look up the Key Terms in the glossary.
4. Review the prohibited abbreviations listed in Table 2-2.
5. Review the list of approved abbreviations from the facility where you will have clinical experience.
6. Read through this module, and mentally practice the documentation techniques described. Study so that you would be able to teach these skills to another person.

DEVELOP YOUR SKILLS

1. If charting samples are available in your practice setting, review them.
2. Practice charting, using the situations provided in the module. Make a sample form for practice charting that is similar to the one used in your facility.
3. Exchange your practice charting with another student, and check each other's work. Review and rewrite your own charting based on this critique.
4. Have your instructor review your practice charting.
5. Review your instructor's comments, and rewrite your practice charting if necessary.

PRACTICE YOUR SKILLS

The following are clinical situations to be used for practicing documentation. Each focuses on a situation in which you are providing bedside care and assistance. You can use these situations on your own to practice writing various styles of progress notes, filling in forms used in your facility, or designing flow sheets. Alternatively, your instructor may direct you to other activities based on these situations. Evaluate your own documentation based on the instructions given in the module.

Situation 1: You worked as a nursing student from 7:00 a.m. until 10:30 a.m. During that time, you cared for Mr. Oscar Johanson. He is 66 years old and is in the hospital for bronchial pneumonia. This is his third hospital day. You assisted him with a bed bath; you washed his back and legs, and he did the rest. He sat in a chair while you made his bed. At the end of 15 minutes, he felt tired and asked to return to bed. For breakfast, he was served and ate hot cereal with cream, toast with margarine and jelly, orange juice, and coffee. His blood pressure was 146/84, his pulse rate was 78, and his respiratory rate was 22. He coughed intermittently, but the cough was nonproductive.

Situation 2: You worked as a nursing student from 7:00 a.m. until 11:00 a.m. at Cascade Vista Nursing

Home, caring for Paulina Munsch. She is 84 years old and has mild congestive heart failure. She is somewhat unsteady on her feet but can usually ambulate from her room to the dining room, the chapel, and the activities room. She is normally cheerful, cooperative, and interested in the scheduled activities at Cascade Vista. Today, you noticed that she was slow to wake up and reluctant to participate in her care. Although she normally eats all of her breakfast, today she ate only a few bites of cereal and refused the rest of the meal. On the way back to her room, she asked to stop to rest twice. At 10:30 a.m., when it was time to bake cookies, she stated that she wished to stay in her room and rest. She had an occasional nonproductive cough, and vital signs were as follows: T, 97.88°F; P, 88; R, 22; BP, 148/86.

Situation 3: You worked as a nursing student from 4:30 p.m. to 8:30 p.m., caring for Mrs. Effie Sturdevan, who is 45 years old and who had a hysterectomy 2 days ago. Her postoperative course has proceeded smoothly. She had a soft diet for dinner and had a large, soft bowel movement after dinner. She complained of abdominal pain, noted as 7 on a scale of 0 to 10 and was given a pain pill by the medication nurse at 7:00 p.m. At 7:30 p.m., she stated that the pain was now reduced to a 3 on the same scale. During visiting hours, her husband and daughter were present. After they left, you observed that she was quiet, did not speak, and had tear-stained cheeks.

You helped her to ambulate at 4:30 p.m. and again at 8:00 p.m. Then you helped her get ready for bed and gave her a back rub. While you were giving her the back rub, she said that she knew the surgery had been necessary, but she somehow felt like a different person. After you listened to her for 10 minutes, she seemed more relaxed and said she felt she would be able to sleep.

Situation 4: You worked as a student nurse from 0700 to 1200, caring for Mr. John Steiner, 36 years old. He is recovering from abdominal surgery to remove his gallbladder, which had been filled with large gallstones. This is his second postoperative day, and you helped him bathe himself and gave him back care. For breakfast, he ate a small serving of cooked cereal with milk and drank a small glass of apple juice and a cup of tea. You assisted him in ambulating the length of the hall and back, after which he asked for and was given his pain medication. His vital signs were as follows: T, 98.88°F; P, 78; R, 14; BP, 134/86. His pulse and respiration were unchanged after ambulation.

Situation 5: During clinical laboratory practice, from 1300 to 1600, you cared for Mrs. Jennie Johnson, 77 years old. She had a mild stroke 2 weeks ago and is now on the transitional care unit. She has some difficulty speaking and cannot use her right arm. You washed her hair and set it, read a newspaper article to her, and helped her select her menu for the next day. She understood what you asked her about the menu and nodded yes or no about food selection. She could not comb her hair with her left hand; she held the comb awkwardly and kept dropping it. Her speech was not clear, but with enough time, she made some appropriate verbal responses. She said "toilet" and urinated when taken to the bathroom. Her right arm was in a supportive sling. When you took her arm out to exercise it, her elbow flexed easily, but her shoulder was stiff.

Situation 6: Your clinical time as a nursing student was from 0700 to 1100. You were assigned to care for Mrs. Dorothy Wu, 88 years old. Mrs. Wu was transferred from a nursing home for diagnostic studies related to decreasing functional ability. She is totally dependent and on complete bed rest. You did complete morning hygiene, including a bed bath and oral, nail, and hair care. You turned her every 2 hours and gave her a back massage each time you turned her. At 0800, you fed her breakfast. She ate a bowl of oatmeal, a dish of applesauce, and a glass of milk (240 mL); she would not take coffee and could not chew toast because she had no dentures. She was incontinent of urine twice and had an incontinent stool after breakfast.

Situation 7: In your role as a nursing student, between the hours of 3:00 p.m. and 7:00 p.m., you cared for Mr. Joseph Gonzales, 38 years old. He had surgery to repair a right inguinal hernia at 8:00 a.m. today. He returned to the surgical nursing unit from the postanesthesia room at 12:00 noon.

You took his blood pressure, pulse, and respiration every 2 hours, and they were as follows: 4:00 p.m., 130/82, 68, 14; 6:00 p.m., 128/82, 66, 16. He took 200 mL of liquid during the 4 hours you were present and had no nausea. You helped him walk to the bathroom and stand to void. He voided 150 mL. When you examined his dressing, you noted that there was no drainage, and the dressing was clean. He had pain in the incisional area that he indicated was a 4 on a scale of 0 to 5. You gave him 50 mg of meperidine (Demerol) IM at 6:00 p.m. He stated that this reduced his pain to about a 2 out of 5. He moved around in bed with ease and performed deep-breathing exercises well when directed to do so.

Situation 8: From 7:00 a.m. to 3:30 p.m., you were on a general medical unit as a nursing student.

You cared for Mr. Thomas Brown, 32 years old. Mr. Brown has been diagnosed as having severe hypertension and is hospitalized to establish control of his blood pressure through an appropriate medication regimen. He is on a 500-mg sodium diet and allowed up ad lib. He had routine morning care. He ate all of his breakfast and borrowed salt from his roommate, which he used liberally on his eggs. He complained that the food was tasteless. He was dizzy when he got up to go to the shower. His blood pressure at 9:00 a.m. was 180/100 while lying, 130/80 while sitting, and 118/70 when standing. His pulse was 72, respirations 20, and temperature 98.48°F. At noon, he ate all of his lunch plus some potato chips brought in by a friend. He rested in the afternoon. At 1:00 p.m., his blood pressure was 176/98 lying, 128/76 sitting, and 122/70 standing.

Situation 9: You cared for Mr. Wayne Jefferson this morning. He is 90 years old and had bilateral inguinal hernias repaired. He ate all of a general diet for breakfast. He has been constipated, and you gave him a Fleet enema at 8:30 a.m. He then had a large, formed, brown stool. He bathed himself at the bedside. You washed his back and gave him a back rub. Vital signs checked at 7:30 a.m. were as follows: T, 97.88°F; P, 62; R, 18; BP, 144/90. He has had no incisional pain. He walked around the room and down the hall twice. He napped for an hour from 11:00 a.m. until noon, when you left.

Situation 10: From 3:00 p.m. to 7:00 p.m., you cared for Mrs. Bessie McDonald, who was admitted 4 days ago with mild heart failure. At 4:00 p.m., you assisted her to walk to the bathroom, where she urinated 250 mL clear urine. She then sat in a chair until after she had eaten all of her dinner. She said, "I'm so glad I can get around some now. I was so short of breath when I came in." You noted that there was no shortness of breath and that she did not seem fatigued from her activity. She returned to bed after dinner and rested quietly. As you were leaving at 7:00 p.m., her husband arrived to visit.

DEMONSTRATE YOUR SKILLS

In the clinical setting:

1. Consult with your instructor regarding the opportunity to document data regarding a patient to whom you are assigned. Make a first draft on a piece of paper, and have your clinical instructor review it before you write or keyboard it into the patient's record.

2. Continue to chart on patients assigned in the clinical area. Have your first draft reviewed before writing in patients' records until your instructor directs you to do otherwise.

3. Evaluate your performance with the instructor.

CRITICAL THINKING EXERCISES

1. You are working in a facility that uses a POR system for charting. Mr. J. W., 78 years old, was admitted for a treatment of his broken hip. Since his admission 4 hours ago, he has been lying in bed. You have noted that Mr. W. is very thin, and a bright red area has developed over his coccyx. Design a flow sheet to monitor his skin condition and to record actions taken to prevent skin breakdown.

2. You will be assessing pulse, respiratory rate, and blood pressure every 15 minutes after a patient returns from a procedure. In addition, your instructor has stated that every 5 minutes, you should assess popliteal and pedal pulses on the right leg, and make sure that a sandbag stays in place over the right groin to prevent bleeding where an arterial catheter was removed. To ensure that you do all of this correctly, design a working form for the bedside to help you remember all details and keep records as you care for the patient.

SELF-QUIZ
SHORT-ANSWER QUESTIONS

1. List two systems for organizing the contents of a chart.

   a. _____

   b. _____

2. What are two methods of writing progress notes?

   a. _____

   b. _____

3. Why should objective terminology be used in charting?

   _____

4. In the following sample, underline the subjective terms:

   "Crying. States upset over upcoming surgery. Paced the room for 1 hour before bedtime."

5. On the following charting sample, an error was made in the quantity of urine. The correct amount was 175 mL. Correct the sample as if it were a real chart.

"Up in chair for 30 min. No sign of fatigue. Assisted to BR to urinate. 225 mL clear yellow urine."

6. To whom does the physical chart or medical record belong?

_____

7. Discuss the patient's right to the information contained in his or her own chart.

_____

_____

_____

MULTIPLE CHOICE

_____ **8.** Ink is used for all charting primarily because
    a. it looks neater.
    b. it is more permanent.
    c. changes or erasures can be seen.
    d. it is a custom.

_____ **9.** If a 24-hour clock is in use, the correct term for 4:00 p.m. would be
    a. 0400
    b. 0800
    c. 1600
    d. 2000

_____ **10.** In problem-oriented medical records, the progress notes are often written in a standard form. This form is abbreviated as
    a. SOAP
    b. SOLD
    c. COAP
    d. PROP

Answers to Self-Quiz questions appear in the back of this book.

MODULE

3

Basic Body Mechanics

KEY TERMS

base of support	gait (transfer) belt
body mechanics	repetitive strain
center of gravity	injury
counterbalance	supporting muscles
ergonomics	

OVERALL OBJECTIVES

▸ To apply the principles of body mechanics to conserve energy.
▸ To decrease the potential for strain, injury, and fatigue.
▸ To promote safety.

LEARNING OUTCOMES

The student will be able to

1. Examine each physical task encountered to determine the most appropriate way to accomplish it for the safety of the nurse and that of the patient.
2. Apply principles of body mechanics appropriately.
3. Determine appropriate nurse/patient outcomes, and recognize the potential for adverse outcomes.
4. Prevent adverse outcomes (musculoskeletal injuries) through diligent use of body mechanics, adequate staff, and appropriate equipment.
5. Teach use of body mechanics to patients, family members, and assistive personnel to ensure correct body movement and to prevent musculoskeletal injury.
6. Analyze the use of body mechanics during activity.
7. Evaluate own or patient body movement in specific situations.

A nurse engaged in clinical practice performs a variety of physical tasks daily, including reaching, stooping, lifting, carrying, pushing, and pulling. Practiced incorrectly, any of these has the potential to cause strain, fatigue, or injury to the nurse or patient. Some injuries occur as a result of a single action. Far more injuries result from multiple strains. A **repetitive strain injury** is characterized by tissue damage caused by repeated trauma to an area. Many back and shoulder injuries in healthcare workers are the result of the repetitive strain involved in moving patients. To prevent these injuries, attention to posture and body mechanics is essential.

OSHA (U.S. Dept of Labor, 2005) has identified several aspects of the work environment that create hazards for musculoskeletal injury. These are

- Force—the amount of physical effort required to perform a task (such as heavy lifting) or to maintain control of equipment or tools
- Repetition—performing the same motion or series of motions continually or frequently
- Awkward postures—assuming positions that place stress on the body, such as reaching above shoulder height, kneeling, squatting, leaning over a bed, or twisting the torso while lifting

The physical risk of a task causing an injury can be related to multiple factors. For assessment purposes, these have been categorized as (1) exposure—the number of times the task is performed in a day, (2) duration—the length of time the task takes, (3) cycle—the number of times the task is repeated without rest, (4) force applied, (5) speed at which it occurs, (6) awkwardness, and (7) vibration (Burgess-Limerick, Straker, Pollack, et al., 2004). When determining whether actions have the potential for injury, all these factors must be considered.

PREVENTING MUSCULOSKELETAL INJURY

Ergonomics is the science of designing the objects and systems to accommodate a person's physical characteristics to enhance safety, efficiency, and well-being. Ergonomics is important for all healthcare providers because the healthcare environment is one in which musculoskeletal injuries are common. In the healthcare environment, ergonomics is resulting in changes in the ways that facilities are constructed, how patients are moved, and how workers do their jobs. Some facilities use lifting devices and/or lift teams to decrease the potential for repetitive strain injuries to backs of employees. An ergonomic approach is essential to decreasing the incidence of musculoskeletal injuries. This must be a system-wide approach supported by the purchase of mechanical lifting and moving devices.

In addition to changing the physical environment and the systems for work to protect against injury, healthcare workers can add to their own safety and well-being by using correct body mechanics in their work. **Body mechanics** involves the analysis of the action of forces on the body parts during activity. Using these forces effectively can help to prevent injury. However, no attempt at correct body mechanics can compensate for undertaking actions that put excessive strain on the body. Nurses must vigilantly protect themselves and assistive personnel against injuries related to moving and lifting patients. Strategies for moving and transferring patients are found in Modules 6 and 18.

Rickover and Rickover (2005, p. 1) have suggested that injuries are minimized when the following principles are maintained:

- "All work activities should permit the worker to adopt several different, but equally healthy and safe postures.

- "Where muscular force has to be exerted, it should be done by the largest appropriate muscle groups available."
- "Work activities should be performed with the joints at about midpoint of their range of movement. This applies particularly to the head, trunk, and upper limbs."

Additionally, OSHA recommends that manual lifting of residents in nursing homes be minimized in all cases and eliminated when feasible (U.S. Dept of Labor, 2005). Many hospitals are adopting this same recommendation. Keeping these principles of body mechanics in mind is a constant challenge for the nurse. These principles are often taught to patients. The promotion of proper body mechanics is, in itself, a valid nursing intervention.

USING PRINCIPLES OF BASIC BODY MECHANICS

Examine each physical task encountered to determine the most appropriate way to accomplish it for your own safety and that of the patient. When moving or transferring patients, you may need to obtain supplies, such as a lift sheet (also called a turn or pull sheet) or a **gait (transfer) belt,** before you undertake the necessary task. You may also need another staff person or a mechanical lift to ensure safety for all involved. The following strategies have been selected because of their applicability to commonly encountered nursing situations. Examples of how they can be applied are included as illustrations.

1. Stand with the **center of gravity** (the point in an object or person at which gravitational pull functions as if the entire weight of the object or person were at that single point) directly above the base provided by the feet. **R:** This maintains balance and stability with the least amount of effort and thereby decreases the potential for strain, fatigue, and poor balance.
2. When moving from one position to another or lifting, first make sure that you have enlarged the **base of support** by moving the feet apart. **R:** Changes in position move the center of gravity, and if the base of support is narrow, it may fall beyond the edge of the base and thus create instability.
3. When picking up an object from the floor, bend your knees, and keep your back straight, rather than bending forward at the waist. **R:** Bent knees and a straight back will maintain your center of gravity close to the base of support and prevent back strain. Bending over places a mechanical strain on the lower back from the weight of the head and shoulders at the end of the spine.
4. Place one foot forward when you push a heavy object (such as a bed with a patient in it), or place one foot back when you move a patient toward the side of the bed. **R:** This enlarges the base of support in the direction of the force to be applied, thereby increasing the amount of force that can be applied.
5. Tighten or contract your supporting muscles before beginning a lifting task to support your joints and prevent injury to the muscles. **R:** Supporting muscles are the muscles of the abdomen and lower back that provide stability and support to the lower spine, decreasing the potential for strain. Muscles that have been contracted before beginning are less likely to tear with strain. If you practice tightening the supporting muscles continually, you will eventually do it automatically when you prepare for any activity.
6. Face in the direction of the task to be performed, and turn the entire body in one plane (rather than twisting) (Fig. 3-1). **R:** To lessen the susceptibility of the back to injury. When the back is twisted, one group of muscles is stretched, while the other is contracted. Muscles that are stretched are weaker and more susceptible to injury. Also, the spine functions less effectively when it is twisted due to the balance of the spinal vertebrae upon one another.
7. Lift by bending the legs and using the leg muscles rather than by using the back muscles (see Fig. 3-2).

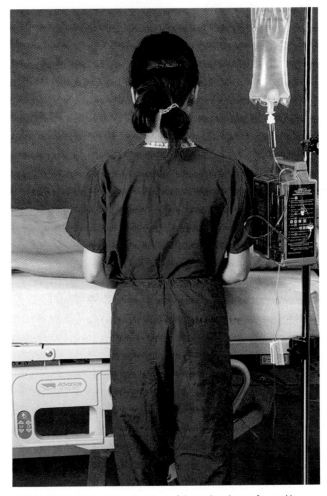

FIGURE 3-1 Facing in the direction of the task to be performed lessens the susceptibility of the back to injury.

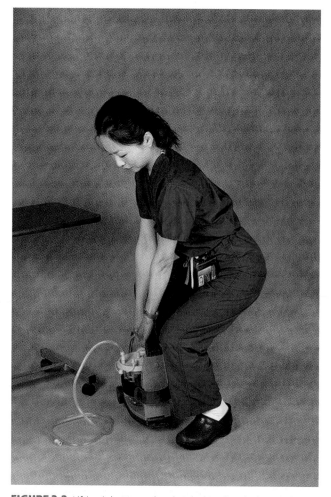

FIGURE 3-2 Lifting is better undertaken by bending the legs and using the large muscles of the legs.

R: The large, compact muscles of the legs are stronger and less prone to injury than the broad, flat muscles of the back. Because large muscles tire less quickly than small muscles, use the large gluteal and femoral muscles rather than the smaller muscles of the back. In addition, if the back muscles are strained, they may be injured. Repeated injuries can lead to repetitive strain injury. Ligaments, tendons, and even the intervertebral disks may be injured as well. Back injuries are one of the major health problems in adult workers, resulting in pain, disability, and economic loss to the individual, the employer, and society.

8. If the patient can tolerate being in a flat position, lower the head of the bed before moving him or her up toward the head of the bed. **R:** It takes less effort to move an object or person on a level surface rather than up a slanted surface against the force of gravity. Patients also can apply this principle to moving themselves up in the bed.

9. When moving a patient in bed, work on a smooth surface, such as a taut sheet. A smooth sheet also allows patients to move themselves more easily. **R:** Friction opposes motion; therefore, less energy is required to move an object when the friction between the object and the surface on which it rests is minimized.

10. Hold heavy objects close to your body, and move the patient near to your side of the bed when providing care (Fig. 3-3). Instruct patients walking with equipment, such as an intravenous pole or walker, to keep the equipment close to the body. **R:** It takes less energy to hold an object close to the body than at a distance from the body; it also is easier to move an object that is close. Muscles are strongest when contracted and weakest when stretched.

11. When assisting a patient to stand, use the weight of your body by rocking backward, counterbalancing the patient's weight. Use the patient's weight by placing his or her legs in a knees-up position before moving him or her from side to side or up in bed. Teach patients to move themselves more easily by using their body weight to facilitate turning. **R:** The weight of the body can be used as a force to assist in lifting or moving.

12. When working with patients, use smooth, rhythmic movements at moderate speed rather than rapid, jerky ones. Caution patients not to move rapidly. **R:** Smooth, continuous motions also are more accurate, safer, and better controlled than sudden, jerky movements. You will work more effectively if not hurried.

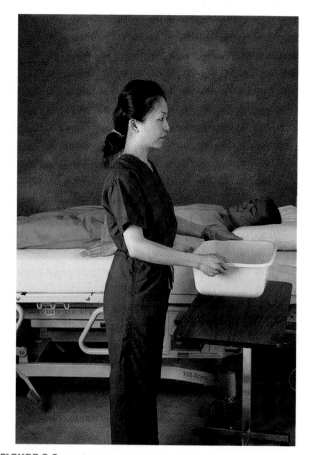

FIGURE 3-3 It takes less energy to hold an object close to the body than at a distance from the body.

13. When moving patients, pull steadily rather than pushing. **R:** When an object is pushed, it absorbs part of the force being exerted, leaving less force available to move the object. When an object is pulled, all of the force exerted is available for the task of moving.

14. Raise the bed or overbed table to an appropriate height for maximum working comfort. Also instruct patients using a working surface of any type to be sure that the surface is at an appropriate height. **R:** It takes less energy to work on a surface at an appropriate height (usually waist level) than it does to stoop or stretch to reach the surface. The back is susceptible to injury and fatigue from excessive bending.

Acute Care

Many patients in acute care are extremely weak, either because of an acute infectious process or because they are in the beginning stages of recovery from another major illness or surgery. In such instances, it will be extremely important for you to use excellent body mechanics to protect yourself and to conserve energy. In addition, it will be important for you to teach patients to use good body mechanics to facilitate their recovery.

Long-Term Care

The same principles of basic body mechanics apply in the long-term care setting as in the acute care setting. However, the residents in this setting may need more assistance from you, and you may need to secure more help before attempting a task. In addition, because many caregivers in long-term settings are nursing assistants, you may need to teach these principles to them. The example you set by the body mechanics you use is important to those with whom you work.

Home Care

The client receiving care at home, the family, and other caregivers will need to learn appropriate principles of body mechanics to ensure safety for all concerned. You may need to assess family members and caregivers for adequacy of knowledge, skill, and equipment to handle a client in a particular situation. The height of the chair or bed, the distance to the bathroom or kitchen, the size of the client and the caregiver, and the availability of mechanical assistive devices should be considered during this assessment.

LEARNING TOOLS

DEVELOP YOUR BACKGROUND KNOWLEDGE

1. Review the Learning Outcomes.

2. Read the section on posture and body mechanics in your assigned text.

3. Look up the Key Terms in the glossary.

4. Review the module as though you were preparing to teach the contents to another person. Mentally practice the techniques.

5. Pay attention to your habitual posture as well as the way you perform routine tasks of lifting and moving. Are you using good body mechanics?

DEVELOP YOUR SKILLS

1. In the practice setting, with a partner observing

   a. Stand with your weight balanced over your base of support.

   b. Stand 3 feet from a table or counter. Try to place a book on the table without enlarging your base of support. Begin again, and place the book on the table using an enlarged base of support. Compare your stability in the two situations.

   c. Stand in a normal position. Have your partner take your arms and pull until you begin to tip forward. Using the same base of support, squat low, and have your partner pull again. Compare the force needed to disrupt your stability in the two positions.

   d. Stand with your feet 8 inches apart, but side by side, and try to push a bed. Now enlarge your base of support in the direction in which you are pushing, and note the difference.

   e. Practice tightening your abdominal muscles upward and your gluteal muscles downward. Relax. Tighten the muscles again. Do this before you attempt any task.

   f. Face the bed. While keeping your feet in the same position, turn your upper body 90 degrees to the right as if reaching for something; note the feeling of strain and pull on your back muscles. Try bending from this position; note the lack of stability.

   g. Face the bed. Turn 90 degrees to the right by moving your right foot and turning your whole body; note that your back is straight. Now try bending and reaching; note the increased stability in this position.

   h. Pick up an object from the floor or other low surface, bending your knees and keeping your back straight. Use this posture whenever you need to reach something on the floor.

i. With your partner assisting, try to move another person up in bed with the head of the bed at a 30-degree angle. Now place the bed in a flat position, and repeat the activity. Compare the amount of energy required. Have your "patient" evaluate the experience.

j. Again, with your partner assisting and with the bed in a flat position, move your "patient" up in bed without a turn sheet and against a wrinkled bottom sheet. Now tighten the bottom sheet, and use a turn sheet for the same activity. Compare the experiences. Ask your "patient" to comment.

k. Hold a 10-lb object (brick, book) with both hands directly in front of and close to your body for 3 minutes. Now do the same thing holding the object at arm's length from your body. Compare the amount of energy required for each task.

l. With a turn sheet, turn your "patient" from a supine position to a lateral position, using your weight as a **counterbalance.** Note the ease with which you can do this.

m. Have one person lie in the bed and act like a patient. Try to move the "patient's" shoulders closer to the far edge of the bed by pushing. Then push the hips and feet toward the far side of the bed. Next, move the patient's shoulders toward you by slipping your arms under the shoulders and pulling. Do the same for the hips and feet. Note the difference in ease of movement when pushing and pulling.

n. Trade places with the person in the bed, and repeat the exercise of pushing and pulling. Compare how it felt to be pulled and how it felt to be pushed.

2. When you think you have practiced enough, perform all the above tasks correctly for your instructor, using your partner as a "patient" when necessary.

DEMONSTRATE YOUR SKILLS

In the clinical setting
1. Apply basic body mechanics whenever possible. If you are unsure or need help, consult your instructor.

2. Identify a patient who would gain by using body mechanics principles. This may be a patient with limitations in one or both lower extremities. Instruct the patient in the correct use of body mechanics with the help of your instructor.

CRITICAL THINKING EXERCISES

1. You are to transfer 86-year-old Mabel Seeland, who has an abdominal wound, from a chair to a standing position. Review the principles presented in the

module and then determine which ones are essential for this task. Identify the rationale for each principle you will follow. After planning for the task, state the directions you will give the patient so that she can assist you.

2. Mr. James Smithhart is lying on his back in bed. He is 35 years old, 6 feet tall, and weighs 210 lb. The head of his bed is elevated to 30 degrees, and he needs to be moved up toward the head of the bed. At this time, he is unable to help in any way. Plan how you will move him up in bed. Include all principles you will use, and support your choices.

SELF-QUIZ
TRUE-FALSE

_____ 1. The body is less stable when the center of gravity falls beyond the edge of the base of support.

_____ 2. Stability is increased when the center of gravity is close to the base of support.

_____ 3. Facing in the direction of the task to be performed is not recommended.

_____ 4. Friction enhances movement.

_____ 5. It takes less energy to hold an object close to the body than at a distance from the body.

_____ 6. When carrying out a task, the faster one moves, the better.

SHORT-ANSWER QUESTIONS

7. Why is lifting or pulling using the back muscles contraindicated?

_____

8. Which principle of body mechanics is the basis for a decision to put the head of the bed down before moving the patient?

_____

9. Which principle of body mechanics is the basis for a decision to spread your feet farther apart before trying to lift a patient?

_____

10. Which principle of body mechanics is the basis for a decision to move closer to the patient's bed before attempting to move the patient?

_____

Answers to Self-Quiz questions appear in the back of this book.

MODULE
4

Basic Infection Control

SKILLS INCLUDED IN THIS MODULE

General Approaches and Principles of Medical Asepsis
Using Standard Precautions for Preventing Infection
General Procedure for Standard Precautions
Procedure for Handwashing
Procedure for Using an Alcohol-Based Hand Disinfectant
Procedure for Putting On and Removing Clean Gloves

PREREQUISITE MODULE

Module 1   An Approach to Nursing
             Skills

KEY TERMS

bacteria	invasive
barrier	medical asepsis
blood-borne	microorganism
body substances	nosocomial
contamination	pathogens
droplet nuclei	post-exposure
face shield	prophylaxis (PEP)
friction	Standard
goggles	Precautions
immunosuppression	subungual
interdigital	surgical asepsis

OVERALL OBJECTIVE

▸ To apply principles of basic infection control when practicing all aspects of nursing, with particular emphasis on hand hygiene.

LEARNING OUTCOMES

The student will be able to

1. Describe the requirements for Standard Precautions as identified by the Centers for Disease Control and Prevention (CDC).
2. Assess the healthcare environment in order to identify possible sources of transmission of microorganisms.
3. Analyze situations to identify those in which handwashing is essential and when hand anti-sepsis may be accomplished by using a hand disinfectant.
4. Analyze situations to accurately determine when specific personal protective equipment (PPE), such as gloves, eye protection, masks, gowns, or aprons, are needed.
5. Implement actions to prevent microorganisms from moving from one area or item to another.
6. Wash hands correctly.
7. Use hand disinfectant correctly.
8. Put on and remove PPE correctly so as to avoid contaminating own body or clothing.
9. Maintain personal hygiene appropriately for the clinical setting.
10. Evaluate own performance in relation to maintaining Standard Precautions and protecting both the patient and self from the transmission of microorganisms.

Infection control includes all of the practices used to prevent the spread of any **microorganism** (or germ) that could cause disease in a person. Traditionally, infection control procedures have been classified as medical asepsis and surgical asepsis.

ASEPSIS

Medical asepsis is the practice of techniques and procedures designed to reduce the number of microorganisms in an area or on an object and to decrease the likelihood of their transfer. Medical asepsis is sometimes referred to as "clean technique." The practice of medical asepsis takes on added importance in individuals who are more susceptible to infection because of illness, surgery, or **immunosuppression.**

Because the nurse may be in contact with a number of patients during any day, he or she must be aware of the principles of medical asepsis to avoid transferring microorganisms from a patient to the nurse, from the nurse to a patient, from the nurse to a coworker, or from one patient to another. Microorganisms can also be transferred in a wide variety of ways.

Intact skin is an effective **barrier** to microorganisms. Skin that is not intact and areas of the body that are normally sterile (such as the eyes and inside of the bladder) require additional precautions to prevent the entry of infection-causing microorganisms. These additional precautions are called surgical asepsis.

Surgical asepsis includes all the sterile procedures and techniques used to exclude all microorganisms from

an area. Surgical asepsis is described in Module 24 and Module 25.

NURSING DIAGNOSIS

Risk for Infection: Infection control measures are used for all patients in all settings. However, some patients are more susceptible to infection because of compromised immune systems, breaks in the normal defense barrier of the intact skin, or **invasive** devices, such as IV lines. For these patients, the nursing diagnosis Risk for Infection is appropriate.

GENERAL APPROACHES AND PRINCIPLES OF MEDICAL ASEPSIS

The first step in infection control is preventing the spread of microorganisms from one place in the environment to another.

1. Avoid shaking or tossing linens, which can create air currents. Be sure that all doors leading to rooms used for respiratory isolation are kept closed to stop air currents. **R:** Microorganisms move on air currents.

   Note: Most hospitals are built in such a way that the ventilation system does not circulate air from one section to another. Rooms designed to be used for patients with airborne infections, such as tuberculosis, have air systems that create negative pressure in the room. When the door is opened, air from the corridor moves into the room, and potentially contaminated air from the room does not move outward. In operating rooms, the air systems are designed to provide positive pressure. When the door is opened, potentially contaminated air does not move into the operating room. Instead, air from the extra-clean environment tends to move out into the corridor.

2. Always keep clean items separate from dirty ones. Do not allow items that have touched one patient or patient's environment to touch another patient or patient's environment. Keep your hands away from your own hair and face. Keep linens away from your uniform. If you drop anything on the floor, consider it dirty. **R:** Microorganisms are transferred from one surface to another whenever objects touch. The patient and the patient's environment all contain microorganisms, some of which may produce disease in another patient or in you as a care provider. Microorganisms from one area of the body may be disease producing in another area of the body.

3. Avoid passing dirty items over clean items or areas because it is possible for microorganisms to drop off onto a clean item or area. When storing items in a bedside stand, place clean items on upper shelves and potentially dirty items, such as bedpans, on lower shelves. **R:** Microorganisms are transferred by gravity when one item is held above another.

4. Avoid having a patient breathe directly into your face, and avoid breathing directly into a patient's face. If the patient has a cough, wear a mask when giving care. Whenever you cough or sneeze, cover your nose and mouth with a tissue, and discard it immediately in an appropriate container. **R:** Microorganisms are released into the air on droplet nuclei whenever a person breathes or speaks. Coughing or sneezing dramatically increases the number of microorganisms released from the mouth and nose. A tissue confines the droplets for disposal.

5. Whenever you have coughed, sneezed, or blown your nose, wash your hands before you touch anything else. Teach the patient to handle coughing and sneezing in the same way. If you handle tissues that a patient has used when coughing or sneezing, always wash your hands thoroughly. **R:** Handwashing removes both secretions and microorganisms that have been transferred to the hands.

6. To prevent ongoing **contamination,** use a dry paper towel when you turn off faucets. **R:** The faucet handle became contaminated when the water was turned on. Touching the handle with clean hands will transfer microorganisms from the handle back to your hands. The dry paper towel provides a barrier to the transfer of microorganisms.

7. Dry a bath basin before you return it to a bedside stand for storage. **R:** Microorganisms multiply more rapidly in moist environments than in dry environments.

8. Wash your hands or use an alcohol-based hand disinfectant when hands are obviously soiled and also whenever you move from one patient to another or from patient contact to contact with the general environment or vice versa. **R:** Proper hand hygiene removes many of the microorganisms that can be transferred by the hands from one item or one person to another.

USING STANDARD PRECAUTIONS FOR PREVENTING INFECTION

Blood-borne infections, especially human immunodeficiency virus (HIV), which causes acquired immunodeficiency syndrome (AIDS), and hepatitis B and C viruses, may be spread to another person through contact between blood and **body substances** that contain the blood-borne organism and open wounds, sores, or mucous membranes. Infection may also be spread between penetrating injuries (such as those caused by needle sticks or cuts) and contaminated items. The body substances that transmit blood-borne **pathogens** (disease-causing agents) include amniotic fluid, blood, cerebrospinal fluid, pericardial fluid, peritoneal fluid, pleural fluid, semen, synovial fluid, and vaginal secretions (Box 4-1). In 1987, the CDC of the U.S. Department of Health and Human Services developed a set of guidelines to prevent the transmission of blood-borne pathogens. These guidelines are called *Universal Precautions for Blood and Body Fluids* (Mason, 1988).

The Occupational Health and Safety Administration (OSHA) has mandated that healthcare agencies provide educational sessions regarding Universal Precautions

---

box 4-1   *Infection Sources of Concern in Standard Precautions*

1. Blood
2. All body fluids, secretions, and excretions regardless of whether or not they contain visible blood:

Amniotic fluid	Semen
Cerebrospinal fluid	Sputum
Feces	Synovial fluid
Nasal secretions	Urine
Pericardial fluid	Vaginal secretions
Peritoneal fluid	Vomitus
Pleural fluid	

3. Nonintact skin
4. Mucous membranes

Note: Universal Precautions for Blood-borne Pathogens do not apply to nasal secretions, sputum, urine, feces, saliva, sweat, tears, or vomit unless there is visible blood in them because those substances do not transmit blood-borne pathogens.

before any employee comes in contact with patients. In addition, OSHA regulations require that agencies provide an annual review of these practices for every employee. Every agency must provide the supplies needed to enable employees to carry out Universal Precautions. Any agency that does not provide appropriate supplies or in which personnel are violating these standards is subject to a substantial fine.

Although blood-borne pathogens are a great concern, many other pathogens exist in the healthcare environment. Some body substances, such as feces, urine, nasal secretions, vomit, and sputum, do not contain blood-borne organisms, but they may contain such large quantities of **bacteria** that their removal through normal hand hygiene is difficult. Additionally there are drug-resistant organisms present in the healthcare environment.

Therefore, in 1994, the CDC released a draft of new infection control guidelines termed **Standard Precautions.** These guidelines have sometimes been referred to as Body Substance Precautions. These guidelines are considered the Tier 1 precautions and include all those in Universal Precautions and then expand to precautions that prevent all contact with any moist body substance including feces, urine, nasal secretions, vomit, and sputum to decrease the potential for transmission of bacteria found in these substances. Although OSHA has not revised its regulations to require the use of Standard Precautions, their use is required by the Joint Commission for the Accreditation of Healthcare Organizations (JCAHO) and Medicare and Medicaid Conditions of Participation. Because of these requirements and the CDC recommendations, Standard Precautions are emphasized here and throughout the text. Remember that Standard Precautions include all of the measures that are a part of Universal Precautions (Garner & HICPAC, 1996). Appendix A provides an overview of Standard Precautions for easy reference.

The Tier 2 "Transmission-Based Precautions" were designed for patients known to be or suspected of being infected or colonized with highly transmissible or important microorganisms. These precautions are discussed in Module 23.

GENERAL PROCEDURE FOR STANDARD PRECAUTIONS

1. Wear clean latex or vinyl gloves whenever there is potential for contact with any of the body fluids listed in Box 4-2. Other nonlatex gloves, such as nitrile rubber gloves, are now available in some settings for use by personnel who are allergic to latex (see Box 4-3 for more information). **R:** This protects you by preventing any accidental contact of a substance that could carry a pathogen through breaks

---

box 4-2 *Actions Requiring Glove Use for Personal Protection*

1. Performing phlebotomy (if the nurse is learning phlebotomy technique; if the nurse has cuts, scratches, or other breaks in the skin; and when hand contamination with blood may occur)
2. Performing finger or heel sticks on infants and children. *Note:* It is the performing that is key to the requirement. If you are not the person performing the needle stick (just holding the child for example), you do not need gloves.
3. Throughout procedures involving contact with mucous membranes and diagnostic procedures that do not require sterile gloves
4. Changing or manipulating intravenous lines when blood contamination is possible
5. Handling dressings soiled with body fluids
6. Giving care (such as perineal care) that could result in contact with body fluids that transmit blood-borne pathogens
7. Handling urine or feces
8. Giving mouth care or handling nasal secretions and sputum

Note: Items 1 to 6 are required in Universal Precautions and items 7 to 8 comply with Standard Precautions.

---

box 4-3 *Concerns and Cautions Regarding Latex*

Latex allergies are an increasing problem in healthcare because of the high exposure to latex gloves and latex in medical supplies. Latex allergies may begin as localized sensitivity reactions on the hands; however, latex allergy can develop into potentially life-threatening anaphylaxis. Even a local sensitivity reaction on the hands would prevent a healthcare worker from providing care if a substitute type of gloves was not available. Therefore, efforts are being made to decrease the potential for latex exposure; some environments are latex-free.

Latex gloves without powder are less likely to cause allergy to develop because the powder carries microscopic latex particles into the air where it can be inhaled. This inhalation increases the potential for systemic allergy. Therefore, unpowdered gloves are one avenue of prevention of latex allergies. The use of nonlatex gloves and medical supplies are essential for those healthcare providers and patients who already have a latex allergy. When the patient has a latex allergy, everyone on the healthcare team must be aware of that allergy and protect the patient from any latex contact. Many facilities are making nonlatex gloves a standard to prevent the development of latex allergies.

in your skin and decreases the potential for your acquiring pathogens on your hands.

2. Wear gloves in the specific situations in which gloves are recommended by the CDC because the potential for contact with pathogens is high. **R:** Knowing specific requirements enables you to protect yourself and supports your compliance with regulatory requirements.

3. Change gloves between patient contacts. **R:** Gloves can carry pathogens from one patient to another.

4. Do not wash or clean examination gloves. **R:** Examination gloves are not designed for heavy use, and washing them creates small holes and weakened areas that diminish their effectiveness and allow microorganisms to enter.

5. Wash your hands thoroughly with soap and water when the hands are visibly soiled and immediately after accidental contact with body substances. **R:** Washing with soap and water removes foreign material and microorganisms.

6. Wash hands or use disinfectant alcohol-based hand rub:
   a. between patients
   b. immediately after gloves are removed. **R:** Microorganisms are always acquired when touching a patient. Gloves may contain microscopic holes that allow some microorganisms to enter. Microorganisms multiply rapidly on the warm, moist skin under gloves. Handwashing removes visible soil and microorganisms from intact skin. Disinfectant alcohol-based hand rubs remove microorganisms and slow microbial regrowth on hands.

7. Wear masks and protective eyewear or **face shields** during procedures that may generate droplets or splashes of blood or other body fluids. **Goggles,** plastic eyeglasses, or shields that fit over eyeglass frames may be used as protective eyewear. A face shield may be attached to the top of a mask or to a headband. **R:** Blood-borne pathogens may enter the body through mucous membranes. Masks protect the mouth and nose. Protective eyewear will protect the mucous membranes of the healthcare worker's eyes. A face shield protects the mouth and nose as well as the eyes.

8. Wear a disposable, moisture-proof apron or gown during procedures likely to soil your clothing or generate splatters of body fluid. **R:** This protects your body from accidental contact with pathogens and prevents you from carrying contaminated substances to others on your clothing.

9. Wear general purpose utility gloves (such as rubber household gloves) for housekeeping chores and instrument cleaning. **R:** Utility gloves are thicker and stronger and provide better protection against accidental glove breaks than patient care gloves in situations where dexterity and touch are not concerns. Utility gloves are less likely to have microscopic holes because of their thickness.

10. General purpose utility gloves may be decontaminated and reused. **R:** These gloves are strong enough to remain intact when cleaned; however, they should be discarded if they are peeling, cracked, or discolored or if they have punctures, tears, or other evidence of deterioration because they will no longer provide an effective barrier.

11. Wear sterile gloves for procedures involving contact with normally sterile areas of the body (see Module 24). **R:** The sterile gloves protect the patient from environmental microorganisms while protecting you from the patient's microorganisms.

12. Dispose of sharp equipment (such as needles, disposable syringes, scalpel blades, and the like) and secretions properly. Place sharp instruments in puncture-resistant containers for disposal. These items should not be recapped, broken, or carried from one area to another but disposed of directly in an appropriate container in the area where used. **R:** Accidental penetrating injuries and contact with contaminated substances are serious occupational hazards for healthcare workers as well as for patients and visitors in the environment. Puncture-resistant containers protect maintenance workers who remove trash. Any manipulation or uncovered transporting of the sharp object increases the potential for accidental injury.

13. Carefully pour bulk blood, suctioned fluids, and excretions that contain blood and listed body fluids down drains to the sewer. **R:** The sanitary sewer system is designed to prevent pathogens from contact with people in the community.

14. Put all specimens of blood and listed fluids in moisture-proof containers with secure lids. Avoid contaminating the outside of the container. In many settings, specimen containers are placed inside a plastic bag for further protection against potential leakage. **R:** This prevents leakage during transport and protects transporters and laboratory personnel from accidental contamination.

15. Handle soiled linen correctly.
    a. Hold linen away from your uniform. **R:** This prevents contaminating your uniform.
    b. Do not shake or toss linen. **R:** Shaking and tossing linens creates contaminated air currents.
    c. Place and transport linen soiled with blood or body fluids in leakage-resistant bags. **R:** This prevents accidental contamination of those who handle soiled linens.

16. Follow your facility's policies for cleaning contaminated surfaces and materials and for disposing of infective wastes.
    a. Clean visible soil from objects and surfaces before disinfection. **R:** Pathogens can live inside of or under visible soil despite contact with disinfectants.

b. Use a commercial germicide solution for cleaning. In the absence of a commercial germicide, household bleach in a 1:10 dilution is an effective disinfectant. **R:** These solutions can destroy all blood-borne pathogens and most other microorganisms.

17. Use mouthpieces, resuscitation bags, or other ventilation devices for cardiopulmonary resuscitation whenever possible. Facilities are urged to place these devices in areas where their need is predictable. **R:** Although saliva has not been implicated in HIV transmission, other infections are transmitted by saliva.

18. Healthcare workers with open or draining lesions should refrain from all direct patient care and from handling patient care equipment until the lesions heal. **R:** This prevents any possible contact between contaminated substances and the lesions of the healthcare worker who is at high risk if accidental contact occurs. This also protects the patient from a healthcare worker who may have a blood-borne infection.

POST-EXPOSURE PROPHYLAXIS

Post-exposure prophylaxis (PEP) refers to providing medical treatment of an individual for a serious communicable disease after known exposure, before any disease has developed. In some diseases such as rabies, PEP involves immunization, which is effective because the disease has a long incubation period. For many communicable diseases, PEP involves providing specific drug treatment of the disease-producing organism. PEP has both benefits and adverse effects. In many cases, PEP may completely eliminate the potential for the disease; in others, PEP sets the stage for a mild rather than severe illness. The adverse effects are those of the side effects of the drugs. When side effects are very mild, this may not be a concern; however, in some instances, side effects are potentially very serious (CDC, 2001a).

PEP is available for those exposed to the blood-borne pathogens of hepatitis B and C and HIV (CDC, 2001b). The decision to use PEP is made with the individual exposed and the healthcare provider determining the risks and benefits. Whenever exposure to a blood-borne pathogen occurs in the healthcare setting, the exposed employee must be provided counseling regarding the PEP available, the risks and benefits, and the relevant medication. Students are not employees of healthcare institutions and are therefore not covered by regulations that require employer coverage of injuries on the job, although some institutions may choose to treat students. In the case of exposure, a student may be covered by personal health insurance or by a student health plan for PEP. Students are encouraged to learn about relevant policies.

HAND HYGIENE

The most important procedure for preventing the transfer of microorganisms, and therefore **nosocomial** infection (infection acquired in a healthcare facility) is correct and frequent hand hygiene. Proper hand hygiene protects the patient, your coworkers, you, and your family. Hand hygiene should be performed in all of the instances listed in Box 4-4. Hand hygiene may consist of handwashing or the use of a disinfectant alcohol-based hand rub. Handwashing is essential if there is visible soil on the hands. When no visible soil exists, alcohol-based hand rub provides excellent hand hygiene (Boyce & Pittet, 2002).

For medical asepsis, the CDC recommends at least a vigorous 10-second handwashing procedure that includes "a rubbing together of all surfaces of lathered hands followed by rinsing under a stream of water." Further, they comment that in situations in which hands are visibly soiled, "more time" may be required (Boyce & Pittet, 2002). Some nurses prefer to use a 30-second handwash all of the time as an extra safety precaution. Current recommendations for safety suggest that you always wash or disinfect your hands where the patient can see your actions and be reassured that he or she is being protected from infection.

PROCEDURE FOR HANDWASHING

ASSESSMENT

1. Assess your hands. **R:** To determine the soil present.

ANALYSIS

2. Analyze your data to determine whether handwashing is needed or a hand disinfectant can be used. **R:** Visible soil requires handwashing. Hand hygiene with a skin disinfectant may be used if no visible soil is present.

PLANNING

3. Note where the nearest sink is located in relation to the tasks you have before you. **R:** Washing hands close to the site of activities lessens the potential for hand contamination before you begin.

---

box 4-4 *Situations Requiring Hand Hygiene*

At the beginning of every work shift
Before and after contact with each patient
Immediately before invasive procedures
Before and after touching dressings
Whenever gloves are removed
Any time you question whether hand hygiene is needed
At the end of every shift before leaving the healthcare facility

IMPLEMENTATION

Action	Rationale
4. Roll your sleeves above your elbows, and remove your watch and all other hand and wrist jewelry. If your watch has an expansion band, move it up above your elbow to allow you to wash well up your arms. After the initial handwash of the shift, wash your hands well above the wrists, unless you have been in a situation that you feel necessitates more thorough washing.	This exposes your hands and ensures that you can complete thorough washing without soiling your uniform or damaging your watch.
5. Do not touch the sink, and avoid splashing dirty water on your uniform.	The handwashing procedure causes microorganisms to accumulate in the sink.
6. Turn on the water, adjust the temperature, and leave it running during the procedure.	Warm water removes fewer oils from the skin than hot water and removes microorganisms more effectively than cold water.
7. Dispense liquid or powdered soap, preferably with a foot control.	The CDC recommends that the cleansing agent may be plain soap in all situations except those involving the care of newborns, between patients in high-risk units, and before the care of immunosuppressed patients. In these situations, antimicrobial products should be used. Bar soap is not recommended because it may harbor microorganisms. If only bar soap is available, lather and rinse the bar thoroughly to remove the outside layer of soap before you use it.
8. Lather your hands and arms well.	The lather emulsifies skin oils and picks up microorganisms.
9. Clean your fingernails as needed with a nail file or other nail-cleaning utensil. (If these utensils are not provided, do this before you leave home.) It is only necessary to do this once at the beginning of the shift.	The **subungual** (under the fingernails) area is an area where bacteria multiply and is frequently missed in handwashing.
10. Using a rotary motion and **friction,** wash your hands and arms up to your elbows, adding soap as needed to maintain a lather. Hold hands and forearms lower than elbows (Fig. 4-1).	A rotary motion removes microorganisms from the creases in the skin. Friction displaces skin debris and microorganisms into the lather. Microorganisms are suspended in the lather and can be rinsed off. Holding the hands down causes the soiled water to run off into the sink so that it does not run back up your arms or onto your uniform.

(continued)

Action	Rationale

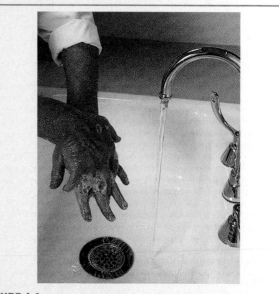

FIGURE 4-1 Handwashing with hands lower than elbows and fingers intertwined to promote sudsing.

Action	Rationale
11. Pay particular attention to the **interdigital** spaces (between your fingers), your knuckles, and the outside surfaces of the fifth or "little" fingers.	The area between the fingers is easily overlooked.
12. Holding your hands and forearms lower than your elbows, rinse thoroughly, starting at one elbow and moving down the arm (see Fig. 4-1). Then repeat this step for the other arm.	This position prevents microorganisms from being rinsed up your arms from your hands, which are frequently the most contaminated.
13. Blot your hands dry from fingers to forearms. Most facilities provide paper towels for this purpose.	Blotting with a paper towel is easier on the skin than rubbing.
14. Turn off the water with a dry paper towel if the faucet is hand operated.	The dry paper towel protects your hands from the microorganisms that are on the faucet.
15. Use lotion if appropriate.	Because frequent handwashing can lead to dry, cracked skin in some individuals, the use of lotion may be encouraged to help keep skin intact, thus preventing possible invasion by microorganisms. In some settings, however, you may be asked not to use lotion during the workday because it can be an excellent medium for bacterial growth.

EVALUATION

16. Evaluate the condition of your hands and whether you have disinfected all surfaces.

PROCEDURE FOR USING AN ALCOHOL-BASED HAND DISINFECTANT

ASSESSMENT

1. Assess your hands. **R:** To determine the soil present.

ANALYSIS

2. Analyze your data to determine whether handwashing is needed or a hand disinfectant can be used. **R:** Visible soil requires handwashing. Hand hygiene with a skin disinfectant may be used if no visible soil is present.

PLANNING

3. Note where the hand disinfectant is located in relation to the place where you will perform your task. **R:** Washing hands close to the site of activities lessens the potential for hand contamination before you begin.

IMPLEMENTATION

Action	Rationale
4. Release approximately 1 tablespoon of disinfectant into the palm of your hand.	This amount will allow you to thoroughly disinfect all surfaces of both hands.
5. Rub the disinfectant thoroughly over all surfaces of your hands including the interdigital spaces, around the nails, and the backs of your hands. Rub until the gel disappears.	All surfaces must be in contact with the disinfectant for it to be effective.

EVALUATION

6. Evaluate the condition of your hands and whether you have disinfected all surfaces (Fig. 4-2).

PLANNING

4. Identify the location of the type of gloves you need. **R:** Nonlatex gloves may need to be obtained from central supplies.

PROCEDURE FOR PUTTING ON AND REMOVING CLEAN GLOVES

ASSESSMENT

1. Assess the situation. **R:** To determine whether clean gloves are required.
2. Check patient allergies. **R:** Latex allergies are increasingly common.

ANALYSIS

3. Analyze your information **R:** To determine whether latex gloves are acceptable or whether a latex substitute is needed.

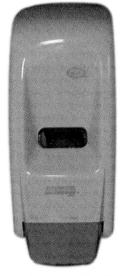

FIGURE 4-2 Disinfectant alcohol-based hand rub.

IMPLEMENTATION

Action	Rationale
5. Wash or disinfect your hands.	Hands are washed or disinfected before putting on gloves to decrease the microbial growth in the warm environment under the gloves.
6. Remove two gloves from box.	Removing both gloves at once allows you to proceed more efficiently.
7. Pull each glove on, being sure that you have extended them up your wrists.	For maximum protection of your skin.
8. Press the gloves down between the fingers.	This provides a better fit over the fingers and improves dexterity.
9. To remove the glove, grasp the outside cuff edge of one glove with the other still-gloved hand, and turn the glove inside out as you pull it off.	The outsides of both gloves are soiled, and touching your skin with the outside of a glove will contaminate your skin. Turning the glove inside out as you remove it confines most contamination inside of the glove (Fig. 4-3).

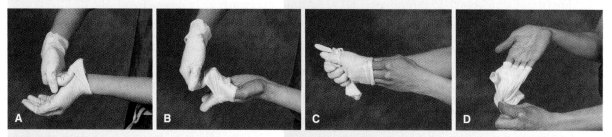

FIGURE 4-3 (**A**) Removing clean gloves. (**B**) Remove the first glove by touching the outside with the still-gloved other hand. (**C**) Remove the second glove by sliding the fingers inside the glove to avoid touching the outside of the glove with the hand. (**D**) Turn the glove inside out and slide off.

Action	Rationale
10. Slide your ungloved hand inside the remaining glove and remove it by turning it inside out.	By touching skin to skin, you are preventing the contamination of one hand by the contaminated glove.
11. Dispose of both gloves in the waste receptacle closest to where you took them off.	Soiled items remain a source of contamination, and proper disposal prevents further transfer of microbes.
12. Wash or disinfect your hands.	Cleaning your hands removes the microbial growth that occurred in the warm environment under the gloves.

EVALUATION

13. Evaluate. **R:** To determine that you have not contaminated your hands, uniform, or any object in the environment.

PERSONAL HYGIENE

Obviously, to enhance infection control, you must practice good personal hygiene. In addition, the personal hygiene of the nurse is important to the perception of the nurse as a competent professional. In situations where these guidelines are not enforced by employers, your knowledge of the rationale for such guidelines and your conscience must guide your actions. The following are guidelines for personal hygiene:

- Arrange your hair in a way that does not contribute to contaminating the patient or the environment and that will protect you from contaminating your hair with microbes you may have contacted with your hands. Hair should not fall forward when you lean forward (for example, when you examine a patient). When hair falls over an area, microorganisms can drop from the hair (by gravity) onto the patient, or the hair itself may fall onto trays or wounds. Keep your hair short, or restrain it in some way so that it does not fall forward.

- Also avoid any hairstyle that requires you to constantly brush your hair out of your eyes or back from your face. If your hands have just been washed, you may transfer microorganisms from your hair to your hands. If your hands have not just been washed, you may transfer microorganisms from your hands to your hair.

- Keep your fingernails clean, trimmed, and filed short, so you do not endanger patients by scratching them or by harboring bacteria.

- If you use nail polish, it must be intact; chipped polish also is a place for bacteria to lodge.

- Do not wear artificial nails or nail tips. These very hard nails can easily scratch a patient or create a tear in fragile skin. Additionally, research demonstrates that there are small spaces between the artificial nail and the nail bed that harbor pathogens and increase the potential for transmission of infection (Larson, 1995).

- Wear minimal jewelry, because jewelry is a place for microorganisms to lodge. Plain studs or posts for pierced ears and plain wedding bands or other plain rings are the most jewelry you should wear in a clinical setting. Necklaces and large hoop or dangling earrings are a hazard not only in terms of infection control but also because a patient can grab them and hurt you and the jewelry.

LEARNING TOOLS

1. Review the Learning Outcomes.

2. Read the section on asepsis (in Modules 24 and 25), and focus especially on the chain of infection in your assigned textbook.

3. Look up the Key Terms in the glossary.

4. Review the module and mentally practice the skills. Study the material, so you will be able to teach it to others.

5. Practice putting on clean gloves and taking them off in a way that protects you from contamination.

6. Practice handwashing techniques.

7. Practice using disinfectant hand rub.

8. In the practice setting, practice safe handwashing techniques, using the procedure as a guide and the Performance Checklist (on the CD-ROM that accompanies this book) as an evaluation tool. When you are satisfied with your ability, have your instructor evaluate you.

9. In the clinical setting, demonstrate handwashing to your clinical instructor.

10. In the clinical setting, use Standard Precautions, and demonstrate this to your clinical instructor.

CRITICAL THINKING EXERCISES

1. You entered the patient's room to answer a call light. While there, you retrieved his urinal from the bathroom. You helped him use the urinal and took it to the bathroom to empty it. Before leaving, you poured a glass of water for him and then returned to the nurses' station to chart. Identify all the times when you should have used Standard Precautions in this situation and the specific actions needed. Give the rationale for the actions you decided to perform.

2. Mr. Smith is a resident in a long-term care facility where you are having clinical experience. You note that he has a cough. Identify the specific infection control measures you should institute with Mr. Smith. Determine which infection control measures you should teach him.

3. You are in a hospital room, and the patient cries out, "I just caught my IV tubing in the bed rail, and I've pulled it out. I'm bleeding! Do something!" Identify the infection control principles and directives that apply in this situation. Explain your concerns, and describe the actions you should take to protect yourself.

SELF-QUIZ
SHORT-ANSWER QUESTIONS

State the rationale for the following actions.

1. Avoid shaking or tossing linens.

_____

2. Keep your hands away from your hair and face.

_____

3. Avoid passing dirty items over clean items or areas.

_____

4. Use a dry paper towel when you turn off faucets.

_____

5. Wear goggles and mask or face shield when there is a potential for blood splashes.

_____

6. Do not recap or break contaminated needles.

_____

7. Wear gloves when handling feces.

_____

8. Wear goggles or face shield when irrigating a wound.

_____

9. Use a hand disinfectant when hands are not visibly soiled.

_____

10. Remove gloves by turning them inside out.

_____

11. Wash your hands when you have gotten food on them while assisting a patient with eating.

_____

MULTIPLE CHOICE

_____ **12.** In which of the following situations should nurses wash or disinfect their hands? (Choose all that apply.)
a. At the beginning of the shift
b. Before going to lunch
c. After removing gloves used while handling body substances
d. Before putting on gloves

_____ **13.** Which of the following are essential components of the handwashing procedure? (Choose all that apply.)
a. Friction
b. Running water
c. Foot-operated water controls
d. Cleansing agent

_____ **14.** Which of the following areas should the nurse not touch during the handwashing procedure? (Choose all that apply.)
a. The inside of the sink
b. The outside of the sink
c. A hand-controlled faucet
d. Own hair

_____ **15.** Which of the following should receive attention during the handwashing procedures? (Choose all that apply.)
a. Palms
b. Elbows
c. Spaces between the fingers
d. Fingernails

_____ **16.** Which body substance transmits blood-borne pathogens, such as human immunodeficiency virus and hepatitis B virus?
a. Feces
b. Sputum
c. Urine
d. Vaginal secretions

_____ **17.** How may blood-borne pathogens enter the body?
a. Through breathing contaminated droplet nuclei
b. By skin-to-skin contact with the infected person
c. Through open wounds and mucous membranes that have been contacted by blood and certain body substances
d. By contact with objects that have been handled by the infected person

_____ **18.** When can you use a disinfectant alcohol-based hand rub instead of washing your hands?
a. At any time; it is always appropriate
b. Only if the patient is not immunocompromised
c. Only when putting on gloves
d. Any time if there is no visible soil on the hands

Answers to Self-Quiz questions appear in the back of this book.

Safety in the Healthcare Environment

SKILLS INCLUDED IN THIS MODULE

Procedure for Responding to Fire Codes
Procedure for the Use of Safety Devices and Restraints

PREREQUISITE MODULES

Module 1	An Approach to Nursing Skills
Module 2	Documentation
Module 3	Basic Body Mechanics
Module 4	Basic Infection Control

KEY TERMS

critical care
external disaster
internal disaster
JCAHO
triage

OVERALL OBJECTIVES

‣ To provide a safe environment for staff, visitors, and all people receiving care in healthcare settings by being constantly vigilant for unsafe conditions.
‣ To respond effectively to a fire code.
‣ To apply a variety of safety devices or physical restraints, taking into account the comfort and safety of the patient.

LEARNING OUTCOMES

The student will be able to

1. Assess the environment for basic safety for all patients.
2. Assess the patient for potential threats to individual safety.
3. Analyze the data to determine whether the environment should be modified or if safety measures should be initiated for the individual patient.
4. Determine appropriate patient outcomes in terms of safety and individual autonomy, and recognize the potential for adverse outcomes.
5. Plan safety measures for individual patients as well as for groups of patients.
6. Implement safety measures, meeting regulatory standards such as those governing the use of restraints.
7. Evaluate the effectiveness of implemented measures.
8. Document assessment in relation to safety, safety measures used, and evaluation of the effectiveness of measures used.

Because of its complexity, the healthcare setting is potentially dangerous. Facilities built with many floors have special problems when elevators cannot be used, and disabled individuals must be moved. The structure may have heavily traveled hallways, steps, and elevators. Monitoring areas for unsafe conditions and needed maintenance is a constant challenge and requires the vigilance and assistance of staff.

Patients' rooms are often small and confining—even more so if special equipment is needed for care. The space provided for nurses' stations has become increasingly crowded by records, monitoring equipment, and computer terminals that have been added as nursing and medical practices have grown more sophisticated.

The variety of equipment used within the modern healthcare environment adds to the difficulty of maintaining safety. Equipment as diverse as a simple thermometer and a complicated ventilator are included in the repertoire of practicing nurses today. The nurse must be skilled not only in operating equipment but also in detecting and correcting any problems that arise.

The unfamiliarity of the healthcare facility for most individuals adds to the potential for accident or injury. Members of the nursing staff should have the knowledge to protect themselves and act as advocates for others regarding safety. Nurses should be aware of the ethical and legal issues as well as the skills needed for applying safety devices and restraints. It is part of the nursing role to protect patients who are partially or completely unable to protect themselves. Patients at special risk for falls and injury include children; those who are elderly or confused; those who have sensory deficits, impaired mobility, a history of falls, or a history of substance abuse; and those who are receiving medications that interfere with normal functioning.

Fire and natural disasters pose an especially serious threat in any facility containing a large number of people, especially when many of these people are ill or dependent. An important goal for every practicing nurse is to be knowledgeable and prepared in all aspects of safety.

In long-term care facilities, providing a safe environment is particularly important because of the fragility and advanced age of most of the residents. In addition, the increasing numbers of nurses involved in home care have the responsibility of monitoring the home environment for safety hazards.

The Joint Commission on Accreditation of Healthcare Organizations (**JCAHO**) adopts National Patient Safety Goals each year (JCAHO, 2005). These goals focus on the issues that have created the most serious injuries to patients. The assumption of JCAHO is that routine safety measures are in place in healthcare facilities, but extra vigilance is warranted in situations of high risk. These patient safety goals are presented in Box 5-1.

Of these goals, three can be directly affected by even the beginning nursing student. *Improving communication* is a goal that requires the efforts of every individual in the healthcare setting. You will be learning specific communication strategies, but you can always be respectful, ask for clarification if you do not understand, and communicate what you have learned about the patient to the appropriate person. Throughout the modules, we emphasize the importance of communicating with the patient.

Improving the accuracy of patient identification is emphasized in each procedure. The standard expects that two identifiers will be used each time a procedure, treatment, test, or other aspect of care is done for a patient. Those two identifiers might be any two of the following: the patient's full name from the name band, the patient's identification number from the name band, the patient stating his or her full name, and a family member stating the name of an unresponsive patient. In the busy

box 5-1 *2006 JCAHO National Patient Safety Goals*

Goal 1 Improve the accuracy of patient identification.

Goal 2 Improve the effectiveness of communication among caregivers.

Goal 3 Improve the safety of using medications.

Goals 4, 5, and 6 from previous years were incorporated into other goals.

Goal 7 Reduce the risk of health care-associated infections.

Goal 8 Accurately and completely reconcile medications across the continuum of care.

Goal 9 Reduce the risk of patient harm resulting from falls.

Goal 10 Reduce the risk of influenza and pneumococcal disease in institutionalized older adults.

Goal 11 Reduce the risk of surgical fires.

Goal 12 Implementation of applicable National Patient Safety Goals and associated requirements by components and practitioner sites.

Goal 13 Encourage the active involvement of patients and their families in the patient's care as a patient safety strategy.

Goal 14 Prevent health care-associated pressure ulcers (decubitus ulcers).

Note: These general goals are the basis for site-specific safety goals being used by JCAHO. Greater detail is provided in subsections and explanatory notes on the JCAHO web site: *www.jcaho.org/accredited+organizations/ patient+safety*

healthcare environment, even when a patient is well known, it is all too easy to make a mistake in regard to care. Therefore, this must never be omitted.

Another goal that is directly affected by everyone in healthcare is *to reduce the risk of infection*. In Module 4, the essential requirements for infection control in healthcare settings were presented. Again, these practices must be followed meticulously.

NURSING DIAGNOSES

Risk for Injury related to impaired sensory function, altered cerebral function, altered mobility, and specific disturbances to function that affect ability to perceive or respond to the environment.

AGENCIES THAT GOVERN SAFETY STRATEGIES IN HEALTHCARE INSTITUTIONS

A number of agencies are concerned with maintaining safety for staff and patients in healthcare facilities. Some have a regulatory function, whereas others are advisory. These agencies also conduct or support research to understand better what hazards exist and how to diminish them. Table 5-1 identifies some of these important agencies. Some of these agencies have the ability to fine or even close a healthcare facility for violations of their standards.

MAINTAINING A SAFE ENVIRONMENT

What the agencies presented in Table 5-1 have in common are standards regarding a safe environment, and these standards relate to many different aspects of safety. Table 5-2 identifies common standards of a safe environment, and Table 5-3 identifies safe staff behaviors.

table 5-1. Agencies That Govern Safety

Agency	Role
Joint Commission for the Accreditation of Healthcare Organizations (JCAHO)	This organization sets standards for a voluntary accreditation process for all types of healthcare agencies. Many of their structural and process standards are designed to ensure safety outcomes of care. Each year, the JCAHO adopts safety goals that address areas of high risk in healthcare.
National Institute for Occupational Safety and Health (NIOSH)	NIOSH gathers and interprets data regarding safety collected by other organizations so that changes in practice can be made to ensure safety.
Occupational Safety and Health Administration (OSHA)	OSHA is a federal agency with regulatory powers allowing fines to be imposed on institutions that violate safety regulations for workers in all businesses that engage in interstate commerce. Because the federal government pays for care in healthcare institutions, the institutions are considered to be engaged in interstate commerce.
State Safety and Health Agencies	These are state counterparts to OSHA. State agency regulations may be stricter than national regulations but not more lenient. Safety regulations stemming from these agencies are written into the state administrative codes.
Centers for Disease Control and Prevention (CDC)	This is an advisory organization, largely concerned with preventing the spread of infection.
State Level Department of Health and Human Services or comparable agency.	State health departments inspect facilities for basic safety in areas such as fire safety, water, sewage, storage of hazardous materials, and hygiene.

table 5-2. Safe Environments for Care

Environmental Safety Concern	Standards
Lighting	Ensure that working spaces are lighted well enough to allow objects and people to be seen clearly. During the late evening hours, hallways are sometimes dimmed so that patients can rest more comfortably, but lighting should always be at a level that will ensure clear visibility.
Floor surfaces	Whether the flooring is covered with tile, linoleum, or carpet, surfaces should be smooth. Cracked tiles, raised linoleum, or torn carpeting can easily lead to falls. Highly polished floors can be slippery, thereby causing skids, falls, and injury. Anything on the floor increases the potential for falls. Wipe up liquid spills immediately. Calling a custodian or maintenance person could cause a delay long enough to expose someone to the danger of a fall. If mopping is in progress, always post a "Danger, Wet Floor" sign.
Electrical appliances	Electrical appliances must be in good working order and have a cord weight that is adequate for the appliance. Never use a frayed or damaged cord or plug because it may spark and cause a fire, injuring the operator or endangering the surrounding area. All plugs should be the three-pronged type with the third prong grounding the electrical circuits to prevent shocks and possibly electrocution.

When an appliance, such as an electric floor polisher, is being used in a hallway or work area, the cord should not lie where people can trip over it. The policy of most healthcare facilities is to prohibit any electrical appliance that is brought into the facility from home or to require that such appliances be inspected by an electrician. Unused electrical outlets in settings where young children are present should have a safety cover in place to protect children from electrical shocks. |
Needles and other sharp objects	Most needle sticks are sustained when the nurse is attempting to recap a needle. Based on CDC recommendations and OSHA mandates, hospital personnel should never manually recap contaminated needles. A nurse doing so is considered in violation of the regulation, and the employing agency could be cited and fined if this action were documented by an inspector. After use, any sharp object should be instantly deposited into a bedside "sharps" receptacle after use. Directions for safe handling of contaminated needles are provided in Module 46.
Dangerous or caustic substances or materials	Nurses are increasingly exposed to potentially hazardous procedures and substances. These range from disinfectants to chemotherapeutic drugs. OSHA's Hazard Communication Standard of August 1988 directed all industries, including healthcare facilities, to provide workers who handle hazardous substances with guidelines for minimizing risks. All products, regardless of where they are used, should be clearly labeled to warn of any risks or dangers. They should never be left within easy reach of others in hallways or work spaces, including nurses' stations. They could be ingested by children or by people who are confused or incompetent. A liquid substance could be spilled, causing burns or injury. Workers who need to wear protective equipment, such as gloves or masks, must be clearly designated.
Cluttered hallways	In a fire or emergency, furniture or equipment in hallways could block the access of emergency personnel and equipment and interfere with the evacuation of patients and staff.
Medications and treatment solutions	Remove medications from the bedside to prevent a visitor or someone for whom they were not intended from ingesting them. If a liquid used in treatment, such as a saline or hydrogen peroxide solution, is to remain at the bedside, the container should be clearly marked.

A three-pronged plug provides grounding for electrical current.

An uncluttered corridor in the institution allows safe movement for patients and staff.

table 5-3. **Safe Staff Behaviors**

Behavior	Rationale
Use correct body mechanics.	Injuries to staff are a costly safety hazard in healthcare. Excessive stretching, reaching, and carrying or moving heavy objects can create sudden injury or injury from repetitive strain. Using good body mechanics and reminding others of their importance contributes to a safe work environment. See Modules 3, 6, and 18 for information on protecting oneself.
Avoid falls and collisions with others by walking and turning corners carefully and by wearing appropriate footwear.	Running may lead to falls and/or collisions with others. Often the same task can be accomplished just as rapidly by brisk walking, which is much safer. Some types of shoes contribute to tripping, such as those without backs that can come off. Open-toed shoes present a hazard to feet from collisions with equipment or being stepped on by others. Most collisions take place when two people are rounding a corner. Always keep to the right, slow your pace, and turn corners carefully. This is of particular importance when you are pushing a stretcher or cart. Safety organizations have mandated the placement near the ceiling of mirrors on intersecting walls to allow you to see around the corner and avoid such collisions.
Keep to the right in hallways.	In U.S. traffic, the pattern is to keep to the right. Conforming to this pattern results in reducing the opportunity for collisions with others. It is easy to run into someone else whose attention is diverted.
Open doors with care.	An opening door may easily strike someone on the other side. If it is opened slowly, it is less likely to cause injury. With swinging doors that have a glass insert, it is possible to see whether anyone is on the other side of the door. Even with this safety precaution, however, distractions can interfere with full vision, and a door can strike another person.
Move stretchers (gurneys) with care for the patient.	When pushing a patient on a stretcher, keep the patient's head toward your body. This is done so that the head, which is highly vulnerable to impact injury, is protected, and the feet, which are less vulnerable, are outward. When pushing a stretcher, occupied or unoccupied, or a cart or conveyance of any kind, keep your eyes to the front at all times. Looking away for even a second can result in a collision and possible injury to another.
Use brakes on beds, wheelchairs, and stretchers.	When beds, wheelchairs, and stretchers are stationary, applying the brake or brakes prevents accidental movement that may lead to injury. On beds and stretchers, the brake is usually a flat metal "rocking" bar near the wheels. Pushing down on one side of the bar with your foot applies the brake, and pushing on the opposite side releases it. On wheelchairs, the brake is usually a small handle near the wheel. Moving the handle toward the occupant causes a bar to compress the rubber wheel and prevent it from moving.
When using elevators, place elevators on "Hold" and back in when loading or unloading.	This will keep the doors open until you and the patient are safely in or out of the elevator. Facing the front of the elevator helps the patient to feel more oriented to what is happening.

For safety, back the patient in a wheelchair into an elevator, so that the patient can face the front of the elevator.

SMOKELESS ENVIRONMENT

Most healthcare facilities maintain a strict nonsmoking policy for patients, visitors, and staff. Smoking in healthcare environments presents hazards for the respiratory health of other patients and staff as well as for the person who smokes. Smoking increases the risk for respiratory complications in individuals who are hospitalized with illness. In addition, smoking presents a particularly dangerous fire hazard in a place where many individuals are incapacitated and unable to rescue themselves from fire and smoke. Smokers receiving medications that alter alertness are more likely to drop cigarettes or not extinguish them fully. In deference to the serious nature of nicotine addiction, physicians may prescribe nicotine patches and other drugs to help the patient stop smoking while hospitalized. Patients who are unwilling or who cannot stop smoking may be escorted to an outdoor area where the smoke will not jeopardize the health of others.

FIRE PREVENTION

All large institutions are required to have specific procedures in place for fire safety. Learning those procedures should be one of your first actions when beginning clinical experience or working in a new facility. A "fire code" is the nature of the announcement or sound that is broadcast in the event of a potential fire.

PROCEDURE FOR RESPONDING TO FIRE CODES

Because fire in a healthcare facility is such a serious emergency, personnel must respond based on specific planned actions.

1. When a fire alarm sounds or a fire code is broadcast
   a. If you are not near the fire, return immediately to your unit. **R:** You will be needed to assist the patients.
   b. Do not use elevators. **R:** Elevator shafts become conduits for smoke in fires, and electrical power may be shut off, trapping people in the elevator.
   c. Return patients to their rooms. **R:** Patients in their rooms can be protected from smoke and are out of the way of personnel managing the crisis.
   d. Close all doors. **R:** Closed doors prevent the circulation of smoke in the building.
   e. Be available to calm patients. **R:** Patients are often very anxious and fearful because of their dependency on others in a crisis.
   f. Follow directions of persons in charge. **R:** Efforts at fighting the fire or evacuation must be coordinated to proceed in the most efficient and effective manner.
   g. Stand quietly in the hallway, waiting for further directions or listening for the "all clear" signal. **R:** Most fire alarms do not require further action, but this ensures that you are available if action needs to be delegated or if a patient has a need.
   h. If there is an evacuation, move patients according to the facility procedure. **R:** Facility procedures are based on an understanding of where fire barriers are located and where air circulates. Following the established procedures ensures maximum safety for staff and patients.
2. When you discover a fire or potential fire (such as smoke emanating from an electrical device)
   a. Call the fire code. **R:** Immediately activating the fire code ensures that all patients and staff can be safeguarded and that emergency personnel are dispatched rapidly.
   b. Remove any patient in the vicinity of the fire. **R:** Patient safety must always be the first priority.
   c. Use the appropriate local fire extinguisher if the fire is small, and you can do so without personal danger. Under no circumstances should you endanger yourself or others in an attempt to fight a fire. **R:** A small fire may be extinguished by appropriate action before it becomes large enough to create a serious problem. However,

table 5-4. Types of Fire Extinguishers

Type	Use
Class A	Water or solution type, designed to be used on paper and linens
Class B	Foam extinguisher, designed to be used on grease and other chemicals as well as papers and linens
Class C	Carbon dioxide or a dry chemical type, designed to be used on electrical fires. May be used on others sources as well. Many facilities keep a Class C extinguisher on all patient care units.

because healthcare personnel have not been trained as firefighters and do not have the skills or the equipment to deal with a more serious situation, their actions are more effectively directed toward patient safety. Many facilities have classes where employees learn how to use the different types of fire extinguishers (Table 5-4). If your facility has such a class, be sure to take advantage of the opportunity.

   d. If the fire is extinguished, close the door, and assist with managing the unit as above. **R:** Fire personnel will inspect the site to determine the origin of the problem and to assure that no further danger exists. Meanwhile, you can be assisting patients.
   e. If the fire continues to burn, close the door, and assist with further evacuation of patients in the vicinity. The goal is to move the most patients in the least time. Remaining calm is essential. To accomplish this
      (1) Direct those who are ambulatory to exit first. **R:** Because they can move more rapidly, and this maximizes the number evacuated.
      (2) Then help those in wheelchairs or using assistive devices. **R:** These individuals will need help but can be moved more quickly than the bedridden patients.
      (3) Finally, move those who are bedridden and who need transfer. If stretchers (gurneys) are not available, simply lower patients to blankets on the floor, and pull them to safety. **R:** Lifting patients may create back injuries for the nurse and may result in a patient being dropped. Greater safety for all is maintained by pulling them on the floor.
      (4) Assure people who are restrained or in a confining device such as a cast that they will be promptly evacuated. **R:** To alleviate their fears.
      (5) Remember that your actions during this time will depend on those in charge and on your own decision-making ability. **R:** Being prepared can be comforting and useful should

the need arise. Again, healthcare personnel are not firefighters and are not expected to act as such.

(6) Follow instructions from fire personnel. **R:** Firefighters have training in evacuation and safety as well as in fire fighting. They understand the nature of fires and have the most training to ensure maximum safety of all.

DISASTER PLANS

Other types of disasters may also occur in a healthcare facility or in the surrounding community. Each facility has policies and procedures in place as to how to manage disasters. Disaster planning is often a community-wide endeavor that is coordinated with police and fire personnel, other healthcare facilities, and governmental agencies.

Disaster plans are of two types: internal and external. An **internal disaster** involves explosions, collapse of a part of the building, or damage to the building as a result of earthquake, flood, or toxic fumes. An **external disaster** may affect the facility but has more to do with disasters in the community. This category includes aircraft, train, and transit crashes; earthquakes; building collapses; uncontained fires involving sections of a city; extensive flooding; landslides; and widespread toxic fumes. Disaster plans are often reflective of local potential, such as plans for tornado response in the Midwest and South, floods in river areas, and earthquakes on the West Coast.

To differentiate between external and internal disaster codes, facilities use one of several methods. Some call them by color (e.g., a red or green disaster code); others may call the internal code "A" and the external one "B." Be familiar with the system used in your facility before the need arises to use it.

INTERNAL DISASTER CODES

Just like fire plans, disaster plans assign a specific role to each staff person in the event of a disaster. Usually, this involves a return to the unit, where further assignments may be given. A special part of the facility is designated as a "triage" area. **Triage** means prioritization of patients according to their injuries so that the most expedient and appropriate treatment can be given to a large number of people.

Personnel with special skills, such as starting intravenous therapy or suturing wounds, for example, may have specific assignments. Others may transport or maintain patients who are injured or emotionally upset. Because internal disaster plans vary, you should carefully read and become knowledgeable about the specific plan of the facility in which you practice.

EXTERNAL DISASTER CODES

External disaster plans are regional so that several facilities within the community can respond. In large urban areas, one hospital takes responsibility for continually monitoring the availability of **critical care** beds for those who need immediate lifesaving medical intervention and acute care beds for those who need close monitoring and more intensive nursing care. The hospital supervisor or coordinator, after notifying the administrator, usually has the responsibility of activating the plan within the facility. All personnel are categorized according to their skills, and travel times from home are catalogued so that additional personnel can be summoned quickly. Different facilities may take on responsibility for different types of care; a hospital with a burn unit, for example, may receive patients with burns, while other facilities receive patients with other types of injuries. Again, become acquainted with the policy in your facility and community.

INJURY PREVENTION

Falls in the healthcare environment continue to be a source of serious complications for patients. Individuals receiving healthcare have many illnesses that impair balance, cause weakness, and interfere with judgment. These all contribute to falls. Many safety devices are aimed at fall prevention, and most institutions have instituted fall prevention programs. Home care nurses must plan with clients for safety in the home (Box 5-2).

Another source of injury is created by the patient who pulls out tubes or devices that are essential for therapy. This may occur due to confusion and discomfort but may also happen accidentally when tubes become caught in bedrails and on chairs. Devising ways to prevent this occurrence is an important nursing function.

---

box 5-2 *Fall-Prevention Strategies for Elders at Home*

Remove tripping hazards such as throw rugs and clutter in walkways.
Use nonslip mats in the bathtub and on shower floors.
Have grab bars put in next to the toilet and in the tub or shower.
Have handrails put in on both sides of stairways.
Improve lighting throughout the home.

Source: National Center for Injury Prevention and Control. (2004). (Online.) Available at www.cdc.gov.

SAFETY DEVICES AND RESTRAINTS

A variety of safety devices and restraints are available in most clinical settings (see Table 5-5). Restraints are defined by the Center for Medicare and Medicaid Services (formerly the Healthcare Finance Administration—HCFA) as "any manual method or physical or mechanical device, material, or equipment attached or adjacent to the resident's body that the individual cannot remove easily that restricts freedom of movement or normal access to one's body." The same device may be considered a safety device for one patient and a restraint for another, depending upon the individual's ability to manipulate the device. Because restraints interfere with the right of the patient to be free of restriction and coercion, the use of restraints is highly regulated by both governmental funding agencies and by accrediting agencies such as JCAHO.

While safety devices and restraints are used with safety for the patient or staff as a goal, the restrained patient may feel punished rather than safe and may react by becoming more distressed and angry. This increased agitation can lead to falls or other injuries (bruises, lacerations) that occur when the patient attempts to "escape." The agitation created by restraints can increase risk in patients who have elevated blood pressure or increased intracranial pressure. Later, resignation and withdrawal may set in.

All safety devices or restraints impose some degree of immobility, which can be hazardous. Contractures, pressure ulcers, dehydration, chronic constipation, functional incontinence, loss of bone mass, muscle tone, and the ability to move about independently have all been known to occur at least partially as the result of safety devices or restraints being applied to provide safety.

SIDE RAILS

Side rails are used in many different ways to protect patients. However, side rails can also be considered restraints in some instances. When a patient is unconscious, paralyzed, or otherwise unable to move independently, then side rails are not considered restraints. They are not restricting voluntary action on the part of the patient. In these instances, side rails should always be up to prevent the potential for the patient to fall out of bed.

Half side rails on the top half of the bed often hold bed controls, the call signal, and even the television control. These half rails are also used by the patient to help in turning and to help when getting out of bed. Used in this manner, half side rails are not considered restraints, and many facilities encourage their use at all times.

Full side rails, often accomplished by two half rails on the bed, do have the potential to restrict desired mobility of a patient; therefore, they come under the definition of a restraint. When in place for the physically able patient who is confused or disoriented, the result may be that the patient attempts to climb over the rail and may fall from an even greater height. It is also possible for patients to get caught between the upper and lower rails and experience injuries. Side rails must often be padded to prevent injury to a disoriented patient who bangs his or her arms and legs against them. If side rails are used, then the nurse must consider the potential injuries from them and make plans to prevent injuries. This might include a bed alarm (Fig. 5-1) to alert staff to a patient climbing out of bed, placing the bed in a low position, and frequent toileting.

USE OF RESTRAINTS AND THE LAW

The federal Omnibus Budget Reconciliation Act (OBRA) of 1987 included a provision that patients in healthcare settings have the right to be free from unnecessary physical and chemical restraints. To ensure patients' rights, all healthcare facilities are mandated to meet strict guidelines regarding the use of any type of restraint in order to qualify for Medicare and Medicaid reimbursement. Since this act was implemented in 1991, some healthcare facilities have adopted a "restraint-free environment" policy. To support these actions, many nonrestraint safety devices have been developed. Although acute care facilities were not initially included in these regulations, they are now required to meet these standards. Alternatives to restraints are listed in Box 5-3, and types of restraints are listed in Table 5-5.

All facilities must have established policies and protocols regarding the use of restraints. The general content of these policies and protocols must conform to the regulatory and accreditation standards. These requirements are listed in Box 5-4. If you are involved in a situation in which restraints are being considered, you must follow the facility's policies and protocols.

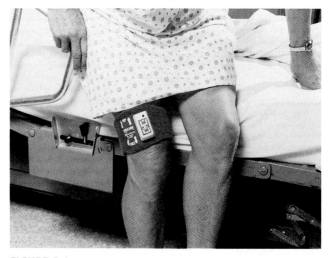

FIGURE 5-1 Bed and chair alarms can alert the staff to a patient's attempt to get up unaided. (Photo courtesy of AlertCare, Inc.)

---

box 5-3 *Alternatives to Restraints*

Addressing Other Patient Needs

Does the patient need toileting now and on a regular schedule?

Does the patient need a diversional activity?

Does the patient have pain that needs treatment?

Does the patient need an opportunity to change position or ambulate?

Does the patient have another physical problem that needs attention (e.g., constipation, hunger, infection)?

Decreasing Confusion

Provide adequate lighting.

Put personal items within easy reach.

Speak to the person by name.

Move slowly, and explain all actions in simple words.

Distract the person by changing the subject.

Do not argue.

Reducing the Risk of Unassisted Bed Exit

Use the following devices as appropriate:

A bed alarm to notify staff when weight is lifted off the bed

Cushioned pads that are placed on the floor beside a low bed to cushion falls

Floor beds that allow the patient to be down where they cannot fall

Family member or "sitter" at the bedside

*Side-rails (half rails that are used by the patient for turning or stability when getting up are not considered restraints)

*Cushioned pads that block the gap between short side rails

*Wedges that fit between the side rail and the mattress to prevent the patient slipping into the gap

*Soft cushions and wedge cushions designed to be placed on each side of the patient to make it difficult to get over the side rail

Reducing the Risk of Unassisted Chair Exit

Use the following devices as appropriate:

Chair alarm that signals when the patient starts to arise

*Safety belts with a buckle that the patient can release but that emits a signal to warn the staff when it is released

*Safety belts that overlap in the front with a hook and loop closure that the patient could pull open

*Wedge cushions that shift a person's weight to the back of the chair.

*Lapboards that provide a place for books and other personal items and encourage the person to stay in the chair

Wheelchair kept near the nurses' station

Reducing the Risk of Tube Pulling

Use the following items of clothing as appropriate:

Long sleeves that cover an intravenous line and keep it out of sight

Fitted shirt that covers a percutaneous gastrostomy tube

Pajama bottoms to cover a catheter

---

*These items may be considered restraints if the patient is restricted from movement; however, because they do not involve devices attached to the patient's body, they are considered more desirable alternatives.

A wide variety of medications can be used to restrict an individual's behavior or activity. These medications are sometimes referred to as chemical restraints. Although valuable in some situations, there is a great potential for abuse of these drugs by caregivers who use chemical restraints as a substitute for personal attention and care for the patient.

PROCEDURE FOR THE USE OF SAFETY DEVICES AND RESTRAINTS

ASSESSMENT

1. Assess the patient. **R:** To identify all factors that may be contributing to the patient's risk for injury or the risk that the patient will injure others.
2. Assess the environment. **R:** To determine what hazards are present for the patient.
3. Identify all types of safety actions that might meet the patient's need for safety and the staff need for safety, include both nonrestraint alternatives and restraints. **R:** To provide a basis for planning.
4. If the patient already has a safety device or restraint in place, reassess the need for the device. **R:** The situation that made the device necessary may have changed, or the patient may need a different type of restraint.

ANALYSIS

5. Critically think through your data, carefully evaluating each aspect and its relationship to other data. **R:** This enables you to determine specific problems for this individual in relation to the need for safety devices or restraints. The decision to apply a safety device or to restrain a patient physically must always be made after careful assessment and analysis of your data.
6. Identify specific safety problems of the patient and modifications of the procedure needed for this individual. **R:** Restraints must never be used for staff convenience. Safety of the patient or staff is the

table 5-5. Types of Restraints

Type of Restraint		Purpose
Belt restraints	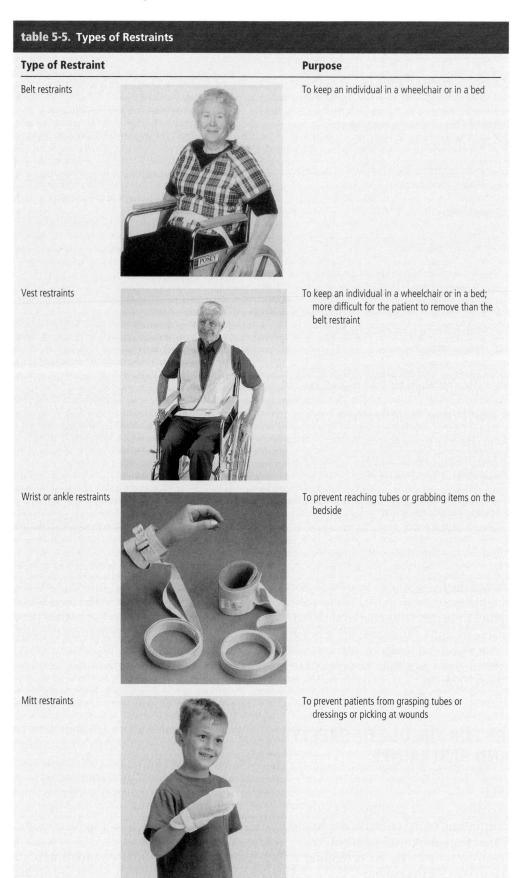	To keep an individual in a wheelchair or in a bed
Vest restraints		To keep an individual in a wheelchair or in a bed; more difficult for the patient to remove than the belt restraint
Wrist or ankle restraints		To prevent reaching tubes or grabbing items on the bedside
Mitt restraints		To prevent patients from grasping tubes or dressings or picking at wounds

box 5-4	*Required Standards for Policies and Protocols Regarding Restraints*

1. Situations in which the use of restraints may be considered, such as
   a. the patient exhibiting irrational or uncooperative behavior that could seriously interfere with a physical treatment or device, such as an IV line, other indwelling lines, respirator, or a dressing, or could seriously injure self or others AND
   b. less restrictive approaches don't work.
2. Guidelines for assessing the patient
3. Guidelines governing obtaining medical orders for restraint use
4. Guidelines for applying the restraint
5. Criteria for monitoring the patient and reassessing the need for restraint
6. Criteria for terminating the restraint
7. Documentation required

only reason for the use of restraints. **R:** Planning for the individual must take into consideration the individual's abilities, specific safety problems, and risks. Restrict the patient's movements as little as possible to accomplish your purpose.

PLANNING

7. Plan for the least restrictive strategies and devices that will protect the patient. **R:** Planning ahead allows you to proceed more safely and effectively. Both good nursing practice and the law mandate that the least-restrictive strategies be used to preserve personal autonomy and dignity. Many types of safety devices are available as alternatives to restraints (see Box 5-3). Nonrestraint alternatives must be tried before restraints are used.

8. If you determine that a restraint is needed, consult with a physician regarding an order for a restraint if possible. A physician's order must be secured before the device is applied unless the safety consideration is an emergency. If the immediate safety of a patient or of the staff is in question, apply restraints at once, and secure an order as soon as possible. **R:** A standard of JCAHO is that of a "time-limited" physician's order for any type of restraint used. This means that a physician's order for this action must be obtained by the nurse within a reasonable period of time, and the order may only be effective for a limited number of days. The specific timelines would be found in the protocol. This forces reassessment and reconsideration of the use of the restraint. Nonrestraint safety devices do not need a physician's order.

IMPLEMENTATION

Action	Rationale
9. Wash or disinfect your hands.	To decrease the transfer of microorganisms that could cause infection.
10. Obtain needed protective devices and assistance if needed.	To save time and promote efficiency.
11. Identify the patient using two identifiers.	Verifying the patient's identity helps ensure that you are performing the right skill for the right patient.
12. Explain the procedure you are about to perform. Emphasize the devices as safety devices rather than as restraints.	Explaining the procedure helps relieve anxiety or misperceptions that the patient may have about a procedure or activity and sets the stage for patient participation. Avoid any indication that the device is punishment or meant to imprison the patient. For example, you might say that the device is to "remind" the patient not to lean too far forward in the chair. This often makes the device more acceptable.
13. When possible, provide for the patient's elimination needs before applying any device.	This adds to the patient's comfort and lessens the chance that you will have to remove the safety device or restraint to provide for elimination immediately after it is in place.

(continued)

Action	Rationale
14. Raise the bed to convenient working height.	To allow you to use correct body mechanics and protect yourself from back injury.
15. Apply the device, using an easy release device or an appropriate knot if needed. Knot the ties to the bed frame.	Knots must be a quick-release type (Fig. 5-2) in case the patient must be quickly released for care or in an emergency. Never knot the ties to the side rails because if the rails were suddenly lowered, the patient could be injured.

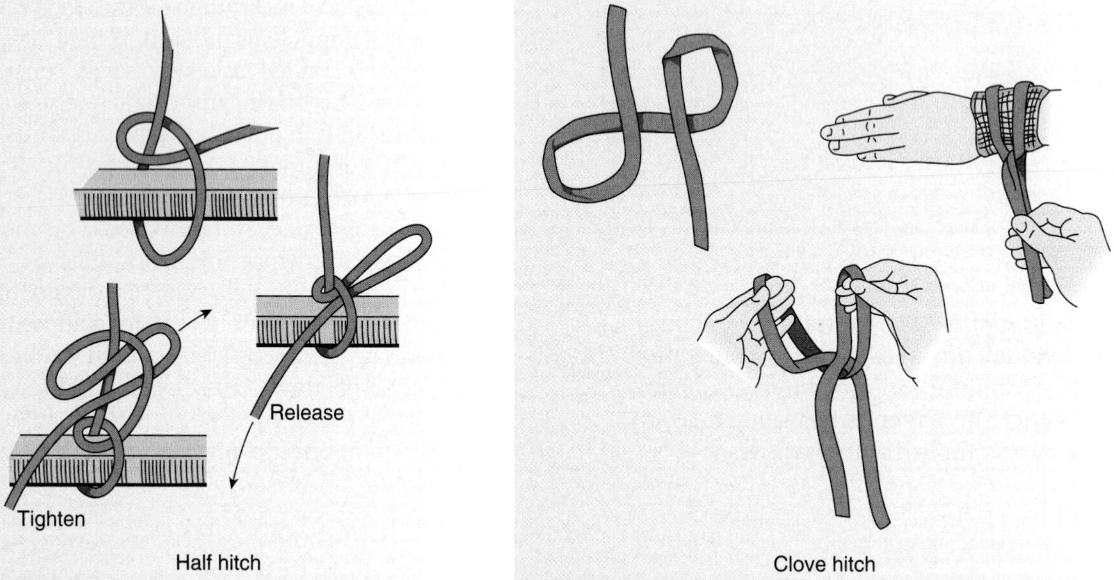

Release

Tighten

Half hitch

Clove hitch

FIGURE 5-2 The "quick release" knot provides safety for the patient in the event of an emergency.

Action	Rationale
16. Check for adequate "slack" in the restraint to allow for circulation.	A tight restraint may cause the patient discomfort, impair circulation, or restrict function. For example, a vest restraint that is too tight could restrict breathing.
17. If the patient is extremely restless or has fragile skin, add extra padding to the restraint. You can use clean cloths, stockinette, or gauze padding.	To protect the tissues from abrasion.
18. Remove any safety device or restraint every 2 hours or less, and check for abrasion and for circulation distal to the restraint, provide for toileting, and encourage movement.	To prevent an injury from developing.
19. Reassess the need for the device, and reapply the safety device or restraint if necessary.	This meets the regulatory requirement and ensures that the use of restraints is minimized.
20. Wash or disinfect your hands.	To decrease the transfer of microorganisms that could cause infection.

EVALUATION

21. Evaluate using the following criteria. **R:** To determine whether desired outcomes have been met.
    a. The patient did not experience any injury from inappropriate behavior.
    b. The safety device did not cause discomfort or injury.
    c. The patient had the least-restrictive alternative applied.

DOCUMENTATION

22. Document the following to communicate the care provided. **R:** Documentation is a legal record of the patient's care and therapy and communicates nursing activities to other nurses and caregivers.
    a. Assessment that demonstrated the safety hazard
    b. All attempts to use a nonrestraint alternative and the evaluation of effectiveness
    c. The consultation with the physician
    d. The time and exact nature of the device applied
    e. The every-2-hour assessment including evaluation of effectiveness and need

POTENTIAL ADVERSE OUTCOMES AND RELATED INTERVENTIONS

1. The patient may struggle to escape a restraint and create the potential for serious injury such as getting a vest restraint around the neck.
Intervention: Remove the restraint, and reassess for the potential use of a nonrestraint alternative.

2. The patient develops skin abrasions under a restraint.
Intervention: Treat the skin abrasion, and reassess for the potential use of a nonrestraint alternative. If the restraint is essential, pad the restraint more effectively.

3. The patient succeeds in pulling out a tube.
Intervention: Consult with the physician about replacing the tube. Identify a different alternative for securing the tube and preventing the patient from pulling it out.

4. The patient falls in spite of the safety devices used.
Intervention: Respond to the fall with appropriate assessment and care and re-examine the safety devices used.

Acute Care

The acute care environment is very complex, with much equipment, and many staff and patients. Because of its constantly changing status, the acute care environment requires extra vigilance for maintaining patient safety. The patient in acute care is much more likely to have a wide array of tubes that could easily be pulled out, creating injury or the need for a procedure to replace the tube. The use of restraints may be needed for a short-term acute situation.

Long-Term Care

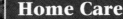

It is particularly important that precautions be taken to protect residents in long-term care facilities. Many are elderly, with impaired mobility and problems with neurosensory function. As you review the various precautions for patients, remember the many limitations of those in long-term care. For example, elderly people may fall because of disturbances in balance and gait. These people also may have difficulty feeling hot and cold temperatures and sharp objects, and the use of safety devices may not always prevent falls. Because the needs of each resident are different, thorough assessment is essential. The dignity as well as the safety of the person in long-term care is often best maintained by a restraint-free environment.

Home Care

Because many elderly and incapacitated people reside in private homes, home safety becomes an issue. Nurses practicing in hospitals or long-term care facilities can review with the family and significant other caregivers a list of precautions to be taken when the patient is discharged. Attention should be given to providing adequate lighting, eliminating physical obstacles, and providing smooth floors. Many other precautions can be taken. One example is the simple but important elimination of small floor rugs, which can cause falls. Homes should be evaluated for electrical safety before medical equipment is put into use. If the application of any safety device becomes necessary, the nurse should carefully instruct the care providers in its use.

The nurse who provides care in the home can also be effective in assessing the home environment for safety and acting as a valuable resource to the family. Suggestions can be made concerning specific changes to minimize hazards. Public funds are available in some states to alter the environment of those who are disabled to provide the maximum in safety.

Ambulatory Care

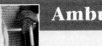

The nurse in ambulatory care may identify individuals with a greater risk for injury at home because of medical conditions or ability to manage self-care. By assessing for home safety with the patient, the nurse may be able to help the patient develop a plan for maintaining safety in the home. Box 5-2 lists the National Center for Injury Prevention and Control–recommended fall-prevention strategies for elders at home.

LEARNING TOOLS

DEVELOP YOUR BACKGROUND KNOWLEDGE

1. Review the Learning Outcomes.

2. Read the appropriate section in your assigned text.

3. Look up the Key Terms in the glossary.

4. Read through this module, and mentally practice the techniques described. Study so that you would be able to teach these skills to another person.

DEVELOP YOUR SKILLS

1. In the practice setting, select a partner, and work together.

2. Inspect the various safety devices and restraints, and check on the fastening devices.

3. Have a partner apply various safety devices and restraints to you. Answer the following:
Which are the most comfortable?
Which are the least comfortable?
Why?
Describe some of your feelings regarding the experience.

4. Apply the various safety devices and restraints to your partner. Check them for comfort and safety.

5. Evaluate your own performance using the Performance Checklist on the CD-ROM in the front of this book.

DEMONSTRATE YOUR SKILLS

In the clinical setting
1. Familiarize yourself with the types of safety devices (restraints and restraint alternatives) used in the facility.

2. Review the policies and procedures for the use of restraints.

3. Observe any safety devices or restraints being used. Have they been applied correctly and safely?

4. Consult with your instructor regarding the opportunity to apply an appropriate safety device or restraint with your instructor's supervision.

5. Evaluate your performance with the instructor.

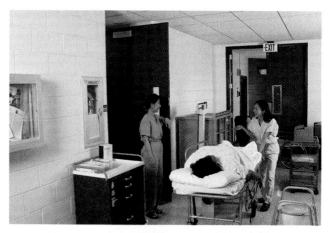

FIGURE 5-3 Critical thinking exercise: Identify the unsafe practices in this photograph.

CRITICAL THINKING EXERCISES

1. Your patient is an elderly woman who suffered a stroke a few days ago. She is semiconscious and slumped in a wheelchair. Her right side is flaccid with her right hand hanging over the arm of the chair and her right foot positioned between the footrests. Identify the safety hazards that are present. Describe the nursing actions you might take to protect the patient. For each nursing action, explain the rationale.

2. Examine the photograph (Fig. 5-3) here, and identify the unsafe practices that you observe.

SELF-QUIZ
SHORT-ANSWER QUESTIONS

1. Give three reasons why providing a safe environment in the healthcare facility is important.

a. _____

b. _____

c. _____

2. List five behaviors that support a safe environment.

a. _____

b. _____

c. _____

d. _____

e. _____

3. List three actions other than restraints that can be used to prevent falls.

a. _____

b. _____

c. _____

4. Discuss electrical safety precautions.

_____

5. List three adverse effects that can result from restraining a patient.

a. _____

b. _____

c. _____

6. What is the most important safety precaution for the dependent patient in your care?

_____

_____

7. What rules or policies do healthcare facilities have about smoking?

_____

_____

8. Briefly, give the steps of responding to a fire code.

a. _____
b. _____
c. _____
d. _____
e. _____
f. _____
g. _____
h. _____
i. _____
j. _____
k. _____
l. _____

9. What might be the role of the staff nurse in a disaster plan?

_____

MULTIPLE CHOICE

_____ 10. What are adverse effects of the use of restraints?
a. Emotional concerns only
b. Potential for injury only
c. Both emotional concerns and potential for injury

_____ 11. Which actions are related to the JCAHO National Patient Safety Goals for 2005? (Choose all that apply.)
a. Use two identifiers before any procedure.
b. Communicate clearly within the healthcare team.
c. Use restraints as needed to prevent falls.
d. Wash or disinfect your hands after any patient contact.

_____ 12. What steps will help the family ensure safety for the person residing in a private home? (Choose all that apply.)
a. Assess the current environment.
b. Install a handrail in the bathroom.
c. Eliminate small rugs in the home.
d. Add lighting.

Answers to Self-Quiz questions appear in the back of this book.

REFERENCES AND SUGGESTED RESOURCES: UNIT 1

Boyce, J. & Pittet, D. (2002). Guideline for hand hygiene in health care settings: Recommendations of the Healthcare Infection Control Practices Advisory Committee and the HICPAC/SHEA/APIC/IDSA Hand Hygiene Task Force. _MMWR, 51_ (16), 1–44. (Online.) Available at http://www.cdc.gov. Retrieved July 1, 2005.

Bucher, L. (1993). The effects of imagery abilities and mental rehearsal on learning a nursing skill. _Journal of Nursing Education, 32_ (7), 318–324.

Bucher, L., & Melander, S. (1999). _Critical care nursing._ Philadelphia: W. B. Saunders.

Burgess-Limerick, R., Straker, L., Pollack, C., et al. (2004). _Manual tasks risk assessment tool (ManTRA) v 2.0._ (Online.) Available at http://ergonomics.uq.edu.au/download/mantra2.pdf. Retrieved February 1, 2005.

Centers for Disease Control and Prevention, National Center for Injury Prevention and Control. (2003). Web-Based Injury Statistics Query and Reporting System (WISQARS). (Online.) Available at www.cdc.gov/ncipc/wisqars. Retrieved July 6, 2004.

Centers for Disease Control and Prevention. (2001a). Serious adverse events attributed to nevirapine regimens for postexposure prophylaxis after HIV exposures—worldwide, 1997–2000. _MMWR, 49_(51), 1153–6. (Online.) Available at http://www.cdc.gov/mmwr/preview/mmwrhtml/rr5011a1.htm. Retrieved January 18, 2005.

Centers for Disease Control and Prevention. (2001b). Updated U.S. Public Health Service guidelines for the management of occupational exposures to HBV, HCV, and HIV and recommendations for postexposure prophylaxis. _MMWR, 50_ (RR-11), 1-42. (Online.) Available at http://www.cdc.gov/mmwr/preview/mmwrhtml/rr5011a1.htm. Retrieved August 20, 2005.

Centers for Medicare & Medicaid Services. (2004). CMS Manuals. (Online.) Available at http://www.cms.hhs.gov/manuals/cmsindex.asp. Retrieved January 20, 2005.

Dave, R. (1970). Psychomotor levels. In R. J. Armstrong (Ed.), *Developing and writing behavioral objectives*. Tucson, AZ: Educational Innovators Press.

Doheny, M. (1993). Mental practice: An alternative approach to teaching motor skills. *Journal of Nursing Education, 32* (6), 260–264.

Ennis, R. (1985). A logical basis for measuring critical thinking skills. *Educational Leadership, 43,* 44–48.

Garner, J. S., & Hospital Infection Control Practices Advisory Committee. (1996). Guideline for isolation precautions in hospitals. *Infect Control Hosp Epidemiol, 17,* 53–80, and *Am J Infect Control, 24,* 24–52. (Online.) Available at http://www.cdc.gov. Retrieved July 1, 2004.

Goode, C. J., & Piedalue, F. (1999). Evidence-based clinical practice. *Journal of Nursing Administration, 29* (6), 15–21.

Joint Commission on Accreditation of Healthcare Organizations. (2004). *Accreditation manual for hospitals.* Chicago: Author.

Joint Commission on Accreditation of Healthcare Organizations. (2005). 2005 National Safety Goals. (Online.) Available at http://www.jcaho.org. Retrieved January 20, 2005.

Larson, E. (1995). *APIC Guidelines for Infection Control Practice: Guideline for hand washing and hand antisepsis in health care settings.* Washington, DC: APIC (Association for Professionals in Infection Control and Epidemiology, Inc.).

Lee, L. (2003). Evidence-based practice in Hong Kong: Issues and implications in its establishment. *Journal of Clinical Nursing, 12,* 618–624.

Mason, J. O. (1988). Centers for Disease Control recommendations for prevention of HIV transmission in health care settings. *MMWR Supplement, 2*S, 36, 25–185. (Online.) Available at http://www.cdc.gov. Retrieved July 1, 2004.

Morris, C., & Harr, J. (2004). *Self-evaluation of health assessment skills in laboratory and clinical settings.* Paper presented at the 10th Biennial North American Learning Resources Center Conference, Spokane, WA.

National Center for Injury Prevention and Control. (2004). *Falls and hip fractures among older adults.* (Online.) Available at http://www.cdc.gov/ncipc/factsheets/falls.htm. Retrieved August 20, 2005.

National Council of State Boards of Nursing (NCSBN). (1995). *Delegation: Concepts and decision-making process.* Chicago: Author.

Oermann, M. (1990). Psychomotor skill development. *Journal of Continuing Education in Nursing, 21* (5), 202–204.

Reilly, D., & Oermann, M. (1992). *Clinical teaching in nursing education* (2nd ed.). New York: National League for Nursing.

Rickover, R., & Rickover, A. (2005). *Posture.* (Online.) Available at www.ergonomics.org. Retrieved February 1, 2005.

U.S. Department of Labor, Occupational Safety and Health Administration. (2005). Safety and health topics: Ergonomics guidelines for nursing homes. (Online.) Available at http://www.osha.gov/ergonomics/guidelines/nursinghome. Retrieved February 1, 2005.

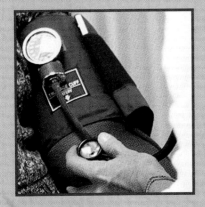

U N I T 2

Providing Basic Patient Care

MODULES

MODULE 6

Moving the Patient in Bed and Positioning

SKILLS INCLUDED IN THIS MODULE

General Procedure for Moving and Positioning a Patient
Specific Procedures for Moving a Patient in Bed
  Moving a Patient Closer to One Side of the Bed
  Moving a Patient Up in Bed: One-Person Assist
  Moving a Patient Up in Bed: Two- or
    Three-Person Assist
  Turning a Patient in Bed: Back to Side
  Turning a Patient in Bed: Back to Abdomen
  Turning a Patient in Bed: Logrolling
  Turning a Patient in Bed: Using a Turn or Pull Sheet
Specific Procedures for Positioning a Patient in Bed
  Supine Position
  Side-Lying Position
  Prone Position
Positioning a Patient in a Chair
Positioning a Patient for Therapy
  Fowler's, High Fowler's, and Semi-Fowler's Positions
  Orthopneic Position
  Dorsal Recumbent Position
  Lithotomy Position
  Sims' Position
  Knee-Chest Position (Genupectoral)
  Trendelenburg Position

PREREQUISITE MODULES

Module 1   An Approach to Nursing
            Skills
Module 2   Documentation
Module 3   Basic Body Mechanics
Module 4   Basic Infection Control
Module 14   Nursing Physical Assessment

KEY TERMS

alignment
anatomic position
axillae
extension
external rotation
flexion
footdrop
gravity
increased
  intracranial
  pressure

orthopneic
paralysis
plantar flexion
pronation
thoracentesis
trapeze
trochanter

OVERALL OBJECTIVES

▸ To move a patient in bed, using good body mechanics.
▸ To place a patient in positions that are anatomically correct as well as comfortable.
▸ To place a patient in the special positions required for examination and therapy.

LEARNING OUTCOMES

The student will be able to

1. Assess the patient effectively to determine the appropriate transfer technique or positioning needed.
2. Analyze assessment data to determine special problems or concerns that must be addressed to successfully transfer or position the patient.
3. Determine appropriate patient outcomes of the transfer process or positioning and recognize the potential for adverse outcomes.
4. Choose an appropriate transfer or positioning technique, including equipment and assistance to be utilized.
5. Transfer the patient, maintaining body mechanics and safety for the nurse and comfort and safety for the patient.
6. Position the patient in anatomically correct and effective positions for therapeutic purposes or for examinations.
7. Evaluate the effectiveness of the transfer process or the position for the specific patient.
8. Document the transfer technique or positioning in the patient's plan of care and the activity in the patient's record as appropriate.

Maintaining the correct position of the body while it is at rest contributes to comfort and rest and prevents strain on muscles. A regimen of good positioning prevents pressure ulcers (decubitus ulcers) and joint contractures. Frequent movement also improves muscle tone, respiration, and circulation.

To position a patient properly, the nurse must have knowledge of anatomy and good body **alignment.** The nurse needs to learn a number of positions so that patients can be repositioned approximately every 2 hours. Patient positioning is designed to maintain body parts in correct alignment so that they remain functional and unstressed.

Additionally, many examinations and other procedures require special positioning of the patient for improved visualization of the examined area. It is usually the nurse's responsibility to assist patients into these positions and to make them as comfortable as possible.

When you must move a patient in bed, correct body mechanics are essential for both you and the patient because correct body mechanics and moving techniques can keep you from injuring your back. Also, correct body mechanics for the patient prevents excessive stress on the joints and severe discomfort. The aim in moving the patient is to put the least possible stress on the patient's joints and skin.

Moving and positioning skills are especially important in the home or in settings where people with limited mobility are receiving long-term care. Teaching other staff members and caregivers are added responsibilities of your nursing role.

NURSING DIAGNOSES

Patients who cannot move themselves in bed or need assistance in getting out of bed may have a variety of nursing diagnoses concerning activity. Examples are

■ Impaired Physical Mobility: inability to turn self in bed related to immediate postoperative state
■ Activity Intolerance: unsteadiness in getting out of bed related to anemia
■ Bathing/Hygiene Self-Care Deficit: related to inability to move self
■ Dressing/Grooming Self-Care Deficit: related to inability to maintain upright position

DELEGATION

The nurse often delegates routine needs for moving and positioning to assistive personnel. When this is done, the nurse must be sure that the person to whom this is delegated has the necessary skill and understands any modifications needed for the individual. Evaluation of positioning and moving continues to be a nursing responsibility when the task itself is delegated.

GENERAL PROCEDURE FOR MOVING AND POSITIONING A PATIENT IN BED

The instructions in the general procedure that follows include the fundamental nursing actions needed to correctly move and position a patient in bed. The specific procedures that follow the general procedure call for the nurse to use many steps of the general procedure and to vary others. The steps of the general procedure are numbered sequentially. They are grouped according to the steps of the nursing process.

ASSESSMENT

1. Assess the patient's need to move. **R:** To determine whether there are any restrictions on movement or specific concerns related to movement. Consider such things as **paralysis,** impaired circulation, recent surgery, and disabilities.
2. Assess the patient's ability to move unaided. **R:** To determine how much assistance the patient will need and how much the patient can participate in moving.
3. Identify whether assistive devices are available. **R:** Assistive devices help prevent injury to staff members when moving and transferring patients.

ANALYSIS

4. Critically think through your data, carefully evaluating each aspect and its relation to other data. **R:** To determine specific problems for this individual in relation to transfer and positioning.
5. Identify specific problems and modifications of the procedure needed for this individual. **R:** Planning for the individual must take into consideration the individual's problems.

PLANNING

6. Determine individualized patient outcomes in relation to moving the patient, including the following. **R:** Identification of outcomes guides planning and evaluation.
   a. The patient is correctly aligned with no abnormal stress on muscles and joints.
   b. The patient states he or she is comfortable.
7. Plan the moving technique. **R:** Planning ahead allows you to proceed more safely and effectively.

IMPLEMENTATION

Action	Rationale
8. Wash or disinfect your hands.	To decrease the transfer of microorganisms that could cause infection.
9. Obtain any needed supportive devices and/or additional personnel.	To save time and promote efficiency.
10. Identify the patient, using two identifiers.	Verifying the patient's identity helps ensure that you are performing the right skill for the right patient.
11. Explain the procedure you are about to perform.	Explaining the procedure helps relieve anxiety or misperceptions that the patient may have about a procedure or activity and sets the stage for patient participation.
12. Raise the bed to an appropriate working position based on your height.	To allow you to use correct body mechanics and protect yourself from back injury.
13. Put the bed in the flat position. If the patient is medically unable to lie flat, you will have to alter the technique, possibly with the help of an assistant.	A flat position helps you to avoid working against **gravity.**

(continued)

Action	Rationale
14. Move the patient according to one of the specific procedures described in the following pages. Remember to use smooth, coordinated movements.	Smooth, coordinated movements are more comfortable for the patient and less likely to cause injury to the caregiver than jerking movements.
15. Correctly position the patient, using one of the specific positions described in the following pages.	Correct position preserves function as well as ensures comfort for the patient.
16. Make sure all safety devices (side rails, pillows, protective restraints, call light) are in place.	To protect the patient from potential falls and ensure that the patient can call for help if needed.
17. Wash or disinfect your hands.	To decrease the transfer of microorganisms that could cause infection.

EVALUATION

18. Evaluate using the individualized patient outcomes previously identified. **R:** Evaluation in relationship to desired outcomes is essential for planning future care.
  a. The patient is correctly aligned with no abnormal stress on muscles and joints.
  b. The patient states he or she is comfortable.

DOCUMENTATION

19. Document the patient's activity as required by your facility. Usually position changes from side to side or from back to abdomen are noted on a flow sheet. If your facility does not use a flow sheet, document this activity in the narrative nurses' notes. Simply assisting a patient to move up in bed is not usually recorded.

20. On a nursing care plan, note the techniques used for moving the patient. If the patient's ability to move is a significant part of the general assessment, you may have to write a progress note about the patient's activity. **R:** Documentation is a legal record of the patient's care and therapy and communicates nursing activities to other nurses and caregivers.

■ POTENTIAL ADVERSE OUTCOMES AND RELATED INTERVENTIONS

1. The patient experiences severe pain with moving. *Intervention:* Stop the procedure, and reassess the patient. Determine the cause and location of the pain if possible. Modify the plan for moving, or seek pain management before moving the patient.

2. The patient is unable to tolerate the new position. *Intervention:* Return the patient to the previous position, and determine what modifications might support the patient's comfort in the new position.

SPECIFIC PROCEDURES FOR MOVING A PATIENT IN BED

Moving a Patient Closer to One Side of the Bed

This activity is needed in many other moves; therefore, it is being presented separately (Fig. 6-1). Most of the time, you will use this technique in conjunction with another type of movement.

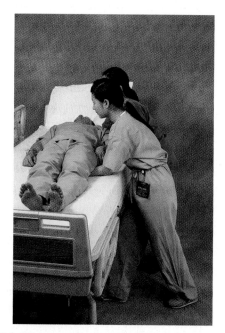

FIGURE 6-1 Moving a patient to one side of a bed: Two-person assist. The nurses role the turn sheet close to the patient. The nurses slide their arms under the patient (one at the shoulders, one at the hips) and pull toward themselves.

ASSESSMENT

1-3. Follow steps 1 to 3 of the General Procedure: Assess need to move, ability to move, and assistive devices available.

ANALYSIS

4-5. Follow steps 4 and 5 of the General Procedure: Think through your data, and identify specific problems and modifications.

PLANNING

6-7. Follow steps 6 and 7 of the General Procedure: Determine individualized patient outcomes in relationship to alignment and comfort and plan the moving technique.

IMPLEMENTATION

Action	*Rationale*
8-13. Follow steps 8 to 13 of the General Procedure: Wash or disinfect your hands, obtain assistive devices, identify the patient (two identifiers), explain the procedure, raise the bed, put the bed in the flat position.	
14. Move the patient to the side of the bed:	
a. Slide your hands and arms under the patient's head and shoulders, and pull that section of the body toward you. Keep your back straight and your hips and knees flexed. Keep one foot forward.	This stance gives you a broad base of support that can withstand a shift in weight as the patient is pulled toward the side of the bed. Pulling while shifting your weight uses your strong large muscles and helps overcome resistance from the soft bed surface. Good body mechanics will help you avoid injuring yourself.
b. Move your hands and arms down under the patient's hips, and pull that section of the body toward you.	Use the body mechanics described in 14a to protect yourself from injury.
c. Slide your hands and arms under the patient's legs, and pull them toward you.	Use the body mechanics described in 14a to protect yourself from injury.
d. Repeat steps a through c in sequence as needed to move the patient to the desired place. If two people are available, the same general technique is used, but two sections of the body are moved at the same time. One nurse slides hands and arms under the patient's shoulders; the other nurse slides hands and arms under the patient's hips (see Fig. 6-1). One nurse signals the move by saying, "One, two, three, pull!"	Counting steps aloud helps everyone work together as a team.
15-17. Follow steps 15 to 17 of the General Procedure: Position the patient, place appropriate safety devices, wash or disinfect your hands.	

EVALUATION

18. Follow step 18 of the General Procedure: Evaluate using the individualized patient outcomes regarding alignment and comfort.

DOCUMENTATION

19-20. Follow steps 19 and 20 of the General Procedure: Document position as appropriate, and document techniques on the nursing care plan and/or patient's activity record.

Moving a Patient Up in Bed: One-Person Assist

Keep in mind that the following technique is used for the patient who is alert and able to cooperate and help.

ASSESSMENT

1-3. Follow steps 1 to 3 of the General Procedure: Assess need to move, ability to move, and assistive devices available.

ANALYSIS

4-5. Follow steps 4 and 5 of the General Procedure: Think through your data, and identify specific problems and modifications.

PLANNING

6-7. Follow steps 6 and 7 of the General Procedure: Determine individualized patient outcomes in relationship to alignment and comfort and plan the moving technique.

IMPLEMENTATION

Action	Rationale
8-13. Follow steps 8 to 13 of the General Procedure: Wash or disinfect your hands, obtain assistive devices, identify the patient (two identifiers), explain the procedure, raise the bed, put the bed in the flat position.	
14. Move the patient as follows:	
a. Move the patient close to one side of the bed, following the procedure above.	Moving the patient close to the side of the bed where you are standing helps you maintain firm support with the legs, keeping your center of gravity over your base of support and working close to your body.
b. Have the patient bend the knees and place the soles of the feet firmly on the surface of the bed, or help the patient place the feet in this position.	Even if the patient is unable to push with the feet and legs, this positioning of the knees and soles eliminates the need to pull the weight of the legs as well as the weight of the trunk.
c. Have the patient grasp the overhead **trapeze,** if one is in place, or the side rails at shoulder level.	Encouraging patients to participate in self-care promotes independence and self-esteem and may speed recovery.
d. Slide your hands and arms under the patient's hips. You should be turned slightly toward the foot of the bed with your outside foot slightly ahead of your inside foot (Fig. 6-2). Keep your back straight, bend at the hips and the knees, and keep your elbows bent.	This stance puts you in a position to pull, which overcomes resistance from the soft bed, and allows you to use your strong leg muscles (rather than your back) for force.

(continued)

Action	Rationale
	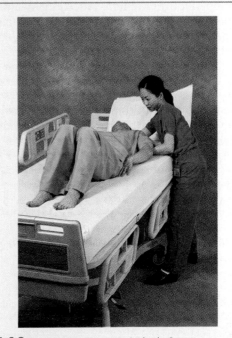 **FIGURE 6-2** Moving a person up in bed: One-person assist. The patient pushes with feet flat on the bed. Although the side rails and trapeze are omitted from the photo for clarity, the patient uses them to push up on the bed. Without the rails or a trapeze, the patient places the palms of the hands flat on the bed and pushes.

Safety Alert   *Under no circumstances should a nurse pull a patient up in bed by grasping the patient under the **axillae** and pulling. This may work well for the nurse, but it is very uncomfortable for the patient and can cause a shoulder dislocation, especially for a person with extremely weak muscles or paralysis.*

Action	Rationale
e. Instruct the patient to move with you on the count "One, two, three, up!" All effort should be simultaneous.	Instructing the patient enables the patient to participate effectively in the process.
f. Count, "One, two, three, up!" The patient should pull with the arms and push with the feet. From your position, you will pull the patient up in bed.	Counting prompts simultaneous action, thereby applying the most combined energy to the task. *Note:* Many people carry out this maneuver by facing the head of the bed and pushing the patient up. This method has two drawbacks: first, you cannot move as much weight this way; second, you meet greater resistance from the bed surface in pushing along it rather than in pulling along it.
15-17. Follow steps 15 to 17 of the General Procedure: Position the patient, place appropriate safety devices, wash or disinfect your hands.	

EVALUATION

18. Follow step 18 of the General Procedure: Evaluate using the individualized patient outcomes regarding alignment and comfort.

DOCUMENTATION

19-20. Follow steps 19 and 20 of the General Procedure: Document the position as appropriate, and document the techniques on the nursing care plan and/or the patient's activity record.

Moving a Patient Up in Bed: Two- or Three-Person Assist

When you must move a heavy patient or one who is unable to help, you will find assistants useful.

ASSESSMENT

1-3. Follow steps 1 to 3 of the General Procedure: Assess need to move, ability to move, and assistive devices available.

ANALYSIS

4-5. Follow steps 4 and 5 of the General Procedure: Think through your data, and identify specific problems and modifications.

PLANNING

6-7. Follow steps 6 and 7 of the General Procedure: Determine individualized patient outcomes in relationship to alignment and comfort and plan the moving technique.

IMPLEMENTATION

Action	Rationale
8-13. Follow steps 8 to 13 of the General Procedure: Wash or disinfect your hands, obtain assistive devices, identify the patient (two identifiers), explain the procedure, raise the bed, put the bed in the flat position.	
14. Move the patient:	
a. Move the patient close to one side of the bed, following the procedure above.	Moving the patient close to the side of the bed where you are standing helps you maintain firm support with the legs, keeping your center of gravity over your base of support and working close to your body.
b. If possible, have the patient bend the knees and plant the soles of the feet firmly on the bed, or help the patient place the feet in this position.	Even if the patient is unable to push with the feet and legs, this positioning of the knees and soles eliminates the need to pull the weight of the legs as well as the weight of the trunk.
c. The first nurse (nurse 1) slides his or her arms under the patient's head and shoulders. This nurse faces the foot of the bed.	This puts nurse 1 in a position to pull strongly.
d. The second nurse (nurse 2) slides his or her arms under the patient's hips from the same side of the bed. This nurse also faces the foot of the bed (Fig. 6-3).	This puts nurse 2 in a position to pull strongly also.

(continued)

Action	Rationale
	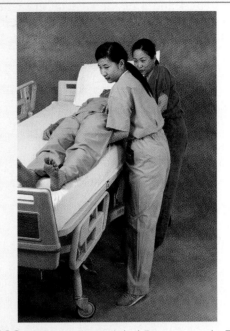 **FIGURE 6-3** Moving a patient up in bed: Two-person assist. The nurses face toward the foot of the bed. The outside foot (left, in this instance) is placed more toward the foot of the bed to provide a wide stance. The back is straight and knees and hips are slightly bent.
e. The nurse with the heavier burden (usually nurse 2) counts, "One, two, three, up!" If a third nurse is needed, all three should position themselves on the same side of the bed.	Counting helps both nurses to pull the patient up in bed at the same time. This procedure can be repeated several times until the patient is in the correct position. In addition, lining up on the same side of the bed helps distribute the patient's weight evenly among the nurses for the most efficient use of muscle power. *Note:* On occasion, it will be necessary to leave a patient in the middle of the bed. In that case, the lifters should position themselves on each side of the bed, paying close attention to their body mechanics.
15-17. Follow steps 15 to 17 of the General Procedure: Position the patient, place appropriate safety devices, wash or disinfect your hands.	

EVALUATION

18. Follow step 18 of the General Procedure: Evaluate using the individualized patient outcomes regarding alignment and comfort.

DOCUMENTATION

19-20. Follow steps 19 and 20 of the General Procedure: Document position as appropriate, and document techniques on the nursing care plan and/or patient's activity record.

Turning a Patient in Bed: Back to Side

ASSESSMENT

1-3. Follow steps 1 to 3 of the General Procedure: Assess need to move, ability to move, and assistive devices available.

ANALYSIS

4-5. Follow steps 4 and 5 of the General Procedure: Think through your data, and identify specific problems and modifications.

PLANNING

6-7. Follow steps 6 and 7 of the General Procedure: Determine individualized patient outcomes in relationship to alignment and comfort and plan the moving technique.

IMPLEMENTATION

Action	Rationale
8-13. Follow steps 8 to 13 of the General Procedure: Wash or disinfect your hands, obtain pillows for support, identify the patient (two identifiers), explain the procedure, raise the bed, put the bed in the flat position.	
14. Move the patient as follows:	
a. Move the patient close to one side of the bed, following the procedure above.	Moving the patient close to the side of the bed provides space so that the patient is in the center of the bed when the move is complete.
b. Raise the side rail nearest you, and move to the other side of the bed. You will be rolling the patient toward you.	Raising the side rail prevents the patient from rolling off the side of the bed after you have left it.
c. Prepare the pillows needed for support (see Side-Lying Position, discussed later).	Pillows will help the patient to remain in the appropriate position.
d. Position the patient for turning:	
(1) Move the patient's near arm out away from the patient's body.	To prevent trapping the arm under the body.
(2) Place the patient's far arm across the chest.	To allow the arm to be used as leverage for the body.
(3) Cross the patient's far ankle over the near ankle, and grasp the patient with one hand behind the far hip. Alternatively, raise the knee on the far leg, and grasp the far side of the knee.	To use the weight of the legs to help turn the body.
e. Grasp the patient behind the far shoulder, and roll the patient toward you (the hips and shoulders may be turned as one unit) (Fig. 6-4).	To maintain the body's alignment as the patient is turned.

(continued)

Action	Rationale
	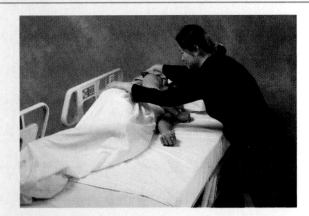 **FIGURE 6-4** Turning a patient from back to side. The nurse uses a wide base of support with back straight and knees slightly bent to grasp the patient behind the shoulder. Then, she rocks backward, using the entire weight of the body to turn the patient. (Side rails omitted for clarity.)
15-17. Follow steps 15 to 17 of the General Procedure: Position the patient, place appropriate safety devices, wash or disinfect your hands.	

EVALUATION

18. Follow step 18 of the General Procedure: Evaluate using the individualized patient outcomes regarding alignment and comfort.

DOCUMENTATION

19-20. Follow steps 19 and 20 of the General Procedure: Document the position as appropriate, and document the techniques on the nursing care plan and/or patient's activity record.

Turning a Patient in Bed: Back to Abdomen

ASSESSMENT

1-3. Follow steps 1 to 3 of the General Procedure: Assess need to move, ability to move, and pillows available.

IMPLEMENTATION

ANALYSIS

4-5. Follow steps 4 and 5 of the General Procedure: Think through your data, and identify specific problems and modifications.

PLANNING

6-7. Follow steps 6 and 7 of the General Procedure: Determine individualized patient outcomes in relationship to alignment and comfort and plan the moving technique.

Action	Rationale
8-13. Follow steps 8 to 13 of the General Procedure: Wash or disinfect your hands, obtain pillows for support, identify the patient (two identifiers), explain the procedure, raise the bed, put the bed in the flat position.	

(continued)

Action	Rationale
14. Move the patient as follows:	
a. Move the patient close to one side of the bed, following the procedure above.	Moving the patient close to the side of the bed provides space for the patient to lie in the center of the bed after turning is completed.
b. Raise the side rail nearest you, and move to the other side of the bed. You will be rolling the patient toward you.	Raising the side rail prevents the patient from rolling off the side of the bed after you have left it.
c. Prepare the pillows needed for support (see Abdomen-Lying Position, discussed later). *Note:* Frequently, a heavy-breasted patient will need a pillow under the abdomen for comfort. A very thin patient may be more comfortable with a small pillow under the iliac crests.	Pillows will assist the patient to be comfortable in the position.
d. Place the patient's near arm over the head.	To keep the patient's arm out of the way as the patient rolls.
e. Turn the patient's face away from you.	To prevent the patient from rolling onto his or her face during the turning procedure (Fig. 6-5).

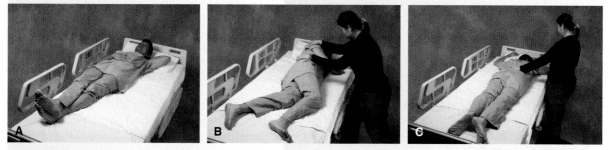

FIGURE 6-5 Turning a patient to the abdomen. (**A**) Patient positioned for turn. (**B**) Turning the patient. (**C**) Patient positioned on the abdomen.

Action	Rationale
f. Roll the patient onto the side by grasping the shoulder and bent far knee, using the technique described under "Turning a Patient in Bed: Back to Side" above.	This technique uses the weight of the leg to help turn the body.
g. Once the patient is on the side, check the arm and face carefully to see that they are correctly positioned.	To ensure that the pillow will provide correct support, and the arm is not twisted under.
h. Roll the patient over onto the abdomen with pillows appropriately placed.	Rolling prevents injury to your back and is comfortable for the patient.

(continued)

Action	Rationale
15-17. Follow steps 15 to 17 of the General Procedure: Position the patient, place appropriate safety devices, wash or disinfect your hands.	

EVALUATION

18. Follow step 18 of the General Procedure: Evaluate using the individualized patient outcomes regarding alignment and comfort.

DOCUMENTATION

19-20. Follow steps 19 and 20 of the General Procedure: Document position as appropriate, and document techniques on the nursing care plan and/or the patient's activity record.

Turning a Patient in Bed: Logrolling

Patients who must maintain a straight (when viewed from the front or back) alignment at all times are turned by a technique called logrolling. The technique requires at least two nurses, and sometimes three

if the patient is very large. The normal S curvature of the spine is supported, and there is no twisting or bending.

ASSESSMENT

1-3. Follow steps 1 to 3 of the General Procedure: Assess need to move, ability to move, and pillows available.

ANALYSIS

4-5. Follow steps 4 and 5 of the General Procedure: Think through your data, and identify specific problems and modifications.

PLANNING

6-7. Follow steps 6 and 7 of the General Procedure: Determine individualized patient outcomes in relationship to alignment and comfort and plan the moving technique.

IMPLEMENTATION

Action	Rationale
8-13. Follow steps 8 to 13 of the General Procedure: Wash or disinfect your hands, obtain supportive devices or additional personnel, identify the patient (two identifiers), explain the procedure, raise the bed, place the bed in the flat position.	
14. Move the patient as follows:	
a. Move the patient to one side of the bed as a single unit. Each person assisting with the turn slides his or her arms under the patient. At a signal ("One, two, three, move!"), all pull the patient, making sure that the patient's body stays correctly aligned at all times.	To keep the body aligned during the entire time of movement.
b. Raise the side rail on that side of the bed.	To maintain safety.
c. All assistants move to the other side of the bed.	To position themselves where they can turn the patient toward them.

(continued)

Action	Rationale
d. Place the pillows where they will be needed for support after the patient has been turned. One is needed to support the head with the spine straight. Another is needed between the legs (in fact, two may be needed here).	To support the legs and prevent twisting of the hips.
e. All assistants reach across and grasp the far side of the patient's body.	To enable them to pull the patient's weight as a unit.
f. At the signal ("One, two, three, turn!"), all turn the patient smoothly.	To keep the patient's body perfectly straight, like a log (Fig. 6-6). **FIGURE 6-6** Logrolling: The patient is rolled as a unit. The legs remain parallel, and a pillow is placed between them to keep the upper leg from dropping and twisting the spine. A pillow is placed to support the head. At least two nurses are essential for this procedure.
15-17. Follow steps 15 to 17 of the General Procedure: Correctly position the patient, ensure that safety devices are in place, and wash or disinfect your hands.	

EVALUATION

18. Follow step 18 of the General Procedure: Evaluate using the individualized patient outcomes regarding alignment and comfort.

DOCUMENTATION

19-20. Follow steps 19 and 20 of the General Procedure: Document the procedure on a flow sheet and the nursing plan as appropriate.

Turning a Patient in Bed: Using a Turn or Pull Sheet

A sheet can be used as an aid in turning and moving a patient in bed. One advantage of using a turn or pull sheet is that the movement takes place between two layers of dry cloth, which produces less friction than does skin on cloth. Another advantage is that it is much easier to grasp a sheet firmly than it is to hold a patient's body. Your hands can slip off the patient if you do not grasp hard enough; if you grasp too hard, you can cause discomfort or even bruising. A third advantage is that the turn sheet supports the patient's entire body and makes it easier to keep the patient straight.

A draw sheet or a flat sheet folded in half may be used as a turn or pull sheet. Place the turn sheet under the patient's trunk, with the bottom edge below the patient's buttocks and the top edge at the top of the patient's shoulders. The sheet will then support the heaviest part of the patient's body. Do not tuck in the sides; fanfold or roll them along the patient on each side. To move the patient up in bed or to turn the patient, follow the general procedures as described above, but rather than grasping the patient, grasp the fanfolded or rolled edges of the sheet, and move the patient up as depicted in Figure 6-7. Do not lift the patient with the pull sheet;

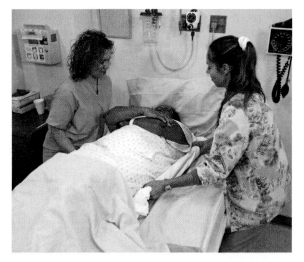

FIGURE 6-7 Moving a patient up in bed using a turn sheet. Both nurses will face the foot of the bed; knees and hips are slightly bent and backs are straight. Feet are spread to form a wide base of support. The nurses roll the turn sheet close to the patient before lifting and moving.

always slide the patient to lessen strain on your back. When a turn sheet is needed, it is usually placed on the bed at the time that the bed is made. However, it can be placed just before moving the patient if the need is identified at that time.

POSITIONING THE PATIENT IN BED

Positioning patients in bed in proper body alignment and changing their positions frequently are important nursing functions. Many alert patients automatically reposition themselves and readily move about in bed. They may not need special attention, but they often need a reminder that comfort and good body align-

ment are sometimes not the same. For example, two large pillows under the head may be comfortable, but when the neck is in constant **flexion,** spasms and contractures can develop. Patients must be repositioned during the night as well.

Keep in mind that healthy people turn many times and adopt many positions during sleep. Repositioning is usually done every 2 hours. For some patients, more frequent turning is needed to prevent skin breakdown. Without a 24-hour repositioning schedule, positioning may be inadvertently omitted. Patients will develop pressure ulcers readily if pressure on bony prominences is not relieved. It is helpful to give range-of-motion exercises (ROM) to patients when they are repositioned to maintain joint flexibility. (See Module 20, Range-of-Motion Exercises.)

Positioning aids are devices used to maintain the patient in the correct position. You can make positioning aids easily from ordinary items found in your facility. Pillows, towels, washcloths, blankets, sandbags, footboards, and strong cardboard cartons can all be used to help maintain a position (Fig. 6-8).

SPECIFIC PROCEDURES FOR POSITIONING A PATIENT IN BED

Use the following directions to position the patient as indicated in step 14 of the General Procedure for Moving a Patient in Bed and Positioning.

Procedure for the Supine Position

The supine position (Fig. 6-9) is frequently used for examining the patient and performing procedures. Some pa-

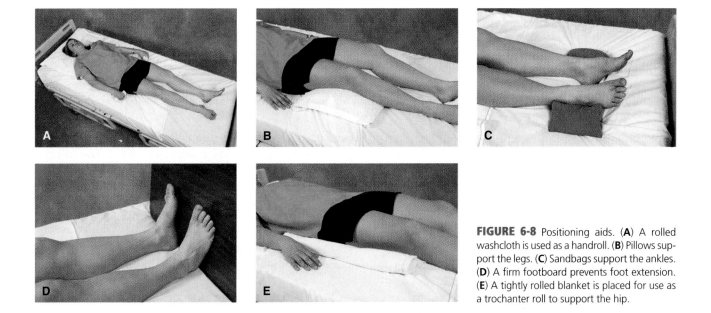

FIGURE 6-8 Positioning aids. (**A**) A rolled washcloth is used as a handroll. (**B**) Pillows support the legs. (**C**) Sandbags support the ankles. (**D**) A firm footboard prevents foot extension. (**E**) A tightly rolled blanket is placed for use as a trochanter roll to support the hip.

tients may rest comfortably in the supine position, while others may not be able to remain in this position for long periods.

ASSESSMENT

1-3. Follow steps 1 to 3 of the General Procedure: Assess need to move, ability to move, and assistive devices available.

ANALYSIS

4-5. Follow steps 4 and 5 of the General Procedure: Think through your data, and identify specific problems and modifications.

PLANNING

6-7. Follow steps 6 and 7 of the General Procedure: Determine individualized patient outcomes in relationship to alignment and comfort and plan the positioning technique.

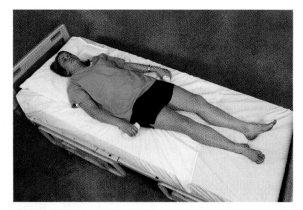

FIGURE 6-9 Supine position. In this position, patients with mobility problems could have a footboard (such as the one in Figure 6-8) to prevent footdrop. Handrolls would help to maintain functional position for patients with paralysis.

IMPLEMENTATION

Action	Rationale
8-13. Follow steps 8 to 13 of the General Procedure: Wash or disinfect your hands, obtain pillows for support, identify the patient (two identifiers), explain the procedure, raise the bed, put the bed in the flat position.	
14. Turn the patient to his or her back using correct body mechanics.	To prevent injury to the caregiver.
15. Position the patient as follows:	
a. Check that the spine is in correct alignment.	To prevent stress on the back and joints.
b. Place a low pillow under the head.	To prevent neck hyperextension.
c. Place the patient's arms at the patient's sides with the hands pronated. The forearms can also be elevated on pillows.	To provide support for the joints and prevent torsion on the shoulder joint.
d. If the patient's hands are paralyzed, use handrolls. Place the handroll in the palm of the patient's hand.	To maintain the hands in functional positions. The fingers and thumb should be flexed around it. The roll should be large enough so that the fingers are only slightly flexed. A handroll may have to be secured to the hand with paper tape. Handrolls can be made of several washcloths (or other linen) that have been rolled and taped. Commercial handrolls are also available, usually through the physical therapy department. *(continued)*

Action	Rationale
e. Position the legs with toes pointing ventrally and the leg lying straight. A **trochanter** roll provides support to the hip joint to maintain its position and is effective in preventing **external rotation** of the hip. (This roll can be made from a sheet, bath towel, or pad.) Place one end flat under the patient's hip, centered where the trochanter is located. Roll the linen under to form a roll that stabilizes the hip and prevents it from turning outward. An ankle roll, which is made in the same way but is smaller than a trochanter roll, may be used for the same purpose but is less effective due to the weight of the leg. If both legs are paralyzed, place a roll on either side at the hip.	Allowing the feet to turn to the outside externally rotates the hip joint. Externally rotated hips become less functional and do not support a patient who is trying to regain function.
f. Support the foot so that the toes point upward in **anatomic position** and do not fall into **plantar flexion.** High-topped athletic shoes are very effective in maintaining a functional foot position. Special splints may also be used to maintain position. Although a manufactured footboard, sandbags, or a strong cardboard carton can be used to maintain the feet at right angles to the legs thereby preventing foot **extension,** these are less effective because the feet slip out of the right-angle position.	When plantar flexion is maintained for a long time, a permanent deformity called **footdrop** develops. The foot becomes unable to dorsiflex and ceases to be functional.
16-17. Follow steps 16 and 17 of the General Procedure: Place appropriate safety devices; wash or disinfect your hands.	

EVALUATION

18. Evaluate using the individualized patient outcomes in relationship to alignment and comfort

DOCUMENTATION

19-20. Follow steps 19 and 20 of the General Procedure: Document the position as appropriate, and document the techniques on the nursing care plan and/or patient's activity record.

Procedure for the Side-Lying Position

The side-lying position can be particularly comfortable for the patient when attention is given to good body alignment (Fig. 6-10). A patient who is paralyzed on one side can be placed on that side as well as on the unaffected side. Pain of the affected joints due to muscle relaxation may lead to dislocation of the joints; therefore, special consideration should be taken when moving or positioning these persons. To avoid dislocation, never pull on the affected extremities. Any pain in the joint should always be reported to the team leader or physician.

ASSESSMENT

1-3. Follow steps 1 to 3 of the General Procedure: Assess need to move, ability to move, and assistive devices available.

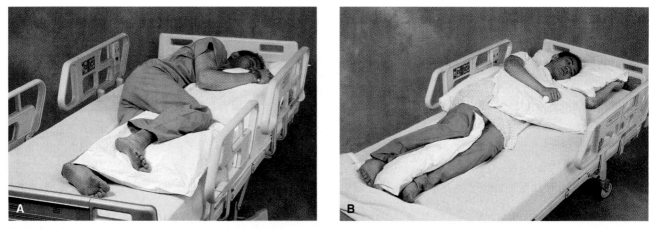

FIGURE 6-10 Side-lying position. (**A**) Traditional, fully side-lying supported position. (**B**) Tilted side-lying position to decrease pressure on bony prominences (trochanter and acromion process) for the patient at risk of skin breakdown.

ANALYSIS

4-5. Follow steps 4 and 5 of the General Procedure: Think through your data, and identify specific problems and modifications.

PLANNING

6-7. Follow steps 6 and 7 of the General Procedure: Determine individualized patient outcomes in relationship to alignment and comfort, and plan the positioning technique.

IMPLEMENTATION

Action	Rationale
8-13. Follow steps 8 to 13 of the General Procedure: Wash or disinfect your hands, obtain pillows for support, identify the patient (two identifiers), explain the procedure, raise the bed, put the bed in the flat position.	
14. Turn the patient to his or her side, using correct body mechanics.	To prevent injury to the caregiver.
15. Position the patient on his or her side as follows:	
a. Check that the spine is in correct alignment.	To prevent stress on the back and joints.
b. Place a low pillow under the head.	To prevent neck hyperextension to one side.
c. Place the patient's arms to the front of the body. Support the entire upper arm on pillows with the elbow slightly flexed. Position the lower arm with the elbow flexed and the hand supported by the pillow that is under the head.	To prevent pressure of the body lying on the arm and prevent torsion of the shoulder and back from the arm pulling down.
d. If the patient's hands are paralyzed, use handrolls as outlined in the General Procedure.	To maintain a functional alignment of the hands.

(continued)

Action	Rationale
e. Position the legs with the lower leg lying straight. The upper leg should be flexed forward and supported along its whole length with pillows.	Extending the lower leg provides a period with the joint extended, and then when the patient is turned, that joint will be flexed. This prevents stiffness of the joints, preserves range of motion, and provides a functional basis for restoration of function.
f. Support the foot so that the toes point dorsally in anatomic position and do not extend into plantar flexion as described in the General Procedure.	To prevent footdrop and preserve the functional ability of the foot.
16-17. Follow steps 16 and 17 of the General Procedure: Place appropriate safety devices; wash or disinfect your hands.	

EVALUATION

18. Follow step 18 of the General Procedure: Evaluate using the individualized patient outcomes in relationship to alignment and comfort.

DOCUMENTATION

19-20. Follow steps 19 and 20 of the General Procedure: Document the position as appropriate, and document the techniques on the nursing care plan and/or patient's activity record.

Procedure for the Prone Position

The prone position (Fig. 6-11) is used infrequently because for some patients, respiration may be compromised in this position. However, a number of patients can tolerate **pronation** if the position is accomplished correctly.

ASSESSMENT

1-3. Follow steps 1 to 3 of the General Procedure: Assess need to move, ability to move, and assistive devices available.

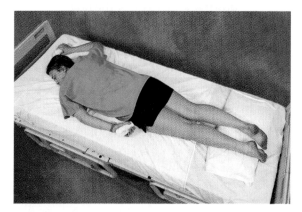

FIGURE 6-11 Prone position. A small pillow supports the patient's ankles. The patient's arms bend upward toward the shoulders or remain at the sides. A small pillow may be used under the head. A few patients may need handrolls to maintain hands in functional position.

ANALYSIS

4-5. Follow steps 4 and 5 of the General Procedure: Think through your data, and identify specific problems and modifications.

PLANNING

6-7. Follow steps 6 and 7 of the General Procedure: Determine individualized patient outcomes in relationship to alignment and comfort and plan the positioning technique.

IMPLEMENTATION

Action	Rationale
8-13. Follow steps 8 to 13 of the General Procedure: Wash or disinfect your hands, obtain pillows for support, identify the patient (two identifiers), explain the pro-	

(continued)

Action	Rationale
cedure, raise the bed, put the bed in the flat position.	
14. Turn the patient to his or her abdomen using correct body mechanics.	
15. Position the patient on his or her abdomen as follows:	
a. Check that the spine is in correct alignment.	To prevent stress on the back and joints.
b. Turn the head to the side.	To facilitate respiration and expectoration of sputum, saliva, or vomitus.
c. Place the patient's arms thumb side down on each side of the body.	To prevent pressure of the body lying on the arm and prevent torsion of the shoulder and back.
d. If the patient's hands are paralyzed, use handrolls as outlined in the General Procedure.	To maintain a functional alignment of the hands.
e. Position the legs with the lower leg lying straight. The lower leg may be positioned with a flat pillow or folded blanket under the ankles.	Supporting the ankles takes the pressure off the toes and allows the foot to remain in a functional position.
16-17. Follow steps 16 and 17 of the General Procedure: Place appropriate safety devices; wash or disinfect your hands.	

EVALUATION

18. Follow step 18 of the General Procedure: Evaluate using the individualized patient outcomes in relationship to alignment and comfort.

DOCUMENTATION

19-20. Follow steps 19 and 20 of the General Procedure: Document position as appropriate, and document techniques on the nursing care plan and/or patient's activity record.

POSITIONING A PATIENT IN A CHAIR

Transferring the patient into a chair is discussed in Module 18. The following discussion will guide you in assisting the patient who is in a chair into a correct sitting position in the chair. Remember that the patient who is physically able to change positions may sit in what would be an uncomfortable position for a short

time and will then move. The incapacitated patient must rely on your careful judgment to be in a seated position that provides comfort.

ASSESSMENT

1-2. Follow steps 1 and 2 of the General Procedure: Assess need to move and ability to move.

3. Assess strength to determine the patient's ability to maintain stability of the trunk while sitting.

ANALYSIS

4-5. Follow steps 4 and 5 of the General Procedure: Think through your data, and identify specific problems and modifications.

PLANNING

6-7. Follow steps 6 and 7 of the General Procedure: Determine individualized patient outcomes in relationship to alignment and comfort and plan the positioning technique.

IMPLEMENTATION

Action	Rationale
8-11. Follow steps 8 to 11 of the General Procedure: Wash or disinfect your hands, obtain pillows or bolsters for support if needed, identify the patient (two identifiers), and explain the procedure. (Omit steps 12 and 13.)	
14. Assist the patient to move to the chair. If the patient needs more than general balance in moving, consult Module 18.	
15. Position the patient in the sitting position as follows:	
a. Place feet flat against the floor.	To maintain a functional position of the foot for future walking.
b. Position knees and hips at right angles, and straighten the spine.	To provide an upright position with weight over the sitting base and avoid stress on the spine.
c. Support elbows on armrests.	To prevent stress from the weight of the arms pulling down on the shoulders.
d. Place handrolls, footrest, or bolsters if needed.	To assist the patient to remain in the position.
16-17. Follow steps 16 and 17 of the General Procedure: Place appropriate safety devices; wash or disinfect your hands.	

EVALUATION

18. Follow step 18 of the General Procedure: Evaluate using the individualized patient outcomes in relationship to alignment and comfort.

DOCUMENTATION

19-20. Follow steps 19 and 20 of the General Procedure: Document position as appropriate, and document techniques on the nursing care plan and/or patient's activity record (Fig. 6-12).

POSITIONING A PATIENT FOR THERAPY

In addition to the resting positions described on these pages, a variety of special positions are used for therapeutic reasons. The reasons and detailed explanations of their use can be found in a medical-surgical textbook. Among the positions highlighted here are Fowler's, high Fowler's, and semi-Fowler's; **orthopneic**; dorsal recum-

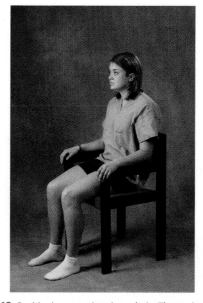

FIGURE 6-12 Positioning a patient in a chair. The patient's buttocks should fit well back into the seat of the chair. The back is straight, the knees are bent, and the feet are flat on the floor. The elbows are supported by armrests.

bent; lithotomy; Sims'; knee-chest (genupectoral); and Trendelenburg's positions.

THERAPEUTIC POSITIONS

FOWLER'S, HIGH FOWLER'S, AND SEMI-FOWLER'S POSITIONS

The Fowler's position promotes lung expansion and decreases the potential for **increased intracranial pressure** for the patient with neurologic problems. It can be used to perform certain procedures such as oral care, insertion of a nasogastric tube, or eating. The patient lies in supine position with the head of the bed elevated 18 to 20 inches (approximately 45 degrees). In high Fowler's position, the patient lies supine with head of the bed elevated more than 45 degrees; in semi-Fowler's position, the patient lies supine with the head of the bed raised less than 45 degrees (usually 20 to 30 degrees) (Figs. 6-13 and 6-14).

ORTHOPNEIC POSITION

This position (Fig. 6-15) promotes lung expansion for the patient who has extreme difficulty breathing and who is unable to lie flat or with the head only moderately elevated. It is also used to perform **thoracentesis** (see Module 17, Assisting With Diagnostic and Therapeutic Procedures). The patient sits upright with overbed table across the lap. A pillow pads the table, and the table is raised to a comfortable level, allowing the patient to lean forward and rest the head and arms on the table for support.

DORSAL RECUMBENT POSITION

The dorsal recumbent position is often used as a position of comfort for patients with back strain. In this position, the patient lies supine with knees raised and

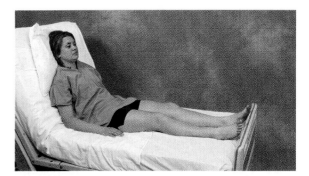

FIGURE 6-14 High Fowler's position.

legs separated (Fig. 6-16). The knee gatch on the bed can be used to elevate the knees for comfort.

LITHOTOMY POSITION

The lithotomy position (Fig. 6-17) is used for perineal and vaginal examinations as well as for some treatments. The patient lies supine with both knees flexed, feet close to the hips, and legs widely separated or with feet in stirrups on an examination table. The patient is draped (not shown for purpose of clarity) so that the perineal area is visible for examination while legs and body remain covered for warmth and modesty.

SIMS' POSITION

The Sims' position is used for administering enemas or for examining the rectal area. It may also be used for catheterization in the patient who is unable to be in the lithotomy position. The patient is in a side-lying position with a small pillow supporting the head. The patient is turned onto the abdomen so that the lower arm is extended behind the back, and both knees are slightly flexed. The upper leg is flexed farther forward than the lower leg, and the upper leg also rests on the bed (Fig. 6-18).

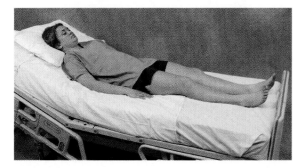

FIGURE 6-13 In the Fowler's position, the head is up approximately 45 degrees. The knees are not elevated to avoid putting pressure on the popliteal areas.

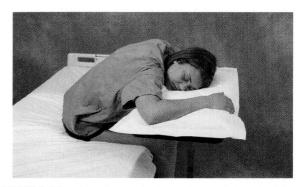

FIGURE 6-15 In the orthopneic position, the patient rests the elbows on a pillow on the overbed table.

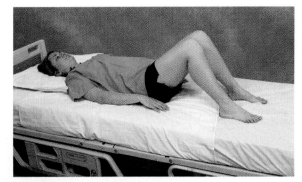

FIGURE 6-16 Dorsal recumbent position.

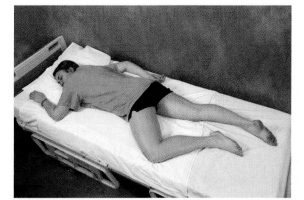

FIGURE 6-18 Sims' position.

KNEE-CHEST POSITION (GENUPECTORAL)

The knee-chest position is used for rectal procedures such as sigmoidoscopy. The patient kneels on the bed or table, and then leans forward with the hips in the air and the chest and arms on the bed or table. A pillow can be placed under the patient's head. If a special examination table is available, have the patient kneel on a platform and lean on the table. The patient is draped (not shown) so that the rectal area is visible, and the rest of the body is covered for warmth and modesty (Fig. 6-19).

TRENDELENBURG POSITION

The Trendelenburg position (Fig. 6-20) is sometimes used for postural drainage (a procedure for draining secretions from certain segments of the lungs) and for promoting venous return in patients with problems in tissue perfusion. The patient lies in a supine position with the head of the bed flat and the bed frame tilted downward so that the head is approximately 30 degrees below horizontal level. A pillow protects the head from the headboard. Reverse Trendelenburg position (see Fig 6-20) is useful for procedures such as tube feeding.

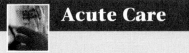

Acute Care

Many individuals in acute care settings rely upon caregivers for moving and positioning. Moving and positioning must frequently be modified based upon the diagnosis or surgical procedure. When planning for discharge, patients and families may need to be taught effective moving and positioning strategies.

Long-Term Care

Moving the resident in bed and positioning is a frequent and essential task for caregivers in long-term care settings. This is because physical limitations prevent many of the residents from adequately moving themselves. It is essential that you have knowledge of these skills because the registered nurse or licensed practical nurse is always in the position of leading the team or supervising others in the long-term care setting.

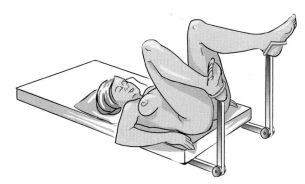

FIGURE 6-17 Lithotomy position.

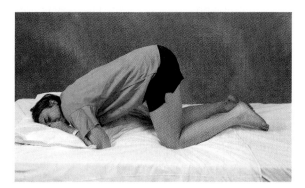

FIGURE 6-19 Knee-chest position.

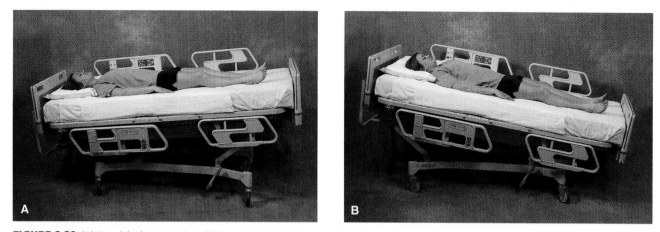

FIGURE 6-20 (**A**) Trendelenburg position. (**B**) Reverse Trendelenburg position.

Assessment of the resident in the long-term care facility is crucial so that proper and safe positioning and transfer occur. Knowing the physical effects of diseases (such as stroke and Parkinson's disease) as well as the more normal changes brought on by the aging process is essential for assessing the physically limited resident. Maintaining good body alignment at all times and avoiding undue pressure on the body parts and limbs of elderly residents are important safety concerns.

Home Care

Caregiving families and the people who are cared for in their homes with health problems that require assistance in moving and changing position usually benefit from health teaching. Family members will want to become proficient in moving and positioning skills, so they can provide better care for their family member. Assisting the caregivers to learn these techniques may require a teaching plan involving demonstration and feedback on your part and a return demonstration by the caregivers. At first, positioning and moving a loved one with physical limitations may be awkward and may create anxiety. With repetition and the nurse's encouragement and praise, this will soon become more comfortable for both the client and the caregivers.

LEARNING TOOLS

DEVELOP YOUR BACKGROUND KNOWLEDGE

1. Review the Learning Outcomes.

2. Read the section on the effects of immobility in your assigned text.

3. Look up the Key Terms in the glossary.

4. Read through this module, and mentally practice the techniques described. Study so that you would be able to teach these skills to another person.

5. Note the different positions you assume during a normal night's sleep. Is one particular position more comfortable for you than others? How often do you estimate you change your position during the night?

DEVELOP YOUR SKILLS

1. In the practice setting, select three other students, and form a group of four.

2. Changing so that each has the opportunity to play the role of the patient, perform each of the following procedures for moving the patient in bed. Use the Performance Checklists on the CD-ROM in the front of this book to check yourself. Those who are not participating at a given time can observe and evaluate the performances of the others.
   a. Move the "patient" closer to one side of the bed.
   b. Move the "patient" up in bed: one-person assist.
   c. Move the "patient" up in bed: two- or three-person assist.
   d. Turn the "patient" in bed: back to side.
   e. Turn the "patient" in bed: back to abdomen.
   f. Turn the "patient" in bed: logrolling.
   g. Perform two of the above using a turn (or pull) sheet. Does this make the task easier? How? Why?

3. With the same group, change roles as you did before, and position the "patient" in the following ways:
   a. supine position
   b. side-lying position
   c. prone position
   d. sitting position (in a chair)
   e. Fowler's position
   f. high Fowler's position
   g. semi-Fowler's position
   h. orthopneic position
   i. dorsal recumbent position

j. lithotomy position
k. Sims' position
l. knee-chest position
m. Trendelenburg position

DEMONSTRATE YOUR SKILLS

In the clinical setting

1. Consult with your instructor regarding the opportunity to move patients using a variety of techniques. Evaluate your performance with the instructor.

2. Consult with your instructor regarding the opportunity to position patients in a variety of appropriate positions. Evaluate your performance with the instructor.

CRITICAL THINKING EXERCISES

1. Martha Smith, a resident in a long-term care facility, had a stroke that left her left arm weak and her left leg paralyzed. The plan is for her to sit up in a chair three times a day. Identify the concerns you have and the assessment that you need. What challenges do you envision in positioning her comfortably? Devise several alternative strategies for making her comfortable in a chair.

2. Marvin Jones is hospitalized after a severe head injury. He is unresponsive and does not move at all. His head must be kept at a 35-degree elevation. Identify the concerns you would have and the assessment that you need. Develop a plan for turning and positioning this patient in bed.

SELF-QUIZ

SHORT-ANSWER QUESTIONS

1. What is the primary reason for having the bed in the flat position when moving a patient?

_____

2. What two important functions are fulfilled by having the patient assist you whenever possible?

a. _____

b. _____

3. If a nurse attempts to move a patient by grasping him or her under the axillae, what may occur?

_____

4. A turn sheet should be placed under which part of a patient's body?

_____

5. List two reasons why patients should be checked after moving.

a. _____

b. _____

6. List three reasons for proper and frequent positioning of a patient in bed.

a. _____

b. _____

c. _____

7. To prevent external rotation of the leg when a patient is in the supine position, what might you use?

_____

8. When a patient is in a side-lying position, where is the top leg placed?

_____

9. When a patient is in the prone position, two methods can be used to keep the feet from plantar flexion and possible development of footdrop. What are these two methods?

a. _____

b. _____

10. When working in long-term care or home care, how could you facilitate the proper moving and positioning of residents or clients by staff and families?

_____

_____

_____

MULTIPLE CHOICE

_____ 11. In all positions, the spine should be
a. slightly flexed.
b. straight.
c. slightly extended.
d. curved.

_____ 12. A patient's position should usually be changed
a. every hour.
b. every 2 hours.
c. every 4 hours.
d. once per shift.

_____ 13. Sims' position is one in which the patient
a. has the feet and legs elevated.
b. has the head elevated at a 30-degree angle.
c. is on the left side with both knees flexed, the right higher than the left.
d. is in a kneeling position.

Answers to Self-Quiz questions appear in the back of this book.

MODULE 7

Providing Hygiene

SKILLS INCLUDED IN THIS MODULE

General Procedure for Hygiene
Specific Procedures for Hygiene
   Procedure for Bed Bath
   Procedure for Shower
   Procedure for Tub Bath
   Partial Bed Bath, Self-Bed Bath, Towel Bath,
     and Bag Bath
   Procedure for Giving a Back Rub
   Procedure for Oral Care
   Procedure for Oral Care for the Unconscious Patient
   Procedure for Denture Care
   Procedures for Brushing and Combing Hair
   Procedure for Shampooing Hair
   Procedure for Eye Care
   Procedures for Contact Lens Removal, Care,
     and Insertion
   Hearing Aid Care

PREREQUISITE MODULES

Module 1	An Approach to Nursing Skills
Module 2	Documentation
Module 3	Basic Body Mechanics
Module 4	Basic Infection Control
Module 6	Moving the Patient in Bed and Positioning

The following may be needed in some instances:

Module 14	Nursing Physical Assessment
Module 18	Transfer
Module 19	Ambulation: Simple Assisted and Using Cane, Walker, or Crutches

KEY TERMS

aspirate	semi-Fowler's position
axilla(e)	
canthus	sordes
expectorate	stomatitis
Fowler's position	supine
genitalia	umbilicus

OVERALL OBJECTIVES

▸ To provide each patient with hygiene according to individual needs, conditions, and preferences.
▸ To promote comfort and stimulate circulation.
▸ To prevent or eliminate body odors through hygiene.

LEARNING OUTCOMES

The student will be able to

1. Assess the patient effectively to determine the appropriate method for hygiene, considering culture, developmental level, financial status, health status, and personal preferences.
2. Analyze assessment data to determine special problems or concerns regarding hygiene that must be addressed to successfully complete hygiene practices.
3. Determine appropriate patient outcomes of the hygiene procedures, and recognize the potential for adverse outcomes.
4. Plan the individual hygienic procedures needed for a specific patient, and choose the equipment needed.
5. Implement and complete the hygiene procedures for a specific patient according to the cultural preferences, developmental level, health status of the patient, and patient preferences.
6. Apply the General Procedure when performing personal hygiene for a patient according to the patient needs.
7. Evaluate the effectiveness of the hygiene procedures carried out and the patient's comfort level.
8. Document the hygiene practices completed, any special preferences or specific cultural practices, and any abnormal findings noted while performing hygiene for the patient.

Patients in healthcare facilities have at least as many needs for hygiene measures in their daily lives as you do in yours. The practices of personal hygiene are varied and individualized according to personal values, cultural practices, socioeconomic status, and developmental levels. Patients may have considerably more need for hygiene measures because of perspiration from fever, drainage from wounds, odor from emesis, physical limitations, and other influences of illness. Often, they are unable to attend to those needs without help. It becomes the responsibility of the nurse to provide the hygiene a patient needs and desires. The nurse may delegate hygiene procedures to unlicensed personnel, but the nurse maintains responsibility for assessment and patient care.

NURSING DIAGNOSES

When providing hygiene for patients, self-care deficient nursing diagnoses are specified in different ways. Etiologies of self-care deficits are numerous and vary according to each patient. Examples include pain, restrained mobility from therapeutic equipment (cast, IV, and so forth), or decreased motivation. Some examples of self-care deficits are

- Bathing/Hygiene Self-Care Deficit: related to immobility. Encompasses all deficits in the ability to perform one's own hygiene such as oral care
- Dressing/Grooming Self-Care Deficit: related to cognitive impairment

- Bathing Self-Care Deficit: related to right upper extremity paralysis
- Toileting Self-Care Deficit: inability to ambulate to the toilet

Associated diagnoses may include

- Risk for Impaired Skin Integrity related to urinary and fecal incontinence and inability to perform own hygiene
- Impaired Oral Mucous Membrane related to ineffective oral hygiene

DELEGATION

Hygiene is frequently delegated to assistive personnel. The nurse remains accountable for assessing the patient and determining appropriate hygiene procedures. The nurse also must evaluate the patient's response to hygiene procedures. For the very fragile or critical patient, hygiene procedures may be performed by the nurse in order to assess throughout the procedure to ensure that the patient is not compromised by the activity.

GENERAL PROCEDURE FOR HYGIENE

The nurse assists the patient with various aspects of hygiene, which can be modified according to the particular aspect of hygiene involved. The patient should be encouraged to do as much as possible, with the nurse providing assistance as needed to meet hygiene needs. Although the bed bath is described here as one that the nurse provides for the patient, keep in mind that the patient may perform portions of the bath even when not able to perform the entire procedure. As the patient gains strength, there should be a gradual shift from personal hygiene performed by the nurse to hygiene performed by the patient. Promoting independence and self-care supports self-esteem and leads toward health.

Cultural practices need to be considered because variations are great in this aspect of daily care. For example, in some cultures, bathing occurs on a weekly basis rather than daily.

ASSESSMENT

1. Review the patient's record and plan of care regarding the patient's ability to participate in the procedure; include medical diagnoses, activity order, or any orders specific to hygiene and type of bath. **R:** To determine the amount of assistance the patient may need with hygiene.

2. Assess the patient to determine if there are other concerns of a higher priority than hygiene. These might be related to other basic needs, such as toileting, current symptoms related to the medical diagnosis, fatigue, pain, and level of sedation. Assess skin care and other hygienic practices and any specific concerns that might affect hygiene needs, such as the presence of a catheter, excessive perspiration from fever, or dry skin. **R:** Hygiene may be a lower priority than rest for the patient who is short of breath or experiencing pain. Higher priority problems need to be addressed before hygiene. Hygiene is planned to meet identified needs.

3. Check to see whether special supplies or equipment needed are in the patient's room. **R:** Having equipment and supplies available and ready saves time. It is not cost effective to obtain unneeded supplies.

ANALYSIS

4. Critically think through your data, carefully evaluating each aspect and its relation to other data. **R:** This enables you to determine specific problems for this individual in relation to hygiene practices.

5. Identify specific problems and modifications of the procedure needed for this individual. **R:** Planning for the individual must take into consideration the individual's problems.

PLANNING

6. Determine the following individualized patient outcomes in relation to hygiene. **R:** Identifying outcomes facilitates evaluation.
   a. Skin and nails clean
   b. Absence of offensive odor
   c. Skin and mucous membranes intact
   d. Patient expresses comfort

7. Plan the procedure, considering
   a. type of hygiene needed; this might include the type of bath, oral care, hair care, and care for eyeglasses, contact lenses, and hearing aids.
   b. supplies needed; collecting those that are not in the room
   c. assistance needed to accomplish the planned hygiene. **R:** Planning ahead allows you to proceed more safely and effectively.

IMPLEMENTATION

Action	Rationale
8. Wash or disinfect your hands.	Handwashing decreases the transfer of microorganisms that could cause infection.
9. Identify the patient using two identifiers.	Verifying the patient's identity helps ensure that you are performing the right skill for the right patient.
10. Explain the procedure you are about to perform.	Explaining the procedure helps relieve anxiety or misperceptions that the patient may have about a procedure or activity and sets the stage for patient participation.
11. Close the door, and pull the curtains around the bed.	To provide privacy.
12. Raise the bed to an appropriate working position based on your height.	Allows you to use correct body mechanics and protect yourself from back injury.

(continued)

Action	Rationale
13. Carry out the hygiene procedure planned.	To support the patient's well-being.
14. Observe the patient carefully for signs of fatigue or other adverse responses. While giving the bath, you will have an opportunity to focus on other assessments, such as inspection of the skin or evaluation of the patient's cognitive ability and psychosocial concerns.	A more relaxed environment allows time for more detailed assessments.
15. Care for all equipment and supplies used. Bathing equipment is generally cleaned and stored in the patient's unit for reuse.	Proper care and storage of equipment is cost effective.
16. Wash or disinfect your hands.	Washing decreases the transfer of microorganisms that could cause infection.

EVALUATION

17. Evaluate in terms of the individualized outcome criteria:
    a. skin and nails clean
    b. absence of offensive odor
    c. skin and mucous membranes intact
    d. patient expresses comfort

Note any adverse outcomes observed. **R:** Evaluation in relation to desired outcomes is essential for planning future care needs.

DOCUMENTATION

18. Document the hygiene measures as appropriate for your facility. Most agencies use a flow sheet for hygiene care. **R:** Documentation is a legal record of the patient's care and therapy and communicates nursing activities to other nurses and caregivers.

19. Record the patient's preferences and ability to participate on the nursing care plan. Any information about physical signs and symptoms identified during the procedure can be recorded either on a flow sheet or on the progress notes. See Figure 7-1 for an example of flow sheet entries. Table 7-1 identifies some common abbreviations used for hygiene procedures. **R:** The nursing care plan promotes a systematic approach to patient care.

POTENTIAL ADVERSE OUTCOMES AND RELATED INTERVENTIONS

1. Dry skin results from the normal aging process and may be increased with frequent bathing and contact with soap.

Intervention: For elderly patients, decrease bathing frequency to two or three times weekly with partial bathing in between. Because the skin is the first line of defense against harmful bacteria, keep the skin hydrated and moisturized, using nonperfumed lotions or soap to prevent breaks in the skin.

2. Excessive fatigue may occur when the patient's condition is fragile.

Intervention: Provide rest after hygiene has been completed, and make plans to perform hygiene in a manner that will not create excess fatigue.

3. The patient experiences shortness of breath and increased heart rate from participating in hygiene procedure.

Intervention: Have the patient rest, and resume the hygiene procedure later without patient participation.

SPECIFIC PROCEDURES FOR HYGIENE

When providing hygiene, the various procedures below may be combined and performed at the same time. For example, a bed bath, oral care, and a back rub may all be done at the same time with the steps intertwined. For instructional purposes, they are presented separately.

Procedure for Bed Bath

ASSESSMENT

1-3. Follow steps 1 to 3 of the General Procedure for Hygiene: Review the record and plan of care, assess the patient related to priority concerns, and check for supplies and equipment in the room.

SHIFT	23–07	07–15	15–23	23–07	07–15	15–23	23–07	07–15	15–23	23–07	07–15	15–23
PERSONAL HYGIENE: BATH: Complete Bed Bath, Shower $\bar{c}$/$\bar{s}$ help, Sit Shower, Bath $\bar{c}$	A.M. care	CBB $\bar{c}$ assist	P.M. care									
ORAL:	self	self	self									
BACK CARE:		Lotion rub	Lotion rub									
PERI-CARE:		self										
CATH CARE:		N/A										
ACTIVITY: (Bedrest, Amb $\bar{c}$ help, Dangle, Chair $\bar{c}$/$\bar{s}$ help, Up Ad Lib, BR $\bar{c}$ BRP)		Chair x2 15"	Chair x1 20"									
TURNED & POSITIONED	q2h	q2h when in bed	q2h when in bed									
DEEP BREATHE & COUGH	q2h	q2h	q2h									
ELIMINATION: BM (Number & Description)		$\frac{\bullet}{1}$ formed										
SLEEP PATTERNS: (Naps, 1 hour intervals, etc.)	Restless	Naps at intervals	Asleep @ 2200									
DIET:	Breakfast	Lunch	Dinner	Breakfast	Lunch	Dinner	Breakfast	Lunch	Dinner	Breakfast	Lunch	Dinner
Type	2 Gm Na											
Amount taken (All, none, fraction)	All	3/4	All									
Calorie Count												
SIGNATURES: 23–07	M. Johnson RN											
07–15	B. Kucinski RN											
15–23	D. Aquaro RN											
DATE:	2–22–06			2-23			2-24			2-25		

ADDRESSOGRAPH:

HOSPITAL MEDICAL CENTER
Seattle, Washington

FIGURE 7-1 Flow sheet entries for hygiene procedures and activities of daily living.

table 7-1.	Common Abbreviations Used for Charting Hygiene Procedures on Flow Sheets
Abbreviations	**Definition**
CBB	Complete bed bath
PBB	Partial bed bath
Self	Patient bathed self
N/A	Not applicable
X2	Done twice (times 2)
X3	Done three times (and so forth)

ANALYSIS

4-5. Follow steps 4 and 5 of the General Procedure for Hygiene: Think through your data, and identify specific problems and modifications.

PLANNING

6. Follow step 6 of the General Procedure for Hygiene: Determine individualized patient outcomes:

    a. skin and nails clean

    b. absence of offensive odor

    c. intact skin and mucous membranes

    d. patient expresses comfort

7. Plan the bathing procedure, and determine the supplies that will be needed for a bed bath.

    a. basin for water

    b. soap (some patients may have their own as a preference) and dish

    c. laundry hamper or bag

    d. bath blanket, towels, and washcloths as needed (Include enough to leave a fresh, unused towel and washcloth at the bedside for use during the day.)

    e. clean gown or pajamas

    f. necessary toiletries, such as toothpaste, toothbrush, deodorant, comb, shaving equipment

    g. clean gloves for perineal care (optional for remainder of bath if contact with body secretions is expected)

    h. clean linen if you plan to make the bed

IMPLEMENTATION

Action	*Rationale*
8-12. Follow steps 8 to 12 of the General Procedure for Hygiene: Wash or disinfect your hands, identify the patient (two identifiers), explain the procedure, close the door, pull the curtains around the bed, and raise the bed to an appropriate working position based on your height.	
13. Carry out the bed bath as follows:	
a. Cover the patient with a bath blanket placed over the top linen. If a bath blanket is not available, use the top sheet for a cover during the bath. Remove the top sheet and bedspread, leaving only the bath blanket covering the patient. Have the patient hold the top edge of the blanket while you pull the sheet down toward the patient's feet.	The flannel blanket helps to prevent chilling and does not adhere to the patient should it become wet during the bath.
b. Offer to assist the patient with oral hygiene as described in the Procedure for Oral Care (below). Some patients may prefer oral care after the bath.	Maintains teeth and gums in good condition, and eliminates unpleasant tastes and odors in the mouth.
c. Fill the basin with comfortably warm water for the bath.	Warm water is comfortable and relaxing to the patient and provides for more effective cleansing.

(continued)

Action	*Rationale*
d. Position the patient for the bath. Usually the **supine** (face-up) position is used unless the patient cannot tolerate it. In some cases, it may be necessary to use a **semi-Fowler's** or even **Fowler's position.** Lower the side rail, and move the patient to your side of the bed.	The position used must first accommodate the comfort and well-being of the patient and, second, make it easy to carry out the bath. The Fowler's positions facilitate respiratory function. The supine position facilitates access to most of the body for bathing. Lowering the side rail helps to decrease the need for the nurse to reach across the bed.
e. Remove the patient's gown. Keep the patient covered with the bath blanket.	To facilitate access to the areas to be bathed and respect the privacy and comfort of the patient.
f. Continue with the bath procedure as follows:	
(1) Spread a towel across the patient's chest on top of the bath blanket.	This keeps the bath blanket dry and prevents chilling.
(2) Make a mitt with the washcloth as shown in Figure 7-2.	Using a mitt prevents loose, cool ends of the cloth from dragging across the patient and causing discomfort.

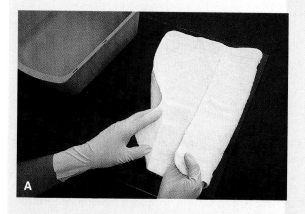

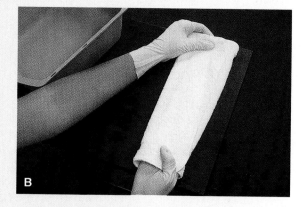

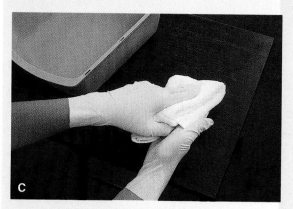

FIGURE 7-2 (**A**) Folding a mitt for bathing. (**B**) Fold washcloth lengthwise in thirds around your hand. (**C**) Then, fold top end of cloth down and tuck under bottom end.

(continued)

Action	Rationale
(3) Without using soap, wipe one eye from the inner **canthus** to the outer canthus. Rinse or use another part of the washcloth to wash the other eye.	Rinsing or changing portions of the washcloth prevents spreading organisms from one eye to the other. The movement of cleansing from the inner canthus to the outer canthus prevents secretions from entering the nasolacrimal duct.
(4) Wash the patient's face. Ask the patient about using soap on the face. Many people do not. Use gentle strokes to wash the face. Use soap to wash behind the ears and the neck. Rinse well. *Note:* Many patients can do this portion of the bath themselves.	Soap can be drying to the skin.
(5) Expose the far arm of the patient, and place a towel lengthwise under the arm (Fig. 7-3). Using long, firm strokes toward the center of the body, wash the hand, arm, and **axilla** (the underarm) while providing support to the patient's wrist and elbow. Cover the arm with half of the towel while rinsing out the washcloth. Rinse and dry the arm thoroughly.	Washing the farther arm prevents contaminating a clean part by leaning over it once it is washed. Long strokes toward the center of the body promote venous return. Covering the arm before rinsing prevents chilling when water evaporates from the skin (see Figure 7-3).

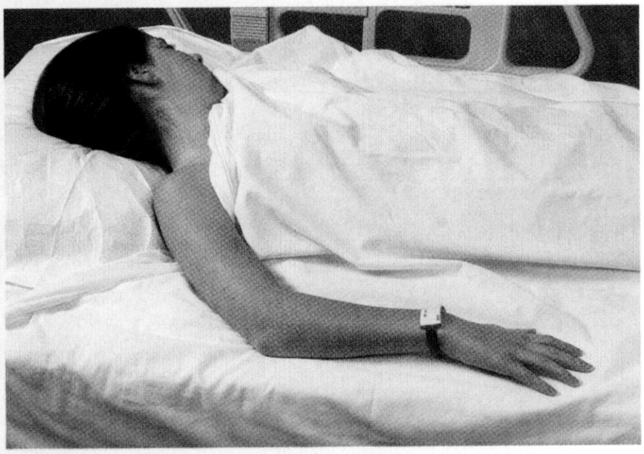

FIGURE 7-3 Positioning for washing a patient's arm. Position patient's arm across body or lengthwise, with towel lengthwise underneath and the nurse holding the arm to bathe it. Fold drape back to wash arm and underarm area.

Action	Rationale
(6) Optional: Place a folded towel on the bed next to the patient's hand, place the basin on the towel, and soak the hand. Wash the hand, rinse, and dry.	Soaking can loosen dirt under the nails.
(7) Place the towel under the near arm, and wash the hand, arm, and axilla in the same way. Rinse and dry.	Bathing the closer arm last prevents contamination from leaning over the clean arm to bathe the opposite arm.

(continued)

Action	*Rationale*
(8) Place a towel over the patient's chest. Fold the bath blanket down to the waist. Wash, rinse, and dry the patient's chest, keeping the patient covered with the towel between washing and rinsing. Pay particular attention to areas under the female breasts.	Exposing one area at a time for cleansing prevents chilling of the patient and promotes privacy. Areas under the breasts may be prone to skin breakdown if not cleansed and dried thoroughly.
(9) Fold the bath blanket down to the pubic bone, leaving the towel over the chest. Wash, rinse, and dry the lower abdomen, paying particular attention to the **umbilicus** (navel). Remove the towel, and replace the bath blanket over the chest and arms.	Keeping the towel in place prevents chilling and respects privacy.
(10) Remove the bath blanket from the far leg only. Place the towel length-wise under the leg. Bending the leg at the knee and supporting the knee joint, wash the leg using long, firm strokes toward the center of the body (Fig. 7-4). Rinse and dry the leg.	Washing from the distal to proximal areas promotes venous blood return and stimulates circulation. 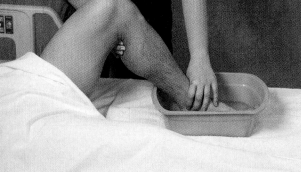 **FIGURE 7-4** Draping for washing the patient's leg. Uncover only one leg at a time, keeping the rest of the patient's body covered.
(11) Place a towel near the patient's foot, and place the basin on it. Put the patient's foot in the basin, and support the ankle and heel in your hand while supporting the leg on your arm. Wash, rinse, and dry the foot, paying attention to the toes and between the toes. Be sure to dry the toes thoroughly.	Placing the patient's foot in the basin is relaxing, and it promotes a more-thorough cleaning of the foot and the areas between the toes. Cleaning and drying between the toes prevents skin irritation and injury.

(continued)

Action	Rationale
(12) Wash the near leg and foot in the same way	Washing the closer leg last prevents contamination.
(13) Change the bathwater at this point or sooner if needed. Make sure the bed's side rails are up while you change the bathwater.	Changing the bathwater keeps it warm and clean. Side rails promote safety.
(14) Assist the patient to a side-lying position, facing away from you. Some patients will turn to a prone position, but for many patients, this position is not comfortable or may be difficult to obtain. Place a towel lengthwise along the back and buttocks, keeping the patient covered with the bath blanket and exposing the back. Wash, rinse, and dry the back of the neck and the back, using long, firm strokes (Fig. 7-5).	Draping prevents unnecessary exposure of the patient, and the towel protects the bedding from dripping water. Long firm strokes promote circulation.

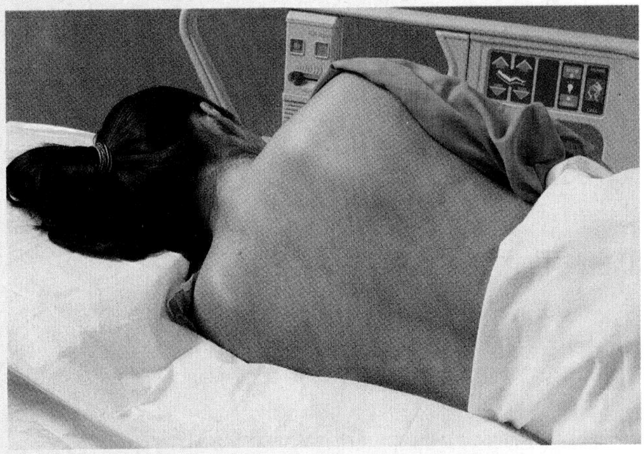

FIGURE 7-5 Draping for washing the patient's back.

Action	Rationale
(15) Put on clean gloves, and wash the buttocks and perianal area. Pay attention to the sacral area by checking for redness and the gluteal folds. Remove gloves and discard.	Gloves protect you from potential contact with fecal material and microorganisms. Any fecal material near the anus is irritating to the skin and a source of microorganisms that can be spread.
(16) Give a back rub at this point, or wait until after all care is completed (see Procedure for Giving a Back Rub).	Back rubs improve circulation to the area and are relaxing.
(17) Change the bathwater.	To prevent the spread of fecal organisms elsewhere on the body.

(continued)

Action	Rationale
(18) Assist the patient to a supine position to wash the perineal area. If patients cannot wash their own **genitalia,** you must do so for them. Put on clean gloves. Wash, moving gently from front to back (clean to dirty), making certain to wash and dry carefully (see Module 8, Assisting with Elimination and Perineal Care). Discard water and gloves. In many cases, the patient can wash the perineal area. If so, make sure that everything is within reach of the patient. Provide privacy but stay within hearing distance, or instruct the patient to use the call light.	Gloves protect you from potential contact with microorganisms. Perineal care decreases odor and contamination from the rectal area.
(19) Assist the patient in applying deodorant if used and applying clean pajamas or gown.	Deodorant decreases body odor, and clean pajamas or gown promotes warmth and general comfort for the patient.
g. Comb or brush and arrange the patient's hair (see Procedures for Brushing and Combing Hair).	This enhances the patient's self-image.
h. Attend to any other personal hygiene needs. Assist the male patient with shaving at this point. You may have to assemble his shaving equipment, which will vary, depending on the type of razor he prefers. If he is unable to shave himself, this task is also your responsibility. Some facilities have an electric razor you can use. Be sure to review the procedure for cleaning the razor after use and infection control procedures related to using the razor.	Shaving promotes comfort and enhances personal image.
i. Change bed linens as described in Module 9.	For comfort and infection control.
j. Return the bed to the low position, and be sure the call light and other items the patient will need are within close reach.	This promotes patient safety.
14-16. Follow steps 14 to 16 of the General Procedure for Hygiene: Observe the patient for adverse responses, provide appropriate care for all equipment and supplies used, and wash or disinfect your hands before leaving the room.	

EVALUATION

17. Follow step 17 of the General Procedure for Hygiene: Evaluate using the individualized patient outcomes previously identified: skin and nails clean, absence of offensive odor, intact skin and mucous membranes, and patient expresses comfort. Note any adverse outcomes.

DOCUMENTATION

18-19. Follow steps 18 and 19 of the General Procedure: Document the hygiene measure as appropriate, and document preferences and ability to participate on the nursing care plan and/or any physical signs or symptoms identified during the procedure.

Procedure for Shower

A shower is the preferred method of bathing for the ambulatory patient who is independent, or it can be given using a shower chair. Most patients prefer a shower to a bed bath. Be sure you have a physician's order for activity that would include showering. Taking a shower requires both energy and balance and could increase the potential for falling.

ASSESSMENT

1-3. Follow steps 1 to 3 of the General Procedure for Hygiene: Review the record and plan of care, assess the patient related to priority concerns, and check for supplies and equipment in the room.

ANALYSIS

4-5. Follow steps 4 and 5 of the General Procedure for Hygiene: Think through your data, and determine if there are modifications needed for the shower.

PLANNING

6. Follow step 6 of the General Procedure for Hygiene: Determine individualized patient outcomes for the bath: skin and nails clean, absence of offensive odor, intact skin and mucous membranes, and patient expresses comfort.
7. Plan the bathing procedure, and determine and obtain the supplies that will be needed for a shower and equipment (wheelchair, walker, wheeled shower chair) needed for transporting the patient to the shower.

IMPLEMENTATION

Action	Rationale
8-10. Follow steps 8 to 10 of the General Procedure for Hygiene: Wash or disinfect your hands, identify the patient (two identifiers), and explain the process for taking a shower.	
11. Assist the patient to the shower stall or to the shower room if the shower is located outside the patient's room. If the patient will walk, be sure you have provided slip-proof slippers or shoes. If a chair shower is to be given, you can transport the patient to the shower room in the shower chair.	These measures promote patient safety.
12. If the shower is located outside the patient's room, hang a sign on the door indicating that the room is occupied. If it's inside the patient's room, close the door to the room.	To provide for the patient's privacy.
13. Carry out the shower as follows, assisting the patient as necessary:	

(continued)

Action	Rationale
a. Prepare the shower. Place a shower mat or bath towel on the floor of the shower. Place the shower chair in the shower (if needed). Run the shower until the water is warm (100° to 115°); then adjust it to the patient's preference.	The shower mat promotes safety and prevents the patient from slipping on the wet floor. The chair assists the patient who may become fatigued or who cannot stand. Appropriate water temperature prevents burns or chilling.
b. If the patient can shower independently, leave the patient alone, explaining how to use the bathroom call light and making sure it is within reach. Leave the towel where the patient can reach it easily. Check with the patient frequently. If the patient is receiving a chair shower, you may have to provide assistance as needed.	Allowing the patient to shower promotes independence and self-reliance. Assisting ensures that needs are met safely when the patient is unable to manage independently.
c. Help the patient put on a clean gown or pajamas.	Assisting the patient with dressing helps ensure that the patient will not fall.
d. Assist the patient to the room.	Promotes patient safety.
14-15. Follow steps 14 and 15 of the General Procedure for Hygiene: Assess the patient during the procedure, and provide appropriate care for all equipment and supplies used. *Note:* If the shower is a shared facility, you may need to return to the shower room and ensure that it is ready for the next patient.	
a. Clean the stall and shower chair in the manner prescribed by your facility.	
b. Discard any used linen.	
c. Put the "unoccupied" sign on the door.	
16. Wash or disinfect your hands.	Decreases the transfer of microorganisms that could cause infection.

EVALUATION

17. Follow step 17 of the General Procedure for Hygiene: Evaluate using the individualized patient outcomes previously identified: skin and nails clean, absence of offensive odor, intact skin and mucous membranes, and patient expresses comfort. Note any adverse outcomes.

DOCUMENTATION

18-19. Follow steps 18 and 19 of the General Procedure for Hygiene: Document the shower as appropriate on the nursing care plan and/or activity record.

Document any physical signs or symptoms identified during the procedure.

Procedure for Tub Bath

Tub baths are used for hygiene if the patient is independent and ambulatory. Some facilities may have a tub room. A doctor's order may be needed for a tub bath because of the energy and agility required. Check for special instructions regarding tub baths and for the method of cleaning and disinfecting the tub between patients. Some long-term care facilities use a specialized bathtub that has an attached chair and mechanical lift for moving the patient into and out of the tub or that has a door in the side for entrance and exit. Familiarize yourself with how specialty tubs operate before using one.

ASSESSMENT

1-3. Follow steps 1 to 3 of the General Procedure for Hygiene: Review the record and plan of care, assess the patient related to priority concerns, and check for supplies and equipment in the room.

ANALYSIS

4-5. Follow steps 4 and 5 of the General Procedure: Think through your data, and identify specific prob-

lems and modifications needed in order to facilitate a tub bath. Gather your supplies (towels, soap, clean gown, bath mat).

PLANNING

6. Follow step 6 of the General Procedure: Determine individualized patient outcomes: skin and nails clean, absence of offensive odor, intact skin and mucous membranes, and patient expresses comfort.

7. Plan the bathing procedure, and determine and obtain the supplies (towels, soap, clean gown, bath mat) that will be needed for a tub bath and equipment (wheelchair or walker) needed for transporting the patient to the tub.

IMPLEMENTATION

Action	Rationale
8-10. Follow steps 8 to 10 of the General Procedure: Wash or disinfect your hands, identify the patient (two identifiers), and explain the procedure for taking a tub bath.	
11. Assist the patient to the tub room either walking or using a wheelchair.	Accompanying the patient is a safety measure.
12. Hang a sign on the door indicating that the room is occupied, or close the door to the patient's room if the tub is located in the patient's bathroom.	To provide privacy.
13. Carry out the tub bath as follows:	
a. Place a towel or rubber mat in the bottom of the tub. Fill tub one-half full with water at 110° to 115°.	Bath mat and water temperature are safety measures to prevent falls and scalds.
b. Help the patient into the tub.	Promotes patient safety.
c. Assist the patient as needed. If the patient is helpless, you may need assistance with the bath. Some patients are independent and may be left for a few minutes while the bath is being taken. Be sure to tell the patient how to use the emergency call signal before leaving the patient unattended. If the patient appears weak, do not leave. An independent patient may need help with washing his or her back.	Promotes patient safety.
d. Drain the water, and assist the patient out of the tub. Get help if you think you might need it.	Draining the water first decreases the chance of a fall. Soaking in warm water may cause pooling of blood in the lower part of the body so that when the patient

(continued)

Action	Rationale
	rises, the blood pressure may drop, causing dizziness and instability.
e. Assist the patient with drying if needed.	Promotes safety by preventing the patient from falling while leaning over and drying some areas of the body.
f. Help the patient put on clean bedclothes.	Clean clothes promote physical well-being and comfort.
g. Assist the patient to the room, being sure to take patient's personal things with you.	Promotes patient safety.
14-15. Follow steps 14 and 15 of the General Procedure: Assess the patient for fatigue, dizziness, or other adverse responses during the procedure, and provide appropriate care for all equipment and supplies used. *Note:* If the tub is a shared facility, you may need to return to the tub room to clean the tub and ensure that it is ready for the next patient.	
16. Follow step 16 of the General Procedure: Wash or disinfect your hands.	

EVALUATION

17. Follow step 17 of the General Procedure: Evaluate using the individualized patient outcomes previously identified: skin and nails clean, absence of offensive odor, intact skin and mucous membranes, and patient expresses comfort. Note any adverse outcomes.

DOCUMENTATION

18-19. Follow steps 18 and 19 of the General Procedure: Document the tub bath as appropriate, and document techniques on the nursing care plan and/or the patient's flow sheet.

Partial Bed Bath, Self-Bed Bath, Towel Bath, and Bag Bath

The partial bed bath and self-bed bath are often appropriate options for the patient (Box 7-1).

The towel bath and bag bath save time as compared with the usual methods of bathing and decrease the chance of skin dryness because the cleansers lubricate instead of removing natural oils from the skin. The towel or cloths stay warmer and are comfortable to the patient. These methods are especially useful in a critical care area where they minimize the energy required of the patient. They conserve time for the nurse as well. See Box 7-1 for directions.

---

box 7-1   *Variations of the Bed Bath*

Partial Bed Bath

A partial bed bath is given for several reasons, including a patient's inability to tolerate a full bath and a lack of need or desire for a full daily bath. A partial bed bath usually includes the face, neck, hands, **axillae,** and the perineum. The back may also be included if the patient can tolerate it, and offer a back rub when the bath is completed. A partial bed bath may be completed by the patient or the nurse.

Self–Bed Bath

This type of bath is given when a patient is unable to take a shower or a tub bath but can move about freely in bed and in the room. The self–bed bath is usually a complete bath. Your responsibility is to provide the basin of water, bath blanket, towels, washcloths, and any other necessary articles. You must be ready to assist the patient with areas such as the feet and legs, and back and buttocks. Offer a back rub when the bath is completed.

Moving the patient to a sink and bathing using running water is often allowed. Place all supplies close to the sink, and arrange for the patient to have some privacy for bathing. A bath blanket is used to drape the legs or shoulders as needed to prevent chilling and to give privacy.

Towel Bath

A towel bath uses a single large towel to cover and wash the patient. The towel must be 3 × 7 feet or a bath sheet. Rather than soap, the patient uses a cleanser that does not need to be rinsed and leaves a softening agent on the skin.

1. Fold the towel and moisten with 2 liters of water heated to between 115° and 120° F and 1 oz of no-rinse liquid cleanser.
2. Unfold the towel to cover the patient and use a section of the towel to wipe each part of the body.
3. Begin at the feet and work upward.
4. As the towel becomes soiled, fold that section to the inside, and allow the skin to air-dry for a few seconds.
5. When the front of the body is bathed, turn the patient on one side and repeat the procedure for the back of the body so that as the towel is unfolded, a clean section covers the patient.
6. Bathe the back and then the buttocks.

Bag Bath

A bag bath is composed of 8 to 10 premoistened, warmed, disposable cleaning cloths. The cloths are premoistened with an aloe and vitamin E formula, which provides lubrication to the skin. Heat the pack of cloths in a microwave for 30 to 45 seconds. If you heat the cloths for any longer, the cloths may burn the skin.

The procedure is as follows:
1. Cover the patient with a bath blanket.
2. Open the package and remove one cloth at a time.
3. Clean different sections of the body with one cloth and discard it.
4. Use a new cloth for each section of the body as follows:
   ■ face, neck, and chest
   ■ right arm and axilla
   ■ left arm and axilla
   ■ perineum
   ■ right leg
   ■ left leg
   ■ back
   ■ buttocks
5. As an area is cleaned, cover the area with the bath blanket.
6. Do not rinse.
7. The cloths are disposable and are not to be reused. Discard them.

Procedure for Giving a Back Rub

The back rub may decrease anxiety, help alleviate pain perception, decrease muscle tension and fatigue, stimulate circulation, and enhance immune system function. Unfortunately, time pressures often have caused nurses to consider back rubs a low priority, omitting them from care. Traditionally, a back rub is given after the bath and at bedtime but should not be limited to these times. If a person is confined to bed, the patient is turned every 2 hours to redistribute pressure. This is an optimum time to assess the skin and massage over pressure areas. If an area is reddened, rub gently around it to stimulate circulation. Do not rub the reddened area because it may increase tissue damage. If a reddened area does not subside quickly, the tissue beneath may be in the beginning stages of breakdown. For the person experiencing pain, the back rub may be scheduled with the pain medication to enhance its effectiveness.

Use lotion to decrease friction on the skin. Lotion also counteracts the potential for dry skin in the institutional setting. A nice touch is to warm the lotion under warm running water prior to using. Once the back rub is initiated, it is more pleasant and relaxing for the patient if one hand remains in contact with the patient's back until the back rub is completed.

Many methods are acceptable for giving a back rub. Long, smooth flowing movements over the length of the back are relaxing. A kneading motion will often relax tight muscle groups. Circular motions stimulate circulation in a specific area. The following is a suggested procedure for general use.

ASSESSMENT

1-3. Follow steps 1 to 3 of the General Procedure for Hygiene: Review the record and plan of care, assess the patient related to priority concerns, and check for supplies and equipment in the room.

ANALYSIS

4-5. Follow steps 4 and 5 of the General Procedure: Critically think through your data, and identify specific problems and modifications to the back rub procedure.

PLANNING

6. Determine individualized patient outcomes related to the back rub:
   a. patient relaxed and comfortable
   b. skin moist and intact without areas of redness
7. Plan the back rub procedure, and determine and obtain the supplies that will be needed.

IMPLEMENTATION

Action	Rationale
8-12. Follow the steps 8 to 12 of the General Procedure: Wash or disinfect your hands, identify the patient (two identifiers), explain what you plan to do, pull the curtains around the bed, close the door, and raise the bed to an appropriate working position.	
13. Follow the procedure for a back rub:	
a. Move the patient close to your side of the bed, and position either on the abdomen or a side-lying position with the patient facing away from you. Pull the covers down below the buttocks.	Moving the patient decreases the distance you need to reach, preventing muscle strain.
b. Pour a small amount of lotion into your hand, and rub your palms together.	Placing lotion on both hands warms it slightly, so it is not cold on the patient's back.
c. With your feet apart, place your hands at the sacral area, one on either side of the spinal column (Fig. 7-6).	Having the feet apart allows you to rock back and forth while maintaining good posture and body mechanics. See Figure 7-6 for an illustration of retaining touch during the back rub.

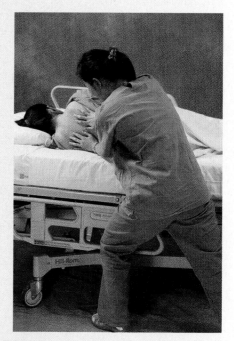

FIGURE 7-6 Maintain your own body mechanics and posture as you give the back rub.

(continued)

Action	Rationale
d. Beginning at the lumbosacral area, rub toward the neckline, using long, firm, smooth strokes along the side of the patient's spine, over the scapular areas, decreasing the pressure over the neck area and then down the lateral aspects of the back, applying firm, continuous pressure and maintaining contact with the skin.	Long, smooth strokes are relaxing to the patient.
e. At the neckline, use your thumbs to rub into the hairline, and use your fingers to massage the sides of the neck.	Using the fingers minimizes pressure to the neck, which is a more tender area but is often strained by being in bed.
f. With a kneading motion, rub along the shoulders. Continue the kneading motion, and move down one side of the trunk with both hands until you are at the sacral area, then do the same on the other side.	Kneading stimulates circulation and is a relaxing maneuver.
g. Placing your hands side by side with the palms down, rub in a figure eight pattern over the buttocks and sacral area (Fig. 7-7). Move the figure eight back and forth to include the entire buttocks area.	The buttocks area and lower back are subject to ongoing pressure if the patient is confined to bed.

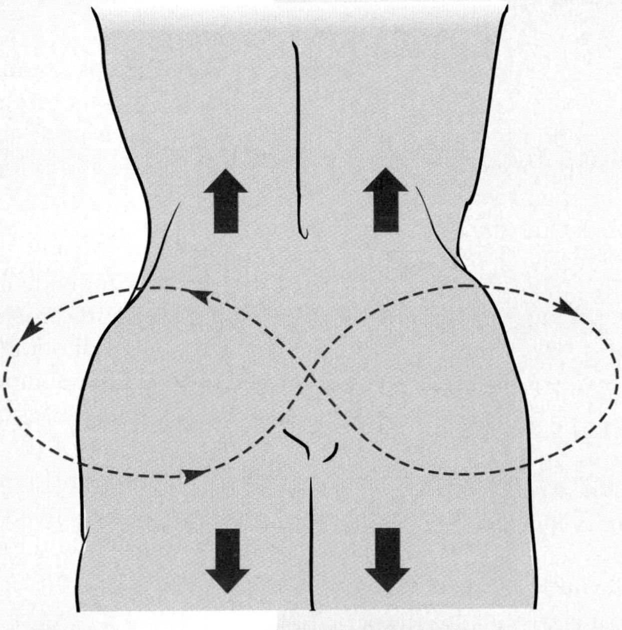

FIGURE 7-7 Figure eight technique in the back rub.

(continued)

Action	Rationale
h. Repeat the motions for about 3 to 5 minutes. To remove excess lotion, pat the back with a towel.	The time allows for relaxation of muscles and stimulates circulation.
i. Return the bed to the low position, and put the call device within reach.	For patient safety.
14. Follow step 14 of the General Procedure: Assess the back for any areas of redness or breakdown.	To detect signs of impending infection or other problems.
15. Return the lotion to the bedside stand.	To make it available for the next time it is needed.
16. Follow step 16 of the General Procedure: Wash or disinfect your hands.	Washing decreases the transfer of organisms that could cause infection.

EVALUATION

17. Evaluate in terms of the individualized outcome criteria related to the back rub: patient relaxed and comfortable and skin moist and intact without areas of redness. Note any adverse outcomes.

DOCUMENTATION

18-19. Follow steps 18 and 19 of the General Procedure: Document the back rub on the flow sheet. Note any information about physical signs and symptoms identified during the back rub.

Procedure for Oral Care

Oral care should be offered before breakfast, after all meals, and at bedtime. Not all patients want oral care this often, but it should be offered. Oral care is especially important for patients who are receiving oxygen, who have nasogastric tubes, and who are fasting or on NPO (nothing by mouth) status because these may increase drying and the formation of **sordes** (a collection of bacteria and residue of mucus and other mouth secretions that collect on the tongue, teeth, and lips) in the mouth. Patients who can sit in Fowler's or even semi-Fowler's position can perform most of their oral care independently, provided the equipment is conveniently placed. For the patient who is unable to request oral care, the nurse should add oral care to the nursing care plan, so it is not overlooked. When the patient is not able to perform oral care independently, the caregiver must do it.

Many dentists recommend a small, soft-bristled toothbrush and fluoride toothpaste. Flossing is recommended daily to remove plaque and food particles that brushing does not reach. Many people use a mouthwash as part of their oral care. An oral rinse of normal saline or sodium bicarbonate solution is safe and gentle to the oral mucosa.

ASSESSMENT

1-3. Follow steps 1 to 3 of the General Procedure for Hygiene: Review the record and plan of care, assess the patient related to priority concerns, and check for supplies and equipment in the room.

ANALYSIS

4-5. Follow steps 4 and 5 of the General Procedure: Critically think through your data, carefully evaluating each aspect, and identify specific problems and modifications for providing oral care.

PLANNING

6. Determine individualized patient outcomes in relation to mouth care. Include
   a. no sordes or odor present
   b. mucous membranes pink and intact
   c. patient expresses comfort
7. Follow step 7 of the General Procedure: Plan the actual procedure for providing oral care, and obtain the needed equipment:
   a. toothbrush and toothpaste
   b. dental floss
   c. cup of water
   d. emesis basin
   e. face towel

Patients may provide their own toothbrush, toothpaste, and floss.

IMPLEMENTATION

Action	Rationale
8-12. Follow steps 8 to 12 of the General Procedure: Wash or disinfect your hands, identify the patient (two identifiers), explain the procedure, provide for privacy, and raise the bed to an appropriate working height.	
13. Provide oral care.	
a. Place a towel under the patient's chin across the chest.	For patient comfort and to keep the gown or pajamas dry.
b. Put on clean gloves.	For infection control.
c. Moisten the toothbrush with water, and spread a small amount of toothpaste on it. If no cleansing agent is available, plain water is adequate. Mouthwash is a substitute that also freshens the breath, or an oral rinse of normal saline or sodium bicarbonate (baking soda) can be used.	These agents freshen the breath. Toothpaste is a cleansing agent.
d. Brush the teeth, allowing the patient to **expectorate** (spit) into the emesis basin.	
(1) Holding the brush at a 45-degree angle, use a small, vibrating, circular motion with the bristles at the junction of the teeth and gums. Use the same action on the front and back of the teeth.	To remove the plaque that forms at the base of the tooth.
(2) Use a back-and-forth brushing motion over the biting surfaces of the teeth.	To remove food particles and plaque from tooth crevices.
(3) Brush the tongue, and rinse the mouth.	To decrease sordes and the bacterial count.
e. Allow the patient to rinse the mouth with water, followed by flossing and mouthwash if desired. For tips on assisting a patient with flossing, see Box 7-2.	To remove any debris and/or food particles and to freshen the breath.
f. Wipe the patient's mouth.	For patient comfort and appearance.
g. Return the bed to the low position.	For patient safety.
14. Follow step 14 of the General Procedure: Assess the patient's mucous membranes during the procedure.	The period of time used for care provides an opportunity for careful observation.

(continued)

box 7-2 *Flossing*

Flossing should be done once daily to remove plaque (microorganisms trapped in a mucous base) that is not reached by brushing and which, if not removed, causes tooth and gum disease. Plaque forms in 24 hours and eventually becomes impossible to remove without dental instruments. Floss is correctly held as demonstrated here.

1. Wrap one end of the floss around your third finger of each hand.
2. Use your thumb and index finger to pull the floss taut, moving the floss up and down between the teeth to the gum line.
3. Floss both between teeth and between the gums and each individual tooth, taking care not to injure the delicate mucous membranes.
4. Rinse the mouth after flossing to remove debris.

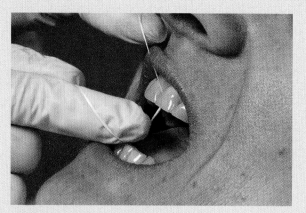

Flossing the teeth.

Action	Rationale
15. Care for equipment:	
a. Rinse equipment, and return it to the appropriate place.	So that equipment is ready for its next use.
b. Remove and dispose of gloves.	For infection control.
16. Wash or disinfect your hands.	Washing decreases the transfer of organisms that could cause infection.

EVALUATION

17. Follow step 17 of the General Procedure: Evaluate individualized patient outcomes in relation to sordes, odor, and comfort. Note any adverse outcomes.

DOCUMENTATION

18-19. Follow steps 18 and 19 of the General Procedure: Document on the nursing care flow sheet that oral care was provided, and note any abnormal condition of the mouth.

Procedure for Oral Care for the Unconscious Patient

Unconscious patients are completely dependent on you for their oral care. Because these persons may be "mouth breathers" and are not taking food or fluids by mouth, sordes accumulates rapidly. They are also in danger of aspirating the liquid used for mouth care. A suitable procedure for the oral care of unconscious patients is as follows:

ASSESSMENT

1-3. Follow steps 1 to 3 of the General Procedure for Hygiene: Review the record and plan of care, assess the patient related to priority concerns, and check for supplies and equipment in the room.

ANALYSIS

4-5. Follow steps 4 and 5 of the General Procedure: Think through your data, and identify specific problems and modifications.

PLANNING

6. Determine individualized patient outcomes in relation to mouth care. Include
   a. no sordes or odor
   b. mucous membranes pink and intact
7. Plan the actual procedure for providing oral care, and obtain the needed equipment, which includes
   a. tongue blade wrapped in gauze
   b. toothbrush or toothette

c. toothpaste, cleansing agent, or mouthwash (Regular toothpaste or mouthwash is preferred.) Do not use solutions containing lemon juice because it etches the enamel and therefore is cariogenic (causes cavities).

d. water-soluble lip lubricant

e. towel

f. clean gloves

g. cotton-tipped applicators or clean gauze squares

h. large bulb syringe (often referred to as an Asepto syringe) with a soft tip

i. emesis basin

j. optional: large-diameter suction catheter (such as a Yankauer suction tip)

IMPLEMENTATION

Action	Rationale
8-12. Follow steps 8 to 12 of the General Procedure: Wash or disinfect hands; identify the patient (two identifiers), explain the procedure, provide for privacy, and raise the bed to a working height.	
13. Provide oral care (Figs. 7-8A & B).	

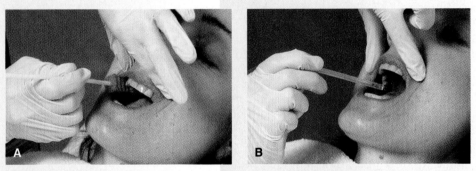

FIGURE 7-8 Oral care of the unconscious patient includes (**A**) gentle brushing, (**B**) rinsing, and suctioning to remove residual fluid.

Action	Rationale
a. Place the unconscious patient in a side-lying position with the head of the bed in a semi-Fowler's position and with the patient's head turned toward you. If the patient's head cannot be raised, leave the patient flat, and turn the head toward you.	In this position, the fluids used for mouth care will drain out of the mouth by gravity and decrease the chance of aspiration.
b. Place a towel under the patient's chin, tucking it in beneath the shoulders.	To prevent the gown or pajamas from becoming damp.
c. Put on clean gloves.	For infection control.
d. Place a padded tongue blade (made by wrapping 4- × 4-inch gauze squares around a tongue blade and taping them securely) in the patient's mouth. Use this to hold the mouth open.	To prevent patient from biting down on the equipment or your hands.
e. Moisten the toothbrush or toothette very lightly, and apply cleansing agent.	Cleansing agent removes debris and microorganisms from the teeth.

(continued)

Action	Rationale
f. Brush all tooth, tongue, and mouth surfaces.	Brushing removes the plaque that forms at the base of the tooth. Brushing the tongue decreases sordes on the tongue and the resident bacterial count.
g. Using oversized cotton-tipped applicators or other substitute, clean all surfaces of the mouth, including the palate, inner cheeks, and tongue. If a large accumulation of sordes is present, it may be necessary to remove the sordes in stages.	To remove sordes and decrease the resident bacterial count. Removing sordes in stages decreases the damage to tissue.
h. Rinse the patient's mouth, using the rubber-tipped syringe to inject small amounts of water. Allow the water to drain into the emesis basin by gravity, or use the rubber-tipped syringe or suction to **aspirate** it.	Removal of the water from the mouth prevents aspiration by the patient.
i. Wipe the patient's mouth.	To promote patient comfort and appearance.
j. Lubricate the lips as needed.	To prevent the lips from drying and cracking.
k. Return the bed to a low position.	For the safety of the patient.
14-16. Follow steps 14 to 16 of the General Procedure: Assess the patient during the procedure, care appropriately for all equipment, and wash or disinfect your hands.	

EVALUATION

17. Follow step 17 of the General Procedure: Evaluate individualized patient outcomes in relation to sordes and odor. Note any adverse outcomes.

DOCUMENTATION

18-19. Follow steps 18 and 19 of the General Procedure: Document oral care as appropriate, and document technique on the nursing care plan and/or patient's activity record. Document any abnormal findings. **R:** Documentation is a legal record of the patient's care and therapy and communicates nursing activities to other nurses and caregivers.

Procedure for Denture Care

Patients often want to care for their dentures themselves. If so, your responsibility will be to provide them with the necessary articles. A patient may have a denture brush and cleansing agent, but if not, a regular toothbrush and paste will suffice. Provide the patient with a partially filled bath basin over which to wash the dentures, so that if they fall, they will not break. The patient will also need a glass of water for rinsing. If you care for the patient's dentures yourself, keep the following procedures in mind:

ASSESSMENT

1-3. Follow steps 1 to 3 of the General Procedure for Hygiene: Review the record and plan of care, assess the patient related to priority concerns, and check for supplies and equipment in the room.

ANALYSIS

4-5. Follow steps 4 and 5 of the General Procedure: Think through your data, and identify specific problems and modifications.

PLANNING

6. Determine individualized patient outcomes in relation to denture care. Include dentures clean of debris and stains, mouth without odor, clean and comfortable.
7. Plan the procedure for providing denture care, and obtain the needed equipment, which includes
   a. denture brush or regular toothbrush
   b. denture cleaner or toothpaste
   c. clean gloves

IMPLEMENTATION

Action	Rationale
8-12. Follow the steps 8 to 12 of the General Procedure: Wash or disinfect your hands, identify the patient (two identifiers), explain the procedure, provide for privacy, and raise the bed to an appropriate working height.	
13. Clean the dentures.	
a. Put on clean gloves.	For infection control.
b. Assist the patient with removal of the upper plate by applying downward pressure with the index fingers from above the upper denture. It may help if the patient inflates the cheeks. Lower dentures lift out easily (Fig. 7-9). If no assistance is needed, it works well to have the patient remove the dentures, and place them in a denture cup for you.	Slight pressure on the upper denture breaks the suction that holds the plate on the palate.

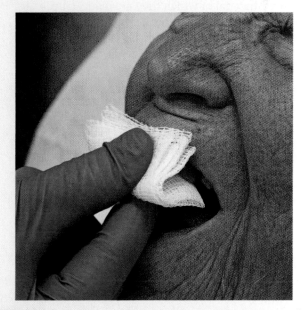

FIGURE 7-9 Denture care. When removing dentures, assist patients by applying downward pressure with the index fingers from above the upper denture. Lower dentures should lift out easily. If no assistance is needed, have patients remove the dentures themselves.

Action	Rationale
c. Take the dentures to the sink in the denture cup, and partially fill the sink with water, or place a towel in sink.	Dentures may break if dropped. Cleaning over a basin of water or towel cushions the fall and may prevent breaking.

(continued)

Action	Rationale
d. Use a denture brush to clean the teeth if the patient has one. Note that the longer side of the brush is used for the tooth surface and the smaller part for brushing the inner surface. Hold the teeth close to the bottom of the sink so if dropped, they do not fall far. Use tepid water for cleaning and rinsing.	Brushing removes food particles from teeth. Water that is too hot may change the shape of some dentures.
e. Have the patient rinse out his or her mouth before reinserting the dentures. Some like to use a soft toothbrush to brush the gums and tongue.	To remove any food particles in the mouth and coating from the tongue; it also freshens the mouth.
f. Return dentures to the patient, fitting the upper dentures in first.	The upper denture is larger and difficult to insert with the lower denture in place.
g. If dentures are to be stored (for an unconscious patient or at night), use a covered container, carefully labeled, and preferably placed in a drawer. Whether they should be stored in water depends on the material of which they are made. Check with the patient or the patient's family. Cool water with mouthwash or a few drops of vinegar is suggested for storage.	To prevent loss or breakage. Mouthwash or vinegar for denture cups prevents odor from clinging to the dentures.
h. Dry the patient's mouth.	For comfort and aesthetic purposes.
14-16. Follow steps 14 to 16 of the General Procedure: Assess the patient as you proceed, care for equipment and supplies appropriately, and wash or disinfect your hands.	

EVALUATION

17. Evaluate individualized patient outcomes in relation to sordes, odor, and comfort. Note any adverse outcomes.

DOCUMENTATION

18-19. Follow steps 18 and 19 of the General Procedure: Document the oral care as appropriate as well as the technique used on the nursing care plan. Also document any abnormal findings.

POTENTIAL ADVERSE OUTCOMES AND RELATED INTERVENTIONS

1. **Stomatitis** is an inflammation of the oral mucosa. Those who are elderly or immunocompromised are especially susceptible to stomatitis; however, it may happen in anyone who does not receive mouth care. It is seen as inflamed areas of the mucous membranes. Open tissue may occur when stomatitis is severe.

Intervention: Cleanliness of the mouth is the first defense. For the person who already has stomatitis, this might be frequent saline mouthwashes to remove mouth debris, dilute bacteria, and soothe tissue. In the immunocompromised patient, stomatitis may be caused by fungal overgrowth in the mouth. The nurse may need to consult with the physician for the antifungal mouth care products needed.

2. Bleeding gums, especially if the person has had poor oral hygiene. The tissues are fragile and easily damaged.

Intervention: A very soft toothbrush and gentle care are needed; however, do not stop mouth care. The condition will become more severe if oral hygiene is neglected. Regular mouth care decreases the fragility of the tissue.

3. Thick sordes in the mouth that cannot be easily removed. This may occur in the person who is NPO for a long period of time and who has not had mouth care.

Intervention: Perform gentle mouth care frequently, removing the sordes in stages. Moistening the sordes with saline or with a moistening agent may make it easier to remove. Aggressive attempts to remove sordes may damage the oral mucosa.

4. Mouth lesions, such as canker sores or herpes simplex, make oral care painful for the patient.

Intervention: Lubricate the lips before beginning to avoid creating tension that will crack the lip. Proceed gently. Do not omit oral care because that may cause more serious adverse outcomes to occur.

Procedures for Brushing and Combing Hair

A patient's hair should be combed and brushed daily. Generally, this is done along with other hygiene activities and at other times throughout the day as necessary. Hair care is especially important to the patient, because morale is often directly related to appearance. Brushing also stimulates circulation of blood to the scalp. Hair care is usually given after the bath. It will vary according to different cultures, which is a consideration in assisting with hair care. Ask the patient or a family member for specific hair care considerations. Whenever you assist with hair care, there are some important points to remember.

ASSESSMENT

1-3. Follow steps 1 to 3 of the General Procedure for Hygiene: Review the record and plan of care, assess the patient related to priority concerns, and check for supplies and equipment in the room.

ANALYSIS

4-5. Follow steps 4 and 5 of the General Procedure: Think through your data, and identify specific problems and modifications.

PLANNING

6. Determine individualized patient outcomes in relation to hair care. Include
   a. hair and scalp are clean
   b. hair has a neat appearance
   c. patient expresses comfort and satisfaction
7. Plan the procedure for hair care, considering
   a. brushing, combing and arranging the hair
   b. supplies needed, obtaining those that are not in the room
   c. assistance needed to accomplish the hair care

IMPLEMENTATION

Action	Rationale
8-12. Follow steps 8 to 12 of the General Procedure: Wash or disinfect your hands, identify the patient (two identifiers), explain the procedure, pull the curtains around the bed, close the door, and raise the bed to an appropriate working position based on your height.	
13. Provide hair care:	
a. Place a face or bath towel over the pillow.	The towel will collect any hair, dandruff, or dirt.
b. Place patients who are able to comb and brush their own hair in a Fowler's position, with the hair care items on the overbed table. Assist as necessary. The helpless or unconscious patient may be flat or in a semi-Fowler's position.	A sitting position facilitates brushing and combing.

(continued)

Action	Rationale
c. Turn the patient's head away from you, and bring the hair back toward you. Brush hair with few tangles in two or three large sections. Matted hair may have to be separated into small sections and treated with a cream rinse, oil (such as mineral oil), or alcohol.	To help loosen the tangles.
d. Hold a section of hair 2 to 3 inches from the end. Gently comb the end until it is free of tangles. Gradually move toward the scalp, combing 2 to 3 inches at a time until the hair is tangle-free.	Working in small sections avoids trauma and pain to the scalp.
e. Turn the patient's head in the opposite direction, and repeat step d.	This provides care for the hair on the opposite side.
f. Arrange the hair as neatly and simply as possible. Braiding may be the most appropriate style for long hair. (Ask the family to bring in clips to make your job easier.) Use hair care products that the patient provides and requests to be used.	To provide for comfort as the patient moves about in bed.
g. Carefully remove the towel.	To contain the hair or dandruff collected there.
14. Follow step 14 of the General Procedure: Assess the patient during the procedure.	
15. Place the towel in a laundry hamper or bag. Clean the comb and brush, and return them, along with the other toilet articles, to the bedside stand.	To provide proper care and storage of equipment for later use.
16. Wash or disinfect your hands.	For infection control.

EVALUATION

17. Follow step 17 of the General Procedure: Evaluate based on individualized desired outcomes: hair and scalp clean, hair has neat appearance, patient expresses comfort and satisfaction. Note any adverse outcomes.

DOCUMENTATION

18-19. Follow steps 18 and 19 of the General Procedure: Document the condition of the hair and scalp on the nursing care plan and/or patient's activity record.

◼ POTENTIAL ADVERSE OUTCOMES AND RELATED INTERVENTIONS

1. Hair is tangled and cannot be combed.
Intervention: Comb small sections of the hair starting from the ends and gradually working toward the roots. This may be time consuming, and a family member might be requested to assist with it. If the tangles are very dense, and it hurts the patient to comb the hair, request that the family bring in hair conditioner. Use small amounts of hair conditioner on the hair, massaging it into the tangles. This then allows combing through small sections.

2. Scalp shows evidence of dry, scaling skin. *Intervention:* In some instances, scales are the result of not shampooing. Mineral oil rubbed into the scalp before shampooing may soften the scales and allow them to be washed out. If the scales are due to a scalp condition such as seborrheic dermatitis, a prescription may be needed for a shampoo that treats the problem.

Procedure for Shampooing Hair

Many patients whose illnesses keep them in the hospital for only a few days do not want or need shampoos during that time. Other patients, however, may need shampoos, not only to remove oil and dirt and to increase circulation to the scalp but to improve appearance and morale as well. A shampoo may be important for the patient who has been confined to bed, who has been in an accident, or who has oily hair.

Generally, a shampoo is not given at the same time as the bath because it is a tiring procedure. The obvious exception is when a patient can shower. The equipment and general procedure you will use for those patients who need a shampoo and cannot shower will vary with the facility. In most facilities, the patient remains in bed, and the shampoo is given using a pitcher of warm water and a trough arrangement to guide the water into a receptacle on the floor or chair beside the bed. Dry or no-rinse shampoos are also available as are shampoo caps, which are heated in the microwave, placed on the head, and massaged into the scalp without having to rinse. These commercial types of shampooing remove some of the dirt, odor, and oil. Often these types of shampoo may cause some drying of the hair and scalp. Use this general procedure for giving a shampoo:

ASSESSMENT

1-3. Follow steps 1 to 3 of the General Procedure for Hygiene: Review the record and plan of care, assess the patient related to priority concerns, and check for supplies and equipment in the room.

ANALYSIS

4-5. Follow steps 4 and 5 of the General Procedure: Think through your data, and identify specific problems and modifications.

PLANNING

6. Determine individualized patient outcomes in relation to the shampoo. Include
   a. hair and scalp clean
   b. hair appears neat
   c. patient expresses comfort
7. Plan the procedure for a shampoo, and gather the equipment:
   a. bath blanket and two towels
   b. shampoo and conditioner (optional)
   c. plastic square or sheet to protect the bed
   d. shampoo basin or trough and receptacle for the shampoo water
   e. pitcher
   f. gloves if the patient has abrasions or open areas on scalp
   g. hair dryer and comb

IMPLEMENTATION

Action	Rationale
8-12. Follow steps 8 to 12 of the General Procedure: Wash or disinfect your hands, identify the patient (two identifiers), explain the procedure, pull the curtains around the bed, close the door, and raise the bed to an appropriate working position based on your height.	
13. Shampoo hair:	
a. Fanfold the top linens to the foot, and place a bath blanket over the patient (see Module 9, Bedmaking and Therapeutic Beds).	To provide warmth for the patient. Folding the linens to the foot will keep them dry.
b. Place the plastic square under the patient's head and shoulders.	To help keep the bedding dry.

(continued)

Action	Rationale
c. Place a towel around the patient's shoulders and neck, with the ends of the towel coming together in front.	To keep the shoulders and chest dry.
d. Place or arrange a trough under the patient's head with one end extending to the receptacle for water.	The trough provides a place to shampoo the hair without getting the bed wet as well as a means of removing the water.
e. Wet the hair, taking care to keep water out of the patient's eyes. Some patients like to hold a folded washcloth over their eyes (Fig. 7-10).	Shampoo in the eyes is irritating.
f. Shampoo and rinse twice, using only a small amount of shampoo and rinsing thoroughly. Use conditioner or rinse (optional).	Massaging the scalp stimulates the circulation to the scalp. Rinse well to remove all shampoo because it may cause drying and irritation if left in the hair.
g. Dry the patient's hair, ears, and neck with a towel. If a hair dryer is available, you may find it helpful, particularly if a patient has long hair.	Thorough drying is for patient comfort.
h. Comb and arrange the hair, allowing the patient to assist if able.	For the comfort and well-being of the patient.
i. Remove the plastic square, towels, trough, pitcher, and basin, and dry the equipment.	The equipment may be returned to a central service for processing or may remain in the patient's room for future use.
j. Replace the top linen, and remove the bath blanket.	For patient comfort.
k. Put the bed in the low position, and make sure the call signal is in place.	To provide safety.
l. Allow the patient to rest.	For patient comfort and conservation of energy.
14-16. Follow steps 14 to 16 of the General Procedure: Assess the patient during the procedure, care for the equipment, and wash or disinfect your hands.	

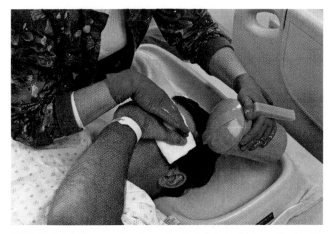

FIGURE 7-10 Shampooing the patient's hair in bed. The patient holds a washcloth over the eyes. Water is poured from the pitcher over the patient's hair, drains down through the trough beneath the patient's head, and falls into the basin below.

EVALUATION

17. Follow step 17 of the General Procedure: Evaluate based on the individualized patient outcomes in relation to the shampoo. Include hair and scalp clean, hair appears neat, patient expresses comfort. Note any adverse outcomes.

DOCUMENTATION

18-19. Follow steps 18 and 19 of the General Procedure: Document the shampoo procedure, and document any abnormal conditions of the hair and scalp.

Procedure for Eye Care

The eyes of the healthy individual need no special care other than that given during the usual bathing procedure. However, if there is a neurologic deficit that prevents the blink reflex from operating, or if the person is comatose, the eyes need special care to prevent drying of the surface, which can lead to ulceration and permanent vision impairment. The physician may order a product known as "artificial tears" to keep the eye surface moist, or he may order the eyes be patched for protection. For information on eyeglass care, see Box 7-3.

ASSESSMENT

1. Assess the patient's ability to blink. **R:** Diminished or absent blink reflex may result in drying of the eye surface and corneal ulceration.
2. Assess the patient's eyes for any abnormalities, such as inflammation, drainage, and encrustations

---

box 7-3   *Care of Eyeglasses*

It is probable that most nursing students have worn some type of eyeglasses, either regular glasses or sunglasses. Therefore, it seems somewhat unnecessary to describe the care of glasses. However, in the busy care environment, it is easy to forget certain essentials.

Cleaning Glasses

1. Wash glasses at the beginning of the day. A soiled surface that is tolerable when it accumulates gradually during the day is disturbing when the glasses are put on at the beginning of the day.
2. Use water and soap to clean the glasses before polishing them dry. This prevents the fine scratches on the surface of glasses that dust particles can cause. Many glasses are now made of plastic, which is much more susceptible to scratching than traditional glass; therefore, extra care is needed.

Protecting Glasses

1. After glasses have been removed, place them in a labeled glasses case for protection if possible.
2. If a case is not available, place the glasses in a bedside drawer, where they are more protected.
3. Always place them with the glass surface up to avoid scratches on the glass. Be careful where glasses are placed so that they do not get accidentally pushed onto the floor.

---

or for special eye care needs. **R:** To determine how much assistance with eye care the patient requires.
3. Identify whether special eye care supplies are available. **R:** Eye care supplies are usually sterile to protect the eyes from microorganisms that might cause infection.

ANALYSIS

4-5. Follow steps 4 and 5 of the General Procedure: Think through your data, and identify any modifications to the eye care procedure.

PLANNING

6. Determine individualized patient outcomes in relation to eye care. Include
 a. eyes are not red, and surface is not dry
 b. eye is held closed by the eye pad (if used)
 c. patient expresses comfort
7. Plan the procedure for eye care, and obtain a clean washcloth and hand towel. Clean cotton balls may be used if there is drainage from the eyes. An eye pad may be used if the blink reflex is not intact.

IMPLEMENTATION

Action	Rationale
8. Wash or disinfect your hands.	Gloves are not usually used for this procedure because it is designed for healthy eyes, which do not contain infectious material. You will be touching only the skin surface of the face, and clean hands will prevent introducing microbes to the patient. According to guidelines posted by the Centers for Disease Control and Prevention (CDC), gloves are not required because tears of healthy eyes do not contain infectious organisms. Gloves may be used as an option if there is any question about infection. If secretions are apparent, or if you have cuts or scratches on your hands, wear clean gloves to decrease the transfer of microorganisms that could cause infection.
9-12. Follow steps 9 to 12 of the General Procedure: Identify the patient (two identifiers), explain the procedure, pull the curtains around the bed, close the door, and raise the bed to an appropriate working position based on your height.	
13. Clean the eyes as follows:	
a. Either elevate the head of the bed to a semi-Fowler's position, or turn the patient's head toward you.	To prevent solution from contaminating the opposite eye by crossing the bridge of the nose.
b. Clean the eyes, using a clean washcloth or cotton ball and clear warm water. Wipe the exterior of each eye from the inner canthus to the outer canthus. Dry the eyes in the same way. Turn the head the other way, and clean the opposite eye, using the same technique, and using another section of the washcloth or a clean cotton ball.	To decrease the amount of debris in the area drained by the nasolacrimal duct and to prevent cross contamination.
c. If artificial tears are ordered, instill them into the eyes at this time (see Module 45 for directions on administering eye drops).	Artificial tears moisten the eye surface to prevent drying.
d. Observe the surface of the eye.	To detect any irritation or inflammation.
e. If the eye is unable to blink, gently close each eyelid, and hold it closed while the eye pad is placed over it.	Covering the eyes prevents drying of the eye surface.
f. Secure the eye pad with tape so that it holds the eye closed.	The eyelid will protect the surface of the eye from foreign bodies and allow tears to keep the surface moist.

(continued)

Action	Rationale
g. Return the bed to the low position, and place the call device within reach.	For the patient's safety.
14. Follow step 14 of the General Procedure: Assess the patient as well as the eye and skin surrounding the eye during the procedure.	To detect emerging or existing problems.
15. Place the washcloth and towel in a laundry hamper or bag.	To prevent the spread of microorganisms.
16. Wash or disinfect your hands.	For infection control.

EVALUATION

17. Evaluate individualized patient outcomes in relation to eye care: Eyes are not red, and surface is not dry; eye is held closed by the eye pad (if used); patient expresses comfort. Note any adverse outcomes observed.

DOCUMENTATION

18-19. Follow steps 18 and 19 of the General Procedure: Document the eye care procedure and any abnormal conditions of the eye. Add eye care to the nursing care plan.

Procedure for Contact Lens Removal, Care, and Insertion

When a patient wears contact lenses, self-care is the best way to ensure proper care. Contact lenses have many variations today and are either hard or soft. The newer hard lenses are gas permeable, allowing oxygen to pass through the lens to the cornea, but are made of a rigid plastic that does not absorb water or saline solutions. Soft lenses are made of a plastic material that absorbs water to become soft and pliable and molds to the eye for a snugger fit and extended wear. The duration of the extended-wear lenses is from 1 to 30 days and varies according to the underlying composition of the lens. An individual who enters a hospital in an emergency may have contact lenses in place that must be removed to prevent complications associated with excessive wear that could lead to permanent damage. During a stay, an incapacitated patient may need assistance with routine care and placement of contact lenses.

ASSESSMENT

1. Assess to see if the patient has contact lenses in place. **R:** Contact lenses may need removal to avoid damage from prolonged wear.

2. Determine what type of lenses is being worn (i.e., soft lenses or hard lenses) and the length of time that this particular lens can be worn. **R:** The specific nature of the lenses will determine how long the lenses can safely be worn before removal.

3. Assess the patient's ability to participate in contact lenses care. **R:** This is to determine how much assistance the patient will need.

ANALYSIS

4. Critically think through your data, carefully evaluating each aspect and its relation to other data. **R:** This enables you to determine specific problems for this individual in relation to contact lens care.

5. Identify specific problems and modifications of the procedure needed for this individual. **R:** Planning for the individual must take into consideration the individual's problems.

PLANNING

6. Determine individualized patient outcomes in relation to contact lens care. Include
   a. contact lenses are clean
   b. patient expresses eye comfort
   c. eyes do not appear irritated or reddened
7. Plan the technique for removing the contact lenses, and obtain the equipment:
   a. A clean container in which to store the contact lenses. If a regular contact lens container is not available, use sterile specimen containers that have been carefully marked with the patient's name. The left and right lenses should be separated and marked as left or right. Hard lenses may be stored dry; however, both hard and soft lenses may be stored in sterile saline solution. Lenses are individually prescribed for each eye, and care needs to be taken to keep them separate and labeled in order to not place them in the

wrong eye. The material of which the lenses are made determines the storage technique. **R:** Planning ahead allows you to proceed more safely and effectively.

b. Clean gloves. **R:** These will facilitate handling the lens and protect the eyes.

c. Flashlight. **R:** This will make the lens visible.

d. Cleaning or saline solution. **R:** This is to clean the surface of the lens.

e. Hand towel to place under the area where the lens is being cleaned. **R:** This will protect the lens if it is accidentally dropped.

IMPLEMENTATION

Action	Rationale
8. Wash or disinfect your hands.	To decrease the transfer of microorganisms that could cause infection.
9–12. Follow steps 9 to 12 in the General Procedure for Hygiene: Identify the patient (two identifiers), explain the procedure, pull the curtains around the bed, close the door, and raise the bed to an appropriate working position based on your height.	
13. Care for contact lenses as follows:	
a. Hard lenses	
(1) Use a flashlight or penlight to examine the eye to determine where the contact lens is resting.	The lens will reflect light and be visible.
(2) Put on snug-fitting clean gloves.	For infection control. Snug gloves are used because of difficulty in handling contact lenses with gloves. The surface of the glove will tend to adhere to the lens.
(3) Place a drop of saline solution or eye drops for contact lenses in the eye.	Moistens the eye surface and facilitates lens removal.
(4) Place one forefinger on the upper lid and one on the lower lid.	To stabilize the head and reduce eyelid movement.
(5) Raise the upper eyelid, and remove the lens by gently pushing in on the lower eyelid at the lower margin of the lens (Fig. 7-11). If unsuccessful, a small contact lens suction device (available in most Emergency Department settings) may be used.	The lower edge of the lens is raised and separated from the cornea, decreasing the surface tension that causes it to stay in place.
(6) Clean each lens by holding it over a basin or sink with water in it in case you drop it. A towel may be placed in the sink to protect the lens. Moisten the lens with cleaning solution, and rub it gently between your fingers. Then rinse the cleaning	Holding the lens over a basin of water helps to avoid losing the lens in the event that it slips from your fingers. Gentle rubbing removes accumulated materials, and rinsing removes any cleaning agent that could cause eye irritation.

(continued)

Action	Rationale

Removing hard contact lenses

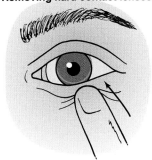

If the lens is not centered over the cornea, apply gentle pressure on the lower eyelid to center the lens.

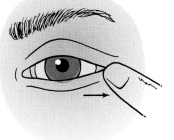

Gently pull the outer corner of the eye toward the ear.

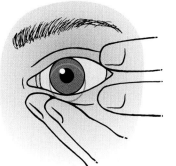

Position the other hand below the lens to receive it and ask the patient to blink.

Or

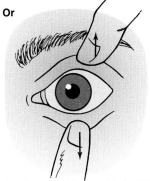

Gently spread the eyelids beyond the top and bottom edges of the lens.

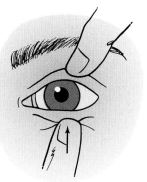

Gently press the lower eyelid up against the bottom of the lens.

After the lens is tipped slightly, move the eyelids toward one another to cause the lens to slide out between the eyelids.

Removing soft contact lenses

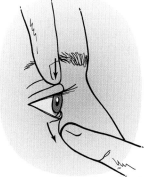

Have the patient look forward. Retract the lower lid with one hand. Using the pad of the index finger of the other hand, move the lens down to the sclera.

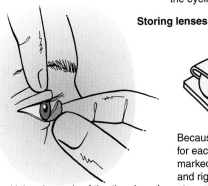

Using the pads of the thumb and index finger, grasp the lens with a gentle pinching motion and remove.

Storing lenses

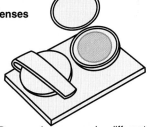

Because lenses may be different for each eye, storage cases are marked L and R, designating left and right lenses. It is important to place the first lens in its designated cup in the storage case before removing the second lens to avoid mixing them up.

FIGURE 7-11 Removing contact lenses requires dexterity.

Action	Rationale
solution off with sterile saline or wetting solution. If contact lens cleaning solution is not available, use saline as a temporary measure for cleaning.	
(7) Replace each lens by placing the lens on the tip of the index finger with the concave surface up and applying wetting or sterile saline solution.	Wetting solution allows the lens to glide over the cornea to reduce risk of injury.
(8) Hold the eye open with the thumb and index finger of the other hand, tip the lens onto the surface of the eye, and then have the patient blink.	Tipping the lens centers it over the cornea for correct placement. Blinking helps position the lens properly.
b. Soft lenses	
(1) Place a drop of saline or lens-wetting solution in the eye.	Moistens the eye surface and facilitates lens removal.
(2) Place the forefinger on the upper eyelid and the thumb on the lower eyelid, and open the eye wide.	Stabilizes the eye and prevents blinking.
(3) Using the other forefinger and thumb, gently pinch up on the lens. (A contact lens suction device can also be used to remove soft lenses.)	Pinching allows air to enter underneath the flexible lens, making it easy to lift out.
(4) To clean each lens, place it in the palm of one hand held over a hand towel. Apply a few drops of cleaning solution, and rub both surfaces of the lens thoroughly. Then rinse with rinsing or sterile saline solution.	Confining the lens to the palm helps keep it from being lost, and the towel provides further protection. Gentle rubbing removes accumulated materials, and rinsing removes any cleaning agent that could cause eye irritation.
(5) Store the lens in saline solution, or replace it in the patient's eye.	Storing in saline solution maintains the soft character of the lens.
(6) Insert the lens by carefully balancing it, concave side up, on the end of a dry finger.	The dry finger prevents the lens from sticking to the finger.
(7) Open the eye with other thumb and forefinger, place the lens on the eye's surface, and hold it in place for a second as it adheres. Have the patient blink.	These measures allow the lens to conform to the shape of the eye and also allow suction to form between the lens and cornea for adherence. Blinking helps position the lens correctly.

(continued)

Action	Rationale
(8) Put the bed in the low position, and position the call device conveniently.	For safety.
14. Follow step 14 of the General Procedure: Assess the patient as well as the eye and skin surrounding the eye during the procedure.	
15. Place the towel in a laundry hamper or bag.	To prevent the spread of microorganisms.
16. Dispose of the glove, and wash or disinfect your hands.	For infection control.

EVALUATION

17. Evaluate individualized patient outcomes in relation to the following: Contact lenses are clean; patient expresses eye comfort; eyes do not appear irritated or reddened. Note any adverse outcomes.

DOCUMENTATION

18-19. Follow steps 18 and 19 of the General Procedure: Document the contact lens care procedure and any abnormal conditions of the eye. Add contact lens care to the nursing care plan.

Hearing Aid Care

Currently available hearing aids are finely adjusted electronic devices that are battery-powered, sound-amplifying devices used for hearing impairment. They can be damaged by rough handling. There are several types of hearing aids, including behind-the-ear, in-the-ear, and body hearing aids (Fig. 7-12). A notation should be made on the nursing care plan or patient's record of the need for a hearing aid and the ear in which it should be placed to facilitate appropriate care by other caregivers. Some individuals may wear hearing aids in or behind both ears. In this case, they need to be carefully marked "left" and "right" because each earpiece is individually molded to fit that ear only.

CLEANING A HEARING AID

When providing care for the patient's hearing aid, gently wipe the hearing aid with a dry tissue. If earwax has become embedded in the small opening in the earpiece, clean it out with a special cleaning instrument that comes with the hearing aid. The patient may have this at home. If this is not available, use a thin needle as a substitute.

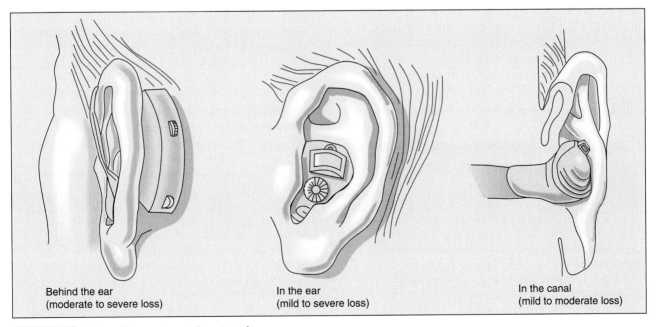

Behind the ear
(moderate to severe loss)

In the ear
(mild to severe loss)

In the canal
(mild to moderate loss)

FIGURE 7-12 Hearing aids come in a wide variety of types.

PROTECTING THE HEARING AID

If the hearing aid will not be used for a period of days, remove the battery for storage. This prolongs the life of the battery and protects the hearing aid. Some individuals remove the battery each evening when the hearing aid is removed. This also prolongs battery life and may be particularly important for the long-term care resident.

Keep the hearing aid dry because any moisture can interfere with its functioning. Place the hearing aid in a bedside drawer or other safe place to prevent its being accidentally pushed onto the floor.

A.M. AND P.M. HYGIENE

In many facilities, a regular routine exists for morning and evening hygiene procedures, usually designated as a.m. (morning) and p.m. (evening) care. The purpose of these procedures is to provide an opportunity for patients to complete those activities that would be done independently if they were at home.

The a.m. care is designed to help the patient be ready to eat breakfast when it is served. Most people would use the toilet, commode, or bedpan, wash their face and hands, and brush their teeth before eating breakfast. At this time, it is appropriate to check the bed of an incontinent patient, and make sure it is clean and dry. Attention to hygiene before meals can greatly enhance the patient's appetite and food intake.

The p.m. care is designed to help patients relax and prepare to sleep. An opportunity to use the toilet, bedpan, or commode, wash their face and hands, and brush their teeth is important. The bed may need straightening, and if the patient has perspired excessively, a clean pillowcase and patient gown may be needed. This is the time when a back rub is especially appropriate to help an individual relax. Careful attention to p.m. care may eliminate the need for sleep medications. The hospital is a strange environment, and many individuals who have no difficulty sleeping at home find themselves having difficulty sleeping in the hospital.

Acute Care

Many factors influence the ability to provide hygiene in an acute care setting. The most common is the medical condition itself. The critically ill patient may only tolerate minimal hygiene because of a precarious status that is easily disrupted by the activity involved in hygiene. The nurse must find ways to provide oral care, perineal care, and back care to this type of patient in order to prevent the development of preventable complication, such as stomatitis of the mouth and skin breakdown in the perineal area or on the back. This might require that each aspect be done at a separate time. The back care might be done when the patient must be moved for another purpose. Many modifications of procedures must be made to accommodate patients with casts, tractions, surgical incisions, various drainage tubes, pain, and fatigue. The nurse must plan for these modifications and often direct assistive personnel in carrying out modified hygiene plans.

Long-Term Care

In long-term care facilities, baths are rarely given every day. A bathing schedule is established that provides for complete baths once or twice a week or as necessary. Because the residents are not physically active and do not perspire as much as younger adults, this kind of schedule usually meets the needs for personal comfort and odor control. Elderly individuals in long-term care may experience excessive drying of the skin, itching, and actual skin breakdown from too frequent bathing. Cognitively impaired individuals may resist bathing because of a variety of fears about the process. Going slowly and making the procedure less frightening are goals (Brawley, 2002).

Chair showers have traditionally been the most common method of bathing in long-term care. Many institutions are now adopting a variety of tub systems that allow residents to be placed in a whirlpool-type tub either by means of an attached mechanically lifted chair or by a door that opens down the side of the tub. Moisturizing skin cleansers are used in these tubs, and the whirlpool action cleans the skin and stimulates circulation while moistening the skin. Bathing in long-term care is delegated to nursing assistants. However, the professional nursing personnel should plan for the hygiene needs of the individual resident.

When individuals enter long-term care, dentures are usually marked with the resident's name by an engraving process. This is especially important in settings where ambulatory, cognitively impaired individuals reside.

Each day, residents who are not scheduled for a bath are assisted with a.m. care. The a.m. care in these situations includes washing under the arms and perineal area as well as face and hands. The resident is then helped with whatever grooming tasks are desired, such as combing hair, shaving, putting on makeup, and so forth, and helped to dress for the day. In long-term care facilities, all residents for whom it is possible are urged to dress for the day. Dress may be adapted for special needs such as being wheelchair bound or incontinent.

The p.m. care in the long-term care facility involves helping the person change from daywear into nightwear. In addition, the individual is helped to complete the regular bedtime hygiene procedures such as oral hygiene and washing the face and hands.

practices of their patients, even offering assistance in bathing clients once or twice a week. During the day, while patients are present, centers will assist with toileting needs, incontinence care, and nutrition. Particular attention is given to skin integrity. Staff are also instructed in caring for patients with hearing and vision losses.

 ## Home Care

When a patient is being discharged or if nursing care is provided in the home, the nurse assesses the person's ability to manage hygiene needs and determines whether adaptations in hygiene procedures are necessary.

Typically, individuals may be able to manage their own hygiene needs if special safety modifications are made. Safety bars and handles in the bathroom are often needed. A nonskid surface may be applied to the bottom of the tub. A bath stool in the tub and a handheld shower may enable an individual who could not climb down into and out of a tub or stand in a shower to be independent. Sometimes, doorways need to be modified to allow a wheelchair to enter.

If the person will need assistance with hygiene after discharge, you may teach a family member how to provide it. If no one in the family is able to provide assistance, you may help the patient arrange for a home health aide.

Home health aides provide personal care and assistance with simple tasks associated with daily living for those whose families or home care providers are not able to manage these tasks. The registered nurse visits the home and does the initial assessment to determine what level of care is needed and to develop the plan for nursing care. The actual care is then delegated to the home health aide with follow-up evaluation by the registered nurse. Home health aides may also do light housekeeping tasks such as making a meal, washing dishes, or running a vacuum cleaner. They do not do heavy housecleaning.

 ## Ambulatory Care

People who are ambulatory are more likely to be independent in their hygiene practices. Some agencies such as adult day centers assist with the hygiene

LEARNING TOOLS

DEVELOP YOUR BACKGROUND KNOWLEDGE

1. Review the Learning Outcomes.

2. Read the section on hygiene in your fundamentals text.

3. Look up the Key Terms in the glossary.

4. Now review this module; mentally practice the techniques described. Study so that you would be able to teach these skills to another person.

5. Consider your personal hygiene habits. At home, give yourself a complete sponge bath using the technique for giving bed baths. This can be done at the bathroom sink, but you should use a basin filled with water (not running water) to simulate the bedside situation. Pay special attention to the following:
   a. the water temperature that feels comfortable to you
   b. possible chilling due to exposure
   c. the amount of pressure or friction that is comfortable
   d. how easily soap can be rinsed off and how much soap should be used
   e. the effect of the "trailing" ends of a washcloth
   f. the need for thorough drying

DEVELOP YOUR SKILLS

1. In the practice setting, select two other students, and form a group of three. Arrive in the lab prepared to put on shorts and sleeveless tops or bathing suits.

2. Changing roles so that each has the opportunity to play the role of the patient, perform each of the following procedures. Those who are not participating at a given time can observe and evaluate the performances of the others.
   a. Practice giving a bed bath (omitting bathing private areas), back rub, oral care, hair care, and eye care, using another student as your patient. Communicate as you would with a real patient.

Have the student comment on his or her comfort and the communication skills you demonstrated. Use the Performance Checklist on the CD-ROM to evaluate yourself. When you are satisfied with your performance, have another student in your group evaluate you.

b. Describe to your group of students what you would do differently to provide a partial bed bath or self–bed bath with assistance.

c. Describe the necessary safety measures for the patient receiving a shower or a tub bath.

d. Practice denture care if dentures are provided in the practice setting. Use the Performance Checklist to evaluate yourself. When you are satisfied with your performance, have another student in your group evaluate you.

e. Practice care of glasses, hearing aids, and contact lenses if they are provided in the practice setting. Use the Performance Checklist to evaluate yourself. When you are satisfied with your performance, have another student in your group evaluate you.

DEMONSTRATE YOUR SKILLS

In the clinical setting

1. Consult with your instructor regarding the opportunity to
   a. assist a patient with a tub bath or a shower and morning care
   b. give a complete bed bath and a.m. care to a patient
   c. provide a.m. and p.m. care
   d. shampoo the hair of a patient confined to bed

2. Evaluate your performance with the instructor.

CRITICAL THINKING EXERCISES

1. Mrs. Wilson is a newly admitted resident to the nursing home. She tells you that she just hates having to bathe in the morning. She is 85 years old and says she bathed every night of her life! She walks with a walker and sits in the shower for baths. You know that she needs help with bathing although she is able to do much of it herself. As a nursing student, how can you serve as her advocate? Determine what further information you need before making any decision. Whom should you consult? Recommend some possible available options.

2. James Wilson, age 74, was admitted 2 days ago with pneumonia associated with chronic obstructive pulmonary disease. His record indicates that he has not been bathed since admission. You note that he

has severe body odor and looks disheveled and unshaven. When you approach him to arrange a bath time, he states, "I told that other nurse that I don't want a bath. It'll just make me short of breath again!" Analyze this situation to determine what concerns are present for both the patient and the staff. Develop a specific approach to Mr. Wilson's situation that you believe will result in his accepting a bath.

SELF-QUIZ
SHORT-ANSWER QUESTIONS

1. Why is a bath blanket used during a bed bath instead of the present linen on the patient's bed?

   _____

2. Why are glasses cleaned with soap and water instead of simply being polished while dry?

   _____

   _____

3. What is usually included in a.m. care?

   _____

   _____

4. What is usually included in p.m. care?

   _____

   _____

5. List the equipment needed to complete a shampoo for a person confined to bed.

   _____

   _____

6. Mr. Jones has hearing aids in both ears. He is going for surgery this morning. How will you care for his hearing aids until he returns?

   _____

   _____

MULTIPLE CHOICE

_____ 7. The temperature of the water for bathing and shampooing has been described as "warm." This means
   a. 75° to 90°.
   b. 90° to 105°.
   c. 100° to 115°.
   d. 110° to 125°.

_____ 8. The preferred position for bathing the patient in bed is
   a. prone.
   b. flat.
   c. semi-Fowler's.
   d. supine.

_____ 9. An elderly patient has very dry skin on her feet and lower legs. To maintain the skin integrity, the nurse should do which of the following for the patient?
   a. Soak her feet frequently.
   b. Put socks on her feet.
   c. Use a foot powder.
   d. Apply a nonperfumed lotion.

_____ 10. Mr. Allen has been hospitalized after an automobile accident. Both legs are in traction, one arm is in a cast, and he has bruises on the other arm. What type of bath will you plan for him?

   a. A shower using a shower chair
   b. A full bed bath
   c. A partial bath
   d. A self-bath

_____ 11. Mrs. Smith is unable to wash her dentures due to a recent stroke. She is asking you to do this for her. How will you perform this procedure?
   a. Hold the dentures under hot water to rinse.
   b. Use dental floss between the teeth.
   c. Fill the sink half-full of water, and brush the dentures.
   d. Place the dentures in a container of mouthwash, and soak them for 30 minutes.

Answers to Self-Quiz questions appear in the back of this book.

MODULE 8

Assisting With Elimination and Perineal Care

KEY TERMS

ADLs	penis
bedpan	perineum
catheter	recumbent
commode	renal calculi
defecation	smegma
foreskin	sutures
fracture pan	trapeze
genital area	urinal
labia	urination
lumbosacral	void

OVERALL OBJECTIVES

▸ To assist patients with the use of bedpans, urinals, or commodes in a hygienic manner, taking into account psychological factors.
▸ To promote patient comfort and hygiene.
▸ To remove excessive secretions by providing appropriate perineal care.

LEARNING OUTCOMES

The student will be able to

1. Assess the patient effectively to determine the need for assistance with elimination and/or perineal care.
2. Analyze data to determine special needs, concerns, and self-care abilities in completing elimination and perineal care.
3. Determine appropriate patient outcomes of the elimination and perineal care procedures, and recognize the potential for adverse outcomes.
4. Choose the appropriate procedure and equipment for the specific elimination and perineal care needed.
5. Determine the assistance needed to complete the procedure.
6. Demonstrate the proper techniques for assisting with elimination and perineal care.
7. Evaluate the effectiveness of the elimination and perineal care techniques for a specific patient.
8. Document the procedure in the patient's plan of care as well as specific observations of any abnormal findings and the patient's comfort level.

Illness, physical disability, and weakness may make it impossible for an individual to go to a bathroom for elimination. Because elimination is a private function in our society and individuals learn to manage this need independently at a very young age, those who require assistance with toileting and perineal care are often embarrassed. In addition, special techniques are required to avoid strain to both the patient and the nurse and to maintain safety. The need for assistance may be temporary or permanent. In either case, the nurse provides support and reassurance by responding promptly and competently to this care need.

NURSING DIAGNOSES

Patients who are confined to bed the majority of the time or require assistance with activities of daily living **(ADLs)** due to weakness or illness may have a variety of nursing diagnoses concerning elimination needs and perineal care. Examples are

■ Toileting Self-Care Deficit: may be due to a lack of neuromuscular control, fatigue and weakness, shortness of breath, or a variety of other disabilities

Special perineal care may be needed with a nursing diagnosis of

■ Bathing/Hygiene Self-Care Deficit: may be due to inability to move, weakness, or as a result of a procedure

DELEGATION

Nurses commonly delegate assisting with elimination and perineal care to assistive personnel. The nurse must plan for appropriate strategies to be used and communicate these strategies to the caregiver carrying out the tasks. If the patient has recently had surgery in the perineal area, the nurse should evaluate the individual patient before delegating the care.

GENERAL PRINCIPLES RELATED TO ELIMINATION AND PERINEAL CARE

Keep several principles in mind when assisting a patient with elimination and/or perineal care. First, observe Standard Precautions (Module 4) for infection control throughout these procedures for your own protection as well as the patient's. When performing these procedures, your hands may come in contact with mucous membrane and body fluids, which may transmit infection. It is also important to protect the patient from the dangers of cross-contamination (contamination from other patients). Follow Standard Precautions by using clean gloves whenever performing any tasks involving the **perineum** and when handling a **urinal** or **bedpan.**

Second, the procedure can be embarrassing to you and to the patient. It is important to recognize these feelings in yourself and to know that with experience, assisting with intimate procedures will become less personal and more routine to you. To reduce a patient's embarrassment or discomfort, maintain a straightforward attitude and respect the patient's privacy, keeping his or her exposure to a minimum.

Third, when you help a patient with any substitution or adaptation of the usual ADLs, it is important—in terms of efficiency and patient comfort—that you approximate the normal as closely as possible. For a female patient, the normal position for **urination** or **defecation** is sitting; a male commonly stands to urinate and sits to defecate. Therefore, having a patient assume these positions when using a bedpan or urinal is helpful and, in some cases, may be a strong factor in whether the patient will be able to eliminate. Provide as much control as possible to patients, for example, by giving them privacy, encouraging them to use tissue by themselves, and to wash their own hands afterward. If patients cannot perform these activities, you should assume this responsibility.

EQUIPMENT

The type of equipment used depends on the health status of the patient. For the patient on strict bed rest, a bedpan is used. Males use a urinal when they need to **void** urine. If activity status permits, a bedside **commode** offers a more relaxed and convenient option. Keep in mind that equipment most closely corresponding to the normal is the better choice.

BEDPANS

Bedpans are made of metal or plastic and come in two sizes, the smaller designed for pediatric patients. Two main types of bedpans are a standard bedpan and a **fracture pan** (Fig. 8-1). Plastic bedpans are disposable and are used by one patient. Metal bedpans are cleaned, disinfected, and reused.

To limit the potential spread of microorganisms, each patient has a personal bedpan that is kept in a

storage unit in the patient's room. A cover should be used to conceal the sight of the contents and to decrease the odor after the patient has used the bedpan and before it is emptied. It should be emptied as soon as possible after it is used. A cover is commonly made of paper and slips easily over the bedpan. When "official" bedpan covers are not available, a disposable incontinence pad or a hand towel can be used for a bedpan cover.

A fracture pan is a type of bedpan used for patients who are unable to raise their buttocks due to physical problems such as a fractured pelvis or as a result of treatments that do not allow such movement. The size is helpful for elderly patients because it is smaller and easier to get onto than a standard bedpan. There is a handle at the front to facilitate placement and removal, but the handle should never be used to just pull the bedpan out. This action may damage fragile skin on the coccyx. Fracture pans also come in two sizes, in plastic or metal, and have a low back.

URINALS

A standard urinal is used by the male patient for urination. It is made of plastic or metal with a bottle-like configuration. A flat side allows it to rest without tipping over. Urinals are available with or without lids. Female urinals are also available for the woman who, because of extreme pain or for a medical reason, should not be raised to bedpan height except for defecation. Female urinals are not common in most healthcare settings, so an emesis basin (Fig. 8-2) can be used as a substitute (Box 8-1). Most patients are grateful for this easy, more comfortable way to urinate.

COMMODES

A commode is a portable toileting device (Fig. 8-3). It resembles a movable chair with a back and arms; some have wheels. The seat lifts up to reveal an opening with

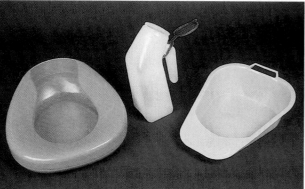

FIGURE 8-1 Standard bedpan (**left**), standard male urinal for nonambulatory patient (**center**), and fracture pan (**right**).

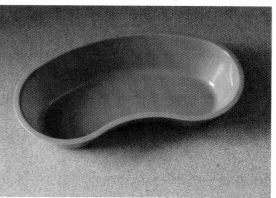

FIGURE 8-2 Emesis basin can be used by the immobile female patient for urine elimination.

1. Place a waterproof pad under the patient to protect the linen.
2. Hold the emesis basin lengthwise between the legs, flat on the bed.
3. Press the rim of the emesis basin firmly against the perineum.
4. Instruct the patient to void. At first a patient may be hesitant, fearing that she will soil the bed. Encourage the patient to void freely. Usually the urine flows into the pan with only a drop or so on the pad.

a sliding container beneath, which serves as a receptacle for urine or feces. The patient uses the open seat as a backrest.

This device is useful for the patient who is able to get out of bed but is unable to walk the distance to the bathroom because of weakness or partial immobilization. Most facilities supply commodes without an order. However, the care plan may read "BSC," which stands for "bedside commode." The same considerations are given to this procedure as are given for getting a patient out of bed or walking a patient to the toilet. (See Module 6, Moving the Patient in Bed and Positioning, and Module 18, Transfer, for proper procedures for getting the patient out of bed and to the bedside commode.) Have sufficient help if the patient requires transfer. Always be sure the wheels are locked on the bedside commode *and* the bed for safety.

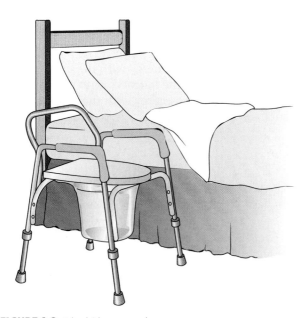

FIGURE 8-3 A bedside commode.

COMFORT CONSIDERATIONS

Although often unavoidable, using any of these devices is not a pleasant experience. A thin, fragile patient may even feel pain from the pressure of the hard surfaces. Fold a soft pad or small towel over the edges of the pan to lessen this discomfort. With metal pans, another source of discomfort is cold. Warm metal pans by holding them under running warm water and then drying them. These simple measures can make the experience less disagreeable. You may also wish to place padding over the edges of a commode for the patient's comfort.

SPECIFIC PROCEDURES FOR ASSISTING WITH ELIMINATION

Assisting With a Bedpan

ASSESSMENT

1. Check the patient's activity order and physical status. **R:** To determine how much assistance is needed and whether a bedpan is necessary.
2. Review the patient's past use of such equipment, and note any problems encountered. **R:** To determine the type of equipment needed according to physical limitations and/or preferences.

ANALYSIS

3. Critically think through your data, carefully evaluating each aspect and its relation to other data. **R:** This allows you to determine any specific problems for this individual regarding the need to eliminate.
4. Identify any specific problems in mobility that may require assistance with elimination needs, and determine equipment and/or personnel that may be needed. **R:** Planning for the individual must take into consideration the individual's problems.

PLANNING

5. Determine individualized patient outcomes in relation to use of the bedpan. **R:** Identifying outcomes facilitates planning and evaluation.
   a. Patient was able to get on the bedpan without difficulty.
   b. Patient was able to urinate or defecate using the bedpan.
   c. Equipment and technique used were appropriate for the patient.
   d. No adverse outcomes were encountered.
6. Plan for the specific procedure or technique to be used, and select the specific type of equipment needed. **R:** Planning allows you to proceed safely and effectively.

IMPLEMENTATION

Action	Rationale
7. Wash or disinfect your hands.	To prevent the spread of microorganisms.
8. Identify the patient, using two identifiers.	Verifying the patient's identity helps to insure that you are performing the procedure for the right patient.
9. Explain in general how you plan to proceed.	Explaining the procedure helps relieve anxiety or misperceptions that the patient may have about a procedure or activity and facilitates patient participation.
10. Close the door, or pull the curtains around the bed.	To provide privacy.
11. Put on clean gloves.	To protect the patient and yourself. Follow the principles of infection control to protect yourself from exposure to body substances.
12. Raise the bed to an appropriate working position according to your height.	This allows you to use correct body mechanics and protect yourself from back injury.
13. Put up the side rail on the opposite side of the bed from where you plan to stand.	Raising the side rail prevents the patient from rolling off the side of the bed.
14. Take the bedpan, cover, and toilet tissue out of the bedside storage unit. Set the cover and tissue aside. A fracture pan or emesis basin, as previously mentioned, can be used in the same way as a conventional bedpan.	To have equipment readily available for use.
15. Assist the patient onto the bedpan, using one of the following methods, depending on the patient's condition and ability to assist you.	
a. With the patient in a **recumbent** position, place your hand under the **lumbosacral** area (the small of the back) and your elbow on the bed, and ask the patient to lift the buttocks by raising up with the feet as you push the pan into position under the patient (Fig. 8-4). For a regular bedpan, place the wide, flat edge toward the patient's back so the buttocks rests on the smooth, rounded rim. For a fracture pan, slide the flat, rimmed edge toward the patient's back with the handle toward the patient's feet (Fig. 8-5).	The patient needs to use less energy with the nurse assisting the patient to lift the buttocks onto the bedpan, and the nurse uses less energy with the assistance of the patient.

(continued)

Action	Rationale

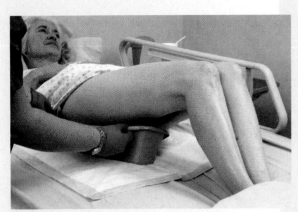

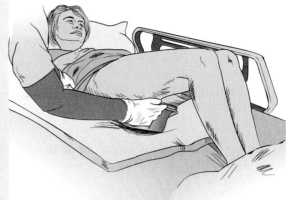

FIGURE 8-4 Place the bedpan under the patient with the wide, flat edge under the buttocks.

FIGURE 8-5 Place the fracture pan under the patient with the handle toward the legs and the low, flat side under the buttocks.

Action	Rationale
b. Ask the patient who is able to assume the sitting position to simply lift the body by pushing down with the hands and feet as you place the pan in position.	The energy of the nurse is preserved with the patient assisting.

Action	Rationale
c. Roll a more immobilized patient onto the pan. For this maneuver, ask the patient to grasp the side rail on the opposite side of the bed (across from where you are standing) for stability as you roll the patient away from you in one plane. Place the pan against the patient. (You may want to pad the pan with a towel to relieve pressure on the patient's buttocks.) Now, hold the pan in place as you roll the patient back (Fig. 8-6). Finally, check the position of the pan. If the patient must remain flat, you may want to place a small pillow above the bedpan under the patient's back for support. *Note:* If the patient's bed has a **trapeze,** make use of this device for placing and removing the bedpan. Have the patient use the trapeze to lift the hips.	Rolling the patient takes less energy than lifting the patient onto a bedpan.

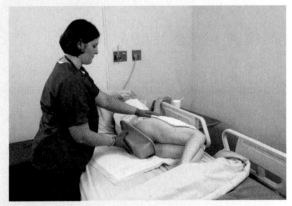

FIGURE 8-6 Rolling technique to place patient on bedpan.

Action	Rationale
16. Raise the side rail nearest you.	To keep the patient from rolling out of bed.
17. Elevate the head of the bed to mid- or high Fowler's position if not contraindicated, while the patient grasps the rails.	This position approximates the normal position for elimination.

(continued)

Action	Rationale
18. Place the toilet tissue and the call bell within the patient's reach.	To prevent the patient from falling while reaching for the tissue or trying to reach the call bell.
19. Leave the patient, or pull the curtain around the bed. Our culture emphasizes privacy during elimination, making it very difficult for some patients to eliminate with a nurse or anyone else in attendance. If the patient is safe, it is best to leave the patient for a time; if this is not possible, you might step just outside to be nearby if the patient suddenly needs assistance.	To provide privacy for elimination needs.
20. When the patient signals, return promptly. If a patient does not signal you within a reasonable amount of time, return to the patient, and check for any problems.	Allowing a patient to remain on a bedpan can be uncomfortable. Checking on the patient frequently ensures safety.
21. Put on clean gloves.	For infection control.
22. If necessary, clean the **genital area** with toilet tissue. Most alert patients will clean themselves adequately. Someone who is incapacitated may need further assistance. Always clean with fresh tissue from the anterior (urinary) region to the posterior (rectal) region. If a specimen is needed, do not place the tissue in the bedpan.	Cleaning in this direction minimizes the chance of contaminating the urinary tract with fecal microorganisms. If a specimen is needed, placing tissue in the bedpan will contaminate the specimen.
23. Remove the bedpan, reversing the method that you used when you placed the patient on it. If you used the rolling technique, hold onto the bedpan firmly, or get help.	Holding the bedpan will prevent unnecessary soiling of linen.
24. Cover the pan.	For aesthetic reasons.
25. Carry the pan to the bathroom, and, if ordered, measure the urine. If a patient is on intake and output, a measuring container is usually kept in the bathroom.	Measure the urine in the bathroom both for aesthetic reasons (it is out of the sight of the patient) and for practical purposes (it is where the measuring container is located).
26. Collect a specimen of urine or feces, if ordered (see Module 15). Even when precise measurements or specimens are not ordered, note the amount, color, consistency, and odor as well as the presence of blood, mucus, or foreign material. A patient who is being observed for **renal calculi** (kidney stones) may have an order to have all	These observations are important data that may contribute to the medical diagnosis.

(continued)

Action	Rationale
urine strained so that the small stones or particles can be retained and examined. If you even suspect that a patient's urine or feces contain blood, in most facilities, you can independently test a specimen to verify your suspicion (see Module 15).	
27. Empty the contents into the toilet and flush.	To facilitate disposal of body wastes.
28. Thoroughly clean the pan with cold water, or pull down the bedpan sprayer over the toilet as you flush it. Health regulations may require that a container of disinfectant solution and a long-handled brush be kept in the bathroom for cleaning bedpans. Wash and rinse the bedpan thoroughly. Use paper towels for drying. Return the bedpan to the patient's storage unit.	Cold water minimizes odors and combines with the contents more effectively than hot water.
29. Remove and dispose of gloves.	To prevent the spread of microorganisms.
30. Give the patient a basin of warm water, a washcloth, soap, and a towel, a packaged moist towelette, or hand sanitizer so that hygiene can be carried out. Allow the patient to wash hands and perineal area, if desired.	To prevent the spread of microorganisms.
31. Place the bed in the low position, and lower the rail on the stand side if appropriate.	Lowering the bed provides a safe environment.
32. Care for the equipment appropriately.	Proper care and storage of equipment is cost effective.
33. Wash or disinfect your hands.	To prevent the spread of microorganisms.

EVALUATION

34. Evaluate using the individualized patient outcomes previously identified. **R:** Evaluation in relation to desired outcomes is essential for planning future care needs.
    a. Patient was able to get on the bedpan without difficulty.
    b. Patient was able to urinate or defecate using the bedpan.
    c. Equipment and technique used were appropriate for the patient.
    d. No adverse outcomes were encountered.
35. Identify any specific problems and possible improvements, and note them on the nursing care plan. **R:** To determine any changes in the procedure that would accommodate a patient's condition.

DOCUMENTATION

36. Record any problems or unusual observations such as painful urination. Routine elimination is usually recorded on a flow sheet or output sheet. Note any of the following: volume of urine, color, unusual odor, presence of blood, and presence of any foreign material. For feces, note appearance, form or consistency, color, unusually foul odor, and presence of mucus or blood. **R:** Adequate documentation includes observations that may assist in identifying a diagnosis.

POTENTIAL ADVERSE OUTCOMES AND RELATED INTERVENTIONS

1. Patient complains of painful urination.
Intervention: Report to physician. Prepare patient to collect "clean catch" sample at next urination (see Module 15).
2. Urine has dark color, an unusual odor, or foreign material in it.
Intervention: Report to physician. Collect 30 mL of urine to send for laboratory analysis if physician orders.
3. Stool has unusual appearance (presence of mucus or blood) and/or unusually foul odor.
Intervention: Report to physician. Collect stool sample to send for laboratory analysis if physician orders.

Assisting With a Urinal

The steps used to assist a male patient in using the urinal are the same as those for a bedpan (see Performance Checklist on the CD-ROM), except for a few adaptations. If a male patient is able to stand alone, he will usually be more successful if he is allowed to stand to urinate. If the patient is unable to stand alone, have him lean on the edge of the bed for stability with his feet on the floor. Always check the patient's activity order and activity tolerance before undertaking this action.

Never place a urinal between a patient's legs for long periods of time in an effort to control incontinence. This can irritate and erode the skin of the **penis.** If a patient is unable to use the urinal himself, protect the linen with a waterproof pad, and place the urinal between the patient's legs so that the flat portion of the receptacle rests on the bed. Place the head of the penis well inside of the urinal opening, and tell the patient he can now urinate. Measure urine if required, and document the volume. Also note the appearance, odor, and color of the urine before emptying the urinal. Rinse the urinal with cold water, and return to the bedside storage.

Assisting With a Commode

ASSESSMENT

1. Check the patient's activity order and physical status to determine whether a commode is necessary. **R:** To promote safety with regard to the patient's ability to ambulate.
2. Assess the patient's ability to ambulate short distances. **R:** To determine how much assistance the patient will need to ambulate to the commode.

ANALYSIS

3. Critically think through your data, and evaluate each aspect and its relation to other data. **R:** To determine specific problems for this patient in relation to ambulation and elimination.
4. Identify any specific problems and modifications of the procedure needed for this individual. **R:** Planning for the individual must take into consideration the individual's problems.

PLANNING

5. Determine individualized patient outcomes in relation to using the commode. **R:** Identifying outcomes facilitates evaluation.
   a. Patient can get on the commode with the amount of assistance provided.
   b. Patient can urinate or defecate using the commode.
   c. No adverse outcomes were encountered.
6. Plan a specific procedure for getting the patient out of bed, using the guidelines described in Module 18. Get additional personnel if indicated. **R:** Planning ahead allows you to proceed more safely and effectively.

IMPLEMENTATION

Action	Rationale
7. Place the bedside commode at the foot of the patient's bed.	To provide for smoother transfer from bed to commode.
8. Wash or disinfect your hands.	To prevent the spread of microorganisms.
9. Identify the patient using two identifiers.	Verifying the patient's identity helps to ensure that this patient is permitted to get out of bed.
10. Tell the patient how you plan to proceed.	Explaining the procedure helps to decrease the patient's apprehension and may facilitate patient participation.
11. Pull the curtains around the bed.	To provide privacy.

(continued)

Action	Rationale
12. Assist the patient out of bed, using proper transfer techniques and body mechanics. Help him or her pivot onto the commode.	To promote safety for the patient and the nurse.
13. Cover the patient's legs with a bath blanket or sheet.	This is for privacy and comfort.
14. Place the call light and toilet tissue within the patient's reach.	To prevent the patient from falling while seeking assistance or reaching needed items.
15. Leave the patient alone, allowing adequate time for elimination.	To respect privacy during elimination.
16. Return to the bedside, and put on clean gloves.	To prevent the spread of microorganisms.
17. Assist the patient in cleaning the perineal area if necessary.	Cleaning reduces odor and irritation to skin.
18. Assist the patient back to bed as needed.	To promote safety with regard to the patient's ability to ambulate.
19. Move the commode to the bathroom, remove the sliding container, and observe and measure or properly dispose of contents.	This is done in the bathroom for odor control and aesthetics. Observation and measurement contributes to assessment.
20. Wash or disinfect your hands.	To decrease the transfer of microorganisms that could cause infection.

EVALUATION

21. Evaluate using the individualized patient outcomes previously identified. **R:** Evaluation in relation to desired outcomes is essential for planning future care needs.
    a. Patient was able to get on the commode with the amount of assistance provided.
    b. Patient was able to urinate or defecate using the commode.
    c. No adverse outcomes were encountered.

DOCUMENTATION

22. Document any problems encountered, such as dizziness, a drop in blood pressure, or discomfort from sitting on a hard surface, in the nursing notes. Record output if indicated. Indicate bowel movement on the correct flow sheet. Describe urine and/or stool appearance if abnormal. **R:** Proper documentation of observations may assist in identifying a patient's diagnosis if abnormalities are noticed.

SPECIFIC PROCEDURE FOR GIVING PERINEAL CARE

In the clinical setting, this procedure is sometimes called "pericare." People who are immobilized or ill may have an increased need for perineal care or will need assistance with it. When ill, the body's defenses against infection may be weakened or impaired, and unless perineal hygiene is meticulous, urinary tract infections can occur. This is especially true if the patient is incontinent or has an indwelling urinary **catheter.** If not promptly removed, urine or feces on the skin of the incontinent patient can result in skin breakdown and infection. The incontinent patient should have perineal care given after each urination and defecation. If the patient has a catheter in place, the catheter itself can be a means for microorganisms to travel upward into the bladder and cause a urinary tract infection. For this reason, patients who have an indwelling catheter should have meticulous perineal care at least every 8 hours. The nurse may provide perineal care to any patient who is assessed as needing it without an order.

ASSESSMENT

1. Determine the condition of the patient's skin and the extent of soiling of the perineal area. **R:** To provide a baseline assessment for planning.
2. Identify the patient's capability. **R:** To determine the amount of assistance that he or she will need with perineal care.

ANALYSIS

3. Critically think through all data, carefully evaluating each aspect and its relation to other data. **R:** To enable you to determine specific problems for this individual in relation to the need for special perineal care.
4. Identify specific problems and modifications of the procedure needed for this individual. **R:** To determine modifications before beginning the procedure.

PLANNING

5. Determine individualized patient outcomes in relation to perineal care. **R:** Identifying outcomes facilitates evaluation.

   a. Perineal area is clean and odor-free.
   b. Patient reports feeling comfortable.
   c. Patient exhibits no areas of redness or tenderness or other adverse outcomes.
6. Plan and select the appropriate equipment needed to perform perineal care. **R:** The equipment used will vary with the needs and problems of the patient receiving care.
   a. Postpartum or surgical patient: bedpan, disposable waterproof pad, plastic peri-bottle or pitcher, tap water or antiseptic solution, cotton balls, gauze squares or "wipes," clean pad or dressing
   b. Nonsurgical patient: disposable waterproof pad, washcloth and towel, mild soap or cleansing agent
   c. Patient with a catheter: Wash around the catheter insertion site with soap and water and rinse thoroughly. Special cleaning procedures are not indicated (Garner, 1996).
7. Decide if you will need additional personnel to assist. **R:** To maintain the safety of the patient and the nurse.

IMPLEMENTATION

Action	Rationale
8. Wash or disinfect your hands.	This decreases the transfer of microorganisms that could cause infection.
9. Identify the patient, using two identifiers.	Verifying the patient's identity helps ensure that you are performing the right skill for the right patient.
10. Pull the curtains around the bed, close the door, and drape the patient as indicated.	Decreasing exposure maintains the patient's modesty and shows respect for the patient's privacy.
11. Explain what you plan to do. Use words the patient understands, such as "washing your genital area" or "washing between your legs." Proceed in a professional manner.	To minimize the embarrassment of the patient by clear and respectful communication.
12. Raise the bed to an appropriate working position based on your height.	This allows you to use correct body mechanics and protect yourself from back injury.
13. Put on clean gloves.	To protect you from body fluids.
14. Cleanse the perineum.	
a. Postpartum or surgical patients: If the patient is able to ambulate to the bathroom, patient may sit on toilet and pour warm water over perineum into toilet.	This allows the warm water to cleanse the perineum and drain into the toilet.

(continued)

Action	Rationale
b. However, if patient is unable to ambulate to the bathroom	
(1) Remove dressing or pads, and dispose of them according to facility policy (usually by placing in a waste bag or plastic bag and depositing in a biohazard container).	To protect the staff from body fluids.
(2) Place a waterproof pad under the patient, and position the bedpan according to the procedure "Assisting With a Bedpan."	The waterproof pad will protect the bed linens, and the bedpan will collect the solution poured over the perineum.
(3) Do not spread the **labia** of the female patient.	Spreading the labia may allow solution to enter the vagina and lead to infection.
(4) Pour tepid tap water or the solution used in your facility over the perineum (Fig 8-7).	The warm water will cleanse the perineum and drain into the bedpan. **FIGURE 8-7** Giving perineal care by pouring water over the perineum.
(5) Rinse with clear water.	Clear water removes soap residue that may be an irritant.
(6) Using cotton balls, gauze, or wipes, wipe gently from anterior (front) to posterior (back), using each one for only one wipe and then discarding. Use extra gauze, cotton balls, or wipes as needed.	Wiping in this direction lessens the possibility of contamination of the urinary tract from the rectal area. Wiping gently prevents pain and pressure on sutures (stitches). Using each cotton ball for only one wipe prevents contamination.
(7) Discard used cotton balls, gauze, or wipes in a waste bag, not the bedpan.	To prevent contamination.
(8) Replace any dressings or pads.	This is for infection control and absorption of drainage.

(continued)

Action	Rationale
c. Nonsurgical patients:	
(1) After placing a waterproof pad under the patient, wash the perineum, using warm water and mild soap and a washcloth.	The waterproof pad will protect the bed linens. Perfumed soap may increase the chances of skin irritation.
(2) Gently separate the labia of the female patient, and clean from front to back on one side using a downward motion. Change areas of washcloth used, and repeat the cleansing stroke on the other side. Repeat as needed. Rinse.	Wiping in this direction lessens the possibility of contamination of the urinary tract from the rectal area. Changing areas of the washcloth prevents cross-contamination. Cleaning removes secretions and **smegma** (an odorous collection of desquamated epithelial cells and mucus), which can build up in this area.
(3) For the male patient, clean beginning with the penile head, and move downward along the shaft (Fig. 8-8). Retract the **foreskin** of the uncircumcised male gently.	Retracting the foreskin allows removal of the smegma that collects under the foreskin and therefore decreases bacterial growth. **FIGURE 8-8** Male perineal care.
(4) Cleanse and rinse the area. Replace the foreskin over the head of the penis when completed.	Replacing the foreskin prevents constriction of the penis, which could cause pain and edema.
(5) Spread the legs, and gently wash the scrotum.	The scrotum is cleaned after the penis because it is closer to the rectum.
(6) Assist the patient to turn away from you. Using another area of the washcloth, clean the anal area. Rinse the area, and dry it well.	Use another area of the washcloth to avoid cross-contamination. Leaving soap on the skin can cause skin irritation. Moisture supports the growth of microorganisms.
d. For patients with a catheter:	
(1) Wash the perineal area thoroughly with soap and warm water. Clean well around the entire insertion site.	To remove secretions and microbial buildup.
(2) Rinse with clear water.	To prevent irritation of the mucosa by soap residue.

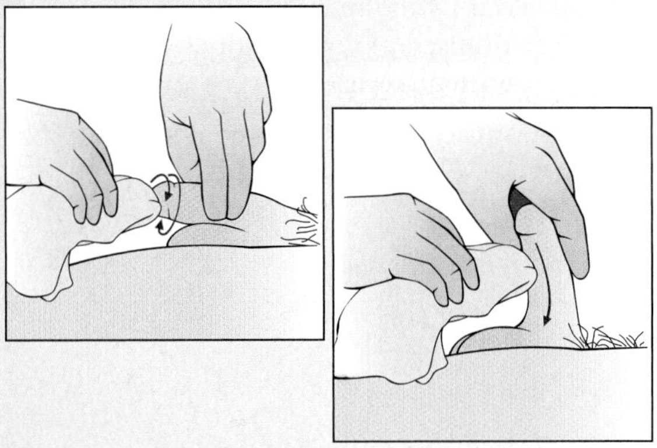

(continued)

Action	Rationale
15. Remove the bedpan, and discard the contents.	To facilitate disposal of body secretions.
16. Replace the bed linens, reposition the patient, and lower the bed.	This is for comfort and safety.
17. Care for equipment appropriately.	Proper care and storage of equipment is cost-effective.
18. Remove gloves, and wash or disinfect your hands.	To prevent the spread of microorganisms.

EVALUATION

19. To plan future care needs, evaluate in terms of the individualized outcome criteria:
    a. Perineal area is clean and odor-free.
    b. Patient reports feeling comfortable.
    c. Patient has no areas of redness or tenderness or other adverse outcomes.

DOCUMENTATION

20. Perineal care is usually documented on a flow sheet. Also record in the narrative notes any pertinent observations, such as residual redness or tenderness of the area, and any unusual drainage (appearance and amount). Any difficulties with carrying out the procedure should be noted on the nursing care plan. **R:** Documentation is a legal record of the patient's care and therapy and communicates nursing activities to other nurses and caregivers.

POTENTIAL ADVERSE OUTCOMES AND RELATED INTERVENTIONS

1. Perineal area is reddened, inflamed, or painful.
Intervention: Report to physician. Do not use any soaps or creams until the area is examined.
2. Patient complains of itching and discomfort in perineal area that was not present previously.
Intervention: Notify physician. Discontinue use of soaps and creams until area is examined.

Long-Term Care

Depending on the limitations of the resident in the long-term care facility, you may have to meet his or her elimination needs by supplying and being able to help with a bedpan, urinal, or bedside commode. Urinary incontinence is often observed in residents with decreased mobility or cognitive levels. Skin care is a primary concern. Often elderly residents are thin with bony prominences near the skin surface. Sharp and hard edges of bedpans may need padding. Older residents may need additional time to urinate or defecate, and you must provide this for successful elimination. Due to decreased bladder muscle tone, responding quickly to a resident's request for elimination is essential.

Persons of advanced age may also be more modest than younger people, so you must also take this into consideration. Accurately assessing the resident, regardless of age, and providing the most appropriate means for elimination is a nursing challenge in long-term care. Perineal care is very important because chronically ill persons may have less reserve to fight off urinary tract infections. A great number of these infections could be prevented with frequent and meticulous care. Should an elderly resident have difficulty with incontinence, many products are available to assist with this problem.

Acute Care

Patients in the acute care setting rely on caregivers to assist them with many hygienic and elimination needs. Often the patient is discharged from the hospital after surgery or an illness and still requires assistance with these daily tasks. The nurse must consider the patient's physical and mental status and include these needs in discharge planning and instructions provided to families and patients.

Home Care

The person being cared for in the home may temporarily or permanently use a bedpan, urinal, or a bedside commode. Bedpans and urinals are inexpensive to buy or may be covered by health insurance. Some home care agencies supply these items. Commodes may be purchased or rented from a medical supply company. Regardless of the equipment used, your role may be that of teaching the care provider in the home the proper procedure and the adaptations that should be made on an individual basis. Giving perineal care may be seen as an invasion of privacy, so your instruction and support in having the care provider carry out this procedure are essential.

Ambulatory Care

Often people with varying types of incontinence isolate themselves socially, fearing an "accident" in public. Many commercial products, such as incontinence pads and pull-up briefs, are available today to assist people experiencing this problem. The nurse can familiarize clients with products and solutions for this problem. Treatment for incontinence is successful for many people and should be encouraged.

LEARNING TOOLS

DEVELOP YOUR BACKGROUND KNOWLEDGE

1. Review the specific Learning Outcomes.

2. Read the sections on elimination and perineal care in your assigned text.

3. Look up the Key Terms in the glossary.

4. Review this module and mentally practice the techniques described. Study so that you would be able to teach these skills to another person.

5. Think of your personal elimination habits and perineal care practices. If you were hospitalized, how would your personal habits be affected? How would you feel if a nurse had to help you with these components of care? How would you feel if the nurse were of the opposite sex?

DEVELOP YOUR SKILLS

In the practice setting
1. Become familiar with the various pieces of available equipment (different types of bedpans, urinals, commodes, perineal care kits).

2. Select a partner, and perform the following:
   a. Act as if you are an incapacitated patient. Without disrobing, have your partner place you on a bedpan.

   b. Remain on the bedpan for 3 minutes in a flat position, then for another 3 minutes in a sitting position.
   c. Have your partner remove the bedpan as though you were incapacitated.
   d. Describe your feelings about the experience.

3. Reverse roles, repeating a, b, c, and d.

4. Using a mannequin, go through the specific procedure for giving perineal care to each of the following:
   a. a postpartum or perineal surgical patient
   b. a nonsurgical patient
   c. a male patient
   d. a patient with an indwelling catheter

DEMONSTRATE YOUR SKILLS

In the clinical setting
1. With your instructor's supervision
   a. Place a patient on a bedpan, using both a lifting and a rolling method.
   b. Give a urinal to a male patient.
   c. Assist a patient to a bedside commode.
   d. Administer perineal care to a postpartum patient or perineal surgical patient, a nonsurgical patient, and a catheterized patient.

2. Evaluate your performance with your instructor.

CRITICAL THINKING EXERCISES

1. Sara Jones is 83 years old. She recently fell in her home and fractured her right hip. She underwent surgery yesterday for a total hip replacement. She has an indwelling catheter. The plans are to begin short periods of ambulation on the second postoperative day, which is today. Mrs. Jones will be discharged in a few days to her daughter's home for recovery and outpatient physical therapy. What assessment data will you need to develop a plan to meet her elimination needs? In meeting this need, what are your plans for Mrs. Jones as she progresses postoperatively? What discharge teaching will her daughter require?

2. Your patient, 89-year-old Robert Aston, has been somewhat confused at times. This afternoon, when you answer his call light, you find him with his lower leg draped over the side rail. He calls out, "Help me! I have to go to the bathroom, and I can't get out of bed!" Analyze the situation. Identify further assessment that is needed immediately. Outline your nursing actions, including the priority order in which you would undertake them. Predict future care needs, and develop a plan to meet this patient's elimination needs.

SELF-QUIZ
SHORT-ANSWER QUESTIONS

1. List three principles to be followed when assisting a patient with a bedpan or urinal.

   a. _____

   b. _____

   c. _____

2. Describe two methods for placing a patient on a bedpan.

   a. _____

   b. _____

3. Identify three categories of patients who may need special perineal care.

   a. _____

   b. _____

   c. _____

4. Describe the procedure for one of the three categories in question 3.

   _____

   _____

   _____

5. Why is all cleansing on the female patient's perineum done from front to back?

   _____

6. Why are infection control principles important when assisting a patient to a bedpan or when providing perineal care?

   _____

MULTIPLE CHOICE

_____ 7. The type of equipment used when assisting a patient with elimination is based on
   a. the patient's preference.
   b. what is available on the nursing unit.
   c. the nurse's preference in what type of equipment to use.
   d. the patient's health status.

_____ 8. When providing perineal care for a patient who had a baby by vaginal delivery, the procedure would include
   a. wiping from back to front.
   b. spreading the labia for better cleaning.
   c. using a new cotton ball or wipe for each stroke.
   d. placing the patient in the lithotomy position.

_____ 9. Infection control principles such as wearing gloves when assisting a patient with elimination or perineal care are important to follow because
   a. the perineal area has moist secretions that support microbes.
   b. they protect the patient from the danger of cross-contamination.
   c. often nurses do not wash their hands between patients.
   d. it is reassuring to the patient that a nurse wears gloves.

_____ 10. A bedside commode is used for a patient who
   a. is on bed rest.
   b. is physically unable to walk to a bathroom commode but able to be out of bed.
   c. shares a bathroom with other patients.
   d. is on intake and output, and the amount of urine must be strictly measured.

_____ 11. An abnormal finding or observation for a patient's urine or feces that requires further documentation would be
   a. urine that is yellow, straw-colored.
   b. stool that is brown, soft, formed.
   c. cloudy appearance of urine.
   d. odor to stool.

_____ 12. A fracture bedpan would be best for which of the following patients?
   a. A recently delivered postpartum patient
   b. A man who had open heart surgery
   c. A frail elderly woman from a nursing home admitted for poor nutrition and dehydration
   d. A middle-aged woman who is on bed rest following an ankle fracture sustained in a motor vehicle accident

Answers to the Self-Quiz questions appear in the back of the book.

Bedmaking and Therapeutic Beds

SKILLS INCLUDED IN THIS MODULE

Procedure for Making an Unoccupied Bed
Procedure for Making the Postoperative Bed
Procedure for Making an Occupied Bed

PREREQUISITE MODULES

Module 1	An Approach to Nursing Skills
Module 2	Documentation
Module 3	Basic Body Mechanics
Module 4	Basic Infection Control
Module 6	Moving the Patient in Bed and Positioning
Module 14	Nursing Physical Assessment

KEY TERMS

bedboard	plantar flexion
bed cradle	postoperative bed
edema	pressure ulcer
fanfolding	surgical bed
footboard	toe pleat
footdrop	trochanter roll
mitered corners	

OVERALL OBJECTIVES

▸ To make beds that are both safe and comfortable for patients in healthcare settings.
▸ To use special mattresses, therapeutic frames, and beds effectively and safely, with emphasis on physical aspects of care.

LEARNING OUTCOMES

The student will be able to

1. Assess the patient and type of bed to determine the appropriate bedmaking procedure.
2. Analyze assessment data to address special problems and concerns and specific equipment that must be utilized to complete appropriate bedmaking procedures.
3. Determine appropriate patient outcomes of bedmaking, special equipment, and any therapeutic bed or mattress modifications, and recognize the potential for adverse outcomes.
4. Determine the appropriate bedmaking procedure and any modifications to the process.
5. Complete the appropriate bedmaking technique, utilizing appropriate body mechanics and safety for the nurse and the patient.
6. Evaluate the effectiveness of the bedmaking procedure, any special equipment, and any therapeutic beds or mattresses utilized for the patient.
7. Document the bedmaking procedure and use of any special equipment or a therapeutic bed or mattress.

BEDMAKING

The bed is one of the most important parts of the patient's environment in the healthcare setting. Knowing how to make various types of beds and how to modify them for special situations is important for the nurse. A clean, wrinkle-free bed that remains intact when a patient moves helps the patient's physical and psychological comfort. The bed becomes the center of activity for all care should a patient be confined to bed for an extended period of time.

NURSING DIAGNOSES

Nursing diagnoses relate to the activity level and safety issues when changing the bed for a patient. Examples are

- Risk for Impaired Skin Integrity related to wrinkled or soiled linens, prolonged immobility, or inability to move
- Risk for Infection related to linen soiled with urine, stool, or wound drainage

INFECTION CONTROL IN BEDMAKING

Apply these principles of basic infection control to all bedmaking procedures:

- Microorganisms move through space on air currents; therefore, handle linen carefully. Avoid shaking it or tossing it into the laundry hamper. (It should be placed in the hamper.)
- Microorganisms are transferred from one surface to another whenever one object touches another.

Therefore, hold both soiled and clean linen away from your uniform to prevent contamination of the clean linen by the uniform and contamination of the uniform by the soiled linen. In addition, avoid placing it on the floor to prevent the spread of any bacteria present either on the linen or on the floor.

- Proper handwashing or disinfection removes many of the microorganisms that would be transferred by the hands from one item to another. Therefore, wash or disinfect your hands before you begin and after you finish bedmaking. Observe Standard Precautions (Module 4 and Appendix A) for infection control throughout these procedures for your own protection as well as that of the patient.
- Wear clean gloves when removing linens soiled with urine, feces, or wound drainage to carry out Standard Precautions (see Box 9-1).

BODY MECHANICS IN BEDMAKING

Apply these principles of body mechanics to all bedmaking procedures:

- A person or an object is more stable if the center of gravity is close to the base of support. Therefore, when you must bend, bend your knees, not your back, to keep the center of gravity directly above and close to the base of support and to help prevent fatigue (Fig. 9-1).
- Facing in the direction of the task to be performed and turning the entire body in one plane (rather than twisting) lessens the susceptibility of the back to injury. Therefore, face your entire body in the direction that you are moving and avoid twisting to prevent back strain or injury.

---

box 9-1   *Infection Control in Bedmaking*

1. Handle linen carefully; do not shake linen; place in hamper.
2. Hold both soiled and clean linen away from your uniform.
3. Wash or disinfect hands before and after bedmaking.
4. Wear gloves to handle linens soiled with body substances, such as urine, feces, vomitus, or drainage.

---

box 9-2   *Body Mechanics in Bedmaking*

1. When you must bend, bend your knees, not your back.
2. Face your entire body in the direction in which you are moving and avoid twisting.
3. Organize your work to conserve steps.
4. Raise the bed to an appropriate height.

- There is less strain on the lower back if you work at waist level height than if you stoop or stretch to reach the surface. Therefore, raise the bed to an appropriate level for your own height for maximum working safety and comfort.
- Fatigue increases the potential for musculoskeletal injury. Decrease energy expenditure by using smooth, rhythmical movements at moderate speed. Organize your work to make as few trips around the bed as possible (see Box 9-2).

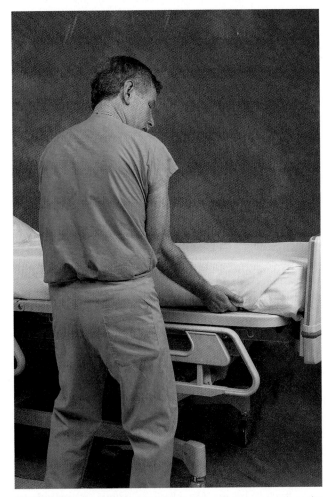

FIGURE 9-1 Correct posture for bedmaking. The nurse bends at the knees, not the back, to keep the center of gravity directly above and close to the base of support.

PROCEDURE FOR MAKING AN UNOCCUPIED BED

ASSESSMENT

1. Assess the patient and the patient's ability to get out of bed during the change of linens. **R:** To determine whether there are factors present (fatigue or pain, for example) that may affect the patient's ability to be out of bed during the bedmaking procedure.
2. Assess the condition of the linen on the bed for soiling or moisture. **R:** To determine which linens need to be replaced or added to complete the bedmaking procedure and to determine the need for gloves.

ANALYSIS

3. Critically think through your data, carefully evaluating each aspect and its relation to other data. **R:** To determine if there are any specific problems regarding making the bed.
4. Identify any problems or special needs that might require extra linen or special equipment for this individual in making the bed. **R:** Planning for the individual requires specific needs to be addressed in procedure.

PLANNING

5. Plan for individualized outcomes for bedmaking and the patient. **R:** Identifying outcomes facilitates evaluation.
   a. Bed has smooth, wrinkle-free surface; tight corners.
   b. Bed correctly positioned (high or low) for the patient's needs.
   c. Call signal attached in appropriate place.
   d. Patient resting comfortably.
6. Gather the linen to be used and place it in order, so that the first item to be used will be on the bottom, the second item next, and so on. Once the linen is gathered, turn the stack over. Items can include the following. **R:** Choose only those items that need to be changed. Remember that preventing excessive use and laundering is part of cost containment in the healthcare environment. Linen placed in order of use promotes efficient use of time. The laundry

hamper prevents environmental contamination from soiled linens.

a. mattress pad

b. bottom sheet (most facilities have fitted bottom sheets)

c. cloth or disposable moisture proof pads (may be optional)

d. one cloth drawsheet (turn or pull sheet); a top sheet folded in half may be used in some settings. The use of a drawsheet may be optional; use one if it is needed to assist with turning or if the patient has drainage or some other condition that may require more frequent linen changing.

It is much easier to change a drawsheet than an entire bottom sheet.

e. one top sheet

f. one blanket (optional)

g. one bedspread

h. one pillowcase for each pillow on the bed

i. laundry bag or hamper

7. Obtain any other needed items or equipment, such as extra pillows or a bed cradle and clean gloves if you will be handling linen soiled with body secretions. **R:** Gathering all equipment before beginning the procedure is more time efficient.

IMPLEMENTATION

Action	Rationale
8. Wash or disinfect your hands.	To decrease the transfer of microorganisms that could cause infection.
9. Raise the bed to an appropriate working height. Be certain the wheels are locked.	Allows you to use correct body mechanics and protects you from back strain. Locked wheels keep the bed from moving, thus preventing injury to the nurse.
10. Remove attached equipment (call light, waste bag, personal items). Place side rails in the down position.	To prevent linen from being torn and personal items from being lost. Having side rails in the down position promotes working comfort for the nurse and prevents strain from reaching over the side rails.
11. Put on gloves before handling linen soiled with body secretions.	To prevent the spread of microorganisms.
12. Remove cases from pillows, and place the pillows on a chair or bedside table	Placing pillows on a clean surface will prevent contamination.
13. Loosen the top and the bottom linen from the mattress, moving around the bed from head to foot on one side and from foot to head on the opposite side.	Loosening linen and moving around the bed prevents muscle strain from reaching across the bed.
14. Remove any clean items to be reused (spread, blankets, sheets) one at a time. Fold each in quarters, and place across the back of a chair.	Folding the linen saves time and energy when reapplying.
15. Remove the remaining linen, and place it in a laundry hamper. If you put on gloves to handle linen soiled with body secretions, remove them, and wash or disinfect your hands before touching any clean items.	Soiled linen has potential for spreading microorganisms to whatever surface it touches. Proper disposal of contaminated gloves prevents spreading microorganisms.
16. Wash or disinfect your hands after handling the soiled bed linens.	To prevent spread of microorganisms.

(continued)

Action	Rationale
17. If your facility uses fitted sheets, first fit diagonal corners over the mattress.	This facilitates getting the corners in place. A fitted sheet stays in place effectively.
18. If your facility uses flat sheets, place a bottom sheet on the bed, with the center fold at the center of the bed, the lower hem even with the edge of the mattress at the foot of the bed, and the seam toward the mattress. Spread the sheet over the bed, tucking it under at the head of the bed using **mitered,** or square, **corners**. See Figure 9-2 for instructions on mitering a corner. A square corner is a modification of that technique with step A modified so that the sheet is picked up to form a 45-degree angle so that when the folded edge is placed on the top of the mattress before tucking, it is even with the bottom edge of the mattress.	Tucking the sheet at the top of the bed keeps it securely in place. A mitered, or square, corner remains tucked better and appears neater.
19. Tuck the remainder of the sheet under the side of the mattress all the way to the foot of the bed, pulling it tightly toward the bottom of the bed as you go to create a smooth surface.	Bottom linens that are free of wrinkles prevent unneeded pressure areas on the skin.
20. Place the cloth drawsheet with its center fold in the center of the bed so that it will be under the patient's midsection. If needed, add a cloth moisture-proof or disposable pad on top of the drawsheet. Tuck the drawsheet under the mattress. Fanfold the sheet toward the far side.	Should soiling occur, the bottom linens are protected, and only the disposable pad would need to be changed, saving time. A drawsheet can also be used as an aid in turning a patient in bed. Fanfolding facilitates extending the sheet across the bed.
21. Place the top sheet on the bed with the center fold at the center of the bed, seam side up. Align the top edge of the sheet with the top edge of the mattress. Unfold it toward the far side of the bed.	Shaking linens will spread organisms into the air.
22. Make a **toe pleat** (optional—follow the procedure at your clinical facility) by folding a 2-inch pleat across the sheet about 6 to 8 inches from the foot of the bed. Tuck the end of the sheet under the mattress.	To prevent impingement of the top linen on the patient's toes.
23. If a blanket is needed for additional warmth, place it on the bed with the fold at the center of the bed, so that the top edge of the blanket is about 6 inches from the top of the mattress. Unfold the blanket	To promote patient comfort.

(continued)

Action	*Rationale*

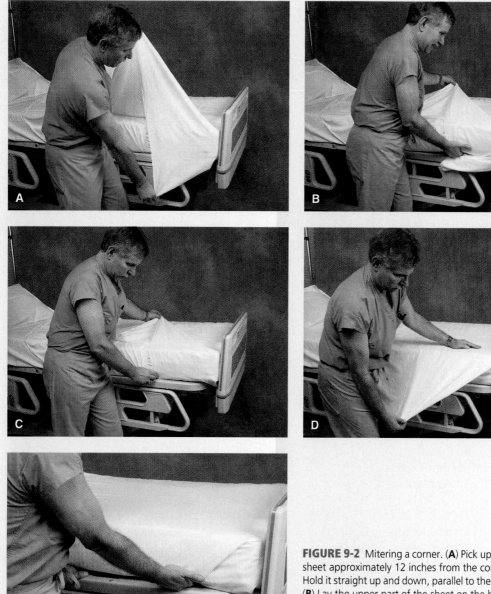

FIGURE 9-2 Mitering a corner. (**A**) Pick up the side edge of the sheet approximately 12 inches from the corner of the mattress. Hold it straight up and down, parallel to the side of the mattress. (**B**) Lay the upper part of the sheet on the bed, and (**C**) tuck the part of the sheet that is hanging below the mattress smoothly under the mattress. (**D**) Holding the sheet in place against the mattress with one hand, use your other hand to lift the folded part of the sheet lying on the bed and bring it down. (**E**) Tuck the remaining sheet firmly under the mattress.

Action	*Rationale*
toward the far side of the bed. In warm weather, or at the patient's request, omit the blanket, or if the patient is cold, use additional blankets. Blankets may be left at the bedside to be added as needed.	
24. Place the bedspread on the bed, with the center fold at the center of the bed. The top edge of the spread should be about 6 inches from the top of the mattress.	To keep the top linen in place.

(continued)

Action	Rationale
Unfold the remainder of the spread toward the far side of the bed. Tuck all three—top sheet, blanket, and spread—together, using a mitered, or square, corner. Some nurses may prefer to tuck each one separately. Either way is appropriate, according to the preference of the nurse.	
25. Miter the corner of the top linen at the foot of the bed. Do not tuck in the upper portion; allow it to hang down smoothly and freely.	To allow free movement of the patient into and out of bed.
26. Move to the other side of the bed. Pull the bottom linen smoothly and tightly across the mattress, and tuck the bottom sheet under the head of the mattress and make a mitered, or square, corner.	To save time and energy by completing one side and then moving to the other.
27. Tuck the bottom sheet along the side of the bed, pulling toward you and slightly toward the bottom of the bed to make the sheet tight as you move toward the foot of the bed.	To create a smooth, comfortable surface for the patient.
28. Pull the center of the drawsheet (if present) toward you. Tuck it under the mattress, as snugly as possible. Grasp the top corner of the drawsheet, pull it diagonally, and tuck it under the mattress snugly. Repeat this activity with the lower corner of the drawsheet.	To obtain an absolutely wrinkle-free surface.
29. Straighten and smooth the top sheet, blanket, and spread, starting at the top of the bed and moving toward the foot of the bed. Tuck the linens under the foot of the mattress. Miter the corners at the foot of the bed either together or one at a time.	Mitered, or square, corners keep the linen secure.
30. Fold the top sheet back over the top edge of the blanket and the spread. If there is more spread than blanket at the top of the bed, fold the excess spread back over the blanket to form an even line. Then fold the top sheet over as described.	
a. *Closed bed:* The upper edge of the spread is left even with the upper edge of the mattress to designate a closed bed.	In healthcare facilities, this may only be done when no patient is assigned to the bed. In long-term care facilities, the bed is usually closed during the day.

(continued)

Action	Rationale
b. *Open bed*: Opening a bed is usually done by grasping the upper edge of the top linen with both hands, bringing it all the way to the foot of the bed, then folding it back toward the center of the bed. This is known as **fanfolding** (Fig. 9-3).	If beds are left open, it is easier to assist patients back to bed when they are ready. Open beds are usually made for patients who are up for a brief period in the room or out of the unit, perhaps for X-ray or laboratory procedures, but who are expected to spend much of the time in bed.

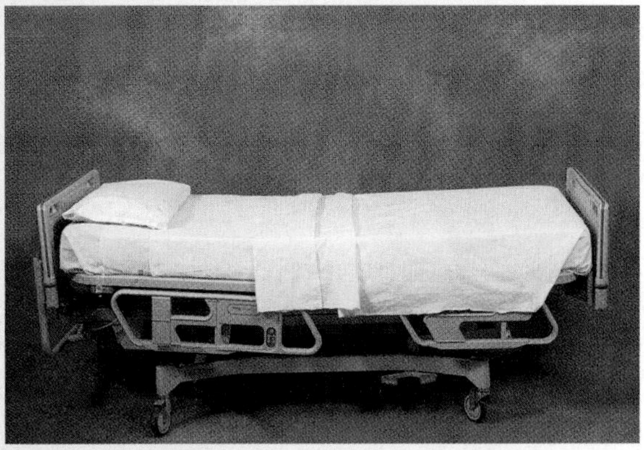

FIGURE 9-3 The open bed, with top linen fanfolded back, is ready for the patient.

Action	Rationale
31. Put a pillowcase on the pillow without shaking the pillow. One way to do this is as follows:	Shaking linens causes organisms to be carried on air currents.
a. Grasp the pillowcase at the center of the closed end of the case (Fig. 9-4).	
b. Gather the case up over that hand and grasp the zipper, or open end of the pillow cover, with the same hand, pulling the case down over the pillow with the other hand.	
c. Straighten and smooth the case over the pillow, and place it at the head of the bed with the open end away from the door (for neater appearance).	
d. Keep the pillow and case away from your uniform as you apply the case.	
32. Replace the call light in an appropriate place, and leave the bed in the low position, ready for the patient who will be returning to the bed from a chair or a walk. If the patient will be returning to bed from a stretcher, leave the bed in the high position.	This promotes patient safety when the patient is getting into bed and eases strain on the person transferring the patient from a stretcher to the bed.

(continued)

Action	*Rationale*

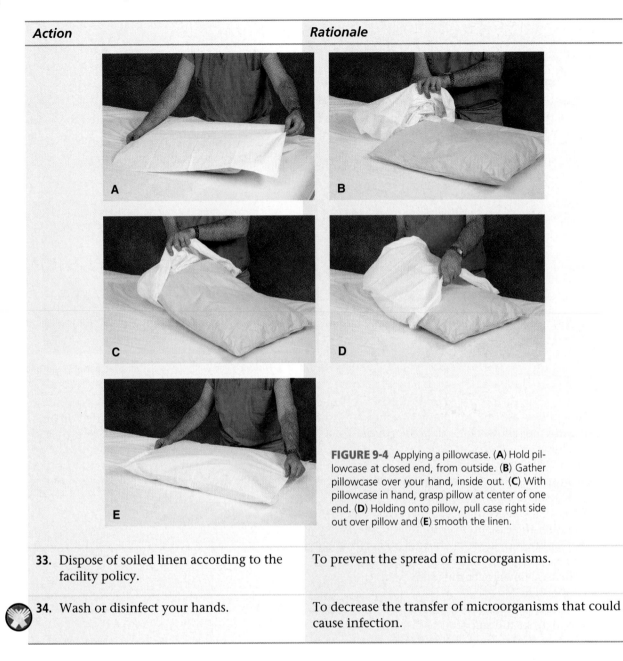

FIGURE 9-4 Applying a pillowcase. (**A**) Hold pillowcase at closed end, from outside. (**B**) Gather pillowcase over your hand, inside out. (**C**) With pillowcase in hand, grasp pillow at center of one end. (**D**) Holding onto pillow, pull case right side out over pillow and (**E**) smooth the linen.

Action	*Rationale*
33. Dispose of soiled linen according to the facility policy.	To prevent the spread of microorganisms.
34. Wash or disinfect your hands.	To decrease the transfer of microorganisms that could cause infection.

EVALUATION

35. Evaluate the unoccupied bed, using the individualized outcomes previously identified: Smooth, wrinkle-free surface and tight corners; correct position (high or low) for the patient's needs; and call signal attached in appropriate place; patient resting comfortably. **R:** Evaluation in relation to desired outcomes is essential for planning future care needs.

DOCUMENTATION

36. Linen changes are not routinely documented, but the tolerance of the patient's being out of bed might be recorded.

PROCEDURE FOR MAKING THE POSTOPERATIVE BED

The **postoperative bed** is also called the **surgical bed** or anesthetic bed. It is made so that the patient can be transferred from a stretcher to the bed with a minimum of motion and discomfort, then covered with the top linen, including the blanket, which is easily within reach, to prevent chilling (Fig. 9-5).

ASSESSMENT

1. Follow step 1 of the Procedure for Making an Unoccupied Bed: Assess the activity orders for the patient.

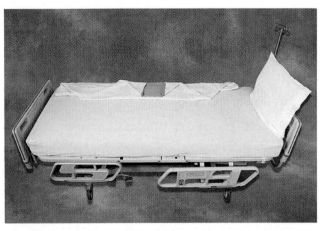

FIGURE 9-5 Postoperative bed. Top sheet, blanket, and spread are fanfolded lengthwise for convenient transfer from stretcher to bed.

ANALYSIS

3-4. Follow steps 3 and 4 of the Procedure for Making the Unoccupied Bed: Think through your data, and identify specific problems and modifications.

PLANNING

5. Determine individualized outcomes for the postoperative bed:
    a. smooth, wrinkle-free surface; tight corners
    b. bed in high position for transferring the patient from the stretcher
    c. call signal attached in appropriate place
    d. patient is transferred into the bed with ease
    e. items needed for patient care immediately after transfer are available

6-7. Follow steps 6 and 7 of the Procedure for Bedmaking: Gather the linen and supplies needed for postoperative care.

2. Consult the patient record regarding the type of surgery the patient is having. **R:** This is to determine the need for any special equipment.

IMPLEMENTATION

Action	Rationale
8-22. Follow steps 8 to 22 of the Procedure for Making an Unoccupied Bed: Wash or disinfect your hands, raise the bed to an appropriate height, put on gloves if needed, remove soiled linen, place soiled linen in laundry hamper, replace bottom sheet with mitered corners, and place top linen on bed.	To decrease the transfer of microorganisms that could cause infection.
23. Complete the top linens as you would for a closed bed, but do not tuck the linens at the foot of the bed. Fold top edges of linen over, and fold the linen from the foot of the bed up toward the center of the bed. Fanfold the top linen to the far side of the bed in a triangular pattern (see Fig. 9-5).	To allow easy transfer of the patient into the bed and the placement of linens over the patient once in the bed.
24. Place each pillow in a pillowcase. Place pillow(s) on a table or chair.	To allow easier transfer of patient into bed without any obstacles.
25. Leave the bed in the high position to receive the patient.	High position facilitates easier movement from the stretcher to the bed.
26. Have equipment readily available: emesis basin, tissues, IV stand, call lights, and any other items indicated according to the type of surgery the patient has had.	Patients usually return with intravenous fluids running, may have some nausea from anesthesia, and may need specialized equipment based on the surgery. Having necessary items readily available facilitates postoperative care.

EVALUATION

27. Evaluate using the individualized outcomes previously identified: smooth, wrinkle-free surface, tight corners, bed in high position for transferring the patient from the stretcher, call signal attached in appropriate place, patient transferred into the bed with ease, and items needed for patient care immediately after transfer are available.

DOCUMENTATION

28. The linen change is usually not specifically included in documentation but is part of the overall hygiene.

PROCEDURE FOR MAKING AN OCCUPIED BED

There are many instances in which a bed must be wholly or partially made with a patient in it. In most cases, this is because the patient is too ill or disabled to get out of bed. When making an occupied bed, keep the patient's safety and comfort foremost in your mind, and take care to avoid bumping the bed or exposing the patient. If the patient cannot participate, you may need another staff member to assist you. The order of activities remains the same; the procedure differs from making an unoccupied bed only because a patient is in the bed (Fig. 9-6).

ASSESSMENT

1. Check the orders. **R:** To verify whether the patient must stay in bed, whether there are restrictions related to position (such as do not adduct leg), or whether a specific position must be maintained (such as the head of bed elevated 30 degrees).

2. Assess the patient to identify any factors (such as fatigue, shortness of breath, or pain, for example) that might affect the ability of the patient to undergo the bedmaking activity. **R:** To determine whether the patient can participate in bedmaking at this time.

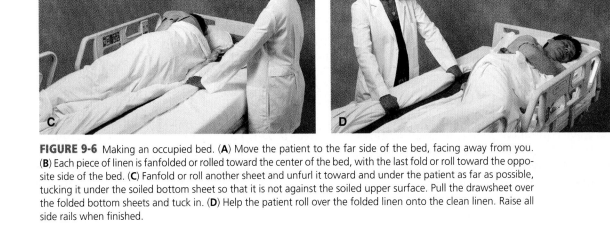

FIGURE 9-6 Making an occupied bed. (**A**) Move the patient to the far side of the bed, facing away from you. (**B**) Each piece of linen is fanfolded or rolled toward the center of the bed, with the last fold or roll toward the opposite side of the bed. (**C**) Fanfold or roll another sheet and unfurl it toward and under the patient as far as possible, tucking it under the soiled bottom sheet so that it is not against the soiled upper surface. Pull the drawsheet over the folded bottom sheets and tuck in. (**D**) Help the patient roll over the folded linen onto the clean linen. Raise all side rails when finished.

ANALYSIS

3-4. Follow steps 3 and 4 of the Procedure for Making an Unoccupied Bed: Think through your data, and identify specific problems and modifications required for the bedmaking procedure.

PLANNING

5. Determine individualized outcomes for the occupied bed and the patient. **R:** Identifying outcomes facilitates evaluation.

a. patient comfortable
b. bed has smooth, wrinkle-free surface
c. bed linens tightly tucked in
d. side rails in correct position
e. bed in the low position for safety
f. call signal and other personal items within patient's reach.

6-7. Follow steps 6 and 7 of the Procedure for Bedmaking: Gather the linen and supplies.

IMPLEMENTATION

Action	Rationale
8-14. Follow steps 8 to 14 of the Procedure for Making an Unoccupied Bed: Wash or disinfect your hands, raise the bed to an appropriate height, remove the attached equipment and place side rails in the down position, put on gloves if handling linen soiled with body secretions, loosen the top and bottom linen from the mattress, remove and fold the bedspread and blanket(s), and put them aside to be reused.	
15. Place a bath blanket over the sheet. Have the patient hold the top edge of the blanket while you remove the sheet from under the blanket. Discard the top sheet.	The bath blanket will provide warmth and respect the privacy of the patient.
16. Elicit the patient's help, and roll the patient to the far side of the bed, making sure to move the pillow also. If possible, the patient should be side-lying, facing away from you. The side rail on the far side of the bed should be up.	To facilitate making the bed on one side. The side rail is up for the safety and comfort of the patient.
17. Loosen the foundation (bottom linen) of the bed on the near side.	To allow the removal of linens without tearing or pulling.
18. Fanfold or roll each piece of linen toward the center of the bed, with the last fold toward the opposite side of the bed and tucked under the patient's back and buttocks. If you put on gloves to handle linen soiled with body secretions, remove them, and wash or disinfect your hands before touching any clean linen.	Tucking linen facilitates reaching it later to pull to the opposite side. Removal of gloves is for infection control.
19. If a flat sheet is used, lay the bottom sheet lengthwise on the bed, and unfold it so	Clean linens are centered for easier pulling through to the opposite side.

(continued)

Action	Rationale
that the center fold of the sheet is at the center of the bed, the bottom hem is at the bottom edge of the mattress, and the top hem of the sheet is over the top of the mattress. Fanfold half the sheet lengthwise toward the center of the bed, allowing the other half to drape over the side toward you. Most agencies use a fitted sheet, so you would pull the sheet over the top and bottom corner on one side of the mattress.	
20. Place the fanfolded sheet under the patient as far as possible, tucking it under the soiled bottom sheet.	So that it is not against the soiled upper surface of the sheet.
21. Tuck the sheet under at the top, miter the top corner, and tuck it in along the side of the mattress to the foot of the bed.	Mitered, or square, corners allow the linen to remain tucked.
22. If a drawsheet is in use, unfold it at this point, pull it over the folded bottom sheets, and tuck it in snugly and smoothly.	Tucking sheets removes wrinkles and promotes comfort.
23. If a waterproof or disposable pad is being used, place it so that the center fold is at the center of the bed.	Centering the waterproof pad places the pad underneath the midsection or buttocks.
24. Help the patient roll over the folded linen toward you and onto the clean linen. Adjust the pillow. Put up the side rail.	To provide for safety and comfort.
25. Move to the other side of the bed. Lower the side rail.	To complete the bed on the opposite side.
26. Put on gloves if the used linen is soiled with body secretions. Loosen the bottom linen. Remove the soiled linen (bottom sheet and cloth drawsheet), and place it in a laundry hamper or bag. Remove gloves, and wash your hands before touching any clean items.	For infection control.
27. Pull the fanfolded bottom sheet, and any drawsheet (if used) out from under the patient. Straighten, pull, and tuck the bottom sheet as if making an unoccupied bed. Pull the sheet tight by bracing against the bed and pulling with both hands to make the sheet smooth and tight under the patient before tucking it.	To remove the wrinkles in the linen.

(continued)

Action	Rationale
28. If a drawsheet is being used, pull and tuck it as you did previously. Pull the waterproof or disposable pads in place under the patient's buttocks or midsection.	To remove the wrinkles in the linen.
29. Move the patient to the center of the bed in a comfortable position.	To provide for patient comfort.
30. Place the top sheet on the bed over the bath blanket. Remove the bath blanket, instructing the patient to hold the sheet as you pull the blanket from the top to the bottom. Place the bath blanket in the laundry hamper, or (if it is unsoiled and dry) fold it, and leave it in the patient's unit for future use.	To provide privacy.
31. Add the blanket and the spread as in the Procedure for Making the Unoccupied Bed, tucking the linens at the end of the bed and mitering the corners. Loosen the linens over the patient's feet, or make a toe pleat by making a fold in the linens and pulling toward the bottom of the bed.	Loosening the linens gives the patient's feet more room to move. Mitering the corners gives a neat appearance to the bed.
32. Remove the pillow, and put on a clean pillowcase. Put the pillow on the bed with the open end away from the door.	For cleanliness and aesthetic purposes.
33. Reattach the call light and any other equipment you removed.	For the patient's safety.
34. Place the bed in the low position, adjusting the side rails according to your facility's policies and the individual situation.	For the patient's safety.
35. Dispose of the soiled linen.	To prevent the spread of microorganisms.
36. Wash or disinfect your hands.	To decrease the transfer of microorganisms that could cause infection.

EVALUATION

37. Evaluate using the individualized outcomes previously identified: patient comfortable, smooth and wrinkle-free surface, linen with tight corners, side rails in correct position, bed in the low position for safety, and call signal and other personal items within patient's reach.

DOCUMENTATION

38. Document any assessment data or change in the patient's clinical status. Changing linens is not documented routinely but is part of the a.m. (morning) care.

ACCESSORIES FOR THE PATIENT ON BED REST

For patients who are confined to bed, comfort is essential for rest and sleep. Because the patient must be in the bed most of the time, the nurse is the person who must consider accessories that facilitate movement and items that prevent skin irritation and breakdown. You must constantly assess the physical status of the patient and determine what special equipment may be required to address the needs. The skin is the largest organ of the body and the first line of defense against infection, so keeping the skin healthy and in good physical status is of utmost importance.

PREVENTING FOOTDROP

Footdrop is an abnormal shortening of the Achilles tendon from a prolonged period of plantar flexion. Footdrop results in the patient's inability to walk normally and requires extensive physical therapy to correct.

A **footboard** may be used to keep the feet at right angles to the legs when the immobilized patient is in the supine position (lying flat on the back) in bed and prevent prolonged **plantar flexion**. The feet are positioned to rest firmly against the footboard and keep them in a functional position. Linen is tucked in around the footboard and is held up off the patient's feet. This prevents the top sheet, blanket, and spread from forcing the feet into plantar flexion. A footboard is only effective if the patient's feet are resting firmly against it. Footboard designs vary according to manufacturers. Often, if the patient is too short to reach the footboard, a footboot may be used (Fig. 9-7). A footboot, which holds the foot at a right angle, looks like a padded boot with interlooping fasteners.

High-top sneakers are also used to prevent plantar flexion. Footboots or high-top sneakers are more effec-

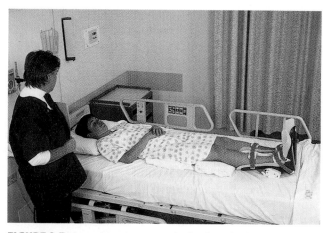

FIGURE 9-7 If a patient cannot use the footboard, a footboot may be used. This device is fastened by interlooping materials and holds the foot comfortably at a right angle to prevent footdrop.

tive than a footboard. The nurse must remember to remove the shoes periodically and provide good foot care. Foot and ankle splints to prevent plantar flexion are available, but these are costly and must be specially ordered for the individual patient. Both footboots and high-top sneakers are effective no matter what the patient's position: supine, prone, or side-lying.

PREVENTING PROLONGED EXTERNAL ROTATION OF THE HIP

When a person lies in a supine position, the hips tend to externally rotate, turning the legs so that the feet point outward. Prolonged external rotation of the hip can create changes in the ligaments that support the hip, making walking more difficult when the patient begins to walk again. A **trochanter roll** may be used to keep the hips from externally rotating. The nurse may place a rolled-up bath blanket or two bath towels at the patient's hip area or trochanter areas. These rolls support the joint and prevent external rotation. See Module 6 for more information about the trochanter roll.

BEDBOARD

A **bedboard** provides additional skeletal support and is used directly under a mattress over a flat spring. Usually bedboards are made of plywood or some other firm type of material. They are most often used with orthopedic patients or those who have a history of back problems. Some patients are simply more comfortable sleeping on a firm surface. Most modern beds in health-care facilities do not need a bedboard to create a firm surface because they are made with flat metal panels under the mattress. A bedboard may be needed in home care. If a bedboard is used on a hospital-type bed, it must have hinged portions to facilitate raising the head of the bed and the foot section.

BED CRADLE

A **bed cradle** is a device designed to keep the linen up off the feet and lower legs of patients, as in cases of **edema** (an accumulation of fluid causing swelling), leg ulcers, surgery on the lower extremities, and burns. There are several kinds of bed cradles, including one called the Anderson frame, which is a simple rod that arches over the bed and is held in place by the mattress (Fig. 9-8). Another type of cradle is a latticework arch. Place the device on the bed over the patient's legs and feet. Arrange the top linen over the device, and tape, clip, or pin it in place. Some facilities do not allow pinning because it can tear the linen. In these situations, linen must simply be tucked as securely as possible around the frame.

TRAPEZE

A trapeze is a triangular piece of metal hung by a chain from a frame over the bed. The patient reaches for the trapeze to lift the body and to move about in bed. A trapeze is most commonly used for the orthopedic patient who cannot use his or her legs and feet to move but has strength in the arms. See Module 22.

THERAPEUTIC BEDS AND MATTRESSES

A variety of special mattresses or mattress overlays are available to relieve pressure on the patient's skin and thus help prevent the formation of **pressure ulcers**. None of these mattresses or overlays takes the place of frequent turning of the patient and meticulous skin care.

MATTRESS OVERLAYS

Mattress overlays are placed over a standard hospital mattress. These items are made of foam, gel, air, or water. Some mattresses have pumps that work to increase and decrease pressure alternately. When making a bed that

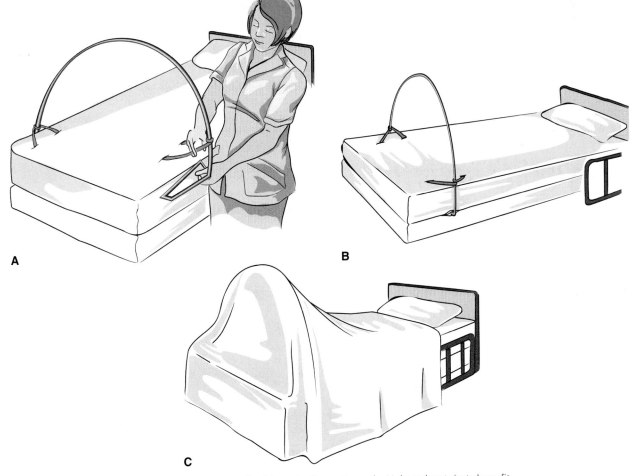

FIGURE 9-8 (**A**) The triangles at the base of the cradle slide under the mattress; the V-shaped parts just above fit over the top of the mattress. (**B**) The cradle in place. (**C**) The top linen is placed over the cradle to keep linen off the feet and legs.

has one or another of these types of mattress, do not tuck the linen tightly under the mattress. Doing so would prevent expansion, thereby defeating the purpose of the special mattress. The manufacturers of many of these special mattresses may recommend that draw-sheets and incontinent pads not be used with their products because the sheet or pad also interferes with the purpose of the mattress.

SPECIALTY BEDS

Patients are placed in specialty beds for a variety of problems including the prevention and treatment of pressure ulcers. Patients who suffer from multiple fractures, extensive burns, spinal cord injury, orthopedic conditions, malnutrition, intractable pain, or immobility may be placed on one of a number of special mattresses, mattress overlays, or therapeutic beds. The device selected varies with the problem of the patient and availability of the device, which is usually ordered by the physician after consultation with healthcare team members such as the wound, ostomy, continence nurse (WOCN) who specializes in wound care treatment; a physical therapist; or other specialists in skin care. See Figure 9-9 for an example of a special bed.

The nurse needs to know what type of mattress, frame, or bed is being used and why it is appropriate in a specific situation. It is also important to know the principles on which it operates and specific operating details, such as attachments or special linens or instructions for adjusting the bed for specific situations, e.g., a cardiopulmonary resuscitation (CPR) procedure.

New types of specialty beds are available to provide care for patients at risk for developing or with pressure

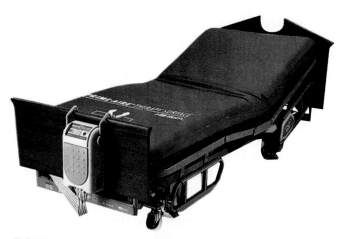

FIGURE 9-9 Primaire Therapy Surface or the First Step Tricell low-air-loss therapeutic mattress. (Courtesy of Hill-Rom Company, Inc.) or (KCI).

ulcers. These beds replace the usual hospital bed, according to the patient's needs and health status. Many of the new beds consider the safety of the nurse and the ease of transfer or position changes. Some beds can be changed into a sitting position for the patient. Bariatric beds are extra-wide for the obese patient and can accommodate weights up to 800 lb. Many critical care areas have beds providing a variety of functions and positions for the immobilized patient and for healthcare staff who must move and lift these patients. The foot of one such bed can become a chair. Another type of bed has a built-in scale; others have bed-exit alarms. In such cases, bed-making for these different beds may require adaptation to the specific bed type. See Table 9-1 for a description of various bed types.

table 9-1. Comparison of the Most Common Therapeutic Frames and Beds			
	Rotation Beds	**Air-Fluidized Bed**	**Static and Active Low-Air-Loss Beds**
Indications for Use	Treatment and prevention of pulmonary complications; mobilizes pulmonary secretions Treatment of wounds and pressure ulcers Used for postural drainage of severely injured patients and for prevention of the complications of immobility (pressure sores, hypostatic pneumonia, deep vein thrombosis, pulmonary embolus)	Used for patients with limited movement, intractable pain, pain with movement, skin flaps, and with significant skin breakdown or at high risk for breakdown	Used for patients with limited movement, pain with movement or handling, or at risk for skin breakdown; also treatment of pressure ulcers Used for patients with orthopedic problems, fractures, amputations, and spinal cord injury Active bed provides gentle pulsations or rotations side to side to promote removal of pulmonary secretions and stimulates circulation. Active uses: pneumonia or other pulmonary problems with skin integrity compromises, congestive heart failure, or massive edema

(continued)

table 9-1. Comparison of the Most Common Therapeutic Frames and Beds (Continued)

	Rotation Beds	Air-Fluidized Bed	Static and Active Low-Air-Loss Beds
Contraindications/ Disadvantages	Constant motion may exacerbate diarrhea and nausea. Bed should be protected, because it is hard to clean. Not for use with unstable cervical, thoracic, and/or lumbar fractures; cervical and/or skeletal traction; or severe agitation/uncontrollable claustrophobia Contraindications include not using percussion therapy for patients with multiple rib fractures, persistent intracranial hypertension, or during postoperative periods following cardiac surgery.	Not for patients with unstable spinal cord injury Constant circulation of warm, dry air may affect temperature and hydration status. Check patient closely. Difficult to elevate head Difficult to transfer patient May cause sagging at the hips Coughing may be inhibited by lack of firm surface. Bed is heavy, but Hill-Rom Services, Inc., has a home model that is safe to use in most homes and is 40% less heavy than institutional models.	Bed does not absorb fluids.
Caring for Equipment	Special linen is needed for bed section.	Special sheets needed The system should be cleaned every week and disinfected between patients.	Special sheets needed. The bed should be cleaned every week and disinfected between patients.
Special Care Techniques	Bed is in constant motion. Posterior hatches open to allow care of cervical, thoracic, and rectal areas. Traction apparatus available Be sure to close any posterior hatches opened while caring for patient.	"Fluidized" temperature-controlled air flows constantly around patient. Standard equipment: foam wedge, turn sheet, IV holder, side rails, and call signal	Air cushions are inflated to meet the needs of the patient. Standard equipment: turn sheet, IV holder, side rails, and call signal

LOW-AIR-LOSS BEDS

A low-air-loss bed contains inflated air sacs or cushions. A motor is constantly blowing air into the cushions, and the air is flowing out of the cushion at a constant rate. Each section of cushion may be filled to a different firmness, supporting the body evenly and decreasing pressure on bony prominences. The low-air-loss beds maintain pressure on the body support surfaces below the level of capillary pressure in order to not interfere with blood flow to the tissue. Regardless of changes in the body position, this type of bed selectively responds by redistributing the air to maintain a low pressure to all skin areas. The cushions can easily be deflated to transfer the patient or to perform CPR. The constant flow of air through the bed surface has a drying effect on the skin (Fig. 9-10). Some low-air-loss beds can rotate from side to side, stimulating capillary blood flow and facilitating movement of pulmonary secretions. The static low-air-loss bed does not move and is firm enough to support a patient with a spinal cord injury.

AIR-FLUIDIZED BED

An air-fluidized bed contains tiny ceramic beads (finer than sand grains) within a mattress cover. Air is forced through the beads and out through the top covering. The warm air keeps the beads in constant motion, resulting in "fluidizing" of the surface, allowing the patient to float. The person lying on this bed has no body surface exposed to pressure greater than capillary pressure, so blood flow in the skin improves. Excretions and secretions drain away from the body and through the beads. The bed can be turned off to make a firm surface should CPR be indicated. The air-fluidized bed is quite heavy, but some companies now offer a home version of the air-fluidized bed that is 40% lighter than the standard one and that can be used for severely impaired patients. See Figures 9-11 and 9-12 for more information.

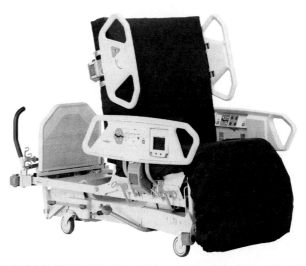

FIGURE 9-10 Total Care Low Air Loss Therapy Bed System. Prevents pressure ulcers by distributing air evenly and provides relief for the nurse by automatically changing to multiple positions. Bariatric beds come in different sizes to accommodate the obese patient of up to 800 pounds.

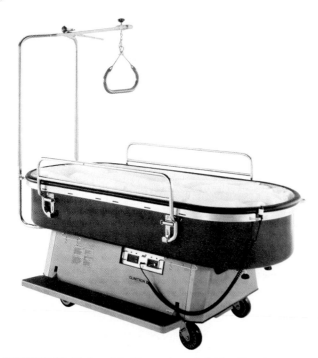

FIGURE 9-11 Clinitron II Bed System is an air-fluidized bed for hospital use. The bed is filled with ceramic beads kept in constant motion by high-level airflow through the beads. (Courtesy of Hill-Rom Company, Inc.)

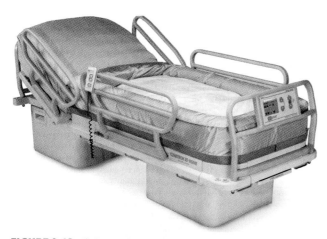

FIGURE 9-12 Clinitron At-Home is an example of the air-fluidized bed that is lighter than the Clinitron II for home use of patients with significantly impaired skin problems (Courtesy of Hill-Rom, Inc., Batesville, IN).

OSCILLATING SUPPORT BED OR ROTATION BED

An oscillating support or rotation bed moves the patient from side to side in a 124-degree arc. This movement relieves and prevents pressure on skin surfaces, helps to mobilize respiratory secretions, stimulates gastrointestinal activity, and promotes circulation (Fig. 9-13). Foam-covered supports are applied to the head, arms, and legs to prevent sliding. Compartments are removable to facilitate elimination or back care.

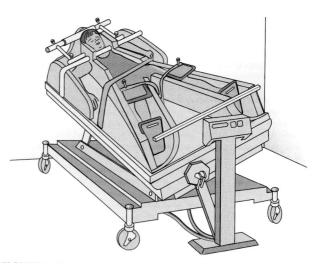

FIGURE 9-13 RotoRest Bed is an example of a rotation bed that facilitates respiratory and circulatory functions by tilting from side to side. (Courtesy of KCI.)

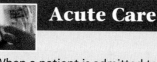
Acute Care

When a patient is admitted to the hospital, many normal activities of daily living change for him or her, making it important at least to provide a clean, safe, and comfortable environment that contributes to a sense of well-being in a strange setting. In acute care, the patient's bed usually becomes the center of activity, with the nurse being responsible for seeing that necessary equipment and items are in their proper place. While there are many variations to bedmaking, according to the patient's health status, safety is a major concern for the patient and the nurse. Positioning the bed at the appropriate height, placing the patient call signal within reach, using side rails safely, and practicing the principles of medical asepsis are standard techniques used to prevent injury to the nurse and the patient. In providing discharge teaching for the patient and home caregivers, the nurse must consider the patient's continuing care needs and the equipment he or she may need at home.

Long-Term Care

The person in a long-term care facility usually spends less time in bed than does the hospitalized patient. Beds are changed less frequently, usually once or twice a week, typically on bath day and as needed. Incontinence is a major concern in long-term care, and drawsheets, disposable pads, and other incontinence products may be used. Mattresses have a moisture-proof covering. Because elderly people may have circulatory problems and thinning skin, there is often a need for extra blankets to maintain warmth, and in many cases, the resident will have a personal warm bedspread. Moreover, beds may be lower in height to take into consideration mobility limitations and safety concerns related to falls. Unlike the bed in acute care, the long-term care bed is usually left in a closed position during the day to encourage residents to stay up.

Skin integrity is of utmost importance with a frail elderly population. Special mattresses may be needed to protect the resident from pressure ulcers or to treat already acquired pressure ulcers. Reimbursement for special pressure-relieving equipment may vary with the insurance or funding for care.

Home Care

If the client in home care spends most of his or her time in bed, is severely disabled, or has skin breakdown, the caregiver may need to make arrangements to rent or buy hospital-type equipment to facilitate caregiving. Hospital beds, side rails, overbed tables, special mattresses, and other equipment are available for rent, lease, or purchase. With a growing trend toward providing more services in the home, the need for specialty mattresses and therapeutic beds is increasing. With a physician's order documenting need, the insurer may reimburse the cost for these devices. Home health nurses need to familiarize themselves with specialty equipment in order to teach the caregivers.

Ambulatory Care

Although beds may not be used in ambulatory care centers for clients, often people such as the elderly are in wheelchairs in adult day care centers. Skin integrity is important to maintain and requires frequent assessment and care. If the majority of time is spent sitting in a wheelchair, some type of pressure-relief cushion, such as a foam or air-inflated one, is recommended. Of course, these cushions do not take the place of having the person redistribute weight from side to side every 2 hours; they are used in addition to moving the person every 2 hours. The nurse needs to instruct the wheelchair-bound client and family members on pressure relief measures.

LEARNING TOOLS

DEVELOP YOUR BACKGROUND KNOWLEDGE

1. Review the Learning Objectives.

2. Read the sections on bedmaking and therapeutic beds in your assigned text.

3. Look up the Key Terms in the glossary.

4. Now review this module, and mentally practice the techniques described. Study so that you would be able to teach these skills to another person.

5. Compare the way you make your bed at home with a hospital-made bed. How does it differ? Could you make your bed using the techniques you've learned?

DEVELOP YOUR SKILLS

1. In the practice setting
   a. Identify the various pieces of linen used to make beds in the facility to which you are assigned.
   b. Partner with one other student. Make an unoccupied, closed bed, using the Performance Checklist on the CD-ROM that accompanies this book as a guide. Have your partner evaluate you. Compare your own evaluation with that of the other student.
   c. Demonstrate how to convert a closed bed to an open bed.
   d. Demonstrate how to convert a closed bed to a postoperative bed.
   e. Make an occupied bed, using your partner as a patient. Pretend that it is a real situation complete with patient communication about the procedure.
   f. Demonstrate the use of a footboard and cradle when making an unoccupied bed.
   g. Reverse positions with your partner, and evaluate his or her performance, completing b through g.

DEMONSTRATE YOUR SKILLS

In the clinical setting, with your instructor's supervision
1. Make an unoccupied bed.

2. Make an occupied bed.

3. Make a postoperative bed.

4. Evaluate your performance with your instructor.

CRITICAL THINKING EXERCISES

1. The long-term care resident you are caring for is an alert, 86-year-old woman with chronic arthritis. You are assigned to change her bed. She reports that she is very tired today, it is painful to move, and the bed "isn't dirty anyway." She suggests that you not

make the bed. What assessment should you make before proceeding with bedmaking? What questions will you ask the resident, and what information will you give? What type of bed should you make? Describe the rationale for your choice.

2. Your patient, a 77-year-old woman, is thin and arthritic. She is out of bed for only a few hours each day. You notice that her sacrum and right hip are reddened and do not blanch with massage. If all special beds and mattresses were available, identify the bed or mattress that would be most effective and appropriate in preventing the formation of pressure ulcers. Determine what additional nursing actions you could carry out to maintain this patient's skin integrity. Describe your rationale for your nursing actions.

SELF-QUIZ

SHORT-ANSWER QUESTIONS

1. What are two goals that should be kept in mind when making the bed of a bedridden patient?

   a. _____

   b. _____

2. Why is it useful to completely finish one side of the unoccupied bed before moving to the other side?

   _____

3. What is the most important safety step when making an occupied bed?

   _____

4. Why is it poor practice to tuck linen tightly over special mattresses?

   _____

5. What provision is made for administering CPR to patients on the low-air-loss bed?

   _____

MULTIPLE CHOICE

_____ 6. Mr. Green is to be up in a chair three times a day for 30 to 45 minutes. Given this information, what type of bed would be most appropriate for you to make for him?
   a. Closed bed
   b. Open bed
   c. Occupied bed
   d. Postoperative bed

_____ 7. Mrs. Pine is going to the radiology department for some special tests. She will arrive back on the floor by stretcher. Under these circumstances, what type of bed would be most appropriate for you to make?
   a. Closed bed
   b. Open bed
   c. Occupied bed
   d. Postoperative bed

_____ 8. A patient who has severe edema of the lower legs should be provided with which accessory device?
   a. Cradle
   b. Bedboard
   c. Footboard
   d. Trapeze

_____ 9. Patients who are confined to bed should be provided with which accessory device to help prevent footdrop?
   a. Cradle
   b. Bedboard
   c. Footboard
   d. Trapeze

_____ 10. Which of the following special beds would be best to use for the patient with an unstable spinal cord injury?
   a. Air-fluidized bed
   b. Air mattress
   c. Low-air-loss mattress
   d. Water-inflated bed

_____ 11. When making an occupied bed, the nurse must remember to
   a. keep the side rails up on both sides.
   b. keep the bed in the high position.
   c. remove all of the top covers before starting the bedmaking procedure.
   d. make the bed before completing the bath.

_____ 12. Which specialty-type bed would be used for a patient who has multiple fractures but also has a history of respiratory problems?
   a. Low-air-loss bed
   b. Air-fluidized bed
   c. Rotation bed
   d. Foam mattress

Answers to Self-Quiz questions appear in the back of this book.

MODULE 10

Assisting Patients With Eating

SKILLS INCLUDED IN THIS MODULE

Procedure for Assisting Patients to Eat
Assisting Patients With Dysphagia to Eat

PREREQUISITE MODULES

Module 1 An Approach to Nursing Skills
Module 2 Documentation
Module 4 Basic Infection Control
Module 5 Safety in the Healthcare Environment

The following modules provide directions on assessment while assisting the patient to eat:
Module 13 Monitoring Intake and Output
Module 14 Nursing Physical Assessment

Also needed is basic information in regard to
Nutrition
Knowledge of the food pyramid
Familiarity with the basic diets used in most healthcare settings

KEY TERMS

anorexia	dysphagia
aspiration	NPO
dexterity	reflux
digestion	tremor

OVERALL OBJECTIVE

▸ To assist patients with a nursing diagnosis of Feeding Self-Care Deficit.

LEARNING OUTCOMES

The student will be able to

1. Assess the patient effectively to determine the amount and type of assistance the patient needs with eating.
2. Analyze assessment data to determine special problems or concerns that must be addressed to successfully assist the patient with eating.
3. Determine appropriate patient outcomes of the eating experience, and recognize the potential for adverse outcomes.
4. Plan preparation, necessary modifications, and equipment or assistance needed to assist the individual patient with eating.
5. Assist the patient to eat, taking into account individual physical difficulties and emotional responses.
6. Evaluate the experience, taking into account the patient's intake, the amount of assistance needed, any difficulties encountered, and the response of the patient.
7. Document the eating experience in the patient's plan of care and the intake in the patient's record as appropriate.

During illness, trauma, or wound healing, the body needs more nutrients than usual. However, many patients, because of weakness, immobility, or inability to use one or both arms, are unable to eat independently. To be sure the patient receives adequate nutrition, the nurse must be knowledgeable, sensitive, and skillful in assisting him or her to eat. To promote well-being, the nurse must also consider the patient's psychological response to being assisted with eating.

FACTORS THAT AFFECT EATING

In a clinical setting, various factors may influence how well the patient eats. Altered mealtimes, unfamiliar foods, or the desire for customary foods also may lead to **anorexia** (lack of appetite). Neuromuscular disturbances can contribute to eating difficulties as well, as can the nature of the patient's illness. Remember that illness interferes with both body and mind, and that most illnesses produce a degree of anxiety within the individual that may diminish or increase appetite or result in erratic eating. An understanding attitude on your part, taking into account all of these factors, promotes a more satisfactory outcome to the mealtime experience.

Physical problems that may affect a person's ability to eat independently include those in which neuromuscular control is impaired, such as stroke or head injury. These individuals may need to receive total assistance with eating for a period of time and then may be partially assisted with eating as they gradually relearn skills. People with movement limited by traction, casts, and special positioning may need assistance with some aspects of a meal, although they may be able to do some

things for themselves. A careful assessment of the precise abilities of each individual patient with regard to independent eating is important to ensuring adequate nutrition.

Being with the patient during a meal and participating in this significant activity also gives you time for several of your most basic and important functions: assessing, analyzing, planning, implementing, and evaluating. At the same time, it is crucial to remember that being assisted with eating can be humiliating to some patients and may give them a feeling that they are now dependent, unable to carry out the simple task of eating independently. The person who is having difficulty eating—someone who dislikes the food, is experiencing nausea and vomiting, or is having other difficulties—may dread mealtime.

NURSING DIAGNOSES

Examples of some nursing diagnoses related to eating and nutrition include

- Imbalanced Nutrition: Less Than Body Requirements related to, for example, nausea and vomiting or inadequate intake
- Imbalanced Nutrition: More Than Body Requirements related to, for example, intake in excess of metabolic requirements or decreased activity patterns
- Feeding Self-Care Deficit related to, for example, right or left upper extremity paralysis
- Impaired Swallowing related to, for example, muscle paralysis or cognitive deficits

DELEGATION

Assisting patients with eating is frequently delegated to assistive personnel. This may be both necessary and appropriate. However, the responsibility for careful assessment and supervision remains with the nurse. Patients with swallowing difficulties are especially vulnerable as are those with poor overall nutritional status. The nurse is responsible for instructing assistive personnel regarding important observations to make when assisting specific patients. When assisting the patient to eat has been delegated to assistive personnel, the nurse should carefully supervise the activity.

PROCEDURE FOR ASSISTING PATIENTS TO EAT

ASSESSMENT

1. Identify the type of diet ordered. **R:** To determine whether the diet is appropriate for the patient in his or her present condition and to determine whether any special eating utensils will be needed.
2. Check to see whether there is any reason why the patient's meal should be delayed or cancelled. **R:** Scheduled laboratory tests, radiologic examinations, and surgery may mean that the patient must fast, taking nothing by mouth (**NPO**) for a period before the test or surgery.
3. Check the nursing care plan, nursing history, or nursing record. **R:** To identify any previous need for assistance or use of modified eating utensils and to note information about allergies, cultural or religious preferences, and specific dietary likes and dislikes.
4. Note any nursing diagnoses related to eating or nutrition. **R:** Knowledge of these, along with the related plan of care, can help you make the eating experience easier and more pleasant for you and the patient.
5. Assess the patient's current condition and ability to eat. **R:** To identify any change in condition that could affect eating.

ANALYSIS

6. Critically think through your data, carefully evaluating each aspect and its relation to other data. **R:** To identify specific problems and modifications of the procedure needed for the individual.

   Here are some examples: If the patient has just developed a high fever and nausea or is in pain, you may wish to change to a lighter meal that the patient can digest more easily or to delay the meal until medications can be given to alleviate the patient's symptoms. If you are aware that there is potential for nausea, vomiting, or pain with a particular patient, it is wise to see that the ordered medication is given 20 to 30 minutes before the meal to enhance the potential for adequate food intake. If the patient has difficulty swallowing, you will need to modify the procedure (see Box 10-1 for suggested foods).

PLANNING

7. Determine individualized patient outcomes in relation to assisting the patient to eat. **R:** Identifying outcomes facilitates evaluation. Long-term care facilities may designate a specific percentage (such as 50%) that triggers further intervention.
   a. The patient will consume at least a specified percentage of each item on the tray.
   b. The patient will not choke or vomit during or after the meal.
   c. The patient will state satisfaction with the eating experience.
8. Consider the time that food trays arrive on the unit. **R:** This is so that tasks and procedures may be scheduled away from mealtime and so that you or the patient are not in the middle of a task or treatment at that time.
9. Allow sufficient time. **R:** This is so that you are free of other tasks and can spend uninterrupted time with the patient. This is important to prevent food from getting cold and the patient from feeling unattended.
10. Obtain specially modified eating utensils if needed (Fig. 10-1). **R:** To foster self-esteem by allowing patients who are partially disabled to eat more independently.

---

box 10-1 *Food Considerations for the Patient Who Has Difficulty Swallowing*

The following list identifies foods and fluids that are usually easy to swallow and those that *in some cases* may cause choking.

Easily Swallowed Food and Fluids

Thickened liquids (milkshakes, slushes)
Hot or cold temperature foods or fluids (hot creamed soup, iced fruit)
Easily chewed foods (cooked vegetables, ground meat)
Soft, smooth foods (pureed fruits, pudding)

Foods That May Cause Choking

Thin, watery liquids (water, tea, coffee, soda)
Neutral temperature foods and fluids (room-temperature water)
Tough, stringy, hard, or dry foods (roast beef, nuts, dry crackers)
Sticky foods (peanut butter and thick mashed potatoes)

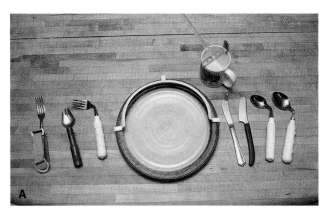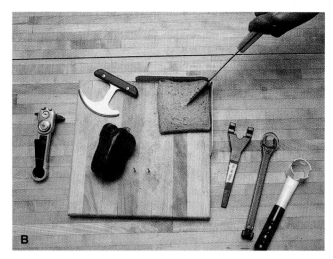

FIGURE 10-1 There are many kinds of utensils to facilitate eating. (**A**) Some forks, knives, and spoons have modified handles and shapes for an easier grip. Plates may have suction cups to secure them to a surface and metal guards to keep food from slipping off, and cups may have straws secured with special clips. (**B**) Other devices have modifications to assist with opening containers and cutting and preparing food.

IMPLEMENTATION

Action	Rationale
11. Wash or disinfect your hands.	To decrease the transfer of microorganisms that could cause infection.
12. Identify the patient using two identifiers.	To be sure that you are carrying out the correct procedure for the correct patient.
13. Greet the patient, and explain what you are going to do.	Communication is a skill that is basic to all interaction with patients. Explaining the procedure helps relieve anxiety or misperceptions that the patient may have and sets the stage for patient participation.
14. Offer the patient the opportunity to use the bathroom, if able, or the bedpan or urinal.	To provide for patient comfort and so that the meal will not have to be interrupted for elimination needs.
15. Assist in washing the patient's hands and face and providing mouth care as indicated.	To ensure comfort and cleanliness.
16. Prepare the eating environment by removing all unsightly equipment, replacing soiled linens, and arranging the bedside table for the meal tray.	A restful, neat, and odor-free environment stimulates appetite, makes eating more pleasant, and aids **digestion**.
17. Wash or disinfect your hands if you handled soiled linens while preparing the environment.	To decrease the transfer of microorganisms.

(continued)

Action	Rationale
18. Position the bed in the low position with the patient comfortably in mid to high Fowler's, if possible.	The low position of the bed allows you to assist the patient from a seated position. The Fowler's position makes swallowing easier and lessens the risk of choking and **aspiration** (inspiration of food into the lungs).
19. If the patient wears eyeglasses, hearing aids, or dentures, be sure they are in place.	This is so that the patient can see, hear, and chew properly.
20. Place a towel or other suitable protective cover over the patient's chest.	To protect the patient's gown and bed linen.
21. Check to be sure that the name on the tray corresponds with the name on the patient's identification bracelet and that the food choices marked on the menu correspond with the food on the tray. If the name on the tray is different from the patient's name, or if the food choices marked on the menu differ from the food on the tray, remove the tray from the room. The correct tray may be immediately available. If it is not, communicate with the Dietary Department, following the procedure in your facility.	To ensure that the patient receives the correct meal.
22. Assist the patient to prepare the food on the tray as needed. For example, cut food into bite-size pieces, open milk cartons and cereal boxes, and butter bread. Encourage independence appropriately. Discard all wrappings and clutter before the patient begins to eat.	Patients with physical or cognitive impairments may need assistance for some or all of these tasks.
23. Position yourself at the patient's eye level by sitting if at all possible (Fig. 10-2).	This establishes an unhurried, social atmosphere for the meal.

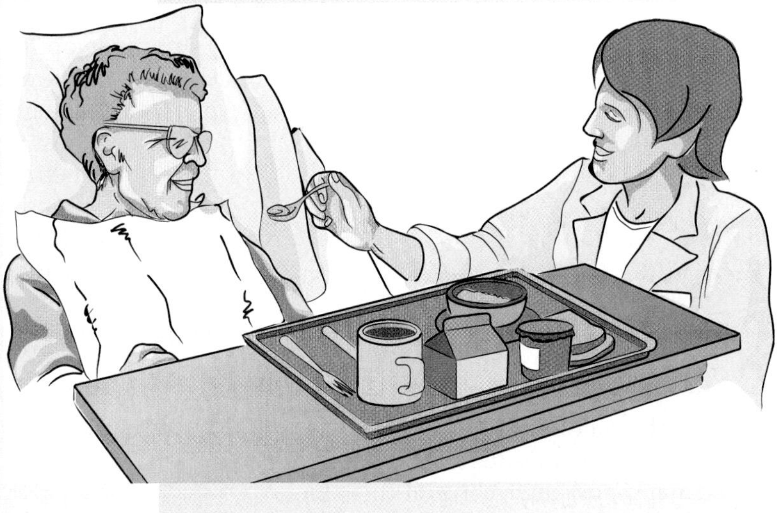

FIGURE 10-2 Assisting the older patient with eating.

(continued)

Action	Rationale
24. Involve the patient as much as possible by working from the unaffected side (the side of the patient least affected by the disease process).	To promote patient participation.
25. Place the tray so that the patient can see the food that is being offered. If the patient is sightless, describing what is on the meal tray is both necessary and helpful. Many visually handicapped patients can manage with very little assistance if they know where food items are located. Often a clock format is used to assist the sightless patient; for example, you may say, "The milk is at 2 o'clock, and the potatoes are at 6 o'clock."	To promote independence.
26. Offer choices.	To promote optimum nutrition and self-esteem.
a. Offer choices regarding the menu when possible.	To promote a sense of control and participation.
b. Offer choices regarding sequence. When possible, find out from the patient what food sequence is preferred. If this is not possible, feed the items in the order in which you would choose to eat them. Provide fluids between bites of solids. If the patient does not respond to being given a choice, feed the more nutritious items of the diet first, in case the patient's intake capacity is limited. For example, if the choice is between broth and tea, broth, which contains protein, is preferable.	To promote optimum intake.
c. Offer choices regarding food preparation.	To promote optimum nutrition and self-esteem. The elderly patient who has difficulty eating because of poorly fitting dentures may prefer to mix eggs, fruit, cereal, and toast together. Although this may strike you as unappetizing, supporting this patient preference may help to build a good nurse/patient relationship. Do not feel compelled to change long-standing eating habits, although you may adopt as a long-term goal, for example, arranging for the patient to be fit with comfortable dentures.
27. Continue assessment as you assist the patient. You can easily and accurately assess the patient's **dexterity** (adroitness), mental status, and feelings at this time. Signs such as skin color, respiratory rate,	Assessment is ongoing; you may gain information during activity that would not be available when the patient is at rest.

(continued)

Action	Rationale
and the presence or absence of **tremor** (trembling or shaking) can also be assessed.	
28. Do not discuss stressful events at mealtime. Try to maintain an open and congenial atmosphere.	Digestion and appetite are enhanced in a stress-free situation.
29. Never hurry a patient's eating.	This not only can cause the patient to feel uncomfortable and fearful of taking up too much of your time, but it can also be dangerous if it causes the patient to choke in an attempt to finish eating quickly. This is especially true if the patient is known to have **dysphagia** (difficulty with swallowing).
30. Allow the patient to determine when enough has been eaten.	To promote a sense of control.
31. Remove the tray, offer the bedpan, or assist to the bathroom as indicated, and provide hygiene as needed.	To promote patient comfort.
32. Reposition the patient. If there have been problems with digestion or vomiting, keep the patient in high Fowler's position for at least 15 minutes following the meal. Turning the head to one side can prevent aspiration if vomiting does occur.	Gravity lessens the pressure of food on the cardiac sphincter and helps to prevent regurgitation and aspiration. If the head is turned to the side, any regurgitation is more likely to drain out of the mouth, lessening the potential for aspiration.
33. Provide quiet so that the patient may relax after the meal.	To promote good digestion.
34. Wash or disinfect your hands.	To decrease the transfer of microorganisms that could cause infection.

EVALUATION

35. Evaluate using the individualized patient outcomes previously identified. **R:** Evaluation in relation to desired outcomes is essential for planning future care needs.
    a. The patient consumed at least the desired percentage of each item on the tray.
    b. The patient did not choke or vomit during or after the meal.
    c. The patient stated satisfaction with the eating experience.

DOCUMENTATION

36. Document the food and fluids consumed as required by the facility, usually either by using the checklist provided by the institution or by charting in more detail on the progress notes (depending on the situation). Include the patient's response, as well. If food intake has previously presented problems, chart the individual food items and the amounts taken. **R:** To provide for greater accuracy.

37. Also document other appropriate information, such as difficulty swallowing or changes in the patient's ability or behavior compared with other eating experiences. Add to the nursing care plan any new information related to the patient's likes and dislikes or methods of assisting that you have noted. **R:** To enhance continuity of care. Documentation is a legal record of the patient's care and therapy and communicates nursing activities to other nurses and caregivers.

POTENTIAL ADVERSE OUTCOMES AND RELATED INTERVENTIONS

1. The patient vomits during or after the meal.
Intervention: Stop the procedure, and assess the patient and situation. Check the record for an order for an antiemetic medication. Seek an order for an antiemetic from the physician if none exists. After administering an antiemetic, wait until it is effective before again attempting to help the patient eat. Check the patient record for food or fluid allergies or both. Suggest an order for a bland or liquid diet until the problem is resolved.

2. The patient chokes or coughs excessively during the meal.
Intervention: Stop the procedure, and assess the patient and situation. Assess the airway and lungs. Determine whether size of bites or talking and laughing during the meal may have contributed to the problem. If the patient is having difficulty swallowing, he or she may have dysphagia and may need a referral to a swallowing specialist (usually a speech therapist) for assessment and planning. Consult with the medical care provider regarding a referral. The nurse may institute some of the strategies for assisting the patient with dysphagia found below.

ASSISTING PATIENTS WITH DYSPHAGIA TO EAT

Dysphagia means difficulty in swallowing. Typically, strokes or other neuromuscular disorders can cause dysphagia. The patient with dysphagia chokes and aspirates food easily. Symptoms of dysphagia include coughing and choking while attempting to eat. However, some less obvious symptoms may also indicate dysphagia. The patient may drool or "pocket" food in the cheek, or simply let food and fluids run out of the mouth. Some people aspirate liquids with no symptoms at all.

Speech therapists are experts on the muscles of the mouth and throat and on techniques for facilitating swallowing. The physician may make a referral to a speech therapist for an evaluation and treatment plan for a dysphagic patient. The nurse who has assessed the patient may bring the need for a referral to the physician's attention. The techniques of assisting the dysphagic patient focus on maintaining safety.

The nurse who is caring for a patient with dysphagia needs to educate both the patient and his or her caregivers about eating despite difficulties. Some suggestions follow:

1. Select appropriate foods, i.e., foods that stimulate the swallowing reflex, that do not move too rapidly through the mouth for the muscles to adapt, and that are easy for the muscles of the mouth to move. Box 10-1 lists foods and fluids that are usually easy to swallow and those that may cause choking.

2. Identify an appropriate position for swallowing. The mouth and throat are in the optimum position when the patient is sitting up straight with the head tilted forward. Figure 10-3 shows how head position can prevent choking and aspiration.

3. Maintain a relaxed pace because hurrying only increases the likelihood of choking.

4. Caution the patient not to try to talk until a few seconds after swallowing. When a person talks, the epiglottis must open for air to exit, and small amounts of food may be aspirated if they are still in the mouth.

5. Suggest taking small bites of food, which are easier for the mouth to control.

6. For patients who are weak or paralyzed on one side, placing the fork or spoon on the unaffected side of

Correct swallowing position

Incorrect swallowing position

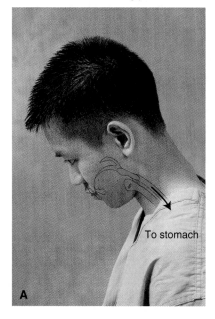
To stomach

A

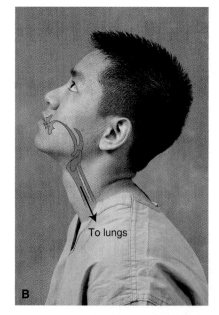
To lungs

B

FIGURE 10-3 (**A** and **B**) The effect of head position on swallowing.

the tongue will be helpful because the muscles and nerves of the unaffected side are better able to control the movement of food through the mouth and pharynx.

7. When placing the food in the mouth, show the patient how to use a rocking motion of the utensil on the tongue. The rocking motion provides greater stimulation to the tongue and will help the patient feel the food more distinctly.

8. Recommend swallowing twice after each bite. The second swallow may prevent food from being left in the mouth.

9. Check for food left in the cheek of the affected side. Teach the patient and caregivers how to check the mouth with a mirror or with a forefinger slipped into the cheek to feel for food left there. "Pocketed" food left in the mouth on a paralyzed side may not be felt and poses an ongoing potential for choking and aspiration as well as mouth odor. If the patient is unable to check independently, show the caregiver how to do so.

10. Caution the patient not to "wash down" food with liquids. Thin liquids such as water, tea, and coffee often cause choking. Liquids may increase the speed with which material moves to the back of the pharynx and increase the likelihood of aspiration.

11. Advise sitting up for 15 minutes after completing the meal to prevent **reflux** (a flowing back) of stomach contents and their possible aspiration.

Acute Care

In the acute care setting, patients who have experienced surgery or trauma to the upper extremities or who have a diagnosis of stroke or another neuromuscular disorder are more likely to need assistance with eating than are other patients. Patients with major surgery and/or trauma may also have difficulty eating and nutritional challenges. Making mealtimes as pleasant as possible under difficult circumstances can be challenging, but also rewarding. You may need to assist patients with the eating process during their hospitalization as well as teach them techniques to use at home. Teaching family and/or friends to assist them during their recovery at home may also be necessary.

Long-Term Care

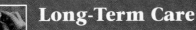

In the long-term care setting, the residents may have many self-care deficits; a feeding deficit is common. These residents often eat in a dining room rather than in their rooms and are grouped at tables with others with whom they can interact. Having residents dressed in day clothing and helping them to be attractively groomed is important for everyone's feelings about the meal. As you plan for assistance with eating for the resident, remember that it should be as unobtrusive as possible so as not to interfere with interactions. In addition, you will be working toward developing independence in the resident whenever that is possible. Sometimes encouragement and "cuing" an individual as to the next step are all that are needed to promote independence in eating.

Nursing assistants usually assist residents with eating in long-term care settings, whereas the nurse is typically involved in teaching the assistants and serving as a role model of how to appropriately assist residents to eat well and enjoy nutritional well-being.

Home Care

Before a patient is discharged, discuss with the patient and his or her caregiver the potential for eating-related difficulties at home. As part of your plan, you may help the family obtain assistive devices and teach family members how to assist the patient with eating. You may also need to address problems related to shopping, storage, refrigeration, and cooking practices. It may be necessary for you to ask for a referral to a community agency to assist the patient and family.

LEARNING TOOLS

DEVELOP YOUR BACKGROUND KNOWLEDGE

1. Review the Learning Outcomes.

2. Read the section on nutrition in your assigned text.

3. Look up the Key Terms in the glossary.

4. Review the module and mentally practice the skills described. Study so that you would be able to teach these concepts and skills to another person.

DEVELOP YOUR SKILLS

1. In the practice setting
   a. Have a classmate assist you with eating lunch as if you were a patient with a feeding self-care deficit. Try eating a portion of the meal in a recumbent position (lying down) and a portion in

a sitting position in bed. Close your eyes for 3 minutes while being assisted to eat. First, have your classmate describe the food to you. Eat a part of the meal with your eyes closed, as though you were blind. Then pretend you are blind but can eat independently. Have your classmate assist you by telling you where various foods are located. Now answer the following questions:

(1) What was pleasant about the experience?
(2) What was unpleasant?
(3) What did you learn?

b. Repeat a, but this time, reverse roles. Discuss with your partner the questions from your point of view as the one assisting with eating.

c. Examine the pictures of eating aids in this module. In your group, determine how you would identify the specific patient problems that the feeding aids are designed to help. Knowing the types of feeding aids available will assist you in more effectively planning for the patient. These aids can be purchased by the institution or in some instances may be constructed by occupational therapy staff. For a patient returning home, the family may be able to purchase the needed feeding aid or construct a substitute.

2. In the clinical setting

a. Observe a patient being assisted with eating. What was done that was helpful to the patient? What might you have done differently?

b. Assist a patient to eat an entire meal. Note the time when you begin and the time the patient completes the meal. Answer the following questions for your own learning, or discuss them with your instructor.

(1) How long did it take the patient to complete the meal?
(2) What conclusions can you draw from the timing?
(3) What were some of the problems that interfered with optimum intake?
(4) What went well?
(5) Were you uncomfortable at any point?
(6) Did the patient appear to be uncomfortable at any point?
(7) Did you use all the steps of the procedure?
(8) Did you make adaptations? If so, what were they, and why did you make them?

c. Observe the amount of food eaten and the patient's response. Share your observations with your instructor. Evaluate your performance with your instructor.

d. Investigate the feeding aids that are available in the institution.

3. Practice your skills, using the Performance Checklist on the CD-ROM that accompanies this book.

CRITICAL THINKING EXERCISES

1. A hospitalized patient for whom you are providing care has just returned from a diagnostic study. He appears upset and tells you he is nauseated and just wants to rest. You are disappointed because the two of you spent considerable time this morning discussing his poor nutritional status and, with the help of the dietitian, ordered special foods from the Dietary Department to encourage optimum intake. His tray has just arrived, and it looks appetizing. In light of the current situation, describe how you will proceed.

2. The 82-year-old woman you have been caring for in the nursing home is going home after rehabilitation following a stroke. She is still having some difficulty with a mild swallowing problem. Identify at least three strategies you will teach her and her primary caregiver to help prevent choking and aspiration.

SELF-QUIZ
SHORT-ANSWER QUESTIONS

1. List four factors that can influence a patient's eating abilities.

a. _____
b. _____
c. _____
d. _____

2. List four easily swallowed foods.

a. _____
b. _____
c. _____
d. _____

3. List four foods that may cause choking.

a. _____
b. _____
c. _____
d. _____

MULTIPLE CHOICE

_____ **4.** Every eating situation presents which of the following opportunities for the nurse?
a. A time for health teaching
b. Determination of the medical diagnosis
c. A time for nursing assessments to be made
d. Repositioning of the patient

Situation: Mr. Swenson, a 63-year-old Scandinavian with right-sided hemiplegia (paralysis on the right side of the body), has been in the hospital for 10 days. His chart states that a soft diet has been ordered and that he is allowed up in a chair for all meals. Lunch trays will be arriving in 20 minutes, and you have been assigned to assist Mr. Swenson with eating. As you enter his room, you see a denture cup on the bedside table and glasses on the overbed table. A urinal is on the floor. Questions 5 to 10 refer to Mr. Swenson.

_____ 5. From the data given, you determine that Mr. Swenson's feeding problem is
   a. lack of ability to swallow food.
   b. not evident from the information available.
   c. lack of ability to use small-muscle groups to eat independently.
   d. depression brought on by dependency.

_____ 6. Your first action in the above situation should be to
   a. introduce yourself, and give the reason for your presence.
   b. empty and put away the urinal.
   c. encourage Mr. Swenson to discuss his feelings about being dependent.
   d. reposition Mr. Swenson in a high Fowler's position for lunch.

TRUE-FALSE

_____ 7. Mr. Swenson should be encouraged to talk about his anxieties while you are at the bedside assisting him to eat.

_____ 8. Because Mr. Swenson is Scandinavian, he will certainly enjoy the fish on the menu.

_____ 9. The goal for Mr. Swenson in regard to eating this meal independently should be established only after you determine his previous abilities.

_____ 10. Mr. Swenson ate only half his meal. This means your nursing care plan was unsuccessful.

Answers to Self-Quiz questions appear in the back of this book.

REFERENCES AND SUGGESTED RESOURCES: UNIT 2

AHCPR. (1992). Pressure ulcers in adults: Prediction and prevention. *AHCPR Clinical Practice Guideline No. 3.* Rockville, MD. Agency for Health Care Policy and Research, Public Health Service, U.S. Department of Health and Human Services Publication No. 92-0047. (Online.) Available at http://www.ncbi.nlm.nih.gov/books/bv.fcgi?rid=hstat2.chapter.4409.

Brawley, E. C. (2002). Bathing environments: How to improve the bathing experience. *Alzheimer's Care Quarterly, 3* (1), 38–41.

Dahlin, C. (2004). Oral complications at the end of life. *AJN 104* (7), 40–47.

Garner, J. S. & Hospital Infection Control Practices Advisory Committee. (1996). Guideline for isolation precautions in hospitals. *Infect Control Hosp Epidemiol, 17,* 53–80, and *Am J Infect Control, 24,* 24–52. (Online.) Available at http://www.cdc.gov. Retrieved July 1, 2004.

Ramponi, D. R. (2001). Eye on contact lens removal. *Nursing2001, 31* (8), 56–57.

Schwartz, M. (2000). The oral health of the long-term care patient. *Annals of Long Term Care, 8* (12), 41–46.

UNIT 3

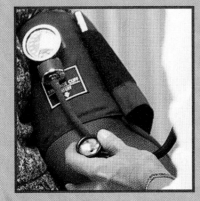

Developing Assessment Skills

MODULES

MODULE 11

Assessing Temperature, Pulse, and Respiration

SKILLS INCLUDED IN THIS MODULE

General Procedure for Measuring Temperature, Pulse, and Respiration
Specific Procedures for Measuring Temperature
  Oral Temperature
  Rectal Temperature
  Axillary Temperature
  Tympanic Temperature
Specific Procedures for Measuring Pulses
  Radial Pulse
  Dorsalis Pedis Pulse
  Posterior Tibial Pulse
  Apical Pulse
  Apical-Radial Pulse
Pulse Rate Using a Doppler Ultrasound Device
Pulse of a Newborn or Infant
Specific Procedure for Measuring Respiration

PREREQUISITE MODULES

Module 1	An Approach to Nursing Skills
Module 2	Documentation
Module 4	Basic Infection Control
Module 5	Safety in the Healthcare Environment

KEY TERMS

afebrile	metabolism
apical pulse	midclavicular line
apnea	orthopnea
asymmetrical	pedal pulse
axilla	popliteal
bounding	posterior tibial
brachial	pulse deficit
bradycardia	radial
bradypnea	reflectance
carotid artery	rhythm
Celsius	Sims' position
Centigrade	supine position
Cheyne-Stokes	symmetry
respirations	tachycardia
dorsalis pedis	tachypnea
dyspnea	temporal
eupnea	thermistor
Fahrenheit	thready pulse
febrile	tympanic
femoral	vital signs
fever	

OVERALL OBJECTIVE

▸ To measure and document patients' temperature, pulse, and respiration (TPR) accurately and safely, recognizing deviations from the norm.

LEARNING OUTCOMES

The student will be able to

1. Assess the patient to determine which method to use for temperature measurement and which pulses should be checked.
2. Assess the patient to determine readiness for the temperature, pulse, and respiration (TPR) procedure.
3. Analyze the assessment data to determine specific concerns that must be addressed prior to taking the TPR or palpating peripheral pulses.
4. Determine appropriate patient outcomes of the TPR process and the potential for adverse outcomes.
5. Choose the appropriate equipment.
6. Position the patient appropriately for the procedure, maintaining principles of body mechanics.
7. Measure the temperature, pulse, and respirations accurately.
8. Evaluate the effectiveness of the process and accuracy of the results.
9. Document the results in the patient record or other agency record as required.

Vital signs is a term that includes temperature, pulse, respiration, and blood pressure. Some facilities are adding assessment for pain to their definition of vital signs and calling it the "fifth vital sign." This practice is to highlight the importance of pain assessment. Accurate measurement and recording of vital signs is basic to the assessment of patients. Temperature, pulse, and respirations will be included in this module. Blood pressure is discussed in Module 12. Pain assessment can be found in a nursing fundamentals text.

The abbreviation "TPR" is used to designate the assessing of temperature, pulse, and respirations. Most institutions have routine times for assessing TPR, but it may be done more frequently if the nurse determines that it is warranted. Depending on institution policy, TPR results are recorded in a variety of places, including on the bedside flow chart, the bedside computer terminal, a central clipboard in the nursing station, and/or the graphic record in the patient's chart (Fig. 11-1). After completing this module, you should be able to define these signs accurately, measure them, and record them. You should also be able to adapt this procedure to both healthy and ill individuals of any age and appropriately interpret your findings.

NURSING DIAGNOSES

- Hyperthermia: elevated body temperature that may be related to illness, exposure to hot environment, excessive clothing, medications, activity, trauma, dehydration, increased metabolic rate, or inability or decreased ability to perspire

- Hypothermia: reduced body temperature that may be related to illness, exposure to cold environment, inadequate clothing, trauma, or aging
- Ineffective Thermoregulation: inability to maintain temperature that may be related to illness, trauma, changing environmental temperatures, immaturity, or aging
- Decreased Cardiac Output: a collaborative diagnosis that may be related to the presence of an excessively slow or excessively rapid pulse rate; the nursing diagnosis would relate to the patient's problems
- Risk for Activity Intolerance: may be related to potential circulatory or respiratory problems
- Disturbed Sleep Pattern or Ineffective Breathing Pattern: may be related to an abnormality in the respiratory rate or pattern

DELEGATION

Temperature, pulse, and respiration are measured by both professional and assistive personnel in healthcare settings. Both can perform the mechanics of the routine procedure equally well. When the **apical pulse** assessment is needed, the nurse is responsible because assistive personnel are rarely taught the skill of listening for the apical pulse. The professional nurse also has the responsibility for determining the appropriate site for measuring temperature and for identifying when specific peripheral pulse must be checked. In addition,

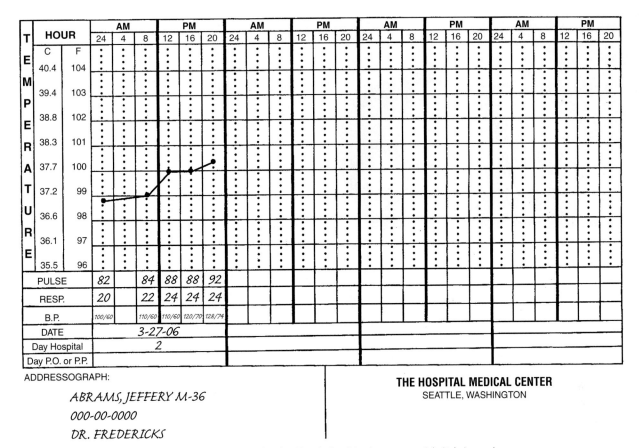

T	HOUR		AM 24	4	8	PM 12	16	20	AM 24	4	8	PM 12	16	20	AM 24	4	8	PM 12	16	20	AM 24	4	8	PM 12	16	20
	PULSE		82		84	88	88	92																		
	RESP.		20		22	24	24	24																		
	B.P.		100/60		110/60	110/60	120/70	128/74																		
	DATE		3-27-06																							
	Day Hospital		2																							
	Day P.O. or P.P.																									

ADDRESSOGRAPH:

ABRAMS, JEFFERY M-36

000-00-0000

DR. FREDERICKS

THE HOSPITAL MEDICAL CENTER
SEATTLE, WASHINGTON

FIGURE 11-1 Vital signs graphic form. You can easily identify relationships between serial vital signs when a graphic flow sheet is used.

the nurse is responsible for understanding deviations from normal on which assessments and interpretations are based. Assistive personnel should be instructed to report any deviations from normal to the nurse.

TEMPERATURE

Body temperature is the balance between heat produced and heat lost by the body. It is surprisingly consistent in healthy individuals; that is, a normal oral reading is 98.6° **Fahrenheit** or (37° **Celsius/centigrade**) with a range of 96.4° to 99.1°F (or 35.8° to 37.3°C). The rectal temperature measures roughly 1°F (0.5°C) higher, as does the tympanic temperature. Both of these reflect core body temperature. The axillary temperature measures roughly 1°F (0.5°C) lower than an oral reading. Because adult temperatures fall within a range of normal values depending upon many factors—age, infection, temperature of environment, amount of exercise, **metabolism**, and emotional status—it is important to know what values are considered "normal" in your facility and for the individual person. For example, an elderly person in a nursing home may always have a

temperature of 96.2°F, and it is considered "normal" for that person.

If a temperature measurement is above normal, the patient is **febrile**, that is, the patient has a **fever**. If the temperature is normal, the patient is considered **afebrile** (without fever).

TYPES OF THERMOMETERS

Glass thermometers containing mercury are no longer the instrument of choice when measuring temperature because of the hazards of mercury. However, since patients may have these in their homes, use the opportunity for teaching the appropriate safety precautions if it arises. All healthcare facilities have procedures in their Material Safety Data Sheet (MSDS) manuals for responding to mercury spills.

Electronic thermometers (Fig. 11-2), are available for oral and rectal use. These thermometers use a component called a **thermistor** at the end of a plastic and stainless steel probe to sense temperature. When the thermometer is in use, the probe is covered with a disposable cover, which is discarded after each use.

The temperature appears on a digital display that resets itself when the probe is replaced in the body of the battery-powered device in which it is stored. Some

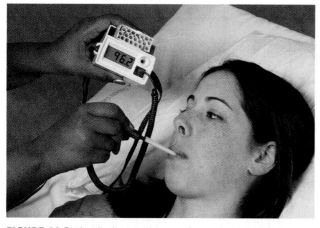

FIGURE 11-2 The display panel on an electronic thermometer registers the temperature reading in 30 to 50 seconds.

electronic thermometers have a timer that may be used when measuring pulse, respiration, intravenous drip rate, or any other timed value. The timer functions like a stopwatch and may be restarted at any time. The electronic thermometer is carried from one patient to another, along with a sufficient supply of disposable probe covers. Therefore, it is not useful for patients with infectious disease, unless it can be used by one patient only. Most facilities do not own enough electronic thermometers to use them in this way, so disposable thermometers are commonly used in such situations.

Another type of electronic thermometer, a **tympanic** thermometer, uses infrared technology (**reflectance**) to measure the temperature on the tympanic membrane. A covered probe is placed at the external opening of the ear canal, where it senses the infrared energy produced by the tympanic membrane, which lies close to the external carotid artery (Fig. 11-3). It is essential that the probe be placed at the proper angle, sealing the ear canal. (Directions from the manufacturer define the correct

angle.) The tympanic temperature registers on a digital display in a few seconds. Because the ear canal has no mucous membranes, it is not easily influenced by evaporation or other ambient changes and has demonstrated reliable correlation with the body's core temperature (Henker & Coyne, 1995). Cerumen (earwax) does not affect the integrity of the readings unless the entire canal is occluded; if one ear shows evidence of otitis (inflammation) or wax impaction, the other ear can be used. The same nonintrusive probe covers may be used for children and adults.

Chemical dot thermometers are for one-time use. They are disposable and consist of a flat plastic device holding many temperature-sensing chemical "dots" that change color when they reach a certain temperature (Fig. 11-4). Advantages of these thermometers include the following: they are inexpensive, unbreakable, and suitable for use in an isolation room.

SITES FOR MEASURING TEMPERATURE

There are four sites for measuring temperature: oral, rectal, axillary, and tympanic (ear canal). A site is chosen based upon the specific needs of the patient and overall facility policy. For information about advantages and disadvantages of the sites, see Table 11-1.

PULSE

As the heart pumps blood through the arteries, an arterial pulse wave is generated. This pulse wave can be palpated at arteries that are close to the surface. These sites are known as peripheral pulse points. A pulse is identified and counted to evaluate the circulation distal to that point and to assess the rate, **rhythm**, and quality of the heartbeat. The nurse uses a variety of techniques to assess the vascular status of the patient. Among these are the interview, inspection, palpation, and auscultation.

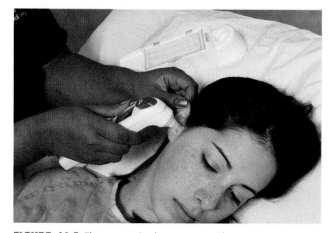

FIGURE 11-3 The tympanic thermometer. The same nonintrusive probe covers may be used for infants and adults.

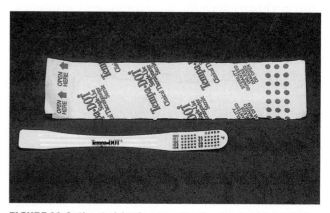

FIGURE 11-4 Chemical dot thermometer. The chemical "dots" change color as the temperature rises.

table 11-1. Temperature Measurement Sites: Advantages and Disadvantages

Site	Advantage	Disadvantage
Mouth	Easy access Commonly used because of rich blood supply Comfortable for most people	Pain if mouth is inflamed or injured Not recommended for confused patients Not recommended for small children Must wait 15 minutes to measure temperature after food or fluid ingestion, which may affect surface temperature of mouth
Rectum	Common site when oral not available Believed most accurate because it reflects core temperature	Requires lubricant Frightening to infants and small children Requires position change and exposure for patient Must be held in place for safety
Axilla	Easy to use on newborns and confused patients Least invasive	Least desirable for adults because the axilla is more likely to be affected by environmental temperatures Must be held in place for accuracy
Tympanic	Easy to use, accessible, and safe for all ages Does not require position change Tympanic membrane lies very close to external carotid artery so it reflects core temperature Reading obtained in as few as 10 seconds	Reading variability depending on placement Total wax buildup occluding ear canal may cause inaccuracy External otitis may cause pain upon insertion of thermometer

table 11-2. Approximate Pulse and Respiration Rates by Age

Age	Pulse (beats/min)	Respiration (breaths/min)
Newborn	120	30–40
4 year old	100	23–30
8 year old	90	20–26
14 year old	85	18–22
Adult	70	12–20

greatly diminished; 2, slightly diminished; 3, normal; 4, bounding.

PERIPHERAL PULSES

Peripheral pulses are palpated using the tips of two or three fingers (never the thumb, which has its own pulse) at the arterial pulse points throughout the body. These pulse points are called the temporal, carotid, brachial, radial, femoral, popliteal, dorsalis pedis, and posterior tibial pulses (Fig. 11-5). It is easiest to assess peripheral pulses with the patient in the **supine position** (face up).

- **Temporal**—located in front of the ear and lateral to eyebrow: Palpate gently for the pulse of the superficial temporal artery (Fig. 11-6). This pulse point is often used in infants or when the radial pulse is not accessible.
- **Carotid**—located beside the larynx (voice box): Slide two or three fingers from the larynx laterally

Pulse rates vary greatly among adults. A pulse rate of around 70 is often considered "normal," although a normal pulse rate may be 60 to 100 beats per minute. In well-conditioned athletes, the resting pulse may be as low as 50. Table 11-2 lists normal pulse rates for infants, children, and adults.

Factors affecting the pulse rate are changes in body temperature, exercise, application of or exposure to heat or cold, medications, emotions, hemorrhage, and heart disease. **Bradycardia** describes an adult pulse rate of fewer than 60 beats/min. **Tachycardia** refers to an adult pulse rate of more than 100 beats/min.

The quality and rhythm of the pulse must also be assessed and described. Terms such as "full" or "**bounding**" are often used to describe a strong pulse, and "**thready**" or "weak" might be used to describe a pulse of diminished strength. In some facilities, "grading" of pulses is done using a 0–4 scale: 0, absent; 1,

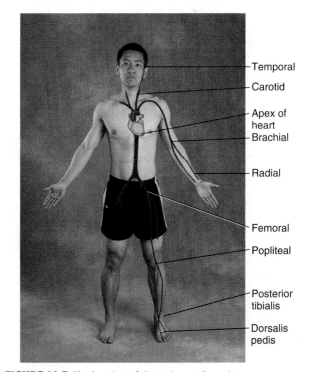

FIGURE 11-5 The location of the various pulse points.

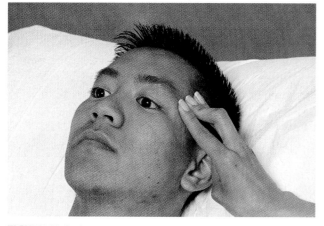

FIGURE 11-6 The temporal pulse is often used in infants and in adults when the radial pulse is not discernible.

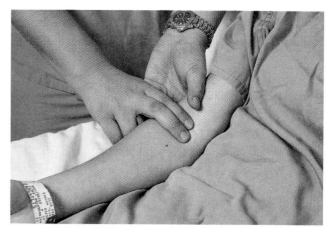

FIGURE 11-8 The brachial pulse site is the access site for blood pressure measurement. This site is also the site used for checking pulse in infant cardiopulmonary resuscitation.

into the groove beside the larynx to palpate the carotid pulse. Be careful to palpate only one side at a time in order to not impede blood flow to the brain. This is the pulse point assessed during adult cardiopulmonary resuscitation (CPR) (Fig. 11-7).

- **Brachial**—located in the medial antecubital fossa (hollow in front of elbow) area: This is the site used to measure the blood pressure as well as the site used during infant CPR (Fig. 11-8).
- **Radial**—located on the thumb side of the forearm at wrist: This site is the most common and convenient site for measuring pulse rate of an adult patient (Fig. 11-9).
- **Femoral**—located halfway between the anterior superior iliac spine and the symphysis pubis, below the inguinal ligament. You may need to press harder to locate this pulse, which is commonly used to assess lower extremity circulation and to evaluate effectiveness of chest compressions during CPR. Keep the genital area covered to safeguard the patient's modesty when assessing this pulse.

- **Popliteal**—located behind the knee in the popliteal fossa with the patient's knee flexed. The popliteal pulse measurement is used in assessing circulation to the lower leg and may be used for measuring blood pressure (Fig. 11-10).
- **Dorsalis pedis**—located on the dorsum of the foot with the foot plantar flexed: Palpate for this pulse halfway between the middle of the patient's ankle and the space between the great toe and the second toe. This pulse is easily obliterated, so palpate lightly (Fig. 11-11).
- **Posterior tibial**—located on the inner side of the ankle slightly below the medial malleolus: This pulse may be difficult to assess in obese patients or in those with considerable edema (Fig. 11-12).

The dorsalis pedis and posterior tibial pulses are used to assess the circulation to the foot. They also may be referred to as **pedal pulses**. If a patient has had surgery on blood vessels leading to the foot, you may be asked

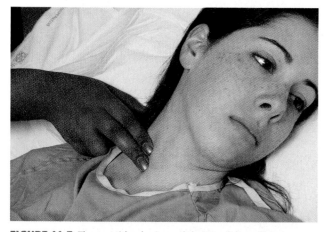

FIGURE 11-7 The carotid pulse is used during adult cardiopulmonary resuscitation and to assess circulation to the head.

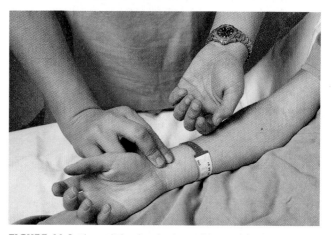

FIGURE 11-9 The radial pulse site is used routinely to measure the pulse rate because of its convenience.

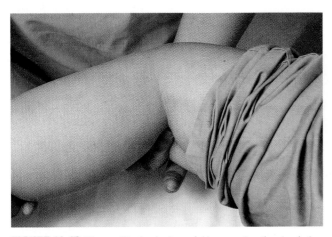

FIGURE 11-10 The popliteal pulse is useful in assessing the circulation to the lower leg and when measuring blood pressure using the leg.

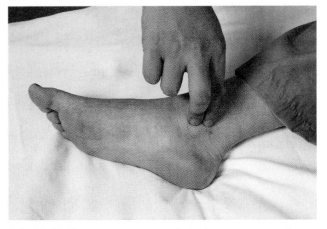

FIGURE 11-12 Locate the posterior tibial pulse by curving your fingers behind and a little below the medial malleolus of the ankle.

to mark the **dorsalis pedis** pulse point or the posterior tibial pulse point with a marking pen so that these can be located more easily by all care providers. If the pedal pulses are not palpable, assess the color and warmth of the foot.

APICAL PULSE

The **apical pulse** is measured by listening over the apex of the heart on the left side of the chest, using a stethoscope. The apex is usually found at the fifth intercostal space just inside the **midclavicular line** (Fig. 11-13).

You may need to move your stethoscope around in this general area to find where the patient's apical pulse is heard most clearly. The elderly individual with some degree of heart failure typically has an enlarged heart. You may need to listen lateral to the midclavicular line to hear the apical pulse in these individuals. The apical pulse is also measured in infants or elderly patients, whose pulse rates are often difficult to determine using peripheral sites. The apical pulse should be counted for

a full 60 seconds. It should also be measured for a full 60 seconds before administering certain heart medications that might be withheld if the pulse rate is too fast or too slow. The apical-radial pulse is sometimes assessed when a patient has a cardiovascular disorder. Two people count the radial pulse and the apical pulse simultaneously and record their results. This allows for exact comparison of the two pulses.

RESPIRATION

The act of breathing is involuntary but can be affected by voluntary control. Respirations are normally regular, even, and quiet, but they can be affected by the same factors that cause the pulse rate to vary. A rate of 12 to 20 breaths/minute is considered "normal" for the adult. The term **eupnea** is used to describe respirations that have normal rate and depth. **Bradypnea** is used to describe abnormally slow respirations, and **tachypnea** to describe rapid respirations that are quick and shallow.

The depth and character of respirations must also be observed and described. Respiratory and metabolic disorders can cause variations as can other acute and chronic problems. The sides of the chest normally rise and fall together. This is termed **symmetry**. If they do not rise and fall together, respirations are termed **asymmetrical**.

The term **dyspnea** may describe any breathing difficulty, but a more specific description that includes depth and any pattern that varies from normal should be included as well. **Orthopnea** refers to a need to sit up in order to breath. The term **Cheyne-Stokes respirations** is used to describe a gradual increase and decrease in the rate and depth of respirations, usually including a period of **apnea** (nonbreathing) at the end of each cycle. Any periods of apnea should be timed.

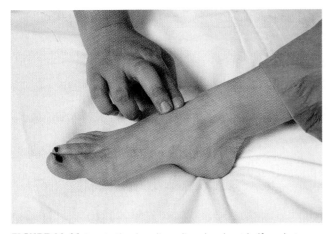

FIGURE 11-11 Locate the dorsalis pedis pulse about halfway between the great toe and the second toe.

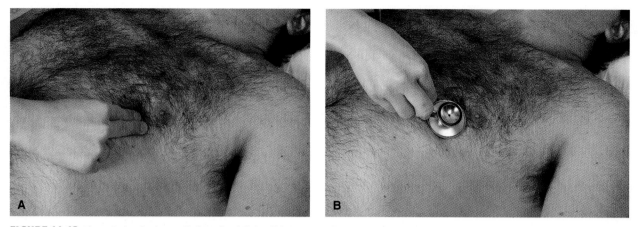

FIGURE 11-13 The apical pulse is usually found at (**A**) the fifth intercostal space just inside the midclavicular line and can be heard (**B**) over the apex of the heart.

GENERAL PROCEDURE FOR MEASURING TEMPERATURE, PULSE, AND RESPIRATION

ASSESSMENT

1. Assess your institution's standard policy and procedures regarding routine times for taking TPR. **R:** The institution's policies and procedures guide the nurse's practice at each institution.
2. Assess the patient's readiness for the procedure. **R:** If the patient is involved in another activity or has just engaged in an activity that could affect the accuracy of the measurement, delay the procedure for 15 to 20 minutes.

ANALYSIS

3. Critically think through your data, carefully evaluating each aspect and its relation to other data. **R:** This enables you to determine specific problems for this individual in relation to assessing TPR.

4. Identify specific problems and modifications of the procedure needed for this individual. **R:** Planning for the individual must take into consideration the individual's problems.

PLANNING

5. Determine individualized patient outcomes in relation to TPR. **R:** Identification of desired outcomes guides planning and evaluation of care.
   a. Temperature, pulse, and respirations are accurately measured.
   b. Results of TPR measurement are within the normal range for this patient.
   c. Patient is comfortable.
6. Select the appropriate equipment including the following. **R:** Planning ahead allows you to proceed more safely and effectively.
   a. Thermometer (include lubricant if the temperature will be measured rectally)
   b. Stethoscope (if an apical pulse is to be measured)
   c. Watch (digital or with a sweep second hand)
   d. Worksheet (to allow immediate recording of the readings).

IMPLEMENTATION

Action	Rationale
7. Wash or disinfect your hands	To decrease the transfer of microorganisms that could cause infection.
8. Identify the patient using two identifiers.	Verifying the patient's identity helps ensure that you are performing the right skill for the right patient.
9. Explain the procedure you are about to perform.	Explaining the procedure helps relieve anxiety or misperceptions that the patient may have about a procedure or activity and sets the stage for patient participation.
10. Raise the bed to an appropriate working position based on your height.	This will allow you to use correct body mechanics and protect yourself from back injury.

(continued)

Action	Rationale
11. Be sure the lighting is adequate.	To ensure accuracy.
12. Assist the patient to a comfortable position.	A comfortable position helps the patient relax during the procedure. Discomfort has the potential to alter some results.
13. Measure the TPR, following the specific procedures described on the following pages.	Accuracy depends on careful attention to detail.
14. Return the patient's bed to the low position, and wash or disinfect your hands.	To maintain safety and to decrease the transfer of microorganisms that could cause infection.

EVALUATION

15. Evaluate using the individualized patient outcomes previously identified. **R:** Evaluation in relation to desired outcomes is essential for planning future care.
  a. Temperature, pulse, and respirations are accurately measured.
  b. Results of TPR measurement are within the normal range for this patient.
  c. Patient is comfortable.

DOCUMENTATION

16. Record findings from your worksheet to the graphic record, vital signs board, or bedside computer, depending on the practice in your facility. Unusual findings may need to be recorded further in the nurse's notes, possibly including written data findings and assessments. **R:** Documentation is a legal record of the patient's care and therapy and communicates nursing activities to other nurses and caregivers.
17. Report any abnormal findings to the appropriate person. **R:** Abnormal findings may require immediate intervention.

POTENTIAL ADVERSE OUTCOMES AND RELATED INTERVENTIONS

1. Temperature more than 1°F above normal.
Intervention: Encourage the patient to drink fluids to prevent dehydration. Encourage rest. If temperature continues to rise, notify physician.
2. Respirations below 10 or above 30 in the adult may lead to severe hypoxia.
Intervention: Position the patient for optimum breathing. Administer oxygen per protocol. Notify the physician.
3. Pulse rate below 60 (unless that is the norm for the patient) may result in lightheadedness and fainting when the patient gets up.

Intervention: Prevent falls by assisting the patient. Encourage the patient to get up slowly. Notify the physician if this is a new finding.
4. Pulse rate of more than 100 increases stress on the heart and results in diminished cardiac output.
Intervention: Encourage the patient to rest. Notify the physician.

SPECIFIC PROCEDURES FOR MEASURING TEMPERATURE

Measuring the Oral Temperature

ASSESSMENT

1-2. Follow steps 1 and 2 of the General Procedure for Measuring Temperature, Pulse, and Respiration: Assess institution's policy and procedures and the patient's readiness for the procedure.

ANALYSIS

3-4. Follow steps 3 and 4 of the General Procedure: Think through your data, and identify specific problems and modifications.

PLANNING

5. Determine individualized patient outcomes in relation to temperature. **R:** Identification of desired outcomes guides planning and evaluation of care.
  a. Temperature is accurately measured.
  b. Results of temperature measurement are within the normal range for this patient.
  c. Patient is comfortable.
6. Follow step 6 of the General Procedure: Select the appropriate equipment:
  a. electronic or chemical dot thermometer
  b. disposable probe covers
  c. vital signs worksheet

IMPLEMENTATION

Action	Rationale
7-12. Follow steps 7 through 12 of the General Procedure: Wash or disinfect your hands, identify the patient (two identifiers), explain the procedure, raise the bed, ensure adequate lighting, and position the patient.	
13. Measure the patient's temperature using an oral electronic thermometer or a chemical dot thermometer:	
a. Follow the manufacturer's instructions for using the specific thermometer. Remove the electronic thermometer from the charging unit, making sure to use the oral probe, or obtain the chemical dot thermometer from the package.	Following the manufacturer's instructions ensures optimal results.
b. For the electronic thermometer: Insert the oral probe into a disposable probe cover, locking it in place. For the chemical dot thermometer: Peel off the covering over the dots.	The probe cover provides for infection prevention between patients, and the probe is designed to measure temperature through the cover. The chemical dots must be exposed to register temperature.
c. Have the patient open his or her mouth, and place the thermometer carefully in either the left or right posterior sublingual pocket at the base of the tongue (Fig. 11-14). Have the patient close his or her mouth over the chemical dot thermometer. With the electronic thermometer, there is a minimal change in readings between an open and closed mouth.	Proper placement ensures accuracy. **FIGURE 11-14** The most common site for measuring the patient's temperature in the clinical setting is the oral site, with the thermometer placed in the left or right posterior sublingual pocket.
d. Keep the electronic thermometer in place until the audible signal tells you the process is complete (usually 30 to 50 seconds) (see Fig. 11-2). Keep the chemical dot thermometer in place until the colors change (see Fig. 11-4).	To ensure the accuracy of the reading.

(continued)

Action	Rationale
e. Read the temperature on the display panel on the electronic thermometer. On the chemical dot thermometer, the changed colors of the dots correspond to the temperature. Write down the results on your worksheet.	Accuracy is enhanced when numerical data is written down immediately.
f. Push the button on the probe of the electronic thermometer to release the probe cover, and reinsert the probe into the thermometer. Dispose of the probe cover, and return the electronic thermometer to the charger. Dispose of the chemical dot thermometer.	Proper battery function of the electronic thermometer depends on the use of the charger. The probe cover and chemical dot thermometer are contaminated with oral secretions and must be disposed of for infection control.
14. Follow step 14 of the General Procedure: Return the bed to the low position, and wash or disinfect your hands.	

EVALUATION

15. Follow step 15 of the General Procedure: Evaluate using the individualized patient outcomes previously identified:
    a. Temperature is accurately measured.
    b. Results of temperature measurement are within the normal range for this patient.
    c. Patient is comfortable.

DOCUMENTATION

16-18. Follow steps 16 to 18 of the General Procedure: Record your findings, and report abnormal readings as indicated.

Measuring the Rectal Temperature

ASSESSMENT

1-2. Follow steps 1 and 2 of the General Procedure for Measuring Temperature, Pulse, and Respirations:

Assess institution's policy and procedures and the patient's readiness for the procedure.

ANALYSIS

3-4. Follow steps 3 and 4 of the General Procedure: Think through your data, and identify specific problems and modifications.

PLANNING

5. Determine individualized patient outcomes in relation to rectal temperature:
    a. Temperature is accurately measured.
    b. Results of temperature measurement are within the normal range for this patient.
    c. Patient is comfortable.
6. Follow step 6 of the General Procedure: Select the appropriate equipment:
    a. electronic thermometer
    b. disposable probe covers
    c. lubricant
    d. vital signs worksheet

IMPLEMENTATION

Action	Rationale
7-12. Follow steps 7 through 12 of the General Procedure: Wash or disinfect your hands, identify the patient (two identifiers), explain the procedure, raise the bed, ensure adequate lighting, and position the patient.	

(continued)

Action	Rationale
13. Measure the patient's temperature using an electronic rectal thermometer:	
a. Follow the manufacturer's instructions. Remove electronic thermometer from charging unit, making sure to include the rectal probe for use.	Following the manufacturer's instructions ensures optimal results.
b. Close the door to the patient's room, pull the curtains, and keep the patient covered, exposing only the anal area during the procedure.	To maintain patient privacy.
c. Put on disposable gloves, and position the patient on the left side (**Sims' position**).	For infection control. Sims' position provides access to the anal area.
d. Insert the rectal probe into a disposable probe cover, locking it into place. Liberally apply lubricant, covering 1.5 inches (3.8 cm) of the thermometer, and insert the thermometer into the patient's rectum 1.5 inches (3.8 cm). Always hold the end of the thermometer while it is in place.	This prevents damage to rectal mucosa and prevents displacement of the thermometer if the patient moves.
e. Keep the thermometer in place until the audible signal tells you the process is complete (usually 30 to 50 seconds).	To ensure the accuracy of the reading.
f. Read the display panel on the electronic thermometer, and write down the results on your worksheet. Push the button on the probe of the electronic thermometer to release the probe cover, and reinsert the probe into the thermometer. Dispose of the probe cover and return the electronic thermometer to the charger.	The proper battery function of an electronic thermometer depends on the use of the charger. The probe cover is contaminated and must be disposed of immediately.
g. Wipe the patient's anal area, and discard your gloves.	To remove lubricant and for infection control.
14. Follow step 14 of the General Procedure: Return the patient's bed to the low position, and wash or disinfect your hands.	

EVALUATION

15. Follow step 15 of the General Procedure: Evaluate using the previously identified individualized patient outcomes:
    a. Temperature is accurately measured.
    b. Results of temperature measurement are within the normal range for this patient.
    c. Patient is comfortable.

DOCUMENTATION

16-17. Follow steps 16 and 17 of the General Procedure: Record the result from your worksheet, marked with "(R)" next to it to indicate that it was taken rectally, and report if necessary.

Measuring the Axillary Temperature

ASSESSMENT

1-2. Follow steps 1 and 2 of the General Procedure for Measuring Temperature, Pulse, and Respiration:

Assess institution's policy and procedures and the patient's readiness for the procedure.

ANALYSIS

3-4. Follow steps 3 and 4 of the General Procedure: Think through your data, and identify specific problems and modifications.

PLANNING

5. Determine individualized patient outcomes in relation to measuring the temperature using the axillary site:
    a. Temperature is accurately measured.
    b. Results of temperature measurement are within the normal range for this patient.
    c. Patient is comfortable.
6. Follow step 6 of the General Procedure: Select the appropriate equipment:
    a. electronic thermometer
    b. disposable probe covers
    c. vital signs worksheet

IMPLEMENTATION

Action	Rationale
7-12. Follow steps 7 to 12 of the General Procedure: Wash or disinfect your hands, identify the patient (two identifiers), explain the procedure, raise the bed, ensure adequate lighting, and position the patient.	
13. Measure the patient's temperature using the axillary site.	
a. Follow the manufacturer's instructions. Remove the electronic thermometer from the charging unit, making sure to select the oral probe for use.	Following the manufacturer's instructions ensures optimum results.
b. Close the door to the room, and pull the curtain during the procedure.	To maintain patient privacy.
c. Place the patient in Fowler's position, and arrange the gown so that the **axilla** (armpit) is exposed.	For optimum patient comfort and access to the axilla.
d. Make sure the patient's axilla is dry; then place the tip of the thermometer in the center of the axilla.	Prevents displacement if the patient moves.

(continued)

Action	Rationale
e. Keep the thermometer in place until the audible signal tells you the process is complete (usually 30 to 50 seconds).	To ensure the accuracy of the reading.
f. Read the display panel on the electronic thermometer, and write down the results on your worksheet. Push the button on the probe of the electronic thermometer to release the probe cover, and reinsert the probe into the thermometer. Dispose of the probe cover and return the electronic thermometer to the charger.	The proper battery function of an electronic thermometer depends on the use of the charger. The probe cover is contaminated and must be disposed of immediately.
14. Follow step 14 of the General Procedure: Lower the bed, and wash or disinfect your hands.	

EVALUATION

15. Follow step 15 of the General Procedure: Evaluate using the individualized patient outcomes previously identified:
  a. Temperature is accurately measured.
  b. Results of temperature measurement are within the normal range for this patient.
  c. Patient is comfortable.

DOCUMENTATION

16-17. Follow steps 16 and 17 of the General Procedure: Record the result, write an "(A)" next to it to indicate that it was taken at the axillary site, and report as indicated.

Measuring the Tympanic Temperature

ASSESSMENT

1-2. Follow steps 1 and 2 of the General Procedure for Measuring Temperature, Pulse, and Respiration:

Assess the institution's policy and procedures and the patient's readiness for the procedure.

ANALYSIS

3-4. Follow steps 3 and 4 of the General Procedure: Think through your data, and identify specific problems and modifications.

PLANNING

5. Determine individualized patient outcomes in relation to measuring the temperature using the tympanic site:
  a. Temperature is accurately measured.
  b. Results of temperature measurement are within the normal range for this patient.
  c. Patient is comfortable.
6. Follow step 6 of the General Procedure: Select the appropriate equipment:
  a. tympanic thermometer
  b. disposable probe covers
  c. vital signs worksheet

IMPLEMENTATION

Action	Rationale
7-12. Follow steps 7 through 12 of the General Procedure: Wash or disinfect your hands, identify the patient (two identifiers), explain the procedure, raise the bed, ensure adequate lighting, and position the patient.	

(continued)

Action	Rationale
13. Measure the temperature using the tympanic site:	
a. Follow the manufacturer's instructions. Remove the tympanic thermometer from the charging unit.	Following the manufacturer's instructions ensures optimum results.
b. Place a clean, plastic cover over the tip of the probe. Hold the pinna up and back on an adult. Point the probe toward the eardrum (slightly anteriorly), and insert slowly until the opening of the ear canal is "sealed." Incorrect placement results in errors in temperature measurement (Pullen, 2003).	This position provides optimum exposure of the tympanic membrane.
c. Press the scan button on the thermometer. Hold the probe in place until a signal indicates that the reading is complete.	The signal confirms that the temperature reading is visible on the display.
d. Write down the results on your worksheet. Push the button on the probe of the tympanic thermometer to release the probe cover, and reinsert the probe into the thermometer. Dispose of the probe cover and return the tympanic thermometer to the charger.	Proper battery function of an electronic thermometer is dependent upon the use of the charger. The probe cover is contaminated and should be disposed of immediately.
14. Follow step 14 of the General Procedure: Lower the bed, and wash or disinfect your hands.	

EVALUATION

15. Follow step 15 of the General Procedure: Evaluate using the previously identified individualized patient outcomes:
   a. Temperature is accurately measured.
   b. Results of temperature measurement are within the standard range for this patient.
   c. Patient is comfortable.

Also compare the results to the patient's baseline and normal ranges, and repeat as necessary.

DOCUMENTATION

16-17. Follow steps 16 and 17 of the General Procedure: Record the result from your worksheet.

Mark "(T)" next to the temperature reading to indicate that it was taken tympanically, and report if indicated.

SPECIFIC PROCEDURES FOR MEASURING PULSE

ASSESSMENT

1-2. Follow steps 1 and 2 of the General Procedure for Measuring Temperature, Pulse, and Respiration: Assess the institution's policy and procedures and the patient's readiness for the procedure.

ANALYSIS

3-4. Follow steps 3 and 4 of the General Procedure: Think through your data, and identify specific problems and modifications.

PLANNING

5. Determine individualized patient outcomes in relation to measuring the pulse:

a. Pulse is accurately measured.
b. Results of pulse measurement are within the standard range for this patient.
c. Patient is comfortable.
6. Select any equipment necessary.
a. Vital signs worksheet
b. Stethoscope (if needed)
c. Doppler ultrasound device (if needed)

IMPLEMENTATION

Action	Rationale
7-12. Follow steps 7 to 12 of the General Procedure: Wash or disinfect your hands, identify the patient (two identifiers), explain the procedure, raise the bed, ensure adequate lighting, and position the patient.	
13. Measure the patient's pulse:	
a. *Radial pulse:* Position the patient in the supine position with the arm positioned beside the body, palm downward. Curl two or three fingers around the wrist on the thumb side, and palpate gently. If the pulsations are regular, count the beats for 30 seconds and multiply by 2. If the pulse rate is irregular, count the beats for a full 60 seconds. In addition to the rhythm, also note the quality of the pulse (strong or weak or thready) at this time.	This provides for accurate palpation of the radial artery.
b. *Dorsalis pedis pulse:* Locate the dorsalis pedis pulse on the dorsum (top) of the foot, about halfway between the great toe and the second toe. Palpate lightly with your first three fingers over the dorsalis pedis artery, and count the pulse if it can be palpated. Light touch will not occlude the artery. It may take as much as 30 seconds to locate the patient's pulse. When you need to know whether the arterial circulation is strong enough to project a pulsation, describe the pulse in terms of strength as well as rate.	This provides for accurate palpation of the dorsalis pedis artery. The dorsalis pedis pulse and posterior tibial pulse below may be easily obliterated, so feel gently.
c. *Posterior tibial pulse:* Locate the posterior tibial pulse by curving your fingers behind and a little below the	This provides for accurate palpation of the posterior tibial artery.

(continued)

Action	Rationale
medial malleolus of the ankle. Palpate gently, and count the pulse if it can be palpated. Describe its strength.	
d. *Apical pulse:* Place the diaphragm of the stethoscope over the apex of the heart at the fifth intercostal space just inside the midclavicular line. Listen and count the beats for a full 60 seconds.	The heart is closest to the chest wall at this point and most easily heard here.
e. *Apical-radial pulse* (using two nurses): The first nurse measures the pulse radially, while the second nurse listens with the stethoscope and counts the apical pulse over the apex of the heart. Using the second hand of a single watch placed where both nurses can see it, count the pulses for 60 seconds.	A **pulse deficit** (radial rate is less than the apical rate) means that some of the cardiac contractions do not have the strength to push a wave of blood that can be palpated at the radial site.
f. *Pulse rate using a Doppler ultrasound device:* Place electrode gel on the patient's skin or on the end of the Doppler probe (a transducer in the device will convert ultrasonic vibrations into sounds), and position the probe over the pulse point. Listen with stethoscope earpieces, headphones, or a speaker, depending on the equipment you are using. Note the rate and quality of the pulse if it is audible.	A Doppler device may be used when pulses are either difficult or impossible to palpate.
g. *Pulse of a newborn or infant:* Use a stethoscope, and listen over the apex of the heart for 60 seconds.	Infant heart rates normally vary with respiration, necessitating counting the pulse beats for a full 60 seconds.
14. Follow step 14 of the General Procedure: Lower the bed, and wash or disinfect your hands.	

EVALUATION

15. Follow step 15 of the General Procedure: Evaluate using the individualized patient outcomes previously identified:
   a. Pulse is accurately measured.
   b. Results of pulse measurement are within the normal range for this patient.
   c. Patient is comfortable.

DOCUMENTATION

16-17. Follow steps 16 and 17 of the General Procedure: Record from your worksheet the site, rate, rhythm, and quality of the pulse, and report as necessary.

SPECIFIC PROCEDURE FOR MEASURING RESPIRATION

ASSESSMENT

1-2. Follow steps 1 and 2 of the General Procedure for Measuring Temperature, Pulse, and Respiration: Assess your institution's policy and procedures and the patient's readiness for the procedure.

ANALYSIS

3-4. Follow steps 3 and 4 of the General Procedure: Think through your data, and identify specific problems and modifications.

PLANNING

5. Determine individualized patient outcomes in relation to measuring the respirations:
   a. Respirations are accurately measured and observed.
   b. Results of respiratory observations are within the normal range for this patient.
   c. Patient is comfortable.

6. Follow step 6 of the General Procedure: Select the appropriate equipment. Although no other equipment is needed, you will still need a vital signs worksheet.

IMPLEMENTATION

Action	Rationale
7-12. Follow steps 7 to 12 of the General Procedure: Wash or disinfect your hands, identify the patient (two identifiers), explain the procedure, raise the bed, ensure adequate lighting, and position the patient.	
13. Measure the respiratory rate as follows:	
a. With your fingers still in the same position for taking the radial pulse, look at the patient's chest, and observe and count the respirations.	Observing while still in the pulse-taking position keeps the patient from knowing that you are assessing his or her breathing pattern and therefore altering it.
b. If rhythm of respiration is regular, count the breaths for 30 seconds, and multiply by 2. If rhythm is irregular or less than 12 breaths/minute, count breaths for a full 60 seconds.	It may take at least 30 seconds to assess whether the pattern of respiration is regular.
c. Note the rate, rhythm, and characteristics of respirations and the length of any periods of apnea.	Characteristics of breathing along with rate and rhythm may relay information regarding the status of the patient's pulmonary system.
14. Follow step 14 of the General Procedure: Lower the bed, and wash or disinfect your hands.	

EVALUATION

15. Follow step 15 of the General Procedure: Evaluate using the previously identified individualized patient outcomes:
    a. Respirations are accurately measured and observed.
    b. Results of respiratory observations are within the normal range for this patient.
    c. Patient is comfortable.

DOCUMENTATION

16-17. Follow steps 16 and 17 of the General Procedure: Record the rate, rhythm, and characteristics of the breathing pattern from your worksheet, and report if indicated.

Acute Care

Each facility has routine times established in the policy and procedure for taking patients' TPRs. TPR is always assessed on admission as a baseline. If the situation permits, it is good practice to take this opportunity to ask patients if they know what their temperature, pulse, and respirations measurements usually are. TPR can also be assessed as necessary based upon the nurse's judgment related to changes in the patient's condition.

Long-Term Care

Under ordinary circumstances, TPRs are measured much less frequently in long-term care facilities than they are in acute care settings. However, there is typically a routine policy, such as once or twice weekly, perhaps on bath day. When a change in TPR or other indicators (often a decline in functional abilities) occurs, caregivers are alerted to the necessity of initiating more frequent monitoring of TPR and perhaps blood pressure as well. The older adults who reside in long-term care facilities may typically have a much lower baseline temperature than is found in people of other ages. This is due to the decreased metabolic rate in the very old. If an older person develops an infection that would normally result in an elevated temperature, that person's temperature may rise or change only slightly. Therefore, caregivers of the elderly must be alert to small changes.

Home Care

The individual giving care in the home setting may need to be taught how to measure TPRs accurately. What you teach will depend on the situation, the equipment available, and your assessment of the caregiver's ability. In some cases, heat-sensitive patches may be adequate to measure body temperature. These are reusable and react to heat by changing color. They are often used in home settings if less precise temperature readings are acceptable. If the client has a glass thermometer containing mercury, the nurse needs to teach the client how to store the thermometer safely and what to do if the thermometer breaks and mercury spills out. All home health agencies have MSDS procedures for dealing with mercury spills that can be used for instruction.

At times, people are taught to monitor their own vital signs. Clients who have cardiac pacemakers are usually asked to monitor the pulse to ensure that the device is performing properly. Clients may also monitor their pulse if they are on specific cardiac medicines. A family member or friend may be taught to do this for the client if the client cannot. Assessing respirations in the home is often done for the person who has a respiratory disorder. Therefore, assessing the home environment is also important for the client. Questions to ask may be related to dust, allergies, or environmental hazards, such as smoking.

Ambulatory Care

As in acute and long-term care settings, ambulatory care centers have set policies and procedures for taking TPR. The ambulatory care center is a place where the nurse may need to provide some client and family teaching for assessing TPR in the home after particular procedures. Gathering data about the home's safety and environment is important for any client who has had an anesthetic procedure.

LEARNING TOOLS

DEVELOP YOUR BACKGROUND KNOWLEDGE

1. Review the Learning Outcomes.

2. Read the section on temperature, pulse, and respirations in your assigned text.

3. Look up the Key Terms in the glossary.

4. Review this module, and mentally practice the techniques described. Study so that you feel able to teach these skills to another person.

DEVELOP YOUR SKILLS

1. In the practice setting, select two other students to form a group of three.

2. Alternating so that each has the opportunity to play the role of the patient, perform each of the following procedures for TPR and assessing peripheral pulses. Record each value on a vital signs graphic sheet. Use the Performance Checklists on the CD-ROM in the front of this book to check yourself. The person not participating at a given time can observe and evaluate the performances of the others for the following:

   a. oral, axillary, and tympanic temperatures (compare findings at different sites)
   b. rectal temperature (using a mannequin)
   c. apical and radial pulses at rest
      (1) Two "nurses" measure an apical-radial pulse for the "patient."
      (2) Have the "patient" exercise briskly for 3 minutes.
      (3) Compare the pulse rate and quality with the one taken at rest.
   d. Measure and describe respirations.
   e. Evaluate the vital signs graphic record of another student before submitting it to the instructor.

DEMONSTRATE YOUR SKILLS

In the clinical setting

1. Consult with your instructor regarding the opportunity to measure TPRs for patients.

2. Evaluate your performance with the instructor.

CRITICAL THINKING EXERCISES

1. You are caring for three young patients, Megan, Melissa, and Hanna. All share the same room and are between 5 and 7 years old. You take their 4 p.m. TPR, noting your readings as follows:

   Megan—36.2°C, 88, 29
   Melissa—37°C, 92, 22
   Hanna—37.8°C, 108, 28

   Interpret these readings. Are all of the patients within the normal range for children in their age group? If not, which of these patients has abnormal TPR? Determine whether you should report these findings and, if so, to whom.

2. Your 66-year-old female patient is lying in bed covered with three blankets telling you that she feels cold and sick. She is shivering and appears flushed. Her skin is hot to touch. Vital signs are as follows: T 99.2°F, P 126, R 28. Are these vital signs within the normal ranges? Are these the findings you would expect based upon the clinical data given? What key question related to the patient's temperature might you have missed, and what will your next steps be?

SELF-QUIZ
SHORT-ANSWER QUESTIONS

1. What is the normal oral temperature for the average adult? State your answer in both Fahrenheit and Celsius measurements.

   _____

2. List the four factors that may change body temperature.

   a. _____

   b. _____

   c. _____

   d. _____

3. List the three arteries that can be used for counting the pulse rate.

a. _____

b. _____

c. _____

4. State the normal pulse rate range for a resting adult in beats per minutes.

   _____

5. State the normal respiratory rate for an adult in breaths per minute.

   _____

6. List the four factors that cause changes in respiration.

   a. _____

   b. _____

   c. _____

   d. _____

MULTIPLE CHOICE

_____ 7. The proper time frame for waiting to check a temperature for the patient who has just had a drink of water is
   a. 2 minutes.
   b. 5 minutes.
   c. 10 minutes.
   d. 15 minutes.

_____ 8. The best thing to do when you get a reading on a digital thermometer that does not seem quite right is to
   a. record that temperature.
   b. do nothing.
   c. repeat the temperature measurement.
   d. report the measurement immediately.

_____ 9. The best location for taking the apical pulse is
   a. over the base of the heart.
   b. at the fifth intercostal space just inside the midclavicular line.
   c. upper left chest near nipple.
   d. at the third intercostal space just inside the midclavicular line.

_____ 10. The locations for assessing peripheral pulses are
   a. radial, temporal, carotid, clavicular, femoral, popliteal, pedal, and posterior tibial.
   b. radial, temporal, carotid, brachial, femoral, crucial, pedal, and posterior tibial.

   c. radius, temporal, carotid, brachial, femoral, crucial, pedal, and posterior tibial.

   d. radial, temporal, carotid, brachial, femoral, popliteal, pedal, and posterior tibial.

_____ **11.** A patient who is experiencing eupnea is said to be

   a. breathing slowly.

   b. breathing rapidly.

   c. breathing normally.

   d. not breathing.

_____ **12.** A normal respiratory rate for the adult is

   a. 10 to 20 breaths per minute.

   b. 12 to 20 breaths per minute.

   c. 14 to 20 breaths per minute.

   d. 16 to 20 breaths per minute.

Answers to Self-Quiz questions appear in the back of this book.

MODULE
12
Measuring Blood Pressure

SKILLS INCLUDED IN THIS MODULE

Procedure for Measuring Blood Pressure
Measuring Ankle-Brachial Index

PREREQUISITE MODULES

Module 1	An Approach to Nursing Skills
Module 2	Documentation
Module 4	Basic Infection Control
Module 5	Safety in the Healthcare Environment
Module 11	Assessing Temperature, Pulse, and Respiration

KEY TERMS

aneroid manometer	postural hypotension
antecubital space	pulse pressure
auscultatory gap	radial artery
brachial artery	shock
diaphragm	sphygmomanometer
diastolic blood pressure	stethoscope
	supine
Korotkoff's sounds	systole
palpation	systolic blood pressure
popliteal artery	

OVERALL OBJECTIVE

▸ To accurately measure and document blood pressure using a cuff, sphygmomanometer, stethoscope, and automatic blood pressure monitor.

LEARNING OUTCOMES

The student will be able to

1. Assess the patient to determine which method to use for blood pressure measurement.
2. Assess the patient to determine readiness for the blood pressure measurement.
3. Analyze the assessment data to determine specific concerns that must be addressed prior to measuring the blood pressure.
4. Determine appropriate patient outcomes of the blood pressure measuring process, and recognize the potential for adverse outcomes.
5. Choose the appropriate equipment.
6. Position the patient appropriately for the procedure, maintaining principles of body mechanics.
7. Measure the blood pressure accurately.
8. Evaluate the effectiveness of the process and the accuracy of the results.
9. Document the results in the patient record or other facility documentation as required.

Blood pressure is the force exerted by the blood against the walls of the arteries of the body. The pressure of the blood when the heart beats and forces blood into the vessels (systole) is termed the **systolic blood pressure.** The lowest blood pressure that is present in the vessels between pulses, when the heart is at rest and filling, is termed the **diastolic blood pressure.** Blood pressure is measured as millimeters of mercury (mm Hg).

Blood pressure is an indicator of a patient's circulatory status and is measured as a part of "vital signs," along with temperature, pulse, and respirations. Many complications related to prescribed medications and medical procedures are identified partly through the changes in blood pressure that may occur. Therefore, blood pressure may be measured both before and after specific medications are administered. The nurse must be able to measure and record blood pressure accurately and to interpret that measurement as it relates to the particular patient.

Pulse pressure is the difference between the systolic blood pressure and the diastolic blood pressure. A change in pulse pressure may be an early indicator of certain disease conditions. Therefore, when evaluating blood pressure over time, the pulse pressure should be identified as well as the blood pressure itself.

NURSING DIAGNOSES

Blood pressure measurements are used to assess all patients. Ongoing blood pressure monitoring is part of the nursing and medical plans of care for many clients.

- Decreased Cardiac Output: This is a collaborative diagnosis that may be related to the presence of an excessively slow or excessively rapid pulse rate. The nursing diagnosis would relate to the patient's medical problems. Individuals with decreased cardiac output may have decreased blood pressure or blood pressure that is difficult to measure because the auscultatory sounds are faint.
- Deficient Fluid Volume: This may be related to active fluid loss or failure of regulatory mechanisms. This may cause blood pressure to fall.
- Excess Fluid Volume: This may contribute to high blood pressure.
- Ineffective Tissue Perfusion: This may be related to arterial or venous flow issues, fluid exchange problems, hypervolemia, or hypovolemia.

DELEGATION

Measuring blood pressure is frequently delegated to assistive personnel. One of the concerns in this process is the importance of accuracy and the potential lack of background understanding of the assistive person. The nurse who is delegating must be sure that the assistive person has a clear understanding of correct technique and knows which blood pressure levels, either high or low, must be reported immediately. The nurse should plan to verify any abnormality reported by assistive personnel before taking action.

EVALUATING BLOOD PRESSURE

Blood pressure varies for an individual both throughout the day and from one day to another. Therefore, it is important for the nurse to understand that the trend of the blood pressure over time is more useful in assessing the individual patient than one isolated blood pressure measurement. Blood pressure may differ between arms if there are anatomic differences in vasculature or vessel disease. A baseline assessment for blood pressure calls for readings in both arms. Table 12-1 provides the most current standards for evaluating blood pressure in the adult. Blood pressure standards for children are based on height and weight as well as age with differences for boys and girls. The National Institutes of Health (2004) complete tables are available at http://www.nhlbi.nih. gov/guidelines/hypertension/child_tbl.htm.

FACTORS AFFECTING BLOOD PRESSURE

Blood pressure varies based on age. It is lowest in the newborn and gradually increases to the level of the adult. While many adults continue to exhibit increases in blood pressure as they age, this is evidence of disease and is not simply the result of aging. The healthy older person should have the same blood pressure as the healthy younger adult.

Many factors may cause blood pressure to rise, including activity, anxiety, strong emotion, recent intake of food, disease, pain, fluid retention, and drugs. The two major factors causing the blood pressure to drop are blood loss and anything that causes the blood vessels to dilate.

Postural hypotension (also called orthostatic hypotension), is a drop in blood pressure caused by a change in body position, for example, from lying to sitting or standing. Symptoms may include dizziness, fainting, or falling. An order written for "postural blood pressures" refers to blood pressures taken in the lying, the sitting, and the standing positions in order to compare them. Instructions for making postural blood pressure measurements are discussed later in the module.

EQUIPMENT FOR MEASURING BLOOD PRESSURE

What is commonly referred to as the *blood pressure cuff* consists of an oblong rubber bag, or bladder, covered with a nonexpandable fabric called the cuff. Today, cuffs may be reusable or disposable. Reusable cuffs pose some potential for transmitting microorganisms from one patient to another. For example, some antibiotic-resistant organisms can be transmitted on dry surfaces. Follow your facility's policy and procedure for cleaning nondisposable blood pressure cuffs.

Note: Never use a nondisposable cuff on a sphygmomanometer that is moved from room to room (such as an automatic device) for a patient with an infection.

It is essential that the width of the blood pressure cuff be correct to ensure accurate measurement. According to the American Heart Association (AHA, 2004), the cuff should be 40% of the circumference of the midpoint of the limb on which it is being used. If the cuff is too narrow, the reading may be higher than the correct one; if it is too wide, the reading may be lower than the correct one. The AHA (2004) recommends the availability of several sizes for use with adults, including small adult, adult, and large adult (also used for thigh measurements). These cuff sizes are not available in all settings. Most facilities have at least three sizes: child (which can be used for a very thin adult), adult, and large adult. The circumference of the arm, not the age of the patient, determines cuff size (Table 12-2). A wrist cuff may also be used. This may be best for the very obese patient. Whatever type of cuff is used, it is most accurate if the center of the cuff is at the level of the heart (AHA, 2004).

The **sphygmomanometer** is the device used to measure pressure. All measure blood in millimeters (mm) of mercury. *Mercury manometers* are the most accurate type of blood pressure measuring device. The mercury rises in a calibrated glass tube, registering the pressure as the cuff is inflated with air, then falls as the air is released. Rubber tubing connects the mercury reservoir with the cuff (Fig. 12-1). They are manufactured in

table 12-1. Classification of Hypertension

Blood Pressure Classification	Systolic Blood Pressure (mm Hg)*	Diastolic Blood Pressure (mm Hg)*
Normal	< 120	< 80
Prehypertensive	121–139	81–89
Stage 1 hypertension	140–159	90–99
Stage 2 hypertension	≥ 160	≥ 100

*Classification determined by higher BP category.
Source: Pickering, T. H., Hall, J. E., Appel, L. J., et al. (2004). Recommendations for Blood Pressure Measurement in Humans and Experimental Animals: Part 1: Blood Pressure Measurement in Humans: A Statement for Professionals From the Subcommittee of Professional and Public Education of the American Heart Association Council on High Blood Pressure Research (p. 147). (Online). Available at http://hyper.ahajournals.org.

table 12-2. Choosing the Correct Cuff Size for Blood Pressure Measurement

Arm Circumference	Recommended Cuff Size
22 to 26 cm	Small adult size: 12 to 22 cm
27 to 34 cm	Adult size: 16 to 30 cm
35 to 44 cm	Large adult size: 16 to 36 cm

Source: Pickering, T. H., Hall, J. E., Appel, L. J., et al. (2004). Recommendations for Blood Pressure Measurement in Humans and Experimental Animals: Part 1: Blood Pressure Measurement in Humans: A Statement for Professionals From the Subcommittee of Professional and Public Education of the American Heart Association Council on High Blood Pressure Research (p. 150). (Online). Available at http://hyper.ahajournals.org.

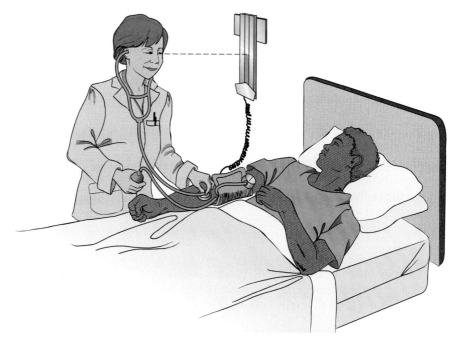

FIGURE 12-1 In a few settings, mercury manometers may still be in use. In such cases, make sure that the manometer is level on the surface and that you read the meniscus of the mercury in the tube from eye level.

a variety of models, including a floor model (which can be moved from one place to another), a portable model (which comes in a box), and a wall model (which is probably the most common). Mercury manometers are used less than in the past because of the dangers associated with mercury spills. Caution needs to be taken when using a mercury manometer to prevent breakage of the tubing and spilling mercury. Follow your facility's Material Safety Data Sheet (MSDS) recommendations located in the appropriate policy and procedure manual for instructions on managing a mercury spill.

The **aneroid manometer** is an air pressure gauge that registers the blood pressure by a pointer on a dial (Fig. 12-2). The dial generally attaches to the outside of the cuff by hooks that fit into a small pocket to make handling easier. The aneroid manometer should be recalibrated approximately every 6 months to ensure accuracy (AHA, 2004).

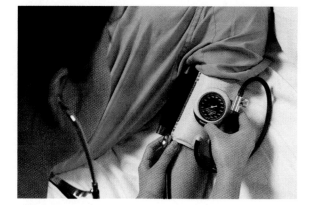

FIGURE 12-2 Equipment for measuring blood pressure with an aneroid sphygmomanometer.

The *hand bulb* is the device attached to the bladder by a rubber tube through which air is pumped (see Fig. 12-1). The hand bulb has a valve, regulated by a thumb-screw, which allows air to escape from the bladder at the desired rate. In automated blood pressure devices, the hand bulb is not needed.

The **stethoscope** is an instrument used for listening to body sounds. The bell head of the stethoscope is usually used for listening when blood pressure is measured (see Fig. 12-1). (The low-pitched sounds associated with blood pressure are heard more easily with the bell head of the stethoscope than with the **diaphragm** on the side opposite the bell.)

PROCEDURE FOR MEASURING BLOOD PRESSURE

ASSESSMENT

1. Examine your institution's standard policy and procedure regarding routine times for taking blood pressure. **R:** The institution's policies and procedures guide the nurse's practice.

2. Assess the patient's readiness for the procedure. Determine any factors present that might affect how the blood pressure is taken. If the patient is receiving an intravenous infusion, has a dialysis cannula in an arm, or has had a mastectomy, the blood pressure should be taken in the opposite arm. In some patients, there are anatomic or physiologic reasons why the blood pressure should not be taken on one arm or the other. This information may be found on

the patient's care plan, or it may even be a part of the physician's orders.

ANALYSIS

3. Critically think through your data, carefully evaluating each aspect and its relation to other data. **R:** To determine specific problems for this individual in relation to measuring blood pressure.
4. Identify specific problems and modifications of the procedure needed for this individual. **R:** Planning for the individual must take into consideration the individual's problems.

PLANNING

5. Identify the individualized patient outcomes, including the following. **R:** Identification of desired outcomes guides planning and evaluation of care.

   a. Blood pressure is accurately measured.
   b. Blood pressure is within the standard range for this patient.
   c. Patient is comfortable.

6. Select the appropriate equipment:
   a. sphygmomanometer; in hospitals, there is often one attached to the wall at each patient unit.
   b. appropriate-size blood pressure cuff; the bladder of the cuff should extend 80% of the way around the arm for an adult and 100% of the arm for a child (AHA, 2004). **R:** Incorrect size will result in an inaccurate reading (see Table 12-2).
   c. stethoscope; if the stethoscope is not your own, disinfect the earpieces with an alcohol wipe.
   d. vital signs worksheet to allow you to write down information immediately to prevent forgetting data when distracted by other patient needs. **R:** Planning ahead allows you to proceed more safely and effectively.

IMPLEMENTATION

Action	Rationale
7. Wash or disinfect your hands.	To decrease the transfer of microorganisms that could cause infection.
8. Identify the patient, using two identifiers.	Verifying the patient's identity helps ensure that you are performing the right skill for the right patient.
9. Explain the procedure you are about to perform.	Explaining the procedure helps relieve anxiety or misperceptions that the patient may have about a procedure or activity and sets the stage for patient participation.
10. Raise the bed to an appropriate working position based on your height.	To allow you to use correct body mechanics and protect yourself from back injury.
11. Be sure the room lighting is adequate.	To allow you to accurately read the sphygmomanometer.
12. Assist the patient into a comfortable position—**supine** or sitting if able. The arm should be fully supported on a flat surface at heart level.	A comfortable position helps the patient relax during the procedure. Discomfort has the potential to alter the blood pressure. Blood pressure readings not taken at heart level will result in an incorrect pressure value.
13. Measure the blood pressure following the specific instructions listed below:	
a. Remove clothing from upper arm.	Clothing that is restrictive may cause a false elevation in the blood pressure value.

(continued)

Action	Rationale
b. With the bladder centered over the **brachial artery,** wrap the blood pressure cuff around the arm above the elbow making sure it is smooth and snug and fastened securely. (Velcro is the most common fastener.) The lower edge of the cuff should be about 1 inch above the **antecubital space** (fossa).	Placement over the artery ensures that pressure exerted by the air-filled bladder during inflation is directed to the artery.
c. Place the gauge at the proper location for correct reading. If an aneroid gauge is attached to the cuff, place the gauge where it can be easily read. If a mercury gauge is used, the manometer should be read at eye level.	To ensure accurate reading.
d. Place the stethoscope earpieces (facing forward) in your ears.	This position more effectively directs the sound into your ears.
e. Palpate the brachial artery, located slightly more medial than the center of the antecubital space.	Improper location may cause an inaccurate reading.
f. Keeping your fingers over the brachial artery, turn the valve on the hand bulb clockwise until it is tight. Pump the hand bulb to fill the rubber bladder in the blood pressure cuff with air. As you pump, the gauge will register the pressure in the cuff. Pump until you no longer feel a pulse, and continue for 30 mm Hg beyond that point. Slowly deflate the cuff, noting the level of pressure at which the pulse reappears. Wait at least 30 to 60 seconds before attempting to re-inflate the cuff.	Using palpation first assures that you do not pump the pressure in the cuff much higher than needed, thereby creating discomfort. It also prevents missing the first Korotkoff sound (Box 12-1) as a result of the **auscultatory gap.** The auscultatory gap is the period between the Phase 1 initial tapping sounds, which may be faint, and the Phase 3 crisp and strong sounds. Failure to hear the sounds above the auscultatory gap will result in an erroneously low blood pressure measurement.

box 12-1 *Korotkoff's Sounds*

- Phase 1: The first faint, clear, repetitive tapping sounds are heard, signifying systolic blood pressure.
- Phase 2: Swishing or murmur sound.
- Phase 3: Sounds are crisper and increase in intensity.
- Phase 4: Sound changes to a muffle, signifying diastolic blood pressure in the child.
- Phase 5: The last sound is heard, signifying diastolic blood pressure in the adult.

Source: Pickering, T. H., Hall, J. E., Appel, L. J., et al. (2004). Recommendations for Blood Pressure Measurement in Humans and Experimental Animals: Part 1: Blood Pressure Measurement in Humans: A Statement for Professionals From the Subcommittee of Professional and Public Education of the American Heart Association Council on High Blood Pressure Research. (Online). Available at http://hyper.ahajournals.org.

(continued)

Action	Rationale
g. Position the bell of the stethoscope over the brachial artery, making good contact with the skin.	Skin contact allows for conduction of sound.
h. Inflate the bladder rapidly and steadily, reaching a pressure of 20 to 30 mm Hg above the previously palpated pressure level.	Rapid inflation allows for maximum accuracy.
i. Open the valve on the hand bulb (turning counterclockwise) to release air from the rubber bladder (no faster than 2 to 3 mm Hg/sec), and watch the pressure registered on the gauge decrease, while listening for **Korotkoff's sounds** (see Box 12-1). The Phase 1 first sound represents systolic blood pressure and the Phase 5 last sound correlates to diastolic blood pressure in the adult. After you hear the last sound, continue deflating the cuff for another 10 mm Hg to ensure that no further sounds are audible before rapidly deflating. If sounds continue all the way to zero, record all three readings, Phase 1, Phase 4, and Phase 5.	Following this process allows optimal transmission of sounds to identify systolic and diastolic blood pressure.
j. To double-check the blood pressure, wait at least 1 full minute, then repeat on same arm. If this is the first assessment, follow the procedure, and check blood pressure on other arm as well.	Waiting 1 minute allows the release of blood trapped in the veins. Checking blood pressure on the opposite arm helps assess potential for circulatory problems.
k. Remove the stethoscope earpieces from your ears.	To allow you to hear the patient speaking.
l. Remove the cuff from the patient's arm.	To give the patient freedom to move.
m. Return the patient's bed to the low position when completed.	For patient safety.
14. Clean the stethoscope earpieces with an alcohol wipe, and wipe the bell head with another alcohol wipe.	To remove any possible source of infection.
15. Wash or disinfect your hands.	To decrease the transfer of microorganisms that could cause infection.

EVALUATION

16. For future planning, evaluate based on the previously established individualized patient outcomes.
    R: Evaluation enables planning for future care.
    a. Blood pressure is accurately measured.
    b. Blood pressure is within the standard range for this patient.
    c. Patient is comfortable.

DOCUMENTATION

17. Record findings from your worksheet on the graphic record, vital signs board, or bedside computer, depending on the practice in your facility. Unusual findings may need to be recorded further in the narrative notes. The blood pressure is written with the systolic pressure (first Korotkoff's sound) followed by a slash and the diastolic pressure, which is usu-

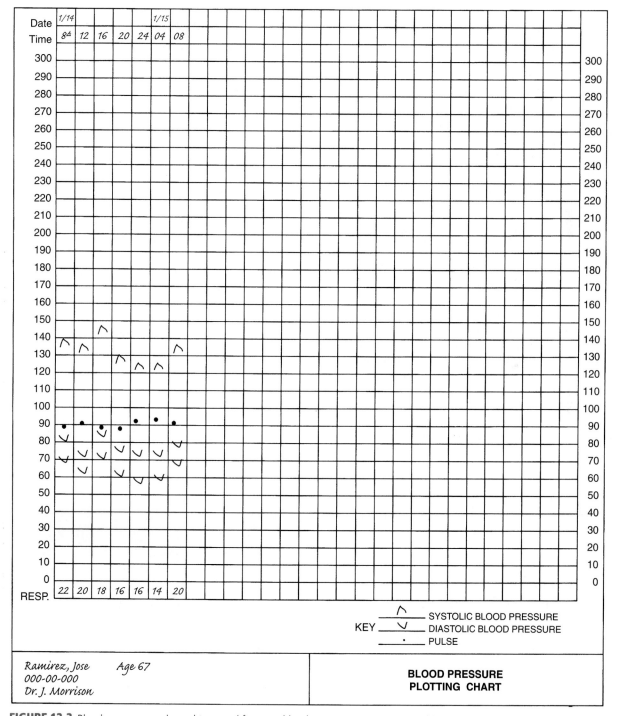

FIGURE 12-3 Blood pressure graph used to record frequent blood pressure measurements. This visual provides for trending over time.

ally the fifth Korotkoff's sound, after the slash (eg, 140/70). When there is muffling (the fourth Korotkoff's sound) heard, that number is placed second followed by another slash and then the fifth Korotkoff's sound (eg, 140/80/70). All three sounds may be recorded on a graphic form (Fig. 12-3).

18. Report any abnormal findings to the appropriate person (instructor, RN, or MD). **R:** Documentation is a legal record of the patient's care and therapy and communicates nursing activities to other nurses and caregivers.

■ POTENTIAL ADVERSE OUTCOMES AND RELATED INTERVENTIONS

1. The patient is not ready for the procedure or a factor is identified that could interfere with obtaining an accurate result.

Intervention: Take care of the patient's needs first, and problem solve for any factors identified. Encourage the patient to rest for 5 minutes, and then take the blood pressure.

2. The patient reports pain with position change or is unable to tolerate the new position for the procedure.

Intervention: Assess the patient, and identify the potential reason for pain with position change. Try again to position the patient, moving slowly and carefully. If standard positioning is still not possible, measure the blood pressure with the patient in a different position, and note it on the record.

3. Korotkoff's sounds cannot be heard.

Intervention: Recheck the blood pressure manually on the other arm. If you're still not successful, switch to palpation, electronic, or Doppler method. (See below for instructions.)

4. Blood pressure is not within normal limits or is too high or low when compared with patient's baseline.

Intervention: Retake the blood pressure after the patient rests for 10 minutes:

a. Assess patient for signs and symptoms of hypo/hypertension and possible contributing factors.

b. Recheck pulse sites.

c. Inform the physician of findings if necessary, and await potential orders.

ALTERNATIVE BLOOD PRESSURE MEASUREMENT TECHNIQUES

A variety of alternative approaches to measuring blood pressure are used in special situations.

THIGH MEASUREMENT

Occasionally, it may be necessary to measure blood pressure on the lower extremity. In such instances, use an appropriately larger thigh cuff (usually 18 to 20 cm,

which is 6 cm wider than the arm cuff), and position the patient on the abdomen. A patient who cannot lie on the abdomen may be placed on the side or in the supine position, with the knee slightly flexed (Fig. 12-4).

Apply the cuff around the midthigh above the knee. Place your stethoscope over the **popliteal artery,** and measure the patient's blood pressure as directed in the procedure above. The diastolic pressure in the legs is usually similar to that in the arms. The systolic pressure may be 20 to 30 mm Hg higher (AHA, 2004).

ELECTRONIC MEASUREMENT

Electronic blood pressure recording devices are used in many healthcare settings (Fig. 12-5). The blood pressure cuff is placed on the patient's arm as in the procedure above. The machine is turned on. It may be used for a single measurement or may be set to take the blood pressure automatically at regular intervals, such as every 5 minutes. Warning alarms can be set to signal if the blood pressure goes above or below the desired range. Electronic devices are most often used when frequent monitoring is needed, and the blood pressure is a critical parameter in determining care and treatment needs. They are becoming more commonly used throughout hospitals. While using an electronic device for blood pressure assessment may be easy and efficient, remember that the equipment may be sensitive to movement and other sounds, which could alter the reading. Before using an electronic device, the nurse should always attempt to do a manual blood pressure assessment to look for consistency between the measurements.

MEASURING BLOOD PRESSURE USING PALPATION

When you cannot hear Korotkoff's sounds, you can measure systolic blood pressure by **palpation.** (The diastolic pressure cannot be measured in this manner.) The procedure is the same except that no stethoscope is used, and the pressure shown when the first pulsation is

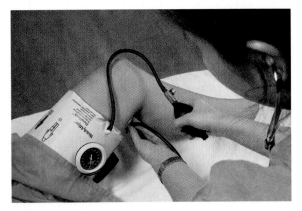

FIGURE 12-4 Thigh-sized blood pressure cuff placed at mid-thigh with the leg flexed for ease of access to the popliteal space.

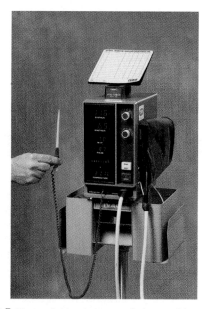

FIGURE 12-5 Electronic blood pressure device provides accurate measurement at predetermined intervals.

felt is considered the systolic pressure. A palpated blood pressure may be recorded as, for example, 80/P. If you find you can measure blood pressure only by palpation, this should be reported to a registered nurse immediately because it may represent a serious problem.

DOPPLER MEASUREMENT

When Korotkoff's sounds are difficult to hear (for example, in cases of shock or with obese patients or infants), a Doppler ultrasound stethoscope can be used. The Doppler, which is used to detect and assess blood flow, consists of a stethoscope or headset attached to a battery-operated ultrasound unit (Fig. 12-6).

To measure systolic blood pressure, use the previous procedure, modifying as follows: Locate the brachial or other pulse point desired, apply electrode or contact gel over the pulse site, and gently place the instrument over

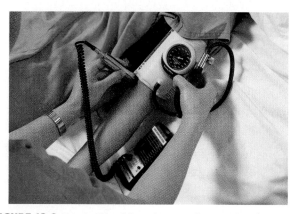

FIGURE 12-6 Doppler blood-flow detector ultrasound stethoscope is used to detect blood flow when a pulse is not palpable.

the pulse point. Pump up the blood pressure cuff, and slowly let the pressure out. The systolic blood pressure is recorded as the first point at which the pulse is audible. (Volume is adjustable on the machine.) Blood pressure obtained by a Doppler device may be recorded with a "D" to indicate it was obtained by using a Doppler.

DIRECT ARTERIAL MEASUREMENT

Direct arterial blood pressure monitoring also is appropriate when blood pressure measurement is critical. This type of blood pressure monitoring requires sophisticated equipment that includes an intra-arterial catheter, which is usually available only in intensive care settings. The blood pressure is provided as a constant readout.

POSTURAL MEASUREMENT

Postural blood pressure measurement is done to assess the patient who may be experiencing postural hypotension (sudden drops in blood pressure in response to position changes). Frequently, this is done when the patient reports dizziness when changing position. Follow the steps in Box 12-2 to take the blood pressure first lying, then sitting, then standing. The blood pressures are recorded in the same order they were taken. The position of the patient during the measurement is often recorded by drawing simple "stick" figures beside the recording.

The desired result is that the blood pressure should decrease by less than 10 mm Hg, and the pulse should increase less than 20 beats per minute. If the patient's blood pressure decreases by 10 or more mm Hg, or the heart rate increases by more than 20 beats per minute when the position is changed, it is considered positive for the presence of postural hypotension. The physician should be informed, and the patient's teaching plan should include information about rising slowly

box 12-2 *Measuring Postural Blood Pressures*

1. Have the patient in the supine position for at least 5 minutes.
2. Measure and record a blood pressure and pulse rate in the lying position.
3. Bring the patient to a sitting position with legs dangling from the bedside or examination table.
4. Wait for 1 to 2 minutes for the circulatory system to stabilize.
5. Measure and record blood pressure and pulse rate in the sitting position.
6. Bring the patient to full standing position.
7. Wait 1 to 2 minutes.
8. Measure and record the blood pressure and pulse rate in the standing position.

Note: If at any time during the procedure the patient complains of feeling weak or dizzy, return him or her to the bed in the supine position.

box 12-3 *Measuring Ankle-Brachial Index*

1. Place the patient in a supine position.
2. Measure the systolic blood pressure in both the right arm and the left arm (brachial blood pressures) and record these readings. Select the higher of these two measures to use as the brachial pressure to use when calculating the index.
3. Right ankle-brachial index
   a. Place a small size blood pressure cuff on the right ankle.
   b. Use the Doppler to measure and record the systolic blood pressure first in the anterior tibial and then the posterior tibial artery. Select the higher of these two pressures as the right ankle measurement.
   c. Divide the selected ankle pressure by the selected brachial pressure. This figure is the right ankle-brachial index.
4. Left ankle-brachial index
   a. Place the small size blood pressure cuff on the left ankle.
   b. Use the Doppler to measure and record the systolic blood pressure first in the anterior tibial and then the posterior tibial artery. Select the higher of these two pressures as the left ankle measurement.
   c. Divide the selected ankle pressure by the selected brachial pressure. This figure is the left ankle-brachial index.

from lying to sitting to standing to avoid dizziness and prevent falls.

MEASURING THE ANKLE-BRACHIAL INDEX

The ankle-brachial index (ABI) compares systolic blood pressures in upper extremities with those in the lower extremities to evaluate for peripheral vascular disease. See Box 12-3 for directions on measuring ABI. Use the procedure above for measuring blood pressures as directed. ABIs as high as 1.10 are normal. An index of less than 1.0 is considered abnormal. An index lower than 0.20 is associated with severely ischemic extremities (Sacks, et al., 2002).

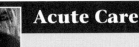 **Acute Care**

Each facility will have routine times established in the policy and procedure for taking patients' blood pressures. Blood pressure is always assessed on admission in both arms to establish a baseline. In performing the baseline assessment, many nurses ask their patients if they know what their blood pressure readings usually are. This assessment gives the nurse valuable information that can later be used in developing a teaching plan for the patient.

Blood pressure is assessed during hospitalization based on the physician's orders and as necessary based upon the nurse's judgment related to changes in patient's condition.

 Long-Term Care

In the long-term care setting, blood pressure is not measured daily as a routine. Instead, blood pressure is monitored as it would be for a person living at home. If a resident is on medications that affect blood pressure, monitoring is more frequent than for a resident who is not on such medications. When medications are changed or dosages altered, monitoring may be more frequent until you determine that the resident is stable. The nurse is responsible for determining that additional monitoring is needed when the situation changes.

Home Care

Blood pressure may be monitored at home by a home healthcare nurse, or the nurse may teach the client and family how to self-monitor blood pressure. Using the directions in this module, demonstrate the procedure to the client, and have the client demonstrate the procedure for you in return. This will allow you and the client to solve problems encountered in blood pressure measurement together. Electronic blood pressure recording devices are available in small units for home use. These enable an individual to monitor personal blood pressure regularly, but they are not usually considered reliable enough for professional use. Equipment for home blood pressure monitoring may include a stethoscope built into the cuff and a digital electronic display that provides the blood pressure reading after the cuff is pumped up and then released. This enables the individual to manage the equipment while measuring his or her own blood pressure. The calibration of these instruments must be checked periodically to ensure that they remain accurate.

When providing information to the client about taking blood pressure at home, be sure that the client has an understanding of what normal is and where he or she falls in that range. Encourage the client to enter blood pressure values in a journal according to time of day so that the information is readily available for the healthcare provider to view during subsequent visits.

Ambulatory Care

The ambulatory care area, such as a physician's office, is the perfect place for the nurse to assess the client's current practice related to self-measurement of blood pressure. Reviewing technique and answering questions the client may have will be helpful.

LEARNING TOOLS

DEVELOP YOUR BACKGROUND KNOWLEDGE

1. Review the Learning Outcomes.

2. Read the section on blood pressure in your assigned text.

3. Look up the Key Terms in the glossary.

4. Review this module, and mentally practice the techniques described. Study so that you can teach these skills to another person.

5. Note the variations in blood pressure values for different age groups.

DEVELOP YOUR SKILLS

1. In the practice setting, select two other students, and form a group of three.

2. Alternating so that each has the opportunity to play the role of the patient, perform each of the following procedures:
   a. manual blood pressure, using the brachial artery
   b. automatic blood pressure measurement
   c. postural blood pressures
   d. ankle-brachial index measurement

3. Use the Performance Checklists on the CD-ROM in the front of this book to check yourself. Those who are not participating at a given time can observe and evaluate the performances of the others.

DEMONSTRATE YOUR SKILLS

In the clinical setting
1. Consult with your instructor regarding the opportunity to take the blood pressures of patients on the clinical unit.

2. Consult with your instructor regarding the opportunity to evaluate your performance with the instructor.

CRITICAL THINKING EXERCISES

1. You are caring for an 84-year-old resident of a nursing home. You try to take her blood pressure but are unable to hear the Korotkoff's sounds. Consider the various factors that might contribute to this situation. Recommend actions you can take to modify the situation, the environment, or your technique to increase your ability to obtain an accurate blood pressure reading.

2. You note on Jack Q's record that he weighs 290 lb. You also note that his blood pressure has been varying widely. Describe the factors that might be contributing to a wide variation in blood pressure. Identify which factors in your technique you should modify to ensure that you obtain an accurate reading.

SELF-QUIZ
SHORT-ANSWER QUESTIONS

1. The systolic pressure is heard at 140 mm Hg, the point of muffling is heard at 80 mm Hg, and the last sound is at 70 mm Hg. Document appropriately.

   _____

2. Why is the bell head of the stethoscope preferred to the diaphragm for measuring blood pressure?

   _____

3. What is the auscultatory gap?

   _____

4. How can you prevent underestimation of the systolic pressure as a result of the auscultatory gap?

   _____

5. What is the result of using a blood pressure cuff that is too narrow for the arm?

   _____

6. What are the two problems that result from deflating the blood pressure cuff too quickly?

   a. _____

   b. _____

MULTIPLE CHOICE

_____ 7. Which of these factors can affect blood pressure? (Choose all that apply.)
   a. Age
   b. Height
   c. Recent activity
   d. Position

_____ 8. The best position for a hospitalized patient to assume during blood pressure measurement is
   a. sitting.
   b. prone.
   c. supine.
   d. lateral.

_____ 9. The bell head of the stethoscope should be placed over which artery to measure blood pressure in the arm?
   a. Radial
   b. Brachial
   c. Femoral
   d. Carotid

_____ 10. What is the first sound you hear as the pressure on the artery decreases?
   a. Systolic pressure
   b. Diastolic pressure
   c. Pulse pressure
   d. Cannot tell by one sound

_____ 11. The point at which the heart is beating and exerting its greatest force is called
   a. systolic pressure.
   b. diastolic pressure.
   c. pulse pressure.
   d. basal pressure.

_____ 12. If you want to double-check a blood pressure measurement, how long should you wait before you assess the pressure in the same arm?
   a. 30 seconds
   b. 1 to 2 minutes
   c. 3 minutes
   d. It makes no difference.

Answers to the Self-Quiz questions appear in the back of this book.

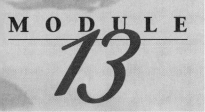

MODULE 13

Monitoring Intake and Output

SKILLS INCLUDED IN THIS MODULE

Procedure for Monitoring Intake and Output

PREREQUISITE MODULES

Module 1	An Approach to Nursing Skills
Module 2	Documentation
Module 4	Basic Infection Control
Module 5	Safety in the Healthcare Environment

KEY TERMS

catheter	fluid balance
diaphoresis	mini–IV bag
diarrhea	parenteral fluids
diuretic	

OVERALL OBJECTIVE

▸ To monitor and keep accurate records of patients' fluid intake and output.

LEARNING OUTCOMES

The student will be able to

1. Assess the patient to determine the need for initiating or continuing to monitor intake and output (I & O).
2. Analyze the assessment data to determine specific concerns that must be addressed prior to initiating I & O.
3. Determine appropriate patient outcomes related to monitoring I & O, and recognize the potential for possible adverse outcomes.
4. Choose the appropriate equipment for measuring I & O.
5. Evaluate the effectiveness of the process, and correlate the results with the patient's status.
6. Document the results on the I & O flow record or other facility documentation as required.
7. Describe the characteristics of the output in the patient's record as necessary.

Many illnesses cause changes in the body's ability to maintain **fluid balance.** Intake can decrease as a result of anorexia, nausea, vomiting, and many other conditions. Output can be changed by various disease processes in the body, especially diabetes and kidney and heart problems. Infants, children, and older adults are particularly susceptible to fluid imbalance. A number of drugs in current use can cause kidney damage and alter urinary elimination. This is why careful monitoring and measurement of intake and output (I & O) is essential to total patient assessment. A record of this measurement is maintained for the use of all healthcare team members.

NURSING DIAGNOSES

A variety of nursing diagnoses are useful for the patient whose I & O must be measured. Some of these are appropriate because of the patient's medical condition, which may alter either intake or output. Medical conditions may also influence electrolyte balance, so that nursing diagnoses related to fluid volume are applicable. If the patient is receiving a medication that changes either intake or output, measurement should be initiated. Other nursing diagnoses are appropriate when assessment detects phenomena such as nausea, vomiting, constipation, or **diarrhea.** The following are examples of nursing diagnoses related to I & O measurement:

- Impaired Urinary Elimination: related to limited fluid intake, obstruction, urinary tract infection (UTI), or sensory motor impairment
- Constipation: related to inactivity, lack of mobility, decreased or limited fluid intake,

privacy issues related to defecating, and low fiber intake
- Diarrhea: related to GI infection or disorders, medication, fecal impaction, dietary changes, or medications
- Deficient Fluid Volume: related to fluid loss, or malfunctioning regulatory mechanisms
- Excess Fluid Volume: related to malfunctioning regulatory mechanisms or increased sodium intake
- Hyperthermia: related to activity, excessive heat exposure, increased metabolism, trauma or illness, dehydration, inability to perspire, or medications
- Impaired Swallowing: related to obstruction or tumor, neuromuscular injury, paralysis, or improper feeding
- Risk for Infection: related to malnutrition, decrease in primary or secondary defenses, tissue destruction, environmental exposure, trauma, or invasive procedures

These nursing diagnoses may also be used when the patient is at risk for the situation.

DELEGATION

Measuring and recording intake is the responsibility of any healthcare team member who provides direct care to the patient. It is important for all team members to be aware of this addition to the plan of care. Generally, during meals, the provider who removes the tray from the bedside should be the one recording the intake. If the patient's I & O status is critical, exact measurements must be recorded. Nurses remain responsible for supervision of this activity and for the interpretation of the data recorded.

ASSESSMENT FOR INITIATING MEASUREMENT OF INTAKE AND OUTPUT

Although a physician's order is commonly written for measuring and monitoring intake and output, usually referred to as I & O, you may also initiate this activity if you determine that these data are important to your assessment. You may initiate I & O measurement to assess whether a patient is receiving adequate fluids or to verify that the output is sufficient for optimal kidney function. In some facilities, to facilitate effective assessment, I & O is routinely monitored for patients receiving medications that have an effect on I & O, postoperative patients, patients with an indwelling urinary **catheter,** and those receiving intravenous (IV) fluids or tube feedings. Other considerations, such as specific illnesses, also indicate the need for monitoring I & O. For patients who are diabetic, have burns or draining wounds, are on steroid therapy, or who have a debilitating disease and inadequate oral fluid intake, I & O monitoring may also be initiated.

Age is also a factor. Infants, children, and elderly adults are at higher risk for fluid imbalance and, therefore, need careful observation to ensure effective hydration and elimination. Many older patients take a **diuretic** or other drugs that increase urinary elimination, putting them at risk for dehydration. In any patient, fluid intake should approximately equal fluid output, and any ratio that is significantly unequal should be reported.

Intake monitored over several days provides more accurate assessment of the patient's fluid status trends. If the total intake is substantially below the total output, the patient is at risk for fluid volume deficit. If the total fluid intake is substantially above the total output, the patient is at risk for fluid volume excess (Ackley & Ladwig, 2004).

Urine output of less than 30 mL/hr may indicate renal disease, inadequate blood flow to the kidneys, or dehydration and should be reported. For the critically ill patient with a urinary catheter in place, urine output may be measured hourly. For some patients whose fluid balance is crucial, I & O will be measured along with daily weight. A rapid change in daily weight is most likely to be related to fluid status (dehydration or fluid retention) rather than nutritional status. When weight increases over time, the nurse must differentiate weight gain that is fluid retention from weight gain that is from an increase in body mass. Measurement of I & O may be inaccurate because of the various estimates used

regarding intake so that the patient's weight becomes even more important assessment data. Some patients for whom fluid balance is important will have their weight measured daily but not their I & O. This is common for the patient at home.

SUBSTANCES MEASURED
INTAKE

It is important to accurately measure all substances considered intake (refer to Box 13-1 for an inclusive list). The rule of thumb is that if a substance is liquid at room temperature, it is considered a liquid and should be included as intake. Thus ice cream and gelatin are considered liquids because at room temperature, they typically melt into liquids.

OUTPUT

Urine is the major output fluid that is measured. In the healthy person, the volume of urine excreted is approximately equal to the volume of oral fluid ingested, and water derived from solid food and from chemical oxidation in the body approximately equals the normal loss of water through the lungs, skin, and stool. If water losses through the skin and stool become excessive, measure them, and add them to the output. For example, this measurement is appropriate for patients with diarrhea or profuse **diaphoresis** (sweating).

---

box 13-1 *Fluid Items Constituting Intake*

- Liquids with meals and snacks—any item that is liquid at room temperature, such as:
  Gelatin
  Custard
  Ice cream
  Sorbet/sherbet
  Popsicles
  Ice chips
  Water
  Juice
  Milk
  Coffee/tea/creamer
  Soda
  Soup
- Liquid medications
  Oral liquid medications
  Any liquid given with medications
- Enteral nutrition
  Tube feedings
  Any irrigation prior to and after feedings and medications
- Parenteral nutrition
  Intravenous fluids
  Blood and blood products
  Flush solutions if more than 100 mL per day

Vomitus, drainage from suction devices, wound drainage, and bleeding are abnormal fluid losses. Always measure or estimate, as well as describe, these kinds of losses. Refer to Box 13-2 for a list of output fluids and their characteristics. In patients for whom maintaining fluid balance is critical and from whom excessive blood loss, perspiration, or drainage onto bed sheets has occurred, weighing the saturated sheet may be necessary. The final weight calculation for that drainage can be done by weighing the wet sheet and then weighing a dry sheet and subtracting the dry weight from the wet weight.

MEASUREMENT DEVICES AND UNITS OF MEASUREMENT

All patients having I & O monitored need to have measuring devices in their rooms. These containers are fairly standard in healthcare environments. A helpful device for measuring urine is a plastic collection basin that is shaped like a hat with a brim. When this "hat" is placed upside down, it fits the seat of the toilet or commode and collects the urine of the female patient who is sitting down to void (Fig. 13-1). A male patient should have a urinal close to the bedside for ease of access. The bathroom should have a graduated container to measure fluids or drainage before discarding. If more than one patient uses the bathroom, each must have a separate

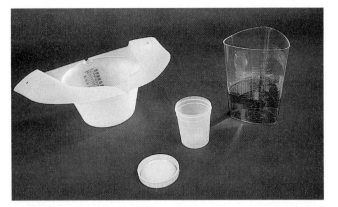

FIGURE 13-1 A specimen "hat" (upper left) is placed under the toilet seat for easy urine collection. Other specimen collection devices include a specimen cup with lid and a larger graduated container.

measuring container clearly marked to prevent potential cross contamination.

All measuring devices are marked in either metric liquid units called milliliters (mL) or cubic centimeters (cc) or both. These two measurement modalities are equivalent. It is preferable to use the milliliter, which is the liquid unit, as a standard because of ease in making calculations that require conversion of liquid and weight measures. Intravenous (IV) fluids are standardized in metric measurement for this reason as well.

PATIENT PARTICIPATION

Accurate I & O records are greatly facilitated when the patient is involved in the process. Patients can become highly motivated to participate when they know the reasons for a procedure. First, make sure the patient knows which fluids are to be measured and the units of measurement. Explain the use of any devices for measuring either intake or output, so the patient is familiar with them.

Show the I & O records to the patient, and demonstrate how to record items. Some patients may prefer to use paper and pencil at the bedside, which is a much simpler method of recording and which can be documented later. If the patient is on restricted or increased fluid intake, develop a plan that is the most acceptable and comfortable for that person. You and the patient may wish to plan water intake with the addition of juices throughout the day to increase oral fluid intake.

Restricting oral fluids is very difficult for most patients. It is helpful to plan one-half or more of the total fluid intake for the day shift when the patient is more active and requires more hydration. One-third should be planned for the evening, with the remainder allocated for night hours. The patient will be more conscientious in complying with measurement of I & O if given this preparation and may even assist with recording as well as alerting other healthcare workers concerning the need for measurement.

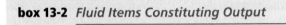

box 13-2 *Fluid Items Constituting Output*

Fluids and their characteristics that should be included in the I & O measurement as output are listed below. (*Note:* Always describe clarity, color, and odor of any drainage output.)

- Urine
  Clarity—clear or cloudy
  Color—pale yellow/straw to amber
  Odor—the more concentrated, the stronger the smell
- Liquid stool—describe what you see and smell
- Emesis—describe what you see and smell
  Green-brown (color of bile)
  Yellow
  Bright red—indicative of new bleeding
  Granular brown (coffee grounds)—indicative of old bleeding
- Wound drainage—describe what you see and smell
  Serous
  Purulent
  Serosanguineous
- Bleeding
- Nasogastric drainage
  Bile
  Yellow
  Green
  Bloody
- Profuse sweating
- Any other drainage of considerable volume

RECORD KEEPING

A variety of forms are used for documenting I & O. Some are completed on paper, and some are computerized. Entries must be timely and accurate.

BEDSIDE RECORDS

An I & O worksheet must be kept at the patient's bedside or in the room to capture the data required for monitoring I & O (Fig. 13-2). Often, the worksheet is taped on a door or placed on a clipboard near the bathroom so that measurements can be recorded immediately.

PERMANENT RECORDS

The patient's record includes a special form for making a permanent record of the patient's I & O (Fig. 13-3). This form may be a separate record or may be incorporated with the graphic record used for documenting vital signs. The I & O record may be a separate screen in a computerized record.

This record is for recording data collected at 8-hour or 24-hour intervals (according to facility procedure) and is not to be confused with the I & O worksheet (see Fig. 13-2). The specific items that are included will vary according to each facility's forms, but the principle is the same, and that is to identify trends from accumulated data.

Parenteral fluids (those given by **infusion**) may be recorded on an independent record as well as on the overall record (Fig. 13-4).

PROCEDURE FOR MONITORING INTAKE AND OUTPUT

ASSESSMENT

1. Assess your institution's policy and procedures for monitoring and recording I & O. **R:** The hospital's policies and procedures guide nursing practice at each institution.
2. Assess the physician's orders and/or need for I & O monitoring. **R:** I & O measurement is initiated by the nurse based either on a physician's order or on the nurse's assessment.
3. Assess the patient's understanding of the I & O monitoring process. **R:** Understanding is basic to cooperation.
4. Assess the patient's ability to participate in this process. **R:** The process promotes independence.

ANALYSIS

5. Critically think through your data, carefully evaluating each aspect of the data and its relation to other data. **R:** To determine specific problems for this individual in relation to monitoring I & O.
6. Identify specific problems and modifications of the procedure needed for this individual. **R:** Planning for the individual must take into consideration the individual's problems.

PLANNING

7. Determine individualized desired patient outcomes in relation to I & O:
   a. Intake and/or output are monitored accurately.
   b. I & O are approximately equal within normal limits for health, or the trend is toward normal expectations.
   c. The patient cooperates in ensuring accuracy of I & O.
8. Select the proper equipment:
   a. graduated measuring container
   b. urine "hat" receptacle for measuring urine in the toilet
   c. bedpan, urinal, or commode as indicated
   d. I & O bedside worksheet
   e. clean disposable gloves

IMPLEMENTATION

Action	Rationale
9. Wash or disinfect your hands.	To decrease the transfer of microorganisms that could cause infection.
10. Identify the patient, using two identifiers.	Verifying the patient's identity helps ensure that you are performing the right skill for the right patient.
11. Explain the procedure you are about to perform.	Explaining the procedure helps relieve anxiety or misperceptions that the patient may have about a procedure or activity and sets the stage for patient participation.

(continued)

HOSPITAL MEDICAL CENTER

FLUID INTAKE FOR STANDARD SERVINGS

Juice glass	100	D'Zerta	100
Milk glass	180	Popsicle	80
Milk carton	240	Jello	150
Coffee pots (sm) 225 (lg.)	300	Ice Cream, Sherbet	120
Coffee cup	150		
Coffee cream	15	Soup	180
Clear Disp. glass (sm) 150 (lg)	275		
Styrofoam cup	150	Cereal cream	120
Paper cup	180		
Plastic bowls	125 & 200	Ice cubes 1/2 of vol.	
		Crushed ice 2/3 of vol.	
		Pitcher c̄ or s̄ ice	900

B E D S I D E
I. & O.
W O R K S H E E T

PATIENT _George Dugan_

RM: _932_   BED: _W_

DATE: _3/16/06_

SHIFT	TIME	INTAKE		OUTPUT				IRRIGATIONS		
		ORAL	TUBE	URINE	GASTRIC			IN	OUT	BALANCE
N I G H T S	2200-2300	240								
	2300-2400									
	2400-0100									
	0100-0200			400						
	0200-0300									
	0300-0400									
	0400-0500									
	0500-0600	75		120						
	TOTAL									
D A Y S	0600-0700									
	0700-0800	ᴮ445								
	0800-0900							100	100	——
	0900-1000	180		300						
	1000-1100									
	1100-1200									
	1200-1300	ᴸ410		360						
	1300-1400									
	TOTAL									
E V E N I N G S	1400-1500	100								
	1500-1600	ᴰ380								
	1600-1700									
	1700-1800									
	1800-1900									
	1900-2000	150						100	100	——
	2000-2100			300						
	2100-2200									
	TOTAL	1980		1480						

FIGURE 13-2 Intake–output worksheet.

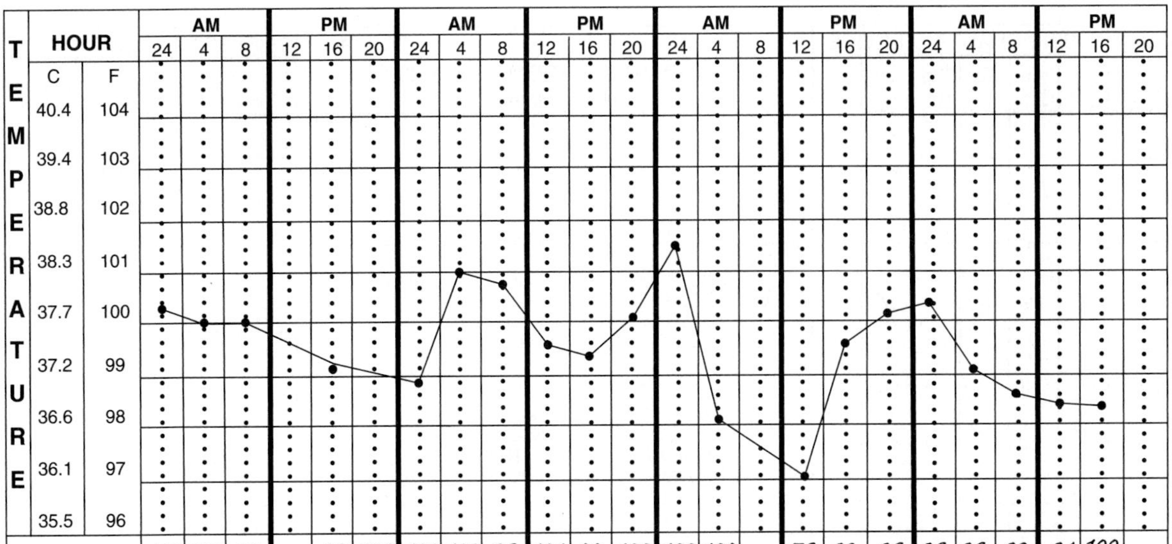

Vital Signs

	AM 24	4	8	PM 12	16	20	AM 24	4	8	PM 12	16	20	AM 24	4	8	PM 12	16	20	AM 24	4	8	PM 12	16	20
PULSE	116	112	92		88	104	100	100	96	104	88	100	100	108		76	92	96	96	96	92	94	100	
RESP.	16	20	18		16	18	18	20	20	20	20	18	20	20		16	20	20	16	16	20	20	16	
B.P.	100/70			88/50	90/50		98/60		90/58	110/60	94/64	90/60	104/64	112/76		94/78	84/52	92/60	96/56	92/64	84/60		86/60	

WEIGHT

Intake and Output

IN	2200 0600	0600 1400	1400 2200	TOTAL	2200 0600	0600 1400	1400 2200	TOTAL	2200 0600	0600 1400	1400 2200	TOTAL	2200 0600	0600 1400	1400 2200	TOTAL
ORAL	Ø	300	400	700	Ø	400	550	950	Ø	500	800	1300	300	500	600	1400
TUBE Formula																
TUBE Water																
PARENTERAL	1601	562	410	2573	1203		461	1664	1069		refused	1069			547	547
MINI-BAGS																
BLOOD & COMPONENTS						500	167	667								
TOTAL				3273				3281				2369	300	500	1147	1947
OUT URINE	700	500	450	1650	550	450	400	1400	450	550	400	1400	400	425	325	1150
OUT GI					100	350		450								
OUT OTHER																
OUT OTHER																
TOTAL				1650				1850				1400				1150

DATE			
Day Hospital	10/15/06	10/16/06	10/17/06	10/18/06
Day P.O. or P.P.	5	6	7	8

ADDRESSOGRAPH:

Williams, Rosemary F-52
000-00-0000
Dr. Connolly

HOSPITAL MEDICAL CENTER
SEATTLE, WASHINGTON

FIGURE 13-3 Intake–output record for patient's chart.

Date and Time	TUBING CHANGE				DEVICE		Initials	AMOUNT-SOLUTION-ADDITIVES (number consecutively)	Rate	SHIFT TOTALS		Solu'	DC'd
	MACRO SET	MICRO SET	PUMP SET	BLOOD SET	PUMP	CONTR-OLLER				Time	Total	Time	Amount Absorb.
Date: 7/18 Time: 1430	✓		✓		✓		F.S.	D5 1/2 c̄ 20 meq KCl	125/hr	22	388	1640	1000
										06	372		
										14	240		
Date: 7/19 Time: 1900	✓		✓		✓		SA	HA# _9_ 1000 DEX. _25_% A.A. _5_% NACL _30_ NA ACET___ KCL _25_ KP0$_4$ _15_ CA GLU _8_ MG S0$_4$ _8_ TR EL___ REG INS___ MVL _1_ VIT.K___	85/hr	22	381	0300	1025
										06	644		
Date: 7/20 Time: 1915	✓		✓		✓		SA	HA# _10_ 1000 DEX. _25_% A.A. _5_% NACL _30_ NA ACET___ KCL _25_ KP0$_4$ _15_ CA GLU _8_ MG S0$_4$ ___ TR EL___ REG INS___ MVL _1_ VIT.K___	85/hr	22	377	0330	1119
										06	742		
Date: 7/21 Time: 0915	✓		✓		✓		F.S.	D5 1/2 c̄ 20 meq KCl	125/hr	22	108	2115	1008
										06	340		
										14	560		
Date: 7/22 Time: 2200	✓		✓		✓		K.R.	D5 1/2 c̄ 20 meq KCl	125/hr	22	124	0900	1034
										06	444		
										14	466		
Date: Time:													
Date: Time:													
Date: Time:													
Date: Time:													

Identify Initials with Signature:
1. Frank Shulz, RN   4.   7.
2. Shelly Atkinson, RN 5.   8.
3. Kerry Rollins, RN   6.   9.

ADDRESSOGRAPH:

Martinelli, Anita F-67
000-00-0000
Dr. Ronderos

CODE: * see Nurses Progress Notes

HOSPITAL MEDICAL CENTER
SEATTLE, WASHINGTON

FIGURE 13-4 Parenteral fluid form.

Action	Rationale
12. Initiate the I & O process, according to the following:	
a. Explain or reinforce the reasons for accurate measurement to the patient to encourage his or her participation if able.	Patients will more likely feel involved in their own care and be more inclined to participate.
b. Incorporate the I & O process into the plan of care.	All team members need to be aware of the need for measurement.
c. Measure all ingested and/or infused fluids as intake (see Box 13-1), noting the amounts on the worksheet. Most I & O worksheets have a "key" that addresses standard container size and amount. For patients on strict measurement, you will need to actually measure and not estimate.	Accuracy is basic to assessment of fluid and electrolyte balance.
d. Prior to measuring output, put on clean gloves.	To protect you from contact with body fluids.
e. Encourage the patient to turn on the call light after elimination so that measuring can occur in a timely manner. Always measure fluids as soon as you become aware of them. A patient who is active in self-care can be taught how to measure and record output if desired.	Prompt measurement alerts the nurse to changes in the patient's pattern.
f. Continue to measure and note the characteristics of all fluid output on your shift (see Box 13-2), and record the volume on the worksheet (see Fig. 13-2). Use the graduated measuring container located in the patient's bathroom, and always be careful to rinse out the container, "hat," commode, or urinal after use.	For accuracy and infection control.
g. At the end of your shift, make sure you have recorded all of your patient's *intake* in the correct columns of the worksheet (see Fig. 13-3), including regular IV fluids, fluids from **mini–IV bags** that have infused (see Fig. 13-4), liquid medications or liquids consumed with medications, and fluids taken in from the bedside water pitcher that have not yet been recorded. Add the columns to obtain intake totals for the shift, and enter on the worksheet.	An accurate account of fluid intake will contribute to a clearer picture of patient fluid balance status.

(continued)

Action	Rationale
h. At the end of your shift, make sure you have recorded all of your patient's *output* in the correct columns of the worksheet (see Fig. 13-3). At this time, also make sure you have included all other forms of output, including any remaining urinary, gastric, wound, liquid stool, or other drainage. Add the columns for output totals, and enter on the worksheet.	An accurate account of fluid output contributes to a clearer picture of patient fluid balance status.
13. Remove gloves, and wash or disinfect your hands every time you measure output.	To decrease the transfer of microorganisms that could cause infection.

EVALUATION

14. Evaluate using the individualized patient outcomes previously identified:
   a. Intake and/or output are monitored accurately.
   b. I & O are approximately equal within normal limits for health, or the trend is toward normal limits.
   c. The patient cooperates in ensuring accuracy of I & O. **R:** Evaluation in relation to desired outcomes is essential for planning future care.

15. Review the data collected related to the descriptions of the output fluids (see Box 13-2), comparing them with previously obtained fluids. Assess for differences, and report changes to physician if necessary. Do not wait until the end of the shift to report any fluid characteristics that represent serious deviations from normal, such as the presence of blood or evidence of pus in urine. **R:** Reporting these deviations supports effective planning to correct problems.

DOCUMENTATION

16. Transfer the 8-hour totals from the I & O worksheet and the parenteral fluid sheet to the I & O record in the patient's record (see Fig. 13-3). If evaluation has resulted in the identification of any problem, record that in the narrative. **R:** Documentation is a legal record of the patient's care and therapy and communicates nursing activities to other nurses and caregivers.

POTENTIAL ADVERSE OUTCOMES AND RELATED INTERVENTIONS

1. Totals for I & O show that the patient has a *fluid intake greater than fluid output.*
Intervention: Assess the patient for signs and symptoms of fluid volume excess, correlating assessment findings with data such as vital signs, I & O totals, and weight. Look for evidence of edema. Also look for trends from

previous data collected over the past 24 to 48 hours. Was there a low intake prior to this day resulting in overall I & O balance?

2. Totals for I & O indicate that the patient may have a *fluid volume deficit.*
Intervention: Assess the patient for signs and symptoms of fluid volume deficit, correlating assessment findings with data such as vital signs, I & O totals, and weight. Also look for trends from previous data collected over the past 24 to 48 hours.

Acute Care

Acute care facilities have procedures in place for monitoring I & O. Patients come to hospitals for nursing care, and it is always the nurse's responsibility to assess the needs of the patient. Patients needing I & O measurement include anyone who has experienced a change in condition, has developed a fever, has a chronic debilitating illness, has surgery or post-procedure status, is receiving IV fluids, has a urinary catheter in place, is on a restricted fluid diet, or is taking a diuretic medication.

Long-Term Care

Most residents in long-term care are elderly, and many have insufficient oral fluid intake. As people get older, fluid intake decreases due to diminished thirst sensation. They may find fluids too filling and avoid taking more than sips. In addition, many residents take diuretic drugs and are more susceptible to dehydration. They incorrectly think they should decrease fluids because they are taking "water pills" to get rid of excess fluid.

Your responsibility includes teaching residents and staff that older people, in general, need to consume sufficient fluid. The amount needed is guided by the person's medical condition. If urine output is much greater than fluid intake over several days or urine is dark and strong, it should be reported. If the resident is incontinent, the best estimate is to record the number of times the person has been incontinent and whether, in your opinion, the amount has been small, moderate, or large.

It is also important to remember that behavioral changes, for example, confusion, can occur because of dehydration. Any resident on diuretic therapy in the long-term care setting should be on regular weight measurement, and if there is an unexplained weight gain, I & O monitoring should begin so that the nurse can accurately assess the resident's fluid status.

Home Care

An increasing number of people are being cared for in the home, particularly elderly people and those with terminal or protracted illnesses. Family care providers may need to know how to monitor weight and, if it is not stable, how to measure I & O. Generally, a computation less rigid than the type done in the acute care setting is sufficient. Studies show that people being cared for in the home drink a greater variety and amount of fluids than do those in the long-term care setting. Despite this, a record is sometimes needed because of debilitation or the serious nature of the individual's illness or condition.

Ambulatory Care

Ambulatory care centers look at I & O differently from acute care or long-term care centers. The staff in a physician's office are interested in knowing the client's previous patterns and noting any differences. They also focus on medications that have an impact on I & O such as diuretics. They correlate findings with patterns of weight as well. The care provider will provide information and teach clients about the medications they are taking so that clients can learn to monitor status at home.

Another type of ambulatory care center, such as an outpatient health center where procedures and day

surgery may be performed, is concerned with I & O as a general (not exact) measurement. This is particularly true with regard to clients who have had bowel preparation through laxatives and enemas before a procedure and who may have been without food or fluids for at least 8 hours or who may have received IV fluids during the procedure. All of these factors contribute to the potential for fluid imbalance. Moreover, anesthetics used may cause nausea and vomiting and urinary retention. Before these clients are discharged, the nurse must make sure that they can drink fluids without vomiting. The nurse also needs to make sure that the client has urine output prior to being discharged.

LEARNING TOOLS

DEVELOP YOUR BACKGROUND KNOWLEDGE

1. Review the Learning Outcomes.

2. Read the section on measuring I & O in your assigned text.

3. Look up the Key Terms in the glossary.

4. Review this module, and mentally practice the techniques described. Study so that you would be able to teach these skills to another person.

DEVELOP YOUR SKILLS

In the practice setting
1. Practice accurately measuring liquids, using containers showing metric measurement.

2. Practice estimating amounts of fluids in various containers. Then measure the fluids to determine your accuracy.

DEMONSTRATE YOUR SKILLS

In the clinical setting
1. Familiarize yourself with the various dietary fluid containers used in your facility and the fluid content of each.

2. Check the forms used to monitor I & O in your facility.

3. Identify three or four patients who are having I & O measured. Determine the rationale for this action. Prepare to teach a patient who is able to participate in I & O measurement.

4. Consult with your instructor regarding the opportunity to monitor I & O for a patient on a clinical unit. Enter data on the appropriate forms. Have your instructor check your accuracy.

CRITICAL THINKING EXERCISES

1. The physician has ordered I & O measurement for your patient. Determine which food items should be included in these measurements. Then use the various containers given on the sample form (see Fig. 13–3) to calculate the I & O for this patient.

   On rising, your patient brushed his teeth. After rinsing his mouth, he drank half a glass (small) of water. He voided 250 mL urine. Breakfast arrived and consisted of

   fruit juice, small glass
   cereal bowl of hot oatmeal with a pitcher of milk
   bacon and soft-boiled egg
   pot of black coffee
   glass of low-fat milk

   Shortly after breakfast, your patient felt nauseated and vomited 75 mL semiliquid emesis. Throughout the morning, he voided two additional times: 50 mL and 225 mL. By lunchtime, your patient was feeling much better, and a light diet was ordered. When lunch arrived, your patient ate a small bowl of broth and half of a small bowl of gelatin. He voided once more after lunch: 125 mL. He was given oral medications twice, each time with 1 oz of water. At the end of the day shift, half of a 1,000-mL bottle of intravenous fluids had been absorbed.

   Submit your calculations to your instructor for evaluation.

2. It is the end of your shift, and despite IV fluids running at 150 mL/hr, your patient, a 40-year-old, otherwise healthy female, has a total urine output of only 350 mL. She also vomited twice, totaling 600 mL and has been unable to keep any fluids down. She tells you that she has no energy. Her mucous membranes appear dry, and her lips are slightly cracked. Her blood pressure is 92/44 mm Hg (lower than normal); her heart rate is 118 beats/min and regular. She does not have a fever. Knowing what you do about I & O, should you be concerned about this? If yes, why? If no, why not? Looking at the nursing diagnoses for this module, what diagnoses might you choose and why? Is there anything else that you would do for this patient?

SELF-QUIZ
SHORT-ANSWER QUESTIONS

1. What common term is used for "diaphoresis"?

2. What is the effect of a diuretic on a patient?

3. List two age groups that are more frail or at risk for fluid imbalance.

   a.

   b.

4. What do daily weights tell you about a patient?

5. List three types of output:

   a.

   b.

   c.

6. What behavioral changes might be seen in an elderly patient who is dehydrated?

MULTIPLE CHOICE

_____ 7. Totals of intake and output (I & O) over 24-hour periods are helpful because
   a. I & O balance usually cannot be identified over shorter periods.
   b. they reduce the time needed for record keeping.
   c. physicians usually check them once every 24 hours.
   d. a 24-hour total is most accurate.

_____ 8. The I & O worksheet is used primarily to
   a. show the patient his or her fluid status.
   b. record amounts of fluid I & O.
   c. record the various items of fluid I & O at the bedside.
   d. provide a permanent record of I & O.

_____ 9. Which of the following items should be included in the total measurement of intake: (1) dietary fluids; (2) irrigation fluids returned; (3) gelatin; (4) fluids at bedside; (5) cereal; (6) ice cream; (7) intravenous fluids; or (8) pureed fruits and vegetables?
   a. 1, 4, 7, and 8
   b. 1, 3, 4, 6, and 7
   c. 1, 2, 4, 5, and 7
   d. All of these

_____ 10. Which of the following items should be included in the total measurement of output: (1) urine; (2) normal stools; (3) diarrhea stools; (4) vomitus; (5) normal perspiration; (6) excessive perspiration; or (7) wound drainage?

a. 1, 3, 4, 6, and 7
b. 1, 4, 5, 6, and 7
c. 1, 3, and 4
d. All of these

_____ 11. Your patient had an output of 400 mL for two shifts. This might indicate
a. that not enough data are given to identify the problem.
b. water intoxication.
c. edema formation.
d. kidney malfunction.

_____ 12. Your patient is a 45-year-old active, male truck driver and father of three who has been admitted with a possible kidney infec-

tion. In planning for accurate measurement, you would
a. measure all urine yourself because this is a critical concern.
b. see that urine is measured by a staff person (aide, LPN, RN), to guarantee accuracy.
c. have him measure his own urine and record it.
d. ask him if he would prefer to measure his output himself or have a staff person do it.

Answers to the Self-Quiz questions appear in the back of this book.

MODULE 14 Nursing Physical Assessment

SKILLS INCLUDED IN THIS MODULE

Basic Techniques for Physical Assessment
  Inspection
  Auscultation
  Percussion
  Palpation
Specific Strategies for Physical Assessment
  Procedure for Neurologic Assessment
  Procedure for Assessing the Heart
  Procedure for Assessing Central Veins and
    Peripheral Circulation
  Procedure for Assessing the Lungs and Respiration
  Procedure for Assessing the Breasts
  Procedure for Assessing the Abdomen and Rectum
  Procedure for Assessing the Testes
  Procedure for Comprehensive Head-to-Toe
    Physical Assessment
  Procedure for Routine Shift Physical Assessment
  Procedure for "Mini" Head-to-Toe Physical Assessment

PREREQUISITE MODULES

Module 1	An Approach to Nursing Skills
Module 2	Documentation
Module 3	Basic Body Mechanics
Module 4	Basic Infection Control
Module 5	Safety in the Healthcare Environment
Module 11	Assessing Temperature, Pulse, and Respiration
Module 12	Measuring Blood Pressure
Module 13	Monitoring Intake and Output

KEY TERMS

accommodation
adventitious sounds
alveoli
apex
apical pulse
ascites
asymmetry
auscultation
base
bell
bronchi
bruit
caries
carotid pulse
cerumen
consensual reaction
consolidation
constriction
convergence
crackles

cranium
dependent edema
diaphragm (of stethoscope)
diastole
distention
dorsiflexion
dullness
edema
flatness
guarding
gurgles
Homans' sign
impaction
inspection
intercostal space
lesions
nare
nasal speculum
nystagmus
objective data

ophthalmoscope
otoscope
palmar
palpation
patellar tendon
pectoralis muscles
percussion
periorbital edema
pinwheel
pitting edema
pleural friction rub
pretibial edema
protuberance
ptosis
rebound tenderness
reflex hammer
resonance
retraction
Snellen chart
stethoscope

subjective data
suprasternal notch
symmetry
symphysis pubis
symptoms
systole
testes
trachea
tremor
tuning fork
turgor
tympany
umbilicus
uvula
venous pressure
vibration
wheezes
xiphoid process

OVERALL OBJECTIVE

▶ To gain an understanding of the components of a complete nursing assessment, which includes developing skills for collecting data via a health history and physical examination, performing beginning-level assessment of individual patients using effective techniques for organizing data, and accurately stating nursing diagnoses based on the data collected.

LEARNING OUTCOMES

The student will be able to

1. Assess generally to obtain brief baseline history or complaint from the patient to determine what types of data, methods, and further assessment techniques are needed.
2. Assess the patient's readiness for the physical assessment.
3. Analyze the initial data to determine specific concerns that must be addressed prior to completing the physical assessment using both objective and subjective data.
4. Determine appropriate patient outcomes of the physical assessment and recognize the potential for adverse outcomes.
5. Plan the appropriate equipment that will aid the assessment process, and organize the process, so it flows efficiently.
6. Position the patient appropriately for the physical assessment while maintaining principles of body mechanics and privacy for the patient.
7. Implement the data collection and physical assessment processes that are appropriate to the situation: comprehensive physical assessment, routine shift assessment, or mini head-to-toe assessment.
8. Evaluate the effectiveness of the process and the accuracy of the results obtained.
9. Begin to formulate nursing diagnoses based on the data collected.
10. Document the results in the patient's record or other facility documentation form as required.

The registered nurse (RN) is responsible for performing patient assessment on a daily basis. In every care setting, the nurse is expected to gather data that will be analyzed to determine patients' problems and strengths, formulate nursing diagnoses, establish treatment priorities, and plan care.

The nurse performs the physical assessment systematically within a framework that is organized and comprehensive. This module introduces you to the process and framework of performing a beginning physical assessment. During this process, physical or physiological problems are identified. Work experience and education will allow you to expand or change it according to the focus of the assessment or your own preferences.

Consultation with other members of the healthcare team, review of the literature, general observation, interview, and physical assessment will all be included in your total nursing assessment. Although all may not be a part of each assessment encounter, the RN tailors the specific assessment process to focus on the needs of the individual patient.

General observations, augmented by skills in inspection, palpation, auscultation, and percussion, give the nurse a better database for nursing care and give the physician valuable input into the medical diagnosis and treatment. Developing the skills presented in this module requires frequent practice. Acquiring these skills forms a foundation from which you can perform a more complete nursing assessment.

Remember to use caution in sharing both verbal and written information about the patient. To protect the patient's privacy, share information only with those who have a need for it within the context of providing healthcare and billing or with those whom the patient has designated to receive the information. The Federal Health Insurance Portability and Accountability Act of 1996 (HIPAA) protects the privacy of the individual's personal health information through mandated procedures and penalties for violation of privacy. You are responsible for following the policies and procedures of the individual facility for ensuring compliance with this act.

NURSING DIAGNOSES

Appropriate nursing diagnoses will be identified after the assessment data have been obtained and analyzed. Every patient presents with a different set of strengths and problems. Refer to your nursing diagnosis, fundamentals, or medical/surgical text for assistance in developing your diagnoses.

DELEGATION

Nurses may delegate specific data collection to assistive personnel who have been taught appropriate skills. This includes weighing and measuring the patient, measuring intake and output, and measuring vital signs. The more comprehensive physical assessment skills in this module are not taught to nursing assistants. When data collection is delegated, the nurse remains accountable for determining what data are needed, how often data must be gathered, and for evaluating and analyzing all data to determine concerns or nursing diagnoses.

GATHERING DATA FOR A COMPREHENSIVE ASSESSMENT

A comprehensive nursing assessment process involves gathering all possible patient data from multiple sources to identify patient problems and strengths (Box 14-1). Every documentation system includes a form for recording the comprehensive assessment. Box 14-2 provides a form for recording all of your assessment data including data gathered in physical assessment. Here, we only briefly review the many sources of assessment data.

CONSULTATION WITH MEMBERS OF THE HEALTHCARE TEAM

The change-of-shift report is the most commonly used method for exchange of information among members of the healthcare team involved in the patient's care.

---

box 14-1 *Sources for Gathering Data*

Consultation with healthcare team members
Review of patient records and reports
Review of literature
Patient interview
General survey or observation
Physical assessment

Additional providers who interact with the patient—such as a physical therapist, occupational therapist, other nurses, dietitians, social worker, and chaplain—will be able to share valuable information with the nurse. Together, all providers contribute information that assists the nurse with developing a plan for effective assessment.

REVIEW OF RECORD AND REPORTS

The patient record contains essential information regarding identified problems. Valuable data can be easily retrieved from the history and physical examination completed by the physician, laboratory and diagnostic reports, the graphic flow record, the nurses' narrative record, and old records if available. This information will help the nurse determine what areas within the physical examination must be emphasized. For example, information indicating a history of cardiac disease would prompt the nurse to do a more comprehensive cardiac assessment even when the admitting problem is a fractured hip.

REVIEW OF THE LITERATURE

Using textbooks and journals to gain information about the patient's medical diagnosis, related diagnostic test results, or medications is an invaluable part of the data gathering process. You will be better able to plan care from the expanded knowledge base this provides. If you are unfamiliar with the patient's diagnosis, you will find it essential to gather this information to be sure that your physical examination includes the appropriate information.

INTERVIEW

The interview is a conversation with the patient through which you can gain information related to the patient's health problem(s), feelings, and perceptions, all of which can assist you as you provide care. Through the interview, the skilled nurse identifies particular aspects of the physical examination that should be expanded. The information provided by the patient is **subjective data.** The patient is always the primary source of data. If the patient is not able to participate fully in the interview because of physical or psychological impairments, include secondary data sources, such as emergency medical service personnel, the family, or those significant to the patient.

The first set of questions focuses on the patient's present health problem and responses to illness. Box 14-3 provides examples of initial interview questions. If a particular symptom is present, you will need to investigate it more thoroughly. See Table 14-1 for a list of questions you can ask the patient to assess specific **symptoms.** Another set of questions establish the patient's or family's perception of the patient's level of wellness before the present health problems. These questions also relate

box 14-2 *Comprehensive Data Gathering Guide*

Patient Initials _____ Room _____ Major Health Problem _____
Physical Needs _____

I. Activity
A. Posture _____
B. Ability to move _____
C. Gait _____
D. Activity ordered _____
E. Abnormalities _____
F. Assistive devices _____
G. Medications _____

II. Circulation
A. Blood pressure _____
B. Pulse
    1. Radial: R _____ L _____
    2. Apical _____
    3. Pedal: R _____ L _____
    4. Rhythm _____
C. Skin and mucous membrane color _____
D. Nail bed color _____
E. Skin temperature _____
F. Diagnostic/laboratory tests _____
G. Cardiac medications _____
H. Cardiac illness risk factors _____

III. Elimination
A. Bowel
    1. Date of last BM _____
        a. Description _____
        b. Stool specimen? _____
    2. Control? _____
    3. Bowel sounds _____
    4. Bowel medications _____
B. Bladder
    1. Urination patterns _____
    2. Appearance/odor of urine _____
    3. Urinary control? _____
    4. Urinalysis results _____
    5. Urinary tract medications _____

IV. Fluid and Electrolyte Balance/Hydration
A. Intake and output _____
B. Intravenous fluids
    1. Type _____
    2. Amount _____
C. Daily weight? _____
D. Skin turgor _____
E. Serum electrolytes _____
F. Electrolyte medications _____

V. Nutrition
A. Height _____ Weight _____
B. Diet ordered _____
C. Likes and dislikes _____
D. Amount eaten _____
E. Medications related to nutrition _____

(continued)

box 14-2 *Comprehensive Data Gathering Guide (Continued)*

VI. **Oxygenation**
   A. Respiration
      1. Rate _____
      2. Rhythm _____
      3. Depth _____
      4. Chest movement _____
   B. Breath sounds _____
   C. Respiratory secretions
      1. Amount _____
      2. Appearance _____
   D. Cough? _____
   E. Diagnostic/laboratory tests related to oxygenation _____
   F. Medications related to oxygenation _____
   G. Respiratory illness risk factors _____

VII. **Protection From Infection/Safety**
   A. Temperature _____
   B. Environment
      1. Side rails _____
      2. Call light _____
      3. Accommodations _____
      4. Room temperature _____
   C. Medications related to infection _____

VIII. **Regulation and Sensation/Comfort**
   A. Speech/communication abilities _____
   B. Level of consciousness _____
   C. Special senses
      1. Vision _____
      2. Hearing _____
      3. Tactile sense _____
   D. Gait _____
   E. Pain
      1. Description _____
      2. Location _____
      3. Duration _____
      4. Medications _____

IX. **Rest and Sleep**
   A. Normal sleep patterns _____
   B. Sleep aids? _____
   C. Appearance _____
   D. Factors interfering with rest/sleep _____

X. **Skin Integrity/Hygiene**
   A. Skin temperature _____
   B. Color _____
   C. Integrity _____
   D. Lesions/wounds/scars? _____
   E. Rash? _____
   F. Hydration _____
   G. Sensitivity to soap/lotion? _____
   H. Hygiene _____
   I. Medications related to skin concerns _____

XI. **Development**
   A. Age _____
   B. Life stage _____

(continued)

box 14-2 *Comprehensive Data Gathering Guide (Continued)*

XII. Mental Health/Psychosocial Needs
  A. Self-esteem
     1. Feelings about self _____
     2. Behaviors exhibited _____
  B. Love and belongingness
     1. Immediate family _____
     2. Help at home _____
     3. Feelings about relationships _____
     4. Behaviors exhibited _____
  C. Relationships and roles
     1. Occupation _____
     2. Role in family unit _____
     3. Immediate family members or significant others _____
     4. Help at home _____
     5. Feelings about relationships _____
     6. Behaviors exhibited _____

XIII. Sexuality
  A. Gender _____
  B. Last menstrual period (LMP); menstrual history _____
  C. Gravida; para _____
  D. Significant other _____
  E. Concerns expressed _____
  F. Diagnostic/laboratory _____
  G. Medications related to sexuality _____

XIV. Social, Cultural, and Ethnic Identity
  A. Country of origin _____
  B. Language used _____
  C. Special needs related to culture _____
  D. Insurance/financial support concerns _____

XV. Values and Beliefs
  A. Religious preference _____
  B. Notification of clergy or other adviser desired _____
  C. Special needs related to religious practices _____

to other aspects of the health history, such as allergies and chronic conditions. In all interviews, you may not need to ask each question specifically to elicit desired information. Using open-ended questions may elicit information about several areas in the answer to one question. Throughout the physical assessment, it is appropriate to continue to ask questions that relate to the examination being done at that time, unless the patient's condition makes it difficult for the patient to respond verbally.

PHYSICAL ASSESSMENT

Nurses must perform some aspects of the physical assessment for most patients. Upon admission to either an acute care or a long-term care facility, the physical assess-

ment may be much more detailed than at other times. When the complete physical assessment is not needed, the nurse determines what aspects of the physical assessment are required and performs a brief physical assessment or a focused physical assessment. Multiple approaches can be used for the comprehensive physical examination including a body systems approach, a head-to-toe approach, a combination of the two, or one you develop yourself. No matter which approach you take, be careful to include all areas. Establishing a pattern and using it consistently will make your examination more thorough.

This module starts with the general survey and techniques used in physical assessment. Then specific assessment strategies for body system areas are introduced. Careful study of each section will facilitate your ability to do a head-to-toe assessment.

GENERAL SURVEY

The first part of any physical examination is a general survey (sometimes referred to as general observation) that takes into consideration the patient as a whole. During the general survey, you will observe the environment of the patient and the patient's response to that environment. While you interview the patient, you can, with practice, make many observations. This includes what is seen, heard, and smelled while standing or sitting at the bedside. The patient's overall physical condition, weight-to-height proportion, relative size, coloring, and fatigue level are all seen in the general survey. Note any medical devices in use and their appropriate functioning. Whenever you contact a patient, observe carefully, and pay close attention to detail (Box 14-4). Your observational skills will improve with practice and experience. Your general observation often will help to guide you in determining when a focused assessment is needed. The information you gather through your senses of sight, hearing, and smell while performing a general survey and physical assessment is called **objective data.**

BASIC TECHNIQUES FOR PHYSICAL ASSESSMENT

Techniques basic to physical assessment include inspection, auscultation, percussion, and palpation. Inspection is always needed. The other techniques may or may not accompany inspection depending upon the organ or system being examined. The physical assessment techniques needed are performed in this sequence to prevent the potential for altered findings (e.g., sounds) based on your manipulation of the patient's body (Mehta, 2003). Terminology and a general overview are included here.

INSPECTION

Inspection is a more specific, precise, and closer examination of the body than occurs during the general survey. Inspection includes assessment of six essential elements: color, odor, size, shape, **symmetry,** and movement (Box 14-5). Inspection may require that clothing or dressings be removed to promote maximum visualization. While primarily visual, it does involve the sense of smell as well.

AUSCULTATION

Auscultation refers to listening with the **stethoscope** to sounds produced by the body. To successfully perform auscultation, you first must be able to recognize the normal variation of sounds. With experience, you will begin to recognize deviations from normal.

Stethoscopes come equipped with a **bell,** a **diaphragm,** or preferably both. With this last type, you

table 14-1. Questions to Explore Symptoms	
Purpose	**Question**
1. To determine the *location* of the problem (such as for pain, pressure, swelling)	"Where is this located? Can you point to where it is most troublesome?"
2. To determine the *onset* and *duration of the problem*	"When did it start?" and "How long has it persisted?"
3. To determine the *quality* (for pain, it might be sharp, dull, piercing, throbbing)	"What word would you use to describe this problem?"
4. To determine the *intensity or severity*	"How big a problem is this for you?" For pain: "Using a scale from 0 (no pain at all) to 10 (worst possible pain), can you rate its intensity?"
5. To determine *other factors affecting* the symptom	"What makes the symptom(s) worse? or better?"
6. To determine *functional effects*	"Does the symptom(s) affect your ability to carry out activities of daily living or to perform other important tasks?"
7. To determine the *patient perception* of the problem or symptom, which may range from insignificant to requiring a career change to life-threatening	"How do you feel about this problem or symptom?" "What is the overall effect of this on you?"

box 14-4 *General Survey Guide*

Lesions, depressions, or protuberances
Facial expressions or gestures
Skin color appropriate for ethnic origin
Body: symmetry, posture and position, movement
Equipment, tubes, drains, and so forth
Sounds of breathing
Speech and its pattern
Patient's breath odor
Odors associated with wounds
Odors associated with hygienic practices

box 14-5 *Essential Elements of Inspection*

Color	Shape
Odor	Symmetry
Size	Movement

can switch from one to the other by turning the chest piece or by flipping a lever. Low-pitched sounds are better heard with the bell placed lightly against the skin. High-pitched sounds are better heard with the diaphragm pressed firmly against the skin. Many nurses purchase their own stethoscopes to ensure quality and consistency. Because stethoscopes come in a wide variety of qualities, you should try one before purchasing to make sure that you can hear well through it. Amplifying stethoscopes are available to assist people with decreased hearing acuity.

A critical aspect of auscultation is the control of the noise level in the environment. This is extremely important for detecting all sounds. To hear well, you may need to close doors, turn off the television set, or ask visitors to pause in their conversations. In addition, instruct the patient not to talk during this aspect of the examination. Along with blood pressure, you will learn to auscultate lung, heart, and bowel sounds.

PERCUSSION

Percussion involves striking a body surface to produce sounds to determine whether the underlying tissues are air-filled, fluid-filled, or solid (Table 14-2). The examiner hears the differences in sounds that are produced by dif-

ferences in the density of the tissue beneath and feels the effects of the percussion. Percussion does not penetrate deeply (5 to 7 cm); therefore, it cannot detect deep **lesions.** To successfully carry out both palpation and percussion, your fingernails should not extend beyond the tips of the fingers.

Follow the steps listed below to begin the percussion process. Understand that to be able to detect abnormal sounds, you will first have to practice on healthy individuals to familiarize yourself with "normal."

- Prepare the patient for the percussion process.
- Place the middle finger of your nondominant hand firmly against the body surface to be percussed, keeping the palm and other fingers off the skin.
- With the tip of the middle finger of your dominant hand, strike the base of the distal phalanx of the stationary finger twice, just behind the nail bed (Fig. 14-1). Using wrist action, make blows brief and even. Remove striking finger immediately to avoid diminishing **vibration.**
- Listen carefully to the sound produced to identify its character.

PALPATION

Palpation involves the sense of touch and may be used simultaneously with inspection. Using the palms, fingers, and tips of the fingers, the nurse can identify softness/rigidity, masses, temperature, position, and size (Box 14-6). You will also use palpation to measure the

table 14-2. Percussion Sounds

Type of Sound	Sound	Example of Where it Is Heard
Resonance	Low-pitched "normal sound," not loud	Over the anterior lung; listen at the third interspace of the anterior right lung
Tympany	Loud and high-pitched (drumlike) resulting from air trapped in an enclosed chamber	Over stomach
Dullness	Short and high-pitched sound	Over solid organs liver, spleen, or diaphragm; or over consolidation (pneumonia) in lung
Flatness	Short and high-pitched sound completely without resonance or vibration	When fluid is in chest or abdomen; thigh

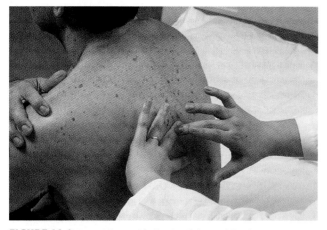

FIGURE 14-1 Percussion. With the tip of the middle of your dominant hand, strike the base of the distal phalanx of the stationary fingers twice, just behind the nail bed.

rate and quality of the peripheral pulses. Explanation is extremely important in gaining the patient's trust and cooperation as you palpate. Explain what it is you are doing, why you are doing it, and what the patient can do to be of assistance.

SPECIFIC STRATEGIES FOR PHYSICAL ASSESSMENT

The following specific strategies are described individually for teaching purposes. You should plan to learn each strategy so that you can perform it accurately. Then you will be able to do each appropriately as part of a comprehensive physical assessment, which is presented later. As each area of assessment is discussed, *only two phases of the nursing process are presented: planning and implementation.* You will be planning the information you want to obtain through the assessment and the equipment needed to obtain that information. You will then be implementing the specific assessment technique. As in all instances, you will be *documenting* appropriately.

---

box 14-6 *Essential Elements of Palpation*

Softness/rigidity
Masses
Temperature
Position
Size

NEUROLOGIC ASSESSMENT

Neurologic assessment is often done first when using a head-to-toe approach. Neurologic assessment includes assessing for the effects of brain function on pupillary responses, sensation, control of body movement, and reflexes. A neurologic assessment is conducted whenever an individual has a head injury or head surgery, a spinal injury or procedure, or disease process that affects the brain or spinal cord. It is also used when an individual has received a medication, such as an anesthetic agent, that affects brain function.

Inspection of the pupils is the first step in neurologic assessment. Pupils that react sluggishly or that show differences between the two pupillary reactions reflect subtle clues of pathology in the very ill (Lower, 2002). If the patient has a brain lesion, the pupil on the same side as the brain lesion will react abnormally. An examination of the optic discs with the **ophthalmoscope** also may disclose a neurologic deficit or disease.

Another part of assessing neurologic function is examining the patient for neuromuscular control. Normal function results in the ability to follow directions and respond equally and strongly with both hands and both legs.

In addition, reflexes are assessed to determine if stimuli can be applied and transmit impulses through the sensory and motor pathways of the reflex arc. Depending on the situation, you may test only a few of the more prominent reflexes or proceed with an abbreviated neurologic examination. Many of the measurements of neurologic functioning will be tested when the other systems or areas are examined. Reflex responses are usually recorded numerically using the following symbols: 0 (no response), 1+ (hypoactive), 2+ (normal), 3+ (hyperactive), and 4+ (very hyperactive).

If you want to check the function of cranial nerves, you can do so during examination of the face by having the patient protrude the tongue, smile, and resist supraorbital pressure. (For a detailed description of a complete neurologic examination, refer to a medical/surgical text or a neurologic nursing text.)

Procedure for Neurologic Assessment

PLANNING

1. Identify the individualized patient outcomes of the neurologic assessment. **R:** Identifying outcomes facilitates planning and evaluation.
   a. Pupils are equal, round, reactive to light and accommodation.
   b. Patient can follow commands for the use of hands and legs and demonstrates muscle strength equally on hands and legs.
   c. Reflex responses tested are present.

d. Patient responds accurately to skin touch.

e. Vision is adequate for self-care.

f. Hearing allows effective communication with others.

2. Obtain the appropriate equipment. **R:** You need this equipment to examine the eyes and reflexes correctly.

a. Flashlight or penlight to examine the pupils

b. Pupillary size chart or neurologic assessment record to compare the pupil size of the patient with a standard

c. Reflex hammer to assess sensory and motor nerve function

d. Database worksheet to record results

IMPLEMENTATION

Action	Rationale
3. Assess the pupils:	
a. Inspect the size, shape, and equality of both pupils.	Normal findings should show round, clear, pupils that are equal in size bilaterally.
b. Inspect pupillary reaction to light on each eye. Holding the eyelid open with one hand, shine a light on the pupil, bringing the light in from the side (Fig. 14-2). Observe what happens to the pupil. Observe what happens to the opposite eye when the light is shined into one pupil. Repeat for the second eye.	The normal pupil should exhibit rapid **constriction** when light shines in it. Normal pupils also exhibit **consensual reaction**; that is, the opposite eye constricts along with the eye that is exposed to light. **FIGURE 14-2** To test the pupillary reactions to light, bring the light source in from the side.
c. Test the pupillary reaction to **accommodation.** Ask the patient to look at an object in the distance and then at your fingers, which you will hold 5 to 10 cm from the bridge of the patient's nose.	Pupils should constrict as they attempt to accommodate to close focus. Pupils should exhibit **convergence**; that is, stay focused on the finger and thus move toward the nose and toward one another.
d. Observe for involuntary, rapid, rhythmic movement of the eyeball.	These movements are called **nystagmus** and are not a normal finding. They should be reported.
4. Assess neuromuscular control:	
a. Ask the patient to grasp both hands and squeeze to evaluate muscle strength and lateral equality.	Grips should be equal and strong. If one is weak, it may represent a problem in the brain on the opposite side of the hand that is affected.

(continued)

Action	Rationale
b. Ask the patient to push both feet against the resistance of your hands.	Normal findings are that the legs are equally strong and able to push straight at your hands. If one is weak, it may represent a problem in the brain on the opposite side of the leg that is affected.
5. Assess reflexes:	
a. Corneal reflex (blink): Touch the cornea with a soft, small wad of cotton.	The normal response is for the eye to blink.
b. Biceps reflex: Place your thumb on the biceps tendon, which is located just above the antecubital fossa. Strike the thumb with the **reflex hammer** (Fig. 14-3A).	The normal response is flexion of the forearm.
c. Triceps reflex: Support the upper arm at a right angle to the body, and allow the forearm to hang freely. Strike the triceps tendon with the reflex hammer (Fig. 14-3B) just above the elbow.	The normal response is extension of the forearm.
d. Brachioradial reflex: Strike the radius slightly above the wrist with the reflex hammer.	The normal response is flexion of the forearm.
e. Quadriceps reflex: Ensure that the patient's lower leg is relaxed and hanging freely from the knee. Strike the **patellar tendon,** which is just below the knee, with the reflex hammer (Fig. 14-3C).	The normal response is extension of the lower leg.
f. Achilles reflex: Hold the foot in a position of **dorsiflexion.** Strike the Achilles tendon at the back of the ankle with the reflex hammer (Fig. 14-3D).	The normal response is plantar flexion of the foot (the toes bend downward).
g. Babinski reflex: Using the end of the reflex hammer or the edge of a tongue depressor, stroke the sole of the foot from heel to toe.	The normal response is plantar flexion (the toes curl downward), which is referred to as a negative Babinski reflex. A negative Babinski is normal from the age of 6 months on (Fig. 14-3E). Failure to demonstrate plantar flexion is referred to as a positive Babinski reflex and is an abnormal finding.
6. Assess skin sensation: You may choose to test sensation to touch by using a **pinwheel** that can be rolled over broad skin areas or by using a cotton-tipped applicator (Fig. 14-4). The patient is asked to report, without looking at the device, whether he or she can feel the sensation.	The normal response is that the patient reports feeling where touch occurred and distinguishes sharp and dull touch.

(continued)

Action	**Rationale**

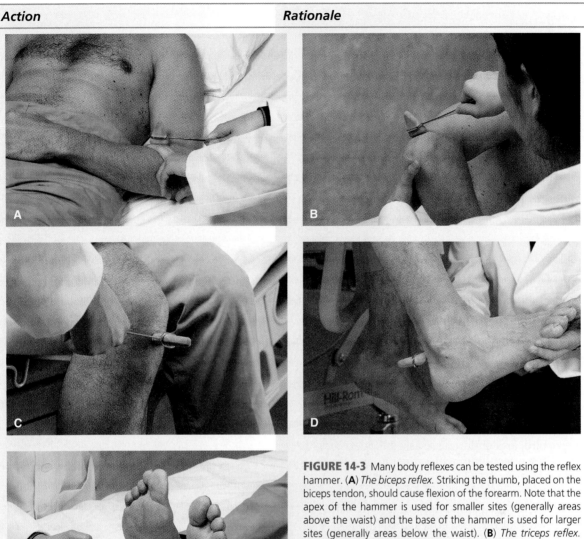

FIGURE 14-3 Many body reflexes can be tested using the reflex hammer. (**A**) *The biceps reflex.* Striking the thumb, placed on the biceps tendon, should cause flexion of the forearm. Note that the apex of the hammer is used for smaller sites (generally areas above the waist) and the base of the hammer is used for larger sites (generally areas below the waist). (**B**) *The triceps reflex.* Extension of the forearm should occur when the triceps tendon is struck with the reflex hammer. (**C**) *The quadriceps reflex.* Extension of the lower leg should occur when the patellar tendon is struck with the reflex hammer. (**D**) *The Achilles reflex.* Plantar flexion of the foot should occur when the Achilles tendon is struck. (**E**) *The Babinski reflex.* The sole of the foot is stroked from heel to toe using the handle of the reflex hammer. A normal result in the adult patient is plantar flexion.

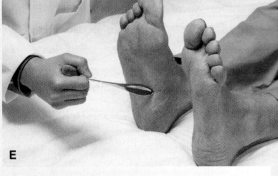

7. Assess visual acuity. Check each eye separately.	The normal response is to be able to describe the environment. The patient may need glasses or lenses for reading small print.
a. Specific charts are not commonly used for hospitalized patients. In the hospital or long-term care facility, you may obtain very general information about visual acuity. You may ask if the patient can read printed material and/or describe objects that are across the room.	

(continued)

Action	Rationale

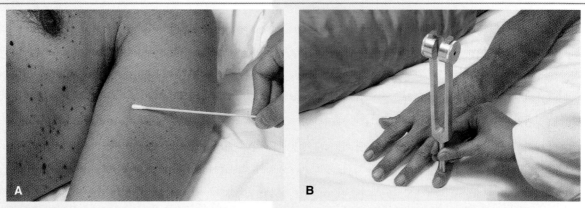

FIGURE 14-4 (**A**) A pinwheel or cotton-tipped applicator is used to test peripheral sensation of the body. (**B**) A tuning fork placed over a bony prominence is used to test the patient's sense of vibration. The patient is asked to indicate when the vibration starts and stops.

Action	Rationale
b. In a school setting or an ambulatory care setting, use a standardized chart. The **Snellen chart** has vertical rows of block letters that become smaller as the reader moves downward. An adaptation of this chart using three-pronged symbols randomly facing in different directions can be used for children and illiterate adults. The blackbird chart uses a modified E to resemble a flying bird, and children are asked to identify the direction in which the bird is flying.	
c. If corrective lenses (glasses or contact lenses) are worn, check vision with and without the corrective lenses in place. Ask the patient if there have been any recent vision changes.	
8. Using the ophthalmoscope to look into each pupil, inspect each eye for corneal, lens, or vitreous abnormalities while the patient gazes straight ahead. Assess the optic disc for shape and color. Retract each eyelid to observe the color and condition of the conjunctiva.	To view the interior of the eye, look through the ophthalmoscope at the patient's eye with your opposite eye. This places your eye in close proximity and allows you to focus the lens of the ophthalmoscope. The normal cornea, lens, and vitreous are clear. The disc should be shaped like the top of a mushroom when viewed from above and a lemon yellow color. The conjunctivae should be pink without lesions or drainage
9. Assess hearing: Ask the patient if there have been any recent changes in hearing ability.	
a. To do a simple hearing assessment for the purposes of care, speak quietly on one side of the patient. Raise your voice	The normal response to the speaking test is to be able to hear a quiet voice in each ear.

(continued)

Action	Rationale
until the patient can hear you. Repeat on the ear on the other side. *Note:* This is a general examination to determine the patient's ability to relate to caregivers.	
b. You can test hearing by striking a **tuning fork** and holding it an equal distance from each ear to test for air conduction of sound (Fig. 14-5). Then place the struck tuning fork on each mastoid process, just below and behind the ears, and on the center top of the **cranium** to test for bone conduction of sound. A more definitive hearing test may be performed using electronic equipment.	The normal response is equal sound detection with air conduction and bone conduction. If the patient experiences bone conduction but does not hear the air conduction, hearing nerves are intact, and the hearing deficit is related to conduction in the ear.

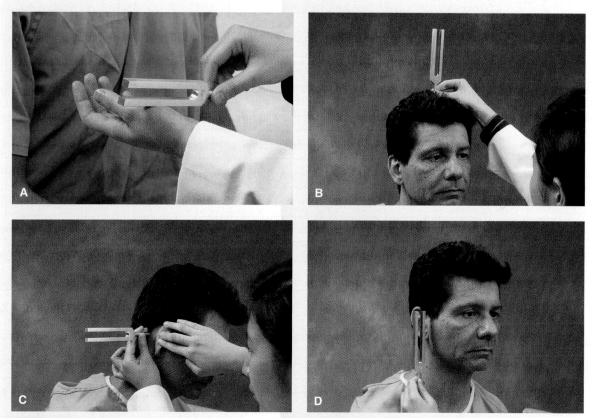

FIGURE 14-5 Testing hearing. (**A**) The nurse activates the tuning fork by striking the tines gently on the hand near the wrist. (**B**) Test for bone conduction of sound by centering the vibrating tuning fork midline over the patient's head or forehead. (**C**) Bone and air conduction are tested using the *Rinne test.* The stem of the vibrating tuning fork is placed on the mastoid process and the patient is asked to signal when sound is no longer heard. (**D**) The two tines of the vibrating tuning fork are then held near the ear. A normal result is that the person will hear by both bone conduction and air conduction.

c. If the patient uses a hearing aid or aids, check to see that they have working batteries, are free from wax buildup, and are properly placed in the ears.

NEUROLOGICAL ASSESSMENT RECORD

DAWSON, HARRY M-24

DR. JORDAN

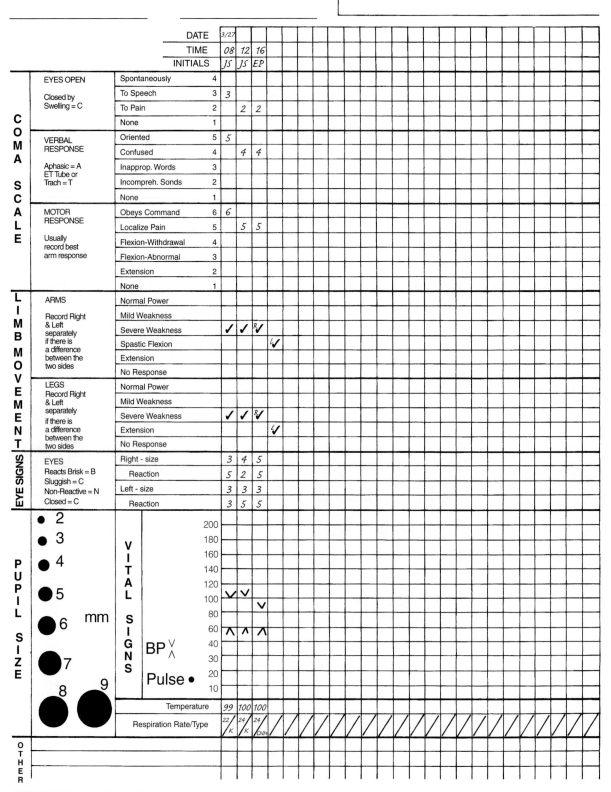

				DATE	3/27			
				TIME	08	12	16	
				INITIALS	JS	JS	EP	
C O M A S C A L E	EYES OPEN Closed by Swelling = C	Spontaneously	4					
		To Speech	3		3			
		To Pain	2			2	2	
		None	1					
	VERBAL RESPONSE Aphasic = A ET Tube or Trach = T	Oriented	5		5			
		Confused	4			4	4	
		Inapprop. Words	3					
		Incompreh. Sonds	2					
		None	1					
	MOTOR RESPONSE Usually record best arm response	Obeys Command	6		6			
		Localize Pain	5			5	5	
		Flexion-Withdrawal	4					
		Flexion-Abnormal	3					
		Extension	2					
		None	1					
L I M B M O V E M E N T	ARMS Record Right & Left separately if there is a difference between the two sides	Normal Power						
		Mild Weakness						
		Severe Weakness			✓	✓	ᴿ✓	
		Spastic Flexion						ᴸ✓
		Extension						
		No Response						
	LEGS Record Right & Left separately if there is a difference between the two sides	Normal Power						
		Mild Weakness						
		Severe Weakness			✓	✓	ᴿ✓	
		Extension						ᴸ✓
		No Response						
EYE SIGNS	EYES Reacts Brisk = B Sluggish = C Non-Reactive = N Closed = C	Right - size			3	4	5	
		Reaction			5	2	5	
		Left - size			3	3	3	
		Reaction			3	5	5	

PUPIL SIZE (mm)
● 2
● 3
● 4
● 5
● 6
● 7
● 8 ● 9

VITAL SIGNS

BP ∨ ∧   Pulse ●

	200				
	180				
	160				
	140				
	120				
	100	∨	∨	∨	
	80				
	60	∧	∧	∧	
	40				
	30				
	20				
	10				

Temperature	99	100	100	
Respiration Rate/Type	22/K	24/K	24/CNH	

OTHER

FIGURE 14-6 Example of a form for recording neurologic observations.

DOCUMENTATION

10. Document your findings in the patient's record. Various forms have been designed for neurologic assessment. Something similar may be in use in your clinical facility. See Figure 14-6 for an example.
    a. Pupillary responses: The abbreviations PERL (pupils equal and reactive to light), PERLA (pupils equal and reactive to light and accommodation), and PERRLA (pupils equal, round, and reactive to light and accommodation) are commonly used in charting pupillary observations.
    b. Neuromuscular control: Describe whether hand grips and leg function are strong and equal. Describe any deviations from normal.
    c. Reflexes: Record reflex results according to the following scale (0 no response, 1+ hypoactive, 2+ normal, 3+ hyperactive, and 4+ very hyperactive).
    d. Touch sensation: Describe any abnormalities in the narrative.
    e. Vision: Describe any problems the patient has in seeing objects within the room or the results of the standardized chart test.
    f. Hearing: Describe any difficulties and which ear has the problem.

NEURO SIGNS

"Neuro signs" are a standard sequence of neurologic assessments in a brief format often used for monitoring patients to detect changes over time. Box 14-7 lists the neurologic assessments that would be included if "neuro signs" were listed on the plan of care or in the physician's orders.

ASSESSMENT OF THE HEART

You will use auscultation as you examine the heart. Evaluate cardiac rate, rhythm, and intensity first. In most facilities, the **apical pulse** is assessed in all patients receiving a digitalis preparation before the administration of the medication. This provides an accurate heart rate for evaluating the patient's response to the drug. Note regular irregularities (those that occur at regular intervals such as every third beat), as well as irregular irregularities (those that occur unpredictably, such as an occasional missed or early beat). Also note abrupt changes in heart rate or rhythm.

You should be able to differentiate between the first and second heart sounds (S_1 and S_2), which is more easily accomplished at normal and slow rates. Heart sounds are created by the closing of valves in the heart. **Systole** occurs between the first and second sounds, and **diastole** between the second and first sounds. The first sound is often more easily heard in the area of the fifth left **intercostal space** near the nipple line (the **apex**); the second sound is more easily heard in the area of the

---

box 14-7 *Assessments Included in "Neuro Signs"*

Level of Consciousness
- To what does the person respond?
- How does the person respond?

Examination of the Pupils
- Equal
- Reactive to light
- Respond with accommodation

Muscle Strength and Control
- Strength of hand grip
- Strength of legs
- Symmetry of strength

Vital Signs

---

second intercostal space immediately to the right of the sternum (the **base**), where the first sound may be heard clearly as well (Fig. 14-7).

Sounds over the apex are usually heard more easily with the bell of the stethoscope; sounds over the base of the heart are usually heard more easily with the diaphragm. You should, however, feel free to experiment with both on any given patient to determine which gives you the best sound.

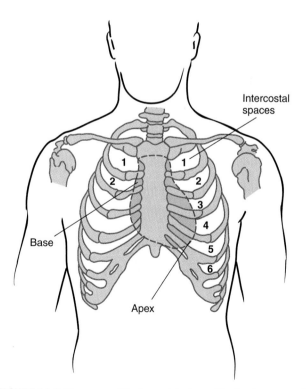

FIGURE 14-7 The apex and the base of the heart. The first heart sound may be clearly heard at either the apex or the base; the second heart sound is more easily heard at the base. The numbers indicate the intercostal spaces.

If you have difficulty distinguishing the sounds, identify the **carotid pulse** while you listen to the heart. The carotid pulse occurs simultaneously with the first heart sound. If the terminology is confusing, just describe what you hear in your own words.

Procedure for Assessing the Heart

PLANNING

1. Identify individualized patient outcomes of the cardiac assessment. **R:** Identifying outcomes facilitates planning and evaluation.

   a. Point of maximal impulse is located at the fifth intercostal space at the left midclavicular line.
   b. Heart rate is between 60 and 100 beats per minute.
   c. The normal S_1 and S_2 heart sounds are audible.
   d. No murmurs are present.
2. Obtain the appropriate equipment. **R:** Obtaining equipment organizes and speeds the assessment process.
   a. Stethoscope
   b. Alcohol wipes
   c. Database worksheet to record results

IMPLEMENTATION

Action	Rationale
3. Examine the heart as follows:	
a. Using an alcohol wipe, clean the chest piece of the stethoscope and the earpieces if the stethoscope is not your own.	To prevent spreading infective agents to others who use the same stethoscope and protect you from bacteria from patients and other staff that might be on the stethoscope.
b. Explain the procedure to the patient.	To relieve patient anxiety, which might alter the heart rate, and to facilitate patient participation.
c. Ask the patient not to speak while you are trying to listen, and control the noise in the environment by turning off the television or radio and closing the door.	Extraneous noise will interfere with your ability to hear the sounds, possibly distorting your findings.
d. With the patient sitting up, remove the gown or pajama top enough to expose the chest. To best hear heart sounds, have the supine patient roll partially over to the left, or have the sitting patient lean slightly forward.	The sounds should be easier to hear because these positions bring the heart closer to the chest wall. Heart sounds that are very difficult to hear are termed distant, and those that are easy to hear are termed clear. The sounds are more difficult to hear in obese or barrel-chested patients.
e. Using a consistent pattern, identify the anatomical landmarks described below, and begin listening for heart sounds.	Correct placement optimizes results. The use of a consistent pattern ensures that you do not inadvertently omit a part of the examination. You will be listening for all heart sounds. The first and second heart sounds (S_1 and S_2), commonly heard as "lub, dub," are normal in children and adults. The third and fourth sounds (S_3 and S_4) are abnormal in adults but may be normal in children and young adults.

(continued)

Action	Rationale
(1) Inspect and palpate the chest carefully. Note whether the chest moves with heartbeats; palpate the intercostal spaces to be sure you can count the heart beats. Note the point of maximal impulse (PMI) where the heartbeat is most strongly felt on the chest wall. The PMI is usually found at the left fifth intercostal space (ICS) at the midclavicular line.	
(2) Start with a warm stethoscope diaphragm (warm the diaphragm by holding it in your hand). Place it and listen at the second ICS at the right of the sternal border (aortic valve area) for S_1 and S_2. The S_2 (second heart sound) "dub" is best heard over the aortic area.	
(3) Move to the second or third ICS at the left sternal border (pulmonic valve area), and listen for S_1 and S_2.	
(4) Move to the fifth ICS near the left sternal border (tricuspid valve), and listen for S_1 and S_2.	
(5) Move to the fifth ICS at the midclavicular line (mitral valve area), and listen for S_1 and S_2. The S_1 (the first heart sound) is best heard at the mitral area and makes the "lub" portion of "lub, dub."	
(6) After identifying S_1 and S_2, listen carefully for additional sounds that may be present. Locate these sounds in relation to S_1 and S_2, and describe them in terms of pitch, loudness, and where they are best heard.	
(i) S_3 occurs just after the S_2 sequence and may create a sound sequence of "Ken-tuc-ky," which is called a gallop.	This is the result of blood rushing from the atrium into the ventricle that is dilated and full of blood.
(ii) S_4 occurs just before S_1 and may create a sound sequence of "Ten-nes-see."	This sound occurs when the atria contract and try to push blood into a ventricle that does not expand.

(continued)

Action	Rationale
(iii) A murmur is a "swishing" or "blowing" sound. Note whether it is low-, medium-, or high-pitched.	A murmur is caused by blood flowing through a valve that does not close completely or by increased blood flow through a normal valve.
(iv) A friction rub is a sandpaper-like sound that occurs in relation to the cardiac cycle.	A friction rub is caused by the movement of the heart muscle rubbing against the pericardial sac.
f. Count the heart rate at the mitral or aortic valve area for one minute by counting each "lub, dub" as one beat. This is the apical heart rate.	The mitral valve area is the place where the heart is closest to the surface and where the heart sound is most distinctly heard. The apical heart rate includes all beats, even those of less force.

DOCUMENTATION

4. Document the pulse rate on the graph or flow sheet. Abnormal cardiac sounds or rhythms are documented on a narrative form.

ASSESSMENT OF CENTRAL VEINS AND PERIPHERAL CIRCULATION

The appearance of the lower extremities, peripheral pulses, blood pressure, edema, and the filling and emptying of veins all provide data regarding circulatory status. Locating and assessing peripheral pulses was described in Module 11. Measuring blood pressure was described in Module 12 as was calculating ankle brachial index for assessing peripheral circulation. Assessing the filling and emptying of veins is described below.

Capillary refill time reflects peripheral arterial flow. **Edema** represents abnormal fluid accumulation. Neck vein **distention** indicates increased central venous pressure. Hand vein emptying time also reflects **venous pressure.** You will use inspection and palpation to detect these indicators. During this part of the assessment, it is also essential to determine whether the patient has any lower extremity pain or cramping in relation to walking and whether the discomfort dissipates with rest (Gehring, 2002).

CAPILLARY REFILL TIME

You can estimate the rate of peripheral blood flow by observing capillary refill time. When you depress the tip of a fingernail, the nail bed blanches. As soon as you release the pressure, the blood should rush back immediately, and the nail bed should become pink again. A more sluggish rate of capillary refill indicates a slower rate of peripheral flow. Normal capillary refill time should be less than 3 seconds. Capillary refill time should be assessed on each extremity.

EDEMA

Edema is the abnormal accumulation of fluid in the intercellular tissues of the body. Edema is often found in dependent areas of the body (hands, feet, ankles, and sacrum), where excess fluids pool as a result of gravity. This is referred to as **dependent edema.**

Periorbital edema is fluid accumulating around the soft tissue of the eyes. This type of edema is usually soft and resilient. It may have diagnostic significance or, in women, it may simply be related to cyclical hormonal changes.

Pitting edema is seen when fingertips pressed into the tissue leave a depression behind. Edema is generally rated on a scale of 1+ to 4+; 1+ is a slight depression that disappears quickly, and 4+ is a deep depression that disappears slowly. Because the scale is subjective, daily weight measurements and circumferential measurements of extremities often provide more objective data about fluid accumulation. A more objective measure of edema of the lower extremities can be obtained by measuring the number of centimeters the edema extends up the tibia (**pretibial edema**) beyond the malleoli (ankle bones).

NECK VEIN DISTENTION

When fluid volume or cardiac problems exist, you may need to inspect the distention of the jugular veins to estimate venous pressure. Normally, when a person is standing, or sitting at an angle greater than 45 degrees to the horizontal, the jugular veins are collapsed. Distention of these veins in a position above 45 degrees indicates abnormally high central venous pressure.

HAND VEIN EMPTYING TIME

Venous pressure is also reflected by distention of the hand veins in nondependent positions. When the hands are allowed to hang freely at the sides, the hand veins will fill and become distended. When the hands are raised to a level above the heart or higher, the veins should be flat. If the hand veins remain distended, the venous pressure is greater than normal. Be careful not to confuse distended hand veins with visible hand veins that often occur in the elderly as subcutaneous tissue in the hands is decreased.

CAROTID ARTERY BLOOD FLOW

A **bruit** is an abnormal blowing sound heard over an artery accompanying each pulse. A bruit in a carotid artery represents turbulent blood flow in the artery and is usually associated with significant atherosclerotic plaques in the artery.

Procedure for Assessing Central Veins and Peripheral Circulation

PLANNING

1. Identify individualized patient outcomes of the venous and peripheral circulation assessment. **R:** Identifying outcomes facilitates planning and evaluation.
   a. Neck veins are flat when the patient's head is above 45 degrees and filled when the patient is lying flat.
   b. Hand veins are filled when down and flat when raised above heart level.
   c. No peripheral or periorbital edema is present.
   d. No bruits are heard over the carotid arteries.
2. Obtain the appropriate equipment:
   a. a centimeter ruler to measure any venous distention noted
   b. database worksheet to record results

IMPLEMENTATION

Action	Rationale
3. Assess neck veins:	To establish a baseline or determine abnormalities.
a. Have the patient lie flat on his or her back. Watch for dyspnea.	In many cases, patients with distended neck veins cannot lie flat without experiencing dyspnea.
b. Identify the jugular veins bilaterally.	Jugular veins are located on each side of the trachea.
c. Gradually elevate the head of the bed to a 45-degree angle, watching to see when the jugular veins collapse.	Pressure in the central veins lowers when the head is elevated, and by the time the head is at 45 degrees, the veins are flat.
d. If the veins remain distended at 45 degrees, estimate venous pressure by measuring the vertical distance (in centimeters) from the right atrium level to the upper level of the distention (Fig. 14-8). Using the sternal angle, which is 5 cm above the right atrium, may work better because the level of the right atrium is difficult to determine. Locate this angle by placing two of your fingers at the **suprasternal notch** and sliding them down the sternum until they reach a bony **protuberance.**	Distended veins when the head is elevated represent an abnormally high venous pressure.

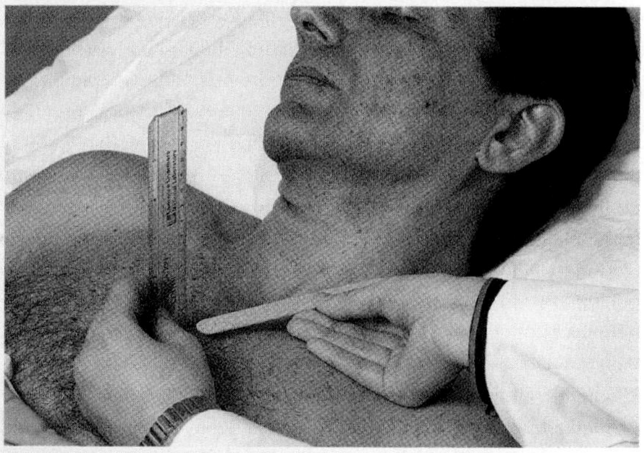

FIGURE 14-8 To estimate venous pressure, measure the vertical distance from the sternal angle to the upper level of distention in the jugular vein.

(continued)

Action	Rationale
4. Assess hand vein emptying:	
a. Inspect hand veins when they are below the level of the heart.	The normal hand vein is filled with blood and appears distended at this level.
b. Lift the hand up, observing the veins as you raise it.	The normal pattern is for the hand veins to empty as they are raised and be flat when above heart level.
5. Assess for edema:	
a. Look at the feet and lower legs for swollen tissue with smooth skin. Note how far above the lateral malleolus the swelling extends. Measure the swelling both in circumference and in distance above the malleolus for an objective measure.	Edema is fluid in the interstitial spaces and accumulates in dependent areas of the body. Objective measures facilitate tracking of improvement or worsening of edema.
b. Palpate the lower legs for edema. To palpate for edema, use the fingertips of the index and middle fingers, pressing firmly over a bony area (Fig. 14-9). When you remove your fingers, observe the area for a depression that remains. Rate the depression as 1+ to 4+. Watch to see how long it takes for the depressed area to disappear.	Increased pitting represents a greater amount of fluid in the tissues.

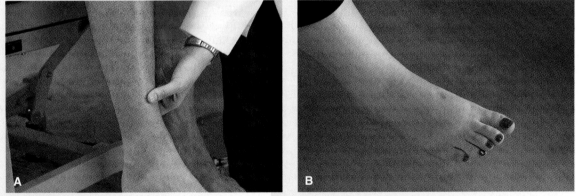

FIGURE 14-9 (**A**) Palpate for pretibial edema by pressing firmly over a bony area. (**B**) Example of pitting edema in the foot of a different patient.

Action	Rationale
6. Ask the patient to hold his or her breath, and assess carotid arteries by placing the stethoscope gently over each carotid artery and listening for a blowing sound.	The normal response is no sound. Carotid arteries should not be pressed firmly because this could block circulation to the brain.

(continued)

Action	Rationale
7. Observe the skin color and texture of the lower extremities.	Smooth, shiny, hairless skin on the legs is often related to a decrease in arterial circulation. Areas of brown discoloration on the lower legs may be related to venous insufficiency. The coloration is due to red cells being forced into the interstitial spaces by high venous pressure. These red cells break down, leaving iron pigments in the tissue.

DOCUMENTATION

8. Document the presence or absence of neck vein distention, distended hand veins above heart level, edema in the lower legs, and carotid bruits. Describe any abnormalities. There may be a special form for these observations in your facility.

LUNG AND RESPIRATORY ASSESSMENT

Both inspection and auscultation are a part of respiratory assessment. As you inspect, look for signs of labored breathing, including the use of accessory muscles and nasal flaring. Also observe the patient's anteroposterior (AP) and transverse chest diameters. Normally, the transverse diameter is roughly twice the AP diameter. Whereas a deep AP diameter may be found in a person with chronic lung disease, it may be a normal finding in an elderly patient or in one who is a professional singer. Watch also to see if chest movements are symmetrical.

As you auscultate the lungs, try to discern normal breath sounds and **adventitious sounds** (abnormal sounds). Remember that to attain any degree of skill, you must practice frequently. Auscultation should be done both anteriorly and posteriorly in a systematic manner, comparing one side with the other. Note the location of the lobes of the lungs in Figure 14-10. The lower lobes are heard only in a very small area on the anterior chest; conversely, the upper lobes are heard only in a small area of the posterior chest.

Breath sounds are created by the movement of air in the **trachea, bronchi,** and **alveoli.** Normally, the expiratory phase is twice as long as the inspiratory phase.

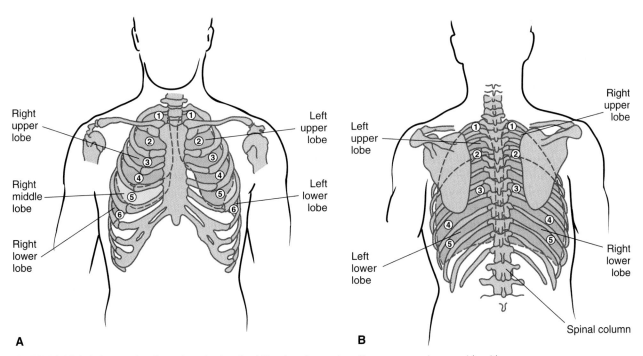

A   **B**

FIGURE 14-10 (**A**) The anterior chest. Auscultation should be done in a systematic way, comparing one side with the other. The numbers indicate a pattern of stethoscope placement: first 1 left, then 1 right; next 2 left, then 2 right, and so on. (**B**) The posterior chest. Note that the upper lobes are heard only in a small area of the posterior chest. The numbers indicate a pattern of stethoscope placement: first 1 left, then 1 right; next 2 left, then 2 right, and so on.

On auscultation, however, you do not hear all of the expiratory phase, so that it seems shorter than the inspiratory phase. In cases of bronchial obstruction, chronic lung disease, or shallow breathing (as might be seen in a patient with incisional pain after abdominal surgery), breath sounds may be absent or decreased. In a condition that causes **consolidation** of lung tissue, such as pneumonia, breath sounds may be louder or increased.

You may hear many adventitious sounds superimposed on the breath sounds. Among these are crackles, gurgles, wheezes, and friction rubs. In most facilities, current practice is to describe what you hear or to describe all abnormal sounds as "adventitious sounds."

Crackles result from air passing through moisture (due to secretions) in the respiratory passages. Usually heard on inspiration, crackles may be fine or coarse. Fine crackles have a high-pitched sound; coarse crackles are louder and tend to have a bubbling quality. If you hear crackles, ask the patient to cough, and listen again. Typically, patients who have been lying quietly have some crackles in the lung bases that clear when they cough. You may occasionally hear crackles referred to as rales; this is an older term that is no longer recommended.

Gurgles are caused by air passing through respiratory passages that are narrowed or partially obstructed by secretions, edema, tumors, and so on. They are usually low-pitched and loud and often change in quality after the patient coughs. They may be heard on both inspiration and expiration. Rhonchi is the older term for gurgles.

Wheezes, like gurgles, are caused by air passing through partially obstructed respiratory passages, but they are higher-pitched because they originate in smaller passages. They have a whistlelike tone. Although they are more commonly heard during expiration, wheezes can be heard during any phase of respiration.

Pleural friction rubs are caused by the rubbing together of inflamed and roughened pleural surfaces. The sound is harsh and scratchy, somewhat like two pieces of sandpaper being rubbed together. Friction rubs are heard on both inspiration and expiration. If this sound correlates with the rate and rhythm of the heartbeat, not the respirations, it is a pericardial friction rub.

Procedure for Assessing the Lungs and Respiration

PLANNING

1. Identify individualized patient outcomes of the lung and respiration examination. **R:** Identifying outcomes facilitates planning and evaluation.
   a. Lungs are clear to auscultation.
   b. Breath sounds are auscultated in all lobes.
2. Obtain the appropriate equipment. **R:** To facilitate organization.
   a. Stethoscope
   b. Alcohol wipes
   c. Database worksheet to record results

IMPLEMENTATION

Action	Rationale
3. Assess the lungs:	To establish baseline information on respiratory function or obtain updated data and compare with norms.
a. Explain the procedure to the patient, asking him or her not to speak while you are trying to listen. Control the noise in the environment by turning off the television and closing the door.	Extraneous noise will interfere with your ability to hear the sounds, possibly distorting findings.
b. Using an alcohol wipe, clean the chest piece of the stethoscope, and clean the earpieces if it is not your own.	To prevent passing infective agents to others who use the same stethoscope.
c. Position the patient to allow you to examine the chest. Sitting on the bed with the feet over the edge is ideal, however, not possible for many	Both anterior and posterior chest will be examined.

(continued)

Action	Rationale
hospitalized patients. The patient can sit up in the bed and lean forward or lie on the side.	
d. Systematically percuss the chest, beginning at the apex of the lungs, comparing one side with the other.	Sounds correlate to underlying density. The normal sound is resonant because of the air filling the lungs.
e. Warm the diaphragm of the stethoscope in your hands, and place the diaphragm at the left apex on the patient's chest. Ask the patient to breathe slowly in and out through an open mouth.	Warming the stethoscope is more comfortable for the patient. The left apex is a standard place to begin the systematic auscultation. A deep breath maximizes air movement into the lungs, making the sounds easier to hear.
f. Using a consistent pattern, listen to the anterior chest by moving the stethoscope from the apex to the base, comparing sounds heard from one side to the other (see Fig. 14-10A).	To assess air movement and detect normal or abnormal sounds.
g. Using a consistent pattern, listen to the posterior chest by moving the stethoscope from the apex to the base to compare sounds heard from one side to the other (see Fig. 14-10B).	To assess air movement and normal or abnormal sounds.
h. If you hear adventitious sounds, ask the patient to cough. Listen again to see if the sounds have cleared.	Clearing after coughing is characteristic of certain adventitious sounds.

DOCUMENTATION

4. Document the breath sounds heard and where they are heard. Adventitious sounds are described using standard terminology above. **R:** Documentation is a legal record of the patient's care and therapy and communicates nursing activities to other nurses and caregivers.

BREAST ASSESSMENT

A common site of cancer in the female is the breast. However, the examination of the breasts in male patients is important, too, because breast cancer does occur in males, although much less frequently than in females. Breast assessment combines both inspection and palpation. The complete breast examination is not a routine part of the nursing physical assessment in the hospital. In the long-term care facility, it may be part of an annual examination.

Procedure for Assessing the Breasts

Nurses working in ambulatory care where patients are taught breast self-examination (BSE) may perform this procedure and also teach the patient how to perform BSE.

PLANNING

1. Identify the individualized patient outcomes of the breast examination. **R:** Identification of outcomes facilitates planning and evaluation.
   a. No abnormal masses identified
   b. No visible abnormalities of the surface of the breasts
   c. No areas of discomfort or tenderness
2. Obtain the appropriate equipment:
   a. a small pillow
   b. database worksheet to record results

IMPLEMENTATION

Action	Rationale
3. Assess the breasts:	To establish baseline information regarding the structure of the breasts or to obtain updated data.
a. Pull the curtain around the bed or examination table and/or close the door to the room. Ask the patient to disrobe to the waist and to be seated with hands in the lap.	To maintain patient privacy. Proper position optimizes obtaining the best results.
b. Observe the nipples for color, discharge, and **retraction** (dimpling).	To identify the signs of underlying problems or disease.
c. Observe breast size, symmetry, skin color, vascularity, and skin retraction while asking the patient to press her hands against her hips.	To establish baseline data and bring out dimpling or retraction that might otherwise go unnoticed.
d. Ask the patient to raise her hands above her head, and particularly observe for irregularities in skin texture or dimpling.	To establish baseline data while looking for underlying disease.
e. Have the patient change her position to supine. Place a small pillow under the patient's shoulder on the side you are examining, and have the patient raise that arm over her head.	This position for palpation allows for full exposure of the underarm as well as the main breast area.
f. Starting with the upper outer quadrant and moving systematically in one direction or the other, use the **palmar** aspect of your fingers to palpate each breast in turn. Palpate the breast by gently compressing the breast tissue against the chest wall. The consistency of breast tissue varies among females, primarily according to age: that of younger women is firm and elastic; that of older women is more stringy and nodular. In addition, be aware of the stage of the menstrual cycle of menstruating females because the breasts can be particularly sensitive at the time of menstruation.	To assess for masses or tenderness that may be related to an inflammatory process.
g. Return the patient to a sitting position, and have her dress.	To allow relaxation and privacy while promoting readiness for the teaching session.

(continued)

Action	Rationale
h. Assess the patient's knowledge of BSE and her family history of cancer. Determine whether the patient performs BSE monthly in mid-menstrual cycle (if applicable) and the technique used. Ask whether the patient marks the date of BSE on a calendar. If the patient finds changes, does she report them to her physician or other healthcare provider? Figure 14-11 shows the usual BSE pattern. Teach the patient to	To determine baseline patient knowledge and create a starting point for teaching.

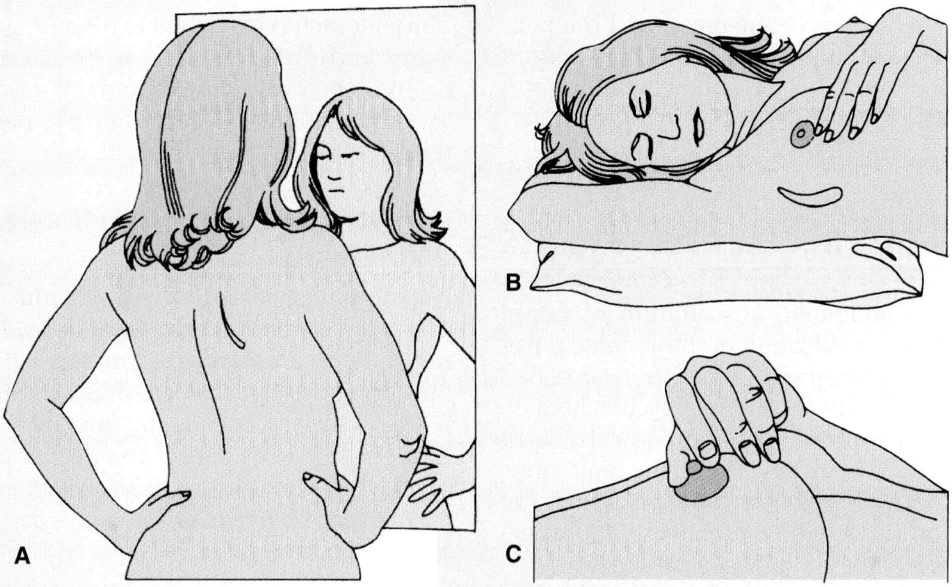

FIGURE 14-11 Examining the breasts. (**A**) Ask the patient to press hands against hips to bring out dimpling or retraction that might otherwise not be noticed. (**B**) Place a small pillow under the patient's shoulder on the side you are examining and have the patient raise that arm over the head. Show the patient how to examine the breast by pressing in a circular or up-and-down or side-to-side manner. (**C**) The patient can complete the examination by squeezing the nipple to detect any abnormal discharge.

(1) Stand in front of a mirror, and observe each breast for **asymmetry,** dimpling, abnormal coloring, or drainage from the nipple.

(2) Lie on a bed with the shoulder raised on a pillow, or stand with the arm raised, and palpate the breast in a consistent circular pattern, and then repeat on the other breast.

(3) Press the nipple area to detect expression of fluid, which may be abnormal.

(continued)

Action	Rationale
i. Use a model to instruct and demonstrate the technique.	Demonstrating proper technique will assist the patient in performing the skill correctly.
j. Have the patient demonstrate the skill in return.	To reinforce learning.
k. Ask questions to assess the patient's learning.	To provide an opportunity to clarify concerns and/or misconceptions.

DOCUMENTATION

4. Document the texture of the breast and the presence or absence of lumps or masses. If any abnormalities were found, document them, and report them immediately.

ABDOMINAL AND RECTAL ASSESSMENTS

Inspection of the abdomen, auscultation of bowel sounds, percussion and palpation of the abdomen, palpation of the liver, assessment for ascites, and digital examination of the rectum are grouped together because aspects of these examinations are commonly considered together. Although all may be done at the same time, they can, of course, be done separately. As indicated, you will use inspection, auscultation, percussion, and palpation when you assess the abdomen and rectum.

Note: Inspect and auscultate the abdomen before carrying out percussion and palpation because percussion and palpation can change the bowel sounds.

BOWEL SOUNDS

Normal bowel sounds, which indicate normal peristaltic activity, are relatively high-pitched and occur every 5 to 15 seconds. They are more frequent immediately before and after eating. The absence of sound or the presence of very soft or infrequent sounds (commonly called hypoactive bowel sounds) indicates decreased motility, as would occur after abdominal surgery or with peritonitis or paralytic ileus. Loud, high-pitched rushing sounds (or hyperactive bowel sounds) indicate increased motility; they occur with gastroenteritis, diarrhea, and laxative use.

VASCULAR SOUNDS

The great arteries in the abdomen are normally characterized by a quiet flow of blood. Bruits are sometimes heard over the aorta, or the renal, iliac, or femoral arteries. They may indicate a narrowed vessel or an aneurysm.

PERCUSSION OF THE ABDOMEN

The abdomen is percussed to disclose patterns of **tympany** and **dullness**—clues to what you can expect to find when palpating. Tympany indicates air in the intestines; dullness occurs when you percuss over a distended bladder, the liver, fluid, or a mass.

PALPATION OF THE ABDOMEN AND LIVER

Palpate the abdomen to evaluate muscle tone and to check for distention and tenderness. If tenderness is noted, assess for **guarding** (muscle rigidity). Guarding may occur because the patient is nervous or ticklish, or it may indicate an acute inflammatory process. Palpation of the liver is part of the overall procedure. Normally, the liver is not palpable. An enlarged nontender liver suggests chronic disease; an enlarged tender liver suggests acute disease.

IDENTIFYING ASCITES

Ascites is a large accumulation of fluid in the peritoneal cavity, which can cause respiratory distress because of the pressure of the fluid on the diaphragm. Ascites can be difficult to identify, especially in an obese person. One way to differentiate between obesity and ascites is to test for a fluid wave indicating fluid in the peritoneal cavity. To do this, place one hand lightly beside the abdomen. With the other hand, tap the other side of the abdomen. If fluid is present, the impact of the tap will be felt by the hand alongside the opposite abdominal wall. Ongoing assessment of ascites usually includes serial measurement of abdominal girth to identify changes that are occurring. You will need a felt-tip marker and a measuring tape to carry out this procedure.

DIGITAL RECTAL EXAMINATION

A digital rectal examination (DRE) is only performed when fecal **impaction** is suspected, based on the patient's complaint of long-term or abnormal constipation, or the leakage of watery stool in the absence of actual bowel movements. This is not a usual part of the physical assessment.

Procedure for Assessing the Abdomen and Rectum

PLANNING

1. Identify individualized patient outcomes of the examination of the abdomen and rectum. **R:** Identifying outcomes facilitates planning and evaluation.

   a. Bowel tones heard in all quadrants
   b. Abdomen soft without masses or presence of fluid
   c. No bruits heard over abdomen
   d. No fecal mass detected in rectum

2. Obtain the appropriate equipment:
   a. stethoscope
   b. tape measure
   c. lubricant (for DRE)
   d. clean gloves (for DRE)
   e. bedpan (for DRE)
   f. database worksheet to record results

IMPLEMENTATION

Action	Rationale
3. Assess the abdomen:	To obtain baseline data or monitor an ongoing area of concern.
a. Pull the curtain and/or close the door to the room. Arrange bed clothing or drape to expose the chest and abdomen. Fanfold the bed linen down to the patient's **symphysis pubis.**	To maintain patient privacy. Proper position optimizes obtaining the best results.
b. Inspect the abdomen, noting scars, rashes, or lesions as well as contour (flat, round, distended); symmetry; and any visible masses or pulsations.	To establish baseline findings while assessing for underlying problems and disease.
c. Auscultate bowel and vascular sounds:	Bowel sounds are often most pronounced (and most easily heard) in the RLQ. Bowel sounds usually occur at 5- to 15-second intervals. Listening for 2 to 5 minutes allows optimum opportunity to hear sounds.
(1) Place the diaphragm of the stethoscope lightly against the skin of the right lower quadrant (RLQ).	
(2) Start in the RLQ, placing the stethoscope systematically to listen to all quadrants. Because bowel sounds are irregular, listen for 4 to 5 minutes before you report absent bowel sounds.	
(3) If you hear no sounds in a quadrant, continue to listen in that quadrant for a minimum of 2 to 5 minutes.	

(continued)

Action	Rationale
d. Continuing to use the diaphragm of the stethoscope, but with firmer pressure, listen over the aorta and the renal, iliac, and femoral arteries for bruits. If you hear any bruits, do not palpate over the area where the abnormal sounds were heard.	This is to enable you to identify abnormal sounds such as bruits, which represent narrowing of the vessels or the possible presence of an aneurysm. Bruits indicate abnormalities of the arteries, and palpation or percussion may cause an aneurysm to rupture.
e. Percuss the abdomen in a systematic fashion, dividing the abdomen into four quadrants. Mentally make a vertical line from the **xiphoid process** to symphysis pubis and a horizontal line across through the **umbilicus.** The four quadrants become right upper quadrant (RUQ), right lower quadrant (RLQ), left upper quadrant (LUQ), and left lower quadrant (LLQ) (Fig. 14-12).	Percussion elicits sounds heard over organs; dullness indicates fluid; tympany indicates air. 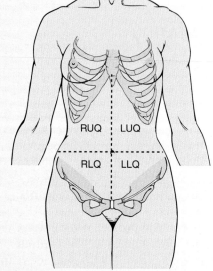 **FIGURE 14-12** The quadrants of the abdomen. The horizontal line extends across through the umbilicus; the vertical line extends downward from the xiphoid process to the symphysis pubis. (RUQ, right upper quadrant; LUQ, left upper quadrant; RLQ, right lower quadrant; LLQ, left lower quadrant.)
f. Palpate the abdomen gently, using the pads of your fingers while moving systematically over each of the quadrants. Assess for tone, swelling, and tenderness. Also assess for **rebound tenderness** (pain elicited when the hand is quickly removed after slow palpation).	Rebound tenderness may suggest underlying masses or peritonitis.
g. Palpate the liver:	
(1) Standing on the right side of the patient, ask the patient to inhale.	

(continued)

Action	Rationale
(2) Place your left hand under the rib cage, and use the palmar surface of the fingers of your right hand to palpate just below the costal margin (Fig. 14-13), as identified by dullness during percussion (Mehta, 2003). Note the number of centimeters the liver descends below that margin.	To outline the borders of the organ and assess for masses. 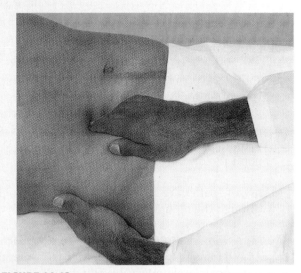 **FIGURE 14-13** To palpate the liver, place your left hand under the rib cage; using the palmar surface of the fingers of your right hand, palpate in and up to feel the liver's edge.
h. Assess for ascites:	
(1) Check for fluid wave. With the patient in a supine position, place the palm of your hand against the lateral abdominal wall. With the opposite hand, gently tap the opposite wall of the abdomen. A fluid wave conducts through the abdomen and can be felt by the opposite hand.	
(2) Check abdominal girth. Identify the area of greatest girth, and using a felt-tip skin marker, place marks at the level of greatest girth on each side of the patient's abdomen. Place the tape measure around the abdomen at the marks, and note the abdominal girth in inches or centimeters.	Girth is the circumference of the body at the level of the abdomen. Marks facilitate consistent measurement. Increasing girth detects the extent of ascites.
4. Perform a digital rectal examination (DRE), if indicated:	
a. Position the patient in a left lateral position with knees bent and drawn up toward the abdomen.	To provide relaxation of the abdomen and expose the anus.

(continued)

Action	Rationale
b. Drape the patient so only the rectal area is exposed.	To preserve the patient's modesty.
c. Put on gloves.	To protect you from contact with feces.
d. Lubricate the gloved index finger.	To prevent injury to the rectal tissue.
e. Spread the patient's buttocks apart with your other hand.	To permit visualizing the anus.
f. Asking the patient to bear down, insert your index finger into the rectum, pointing toward the umbilicus.	Bearing down tends to open the anus.
g. Ask the patient to breathe in and out through the mouth.	To promote relaxation of the bowel.
h. Move the examining finger in a circle. A hard mass that fills the rectum is probably a fecal impaction. You may be able to break it up and remove it with your gloved finger by bending the finger and gently removing small amounts at a time into a bedpan. (An oil-retention enema may be given before attempting to remove a fecal impaction.)	Moving the finger in a circle will allow contact with fecal mass.

DOCUMENTATION

5. Document abdominal assessment: appearance of abdomen, bowel sounds, vascular sounds if heard, any abnormalities detected through percussion or palpation, the position and size of the liver, extent of ascites if present, and results of DRE.

GENITAL ASSESSMENT

Genital examinations include the inspection of external genitalia and the physical examination of the **testes,** penis, and prostate in men and of the vagina and cervix in women. The physical examination of the prostate or of the vagina and cervix is not commonly a responsibility of the RN, although these examinations may be done by advanced practice nurses.

Inspection of the external genitalia is commonly done for patients who have indwelling catheters, those who have had procedures performed on the genital structures or perineum, or for women who are having babies. The examination of the external genitalia in the woman or the testes and penis of the man is not a routine part of the nursing physical assessment for the hospitalized patient who does not have one of the specific indications noted.

The testicular physical examination, which is an external examination, may be done and taught to the patient by nurses working in health promotion settings; therefore, it is presented here. This is of importance because testicular cancer is common in males between the ages of 16 and 35 (Zator-Estes, 2002). While affecting only 1% of all males, it is the number one cancer diagnosis of men in their twenties and thirties. Testicular self-examination (Fig. 14-14) performed monthly can greatly affect outcomes for patients of this cancer, which is curable if caught early.

Procedure for Assessing the Testes

PLANNING

1. Identify individualized patient outcomes of the examination of the testes:
   a. Testes are smooth, firm, and consistent in texture.
2. Obtain clean gloves.

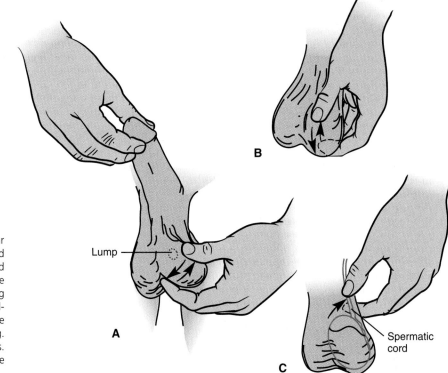

FIGURE 14-14 Teaching testicular examination. (**A**) With the index and middle fingers under the testis and the thumb on top, gently palpate the testicle in a horizontal plane feeling for lumps and abnormalities. (**B**) Palpate upward. (**C**) Locate the cordlike epididymis and continue palpating. Repeat procedure on opposite testis. Report any abnormal findings to the physician.

IMPLEMENTATION

Action	Rationale
3. Pull the curtain, and/or close the door to the room.	To provide for privacy.
4. Inspect external genitalia. Have the patient stand (if able) with genital area exposed.	To establish a baseline, assess maturity, and rule out potential disease or malformation. Proper position optimizes obtaining the best results.
a. Put on gloves.	To protect you from contact with body substances.
b. Drape the patient to expose only the area to be examined.	To respect the patient's modesty.
c. Inspect the area carefully: look at hair distribution, penis, scrotum, urethral meatus, and inguinal area.	
5. Inspect testes.	To establish baseline information regarding testicular tissue and to obtain updated data in response to any patient expressed need.
a. Put on clean gloves.	To protect you from possible contact with body substances.

(continued)

Action	Rationale
b. Observe for swelling on the skin of the scrotum. Observe overall symmetry of the testicles; however, remember that it is normal for one testicle to be slightly larger than the other.	To detect superficial abnormalities.
c. Examine each testicle, gently rolling the testicle between your thumb and fingers.	To assess for size, shape, tenderness, and masses (usually pea-size and painless).
d. Have the patient return to a sitting position; then have him dress.	To allow relaxation and privacy while promoting readiness for the teaching session.
e. Assess the patient's knowledge of testicular self-examination (TSE) and his family history of cancer. Ask whether he examines himself monthly (usually in a warm shower), marks that date on a calendar, and reports any changes to a physician or other health-care provider.	To determine baseline patient knowledge and create a starting point for teaching.
f. Use a model to instruct and demonstrate technique.	Demonstrating proper technique will assist the patient to perform the skill correctly.
g. Have the patient demonstrate the skill in return.	To reinforce learning.
h. Ask questions to assess the patient's learning.	To provide an opportunity to clarify any concerns and/or misconceptions.

DOCUMENTATION

6. Document the size and shape of each testis, and note any tenderness and/or masses. Include the patient's knowledge of testicular self-examination.

COMPREHENSIVE NURSING PHYSICAL ASSESSMENT

After you have made a general survey and have an understanding of the individual assessments presented earlier, the next step is to perform a comprehensive physical assessment. Before beginning, always measure temperature and blood pressure as well as height and weight (if appropriate to the patient's condition); and palpate, count, and describe the pulse. The tools and techniques you will use are the same as when doing an individual assessment. You can do some parts of a nurs-

ing physical assessment while bathing a patient or during other contact. Make sure to observe the patient's response to activities. All information gathered by observation and examination is objective data.

A physical examination is a complex task involving many components. Experience will improve your skill. Still, even at the beginning, you can identify normal and abnormal characteristics in general ways. Later, as you study each system of the body in physiology and learn disease entities and nursing care, you will develop new skills to use in physical examinations. Below is a summary of items by body areas included in a complete nursing physical assessment. Although it is beyond the scope of the beginning student, it exposes you to a comprehensive nursing physical assessment.

You and your instructor can identify which aspects of the assessment are appropriate for you at this point. This format may be the easiest for beginning nursing students. Some nurses prefer a head-to-toe technique somewhat similar to that presented below. Most facilities provide a form outlining the format they prefer for recording the physical assessment findings. When completed, the physical assessment may become a part of, or an addition to, the patient's plan of care. A discussion of all the specific skills needed for a complete physical assessment is beyond the scope of these modules. Many excellent texts on physical examination are available.

The assessment described here may be more comprehensive than that required in your setting, but it is presented to give you an overview of the kind of nursing physical assessment often required of nurses in nursing homes, clinics, and in independent practice.

Procedure for the Comprehensive Head-to-Toe Physical Assessment

ASSESSMENT

1. Review the institution's policies and procedures regarding routine physical assessment. **R:** The hospital's policies and procedures guide the nurse's practice at each institution.
2. Assess the patient's readiness for the procedure. **R:** If the patient is in pain or extremely anxious, this may not be the best time to carry out the procedure.

ANALYSIS

3. Critically think through your data, carefully evaluating each aspect and its relation to other data. **R:** To determine specific problems for this individual in relation to physical assessment.

4. Identify specific problems and modifications of the procedure needed for this individual. **R:** Planning for the individual must take into consideration the individual's problems.

PLANNING

5. Identify individualized patient outcomes of the physical assessment.
   a. Normal findings are desired for all areas. Findings trending toward normal may be appropriate for some individuals.
   b. Note those areas in which problems were previously noted to identify changes. **R:** Identifying outcomes facilitates planning and evaluation.
6. Obtain the appropriate equipment. **R:** This helps to organize the process and to proceed more safely and effectively.
   a. Flashlight to inspect mouth and examine eyes
   b. Tongue depressor to inspect the mouth
   c. Gloves to inspect the genitalia and rectum if genital or rectal exam needed
   d. Lubricant for the rectal examination if needed
   e. Ophthalmoscope to examine the eyes
   f. **Otoscope** to examine the ears
   g. Snellen chart to examine visual acuity
   h. Tuning fork to examine sound perception
   i. Stethoscope for auscultation
   j. Tape measure to measure abdominal girth
   k. Reflex hammer to examine neurological reflexes
   l. Database worksheet to record results

IMPLEMENTATION

	Action	Rationale
	7. Wash or disinfect your hands.	To decrease the transfer of microorganisms that could cause infection.
	8. Identify the patient, using two identifiers.	Verifying the patient's identity helps ensure that you are performing the right skill for the right patient and recording the data in the right record.
	9. Explain the procedure you are about to perform.	Explaining the procedure helps relieve anxiety or misperceptions that the patient may have about a procedure or activity and sets the stage for patient participation.
	10. Raise the bed to an appropriate working position based on your height.	To allow you to use correct body mechanics and protect you from back injury.

(continued)

Action	Rationale
11. Assist the patient to a comfortable position with appropriate draping that can be moved as you examine various body parts.	A comfortable position helps the patient to relax during the procedure. Discomfort has the potential to alter results. Draping keeps the patient from chilling and preserves modesty.
12. Perform an overall inspection of the patient including posture, skin color, alertness, and indications of fatigue or distress.	This information will be used to modify your approach and to identify the need for specific data collection.
13. Examine the arms, hands, and fingers:	
a. Ask the patient to extend both arms out in front of his or her body. Inspect the musculature for asymmetry, and palpate for **turgor.** Move the arms, hands, and fingers to assess range of motion.	
b. Inspect the skin for lesions, spotting, and general color.	
c. Inspect the hands and fingers for color, and palpate for temperature.	
d. Inspect and palpate the joints for nodules and enlargements. Observe the hands for **tremor.** Note any deviation of alignment in the fingers.	
e. Inspect the nails for hardness and general condition, and assess for capillary refill.	
f. Test the grip of each hand.	
14. Examine the head and neck:	
a. Head	
(1) Using your fingers, palpate the cranium for lumps, abrasions, and asymmetry.	
(2) Inspect the condition of the hair. It should be shiny, with distribution appropriate to the age and sex of the person.	
b. Neck	
(1) Palpate the neck for asymmetry, abnormal lymph nodes, and enlarged thyroid.	

(continued)

Action	Rationale
(2) Perform range of motion of the neck to detect any limitations.	
(3) Inspect neck veins for distention.	
(4) Auscultate over the carotid artery to listen for bruits (abnormal sounds resulting from circulatory turbulence).	
c. Face	
(1) Inspect facial skin for moisture, lesions, and ecchymosis (bruising).	
(2) Inspect the face for asymmetry.	
(3) Ask the patient to smile, and then to stick out the tongue. The smile should be generally equal on each side, and the tongue should not deviate to one side.	
(4) Note any **ptosis** (drooping of the eyelids) along with any conditions such as inflammation of the eyelids or periorbital edema.	
d. Eyes	
(1) If inspecting the pupils, do so at this time. Use a flashlight or ophthalmoscope (Fig. 14-15) to observe for pupillary response, size, and movement as described above.	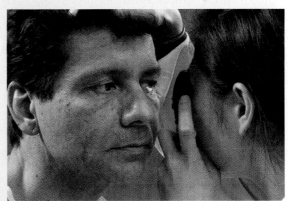 **FIGURE 14-15** Inspecting the eyes. The nurse holds the ophthalmoscope with the finger on the lens selector dial and examines the interior of the eye.
(2) Using the ophthalmoscope, inspect each eye for corneal, lens, or vitreous abnormalities while the patient gazes straight ahead.	

(continued)

Action	Rationale
(3) Assess the optic disc for shape and color.	
(4) Check visual acuity as previously described.	
e. Nose	
(1) With the patient's head tilted slightly back and with a **nasal speculum,** inspect each **nare** (nostril) for color and condition of the mucosa, bleeding, and foreign bodies or masses (Fig. 14-16). *Note:* Some examiners use the light from the ophthalmoscope instead of room light or a flashlight.	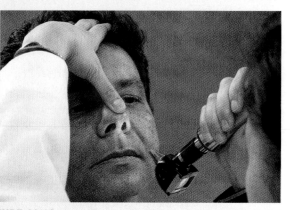 **FIGURE 14-16** The nasal passages can be inspected or treated when dilated with a nasal speculum.
f. Ears	
(1) With the patient's head turned, examine each ear with the otoscope for evidence of excess **cerumen** (earwax), growths, or redness (Fig. 14-17). Assess the eardrum (tympanic membrane) for signs of swelling or color change and for perforations. Palpate the area around the outer ear for tenderness.	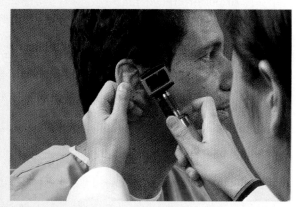 **FIGURE 14-17** The otoscope head is used to inspect the ears.
(2) Assess hearing as previously described.	
(3) Check for hearing aids.	
g. Mouth	
(1) Ask the patient to open his or her mouth, and inspect it with a flashlight and tongue depressor. The	

(continued)

Action	**Rationale**
tongue should be medium red and appear smooth at the margins and rough in the center. When the tongue is lifted, inspect carefully because this area is often the site of cancerous lesions. Examine the back of the throat for swelling, redness, bacterial or viral patches, and the position and size of the **uvula.** Have the patient say "ah," and inspect the tonsils for redness and swelling.	
(2) Inspect the teeth for looseness and **caries** (cavities). Observe the mucosa of the inner mouth for color and lesions. Ask the patient to clench his or her teeth and smile, which helps in assessing bite and facial musculature. Note the color and smoothness of the lips.	
15. Examine the thorax:	
a. Back	
(1) Place the patient in the prone position or in a sitting position in bed with the back facing you. Expose the back, and examine the skin for spots or lesions.	
(2) Note the curvature of the spine, and palpate the vertebral column. Palpate the sacrum for presence of sacral edema.	
Note: Check school-age children for scoliosis (lateral curvature of the spine) by looking for asymmetry of shoulders and hips while observing the standing child from behind and by observing for asymmetry or prominence of the rib cage while watching the child bend over, so the back is parallel to the floor (Fig. 14-18).	

(continued)

Action	*Rationale*

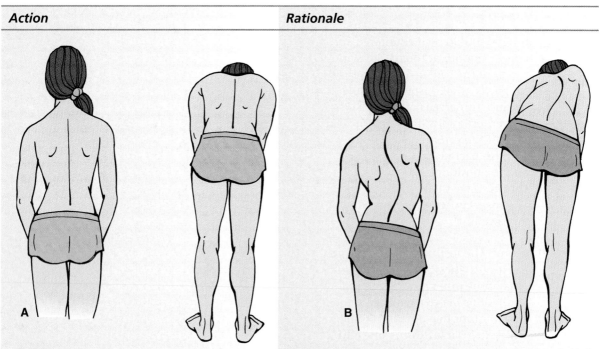

FIGURE 14-18 The nurse assesses the school-age young person for scoliosis by observing the symmetry of the spine from behind and the symmetry of the rib cage as the child bends forward. (**A**) Normally the spine is aligned straight under the head and the shoulders are the same height. (**B**) In scoliosis, the hips are angled at different levels and the spine twists in a serpentine configuration.

(3) With the stethoscope, auscultate all lobes of the lungs, anteriorly and posteriorly. (See the individual procedure for assessment of the lungs.) Ask the patient about and observe for a cough, sputum, and dyspnea on exertion (DOE).

b. Chest

(1) Remove the gown or pajama top from the male patient. Because a female patient may feel modest about exposing her breasts, untie and part her gown for the chest examination. If more exposure is needed, drop the gown to the waist.

(2) With either a male or female patient, observe the levels of the shoulders for equality while the patient is sitting and facing you. Inspect the **pectoralis muscles** of each side of the chest for symmetry as the patient presses his or her palms together and lifts the

(continued)

Action	Rationale
hands over the head. Note any abnormal dimpling, color, or discharge of the nipples.	
(3) Ask the female patient to lie supine. Examine each breast as previously described. A male patient should also have his breasts examined for lumps and masses.	
c. Heart	
(1) With the patient supine, inspect the neck veins for normal filling.	
(2) Auscultate the heart sounds, using the standard pattern as discussed earlier in this module.	
(3) Count the apical heart rate. Replace the gown.	
16. Examine the abdomen:	
a. Keep the patient in the supine position for this assessment.	
(1) Inspect the abdomen for general contour, distention, and asymmetry. Grasp the skin between the fingers to test for turgor.	
(2) Ask the patient about frequency of bowel movements, any recent changes in bowel habits, and when the last bowel movement occurred.	
(3) Auscultate the abdomen in all four quadrants for bowel and vascular sounds as described previously.	
(4) Percuss the abdomen for dullness and tympany as discussed earlier in this module.	
(5) With the patient breathing deeply and with the patient's knees flexed, palpate the abdomen and liver for areas of tenderness. Also palpate for tone, swelling, tenderness, fluid, organs, and masses. As the patient exhales, feel for the position of abdominal structures.	

(continued)

Action	*Rationale*
17. Examine the legs, feet, ankles, and toes:	
a. Legs	
(1) With the patient still in the supine position, palpate each leg for muscle bulk.	
(2) Observe for color, temperature, and skin condition. Skin integrity is particularly important in the feet and lower legs, especially if the patient has diabetes.	
(3) Test the strength of the leg by having the patient press the sole of the foot against your palm.	
b. Feet	
(1) Dorsiflex each foot to check for calf pain, known as **Homans' sign.** The sign is positive when the patient reports pain. A positive Homans' sign is a sign of possible thrombophlebitis.	
(2) Palpate and compare pedal pulses on each foot.	
c. Ankles	
(1) Palpate the ankles with the fingers to assess for edema.	
(2) Note the presence and distribution of hair and the appearance of the skin.	
(3) Inspect the malleoli, the bones on each side of the ankle, for enlargement.	
(4) Rotate the ankle to check for mobility.	
d. Toes	
(1) Inspect the toes for proper alignment. Also check for calluses and bunions.	

(continued)

Action	Rationale
(2) Inspect the nails, which should be without ridges. If thickening is present, it could be a sign of a fungal infection.	
(3) Assess capillary refill bilaterally.	
18. Examine the patient's reflexes (Achilles, Babinski, brachioradial, corneal, quadriceps, and triceps) and skin sensation.	
19. Examine genitalia if appropriate:	
a. Female patients: With the patient in the lithotomy position with knees flexed, drape the patient using a clean sheet or bath blanket. Cover both legs, exposing only the perineum. Provide for adequate light. Put on gloves.	
(1) Observe external genitalia for redness or irritation.	
(2) Part the labia, and observe the catheter insertion site if appropriate.	
(3) Observe for any vaginal drainage.	
b. Male patients: *Note:* This would be done only if a surgery or diagnosis required it or as part of a health promotion visit to teach testicular self-exam. Ask the patient to stand if possible.	
(1) Wearing clean gloves, palpate the inguinal ring to check for herniation.	
(2) Retract the foreskin (if any) of the penis and inspect for irritation, ulceration, and lesions.	
(3) Palpate the testicles to assess for size, position, and masses.	
20. Examine the anal area if indicated by a presenting health problem.	
a. Female patients: Evaluate the anal area for the presence of external hemorrhoids.	

(continued)

Action	Rationale
b. Male patients:	
(1) Inspect the anal area for external hemorrhoids.	
(2) Examine the testes for masses, and teach testicular self-examination as appropriate.	
c. Put on gloves, and use lubricant to examine the rectum (as directed above) if fecal impaction is suspected.	
21. Help the patient back to a position of comfort, and return the patient's bed to the low position after completing the examination.	To maintain patient comfort and safety.
22. Wash or disinfect your hands.	To decrease the transfer of microorganisms that could cause infection.

EVALUATION

23. Compare the results with the patient's previous baseline and to normal. **R:** Comparison helps to determine abnormal findings.

24. Validate abnormal findings immediately and during follow-up assessments, usually at least every shift. **R:** This provides information on rate and direction of change as well as the specific abnormality.

DOCUMENTATION

25. Record from your worksheet to the nursing database form or the computerized database, depending on the practice in your facility. Unusual findings may need to be further recorded in the nurses' narrative notes. **R:** Documentation is a legal record of the patient's assessment and communicates information to other nurses and caregivers.

26. Report any abnormal findings to the appropriate person (instructor, RN, or physician). **R:** Reporting promotes appropriate and timely responses.

■ POTENTIAL ADVERSE OUTCOMES AND RELATED INTERVENTIONS

1. Patient's physical findings are abnormal.
Intervention: Identify contributing factors, and report to the appropriate care provider.

2. Patient's physical findings show distress.
Intervention: Respond immediately to the patient need, intervening with appropriate resources, and inform the physician.

3. Patient is uncooperative or is unable to give information or assist in the process.
Intervention: Utilize secondary sources for information. Consult with the family regarding ways to approach a cognitively impaired person for cooperation. Obtain assistance to complete essential assessment.

ROUTINE SHIFT PHYSICAL ASSESSMENT

At the beginning of a shift in an acute care facility, you will need to do a thorough, but abbreviated, physical assessment on each person for whom you will be providing care. In the long-term care facility, this assessment is done when the resident exhibits indications that a problem may be developing. This assessment includes essential baseline information common to most patients and additionally is focused toward the particular problems or concerns of each person. Each assessment can be individualized by omitting some parts or adding special techniques as necessary.

Procedure for Routine Shift Physical Assessment

ASSESSMENT

1-2. Follow steps 1 and 2 of the Procedure for Comprehensive Head-to-Toe Physical Examination: Review the institution's policy and procedure for assessment, and assess the patient's readiness for the procedure.

ANALYSIS

3-4. Follow steps 3 and 4 of the Procedure for Comprehensive Head-to-Toe Physical Assessment: Think through your data and identify specific problems and modifications.

PLANNING

5. Identify individualized patient outcomes of the examination. **R:** Identifying outcomes facilitates planning and evaluation.

a. Normal findings are desired for all areas. Findings trending toward normal may be appropriate for some individuals.
b. Note those areas in which problems were previously noted to identify changes.
6. Obtain the appropriate equipment for the specific aspects of the examination you will be completing:
a. specific assessment tools for the strategies to be used
b. database worksheet to record results

IMPLEMENTATION

Action	Rationale
7-11. Follow steps 7 through 11 of the Procedure for Comprehensive Head-to-Toe Physical Assessment: Wash or disinfect your hands, identify the patient (two identifiers), explain the procedure, ensure adequate lighting, and position the patient. Meet any immediate needs of the patient before beginning the assessment. Explain what you plan to do.	
12. Carry out the Routine Shift Physical Assessment:	
a. Measure the patient's vital signs: temperature and blood pressure; assess the radial pulses bilaterally; and assess respirations. Compare with most recent assessments recorded and baseline.	
b. Inspect and palpate the hands, noting the skin, nails, capillary refill, joints, and range of motion (ROM). Test grips bilaterally. If there is an intravenous (IV) line present, assess the site. Note any cyanosis.	
c. Inspect the head, face, and eyes. Assess facial skin. Note facial symmetry. Note whether the patient looks at you with both eyes, and assess eye movement. Check sclera and conjunctivae and corneal reflexes as necessary. Check pupils for size as well as response to light and accommodation. Note visual acuity and any visual aids necessary.	
d. Inspect the mouth and lips. Note the color and condition of the skin and mucous membranes. Note the presence or absence and condition of the teeth. Assess the gag reflex as necessary.	

(continued)

Action	Rationale
e. Assess the external ears. Note hearing acuity and use of any hearing aid(s).	
f. Assess neck veins for distention.	
g. Assess breathing and lungs. Observe chest expansion and anteroposterior diameter. Auscultate anterior chest. Note whether the patient is a mouth breather (which may indicate an obstructed nasal passage), and assess for shortness of breath or dyspnea. Note presence and character of cough as well as presence, amount, and character of any sputum produced. If oxygen is in use, note route and rate (liters per minute) of delivery. Note whether an incentive spirometer is in use.	
h. Auscultate the heart sounds, and count the apical pulse. Compare the apical pulse with the radial pulse as well as with the most recent apical rate recorded and baseline.	
i. Auscultate the posterior thorax. Note sacral edema.	
j. Inspect, auscultate, and palpate the abdomen. Ask about any difficulty with urination and when the last bowel movement occurred.	
k. Assess the perineal area as needed. Note presence of urinary catheter, condition of skin, and odor. This may be omitted for the continent, aware patient who has no urinary tract or reproductive tract problems.	
l. Assess the lower extremities. Note condition, color, and temperature of skin, especially of heels, feet, and toes. Assess capillary refill, edema, sensation, pedal pulses, and mobility. Note presence and distribution of hair and appearance of skin. Check for Homans' sign and perform strength testing.	
13. Return the patient to a position of comfort, and return the bed to the low position when completed.	To maintain patient comfort and safety.
14. Wash or disinfect your hands.	To decrease the transfer of microorganisms that could cause infection.

EVALUATION

15. Compare the results to the patient's previous baseline and to normal. **R:** This helps detect abnormal findings.
16. Validate abnormal findings immediately and during follow-up assessments, usually at least every shift. **R:** To provide information on rate and direction of change as well as the specific abnormality.

DOCUMENTATION

17. Record from your worksheet to the hard copy nursing database form or the computerized database, depending on the practice in your facility. Unusual findings may need to be further recorded in the nurses' narrative notes. **R:** Documentation is a legal record of the patient's assessment and communicates information to other nurses and caregivers.
18. Report any abnormal findings to the appropriate person (instructor, RN, or physician). **R:** This ensures an appropriate and timely response.

"MINI" HEAD-TO-TOE PHYSICAL ASSESSMENT

It will also be necessary to do a "mini-assessment" or periodic assessments at times other than the beginning of the shift when you are caring for individuals in acute and long-term care facilities. In some situations, this may be near the middle of the shift, and in others, more frequently as circumstances indicate. These assessments contain only a few essential items.

Procedure for "Mini" Head-to-Toe Physical Assessment

ASSESSMENT

1-2. Follow steps 1 and 2 of the Procedure for Comprehensive Head-to-Toe Physical Assessment: Review the institution's policy and procedure for assessment, and assess the patient's readiness for the procedure.

ANALYSIS

3-4. Follow steps 3 and 4 of the Procedure for Comprehensive Head-to-Toe Physical Assessment: Think through your data, and identify specific problems and the related assessments that must be done.

PLANNING

5. Obtain the appropriate equipment for the specific aspects of the examination you will be completing:
   a. specific assessment tools related to strategies to be used
   b. database worksheet to record results

IMPLEMENTATION

Action	*Rationale*
6-11. Follow steps 6 to 11 of the Procedure for Comprehensive Head-to-Toe Physical Assessment: Wash or disinfect your hands, identify the patient (two identifiers), explain the procedure, ensure adequate lighting, position the patient, and explain what you plan to do.	
12. Carry out the "Mini" Head-to-Toe Physical Assessment:	
a. Measure vital signs as indicated.	
b. Assess upper extremities: Note color and temperature of extremities as well as capillary refill, radial pulses, and grips.	

(continued)

Action	Rationale
c. Assess head: Inspect skin and symmetry of face. Check conjunctivae, external ears, lip color, oral mucous membranes, and jugular vein distention. If the patient has an altered level of consciousness (LOC), check pupil size and response to light and accommodation.	
d. Assess anterior chest: Auscultate heart and lung sounds. Check apical pulse, and compare with radial pulse.	
e. Assess anterior torso: Auscultate bowel sounds in all four quadrants, palpate for tenderness and bladder distension.	
f. Assess posterior chest: Auscultate lung sounds, and check for sacral edema.	
g. Assess lower extremities: Note color and temperature of extremities, capillary refill, pedal pulses, edema, Homans' sign, and strength.	
13. Return the patient to a position of comfort and the bed to the low position when completed.	To maintain patient comfort and safety.
14. Wash or disinfect your hands.	To decrease the transfer of microorganisms that could cause infection.

EVALUATION

15. Compare the results with the patient's previous baseline and to normal. **R:** To help determine abnormal findings.

16. Validate abnormal findings by reassessing. This may be done immediately to ensure accuracy and then during follow-up assessments. **R:** To provide information on rate and direction of change as well as the specific abnormality.

DOCUMENTATION

17. Record from your worksheet to the hard copy nursing database form or the computerized database, depending on the practice in your facility. Unusual findings may need to be further recorded in the nurses' narrative notes. **R:** Documentation is a legal record of the patient's assessment and communicates information to other nurses and caregivers.

18. Report any abnormal findings to the appropriate person (instructor, RN, or physician). **R:** To ensure an appropriate and timely response.

FOCUSED ASSESSMENT

A focused assessment is a brief assessment focusing on a specific concern, need, problem area, or health risk. Nursing care areas with high degrees of specialization and short patient stays utilize this assessment approach. Those areas may include day surgery, emergency department (ED), labor and delivery, cardiac catheterization laboratory, and gastrointestinal procedure department to name a few. In addition, a focused assessment is used for the hospitalized patient for rapid assessment of an emerging problem. For example, if a patient has had neurosurgery, the focused assessment might focus on neurologic signs only (Box 14-8).

box 14-8 *Focused Examination*

Example of patient with abdominal pain arriving in the Emergency Department (ED).

1. Establish reason for coming to the ED to enable the nurse to begin to focus area of questioning.
2. Establish a time line for presenting symptom: where located, when did it start, what the person was doing when symptom started, what makes it worse or better, associated symptoms. This allows the nurse to go from large abdominal area to smaller, more precise area and focus further.
3. Follow guide for individualized abdominal assessment. Individual focused detail specific to one system is being looked at based upon original "focused" complaint.

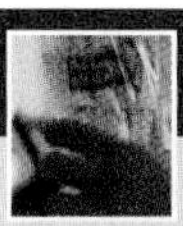

Acute Care

Physical assessment in acute care is an ongoing activity started when the patient arrives and continued until discharge. Patients are hospitalized because they need nursing care, and physical assessment is the mechanism for looking at changes in status and initiating actions in relation to the findings. Each

facility has policies related to assessment times for patients, but the nurse is continually assessing the patient. Each time the nurse provides an intervention for the patient, he or she is going back and reassessing to see what impact the intervention had. The nurse can use the time spent with patients to teach them about the importance of knowing their bodies and of seeking assistance when there is a change.

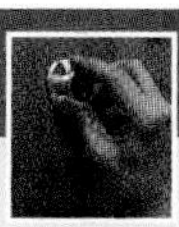

Long-Term Care

Accurate assessment of a resident in a long-term care setting is just as important as it is in the acute care facility. Because the physician generally only visits monthly, the nurse provides the initial assessment for all emerging problems. Unless a thorough assessment is carried out, the resident's problems may either be misinterpreted or undetected. Although most residents in long-term care are elderly, each is a unique individual, and problems cannot be identified without sufficient assessment data.

Some areas should be assessed particularly closely in elderly people (Fig. 14-19). The heart and lungs do

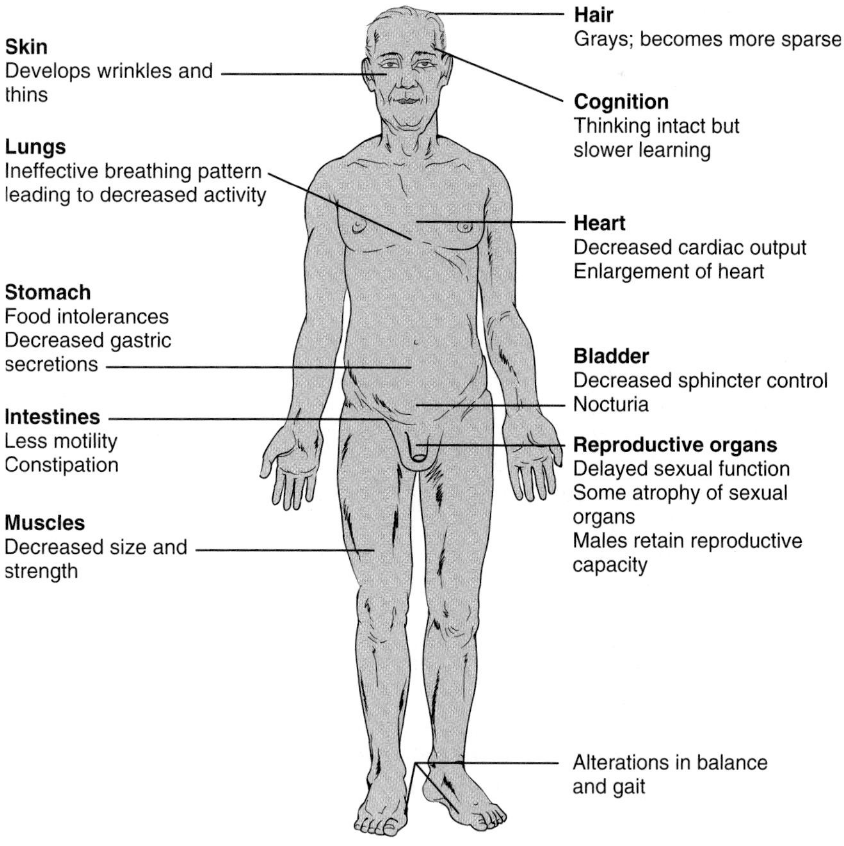

Skin
Develops wrinkles and thins

Lungs
Ineffective breathing pattern leading to decreased activity

Stomach
Food intolerances
Decreased gastric secretions

Intestines
Less motility
Constipation

Muscles
Decreased size and strength

Hair
Grays; becomes more sparse

Cognition
Thinking intact but slower learning

Heart
Decreased cardiac output
Enlargement of heart

Bladder
Decreased sphincter control
Nocturia

Reproductive organs
Delayed sexual function
Some atrophy of sexual organs
Males retain reproductive capacity

Alterations in balance and gait

FIGURE 14-19 Changes in aging that affect assessment in the elderly.

not function as efficiently, resulting in problems with circulation and oxygenation. Mobility may be reduced, and coordination and balance may be impaired. Gastrointestinal disturbances of aging may lead to degrees of food intolerance, urinary incontinence, or constipation. The five senses may not be as acute as they were previously. Cognition and memory function vary with the individual. Certainly, assessment of the environment should not be omitted because safety with this age group is a major concern.

The person entering a long-term care setting is initially assessed for problems and needs using the federally required Minimum Data Set (MDS) form (CMS, 2002). This data set does not contain all the possible assessments needed, but it is designed to provide a common baseline. Individualized assessment should be added as needed. A standard procedure has been established for analyzing the MDS. Certain patterns of information on the MDS are used to identify the need for specific ongoing assessment such as monitoring for possible skin breakdown. The protocols for these specific assessments are called Resident Assessment Protocols (RAPs). The MDS and resulting RAPs must be updated on a regular basis because the resident's condition may change. By doing this, risk factors can be recognized and interventions taken to avoid serious or dangerous situations.

To add to the assessment and gain more complete data, document the perceptions of both the resident and the family. By including the perceptions of the family, you gain insight into problems that may not have been evident on examination. The family also gains a sense of participating in the welfare of the older relative.

Home Care

The nurse in home care must perform a careful and detailed assessment. This represents a baseline to which newer data can be compared as the status of the client changes. The Omaha System is designed for managing data in home care (Omaha System, 2004). Identifying whether the client is home bound is important, because funding for home care often requires that the person be home bound (CMS, 2003). In this setting, the family becomes central in giving information regarding the changing problems and needs of the ill person. It is helpful to use a consistent system for data gathering, which clearly outlines areas where problems exist. These can be updated and deleted, if resolved. Home care does not mean less assessment but a different view toward planning care appropriate to the home.

Ambulatory Care

Depending upon the type of ambulatory care setting, the physical assessment could take on a more focused direction. In ambulatory care areas, clients usually come for a specific procedure that guides the direction of the physical assessment. Background survey data is usually collected related to the problem area, and the physical assessment may be limited or not take place at all. If a procedure that requires anesthesia is completed, the postoperative assessment focuses on vital support systems such as cardiac, respiratory, GI, musculoskeletal, neurologic, and urinary. If the procedure involves simply having an x-ray study, there may be no need for assessment.

The ambulatory care area is an excellent place for focused teaching related to the client's reason for being there. Nurses who work in ambulatory care areas need to possess high-level assessment skills in order to identify problems and act quickly because the client is there only a short time in most instances.

LEARNING TOOLS

DEVELOP YOUR BACKGROUND KNOWLEDGE

1. Review the Learning Outcomes.

2. Read the section on physical assessment in your assigned text.

3. Look up the Key Terms in the glossary.

4. Review this module, and mentally practice the techniques described. Study so that you would be able to teach these skills to another person.

5. Note variations in assessment data for different age groups.

DEVELOP YOUR SKILLS

1. In your home, practice the skills of observation, palpation, and percussion if possible. The more you are able to hear different variations of normal, the easier it will be for you to identify abnormal.
   a. Percussion can be practiced on the thigh, a tabletop, or a hollow container. Listen to the various sounds that are made. Try to distinguish between them based on the whether the object is hollow or dense.
   b. If you have your own stethoscope, you can practice auscultation at home. You may have a family member or friend who will allow you to practice this skill. Although you cannot be as accurate,

you can practice listening to your own heart and lungs and bowels for further experience.

   c. Practice any of the other skills at home that are possible. You can check reflexes on family members, examine their pupils, and practice other assessment to gain experience.

2. In the practice setting

   a. Use simulation equipment that is available. Some skills labs may have simulation equipment to allow listening to various heart sounds, lung sounds, bowel tones, and the like. If these are available, be sure to use all of them to increase your skill level.

   b. Select two other students, and form a group of three, alternating so that each has the opportunity to play the role of the patient. Perform each of the following procedures related to physical assessment techniques. Use the Performance Checklists on the CD-ROM in the front of this book to check yourself. The one who is not participating at a given time can observe and evaluate the performances of the examiner. The "patient" can reflect on the skill with which the "nurse" performs, what is comfortable, and what is not. Specific assessment strategies include

- neurologic assessment
- heart assessment
- peripheral circulatory assessment
- lungs and respiratory assessment
- breast assessment
- genital assessment (perform on mannequin only)
- abdominal and rectal assessment (perform rectal exam on mannequin only)
- comprehensive head-to-toe physical assessment
- routine shift physical assessment
- "mini" head-to-toe physical assessment

   c. Your instructor may have scenarios for you to decide what should be included for a focused assessment for a particular patient situation. These will help you to develop decision-making skills.

DEMONSTRATE YOUR SKILLS

In the clinical setting

1. Consult with your instructor regarding the opportunity to use physical assessment skills.

2. Consult with your instructor regarding the opportunity for evaluation of your performance while doing a physical assessment.

CRITICAL THINKING EXERCISES

1. Tomorrow, you are assigned to care for an 80-year-old male patient in the nursing home who has quite an extensive medical history. In addition to routine care, this patient receives multiple oral medications daily, has a leg ulcer that requires wound care with a dressing change daily, and will need his urinary drainage bag changed. You have an hour at clinical prep this afternoon to collect data that will help you function efficiently tomorrow. Identify your sources of information. Describe the approach will you take to gather the information you need. Identify further activities you will engage in when you leave the nursing home to help you prepare for tomorrow. Share your work with another student in your clinical group, and critique each other's work.

2. You are caring for an 84-year-old woman in the nursing home. You heard in report that at 6:00 a.m., she had a temperature of 100.2°F, a pulse rate of 96 (irregularly irregular), and a respiration rate of 28 and shallow. You know she is scheduled for a chest x-ray at 8:00 a.m.; it is now 7:50 a.m. Determine which areas of assessment are the most important for you to complete before she leaves to have the x-ray study. Give rationale for your choices.

SELF-QUIZ
SHORT-ANSWER QUESTIONS

1. List five elements that should be included in inspection.

   a. _____

   b. _____

   c. _____

   d. _____

   e. _____

2. List three elements that the nurse should include in the explanation to the patient prior to palpation.

   a. _____

   b. _____

   c. _____

3. Before testing the pupillary reaction to light and accommodation, for what three things should the nurse inspect the pupils?

   a. _____

   b. _____

   c. _____

4. In what position are the jugular veins normally collapsed?

_____

5. Why should the nurse be aware of the patient's stage in the menstrual cycle when palpating the breasts of a female?

_____

6. When examining the abdomen, why should auscultation be done before percussion and palpation?

_____

7. Name one situation in which breath sounds might be louder or increased.

_____

8. Name one situation in which breath sounds might be absent or decreased.

_____

9. What is one way to differentiate between a pleural friction rub and a pericardial friction rub?

_____

10. In what area is the first heart sound usually most easily heard?

_____

11. Data are gathered from what sources?

    a. _____

    b. _____

    c. _____

    d. _____

MULTIPLE CHOICE

_____ 12. Of the basic physical assessment techniques listed, which one would the nurse do first?
   a. Percussion
   b. Auscultation
   c. Palpation
   d. Inspection

_____ 13. Which of the following statements is reflective of subjective data?
   a. The patient complains of feeling nauseated.
   b. The patient just vomited.
   c. After ambulating, the patient's heart rate is 92.
   d. The lab report indicates the patient has a hemoglobin level of 8.

_____ 14. Which term describes an essential element of inspection?
   a. Temperature
   b. Size
   c. Masses
   d. Softness

_____ 15. During percussion, the dullness sound represents
   a. a high-pitched normal sound heard over lung tissue.
   b. a short low-pitched sound heard over solid organs.
   c. a short high-pitched sound heard over solid organs.
   d. a high-pitched sound heard over fluid.

Answers to the Self-Quiz questions appear in the back of this book.

Collecting Specimens and Performing Common Laboratory Tests

SKILLS INCLUDED IN THIS MODULE

General Procedure for Collecting Specimens for Testing
Specific Procedures for Collecting Urine Specimens
   Measuring Urine Specific Gravity With a Urinometer
   Measuring Specific Gravity With a Urine Refractometer
   Testing Urine for Glucose
   Testing Urine for Ketone Bodies (Acetone)
   Testing Urine for Occult Blood
   Testing Using a Reagent Strip
Specific Procedure For Measuring Blood Glucose Levels
Procedure for Testing Feces for Occult Blood
Procedure for Obtaining a Specimen for Culture

PREREQUISITE MODULES

Module 1	An Approach to Nursing Skills
Module 2	Documentation
Module 4	Basic Infection Control
Module 24	Basic Sterile Technique: Sterile Field and Sterile Gloves
Module 27	Assisting the Patient Who Requires Urinary Catheterization
Module 29	Inserting and Maintaining a Nasogastric Tube

KEY TERMS

acetone	ketone bodies
acid	lancet
alkaline	meniscus
culture and	occult
sensitivity (C&S)	ova
displacement	parasites
exudate	pH
feces	reagent
gastric secretions	specific gravity
glucose	urine refractometer
guaiac	urinometer
hematuria	

OVERALL OBJECTIVES

▸ To correctly obtain and properly care for specimens collected.
▸ To accurately perform common laboratory tests.

LEARNING OUTCOMES

The student will be able to

1. Assess the patient's understanding of the purpose of the test(s) and his or her ability to carry out the correct procedure to obtain specimens.
2. Analyze assessment data to determine the need for further information about specimen collection.
3. Determine appropriate patient outcomes related to collecting specimens and performing common laboratory tests, and recognize the potential for adverse outcomes.
4. Provide information about the purpose of the test(s) and the correct procedure to the patient.
5. Accurately perform the laboratory test(s), using appropriate equipment.
6. Properly handle the specimens collected.
7. Evaluate the patient's response to the procedure.
8. Document the type of specimen collected, the laboratory test performed, the results of the laboratory test(s) and corresponding intervention(s), and the patient's response to the procedure in the patient's record and on the nursing care plan as appropriate.

Specimens obtained by the nurse, or with the assistance of the nurse, may be the key to the diagnosis and treatment of the patient. To perform the task competently, the nurse must know the rationale for the test(s) involved, necessary teaching and preparation of the patient, correct methods of obtaining and handling specimens, and how to care for patients after the test. Laboratory tests are an important part of establishing a diagnosis. In addition, test results indicate a patient's progress and can be the basis for planning or altering therapy and nursing care.

Modern technology has made many laboratory tests easy to perform, and many are commonly performed at the point of care (POC) on the nursing unit, making the results immediately available. Personnel need to be competent to perform the tests to produce accurate results. This presents an additional challenge to the nurse, who must know the purpose of the tests and the procedures to be followed. Most facilities have policies that require personnel who perform laboratory tests to demonstrate competency in POC testing, in accordance with accreditation standards.

On the nursing unit, equipment for performing tests is usually kept in a central location. Patients who need a specific test done frequently may have individual equipment in their room or bathroom. The equipment needed for cultures is usually kept with other sterile supplies.

The nurse is often responsible for supervising the unit secretary or clerk who orders the specific supplies and should know how those are obtained. Reagent tablets and strips usually come from the pharmacy and may be ordered for the individual patient. Glass urinometers, culture tubes, and swabs are typically ordered from the central supply department.

Tablets and strips have expiration dates, which should be checked carefully. Because exposure of tablets and strips to light or moisture may cause deterioration, many are stored in special containers, such as brown glass bottles and boxes. Be sure to keep containers used for these items tightly capped or closed. To prevent errors, keep all directions, packet inserts, and color charts with the appropriate products. Some **reagent** strips for testing urine have multiple areas on a single strip that can be used to measure a variety of components (Table 15-1).

In addition to performing many laboratory tests yourself, you will also need to teach patients and their families or caregivers how to carry out some tests at home. Diabetic patients, for example, test their blood or urine frequently for **glucose** content and **ketone bodies.**

When collecting specimens, wear clean gloves to protect yourself from contact with body fluids, which can transmit microorganisms. To protect laboratory personnel from exposure to microorganisms, clearly label specimen containers on the jar or tube (not on the lid), tightly seal the container, and place it in a biohazard bag if it is being sent to a laboratory. Some facilities double-bag all specimens for extra protection. Specimens to be tested in the laboratory should be sent promptly to ensure that time and temperature change do not alter the contents.

If you will be doing the testing, keep the specimen in the appropriate area, such as the utility room. If the test must be done in the patient's room, place a paper towel on the working surface to prevent potential contamination. Refer to the specific procedures for further information for collecting specimens.

Any materials collected that are not needed must be disposed of appropriately. Stool and urine are discarded in the toilet. Objects used for collecting specimens

table 15-1. Products Used for Testing Body Substances		
Reagent	**Type**	**Measure or Tests**
Tests for Occult Blood Used on Feces, Gastric Contents, or Urine		
Hemastix	Strip	Occult blood
Hematest	Tablet	Occult blood
Hemoccult	Folder	Occult blood
Tests for Blood Glucose Used on Blood Obtained Through a Finger Stick		
Chemstrip bG	Strip	Blood glucose
Dextrostix	Strip	Blood glucose
Glucostix	Strip	Blood glucose
Tests for Urine Used on Freshly Voided Urine		
Acetest	Tablet	Ketones
Albustix	Strip	Albumin
Bili-Labstix	Strip	Bilirubin
Clinistix	Strip	Glucose
Clinitest	Tablet	All reducing substances, especially sugars
Diastix	Strip	Glucose
Hemastix	Strip	Blood
Ketostix	Strip	Ketones
Multistix	Strip	Produced in several configurations with 10 possibly different: glucose, bilirubin, ketones, specific gravity, blood, pH, protein, urobilinogen, nitrite, leukocytes
Phenistix	Strip	Phenylketones

(such as tongue depressors or swabs) and contaminated specimen containers are discarded in the biohazard waste container.

NURSING DIAGNOSES

Patients undergoing laboratory testing may have a variety of nursing diagnoses related to the actual test, why it is being done, and restrictions before and after the procedure. Examples are

- Anxiety: related to lack of knowledge about test, fear of unwelcome diagnosis and treatment, or perceived necessary changes in lifestyle
- Deficient Knowledge: related to unfamiliar procedure

DELEGATION

The collection of some specimens can be delegated to assistive personnel. They may collect stool and urine specimens as well as sputum specimens. Specimens that require piercing the skin (such as testing for blood glucose) or sterile technique (such as a swab of an open wound) usually are not delegated to assistive personnel.

COLLECTING SPECIMENS FOR TESTING

URINE SPECIMENS

Most urine specimens needed for routine analysis are obtained by having the patient void into a container after cleaning the perineum. These specimens are considered clean, not sterile; however, they are used for urine cultures. See Table 15-2 for directions for obtaining a "clean-catch" urine specimen.

Tests can identify specific abnormal components of the urine and abnormally large amounts of bacteria. Patients are infrequently catheterized for the sole purpose of obtaining urine specimens because of the risk of introducing microorganisms into the normally sterile urinary tract. If the patient already has an indwelling catheter in place, obtain a sterile specimen by clamping the catheter briefly and using a sterile syringe to extract a small amount of urine through the port designed for that purpose (Fig. 15-1). Most indwelling catheters now have a needleless entry port to which a syringe can be attached for obtaining a specimen. Older style catheters have a port that requires a needle for access. Refer to Table 15-2 for how to obtain a urine sample when a catheter is in place.

If a 24-hour specimen is ordered, it is timed to begin in the morning, according to facility policy. Before you begin the timing, the patient should first void and discard this urine because it is urine that has been in the bladder for some time. Then, all urine voided during the next 24 hours is collected in the type of container used in the facility and refrigerated. Some tests require the addition of a preservative to the container. If a preservative is used, it may be a toxic substance and should be treated with care. At the end of the 24-hour period, the patient voids a last specimen, which is added to the rest. The staff and the patient should know that a 24-hour specimen is being collected. A sign posted in the patient's bathroom is useful as a reminder. If the patient has a catheter, the urine is simply collected in one container for 24 hours.

If a voiding is inadvertently discarded, most laboratories can calculate an approximate value for the test based on the specimen that was obtained. However, this lessens accuracy and should be avoided. When a very precise measurement is needed, the test may need to be repeated if a specimen is discarded.

BLOOD SPECIMENS

Simple glucose testing may be performed using a drop of blood obtained through a finger stick on an adult or a heel stick on an infant. Most routine blood specimens are obtained by the hospital laboratory technician or a certified healthcare provider. Venous blood is drawn for most tests, but arterial blood is drawn for blood gas measurement. See Table 15-2 for information on the nurse's role in obtaining routine blood samples.

table 15-2. Quick Reference for Collecting Specimens

Specimen	Preparing the Patient	Positioning the Patient	Role of the Nurse	Special Observations Concerning the Patient	Handling the Specimen

Urine
a. Voided—
"clean catch"
	Instruct how to obtain clean voided specimen.	Up to bathroom or commode or use bedpan or urinal	Obtain specimen.
			Clean voided specimen:
			1. Male
			  a. Clean penis thoroughly with soap and water if needed.
			  b. Cleanse meatus with antiseptic swab, moving from center to outside.
			  c. Begin urine stream and then void 30–60 mL of urine into container.
			  d. Do not allow container to touch body.
			2. Female
			  a. Spread labia apart with nondominant hand.
			  b. Cleanse with antiseptic swab, moving from front to back.
			  c. Begin urine stream and then void 30–60 mL of urine into container.
			  d. Do not allow container to touch body.
				Patient may be embarrassed. Provide privacy and be reassuring.	Specimen is clean. Done for routine urinalysis, and to check for presence of cells for **culture and sensitivity (C&S).** If not sent immediately to laboratory, refrigerate.

b. Catheter in place	Inform patient of procedure.	Supine, with top linen draped back to expose catheter	To remove urine from indwelling catheter: 1. Obtain sterile 5-mL syringe with needleless tip and alcohol swab. 2. Wipe entry port on tubing thoroughly with alcohol swab. 3. Insert needleless tip into port and withdraw urine. If there is no urine in the catheter, clamp it off for 15–20 min before trying to obtain sample. 4. Remove syringe from catheter, and unclamp catheter if it was clamped. 5. Expel urine from syringe into sterile container. 6. Dispose of equipment safely in room receptacle.	Be sure patient is not exposed.	Specimen is sterile. Often done for C&S.
c. Catheter to be inserted	Explain procedure.	See Module 27.	See Module 27 if urine from an indwelling catheter is needed.	See Module 27.	Specimen is sterile. May be done for C&S.
Blood	Instruct as to what to expect and fasting directions if appropriate.		Depending on setting, prepare patient and assist physician or laboratory technician, or prepare patient only.	Apply pressure to puncture site to stop bleeding. If blood is obtained from an artery, apply pressure for 5 min following procedure.	Procedure is sterile. For serology or chemical analysis, or if not immediately examined, refrigerate; for culture, incubate; for other tests, leave at room temperature.

(continued)

table 15-2. Quick Reference for Collecting Specimens (Continued)

Specimen	Preparing the Patient	Positioning the Patient	Role of the Nurse	Special Observations Concerning the Patient	Handling the Specimen
Stool	Provide commode or bedpan. May use paper placed in toilet.		Obtain specimen. Transfer from commode or bedpan to specimen container with tongue blade.	Patient may be embarrassed. Be reassuring, and provide privacy.	Small amount usually adequate. If tests are for ova, parasites, or amoeba, send to laboratory immediately (while it is warm).
Sputum	Explain why specimen is needed, and show container in which to expectorate.	Usually patient will be sitting up; splinting may help. Postural drainage can be used (see Module 32).	Obtain specimen, or assist respiratory therapist to obtain specimen. 1. Remind patient that saliva is not sputum, that sputum is coughed up from lungs. 2. Remind patient not to use mouthwash or toothpaste before sputum collection because they may alter the specimen.	Nausea may occur. Mouth care is indicated after a large amount of sputum is coughed up.	Specimen is clean for cytology; sterile for C&S. Best collected in morning. Send to laboratory as soon as possible.
Gastric secretions	Explain why specimen is needed, and tell patient how you plan to obtain it.	Patient with nasogastric (NG) tube will usually be in mid- to high-Fowler's position.	Obtain specimen. 1. Turn off suction machine. 2. Disconnect distal portion of NG tube from adapter of suction tube. 3. Attach syringe with adapter to NG tube. 4. Gently withdraw secretions for specimen. 5. Turn on suction. 6. Reconnect tubes.	After obtaining specimen, check to be sure that suction is operating and secretions are draining.	Specimen is clean. Tests for blood and pH may be done on unit. Send to laboratory for other ordered tests.

If a patient has a central venous catheter in place, check the facility policy regarding drawing blood from the catheter. This is often a nursing responsibility. In some settings, the nurse must be certified by the facility to perform this function. For the procedure on how to draw blood from a central venous catheter, see Module 49.

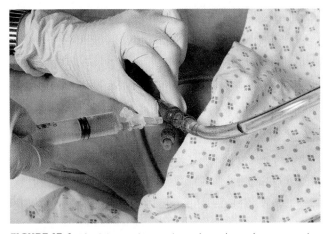

FIGURE 15-1 Obtaining a urine specimen through a catheter port using a syringe. This shows a safety needle used for an older-style catheter.

Arterial blood samples are commonly drawn by a laboratory technician or a respiratory therapy technician. In some settings, such as critical care and long-term care, nurses draw these samples. The facility may certify nurses for this skill.

Procedures for drawing blood vary, but color-coded tubes are used to indicate the type of preservative or anticoagulant that is in the tube. Using the correct tube is essential for accurate test results.

STOOL SPECIMENS

A single stool, or **feces,** specimen may be ordered, or occasionally the physician may want specimens obtained from three subsequent and different defecations. Usually, only a small amount of stool needs to be collected from a bedpan or bedside commode. The collection tool may be a tongue depressor, which is then used to apply the stool to a disposable envelope type of container or to put the stool in a specimen container (see Table 15-2).

Stool can be tested for blood, pus, **ova,** and **parasites.** More stool material is needed for ova and parasite determination than for other tests. The specimen for ova and parasite testing should go to the laboratory before it cools, because cooled organisms are less detectable. A simple test to detect occult (hidden) blood in stool may be done with only a smear of feces on a filter paper or special folder designed for this purpose. A liquid reagent "developer" is added to the smear to determine whether occult blood is present. This is sometimes referred to as a **guaiac** test, although the reagent guaiac is no longer in common use.

SPUTUM SPECIMENS

The examination of sputum is important in diagnosing a variety of conditions. Sputum arises from the tissue of the respiratory tract and should not be confused with saliva, which is excreted by the salivary and mucous glands in the mouth. Collecting a sputum specimen includes teaching the patient the difference between the two.

Because secretions tend to accumulate during the night, the best time to obtain a sputum specimen is first thing in the morning. The amount needed varies with the type of test to be done. Before collection, tell the patient to take several very deep breaths and then cough forcefully. Sputum should be coughed directly into the specimen container to decrease the chance of contaminating the specimen (see Table 15-2).

When the patient cannot raise sputum, the respiratory therapist may use a mist treatment to induce sputum production. In some instances, suctioning may be needed to obtain a sputum specimen (see Module 33).

If the patient is suspected of having tuberculosis and is having a test for acid-fast bacillus, any healthcare provider working with the patient to obtain a specimen must wear a special high-efficiency particulate air filter mask for personal protection from the organism (see Module 23). Collect the specimen in a sterile container, remove the container promptly, and send it to the laboratory. The sight of a container of sputum can be offensive to the patient, visitors, and staff.

GASTRIC SECRETIONS

When a patient has a nasogastric (NG) tube in place, a specimen of **gastric secretions** may be obtained to assess the **pH** (the **acid** or **alkaline** status) and presence or absence of blood or other components. First, the suction should be interrupted. This is done by turning off the suction machine and then, with gloved hands, disconnecting the distal end of the NG tube from the adapter of the suction tube. Using a catheter-tip syringe or a large, regular syringe with an adapter, gently aspirate the amount of gastric secretions needed for testing. Reinstate the suction by reconnecting the tubing and turning the suction back on. If a patient has a copious amount of drainage, a syringe may not be necessary. In this case, simply turn off the suction, disconnect the

tubing, and place the end of the NG tube into a small container. Usually, only a short time is needed to collect the specimen (see Table 15-2).

GENERAL PROCEDURE FOR COLLECTING AND TESTING SPECIMENS

The instructions in the general procedure that follow include the fundamental nursing actions needed to appropriately obtain specimens for testing. The specific procedures that follow the general procedure call for the nurse to use many steps of the general procedure and to vary others. The steps of the general procedure are numbered sequentially. They are grouped according to the steps of the nursing process.

An important aspect of the nurse's role in collecting any specimen involves handling and labeling specimens correctly. For example, the nurse must know which specimens must be placed in a biohazard bag according to the facility policy, whether the specimen should be kept warm or refrigerated, or whether it should be taken immediately to the laboratory or handled in some other special way. In addition, labeling must be complete and accurate. The following information is often included on the specimen container: patient's name, identification number, age, location, and physician's name.

In most cases, a laboratory requisition accompanies the specimen and must also be completely and accurately filled out. In many instances, the requisition is computer generated. Whatever the form, the information must be correct. The patient's identifying information, diagnosis, and the date and time of specimen collection are often included (Fig. 15-2).

ASSESSMENT

1. Determine which tests are to be performed for the patient and the type of specimen required. **R:** Some tests are done only with a physician's order. Others can be done either with a physician's order or when the nurse determines they are needed.
2. Assess the patient to determine the patient's ability to carry out the procedure independently or cooperate during the procedure. **R:** In many cases, the patient can obtain the specimen, such as a urine specimen, independently. If the patient is unable to collect the specimen, the nurse must provide assistance as needed.

ANALYSIS

3. Critically think through your data, carefully evaluating each aspect and its relation to other data. **R:** This enables you to determine specific problems for this individual in relation to the procedure.

Larkin, James   M-47

000-00-0000

Dr. Harrison

ROUTINE BLOOD CHEMISTRY 1

CODE	TEST	NORMALS	RESULTS	CODE		NORMALS	RESULTS
320	AMMONIA			380	CK		
322	AMYLASE			430	LD		
334	BILIRUBIN, T			541	GOT (AST)		
	BILIRUBIN, D			542	GPT (ALT)		
335	MICROBILI, TOTAL ONLY			440	LIPASE		
	MICROBILIRUBIN			245	**PRE ANESTHESIA SURVEY**		
1325	TOTAL			225	ELECTROLYTES		
	DIRECT				SODIUM		
544	BUN (UREA NITROGEN)				POTASSIUM		
410	GLUCOSE FASTING				CHLORIDE		
419	GLUCOSE 2 HR PC				TOTAL CO_2		
1414	GLUCOSE 1 HR PC			377	CREATININE		
233	GLUCOSE RANDOM			494	POTASSIUM		
				313	(PROTEIN TOTAL)		
				301	ALBUMIN		
				496	GLOBULIN		
				496	A/G RATIO		

LABORATORY OF PATHOLOGY
HOSPITAL MEDICAL CENTER.

☐ INFECTIOUS CASE   ☐ LINE DRAW

850
855
866

COLLECT SPECIMEN			
2100 TIME		TIME DRAWN	
7-14-06 DATE			
EN / 35			
NURSE INITIAL & STATION	TECH.	DATE	

NOTE: FOR GROUP CHEMISTRY TESTS SUCH AS:
LIVER PROFILE, PROTEIN ELECTROPHROEIS,
ETC. USE GROUP CHEMISTRY REQUEST FORM.

COMMENTS: *Stat.*

CIRCLE CODE NUMBERS FOR TESTS DESIRED

FIGURE 15-2 Example of a laboratory requisition form. This one is for ordering a routine blood chemistry. Specific test order is circled.

4. Identify specific problems and modifications of the procedure needed for this individual. **R:** Planning for the individual must take into consideration the individual's problems.

PLANNING

5. Determine individualized patient outcomes for collecting and testing the desired specimen including the following. **R:** Identification of outcomes guides planning and evaluation.
   a. Specimen is collected correctly to maximize accuracy of testing.
   b. For specimen to be tested in the laboratory:
      (1) Requisition is completed correctly.
      (2) Specimen is packaged to protect healthcare workers and to support accurate testing.
      (3) Specimen is sent to laboratory in a timely manner.
   c. For specimen to be tested at the point of care: Testing meets standards for accuracy upon which to base patient treatment.
   d. Results of test are within normal limits for this test, indicate progress toward the normal range when compared with previous results, or are within appropriate limits for the individual patient.
6. Review the procedure to determine the equipment needed to collect the specimen and carry out the test when indicated. (See Table 15-2 for a quick reference guide to various tests.) **R:** Planning ahead allows you to proceed more safely and effectively.

IMPLEMENTATION

Action	Rationale
7. Wash or disinfect your hands.	To decrease the transfer of microorganisms that could cause infection.
8. Identify the patient, using two identifiers.	Verifying the patient's identity helps ensure that you are performing the right test for the right patient.
9. Explain the procedure you are about to perform.	Explaining the procedure helps relieve anxiety or misperceptions that the patient may have about a procedure or activity and facilitates patient participation.

(continued)

Action	Rationale
10. Prepare the environment. Depending on the procedure, provide for privacy, adjust the lighting, and assist in positioning and draping as appropriate.	The patient has a right to privacy, and an efficient working environment promotes accuracy.
11. Collect the specimen. Verify that you obtain the right amount of specimen in the right container at the right time from the right patient. Be careful not to get any of the specimen material on the outside of the container.	Accurate test results depend on correct handling of the specimen. If specimens are obtained incorrectly or placed in the wrong container, collection must be repeated and will delay the test results, which may cause the patient undue anxiety and delay therapy.
12. Send the specimen to the laboratory, or perform the test as described in the specific procedures.	Specific procedures for testing are essential to assure accuracy of results.
13. Assess the patient throughout the procedure, and offer reassurance as needed.	Make observations of the patient that are appropriate to the procedure (see column "Special Observations Concerning the Patient" in Table 15-2).
14. Conclude the procedure: This may include repositioning and/or changing or straightening the bedding, depending on the procedure you have performed.	To promote patient comfort.
15. Properly dispose of gloves and specimens that are no longer needed. Place needles in the "sharps" container and contaminated items in the biohazard receptacle. Take care of the equipment, depending on the type of equipment used and the policies of your facility.	To reduce the likelihood of penetrating injuries and contact with contaminated substances.
16. Wash or disinfect your hands.	To decrease the transfer of microorganisms that could cause infection.
17. Record on paper the result of any test you have performed; or label the specimen correctly, and send it to the laboratory for testing; or store it appropriately.	To ensure accuracy when you enter the result in the patient record. Sometimes, nurses attempt to remember test results in an effort to save time, only to have to repeat the procedures later when the recall is not accurate. It is most efficient to record numbers when you first obtain them. Correct labeling and handling are critical to accurate test results.

EVALUATION

18. Evaluate using the desired patient outcomes previously identified. **R:** Evaluation in relation to the desired outcomes is essential for planning future care needs.
   a. Specimen is collected correctly to maximize accuracy of testing.
   b. For specimen to be tested in the laboratory:

(1) Requisition is completed correctly.
(2) Specimen is packaged to protect healthcare workers and to support accurate testing.
(3) Specimen is sent in a timely manner.
   c. For specimen to be tested at the point of care: Testing meets standards for accuracy upon which to base patient treatment.
   d. Results of test are within normal limits for this test, indicate progress toward the normal range

when compared with previous results, or are within appropriate limits for the individual patient.

DOCUMENTATION

19. Document data on the appropriate flowsheet or other patient record according to your facility's policy. **R:** Documentation is a legal record of the patient's care and therapy and communicates nursing activities to other nurses and caregivers.
    a. Procedure completed
    b. Results of any test you performed
    c. Amount, description, and disposition of the specimen obtained
20. Report abnormalities as directed in each specific procedure. **R:** Whether a test result is reported depends on the reason for the test and the patient's medical status.

SPECIFIC PROCEDURES FOR COLLECTING AND TESTING URINE SPECIMENS

Measuring Urine Specific Gravity with a Urinometer

Specific gravity is a measurement of the concentration of urine. Overhydration, or any disease that affects the body's ability to concentrate particles in the urine, leads to a low specific-gravity value. Conversely, dehydration, or any condition that increases water reabsorption in the kidney, results in a high specific-gravity value. The numbers used to delineate the normal range vary slightly, depending on the facility in which you practice or the text that you consult. Generally, the normal specific-gravity range for urine is approximately 1.010 to 1.025 g/mL.

Specific gravity can be measured using a **urinometer,** a **urine refractometer,** or a urine reagent strip. The urinometer uses a **displacement** principle, while the refractometer uses light refraction. The urinometer is more commonly used than is the refractometer. This equipment is often available for use on hospital units, especially critical care, pediatrics, nurseries, and units for those with kidney disease, where specific-gravity measurement may be done on a routine basis.

ASSESSMENT

1-2. Follow steps 1 and 2 of the General Procedure: Confirm the test to be performed, and assess the patient's ability to collect the urine specimen.

ANALYSIS

3-4. Follow steps 3 and 4 of the General Procedure: Critically think through your data, and identify specific problems and modifications.

PLANNING

5. Determine individualized patient outcomes in relation to measuring the specific gravity of the urine. **R:** Identification of outcome guides planning and evaluation.
   a. Specimen is collected correctly to maximize accuracy of testing. Urine collected for specific gravity should be fresh urine that has not had an opportunity for evaporation to change the concentration of solutes.
   b. Testing meets standards for accuracy upon which to base patient treatment.
   c. Results of test are within normal limits, indicate progress toward the normal range when compared with previous results, or are within appropriate limits for the individual patient. **R:** Normal limits for urine specific gravity are 1.010 to 1.025 g/mL.
6. Obtain a urinometer, a urine container, and clean gloves. **R:** The urinometer measures the concentration of the urine by the simple principle of displacement. The particles in the urine displace or push the bulb of the urinometer upward. The specific gravity is read as the number at the **meniscus** of the urine on the urinometer scale. Planning ahead allows you to proceed more safely and effectively.

IMPLEMENTATION

Action	Rationale
7-10. Follow steps 7 to 10 of the General Procedure: Wash or disinfect your hands, identify the patient (two identifiers), explain the procedure you are about to perform, and prepare the environment as appropriate.	

(continued)

Action	Rationale
11. Collect the urine specimen:	
a. Put on clean gloves.	This is to protect you from contact with the urine.
b. Collect at least 20 mL urine, and pour it into a clean container. The urine should be at room temperature for testing.	The container must be clean so that extraneous particles do not alter the true concentration of the urine. Refrigerated urine condenses and therefore has a higher specific gravity.
12. Measure the specific gravity using a urinometer:	
a. Pour at least 20 mL urine into the urinometer so that the base of the bulb floats and does not touch the bottom of the container.	This results in an accurate measurement.
b. Give the stem a slight spin so that the bulb floats freely and is not in contact with the sides of the container.	This contributes to an accurate measurement.
c. Elevate the urinometer to eye level, or place it on a firm surface, and read it at eye level (Fig. 15-3). Read the lowest point of the meniscus. If the meniscus falls directly between two lines, always read to the higher number.	The specific gravity is read as the number at the meniscus of the urine. Because a heavy concentration of particles in the urine pushes the bulb higher, you will find a higher number at the meniscus as the specific gravity increases.

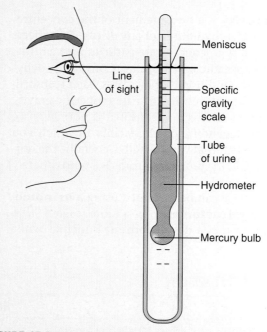

FIGURE 15-3 For accurate reading, the meniscus of the urinometer must be viewed at eye level.

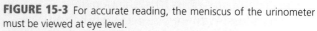

(continued)

Action	Rationale
13-17. Follow steps 13 to 17 of the General Procedure: Make observations as appropriate (see Table 15-2), conclude the procedure, wash or disinfect your hands, record the test result on paper, or label the specimen correctly, and send it to the laboratory if you are not doing the test yourself on the clinical unit.	

EVALUATION

18. As follows, evaluate using the individualized patient outcomes previously identified. **R:** Evaluation in relation to desired outcomes is essential for planning future care.
  a. Specimen was collected correctly to maximize accuracy of testing.
  b. For specimen to be tested at the point of care: Testing meets standards for accuracy upon which to base patient treatment.
  c. Results of test are within normal limits (1.010 to 1.025 g/mL), indicate progress toward the normal range when compared with previous results, or are within appropriate limits for the individual patient.

DOCUMENTATION

19-20. Follow steps 19 and 20 of the General Procedure: Document that the urine was tested for specific gravity and the results in the patient's record or on a flow sheet according to facility policy. Report abnormal results if appropriate.

Measuring Urine Specific Gravity With a Urine Refractometer

ASSESSMENT

1-2. Follow steps 1 and 2 of the General Procedure: Confirm the test to be performed, and assess the patient's ability to collect a urine specimen.

ANALYSIS

3-4. Follow steps 3 and 4 of the General Procedure: Critically think through your data, and identify specific problems and modifications.

PLANNING

5. Determine individualized patient outcomes in relation to measuring the specific gravity of urine. **R:** Identification of outcomes guides planning and evaluation.
  a. Specimen is collected correctly to maximize accuracy of testing.
  b. Testing meets standards for accuracy upon which to base patient treatment.
  c. Results of test are within normal limits (1.010 to 1.025 g/mL), indicate progress toward the normal range when compared with previous results, or are within appropriate limits for the individual patient.

6. Obtain the urine refractometer, a dropper, a urine container, and clean gloves. **R:** When the urine refractometer is used, a beam of light is refracted, or bent, according to the density of the urine and then projected onto a calibrated lens that looks somewhat like a simple microscope. The calibrations are read to identify the density. Planning ahead allows you to proceed more safely and effectively.

IMPLEMENTATION

Action	Rationale
7-10. Follow steps 7 to 10 of the General Procedure: Wash or disinfect your hands, identify the patient (two identifiers), explain the procedure, and prepare the environment as appropriate.	

(continued)

Action	Rationale
11. Collect the urine specimen:	
a. Put on clean gloves.	This is to protect you from contact with the urine.
b. Collect a few drops of urine in a container.	The refractometer can produce an accurate reading from even a drop compressed from a wet diaper.
12. Measure the specific gravity with a refractometer:	The procedure must be performed correctly so that the result will be accurate.
a. Place one drop on the horizontal glass slide at the top of the refractometer scope.	
b. Close the cover over the slide.	
c. Switch on the light.	
d. With both eyes open, look with one eye through the scope.	
e. Read the number at the line where the top black half and the lower white half of the circle meet.	
13-17. Follow steps 13 to 17 of the General Procedure: Make observations as appropriate (see Table 15-2), conclude the procedure, wash or disinfect your hands, and record the result on paper, or label the specimen correctly, and send it to the laboratory if you are not doing the test yourself on the clinical unit.	

EVALUATION

18. Follow step 18 of the General Procedure: Evaluate using the individualized patient outcomes previously identified:
   a. Specimen was collected correctly to maximize accuracy of testing.
   b. Testing met standards for accuracy upon which to base patient treatment.
   c. Results of test are within normal limits (1.010–1.025 g/mL), indicate progress toward the normal range when compared with previous results, or are within appropriate limits for the individual patient.

DOCUMENTATION

19-20. Follow steps 19 and 20 of the General Procedure: Document that the urine was tested for specific gravity and the results in the patient's record or on a flow sheet according to facility policy. Report abnormal results if appropriate.

Testing Urine for Glucose

Patients with elevated levels of glucose in the blood often have some glucose content in the urine. Testing the urine for glucose has long been a nursing function. Sometimes this is done to compare with the blood glucose level to determine if a urine glucose measurement is an accurate reflection of the blood glucose level. It can also be used in other instances to avoid repeated finger sticks. Teaching these procedures to patients and families is a part of the nursing role. Although urine tests have disadvantages because of variations in the filtering ability of the kidneys, urine testing provides a rough estimate of prevailing blood glucose levels and may be important to determining the patient's medical status.

Many commercial products that test for glucose in the urine are available. Most people who test their urine at home use reagent strips, but both tablets and strips may be found within healthcare facilities. Most facilities keep at least two products available. Among the most common are Chemstrip, Diastix, and Clinitest. Each has advantages and disadvantages. Improper handling and storage can cause false readings, so it is important to follow manufacturer recommendations to maintain the integrity of the products. Certain medications and vitamins can also cause false readings. Compare the literature regarding each product with a list of the patient's prescription and over-the-counter drugs so that you can choose an appropriate product for the test. Because the Clinitest requires the use of a reagent tablet that is caustic and that might be mistaken by a child or confused patient for a medication, many facilities have discontinued its use in patient care settings. When it is used, it must be stored with care.

Each product uses a color scale to reflect glucose content. Each color scale is based on the reactions of the chemicals used in that product. Therefore, the color scales are not interchangeable. Once a product has been chosen, use it consistently for that patient. You will compile a more reliable and consistent record if you always use the same product.

In the past, second-voided specimens were used for urine glucose testing. However, according to the American Diabetes Association (2001), second-voided specimens do not offer any appreciable advantage over first-voided specimens. Follow your facility's policy for the appropriate specimen to test.

ASSESSMENT

1-2. Follow steps 1 and 2 of the General Procedure: Confirm the test to be performed, and assess the patient's ability to collect the urine specimen.

ANALYSIS

3-4. Follow steps 3 and 4 of the General Procedure: Critically think through your data, and identify specific problems and modifications.

PLANNING

5. Determine individualized patient outcomes in relation to measuring the level of glucose in the urine:
   a. A fresh urine specimen is collected to maximize accuracy of testing.
   b. Testing meets standards for accuracy upon which to base patient treatment.
   c. Results of testing for urine glucose are within normal limits, indicate progress toward the normal range when compared with previous results, or are within appropriate limits for the individual patient. **R:** Normal urine is negative for glucose content.

6. Obtain the correct product for measuring urine glucose, specimen container(s), and clean gloves. **R:** Planning ahead allows you to proceed more safely and effectively. If you are testing a second-voided specimen, you will need two containers.

IMPLEMENTATION

Action	Rationale
7-10. Follow steps 7 to 10 of the General Procedure: Wash or disinfect your hands, identify the patient (two identifiers), explain the procedure, and prepare the environment as appropriate.	
11. Collect the urine specimen:	
a. Put on clean gloves.	To protect you from contact with the urine.
b. Ask the patient to void and collect a specimen. Use a second-voided specimen if that is the policy at your facility.	If you are using a second-voided specimen, instruct the patient to save the first specimen, and void again in 30 minutes. Test the second specimen. If the patient cannot void a second time, test the first specimen.
12. Measure urine glucose:	
a. Review the directions on the product, and place the correct color scale where it is clearly visible.	To ensure accurate results.

(continued)

Action	*Rationale*
b. *If using Clinitest:* Obtain a clean glass test tube, a test tube holder, a dropper, and tablets. Place the test tube in the holder, and using the dropper, place 5 drops of urine in the test tube. Rinse the dropper, and add 10 drops of water to the test tube. Add one Clinitest tablet to the test tube. Observe the color change as the tablet "bubbles." Fifteen seconds after the bubbling stops, shake the tube gently, and compare the color of the solution with the color chart.	The proper volume of urine and water is necessary for an accurate result. The concentration of glucose determines the color of the solution. Be careful not to touch the tablet with moist fingers because the tablets are caustic when moist and can cause burns.
c. *If testing with a reagent strip:* Remove a strip from the container. Do not touch the area of the strip where the reagent is present. Dip the strip into the urine, then tap it on the inside container edge to remove excess urine. Begin timing according to manufacturer instructions. At the end of the specified time period, compare the color on the strip with the correct color chart (Fig. 15-4).	It is important to follow the manufacturer instructions to obtain accurate test results. **FIGURE 15-4** Reagent strips must be carefully matched to the color chart for accurate results.
13-17. Follow steps 13 to 17 of the General Procedure: Make observations as appropriate (see Table 15-2), conclude the procedure, wash or disinfect your hands, record the test result on paper, or label the specimen correctly, and send it to the laboratory if you are not doing the test yourself on the clinical unit.	

EVALUATION

18. Follow step 18 of the General Procedure: Evaluate using the individualized patient outcomes previously identified:

a. A fresh specimen was used.

b. Testing met standards for accuracy upon which to base patient treatment.

c. Results of test were within normal limits (negative), indicate progress toward the normal range when compared with previous results, or are within appropriate limits for the individual patient.

DOCUMENTATION

19-20. Follow steps 19 and 20 of the General Procedure: Document the test performed and the results in the patient record or on a flow sheet according to facility policy. Report abnormal results if appropriate.

Testing Urine for Ketone Bodies (Acetone)

Ketones are a product of incomplete fat metabolism. They are present in urine when fat is being broken down rapidly and incompletely. This can occur with rigid dieting or with uncontrolled diabetes. Most commonly, tests for ketones are done with diabetic patients to identify lack of control of the disease. Test the urine for ketones at the same time you test it for glucose. Tablets and reagent strips are available to test for ketones. The reagent strips are quicker and require less equipment. Most diabetic patients who test urine for ketones at home use reagent strips. Sometimes this test is called a test for acetone. **Acetone** is one of several ketones that can be produced in the body.

ASSESSMENT

1-2. Follow steps 1 and 2 of the General Procedure: Confirm the test to be performed, and assess the patient's ability to collect the urine specimen.

ANALYSIS

3-4. Follow steps 3 and 4 of the General Procedure: Critically think through your data, and identify specific problems and modifications.

PLANNING

5. Determine individualized patient outcomes in relation to measuring the level of ketone bodies in the urine: **R:** Normal urine is negative for ketones.
   a. A fresh urine specimen is collected.
   b. Testing meets standards for accuracy upon which to base patient treatment.
   c. Results of test are within normal limits, indicate progress toward the normal range when compared with previous results, or are within appropriate limits for the individual patient.
6. Obtain the correct product, a urine specimen container, and clean gloves. **R:** Planning ahead allows you to proceed more safely and effectively.

IMPLEMENTATION

Action	Rationale
7-10. Follow steps 7 to 10 of the General Procedure: Wash or disinfect your hands, identify the patient (two identifiers), explain the procedure you are about to perform, and prepare the environment as appropriate.	
11. Collect the urine specimen:	
a. Put on clean gloves.	To protect you from contact with the urine.
b. Place the color chart where it is clearly visible.	To obtain accurate results.
c. Collect a fresh urine specimen.	If ketones are present in the urine, they will increase as the urine stands at room temperature. *Note:* Testing old urine will produce a false result.
12. Measure urine ketones:	
a. Remove the reagent strip from the bottle, being careful not to touch the area that is impregnated with the reagent.	Doing so may alter the result.
b. Dip the strip into the urine, and tap the strip on the inner edge of the container.	The reagent strip must be thoroughly moistened to activate the chemical reaction and tapped to remove excess urine.

(continued)

Action	Rationale
c. Begin timing for 60 seconds.	Accurate timing is critical for accuracy.
d. Obtain results by comparing the color on the strip with the color chart.	Color changes reflect level of ketones.
13-17. Follow steps 13 to 17 of the General Procedure: Make observations as appropriate (see Table 15-2), conclude the procedure, wash or disinfect your hands, and record the result on paper, or label the specimen correctly, and send it to the laboratory if you are not doing the test yourself on the clinical unit.	

EVALUATION

18. Follow step 18 of the General Procedure: Evaluate using the individualized patient outcomes previously identified:
    a. A fresh urine specimen was collected.
    b. Testing met standards for accuracy upon which to base patient treatment.
    c. Results of test are within normal limits (negative), indicate progress toward the normal range when compared with previous results, or were within appropriate limits for the individual patient.

DOCUMENTATION

19-20. Follow steps 19 and 20 of the General Procedure: Document the results on the patient record or flow sheet. Glucose and ketones are commonly recorded together. The glucose result is given first, then the ketone result. Report abnormal results as appropriate.

Testing Urine for Occult Blood

Normal urine is free of blood. Blood in the urine is called **hematuria** and can result from disease, trauma, or the menstrual flow. Blood can also be present in urine without being visible; for instance, the urine may have only a cloudy or hazy appearance. This is called **occult**, or hidden blood. Urine can be tested for occult blood at the discretion of the nurse, or the physician may order this test.

Reagent strips are used to test for occult blood. A common brand is Hemastix. Collect a urine specimen, and follow the procedure for using urine pH reagent strips. Read the product directions for timing and using the color chart.

MULTIPURPOSE STRIP TESTS FOR URINE

Combination or multipurpose reagent strips that test for several substances at the same time also are available. These strips have a small area of reagent for each test being done. Common reagents included on multipurpose strips are those for testing urine pH, ketones, and occult blood.

Although multipurpose strips are convenient, they do create opportunities for error. For example, there may be confusion as to which area on the strip contains the reagent for each substance. The strip must be read at the appropriate time interval and matched to the color scale according to the manufacturer's directions. Be especially careful about these points. When you use a multipurpose strip, collect a urine specimen, and follow the steps of the procedure for measuring urine pH below.

Testing Urine Using a Reagent Strip

To test urine, use a multipurpose strip or a strip designed for measuring a single substance, following the policy of your facility.

ASSESSMENT

1-2. Follow steps 1 and 2 of the General Procedure: Confirm the test to be performed, and assess the patient's ability to collect the urine specimen.

ANALYSIS

3-4. Follow steps 3 and 4 of the General Procedure: Critically think through your data, and identify specific problems and modifications.

PLANNING

5. Determine individualized patient outcomes in relation to testing the urine:
   a. Specimen is collected correctly to maximize accuracy of testing.
   b. Testing meets standards for accuracy upon which to base patient treatment.
   c. Results of test are within normal limits, indicate progress toward the normal range when compared with previous results, or are within appropriate limits for the individual patient. **R:** Normal urine has a pH of 4.6 to 8.0, protein is absent, and ketones are absent.

6. Obtain the appropriate strip, container, and clean gloves. **R:** Planning ahead allows you to proceed more safely and effectively.

IMPLEMENTATION

Action	Rationale
7-10. Follow steps 7 to 10 of the General Procedure: Wash or disinfect your hands, identify the patient (two identifiers), explain the procedure you are about to perform, and prepare the environment as appropriate.	
11. Collect the specimen:	
a. Put on clean gloves.	To protect you from contact with the urine.
b. Obtain a small amount of urine.	Only enough urine to moisten the reagent section of the strip is needed.
12. Measure substance (pH, glucose, etc.):	
a. Dip the strip into the urine, and tap the strip on the container.	The reagent strip must be thoroughly moistened to activate the chemical reaction and tapped to remove excess urine.
b. Read the strip, comparing it with the color chart on the container.	The color chart is specifically designed for the type of reagent used.
13-17. Follow steps 13 to 17 of the General Procedure: Make observations as appropriate (see Table 15-2), conclude the procedure, wash or disinfect your hands, record the result on paper, or label the specimen correctly, and send it to the laboratory if you are not doing the test yourself on the clinical unit.	

EVALUATION

18. Follow step 18 of the General Procedure: Evaluate using the individualized patient outcomes previously identified:
   a. Specimen was collected correctly to maximize accuracy of testing.
   b. Testing met standards for accuracy upon which to base patient treatment.
   c. Results of test were within normal limits, indicate progress toward the normal range when compared with previous results, or were within appropriate limits for the individual patient based on the individual test.

DOCUMENTATION

19-20. Follow steps 19 and 20 of the General Procedure: Document the test performed and the results. Report abnormal results if appropriate.

SPECIFIC PROCEDURE FOR MEASURING BLOOD GLUCOSE LEVEL

The measurement of blood glucose is performed routinely on the nursing unit, particularly for diabetic patients and others for whom accurate knowledge of glucose levels is important. If measurement of blood glucose is critical, the test may also be done as a laboratory procedure. Blood glucose tests are much more reliable than urine glucose tests and the most commonly used method of monitoring patient glucose levels. The test can be done by visually examining the color of a reagent strip, but in most instances, a portable electronic meter is used. Most clinical agencies require meters in order to obtain the accuracy needed upon which to base treatment decisions. Only the method using an electronic meter is described below. In addition to performing this procedure, you will also be teaching it to patients or their families so that it can be done at home.

The American Diabetes Association (2001) recommends self-monitoring of blood glucose (SMBG) for patients with insulin-treated diabetes. There are various brands of meters on the market to test blood glucose. Some have a computer memory and can store numerous test results. These devices can be purchased for use in the home. Medicare and many health plans pay for glucose monitors to encourage effective management of diabetes. Because the procedure for operating each meter varies in important ways, check the manufacturer's directions carefully before proceeding. Some have built-in timers that automatically manage the entire process. Some even have built-in lancets for collecting the specimen. For visually impaired patients, there are models that have audible signals to manage the process and to provide the result. They also differ in the size of the sample they require (see *http://www.lifeclinic.com/focus/diabetes/supply_meter.asp*).

ASSESSMENT

1-2. Follow steps 1 and 2 of the General Procedure: Confirm the test to be performed, and assess the patient's ability to cooperate during the procedure.

ANALYSIS

3-4. Follow steps 3 and 4 of the General Procedure: Critically think through your data, and identify specific problems and modifications.

PLANNING

5. Determine individualized patient outcomes in relation to measuring blood glucose:

    a. Specimen is collected correctly to maximize accuracy of testing.

    b. Testing meets standards for accuracy upon which to base patient treatment.

    c. Results of test are within normal limits, indicate progress toward the normal range when compared with previous results, or are within appropriate limits for the individual patient. Normal blood glucose concentration ranges between 70 and 105 mg/dL.

6. As follows, obtain appropriate equipment. **R:** Planning ahead allows you to proceed more safely and effectively.

    a. Glucose meter (Fig. 15-5); each brand of glucose meter is standardized and calibrated at regular intervals. Although students do not assume responsibility for this, you should know the policies regarding this procedure in the facility where you practice.

    b. Reagent strip for the specific blood glucose meter that matches any calibration numbers for the meter and has an expiration date after the time of use. **R:** Reagent strips are specific to the meter. Some meters require that recalibration be done for each new supply of strips in order to maintain accuracy. An outdated strip may give inaccurate results.

    c. Tissues to apply pressure to stop bleeding

    d. Clean gloves to protect you from contact with blood

    e. Sterile finger **lancet. R:** A sterile, disposable lancet is used each time the test is performed. Most facilities use a special spring-loaded puncture device that secures the lancet until its release. One puncture device may be used for many patients, but each patient should have a separate end platform that touches the patient's skin and a sterile lancet. The puncture device provides a standardized force and depth of puncture. Because each brand operates differently, read the directions, and practice loading and releasing the device before going to the bedside.

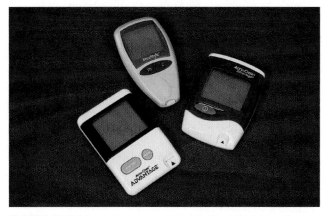

FIGURE 15-5 Many glucometers are available. Follow manufacturer instructions for use.

IMPLEMENTATION

Action	Rationale
7-10. Follow steps 7 to 10 of the General Procedure: Wash or disinfect your hands, identify the patient (two identifiers), explain the procedure you are about to perform, and prepare the environment as appropriate.	

11. Collect the blood specimen (Fig. 15-6):

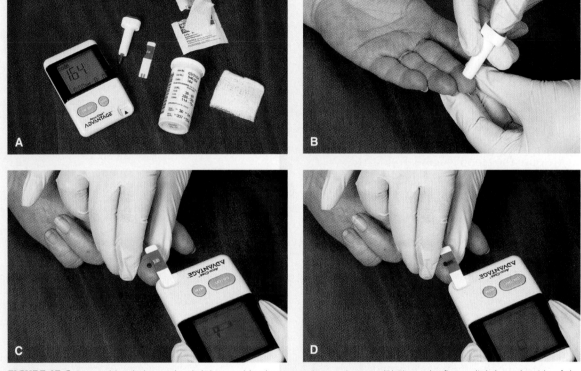

FIGURE 15-6 To test blood glucose level, (**A**) assemble glucose testing equipment. (**B**) Pierce the finger slightly to the side of the fingertip pad for best results. (**C**) Express small drop of blood and (**D**) apply blood to test area of glucometer. Read the blood glucose level that appears on the meter's digital display screen.

Action	Rationale
a. Have the patient wash his or her hands with soap and warm water and dry them.	This cleans the skin and increases blood flow. Alcohol should not be used because it dries and toughens the skin. If alcohol is used, it must be allowed to dry so that it does not compromise test results.
b. Select the location to pierce. Avoid the index finger.	Piercing the index finger causes the patient the most pain. Slightly to the side of the pad on the tip of the chosen finger is usually the best location.
c. Turn on the meter and put on gloves.	To protect you from contact with the patient's blood.

(continued)

Action	Rationale
d. Hold the patient's hand in a dependent position, and massage the base of the chosen finger.	To promote increased blood flow.
e. If using a puncture device, load the lancet. Remove the cover from the point of the lancet, and set the spring. Place the device firmly against the side of the distal portion of the finger. Release the spring to pierce the finger.	The puncture device is set to provide the correct depth to achieve the needed blood specimen when it is pressed firmly against the skin.
f. Allow a drop of blood to form at the site. You may "milk" the base of the finger, but do not put pressure on the site.	This action could alter test results.
g. Drop the blood onto the reagent portion of the strip, covering it completely with the rounded drop.	For accurate results, the reagent must be completely covered.
h. Use a tissue to put pressure on the site.	To stop the bleeding.
12. Measure the blood glucose. Follow the directions for the specific meter. The following are common aspects of the process:	
a. Press the meter start button for the beginning of the timing period.	Accurate timing is critical for accuracy.
b. When the designated time has passed, indicated by an audible signal from the meter, wipe or blot the strip if directed.	
c. Place the strip into the meter, and continue the timing as directed.	
d. When the timing period is ended, an audible signal indicates that the blood glucose measurement has been completed. Read the level from the meter. The readout provides mg/dL.	
13-14. Follow steps 13 and 14 of the General Procedure: Make observations as appropriate (see Table 15-2), and conclude the procedure. If a spring-loaded puncture device was used, dispose of the lancet into the sharps container, clean all parts of the puncture device, and return them to the appropriate storage place.	

(continued)

Action	Rationale
15-17. Follow steps 15 to 17 of the General Procedure: Wash or disinfect your hands, record the test result on paper, or label the specimen correctly, and send it to the laboratory if you are not doing the test yourself on the clinical unit.	

EVALUATION

18. Follow step 18 of the General Procedure: Evaluate using the individualized patient outcomes previously identified:
    a. Specimen was collected correctly to maximize accuracy of testing.
    b. Testing met standards for accuracy upon which to base patient treatment.
    c. Results of blood glucose test were within normal limits (70 to 105 mg/dL), indicate progress toward the normal range when compared with previous results, or were within appropriate limits for the individual patient.

DOCUMENTATION

19-20. Follow steps 19 and 20 of the General Procedure: Document the test performed and the results in the patient record and on the appropriate flow sheet. The flow sheet may also contain other information, such as insulin administered, urine testing results, patient responses, and further nursing action taken. Report abnormal results if appropriate.

SPECIFIC PROCEDURE FOR TESTING FECES FOR OCCULT BLOOD

Blood is not usually as visible in feces as it is in other body tissues and fluids. Blood in feces is commonly occult blood. The undigested portions of oral iron preparations give the stool a black appearance that can be mistaken for blood or can mask the presence of occult blood. Red meat may also give a false positive test result, which is why the patient is instructed to follow a meat-free diet for 24 hours prior to the test (McCormick, Kibbe, & Morgan, 2002). Generally, three separate stools are tested for occult blood. Feces can be tested at the discretion of the nurse if the test materials are available. If the stool must be sent to a laboratory for testing, or the

materials must be ordered and charged to the patient, a physician's order may be needed.

ASSESSMENT

1-2. Follow steps 1 and 2 of the General Procedure: Confirm the test to be performed, and assess the patient's ability to collect a stool specimen.

ANALYSIS

3-4. Follow steps 3 and 4 of the General Procedure: Critically think through your data, and identify specific problems and modifications.

PLANNING

5. Determine the individualized patient outcomes in relation to testing feces for occult blood. Normal stool is negative for occult blood. **R:** Planning ahead allows you to proceed more safely and effectively.
    a. Stool specimen is collected correctly with samples from two different parts of the stool to maximize accuracy of testing.
    b. For specimen to be tested in the laboratory:
       (1) Requisition is completed correctly.
       (2) Specimen is packaged to protect healthcare workers and to support accurate testing.
       (3) Specimen is sent in a timely manner.
    c. For specimen to be tested at the point of care: Testing meets standards for accuracy upon which to base patient treatment.
    d. Test results are negative for occult blood in the stool.
6. Obtain the following supplies:
    a. wooden tongue depressor to collect the specimen
    b. clean gloves to protect you from contact with stool
    c. testing materials
       (1) Hemoccult slide and Hemoccult developing solution. The slide provides a filter paper containing the reagent guaiac to hold the smear and absorb the developer, so it stays in contact with the sample. **R:** The Hemoccult

developing solution causes the guaiac to react with any hemoglobin in the stool. *OR*

(2) Hematest tablets, filter paper, and water. **R:** The Hematest tablet contains the reagent orthotolidine, which is then dissolved by

the water. The paper is a vehicle to hold the smear and absorb the reagent, so it stays in contact with the sample. The supplies may be kept in the patient's bathroom if there is frequent need for them.

IMPLEMENTATION

Action	Rationale
7-10. Follow steps 7 to 10 of the General Procedure: Wash or disinfect your hands, identify the patient (two identifiers), explain the procedure you are about to perform, and prepare the environment as appropriate.	
11. Collect the stool specimen:	
a. Put on clean gloves.	To protect you from contact with the stool.
b. Use a tongue depressor to collect a small amount of stool.	Only a small amount of stool is needed to perform the test.
12. Test the stool:	
a. *If you are using a Hemoccult slide:*	Following the directions precisely is important for an accurate result.
(1) Open the folder flap, and apply a thin smear of fecal material to the filter paper in the first box.	The thin smear will allow the reagent to contact the stool but not be absorbed into the stool.
(2) Apply a thin smear of fecal material from a different part of the stool to the filter paper in the second box (Fig. 15-7).	

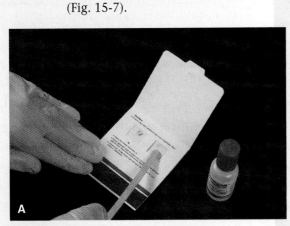
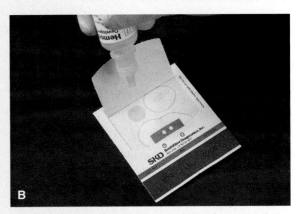

FIGURE 15-7 Testing feces for occult blood. (**A**) Apply thin smear of stool to hemoccult slide. (**B**) Apply drops of reagent solution to the opposite side of the slide.

(continued)

Action	Rationale
(3) Close the folder, and turn to the reverse side.	
(4) Open the flap, and drop two drops of the developing solution onto each sample box, following the manufacturer's instructions.	The solution is the chemical reagent that interacts with hemoglobin to form a blue compound.
(5) Observe the paper for the appearance of blue, which indicates occult blood or a positive test result.	
b. *If you are using a Hematest tablet:*	
(1) Smear a thin layer of fecal material on the filter paper with a tongue depressor.	
(2) Place a Hematest tablet on top of the center of the specimen.	
(3) Apply 2 or 3 drops of water to the tablet, allowing the water to flow onto the filter paper.	The water dissolves the reagent from the Hematest tablet, which will react with hemoglobin to form a blue compound.
(4) Observe the paper for the color blue, which indicates occult blood or a positive test result.	
13-17. Follow steps 13 to 17 of the General Procedure: Make observations as appropriate (see Table 15-2), conclude the procedure, wash or disinfect your hands, record the result on paper, or label the specimen correctly, and send it to the laboratory if you are not doing the test yourself on the clinical unit.	

EVALUATION

18. Follow step 18 of the General Procedure: Evaluate using the individualized patient outcomes previously identified:

a. Stool specimen is collected correctly with samples from two different parts of the stool to maximize accuracy of testing.

b. For specimen to be tested in the laboratory:
  (1) Requisition is completed correctly.
  (2) Specimen is packaged to protect healthcare workers and to support accurate testing.
  (3) Specimen is sent in a timely manner.

c. For specimen to be tested at the point of care: Testing meets standards for accuracy upon which to base patient treatment.

d. Results of test are negative for occult blood.

DOCUMENTATION

19-20. Follow steps 19 and 20 of the General Procedure: Document the test performed and the results in the medical record and on the appropriate flow sheet. It is recorded as negative (–) or positive (+). Report abnormal results as appropriate.

SPECIFIC PROCEDURE FOR OBTAINING A SPECIMEN FOR CULTURE

Culture specimens can be obtained from almost any body surface or orifice. Usually fluids (secretions, **exudates**) are cultured. All culture specimens should be sent to the laboratory promptly so that the character of the specimen does not change with time and produce a false reading.

ASSESSMENT

1-2. Follow steps 1 and 2 of the General Procedure: Confirm the test to be performed, and assess the patient's ability to cooperate with the procedure.

ANALYSIS

3-4. Follow steps 3 and 4 of the General Procedure: Critically think through your data, and identify specific problems and modifications.

PLANNING

5. Determine individualized patient outcomes in relation to obtaining specimens for culture:
   a. Culture specimen is collected correctly to maximize accuracy of testing.
   b. For specimen to be tested in the laboratory:
      (1) Requisition is completed correctly.
      (2) Specimen is packaged to protect healthcare workers and to support accurate testing. **R:** Specimens for culture must be sealed to prevent contamination with microorganisms from the environment. Healthcare workers must be protected from potential pathogens in the specimen.
      (3) Specimen is sent in a timely manner. **R:** If a culture is delayed in getting to the laboratory, microorganism may grow to greater numbers, giving an erroneous view of the concentration of microorganisms.
   c. Results of culture are within normal limits for the area or tissue being cultured, indicate progress toward the normal range when compared with previous results, or are within appropriate limits for the individual patient.

6. Obtain the appropriate culture tube and a pair of clean gloves. Specimens for culture are typically obtained using a sterile cotton swab that is attached to the lid of a flexible sterile culture tube. The culture tube contains a transport medium enclosed in an ampule in the bottom of the tube. After the specimen has been obtained, return the swab to the culture tube, and squeeze the tube to crush the ampule. This action releases the culture medium, which prevents drying of the specimen and maintains the bacterial concentration. Alternatively, you may be using a swab and a sterile test tube with a sealed lid. **R:** Follow the policy in your facility. Planning ahead allows you to proceed more safely and effectively.

IMPLEMENTATION

Action	Rationale
7-10. Follow steps 7 to 10 of the General Procedure: Wash or disinfect your hands, identify the patient (two identifiers), explain the procedure you are about to perform, and prepare the environment as appropriate.	
11. Obtain the culture specimen:	
a. Put on clean gloves.	To protect you from contact with the specimen.
b. Remove the tube from its package, and remove the swab stick from the tube, being careful not to touch the end of the swab against your fingers or any objects.	To prevent contamination with microorganisms.
c. Collect the specimen to be cultured on the cotton end of the swab, saturating the cotton, insert the swab into the tube, and recap.	This releases the transport medium.

(continued)

Action	Rationale
d. With the cap end down, crush the ampule at midpoint.	
e. Push the cap so that the swab moves down, making contact with the medium.	The transport medium prevents drying and maintains the bacterial concentration.
f. In the places designated on the package, note the patient's name, identifying information, physician's name, date, time, and any antibiotics or other anti-infective medications the patient is taking.	Some drugs can affect the result.
g. If you are using a test tube that does not contain a culture medium, swab the area with a sterile cotton swab stick as described above. Place the swab in test tube; recap, and label as in 11f.	This is to prevent contamination with microorganisms and for accurate results.
12. Send the culture specimen to the laboratory immediately in a biohazard bag.	Any bacterial content can change in number or character if left standing.
13-16. Follow steps 13 to 16 of the General Procedure: Make observations as appropriate (see Table 15-2), conclude the procedure, wash or disinfect your hands, and record any special observations on paper.	

EVALUATION

17. Evaluate using the individualized patient outcomes previously identified:
a. Culture specimen was collected correctly to maximize accuracy of testing.
b. For specimen tested in the laboratory:
 (1) Requisition was completed correctly.
 (2) Specimen was packaged to protect health-care workers and to support accurate testing.
 (3) Specimen was sent in a timely manner.
c. Results of culture were within normal limits for the area or tissue being cultured, indicate progress toward the normal range when compared with previous results, or are within appropriate limits for the individual patient. Report results if appropriate. **R:** The culture must be evaluated after the microorganisms have had an opportunity to grow in the laboratory, usually 48 hours or more. Compare results of the culture with information on normal flora of the area being cultured and with information on sensitivity with the drugs being given.

DOCUMENTATION

18. Document that the culture specimen was obtained and sent to the laboratory. If the culture results identify the specimen as positive for pathogenic organisms, notify the physician.

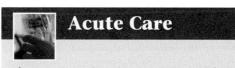

Acute Care

If you are employed in an acute care facility, you may be involved in collecting a variety of specimens and performing some tests on your nursing unit. Most facilities will require that employees demonstrate competency in point of care testing using their equipment and procedures before they are allowed to perform these tests independently. You will also need to prepare patients for the various tests, and at times, explain the test results. You may also be involved in teaching patients and caregivers how to perform some of the tests at home.

Long-Term Care

Long-term care facilities do not have laboratories. Therefore, when specimens must be sent to a laboratory, the nurse must usually make arrangements for transporting the specimen from the facility to the laboratory. This may require extra planning because of the time it will take to transport the specimen. Laboratories that are experienced in meeting the needs of long-term care facilities usually have specific directions to ensure that the specimen is useful when it arrives at the laboratory.

Nurses typically draw all blood samples in long-term care. If the nurses do not, laboratory personnel may come to the facility to draw the sample, or the resident may be sent to a physician's office or to a clinic where there are experienced laboratory personnel.

Home Care

Some of these tests will be done by clients at home to monitor their own therapy and progress. The skill may be taught initially in a hospital or in a clinic, or the home health nurse may teach it when the need arises. After the nurse explains or demonstrates the test procedure, the client is asked to return the demonstration for evaluation of his or her expertise. Also ask clients to demonstrate such skills on a subsequent outpatient visit to verify that their technique continues to be correct. The home health nurse may be responsible for monitoring laboratory results, teaching clients, and evaluating their ability to perform tests independently.

Ambulatory Care

Depending on the specific setting, specimens may be obtained and tested in an office or clinic. In small offices, you may collect the specimen and then send it out to a laboratory for processing. Larger clinics may have a laboratory on site. Even if you are not responsible for obtaining specimens or performing tests, you often will need to explain the reasons for tests to be done elsewhere or to teach clients to do tests at home. Written instructions for clients to take home are helpful in these situations.

LEARNING TOOLS

DEVELOP YOUR BACKGROUND KNOWLEDGE

1. Review the Learning Outcomes.

2. Read the section on collecting specimens and performing common laboratory tests in your assigned text.

3. Look up the Key Terms in the glossary.

4. Review this module, and mentally practice the techniques described. Study so that you would be able to teach these skills to another person.

DEVELOP YOUR SKILLS

1. In the practice setting, join two other students, and form a group of three.

2. Alternating so that each has the opportunity to play the role of the patient, perform each of the following procedures if the equipment is available in your practice laboratory. There may be "substitute" products that are used to teach the testing process while not creating the potential for exposure to actual body substances. Those who are not participating at a given time can observe and evaluate the performances of the others. Include pertinent patient education for each procedure.

   a. Testing specific gravity of urine using a urinometer
   b. Testing urine for glucose, ketones, blood, and pH using test strips
   c. Testing blood glucose level using electronic meter
   d. Testing feces for occult blood
   e. Obtaining culture specimens

DEMONSTRATE YOUR SKILLS

In the clinical setting

1. Consult with your instructor regarding the opportunity to collect specimens and perform common laboratory tests in the clinical setting. Evaluate your performance with the instructor. Use the performance checklist on the CD-ROM in the front of this book as a guide.

2. Consult with your instructor regarding the opportunity to analyze the results of common laboratory tests and the corresponding nursing implications. Discuss with your instructor and clinical group.

CRITICAL THINKING EXERCISES

1. You notice that a patient being treated with large doses of prednisone is complaining of gastric distress. This morning, the patient's stool is dark and

odorous. Synthesize information about this drug, the characteristics of normal stool, and the assessment data you have gathered to identify a potential problem for this patient. Determine what further nursing assessment is indicated, and discuss the rationale.

2. A person with diabetes mellitus has been admitted to your unit in a long-term care facility. The medical orders include insulin daily, plus regular insulin coverage as needed. Identify which common laboratory tests you expect to perform for this resident, and explain why.

SELF-QUIZ
SHORT-ANSWER QUESTIONS

1. What is the nurse's responsibility when an abnormal laboratory test result is identified?

   _____

   _____

   _____

2. Where would you find information on how to perform a laboratory test in the hospital where you have clinical practice?

   _____

   _____

3. Identify four critical aspects of any laboratory testing performed by the nurse.

   a. _____

   b. _____

   c. _____

   d. _____

4. When should gloves be worn when collecting specimens?

   _____

5. How can you protect yourself and other staff when transporting laboratory specimens?

   _____

TRUE-FALSE

_____ 6. Sputum specimens are best obtained first thing in the morning.

_____ 7. When obtaining a 24-hour urine specimen, the last voiding is discarded.

_____ 8. Alcohol is recommended for cleansing a finger when performing a finger stick to measure blood glucose.

_____ 9. All urine glucose–testing products are completely interchangeable.

_____ 10. To obtain a urine specimen from a catheterized patient, drain the specimen from the bottom of the drainage bag.

Answers to Self-Quiz questions appear in the back of this book.

Admission, Transfer, and Discharge

SKILLS INCLUDED IN THIS MODULE

Procedure for Admission
Procedure for Transfer
Procedure for Discharge

PREREQUISITE MODULES

Module 1	An Approach to Nursing Skills
Module 2	Documentation
Module 3	Basic Body Mechanics
Module 4	Basic Infection Control
Module 5	Safety in the Healthcare Environment
Module 11	Assessing Temperature, Pulse, and Respiration
Module 12	Measuring Blood Pressure
Module 14	Nursing Physical Assessment

The following modules may be needed in some situations:

Module 15	Collecting Specimens and Performing Common Laboratory Tests
Module 18	Transfer
Module 19	Ambulation: Simple Assisted and Using Cane, Walker, or Crutches

KEY TERMS

acuity	discharge planner
AMA	nursing history
assessment	protocol
chart	referral

OVERALL OBJECTIVE

▸ To admit, transfer, and discharge patients, taking into consideration both the needs of individual patients and the needs of the healthcare agency.

LEARNING OUTCOMES

The student will be able to

1. Assess patients appropriately in relation to admission, transfer, and discharge.
2. Analyze data, and determine whether concerns are present that must be addressed immediately.
3. Determine appropriate outcomes for the patient being admitted, transferred, or discharged and recognize the patient for adverse outcomes.
4. Develop initial plans for the newly admitted patient.
5. Make certain that there are plans to ensure continuity of care for those being transferred within the facility and those being discharged.
6. Evaluate the effectiveness of actions taken to ensure continuity of care.
7. Document admission, transfer, and discharge processes according to facility policies.

A key nursing focus is continuity of care, wherever that care occurs. This means making sure that, as the patient moves between home, acute care, and long-term care, healthcare needs are identified, nursing care is appropriately planned, and support services are continued. To effectively ensure a smooth progression, the nurse must give careful attention to the processes involved in admission, transfer, and discharge. Many facilities have developed plans for continuous progress called "care pathways," "critical paths," or "clinical pathways." These plans are guidelines for monitoring the patient's progress, and all staff use them.

For most people, entering a healthcare facility is a major crisis. Individuals have many needs and concerns that must be identified and for which action must be taken. In addition, each healthcare facility must maintain certain routine procedures and gather specific information about incoming patients that will help the facility perform its functions. Identifying and meeting both sets of needs is a challenging task for the nurse. The person entering the hospital may be coming from a long-term care facility or home. The person entering long-term care may likewise be moving from home or from an acute care setting. Admission information must be complete and accurate. A care provider in the family or a home care nurse is often appropriately involved in this transition; his or her perceptions may provide valuable information.

Units within the hospital may be specialized, and this means that a patient may sometimes need to be transferred from one unit to another within the facility. Also, health insurance plans, including Medicare and Medicaid, usually restrict the number of reimbursable acute care hospital days; therefore, patients are being transferred to long-term care facilities or home for continued treatment and convalescence. Consequently, the transfer procedure is of great importance. If it is done carefully, the relocation will have minimal impact on the patient, and the receiving staff or family caregivers will receive adequate information on which to base thorough nursing care.

Whenever a patient enters any healthcare facility, the nurse should keep that person's possible transfer and eventual discharge in mind. For most patients, the nurse should begin planning for eventual transfer or discharge at the time the patient is admitted. When patients leave the healthcare facility for home, the nurse has similar responsibilities, which include instructing the patient in any aspect of care to be provided on a continuing basis involving the patient or family, answering questions to decrease anxiety, and sharing any resources that may be useful.

NURSING DIAGNOSES

- Anxiety related to health status and admission to a healthcare facility. Almost all newly admitted patients may present with this diagnosis.
- Health-Seeking Behaviors related to desire for continued improvement in health status. Patients being discharged may be motivated to improve health.
- Impaired Home Maintenance related to inability to engage in activity and restricted mobility. This diagnosis is present for many newly discharged patients and requires that the nurse plan with the patient for management at home.
- Readiness for Enhanced Knowledge related to the patient's own health problems and self-care needs. This occurs when individuals have new insights into what may be interfering with health and an interest in learning more about their health problem.

DELEGATION

Some aspects of the admission procedure are commonly delegated to assistive personnel. Routine tasks associated with the skills the nursing assistant has been taught may include measuring vital signs, assisting with care of possessions, and assisting the patient into bed. The nurse must remain responsible for the baseline **assessment** that will be done and for initiating the plans for care. Final assessment and discharge teaching are nursing functions that do not lend themselves to delegation. At the time of discharge, the assistant may provide transport to a new unit or escort the patient to a car. Volunteers also may be asked to transport individuals out of the facility to a car at the time of discharge. If the person is being transported by ambulance, the ambulance attendants come to the unit to transport the patient.

PLACEMENT OF ADMITTED PATIENTS

The placement of patients who are admitted to the facility is usually a cooperative effort between the admitting department and the individual unit. The individual unit must make sure that there is adequate staffing for the number of patients who will be on the unit and that the staff members have the expertise to meet the patient's needs. Placement also depends on the condition of the patient, the size of the facility, and whether it has specialty units.

In larger hospitals, patients are admitted to units that specialize in treatment of their condition. For example, surgical patients are admitted to a surgical unit. A hospital may be large enough that there is even specialization within the units; patients having abdominal surgery are admitted to one unit and patients having facial surgery are admitted to another. In smaller hospitals, rather than being admitted to specialized units, patients may be admitted strictly on the basis of empty beds.

Acuity (the seriousness of the patient's condition) is another factor that determines where patients are placed. Very ill patients need a higher staff-to-patient ratio than patients who are in the recovery or rehabilitation phase of their illness. If a private room is not available, every attempt is made to place the patient with an appropriate roommate.

ADMISSION

The nurse has many responsibilities in the admission process. When assessing a person being admitted to a healthcare facility, the patient should be your primary source of information if at all possible. However, the family or caregiver may provide useful information that will help you carry out your assessment. You may need to be flexible in your approach to nursing process. Admission activities will not always be done in the same order. For example, a portion of a baseline assessment may conveniently be addressed at the same time that you begin documentation. The needs of the individual patient and your own time organization will guide you.

PROCEDURE FOR ADMISSION TO A HOSPITAL OR NURSING HOME

ASSESSMENT

1. Review the physician's admitting orders. **R:** This will provide information for planning for immediate needs and setting up a plan of care.
2. Identify any specialized equipment that will be needed. **R:** To initiate the medical plan of care as soon as possible.

ANALYSIS

3. Critically think through your data, carefully evaluating each aspect and its relation to other data. **R:** To determine specific problems for this individual in relation to the admission process.
4. Identify specific problems and modifications of the procedure needed for this individual. **R:** Planning must consider the individual's problems.

PLANNING

5. Determine the individualized patient outcomes for the admission process. **R:** Identifying outcomes facilitates planning and evaluation.
   a. Patient is comfortable, with anxiety at a manageable level.
   b. Patient's immediate needs have been met.
   c. All required documentation is in place.
6. Identify the appropriate room placement for the patient. **R:** Room placement needs to match the patient's needs in terms of a variety of factors, including proximity to the nurses' station, the availability of a nurse for care, and appropriate roommate (sex, health condition, and the like).
7. Identify elements of the admission process that could be delegated to a nursing assistant. **R:** Nursing assistants are trained to complete simple procedures that have predictable outcomes and that do not require judgment and decision-making during the procedure. As a student, you may carry out all procedures, but as a registered nurse (RN), you will be able to delegate some aspects.
8. Gather equipment that will be needed for assessment. **R:** Gathering equipment before beginning facilitates an organized process.
   a. Stethoscope
   b. Thermometer
   c. Sphygmomanometer (if not a fixture in the room)

IMPLEMENTATION

Action	Rationale
9. Greet the patient and introduce yourself.	A greeting that conveys interest in and concern for patients provides a foundation for the development of trust in the healthcare team.
10. Wash or disinfect your hands.	To decrease the transfer of microorganisms that could cause infection.
11. Identify the patient, using two identifiers.	Verifying the patient's identity helps ensure that you are initiating actions for the correct patient.

12. Perform a brief focused assessment for immediate needs. Assess particularly for
 	
  a. pain
 	
  b. nausea and vomiting or potential vomiting
 	
  c. need for toileting
 	
  d. severe anxiety
	Patients entering a care facility may be acutely ill and need immediate attention. *Note:* If these problems are identified, then you will need to use the nursing process to address the problems or refer them immediately. This procedure will progress as if there are no immediate concerns.

13. Provide introductions and orientation to the immediate environment. A thorough orientation to the unit includes an explanation of all items for the patient's use, which areas are for personal belongings, and the location of the bathroom. Especially important are directions on how to operate the bed and TV and how to call a nurse. If it is necessary for patients to wait before the rest of the admission process is started, an explanation is appreciated.	An orientation to others and the environment reduces anxiety and allows a patient to participate in his or her own care.

14. Care for the patient's personal property such as clothing and other belongings.	Healthcare facilities have legal obligations for safeguarding personal property of patients.
	
	  a. Send valuables home with the family, or document their placement in a safe (Fig. 16-1).
	
	  b. Place clothing and personal items where they are accessible for discharge or for use during the stay.

(continued)

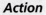

Action	Rationale

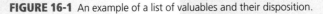

Medical Center
SEATTLE, WASHINGTON 98133

**PATIENT'S VALUABLE
ENVELOPE**

Nolan, Christine   DOB 11-27-82
000-00-0000
Dr. Stewart

CONTENTS OF ENVELOPE DEPOSITED WITH HOSPITAL	ARTICLES RETAINED BY PATIENT OR RESPONSIBLE PARTY
☑ CASH — *$50.00*	☑ CASH — *$11.20*
☐ WATCH	☑ WATCH
☐ RINGS	☑ RINGS — *wedding (1)*
☐ WALLET	☐ WALLET
☐ OTHER EXPLAIN	☐ OTHER EXPLAIN
☐ OTHER EXPLAIN	☑ DENTURES PARTIAL — *lower / partial*
☐ OTHER EXPLAIN	☑ GLASSES
☐ OTHER EXPLAIN	☐ RAZOR
☐ OTHER EXPLAIN	☐ OTHER EXPLAIN
☐ OTHER EXPLAIN	☐ OTHER EXPLAIN

NEITHER NORTHWEST HOSPITAL NOR THE MEMBERS OF ITS STAFF SHALL BE
RESPONSIBLE FOR VALUABLES NOT DEPOSITED IN THE BUSINESS OFFICE.

I, THE PATIENT, OR RESPONSIBLE PARTY ASSUME FULL RESPONSIBILITY FOR
THOSE ITEMS RETAINED IN MY POSSESSION DURING MY HOSPITALIZATION.
I HAVE CHECKED THE ABOVE AND ACKNOWLEDGE THE LISTS TO BE CORRECT.

PATIENT'S SIGNATURE
OR
DATE: *4-16-06*   RESPONSIBLE PARTY: *Bella Sutherland*

TIME: *0845*   HOSPITAL EMPLOYEE: *Al Feldon, N.A.*

RECEIVED BY BUSINESS OFFICE: *Karen Jornis, Sec.*

RELEASE OF VALUABLES:

ORIGINAL – PATIENT   Released By:_____ Date___ / /
YELLOW – CHART
ENVELOPE – BUSINESS OFFICE   Patient or Responsible Party: _____

FIGURE 16-1 An example of a list of valuables and their disposition.

15. Perform a baseline assessment. The information to be gathered in baseline assessment varies from one facility to another based on the common needs and problems of the patients. Admission assessment almost always includes measuring temperature, pulse, and respiration (TPR), and blood pressure. Height and weight may also be measured.

To provide a foundation for establishing a nursing plan of care and to enable effective evaluation of care.

a. Observations and physical examination: In some facilities, the nurse does a complete physical examination. In others, the nurse may do a thorough nursing assessment that does not encompass the traditional physical examination. In long-term care facilities, the federally mandated Minimum Data Set (MDS) guides admission assessment.

(continued)

Action	Rationale
	b. Interview and history taking: Even if a formalized **nursing history** is not used, the nurse collects information relating to allergies, current medications, and the patient's perception of the entering problem (often called the chief complaint). An interview is used to gather subjective information regarding the patient (Fig. 16-2).

SLEEP/COMFORT

PAIN: NO/(YES) Location _breathing_
Duration_____ Type _sharp_
Pain Tolerance 1 2 3 4 (5) 6 7 8 9 10
Usual bedtime _____ 2200
Usual awakening _____ 0600
Nap during day: ☐ Yes ☒ No

COMMUNICATION

PRIMARY LANGUAGE: (If not English) _____
Interpreter _N.A._
Phone Number _____
Deficit of Speech/Hearing/Vision/(None)

SOCIAL/EMOTIONAL

AFFECT: Within normal limits/Angry/Anxious/Depressed/Flat/Hostile

LIVES: Alone/With family/With friends _–with wife_

SUPPORT SYSTEMS: Describe _minimal –wife anxious, close to couple from church_

OCCUPATION:
Last Date Worked: _____
Length of Maternity Leave _N.A._

RESPIRATORY

QUALITY: Normal/Labored/Shallow/SOB/SOB c̄ exertion/Orthopnea/Other _____
COUGH: Absent/Non-productive/Productive _mod. amt_
LUNG SOUNDS: _dull in ↓ lobes, wheezes   clear mucus_
TOBACCO USE: (NO)/YES Type and amount _____

CIRCULATORY

HEART RHYTHM: Regular/Irregular
PERIPHERAL PULSES (When Indicated) _present_
Edema (NO)/YES Periorbital Facial/Hands/Lower Extremities
Dehydration (NO)/YES
SKIN COLOR: Normal/Cyanotic/Dusky/Jaundice _mild_
SKIN TEMPERATURE: Normal/Cold/Hot/Diaphoretic
PREVIOUS TRANSFUSIONS (NO)/YES
ACTIVITY LEVEL _bedrest–up as tolerated_
LIMITATIONS IN MOVEMENT (NO)/YES

NEUROSENSORY

LEVEL OF CONSCIOUSNESS: Alert/Lethargic/Restless/Agitated/Coma/Seizure Disorder _Ø_
PUPIL STATUS (when indicated) _N.A._
ORIENTATION: Person/Place/Time/Situation _oriented_

SENSORY DISABILITY: (NO)/YES

DTR'S: RA | LA Clonus (NO) YES ____
             RL | LL

Headache/Visual Disturbances: (NO)/YES

SKIN

SENSITIVITIES: Soap/Tape/Lotion/Iodine/Other _none_
CONDITION: Normal/Dry/Bruises/Abrasions/Open Wounds/Ulcers/Rash
Describe _____

NUTRITION

Pre-Pregnant Weight
RECENT WEIGHT CHANGE: Gain/Loss _none_ Pounds
INTAKE: Normal/Nausea/Vomiting/Malnourished/Indigestion
Other _____
SPECIAL DIET: NO/(YES) Type _4 small meals until breathing improves_
ALCOHOL: Type and amount _occasional_

GI/GU

ABDOMEN: Normal/Tender/Rigid/Distended/Gravid
EPIGASTRIC PAIN (NO) YES
BOWEL TONES: Normal/Hypo-active/Hyper-active/Absent
BOWELS: Usual Pattern _daily_ Last BM _4/12_
Laxatives/Enemas: (NO)/YES
Diarrhea/Constipation/Hemorrhoids/Other
URINARY: No difficulty/Frequency/Urgency/Pain/Burning/Hematuria
Proteinuria/Glucosuria _Ø_

REPRODUCTION/SEXUALITY

LAST MENSTRUAL PERIOD _N.A._ EDC _____

Discharge/Bleeding/Pain _N.A._

SEXUALLY TRANSMITTED DISEASES (NO)/YES Chlamydia/Yeast/Trich/GC/Syphilis/B. Strep/Others _____
Herpes NO/YES Site_____
Last Culture_____ Current Status _____

Date: _4/13/06_   Time: _1300_   RN Signature _S. Martin, R.N._

ROOM # _1402_   NAME: _Williams, Thomas_   _Dr. Bernie Schiff_   CATEGORY: _Medical_

FIGURE 16-2 A form used to record both subjective and objective information related to functional areas obtained during the nursing interview.

EVALUATION

16. Evaluate using the individualized patient outcomes previously identified. **R:** Evaluation in relation to desired outcomes is essential for planning future care.
    a. Patient is comfortable, with anxiety at a manageable level.
    b. Patient's immediate needs have been met.
    c. All required documentation is in place.

DOCUMENTATION

17. Document the assessment. **R:** Documenting all parts of the admission process is essential for legal records. The baseline assessment serves as a reference throughout the period of care. The record of care of personal effects may need to be consulted, especially if an item is reported lost or missing.
18. Complete other required forms. You may be responsible for a variety of other records (notifying the dietary department, starting a nursing plan of care and medication record, filling out forms that indicate the acuity of the patient, and so forth). Consult the procedure book at each facility to determine which forms are your responsibility. **R:** A variety of forms are available for recording both subjective and objective data.

TRANSFER

Some transfers within the hospital are part of an expected progression of care. For example, the surgical patient is transferred from an admitting unit to the operating room, then to the postanesthesia recovery unit, and then to a patient care unit. These standard transfers usually are guided by well-established protocols and procedures. Other transfers are unexpected. For example, the patient begins to develop a cardiac complication and must be immediately transferred to the cardiac care unit. Both the sending unit and the receiving unit have responsibilities in this process. Still other transfers are initiated for convenience or preference, such as the patient who desires to move to a private room. In all cases, the nurse must ensure the well-being of the patient and also communicate effectively with other departments.

PROCEDURE FOR TRANSFER

ASSESSMENT

1. Assess the patient in regard to current problems and medical conditions. **R:** Assessment establishes the patient's functional abilities.
2. Review the **protocol** or the physician's order for a transfer. **R:** This determines that the transfer is appropriate at this time. Protocols outline the criteria for standard transfers. In other instances, the physician determines when the patient's medical needs can be better met in another environment. In an emergency, the nurse may consult with a supervisor and move the patient to a more intensive care setting.

ANALYSIS

3. Critically think through your data, carefully evaluating each aspect and its relation to other data. **R:** To determine whether this patient meets the protocol for transfer or the patient's condition is as expected by the physician who wrote the transfer order.
4. Identify specific problems and modifications of the procedure needed for this individual. **R:** Specific problems may necessitate development of individualized plans for the transfer process.

PLANNING

5. Determine the individualized desired outcomes of the transfer process. **R:** Identifying outcomes facilitates planning and evaluation.
    a. Patient's anxiety is at a manageable level.
    b. Patient experiences continuity of care.
6. Contact the receiving unit. **R:** To ensure that unit staff are ready to care for the patient.
7. Plan the transport method, such as a wheelchair or a stretcher. Some patients may be transferred in their beds under certain conditions. **R:** Planning ahead ensures a smooth and organized transfer.

IMPLEMENTATION

Action	Rationale
8. Wash or disinfect your hands.	To decrease the transfer of microorganisms that could cause infection.
9. Obtain the needed transport, such as a wheelchair or stretcher and transfer device.	To save time and promote efficiency.

(continued)

Action	Rationale
10. Obtain the patient's **chart** if it is a written (paper) record.	The receiving unit will need the record to ensure continuity of care.
11. Identify the patient, using two identifiers.	Verifying the patient's identity helps ensure that you are transferring the correct patient.
12. Explain the transfer process.	Explaining the process helps relieve anxiety or misperceptions that the patient may have and sets the stage for patient participation.
13. Move the patient to the wheelchair or stretcher. Make sure that all equipment is positioned appropriately. When equipment is new to you, be sure to consult with your instructor to determine how it must be transported. Transport the patient to the new unit.	Medical devices and equipment must be transported with the patient to ensure continuity of care. Some devices must remain functional during transport, and others may be disconnected.
14. On arrival, notify the nurse that the patient has arrived.	The care of the patient must be transferred to the responsible person.
15. Transfer the patient into the new bed, and orient the patient if necessary.	The new environment may create anxiety, and explanations will help reassure the patient.
16. Wash or disinfect your hands.	To decrease the transfer of microorganisms that could cause infection.
17. Give a report on the patient's condition to the nurse responsible for the patient.	To ensure continuity of care.

EVALUATION

18. Evaluate using the individualized patient outcomes previously identified. **R:** Evaluation in relation to desired outcomes is essential for planning future care.
    a. Patient's anxiety is at a manageable level.
    b. Patient experiences continuity of care.

DOCUMENTATION

19. Complete documentation. **R:** Documentation is a legal record of the patient's care and therapy and communicates nursing activities to other nurses and caregivers.
    a. Final assessment of the patient
    b. Means of transfer
    c. Receiving unit (Fig. 16-3)
    d. Forms to other departments indicating the transfer; include
       (1) admitting department
       (2) telephone switchboard and information desk
       (3) dietary department
       (4) pharmacy

DISCHARGE

Ideally the nurse begins planning for the patient's discharge as early as admission. This ensures that when the actual time of discharge arrives, many plans for aftercare have been completed. However, no business documents or final papers are started until the discharge order is written and the precise time of discharge is determined. If you have been told verbally that a patient is to be discharged but the order has not yet been written, you may sometimes order take-home medications and make transportation arrangements in anticipation of the order so that the patient's departure is not delayed.

Note: Most facilities have a **discharge planner** who is the professional who takes primary responsibility for planning for referrals needed, such as home care or nursing home placement, and assists with locating resources for care such as equipment for home care.

Occasionally, a patient becomes disgruntled or impatient and demands to leave the facility without the physician's order for discharge. If the patient leaves under these circumstances, the discharge is identified as **AMA** (against medical advice). The patient certainly has

Original Copy Goes To Receiving Facility – Xerox Copy To Be Retained In Patient Record – Attach Xerox Copy Of Patient Admittance Sheet.

Patient's Last Name	First Name	MI
Hogan	*Susan*	*T*

Address, City, State, Zip Code	Phone
1018 Alder St., Blaine, OR 87453	*(503) 788-1011*

Date of Birth	Age	Sex	Marital Status	Church
1-18-59	*46*	*F*	S ⓜ W D Sep.	*C*

Relative or Guardian (specify relationship) name, address   Phone
Jeff   *husb.*   *same*

PHYSICIANS ORDERS

Attending Physician: *Wm. Hawkins, M.D.*

Consulting Physician(s): *Tom Andrews, M.D.*

Physician after transfer: *Donna Wilson, M.D.*

Admitting Diagnosis:

Discharge Diagnosis:
  Primary: *Multiple Sclerosis*

  Secondary: Ⓡ *hip pressure ulcer, stage II*

Course of Treatment: attach copy of Physician's Discharge Summary.
  see attached

Name and Address of Facitlity Transferring:

From: *Mountain View Hospital*

To: *Coast Conval. Center*   Pt. Hosp. No. *6402573*

Family Informed Of Transfer	Yes ☑	No ☐
Does patient know diagnosis	Yes ☑	No ☐
Does family know diagnosis	Yes ☑	No ☐

Date of telephone referral: *5/19* Adm. Date: *4/16* Discharge Date: *5/21/06*

Previous Hospitalization and/or Nursing Home Stay (Within last 90 days):
  none

Health Insurance Info: Soc. Sec. No. *000-00-0000*

  Medicare ———   Medicaid ———

  Other *Loggers Int.*

Any significant changes from intital H & P   ☐ Yes   ☑ No
If Yes, changes are:

MEDICATION ORDER FOR RECEIVING FACILITY   (If PRN, state reason for giving and max, amt. to be given. List discontinuation date, if any, on all medications ordered) Note: Any brand or form of drug identical in form and content may be dispensed unless checked here: ☐

  Ibuprofen 400 mg. PRN for pain

  Multivit. ī daily

  Docusate 100 mg. B.I.D.

DIET ☑ Regular ☐ Sodium Restriction, _____ gm. ☐ Salt Substitute _____ ☐ Diabetic,____calories ☐ Low Residue ☐ Bland

  ☐ Mechanical ☐ Soft ☐ Tube, ____cc per _____hr ☐ Dietary Supplement _____ ☑ Other *added fiber*

ALLERGIES ☑ No ☐ Yes   Type: _____

SPECIAL TREATMENTS (Including Physical Therapy, Speech, O.T., etc.) Specify frequency.

  ↑ *oral fluids to 2600 ml/day*   *Dressing – Opsite over pressure ulcer, change as needed.*

  special air mattress   *saline soaks q. d.*

  assist pt. to turn frequently when in bed.   *Physical therapy: Evaluation and exercises to increase mobility.*

ACTIVITY ORDERS (List activity level, restrictions and/or precautions, etc.)

  Increase activity level – assist with cane walking.

REHABILITATION POTENTIAL   (Describe the highest level of independent, functioning the patient can be expected to achieve.)
  ☐ Independent   Semi-independent: ☑ Assistance for few activities   ☐ Assistance for most activities

ADDITIONAL COMMENTS: *Outcomes — Maintain skin integrity, possible remission of M.S.*

Certification ☑ I certify that post hospital skilled nursing care is medically necessary on a continuing basis for any of the conditions for which he/she received care during this hospitalization. ☐ I certify that my above orders regarding home health services (skilled nursing care, therapy, or others as defined) are medically necessary because my patient is confined to home. These services are related to the condition(s) for which he/she received inpatient hospital or SNF care.

Signature of Physician *Wm. A. Hawkins* _____ MD   Phone: *732-8017*   Date: *5/19/06*

PATIENT TRANSFER FORM

FIGURE 16-3 A narrative note reflecting transfer to another unit.

the legal right to leave at any time, and refusing to allow the patient to leave would be considered false imprisonment. However, the nurse has an obligation to communicate with the patient to try to alleviate the concern and help the patient understand the need for hospitalization. The nurse can also facilitate the patient's communication with the physician.

PROCEDURE FOR DISCHARGE

ASSESSMENT

1. Check for a discharge order. **R:** Orders verify that the patient has been discharged by the medical provider.
2. Perform a final assessment. **R:** Final assessment describes the patient's condition upon leaving and ensures that untoward changes have been identified.
   a. Physical status
   b. Emotional status
3. Assess for the patient's ability to continue self-care and possible need for continued health supervision. **R:** To facilitate post-discharge care planning.

ANALYSIS

4. Critically think through your data, carefully evaluating each aspect and its relation to other data. **R:** To determine whether this patient meets the protocol for discharge, or the condition is as expected by the physician who wrote the discharge order.

5. Identify specific problems and modifications of the procedure needed for this individual. **R:** Specific problems may necessitate development of individualized plans for the discharge process.

PLANNING

6. Determine the individualized desired outcomes of the transfer process. **R:** Identifying outcomes facilitates planning and evaluation.
   a. Patient's condition was stable at the time of discharge.
   b. Patient (or caregiver) was able to explain discharge instructions.
   c. Patient left with all appropriate belongings and supplies.
7. Plan for continuing care including discharge instructions (this planning should start on admission). **R:** To be sure that you have all the information and documentation needed for **referral.** The written discharge instructions are based on the physician's orders for the patient's self-care or care by another if the patient is unable to care for himself or herself.
8. Plan communication of referral information as needed. Final discharge documents may need to be faxed to a receiving facility. **R:** Timely communication ensures uninterrupted quality care.
9. Plan for contacting family or others if needed to arrange transportation. **R:** Most newly discharged patients are not strong enough to manage transportation independently.

IMPLEMENTATION

Action	Rationale
10. Notify family or others who are providing discharge transportation.	Notifying them first ensures that times are coordinated.
11. Wash or disinfect your hands.	To decrease the transfer of microorganisms that could cause infection.
12. Identify the patient, using two identifiers.	Verifying the patient's identity helps ensure that you are discharging the correct patient.
13. Review written home care instructions with the patient and/or the person who will be providing or assisting with care at home. Include diet, activity, medications, treatment, equipment and supplies, symptoms to report to the physician, and any other pertinent instructions (Fig. 16-4).	To be sure that the patient and/or caregivers have the information needed for effective care after discharge.

(continued)

Action	Rationale

HOME CARE INSTRUCTIONS AFTER SURGERY

1. **DISCHARGE PLAN:** **(Please Circle)** ECF   Home Health Agency   Sustaining Care   Other
   Follow-up plan not indicated because: ~~independent~~   ~~family and/or friends will assist~~   refused

2. **DIET:** _Regular_____, Fluid, fiber and fruits in your diet will help prevent constipation. Food rich in protein will aid in wound healing.

3. **ACTIVITY:**   Follow your doctor's instructions regarding activity.
   a. Avoid pushing, pulling, lifting, prolonged standing or sitting until advised by your physician.
   b. Take an hour rest period in the morning and afternoon.
   c. Contact physician prior to driving a car.

4. **MEDICATIONS:**   ~~OWN MEDICATIONS~~_____PHARMACY:_____ ~~PRESCRIPTION:~~_____
   ~~Review Pharmacy~~ handout regarding discharge medications.

   Acetaminophen with oxycodone one – two every four hours if needed for pain.

   Conjugated estrogen 0.625 mg. q. d. (daily)

5. **TREATMENTS/EQUIPMENT AND SUPPLIES:**

   none
   May shower, resume walking to tolerance.

6. **SYMPTOMS TO REPORT TO YOUR DOCTOR:**   Call your doctor with any questions.
   a. Bleeding, drainage, redness or swelling from incisional area.
   b. If feeling chilled or feverish, take temperature and report if over 100.5 degrees.
   c. Nausea and vomiting or abdominal distention.
   d. Pain not relieved by pain medication or rest should be reported to your doctor.
   e. Difficulty with urination - frequency and/or burning.

7. **OTHER INSTRUCTIONS:**
   a. As you increase your activity you may experience some discomfort or moderate pain.
   b. Showers may be taken. Do not tub bathe before checking with doctor.
   c. After gynecological or bladder repairs check with physician prior to resuming intercourse.
   d. Consult with physician if any change from normal bowel functions.

8. **APPOINTMENTS:**   Please call to make appointment.

   With:_Dr. Sue Hancock_____   When: _one week_____

I have received and understand the above instructions:

DATE: _7/2/06_____PATIENT: _Martha Cheavers_____

WITNESS:__Jim Peters, RN_____

PATIENT'S AGENT OR REPRESENTATIVE _____

ADDRESSOGRAPH	MEDICAL CENTER HOSPITAL Seattle, Washington

FIGURE 16-4 A form like this, which contains home care instructions, may be given to a patient upon discharge.

(continued)

Action	Rationale
14. Check and return personal property. Include personal items that are in the patient's room and items that were placed in a safe.	The facility has been the legal guardian of personal property and has an obligation to ensure its return to the patient.
15. Perform business functions. Include business discharge papers; obtain prescriptions and supplies.	The facility is accountable for ensuring that the patient has what is needed to begin self-care.
16. Escort the patient to the door and into the vehicle that is transporting the patient. Some facilities require that the patient be transported to the entrance/exit in a wheelchair for safety.	The facility remains responsible for patients' well-being until they have left the premises.
17. Fax documents to referral agency according to the protocols of the facility.	Referral agencies need the information to begin assuming responsibility for care. Sending of the documents must meet the standards for maintaining confidentiality of the patient's protected health information.

EVALUATION

18. Evaluate using the individualized patient outcomes previously identified. **R:** Evaluation in relation to desired outcomes is essential for planning future care.
   a. Patient's condition was stable at the time of discharge.
   b. Patient (or caregiver) was able to explain discharge instructions.
   c. Patient left with all appropriate belongings and supplies.

DOCUMENTATION

19. Complete a narrative discharge note (if required by the facility) and all special forms for the facility. **R:** Documentation is a legal record of the patient's care and therapy, and discharge forms provide the patient with written directions for care.

■ POTENTIAL ADVERSE OUTCOMES AND RELATED INTERVENTIONS

1. Assessment reveals that the patient has an elevated temperature or other indication of a negative change in status since the discharge order was written.
Intervention: Stop the discharge process, and notify the physician.
2. Loss of personal items.
Intervention: Review the admission record to determine whether the items were placed in a safe, sent home with the family, or kept at the bedside. If kept at the bedside, ask for a second person to double-check closets and drawers for you. Consider whether it is something that could have become entangled in laundry, and ask that the laundry personnel keep unidentified patient items that arrive in their department. Complete appropriate forms indicating missing personal items.

Acute Care

When acute care admissions are planned in advance, the patient may come in several days before the actual admission to complete all business matters and to have any laboratory work completed. The admission assessment and initial plans for care may also be completed at this time. This makes the actual admission less stressful because the patient feels more in control when the environment is more familiar.

The patient with an unexpected admission either for an emergency or acute illness often experiences intense anxiety. The admission process may need to be flexible to meet the acute needs of the patient and the medical or surgical care that is being initiated. The nurse needs to be able to move quickly in completing essential assessment and moving the whole process forward. Anxious family members often accompany the patient, adding to the potential for confusion.

Long-Term Care

The procedures of admission, transfer, and discharge are very important to nurses practicing in long-term care settings. Along with direct admissions from home, many transfers take place between long-term and acute care settings. Residents whose condition requires hospitalization are transferred to hospitals, and chronically ill or recovering patients are transferred from hospitals to long-term care. Increasing numbers of patients are being discharged to long-term care facilities for rehabilitation purposes with home as the eventual destination.

Follow the same principles as those discussed earlier in this module. In the long-term care setting, however, it is essential that you include family members in planning. Clearly communicate information concerning special needs of residents so that the receiving facility is prepared to meet these needs. Close interaction and cooperation between the nursing staffs of the facilities lead to safe and effective care.

Home Care

One of your responsibilities as a nurse is coordinating care between the home and the receiving or discharging facility. Sharing the nursing assessments and other information is crucial to a smooth transition from one setting to another. The hospital-based nurse may be a resource to family members in determining what is important to the client and what support is needed at home. If the client is returning home from a care setting, the nurse can discuss what arrangements need to be made in the home, such as adaptations that will aid the client. A home health nurse may be needed for skilled nursing care in the home. In some cases, the home health nurse will make a visit to the home to assess the environment for care and recommend changes or modifications that will be needed. If being admitted to the hospital or long-term care facility from home, the client needs information regarding what clothing and possessions are appropriate to bring, what to expect in that environment, and what the admission procedures will be.

Ambulatory Care

A nurse in an ambulatory care setting might be responsible for arranging details of a hospital admission for a client who has come to the office or clinic. If this is for a planned surgery or procedure, the nurse may schedule the time and then notify the client of the process. In emergencies, the nurse may arrange for immediate admission and need to explain the process to the client and family members.

LEARNING TOOLS

DEVELOP YOUR BACKGROUND KNOWLEDGE

1. Review the Learning Outcomes.

2. Read the section on admission, transfer, and discharge in your assigned text.

3. Look up the Key Terms in the glossary.

4. Review this module, and mentally practice the processes described. Study so that you would be able to teach these skills to another person.

DEVELOP YOUR SKILLS

1. In the practice setting, select one other student.

2. Alternating, so that each has the opportunity to play the role of the patient, perform each of the following procedures: admission, transfer, and discharge.

DEMONSTRATE YOUR SKILLS

In the clinical setting
1. Consult with your instructor regarding the opportunity to observe or participate in the admission, transfer, or discharge of a patient insofar as you have the skills for care that is needed. Use the Performance Checklists on the CD-ROM in the front of this book as a guide.

2. Evaluate your performance with the instructor.

CRITICAL THINKING EXERCISES

1. Mr. Robert Wagner is scheduled for discharge on the third morning after his cholecystectomy. His surgical wound has an open draining area that will need dressing changes. He will have a prescription for pain medication and an oral antibiotic to take at home. He is to make an appointment to see his physician at the beginning of the next week. Identify the major concerns for this man's self-care at home. How might the nurse facilitate appropriate home care for this patient?

2. Margaret Wilson has resided in a special care unit for those with Alzheimer's disease for almost 1 year. This morning, she collapsed and was found to have

paralysis on her left side. The physician ordered her transfer via ambulance to the hospital for diagnosis and treatment of a possible cerebral vascular accident (brain attack or stroke). What unique problems may this transfer present? What are the special concerns that the nurse should communicate to the admitting hospital? What steps should the nurse take to ensure a smooth transition in this transfer?

3. If you are caring for a patient who demands to leave without a physician's order, what actions should you take? Why?

SELF-QUIZ
SHORT-ANSWER QUESTIONS

1. What is the title of the professional within some facilities whose task it is to facilitate continuity of care after discharge?

_____

2. Identify a patient situation that should be reported to the physician because it requires that discharge be delayed.

_____

3. What is the purpose of teaching the patient and family before discharge?

_____

4. What is the purpose of doing a preliminary brief assessment when first encountering the patient being admitted?

_____

MULTIPLE CHOICE

_____ 5. The first thing you should do when admitting a patient is
   a. orient the patient to the unit.
   b. determine and meet the patient's immediate needs.
   c. measure TPR and BP.
   d. make a baseline assessment.

_____ 6. When orienting a patient to the environment, which of the following are necessary? (Choose all that apply.)
   a. The location of the utility room and kitchenette
   b. How to call a nurse
   c. The location of the bathroom
   d. How to operate the bed

_____ 7. If a patient is very anxious on admission, you should

   a. hurry as quickly as possible.
   b. go slowly to provide calm as you follow the usual routine.
   c. omit as many routine items as possible.
   d. continue with the admission procedure as usual.

_____ 8. If a volunteer is available to assist with admission, which task could most appropriately be delegated to him or her?
   a. Baseline assessment
   b. Determining immediate needs
   c. Orientation to the unit
   d. Documenting data

_____ 9. Which of the following should you consider if you are transferring a patient to another unit? (Choose all that apply.)
   a. Continuing care
   b. Patient teaching
   c. Care of belongings
   d. Final assessment

_____ 10. A patient has a very valuable ring. You should suggest that
   a. the patient wear it.
   b. the patient hide it well in the suitcase.
   c. it be kept at the nursing station.
   d. it be placed in the facility safe.

_____ 11. Which of the following are usually nursing responsibilities related to transfer? (Choose all that apply.)
   a. Planning transfer of needed equipment
   b. Teaching the patient about medications
   c. Making a final assessment
   d. Making sure the patient's property is also transferred

_____ 12. Which of the following are usually nursing responsibilities related to discharge? (Choose all that apply.)
   a. Planning for transportation
   b. Teaching the patient about medications
   c. Making a final assessment
   d. Making sure that the patient's personal property is sent along

_____ 13. Which of the following patients are likely to need a referral to provide continuing care after discharge? (Choose all that apply.)
   a. One who had a routine appendectomy
   b. One who had a stroke and has right-side paralysis
   c. One who had acute respiratory infection
   d. One with a new colostomy

Answers to the Self-Quiz questions appear in the back of this book.

Assisting With Diagnostic and Therapeutic Procedures

SKILLS INCLUDED IN THIS MODULE

General Procedure for Assisting With Diagnostic and Therapeutic Procedures
Specific Procedures for Assisting With Diagnostic and Therapeutic Procedures
Procedure for Assisting With Thoracentesis
Procedure for Assisting With Paracentesis
Procedure for Assisting With Lumbar Puncture (Spinal Tap)
Procedure for Assisting With Liver Biopsy
Procedure for Assisting With Bone Marrow Aspiration and Biopsy
Procedure for Assisting With Proctoscopy, Sigmoidoscopy, and Colonoscopy

PREREQUISITE MODULES

Module 1	An Approach to Nursing Skills
Module 2	Documentation
Module 3	Basic Body Mechanics
Module 4	Basic Infection Control
Module 5	Safety in the Healthcare Environment
Module 6	Moving the Patient in Bed and Positioning
Module 11	Assessing Temperature, Pulse, and Respiration
Module 12	Measuring Blood Pressure
Module 14	Nursing Physical Assessment
Module 15	Collecting Specimens and Performing Common Laboratory Tests

The following modules may be needed in some situations:

Module 24	Basic Sterile Technique: Sterile Field and Sterile Gloves
Module 44	Administering Oral Medications
Module 47	Preparing and Maintaining Intravenous Infusions
Module 48	Administering Intravenous Medications

KEY TERMS

ascites	lumbar puncture
biopsy	(spinal tap)
bone marrow	paracentesis
cerebrospinal	proctoscopy
fluid	sigmoidoscopy
colonoscopy	stopcock
endoscope	stylet
hypovolemic	supine position
shock	thoracentesis
liver biopsy	trocar

OVERALL OBJECTIVES

▸ To assist with diagnostic and therapeutic procedures, with emphasis on the preparation and support of patients.
▸ To properly handle specimens obtained.

LEARNING OUTCOMES

The student will be able to

1. Assess the patient's understanding of the procedure, ability to cooperate, anxiety level, and comfort level before, during, and after the procedure.
2. Analyze assessment data to determine the need for further information and pre- and post-procedure medication.
3. Determine appropriate patient outcomes, and recognize the potential for adverse outcomes.
4. Provide information about the procedure to the patient.
5. Select appropriate equipment for the procedure.
6. Position the patient appropriately for the procedure.
7. Assist with the specific procedure according to facility policies.
8. Properly handle the specimen collected.
9. Provide patient support before, during, and after the procedure.
10. Evaluate the patient's response to the procedure.
11. Document the type of procedure, specimen collected, and patient response to the procedure in the patient's record as appropriate.

A variety of procedures are used not only to obtain specimens for laboratory testing but also to treat patients. To assist effectively, the nurse must know the rationale for the procedure and test(s) involved, how the procedure is performed, the necessary teaching and preparation of the patient, appropriate methods of obtaining and handling specimens, and how to care for the patient after the procedure. Information obtained through these procedures may be the key to the diagnosis and therapeutic decisions for the patients concerned.

Not only do physicians perform the procedures described, they also provide the information needed for the patient to give informed consent for the procedure. The nurse, however, usually assumes responsibility for obtaining the patient's signature on a consent form, gathering the equipment, preparing the patient, supporting the patient during the procedure, and caring for the patient after the procedure. In addition, the nurse may assist in collecting tissue specimens and ensuring that they are sent for testing in the appropriate manner.

In some instances, an advanced practice nurse (APN) may perform the procedure. In this module, the person performing the procedure will be referred to as the "physician" for ease and clarity.

NURSING DIAGNOSES

Patients undergoing diagnostic testing may have a variety of nursing diagnoses related to the actual procedure, why it is being done, and restrictions following the procedure. Examples are

- Anxiety related to lack of knowledge about the procedure, fear of unwelcome diagnosis and treatment, or perceived necessary changes in lifestyle
- Deficient Knowledge related to unfamiliar procedure
- Acute Pain related to tissue trauma from an invasive procedure

DELEGATION

Assisting with diagnostic and therapeutic procedures may be delegated to assistive personnel when the patient is stable and when the policies and procedures in the facility so indicate. Assistive personnel must have knowledge about appropriate positioning and about observations that must be made before, during, and after the procedure. They must also know which observations must be reported to the nurse. The nurse retains the responsibility for supervision and must know that the assistive person has the skills and experience required for assisting with the procedure. Many of these procedures require the ability to maintain sterile technique, and that is not usually taught to or delegated to assistive personnel.

GENERAL PROCEDURE FOR ASSISTING WITH DIAGNOSTIC AND THERAPEUTIC PROCEDURES

The instructions in the general procedure that follows include the fundamental nursing actions needed to appropriately assist with diagnostic procedures. The specific procedures that follow the general procedure call for the nurse to use many steps of the general procedure and to vary others. The steps of the general procedure are numbered sequentially. They are grouped according to the steps of the nursing process.

ASSESSMENT

1. Check the physician's order. **R:** To be sure of the exact procedure to be done and to identify the purpose of the procedure.
2. Check to be sure that a consent form has been signed, if this is necessary. **R:** A patient must give informed consent for any procedure. When the procedure is invasive and has possible adverse consequences, a written form must be signed and placed in the patient's record. Although informing the patient is the physician's responsibility, in many facilities, the nurse obtains the signature on the form and witnesses it. This does not transfer the responsibility for informed consent from the physician to the nurse. In other facilities, the nurse prepares the form for the physician to present to the patient when information is being given. Follow the procedure in your facility.
3. Assess the patient for the ability to assume and maintain the appropriate position for the procedure. **R:** To enable the planning of alternatives if necessary.
4. Assess the need for premedication. **R:** Premedication may decrease the patient's anxiety and the pain experienced during the procedure.

ANALYSIS

5. Critically think through your data, carefully evaluating each aspect and its relation to other data. **R:** To determine specific problems for this individual in relation to the procedure.
6. Identify specific problems and modifications of the procedure needed for this individual. **R:** Planning for the individual must consider the individual's problems.

PLANNING

7. Determine individualized patient outcomes in relation to the diagnostic or therapeutic procedure being done. **R:** Identification of outcomes guides planning and evaluation. Include the following:
   a. The procedure is performed and a specimen, if needed, is obtained.
   b. The patient's physiological responses, such as temperature, pulse, respiration, and blood pressure, remain stable.
   c. The patient's psychological responses, such as anxiety or distress, remain manageable.
   d. The patient is comfortable before, during, and after the procedure.
8. Obtain the appropriate equipment and gloves to protect you from contact with body secretions. Check the contents of any prepared tray to identify if some items must be obtained separately. **R:** Planning ahead allows you to proceed more safely and effectively.

IMPLEMENTATION

Action	Rationale
9. Wash or disinfect your hands.	To decrease the transfer of microorganisms that could cause infection.
10. Identify the patient, using two identifiers.	Verifying the patient's identity helps ensure that the correct procedure is being done for the right patient.
11. Discuss the procedure with the patient. At this time, determine what the physician told the patient and how well the patient understands the information provided.	Explaining the procedure helps relieve anxiety and misperceptions that the patient may have about the procedure.

(continued)

Action	Rationale
Clarify concerns, and explain how the procedure will affect the patient. Avoid graphic descriptions of the procedure. Focus on how the patient will be positioned, what the patient will be asked to do, and what the patient will experience during the procedure. Also emphasize that part of your role is to remain with the patient and help in whatever way is possible.	
12. Obtain any needed supportive devices or assistance.	To save time and promote efficiency.
13. Set up a surface for equipment, and clean the surface if necessary.	For infection control.
14. Premedicate the patient if indicated.	To prepare the patient for the procedure.
15. Position the patient appropriately.	To facilitate the procedure.
16. Drape the patient as needed.	To provide for modesty and warmth.
17. Assist with the procedure (see the specific details for each procedure described below).	
a. Assess the patient throughout the procedure: Observe the patient for adverse signs or reactions to the procedure.	The physician may be preoccupied with performing the procedure, and the nurse can see early signs of impending problems.
(1) Check the patient's pulse and respiration two or three times.	
(2) Ask the patient to tell you about any feelings of distress or peculiar sensations.	
(3) During some procedures, blood pressure may be monitored.	
(4) Notify the physician promptly of any unusual signs.	
b. Reassure the patient, and assist the patient to maintain the appropriate positioning throughout the procedure.	To decrease anxiety during the procedure and maintain the sterile field.
c. Assist with the procedure, providing equipment as needed. Use gloves appropriately.	To decrease the possibility of contamination of the sterile field. Wear gloves if contact with body fluids is likely.

(continued)

Action	Rationale
18. Conclude the procedure:	
a. Restore the patient to a comfortable position or to the ordered therapeutic position, and place the call signal within reach.	To promote comfort and patient safety following the procedure.
b. Dispose of used equipment in the appropriate biohazard waste containers.	To prevent accidental penetrating injuries and contact with contaminated substances.
c. Label and properly care for any specimen obtained. Send the specimen to the laboratory promptly.	Proper handling of laboratory specimens is critical for accurate test results. Prompt delivery to the laboratory reduces the possibility of misplacement of the specimen.
19. Remove gloves, and wash or disinfect your hands.	To decrease the transfer of microorganisms that could cause infection.

EVALUATION

20. Evaluate using the individualized patient outcomes previously identified. **R:** Evaluation in relation to desired outcomes is essential for planning future care. Include the following:
   a. The procedure is performed, and a specimen, if needed, is obtained.
   b. The patient's physiological responses, such as temperature, pulse, respiration, and blood pressure, remain stable.
   c. The patient's psychological responses, such as anxiety or distress, remain manageable.
   d. The patient is comfortable before, during, and after the procedure.

DOCUMENTATION

21. Document the procedure in the patient's record according to facility policy. Include the procedure, the patient's response, and the disposition of any specimen. **R:** Documentation supports continuity of care and enables the entire healthcare team to provide care.

■ POTENTIAL ADVERSE OUTCOMES AND RELATED INTERVENTIONS

1. The patient experiences extreme pain.
Intervention: Reassess the patient. Determine the cause and location of the pain. Determine if additional pain medication is indicated, and administer as ordered by the physician.
  2. The patient exhibits pallor, diaphoresis, and dyspnea.
Intervention: Inform the physician immediately. Check the patient's pulse, respirations, blood pressure, and blood oxygen level (with pulse oximeter). Administer oxygen if indicated.
  3. The patient bleeds after the procedure is completed. *Note:* For these procedures, the small amount of bleeding that results should quickly stop when pressure is applied after the procedure. Bleeding should not begin again.
Intervention: Apply pressure as appropriate, and inform the physician.

SPECIFIC PROCEDURES FOR ASSISTING WITH DIAGNOSTIC AND THERAPEUTIC PROCEDURES

For each procedure discussed, some steps in the General Procedure may be modified. Table 17-1 provides a quick overview of each of the procedures.

Procedure for Assisting With Thoracentesis

A **thoracentesis** is a sterile procedure involving the insertion of a large-bore needle or a **trocar** (a large, sharp metal device that allows insertion of a tube) into the pleural space of the chest. This may be done to remove air or fluid from the pleural space, to enable insertion of a chest tube, or to inject medication. Fluid that is removed from the chest may be sent to the laboratory for analysis of content and cells or for culture and sensitivity.

table 17-1. Overview of Common Diagnostic and Therapeutic Procedures

Test	Specimen	Preparing the Patient	Positioning the Patient	Role of the Nurse	Special Observations Concerning the Patient	Handling the Specimen
Thoracentesis	Fluid from pleural cavity	Explain. Warn patient not to cough or move suddenly during procedure. **R:** Or needle may puncture lungs.	Sitting position with arms over head or in front of chest. **R:** The objective is to increase the size of the intercostal spaces.	Reassure patient. Assist physicians by setting up equipment, measuring fluid, and cleaning up.	Respiratory distress (cyanosis, dyspnea). Blood-tinged sputum. Monitor for 4–8 h after procedure for signs of respiratory distress or shock.	Specimen is sterile. Send to laboratory immediately.
Paracentesis	Ascitic fluid	Explain. Have patient void before procedure to prevent puncture of bladder.	Sitting position	Reassure patient. Assist physician by setting up equipment, measuring fluid, and cleaning up.	Signs of shock. Monitor vital signs for 4–8 h after procedure.	Specimen is sterile. Send to laboratory immediately.
Spinal tap	Cerebrospinal fluid (CSF)	Explain procedure.	On side with back near edge of bed, knees brought up, head forward on chest, or sitting on edge of bed	Assist patient to maintain position. Be reassuring. Assist physician by setting up equipment, holding and labeling tubes for specimens, and cleaning up.	Signs of shock, nausea, and vomiting. Headache occasionally. Physician may order patient to lie flat for 1–24 h after procedure. Monitor for motion and sensation in lower extremities.	Specimen is sterile, usually in several tubes. Be sure to number tubes sequentially (tube 1, tube 2, and so on). Send to laboratory immediately.
Liver biopsy	Liver tissue	Explain. Patient must remain still during procedure.	Supine position	Reassure patient. Assist physically.	Bleeding is the most serious complication. The patient lies on the biopsy site to apply pressure and prevent bleeding. Monitor blood pressure and pulse.	The core of tissue is placed in a container with a preservative and sent to the pathology department for examination.
Bone marrow aspiration or bone marrow biopsy	Bone marrow tissue	Explain. The patient may hear a distressing noise. The procedure will include a local anesthetic but will still be uncomfortable.	Supine for sternal site; abdomen or side for iliac crest site	Reassure patient. Assist by providing supplies and equipment.	Bleeding is a major concern. Put pressure on the site for 5 min after the procedure. Monitor pulse and blood pressure.	The aspirated bone marrow or the core of bone marrow tissue is placed in a container with preservative and sent to the laboratory immediately.
Proctoscopy, sigmoidoscopy, or colonoscopy	The inside of the colon; biopsy may be done.	Explain. Assist physician.	Knee-chest position or left lateral position	Reassure patient. Assist with equipment.	The patient may be somewhat weak and dizzy.	Any specimen is placed in a container with preservative and sent to the laboratory immediately.

ASSESSMENT

1-2. Follow steps 1 and 2 of the General Procedure: Check the order, and check to be sure a consent form has been signed.

3. Assess the patient's ability to sit upright during the procedure. **R:** The patient must sit upright so that the pull of gravity will consolidate the chest fluid in the lower portion of the affected lung.

4. Assess the need for premedication. **R:** Premedications for thoracentesis are usually for pain control, sedation, or cough-suppressant effects.

ANALYSIS

5-6. Follow steps 5 and 6 of the General Procedure: Think through your data, and identify specific problems and modifications.

PLANNING

7. Determine individualized patient outcomes in relation to the thoracentesis. Include the following:

   a. The procedure is performed, and a specimen, if needed, is obtained.

   b. The patient's physiological responses, such as pulse, respiration, and blood pressure, remain stable.

   c. The patient's psychological responses, such as anxiety or distress, remain manageable.

   d. The patient is comfortable before, during, and after the procedure.

8. Obtain the necessary equipment.

   a. Read the label of prepared trays. **R:** This is to determine if anything needs to be added. A sterile thoracentesis set typically contains all needed equipment and is disposable.

   b. You may need to add the following:

     (1) sterile gloves in the size appropriate for the physician doing the procedure

     (2) a basin to receive large quantities of the fluid being removed

     (3) an injectable local anesthetic

     (4) if a chest tube is to be inserted, a chest drainage set and a chest tube (see Module 35)

IMPLEMENTATION

Action	Rationale
9-14. Follow steps 9 to 14 of the General Procedure: Wash or disinfect your hands, identify the patient (two identifiers), discuss the procedure with the patient, obtain needed supportive devices or assistance, set up a surface for equipment, and premedicate the patient if indicated.	
15. Assist the patient to an appropriate sitting position:	The sitting position provides access to the base of the lungs on the back. The side-lying position ensures that the diaphragm is dependent (Fig. 17-1).
a. The patient may sit on the edge of the bed, leaning on an overbed table or may straddle a chair, and lean on its back. Pad the back of the chair or the overbed table for comfort.	
b. If the patient is weak, another person may need to provide support throughout the procedure.	
c. In some instances, positioning the patient on the unaffected side may be satisfactory.	

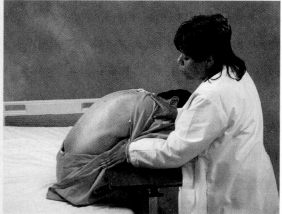

FIGURE 17-1 The patient can sit on the side of the bed for a thoracentesis and the nurse can provide a table for support.

(continued)

Action	Rationale
16. Drape the patient so that the back is exposed.	This facilitates access to the intercostal spaces.
17. Assist with the procedure:	
a. Open the necessary equipment, and set up the sterile field.	This is to prepare for the procedure.
b. Assess the patient especially for skin color, respiratory status, chest pain, and diaphoresis.	The sudden appearance of pallor (seen as a graying in those with dark skin), dyspnea (shortness of breath), cough, chest pain, or diaphoresis (sweating) may indicate that the needle is irritating or even puncturing the pleura. Inform the physician immediately if you observe these signs.
c. Provide the patient with psychological support. If the patient is uncomfortable, reassure him or her that the discomfort will be brief. Tell the patient what is about to take place, and give clear instructions about ways to help. ("Please try not to move for the next few minutes so that we can get the test done quickly.") You may offer to hold the patient's hand for reassurance.	This is for psychological comfort. Patients feel less anxious if they know what is going to happen and how they can help.
d. Be prepared to hold the basin or set up the chest drainage if indicated. The equipment is sterile, and the physician will handle it with sterile-gloved hands.	This is to avoid contamination.
e. The physician will perform the thoracentesis including these steps:	Performing the thoracentesis is a medical procedure.
(1) Clean the area with antiseptic.	
(2) Anesthetize the area using a local anesthetic.	
(3) Insert a 16- or 17-gauge needle with a **stylet** into the pleural space at the level of the seventh intercostal space.	
(4) Remove the stylet, and attach a large syringe with a three-way **stopcock** to the needle (to aspirate fluid from the chest).	
(5) Withdraw the needle (after the fluid has been removed), and place an occlusive dressing over the thoracentesis site.	

(continued)

Action	Rationale
18. Conclude the procedure:	
a. Restore the patient to a comfortable position (semi-Fowler's position is usually used), and place the call signal within reach.	Semi-Fowler's position promotes more effective chest expansion and ventilation. Having the call signal within reach provides for patient safety.
b. Plan a period of undisturbed rest for the patient.	The removal of a large amount of fluid from the chest can result in weakness and fatigue caused by the shift in fluid distribution.
c. Label the specimen, and send it to the laboratory promptly.	Proper handling of specimens is necessary for accurate test results.
d. Dispose of equipment properly. Make sure needles and trocar are discarded in the "sharps" container.	Contaminated articles should be placed in the appropriate biohazard waste containers.
19. Remove gloves if worn, and wash or disinfect your hands.	This is to decrease the transfer of microorganisms that could cause infection.

EVALUATION

20. Follow step 20 of the General Procedure: Evaluate using the individualized patient outcomes previously identified. Include the following:
a. The procedure is performed, and a pleural fluid specimen, if needed, is obtained.
b. The patient's physiologic responses, such as temperature, pulse, respiratory status, and blood pressure, remain stable.
c. The patient's psychological responses, such as anxiety or distress, remain manageable.
d. The patient is comfortable before, during, and after the procedure.

DOCUMENTATION

21. Follow step 21 of the General Procedure: Document the procedure; a brief description of the patient's physiological responses, psychological responses, and comfort; and the disposition of any specimen in the patient's record.

Procedure for Assisting With Paracentesis

A **paracentesis** is the insertion of a large-bore needle or a trocar through the wall of the abdomen into the abdominal cavity to remove fluid (**ascites**) or instill a solution. It is a sterile procedure. A specimen of fluid may be sent to the laboratory for analysis.

ASSESSMENT

1-2. Follow steps 1 and 2 of the General Procedure: Check the physician's order, and check to be sure a consent form has been signed.
3. Assess the patient's ability to sit upright. **R:** The patient usually sits on the edge of the bed for this procedure. Some patients may be unable to do this without assistance. In some cases, it may be possible for the patient to remain in a **supine position,** with the head of the bed elevated. These positions consolidate the fluid in the lower portion of the abdomen.
4. Follow step 4 of the General Procedure: Assess the need for premedication.

ANALYSIS

5-6. Follow steps 5 and 6 of the General Procedure: Think through your data, and identify specific problems and modifications.

PLANNING

7. Determine individualized patient outcomes in relation to the paracentesis. Include the following:
a. The procedure is performed, and a specimen of peritoneal fluid, if needed, is obtained.
b. The patient's physiologic responses, such as pulse, respiration, and blood pressure, remain stable.
c. The patient's psychological responses, such as anxiety or distress, remain manageable.
d. The patient is comfortable before, during, and after the procedure.

8. Obtain the necessary equipment:
   a. Read the label of prepared trays. **R:** This is to determine items that need to be added. A disposable paracentesis set is usually used for this procedure.
   b. You may need to add the following:

   (1) sterile gloves in the appropriate size for the physician
   (2) a large basin or container to hold any fluid removed
   (3) a topical anesthetic agent

IMPLEMENTATION

Action	Rationale
9-14. Follow steps 9 to 14 of the General Procedure: Wash or disinfect your hands, identify the patient (two identifiers), discuss the procedure with the patient, obtain needed supportive devices or assistance, set up a surface for equipment, and premedicate the patient if indicated.	
15. Have the patient void, and measure the abdominal girth before the procedure begins.	This empties the bladder and confines it to the pelvis to prevent accidental bladder perforation during the procedure. It also provides a pre-procedure measure of girth to compare with post-procedure measurement.
16. Assist the patient to a sitting position on the edge of the bed. The patient may need assistance to maintain this position or may be permitted to remain in a supine position with the head of the bed elevated.	These positions consolidate the fluid in the lower portion of the abdomen.
17. Drape the patient's back and legs.	To provide warmth and comfort.
18. Assist with the procedure:	
a. Set up the equipment on a convenient surface; arrange the sterile field.	To prepare for the procedure.
b. Observe the patient for pallor, dizziness, faintness, diaphoresis, rapid pulse and respirations. Assess the patient's blood pressure at 15-minute intervals.	These signs and symptoms can indicate an adverse response to the sudden removal of abdominal pressure from the fluid and the consequent movement of a large quantity of blood into the abdominal circulation. This change in blood flow may create a systemic lack of blood supply and a condition called **hypovolemic shock.**
c. Reassure the patient, and try to relieve anxiety throughout the procedure.	This adds to the patient's psychological comfort. Knowing what to expect and what to do decreases the patient's anxiety.
d. Provide assistance for the physician as needed.	A specimen of the fluid removed may be sent to the laboratory for analysis. It should be sent promptly to prevent the specimen's deterioration.

(continued)

Action	Rationale
19. Conclude the procedure:	
a. Position the patient in bed in a comfortable position, with the call signal within reach.	To promote the patient's comfort and safety.
b. Allow for an undisturbed rest period for the patient.	The removal of large amounts of fluid from the abdomen can result in weakness and fatigue caused by the shift in body fluid distribution.
c. Restore the unit by clearing away equipment.	To promote patient comfort.
d. Label and properly care for any specimen obtained.	Proper handling of laboratory specimens is crucial for accurate test results.
e. Dispose of equipment. Place needles in a "sharps" container. Other contaminated articles should be disposed of in the biohazard waste container.	To prevent accidental penetrating injuries and contact with contaminated substances.
f. Wash or disinfect your hands.	To decrease the transfer of microorganisms that could cause infection.

EVALUATION

20. Follow step 20 of the General Procedure: Evaluate using the individualized patient outcomes previously identified:
   a. The procedure is performed, and a specimen of peritoneal fluid, if needed, is obtained.
   b. The patient's physiologic responses, such as pulse, respiration, and blood pressure, remain stable.
   c. The patient's psychological responses, such as anxiety or distress, remain manageable.
   d. The patient is comfortable before, during, and after the procedure.

DOCUMENTATION

21. Follow step 21 of the General Procedure: Document the procedure, a brief description of the patient's physiological and psychological responses, abdominal girth, and the disposition of any specimen in the patient record and on the intake and output flow sheet as indicated.

Specific Procedure for Assisting With Lumbar Puncture (Spinal Tap)

A **lumbar puncture (spinal tap)** is the introduction of a long needle through the intervertebral space into the subarachnoid space of the spinal canal. This is done to measure the pressure in the subarachnoid space and to collect specimens of **cerebrospinal fluid** (CSF) for examination and diagnosis. The puncture is most commonly performed in the lumbar area.

ASSESSMENT

1-2. Follow steps 1 and 2 of the General Procedure: Check the physician's order, and check to be sure that the patient has signed the consent form.
3. Assess the patient's ability to lie on his or her side in a flexed position. If the patient has arthritis or some other condition that limits the ability to assume this position, consult the physician regarding an alternative position. **R:** Appropriate positioning is necessary to prevent spinal injury during the procedure.
4. Follow step 4 of the General Procedure: Assess the need for premedication.

ANALYSIS

5-6. Follow steps 5 and 6 of the General Procedure: Think through your data, and identify specific problems and modifications.

PLANNING

7. Determine individualized patient outcomes in relation to the lumbar puncture (spinal tap). Include the following:
   a. The procedure is performed, and a specimen of cerebrospinal fluid, if needed, is obtained.

b. The patient's physiological responses, such as pulse, respiration, and blood pressure, remain stable.

c. The patient's psychological responses, such as anxiety or distress, remain manageable.

d. The patient is comfortable before, during, and after the procedure.

8. Obtain the necessary equipment. Read the label of prepared trays. A sterile lumbar puncture tray typically contains all needed equipment and is disposable, but you may need to add sterile gloves in the size appropriate for the physician doing the procedure.

IMPLEMENTATION

Action	Rationale
9-14. Follow steps 9 to 14 of the General Procedure: Wash or disinfect your hands, identify the patient (two identifiers), discuss the procedure with the patient, obtain needed supportive devices or assistance, set up a surface for equipment, and premedicate the patient if indicated.	
15. Position the patient on his or her side with a flat support under the head. Flex the legs and neck, bowing the back toward the side of the bed where the physician will stand or sit (Fig. 17-2).	This keeps the spinal column in horizontal alignment and promotes the flow of spinal fluid. The position of flexion widens the posterior intervertebral spaces.

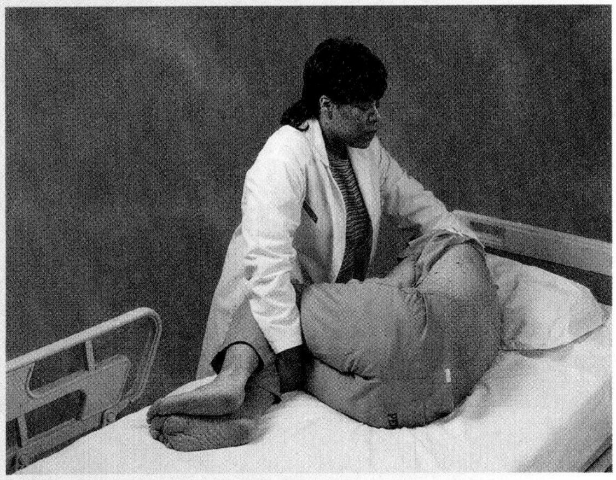

FIGURE 17-2 Nurse holds a patient in position for a lumbar puncture.

Action	Rationale
16. Drape the patient so that the lower spine is exposed, but the rest of the patient is covered.	To provide warmth and privacy.
17. Assist with the procedure.	
a. Open the necessary equipment, and set up the sterile field.	To prepare for the procedure.
b. Assess the patient throughout the procedure. Pay particular attention to comments indicating pain radiating to a leg; sharp, severe back pain; or sudden numbness or tingling of the feet or legs.	The puncture is usually performed below the area where the actual spinal cord is located, but irritation of spinal tissue may create adverse neurologic responses.

(continued)

Action	Rationale
c. Assist the patient to remain still and in the proper position.	The physician will anesthetize the site and then introduce the needle into the subarachnoid space, which is often uncomfortable. It is important that the patient remain still to avoid traumatic injury during the procedure.
d. When the physician attaches the manometer to the needle to measure the pressure, you may be asked to support the top of the manometer to maintain its alignment. If so, be sure you touch only the top.	To prevent contamination of the area that the physician must handle when disconnecting the manometer.
e. If specimens of fluid are needed, you may be asked to hold the tubes while the physician manipulates the manometer. Keep your hands well away from any sterile area.	Maintaining the sterile field prevents introducing microorganisms into the patient.
f. Correctly label the specimens, and send them to the laboratory.	Label the specimens in the order in which they were obtained. Generally, three CSF specimens are obtained; the first and possibly second specimens may be tinged with blood from the puncture itself. The third specimen should be clear; if it is not, this may indicate that the patient's CSF contains blood.
18. Conclude the procedure:	
a. Usually, the patient should remain flat immediately after the procedure and for 4 to 12 hours depending on the physician's directions.	To allow the restoration of spinal fluid before the patient assumes an upright position. This may help to prevent postspinal headache.
b. Encourage the patient to consume increased fluids through a straw.	To restore spinal fluid volume. Drinking through a straw will enable the patient to keep his or her head flat.
c. Restore the unit by clearing away equipment and placing the call signal within reach.	This promotes comfort and patient safety.
d. Label and properly care for any specimen obtained.	Proper handling of specimens is critical for accurate results. Prompt delivery to the laboratory reduces the possibility of misplacement of specimens.
e. Dispose of equipment, placing needles in the "sharps" container and the contaminated articles in the biohazard waste container.	This prevents accidental penetrating injuries and contact with contaminated substances.
19. Remove gloves, and wash and disinfect your hands.	To decrease the transfer of microorganisms.

EVALUATION

20. Follow step 20 of the General Procedure: Evaluate in relation to the individualized outcomes previously identified:
    a. The procedure is performed, and a specimen of cerebrospinal fluid, if needed, is obtained.
    b. The patient's physiological responses, such as pulse, respiration, and blood pressure, remain stable.
    c. The patient's psychological responses, such as anxiety or distress, remain manageable.
    d. The patient is comfortable before, during, and after the procedure.

    Note also any pain, numbness, or tingling in the back and lower extremities. Also evaluate for headache and neurologic changes, including level of consciousness and pupil size. **R:** Postlumbar puncture headaches may occur because of fluid leakage. They are managed with analgesics. Other symptoms may indicate possible spinal nerve irritation, and neurologic changes can indicate possible increased intracranial pressure.

DOCUMENTATION

21. Follow step 21 of the General Procedure: Document in the patient's record a brief description of the procedure, the patient's response, and the disposition of specimens.

Specific Procedure for Assisting With Liver Biopsy

A **liver biopsy** is the removal of a specimen of liver tissue for laboratory examination. It may be done during a surgical procedure when the abdominal cavity is open, but is more commonly done using a fine needle to aspirate tissue for examination. The local anesthetic agent numbs only surface tissue; the entry of the needle into the liver and removal of the liver tissue cause pain.

ASSESSMENT

1-2. Follow steps 1 and 2 of the General Procedure: Check the physician's order, and check to be sure a consent form has been signed.

3. Assess the patient:
    a. Assess the patient's ability to lie still in the supine position during the procedure and in the right lateral position for 2 hours following the procedure. **R:** Lying still is necessary to prevent increased trauma to the liver during the procedure. The position during and post-procedure provides external pressure to control bleeding following the procedure.
    b. Assess the patient's ability to take a deep breath and hold it for a few seconds. **R:** This process will cause the liver to descend and reduces the possibility of a pneumothorax from accidentally puncturing the pleura. It also allows the physician to introduce the biopsy needle into the liver and obtain the tissue specimen.
    c. Assess the patient for risk of bleeding: the use of anticoagulants, prothrombin time, and platelet count. **R:** The liver is vascular and has a high potential for bleeding. These factors will affect the body's clotting ability. Vitamin K may be ordered prior to the biopsy to reduce the risk of bleeding.
4. Follow step 4 of the General Procedure: Assess the need for premedication.

ANALYSIS

5-6. Follow steps 5 and 6 of the General Procedure: Think through your data, and identify specific problems and modifications.

PLANNING

7. Determine individualized patient outcomes in relation to the liver biopsy. Include the following:
    a. The procedure is performed, and a specimen of liver tissue is obtained.
    b. The patient's physiological responses, such as pulse, respiration, and blood pressure, remain stable.
    c. The patient's psychological responses, such as anxiety or distress, remain manageable.
    d. The patient is comfortable before, during, and after the procedure.
8. Obtain the necessary equipment. Read the label of prepared trays. **R:** A prepackaged sterile liver biopsy tray is used for this procedure. Sterile gloves in the appropriate size for the physician may be obtained separately.

IMPLEMENTATION

Action	Rationale
9-14. Follow steps 9 to 14 of the General Procedure: Wash or disinfect your hands, identify the patient (two identifiers), discuss the procedure with the patient, obtain needed supportive devices or	

(continued)

Action	Rationale
assistance, set up a surface for equipment, and premedicate the patient if indicated.	
15. Position the patient in the supine position.	This position helps flatten and expose the liver tissue.
16. Drape the patient so that the lower portion of the patient's chest and the abdomen are exposed.	To facilitate access to the biopsy site and provide for patient privacy.
17. Assist with the procedure:	
a. Assess the patient's vital signs before the procedure.	To establish baseline vital signs. Blood pressure cuff should be left in place in order to monitor blood pressure during the procedure.
b. Reassure the patient, and strive to relieve anxiety throughout the procedure.	The physician will anesthetize a small right subcostal area. The patient is instructed to take a deep breath to lower the diaphragm and push the liver toward the abdomen and hold it while the actual biopsy is being done. This ensures that the liver does not move during insertion. After insertion, the needle is rotated to create a core of tissue inside the biopsy needle, which is then withdrawn.
c. Provide assistance with the procedure as necessary.	Providing assistance allows the physician to proceed more efficiently, decreasing patient distress.
d. Apply pressure over the site.	To control bleeding.
18. Conclude the procedure:	
a. Position the patient on the right side for 1 to 2 hours following the procedure.	The body weight provides continuing pressure to the site to prevent bleeding.
b. Restore the unit by clearing away equipment and placing the call signal within reach.	To promote patient comfort and safety.
c. Label and properly care for any specimen of liver tissue obtained.	The specimen is placed in a preservative solution and promptly sent to the laboratory to ensure accurate results.
19. Dispose of needles in the "sharps" containers. Dispose of contaminated items in the contaminated waste containers.	To prevent accidental penetrating injuries and contact with contaminated substances.

EVALUATION

20. Follow step 20 of the General Procedure: Evaluate using the individualized patient outcomes previously identified:
   a. The procedure is performed, and a specimen of liver tissue is obtained.
   b. The patient's physiological responses, such as pulse, respiration, and blood pressure, remain stable. Measure pulse, respiration, blood pressure, and assess the biopsy site every 15 minutes for the first hour, every 30 minutes for the second hour, every hour for the next 4 hours, and every 4 hours

until stable. **R:** Careful assessment promotes early detection of potential problems. Note, especially, signs of internal bleeding (increased pulse, decreased blood pressure). Bleeding is a rare but potentially serious complication. Liver tissue is very vascular, and internal bleeding may occur from the trauma of the biopsy. If the site becomes infected, peritonitis can occur. This would be evidenced by increased temperature. Also assess breath sounds, and note signs of dyspnea, cyanosis, and restlessness. These are signs of pneumothorax.

  c. The patient's psychological responses, such as anxiety or distress, remain manageable.
  d. The patient is comfortable before, during, and after the procedure.

DOCUMENTATION

21. Follow step 21 of the General Procedure: Document a brief description of the procedure, the patient's response, and the disposition of the specimen in the patient's record. Document assessment of vital signs and biopsy site in the patient's record or on the appropriate flow sheet.

Specific Procedure for Assisting With Bone Marrow Aspiration and Biopsy

A specimen of **bone marrow** may be obtained by aspiration or needle biopsy. The specimen is sent to the laboratory to be examined to establish a diagnosis or to evaluate the patient's response to treatment. In a bone marrow aspiration, marrow is removed through a needle inserted into the marrow cavity of the bone. For a biopsy, a larger bore needle is inserted, and a small, solid core of marrow tissue is obtained. The anterior and posterior iliac crests and the sternum are the most common sites for bone marrow aspiration. The sternum is not usually used for biopsy because it is small and is close to vital organs. The surface tissue is anesthetized, but the patient does feel pressure and a "pulling" sensation when the marrow specimen is removed. In addition, the

puncturing of the bone sounds distressing. For these reasons, a sedative may be given prior to the procedure. When bone marrow is aspirated from a donor for bone marrow transplantation, the marrow is aspirated by needle from multiple sites, and the patient is anesthetized.

ASSESSMENT

1-2. Follow steps 1 and 2 of the General Procedure: Check the physician's order, and check to be sure a consent form has been signed.
3. Assess the patient's ability to cooperate and remain still during the procedure and to assume a lateral position with the knees flexed to provide access to the iliac crest. If the sternal site is used, the patient will lie supine to provide access to the sternum.
4. Follow step 4 of the General Procedure: Assess the need for premedication.

ANALYSIS

5-6. Follow steps 5 and 6 of the General Procedure: Think through your data, and identify specific problems and modifications.
7. Determine individualized patient outcomes in relation to the bone marrow aspiration or biopsy. Include the following:
  a. The procedure is performed, and a specimen of bone marrow is obtained.
  b. The patient's physiological responses, such as pulse, respiration, and blood pressure, remain stable.
  c. The patient's psychological responses, such as anxiety or distress, remain manageable.
  d. The patient is comfortable before, during, and after the procedure.

PLANNING

8. Follow step 8 of the General Procedure: Determine the equipment needed for a bone marrow aspiration and biopsy. A prepackaged sterile tray is usually used for this procedure. Sterile gloves in the appropriate size for the physician may be obtained separately.

IMPLEMENTATION

Action	Rationale
9-14. Follow steps 9 to 14 of the General Procedure: Wash or disinfect your hands, identify the patient (two identifiers), discuss the procedure with the patient, obtain needed supportive devices or assistance, set up a surface for equipment, and premedicate the patient if indicated.	

(continued)

Action	Rationale
15. Position the patient appropriately. If the anterior iliac crest site is to be used, the supine or side-lying position may be used. If the sternal site is to be used, position the patient in the supine position with small pillows beneath the shoulders. When the specimen is obtained from the posterior iliac crest, the patient is placed in either the side-lying or prone position.	To facilitate the procedure.
16. Drape the patient appropriately.	To provide access to the site as well as warmth and comfort for the patient.
17. Assist with the procedure:	
a. Open the pack, and supply sterile gloves. Pour antiseptic solution into a container.	To prepare for the procedure.
b. Assess the patient throughout the procedure.	To identify any problem immediately.
c. Reassure the patient, and maintain a calm environment.	To relieve anxiety throughout the procedure.
d. Assist with the procedure as needed.	You may be asked to hold the specimen containers. If so, be sure not to contaminate the sterile field.
e. After the needle is removed, apply pressure to the site for 5 minutes.	To control the bleeding that occurs. If the patient has a bleeding disorder, you may need to apply pressure for 10 to 15 minutes. In addition, ice packs may be used to increase vasoconstriction and thus control bleeding.
f. In some settings, you will need to apply a pressure dressing and ensure that the patient lies recumbent in bed for 15 to 30 minutes.	To control bleeding and promote patient comfort and safety.
18. Conclude the procedure:	
a. Restore the patient to a comfortable position.	To promote patient comfort.
b. Restore the unit by clearing away equipment and placing the call signal within reach.	To promote patient comfort and safety.
c. Label and properly care for the collected specimen.	The specimen should be placed in a container with preservative and sent to the laboratory immediately for accurate test results.

(continued)

Action	Rationale
d. Dispose of needles in the "sharps" container. Dispose of other articles in the contaminated waste container.	This prevents accidental penetrating injuries and contact with contaminated substances.
19. Follow step 19 of the General Procedure: Remove gloves, and wash and disinfect your hands.	

EVALUATION

20. Follow step 20 of the General Procedure: Evaluate using the individualized patient outcomes previously identified:

  a. The procedure is performed, and a specimen of bone marrow is obtained.

  b. The patient's physiological responses, such as pulse, respiration, and blood pressure, remain stable. Note especially local bleeding at the site.

  c. The patient's psychological responses, such as anxiety or distress, remain manageable.

  d. The patient is comfortable before, during, and after the procedure.

DOCUMENTATION

21. Follow step 21 of the General Procedure: Document a brief description of the procedure, the patient's response, and the disposition of specimens.

Specific Procedure for Assisting With Proctoscopy, Sigmoidoscopy, and Colonoscopy

Various methods are used to view the colon, depending on the extent of visualization needed. A **proctoscopy,** although not as commonly performed today, is the examination of the interior surface of the rectum, using a lighted hollow tube. A **sigmoidoscopy** uses the same principle to examine the interior surface of the bowel as high as the sigmoid colon. A **colonoscopy** involves examination of structures throughout the large intestine. In the sigmoidoscopy and colonoscopy, a flexible fiberoptic **endoscope** is used.

During these examinations, small samples of tissue may be removed (**biopsy**) for laboratory examination, bleeding vessels may be cauterized, and the bowel can be visually examined for abnormalities such as polyps, hemorrhoids, and tumors. The current recommendation for early detection of colon cancer is that persons over age 50 undergo a sigmoidoscopy every 5 years and a colonoscopy every 10 years (American Cancer Society, Inc., 2004). Canadian recommendations are that these tests be included in the "periodic health examination" of asymptomatic individuals of patients over 50 (Canadian Task Force, 2001).

The procedure and position used are uncomfortable and considered embarrassing by most individuals. The more extensive examination, colonoscopy, is the most uncomfortable, although the use of conscious sedation may eliminate this concern. Intravenous access is obtained, and sedation is administered before and during the colonoscopy procedure.

For these procedures, thorough cleansing of the bowel is essential. If feces are present in the bowel, the examiner cannot visualize the tissue. See Module 26 and Module 45 for information about suppositories and other procedures frequently used to cleanse the bowel. Oral laxatives may also be used.

ASSESSMENT

1-2. Follow steps 1 and 2 of the General Procedure: Check the physician's order, and check to be sure a consent form has been signed.

3. Check to see that the appropriate bowel-cleansing regimen has been completed. If it has not been completed or if it has been unsuccessful, notify the physician before proceeding. The patient usually has a liquid diet the day before the examination and is asked to ingest nothing by mouth (NPO) for 8 hours before or from midnight until the examination. **R:** To ensure that the bowel is thoroughly cleansed so the examiner can accurately visualize the tissue. NPO status reduces the likelihood of aspiration of secretions or vomitus during the procedure if sedation is used.

4. Follow step 4 of the General Procedure: Assess the need for premedication.

ANALYSIS

5-6. Follow steps 5 and 6 of the General Procedure: Think through your data, and identify specific problems and modifications.

PLANNING

7. Determine individualized patient outcomes in relation to the proctoscopy, sigmoidoscopy, or colonoscopy. Include the following:

   a. The procedure is performed, and a tissue specimen of any polyp is obtained.

   b. The patient's physiological responses, such as pulse, respiration, and blood pressure, remain stable.

   c. The patient's psychological responses, such as anxiety or distress, remain manageable.

   d. The patient is comfortable before, during, and after the procedure.

8. Follow step 8 of the General Procedure: Determine the equipment needed for the procedure. **R:** Having all equipment and supplies available allows the procedure to be done efficiently, decreasing patient distress. Include the following:

   a. appropriate endoscope

   b. suction machine

   c. clean towels

   d. water-soluble lubricant

   e. long cotton-tipped swabs

   f. slides or containers for tissue specimens

   g. drapes

   h. examination gloves

IMPLEMENTATION

Action	Rationale
9-14. Follow steps 9 to 14 of the General Procedure: Wash or disinfect your hands, identify the patient (two identifiers), discuss the procedure with the patient, obtain needed supportive devices or assistance, set up a surface for equipment, premedicate the patient if indicated.	

15. Position the patient.
 	
  a. For a proctoscopy, position the patient on a special examination table that "breaks" at the hips and has a kneeling platform at the end. This allows the patient to be placed in a knee-chest position. If this examination table is not available, place the patient in a knee-chest position, and use pillows for support. If the patient is unable to attain or sustain this position, have the patient lie on his or her left side.
 	
  b. For a colonoscopy or sigmoidoscopy, the patient is positioned on the left side and turned as needed to visualize different areas of the bowel (Fig. 17-3).
	The knee-chest position allows for easy access of the operator to the anus and the ability to manipulate the equipment. The left lateral position is best for visualization during the sigmoidoscopy and the colonoscopy and is comfortable for the patient.

(continued)

Action	Rationale

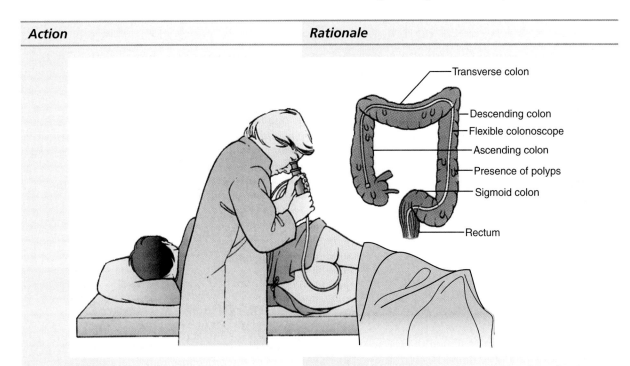

FIGURE 17-3 Flexible fiberoptic colonoscopes permit the examiner to see higher bowel areas with less discomfort to the patient than would result from the use of rigid instruments.

Action	Rationale
16. Drape the patient, exposing only the buttocks.	To facilitate the procedure and limit the exposure of the patient.
17. Assist with the procedure:	
a. Assess the patient throughout the procedure.	To identify any problems or concerns immediately.
b. Reassure the patient, and strive to relieve anxiety throughout the procedure.	The positioning is considered embarrassing by most patients.
c. Assist with the procedure as necessary.	For efficient use of time. You may be asked to provide suction.
d. Encourage the patient to focus on breathing deeply through the mouth when the physician inserts the lubricated endoscope through the anus.	To relax the anal sphincter.
e. When the procedure is completed, assist in cleansing the patient's anal area of the lubricant.	To promote patient comfort.
18. Conclude the procedure:	
a. Assist the patient to rise from the procedure table.	After such a procedure, the patient may feel weak and unsteady and need extra support.

(continued)

Action	Rationale
b. Restore the unit by clearing away equipment and placing the call signal within reach.	This is to promote patient comfort and safety.
c. Label and properly care for the tissue specimen of the polyp if collected.	Place the specimen in a container with preservative, and send it to the laboratory immediately to ensure accurate results.
19. Remove gloves, and wash and disinfect your hands.	This is to decrease the transfer of microorganisms.

EVALUATION

20. Follow step 20 of the General Procedure: Evaluate using the individualized patient outcomes previously identified:

  a. The procedure is performed, and a tissue specimen of any polyp, if obtained, is sent to the laboratory as indicated by policy.

  b. The patient's physiological responses, such as temperature, pulse, respiration, and blood pressure, remain stable. Sudden, acute abdominal pain could indicate the rare complication of perforated colon.

  c. The patient's psychological responses, such as anxiety or distress, remain manageable.

  d. The patient is comfortable before, during, and after the procedure. Discomfort is common but is usually not acute. Because air was insufflated into the bowel, the patient might experience flatulence or gas pains.

DOCUMENTATION

21. Follow step 21 of the General Procedure: Document a brief description of the procedure, the patient's response, and the disposition of any specimen in the patient's record.

Acute Care

In the hospital, many of these procedures are done at the patient's bedside. The nurse must organize the environment to facilitate effective functioning so that the procedure may be accomplished as quickly as possible. Sometimes a treatment or examination room is available for such procedures and must be scheduled in advance.

Long-Term Care

Residents are transferred to another setting for most of these tests. The staff in the facility need to be aware of the procedure to prepare the resident for it and to accurately assess for potential complications after the resident returns.

Home Care

The home health nurse needs to be aware that the client has had the procedure and can reinforce teaching. The nurse can also accurately assess for potential complications following the procedure.

Ambulatory Care

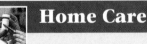

Endoscopic procedures can be done in the ambulatory care setting. If premedication is used, it is imperative that the nurse assesses the client's ability to ambulate and to use transportation. In most cases, the client is instructed to be accompanied by someone who can assist with safe transportation home if premedication is to be used. The nurse must also assess the client's ability to follow postprocedure instructions and especially to recognize signs and symptoms of complications to report to the physician. Telephone follow-up may be indicated to assess for complications. Information on when to expect laboratory examination results is also made available to the client.

LEARNING TOOLS

DEVELOP YOUR BACKGROUND KNOWLEDGE

1. Review the Learning Outcomes.

2. Read the section on diagnostic and therapeutic procedures in your assigned text.

3. Look up the Key Terms in the glossary.

4. Review the module, and mentally practice the techniques described. Use the Performance Checklists on the CD-ROM in the front of this book as a guide. Study so that you would be able to teach these skills to another person.

DEVELOP YOUR SKILLS

1. In the practice setting, select two other students to form a group of three.

2. Changing so that each has the opportunity to play the role of the patient, practice positioning the "patient" for each of the following procedures. The person not participating as patient or nurse at a given time can observe and evaluate the performances of the others. Include pertinent patient education for each procedure: thoracentesis, paracentesis, lumbar puncture, and liver biopsy.

3. In your small group or in the larger class group, discuss the things that the "nurse" said or did that made it easier for the "patient." Also discuss the observations that need to be made by the nurse during and after each of the above procedures as well as with bone marrow aspiration or biopsy, proctoscopy, sigmoidoscopy, and colonoscopy.

DEMONSTRATE YOUR SKILLS

In the clinical setting
1. Consult with your instructor regarding the opportunity to observe a variety of diagnostic and therapeutic procedures. Discuss what you observed with the instructor and clinical group.

2. Consult with your instructor regarding the opportunity to assist with a variety of diagnostic and therapeutic procedures. Evaluate your performance with the instructor.

CRITICAL THINKING EXERCISES

1. Ben Jamerson, age 58, has a family history of colon cancer. His physician has decided that he should have a colonoscopy. As the nurse in the physician's office, you are responsible to schedule the procedure, provide instructions to the patient regarding the procedure, and assist with the procedure when it is performed. Identify what concerns Mr. Jamerson might have, and determine what information he needs. What advice will you give this patient about driving to the office for this procedure?

2. You are preparing a female patient who is 32 years old for a lumbar puncture (spinal tap). What will you include in your discussion? Include information regarding positioning, what signs and symptoms you will ask her to report to you during and after the procedure, and the observations that will be made after the procedure.

SELF-QUIZ

SHORT-ANSWER QUESTIONS

1. What are two important functions of the nurse when assisting with a diagnostic procedure?

   a. _____

   b. _____

2. Why is it necessary to assess for the use of anticoagulants before a diagnostic procedure such as a liver biopsy?

   _____

3. List four aspects that are included in the preparation of the environment for performing a diagnostic procedure.

   a. _____

   b. _____

   c. _____

   d. _____

MULTIPLE CHOICE

_____ 4. The patient about to undergo a paracentesis should be instructed to void first so that
   a. there will be no discomfort from distention.
   b. urine can be tested.
   c. the bladder will not be punctured.
   d. the bladder will not be in the way of the intestines.

_____ 5. The reason for positioning the patient having a lumbar puncture in the flexed position is to
   a. widen the intervertebral spaces to allow entrance of the needle.
   b. attain a position of comfort.
   c. gain exposure of the back.
   d. relax the musculature.

_____ **6.** During a thoracentesis, what complications may be seen? (Choose all that apply.)
  a. Infection
  b. Respiratory arrest
  c. Pleural irritation or puncture
  d. Severe coughing

_____ **7.** Which of the following is (are) true? (Choose all that are true.)
  a. It is important for the patient to void prior to a thoracentesis.
  b. The specimen from a paracentesis is often examined for the presence of abnormal cells.
  c. Headache is a common complication of a lumbar puncture.
  d. Pneumothorax is a common complication of a liver biopsy.

Answers to Self-Quiz questions appear in the back of this book.

REFERENCES AND SUGGESTED RESOURCES: UNIT 3

Ackley, B. J. & Ladwig, G. B. (2004). *Nursing diagnosis handbook. A guide to planning care.* (6th ed.). St. Louis, MO: C. V. Mosby.

American Cancer Society, Inc. (2004). Colon cancer fact sheet. (Online.) Available at http://www.cancer.org/colonmd/pdfs/fact_sheet.pdf. Retrieved March 18, 2005.

American Diabetes Association. (2001). Tests of glycemia in diabetes. *Diabetes Care, 4*(1).

American Diabetes Association. (Online). Available at http://www.lifeclinic.com/focus/diabetes/supply_meter.asp.

Canadian Task Force on Preventative Health Care. (2001). Preventative health care, 2001 update: Colorectal cancer screening. Recommendation statement from the Canadian Task Force on Preventative Health Care, National Guideline Clearinghouse. (Online.) Available at http://www.guideline.gov/summary/summary.aspx?doc_id=2894&nbr=2120. Retrieved March 15, 2005.

Center for Medicare and Medicaid Services. (2003). *Medicare and home health care.* Pub. # CMS 10969. (Online.) Available at http://www.cms.hhs.gov/quality/hhqi/HHBenefits.pdf. Retrieved March 12, 2005.

Center for Medicare and Medicaid Services. (2002). Minimum Data Set (MDS) 2.0 Information Site. (Online.) Available at http://www.cms.hhs.gov/medicaid/mds20/. Retrieved March 10, 2005.

Center for Medicare and Medicaid Services. (2003). Minimum Data Set (MDS) 3.0 Draft Development. (Online.) Available at http://www.cms.hhs.gov/quality/mds30/. Retrieved March 10, 2005.

Gehring, P. E. (2002). Perfecting your skills: Vascular assessment. *RN,* April, 16–24.

Henker, R. & Coyne, C. (1995). Comparison of peripheral temperature measurements with core temperature. *AACN Clinical Issues, 6* (1), 21–30.

JNC-7 (2003). Seventh Report of the Joint National Committee on Prevention, Detection, Evaluation, and Treatment of High Blood Pressure. *JAMA 2003,* 2560–2571. (Online.) Available at http://www.nhlbi.nih.gov/guidelines/hypertension/jnc7full.pdf. Retrieved August, 2004.

Lower, J. (2002). Facing neuro assessment fearlessly. *Nursing02, 32* (2), 58–64.

McCormick, D., Kibbe, P. J., & Morgan, S. W. (2002). Colon cancer: Prevention, diagnosis, treatment. *Gastroenterology Nursing, 25*(5), 204–211.

Mehta, M. (2003). Assessing the abdomen. *Nursing2003, 33*(5), 54–55.

Omaha System. (2004). *The Omaha System: Solving the clinical data-information puzzle.* (Online.) Available at http://www.omahasystem.org/. Retrieved March 12, 2005.

National Institutes of Health, National Heart, Lung, and Blood Institute. (2004). *Fourth Report on the Diagnosis, Evaluation, and Treatment of High Blood Pressure in Children and Adolescents, Blood Pressure Tables for Children and Adolescents.* (Online.) Available at http://www.nhlbi.nih.gov/guidelines/hypertension/child_tbl.htm.

Pickering, T. H., Hall, J. E., Appel, L. J., et al. (2004). Recommendations for Blood Pressure Measurement in Humans and Experimental Animals: Part 1: Blood Pressure Measurement in Humans: A Statement for Professionals From the Subcommittee of Professional and Public Education of the American Heart Association Council on High Blood Pressure Research. (Online). Available at http://hyper.ahajournals.org. Co-published Pickering, T. H., Hall, J. E., Appel, L. J., et al. (2005). *Circulation,* (February 8).

Pullen, R. (2003). Using an ear thermometer. *Nursing2003, 33*(5), 24.

Sacks, D., Bakal, C. W., Beatty, P. T., et al. (2002). Position statement on the use of the ankle brachial index in the evaluation of patients with peripheral vascular disease: A consensus statement developed by the standards division of the Society of Interventional Radiology. *Journal of Vascular Intervention Radiology, 13,* 353.

Zator-Estes, M. A. (2002). *Heath assessment and physical examination* (2nd ed.). Albany, New York: Delmar-Thompson.

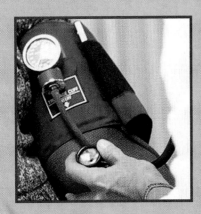

UNIT 4

Assisting With Activity, Mobility, and Musculoskeletal Conditions

MODULES

MODULE 18

Transfer

SKILLS INCLUDED IN THIS MODULE

General Procedure for Transfer
Specific Procedures for Transfer
  Bed to Chair: One-Person Minimal Assist
  Bed to Chair: Two-Person Maximal Assist
  Bed to Chair: Mechanical Lift
  Chair to Chair: Two-Person "Bucket" Lift
  Bed to Chair or Chair to Chair: Two-Person Six-Point Lift
  Horizontal Slide: Using a Transfer Slider Board
  Horizontal Lift: Two- or Three-Person Assist

PREREQUISITE MODULES

Module 1   An Approach to Nursing
            Skills
Module 2   Documentation
Module 3   Basic Body Mechanics
Module 4   Basic Infection Control
Module 5   Safety in the Healthcare
            Environment
Module 6   Moving the Patient in Bed
            and Positioning
The following modules may be needed in some situations:
Module 11   Assessing Temperature,
            Pulse, and Respiration
Module 12   Measuring Blood Pressure
Module 14   Nursing Physical Assessment

KEY TERMS

dangling	out of bed (OOB)
ergonomics	supine
horizontal	weight-bearing
orthostatic	
hypotension	

OVERALL OBJECTIVE

▸ To transfer a patient from a bed to a chair, wheelchair, commode, or stretcher with maximum comfort and safety for the patient and nurse.

LEARNING OUTCOMES

The student will be able to

1. Assess a patient to determine ability to move, bear weight, and maintain balance.
2. Analyze data to identify whether the patient can participate in the transfer process.
3. Determine appropriate patient outcomes related to transfer and recognize the potential for adverse outcomes.
4. Plan an effective transfer technique for the individual patient.
5. Carry out a variety of different transfer techniques safely for the patient and the nurse.
6. Use appropriately selected lift devices to assist in the transfer of patients.
7. Evaluate the effectiveness of the transfer technique used.
8. Document the transfer technique used and the patient's response.

Moving patients **out of bed** is beneficial for them. The movement maintains and restores muscle tone, stimulates the respiratory and circulatory systems, and improves elimination. Patients need only dangle their legs over the side of the bed or sit in a chair at the bedside for a few minutes to improve their physical and psychological well-being. Many patients cannot move at all or need some assistance in moving. It is the nurse's responsibility to help patients move, directing them in the best techniques for self-movement and seeing that enough people are on hand to ensure the safety of the patient and staff during transfer.

Correctly helping a patient from the bed to a chair is an important nursing function in which you play a vital role by giving the patient physical support and encouragement. Pay special attention to safety precautions and to the basics of body mechanics to ensure the safety of all involved. The level of activity is usually determined by a physician's orders, but nursing assessment and judgment are necessary to determine the best method for carrying out the order.

NURSING DIAGNOSES

- Impaired Physical Mobility: related to decreased strength, pain or discomfort, and neuromuscular or musculoskeletal impairment. Patients may be completely unable to move themselves or need assistance in doing so.
- Activity Intolerance: related to poor oxygenation or inadequate perfusion. The person with Activity Intolerance may need assistance to move with safety.

DELEGATION

Nurses routinely delegate to assistive personnel the transfer of the patient for purposes of care, transport for therapies and tests, and change of the patient's position.

Assistive personnel experience a very high incidence of work-related injuries due to lifting and transferring patients. Nurses have a role in teaching correct technique and in advocating for appropriate lifting and transfer devices to prevent injury to staff members. Health promotion for employees in the workplace is partly a nursing responsibility.

ERGONOMICS AND PATIENT TRANSFER

Ergonomics is the science of fitting a job to a person's anatomic and physiologic characteristics to enhance efficiency and well-being. The Occupational Safety and Health Agency (OSHA) has extensive statistical data showing that injuries from lifting patients are excessively high among healthcare workers, especially nurses and nursing assistants. Although teaching proper body mechanics and lifting techniques provides some help related to lifting smaller loads, the major problem is that the average person should not lift more than 51 lb (American Nurses Association, 2002). With the average adult weighing 150 lb, lifting patients clearly has a high potential for causing injury. Even lifting smaller loads continually over the day leads to repetitive strain injuries. Therefore, the techniques outlined below must be used with great care and lifting techniques avoided whenever possible.

Many facilities are responding to this problem for healthcare workers by developing policies for "limited lifting" or "no lifting." Some may have "lift teams" of strong individuals who help with lifting throughout the institution. The difficulty with this is that those on the lift team are also susceptible to injury. To support limited or no lift policies, transfer devices and mechanical lifting devices of various types have been developed. Box 18-1 lists the American Nurses Association (ANA) criteria for selecting lifting and transfer devices. Although these devices are expensive, avoiding back injury makes them cost-effective. In addition, the pregnant, less physically able, or older worker can function in more settings as an effective caregiver when lift devices are available. Table 18-1 identifies various lifts and transfer devices available. Table 18-2 identifies the ANA recommendation for lifting devices for specific patient situations.

PROVIDING ASSISTANCE FOR THE PATIENT'S SELF-TRANSFER

Many patients are able to transfer themselves from the bed to a chair and back but have the potential to become dizzy or unstable. These patients need someone immediately present to prevent falls if the patient loses balance (Fig. 18-1). This is often referred to as "standby assistance." For patients needing this type of assistance, a variety of grab bars are useful in bathrooms next to the toilet or in the shower. Transfer poles may be used by the bed as an assistive device. The use of assistive devices such as these may increase safety without a caregiver present.

GENERAL PROCEDURE FOR TRANSFER

ASSESSMENT

1. Review the patient's record for medical diagnosis, current problems, and physician's orders. Check with other nurses, and consult the patient's record and nursing plan of care to obtain information regarding any transfer techniques that are part of the plan of care. **R:** This information helps to identify any restrictions to be observed. For example, a patient with a recently repaired fractured hip may be allowed to rest only 25% of body weight on the affected side, whereas a postoperative patient who has had an appendectomy may not be restricted in any way.

2. Assess the patient's ability to move. Is the patient capable of moving all extremities? Does the patient have any specific disabilities that affect movement? Is one side stronger? Does the patient have the endurance to sustain activity? How was the patient transferred before? Has the patient received any medication that will affect balance, judgment, or ability to follow directions? **R:** Assessing the patient's abilities facilitates your helping the patient participate in the process.

3. Assess pulse, respirations, and blood pressure before transfer. **R:** These data will help in evaluating the patient's physical response to transfer.

4. Assess the patient for pain to determine whether pain management is needed before moving. **R:** Some patients may need to be medicated for pain before they can move effectively.

5. Assess the patient's ability to cooperate and follow directions. **R:** To plan for patient participation. Asking the patient appropriate questions will usually provide this information, although some patients may be unable to provide accurate information.

6. Assess the patient's need for eyeglasses or a hearing aid. **R:** To ensure maximum ability to cooperate.

7. Identify what equipment is available for moving patients and who is available to assist you.

ANALYSIS

8. Critically think through your data, carefully evaluating each aspect and its relation to other data. **R:** To determine specific problems for this individual in relation to transfer.

9. Identify specific problems and modifications of the procedure needed for this individual. **R:** Planning for the individual must take into consideration the individual's problems.

PLANNING

10. Identify the appropriate individualized outcomes of the transfer as follows. **R:** Identification of desired outcomes guides planning and evaluation of care.
    a. Patient is safely transferred.
    b. Patient's body alignment is correct.
    c. Patient did not experience pain during transfer and is comfortable.
    d. Patient did not experience excess fatigue, and pulse, respiratory rate, and blood pressure remain stable.

11. Devise a plan to transfer the patient in the safest and most convenient manner, taking into account proper body mechanics for you and the patient. Be realistic. You may need more than one person to transfer a heavy or severely disabled patient or to use lifting equipment. **R:** Planning ahead allows you to proceed more safely and effectively.

table 18-1. Types of Transfer and Lift Devices

Device	Description
Transfer belt (gait belt)	Strongly woven of wide canvas, the transfer belt has a large buckle. Placed around the patient's waist, the belt allows the caregiver to get a firm grip. Some transfer belts have built-in handles for even more effective gripping. A belt is used in many transfer situations to provide balance and stability for the patient. It may be used for some lifting, but may cause discomfort when weight is lifted by the belt.
Transfer poles	A transfer pole is placed next to the bed where a patient can grasp it and use upper extremities to rise, balance, and pivot around to the next position. May be used with a transfer board to help a non-weight-bearing patient into a chair.

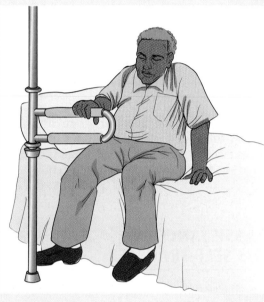

Transfer pole.

Transfer or sliding board (see Fig. 18-7)	Made of a slick plastic that reduces friction as the patient slides across. A large transfer board is designed to help move patients from bed to stretcher and back; smaller boards are designed to help patients slide from a bed into a wheelchair and back.
Inflated lateral transfer device	Made of an air mattress-type fabric, the lateral transfer device is placed under the patient. The air is transferred from one tube to another from in front of the patient to behind the patient. There is a decrease in friction and momentum to facilitate movement.
Transfer disk	This circular disk provides a pivoting base with a place for both feet. It is placed on the floor, and the patient stands on it. The disk swivels so that the person can be swiveled into a chair without moving the feet. The caregiver can apply a transfer belt to facilitate patient balance and movement.
Grab bars and handles	Placed in bathrooms next to showers, tubs, and toilets, grab bars and handles allow the patient to grasp firmly for balance and to use arms to assist with movement; they also assist patients as they transfer.
Transfer or turning sheet	A heavy half sheet or a conventional sheet folded in half and placed under the patient's body, this device facilitates turning and moving the patient in bed.
Mobile mechanical lifts (see Fig 18-4)	These lifts have a wheeled base, an overhead bar with a sling suspension system, and a sling. A variety of sling styles are available for different purposes. They may have manual hydraulic pumps or remote-controlled electrical devices for lifting the bar and attached sling.
Sit-to-stand lifts	Designed for those who can bear weight on the lower extremities, sit-to-stand lifts have a platform for the patient to place feet on when standing. A belt or small sling is placed around the patient, and the patient holds onto handles as the lift pulls the patient to a standing position. The entire lift can be moved with the patient standing on it and used to help lower the patient onto a chair or toilet.
Ceiling lifts	Most commonly seen in critical care units, ceiling lifts are installed on ceiling tracks so that they can move around the room. They are similar to the mobile lifts in the use of a sling for lifting. The sling is attached to the ceiling hoist.
Wall-mounted lifts	Permanently installed next to a bed, these lifts have an arm that can be swiveled to extend out alongside the bed and assist the patient in transferring from bed to chair and back. They are commonly used for patients in long-term care.

(continued)

table 18-1. Types of Transfer and Lift Devices (Continued)

Device	Description

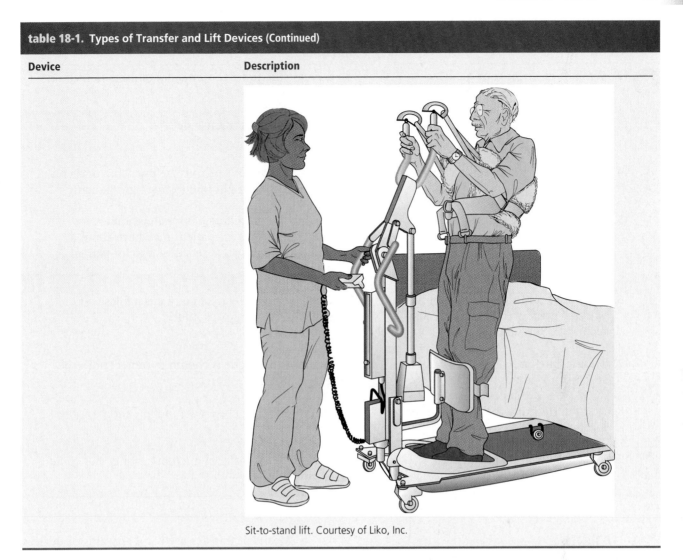

Sit-to-stand lift. Courtesy of Liko, Inc.

table 18-2. Solutions to Lifting Problems

Problem	Suggested Solution
Totally dependent patient	Full sling mechanical lift device
Extensive assistance level	Full sling or sit-to-stand lift
Lift from floor for dependent patient (after patient fall)	Full sling mechanical lift; if manual lift is needed, specify the number of caregivers needed to lift.
Lifts from floor for patient who can assist (after patient fall)	Transfer or gait belt; specify number of caregivers needed to support the person.
Limited patient assistance in moving	Sit-to-stand lift; friction-reducing devices for lateral transfers, transfer disk

American Nurses Association. (2002). *Preventing back injuries: Safe patient handling and movement.* Washington, DC: Author.

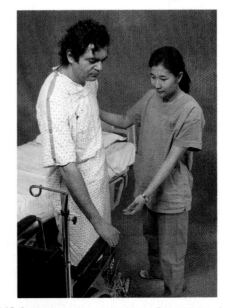

FIGURE 18-1 Most patients need only standby assistance, in which the nurse's function is primarily to provide balance and stand by in case the patient may fall.

IMPLEMENTATION

Action	Rationale
12. Wash or disinfect your hands.	To decrease the transfer of microorganisms that could cause infection.
13. Obtain any needed supportive devices or assistance.	To save time and promote efficiency.
14. Identify the patient, using two identifiers.	Verifying the patient's identity helps ensure that you are performing the right skill for the right patient.
15. Tell the patient about the transfer technique you are about to use.	Explaining the procedure helps relieve anxiety or misperceptions that the patient may have about a procedure or activity and sets the stage for patient participation.
16. Raise or lower the bed to an appropriate working position based on the transfer technique you will be using.	To allow you to use correct body mechanics and protect yourself from back injury.
17. Transfer the patient, using one of the specific procedures below.	The transfer technique is chosen to protect both the patient and staff.
18. Position the patient correctly in the new location.	Correct positioning preserves function and promotes comfort.
19. Wash or disinfect your hands.	To decrease the transfer of microorganisms that could cause infection.

EVALUATION

20. Evaluate in relation to the individualized patient outcomes previously identified. **R:** Evaluation in relation to desired outcomes is essential and enables planning for future care.
   a. Patient is safely transferred.
   b. Patient's body alignment is correct.
   c. Patient did not experience pain during transfer and is comfortable.
   d. Patient did not experience excess fatigue, and pulse, respiratory rate, and blood pressure remain stable.

DOCUMENTATION

21. Document on the nursing plan of care the following essential information about the transfer. In some facilities, documentation of transfers and activity are recorded on the nursing progress notes in a narrative or a SOAP format. Follow the policy in your facility. **R:** Documentation is a legal record of the patient's care and therapy and communicates nursing activities to other nurses and caregivers.

a. Means of transfer used and any aids or devices needed
b. Number of people needed to help
c. Patient's ability to cooperate
d. The exact nature of the activity (such as transfer from bed to chair)
e. The time it was carried out
f. The patient's response to the activity: consider pain, fatigue, pulse, respiratory rate, blood pressure changes, and dizziness.

POTENTIAL ADVERSE OUTCOMES AND RELATED INTERVENTIONS

1. The patient sustains a fall. Falls are the most common hazard to a patient being transferred. The patient may become dizzy or have less strength than expected, or the nurse may not be strong enough to accomplish the task. Additionally, floors may be slippery, creating a hazard. Consider these possibilities carefully before beginning the transfer so that you can plan the specific measures you will take to maintain safety for the patient. For example, if the patient is very large or hard to handle, consider having other nurses assist you, or use a mechanical lift.

Intervention: If a patient begins to fall, lower the patient to the bed, the chair, or the floor in a way that prevents injury. Especially protect the head from a blow. If a patient does fall, complete a thorough assessment before you move the patient to determine if there are any injuries. Moving the patient immediately may increase the severity of a fall-related injury. This assessment may be done by an experienced registered nurse, but in some instances, it should be done by a physician. Consult the policy in your facility.

2. An indwelling tube is pulled loose or pulled out. Another hazard in moving patients is the pull on indwelling tubings (such as catheters or IV tubing) and injuring the patient or dislodging the tubing. Take care to move tubings as necessary without dislodging them.

Intervention: Immediately stop the move. Request assistance if necessary to manage the tubing. If the tubing has pulled out, return the patient to bed and arrange to have the tube reinserted. You may need to notify the physician, who will determine the appropriate course of action.

3. Bruising of arms or legs. Bruising from striking side rails or furniture is another hazard of transferring the patient.

Intervention: Position the patient carefully to prevent him or her from striking against side rails or furniture. Teach the patient to keep hands and arms in the appropriate location. Be sure the patient is wearing shoes or slippers (with firm soles) when stepping onto the floor. If the patient does become bruised, putting an ice pack on the area may diminish the size of the bruise. You may need a physician's order to use an ice pack.

SPECIFIC PROCEDURES FOR TRANSFER

Bed to Chair: One-Person Minimal Assist

This procedure is appropriate for the patient who can bear weight, move with assistance, and needs help with balance and stability.

ASSESSMENT

1-7. Follow steps 1 to 7 of the General Procedure: Review records, assess ability to move, vital signs, pain, ability to cooperate, need for glasses or hearing aid, and identify available equipment.

ANALYSIS

8-9. Follow steps 8 and 9 of the General Procedure: Critically think through your data, and identify specific problems.

PLANNING

10-11. Follow steps 10 and 11 of the General Procedure: Identify the appropriate individualized patient outcomes of the transfer: safe transfer; correct alignment; comfort; no fatigue; pulse, respiratory rate, and blood pressure remain stable; and devise a plan to transfer the patient.

IMPLEMENTATION

Action	Rationale
12-15. Follow steps 12 to 15 of the General Procedure: Wash your hands, obtain needed assistive devices, identify the patient (two identifiers), and explain the transfer technique.	
16. Place the bed in the lowest position so that the patient's feet will reach the floor from the bedside.	To allow you to use correct body mechanics, to protect yourself from back injury, and to enable the patient to participate.
17. Transfer the patient from bed to chair using the following steps.	
a. Angle the wheelchair or armchair at a 45-degree angle to the bed so that the chair is on the patient's stronger side. If the footrests are removable, remove them at this time; otherwise, fold them out of the way.	To allow the patient to pivot on the stronger leg and to move the shortest distance.

(continued)

Action	Rationale
b. Lock the wheels of the bed and wheelchair.	To prevent them from moving during transfer.
c. Begin with the patient in a **supine** position, close to the edge of the bed, with the hips placed where the bed will bend as the head of the bed is raised.	This allows the bed mechanism to be used to lift the patient.
d. Raise the head of the bed slowly until the patient is in a sitting position.	This decreases the effort for you and the patient. Raising the bed slowly helps prevent dizziness from position change.
e. Slide one arm under the patient's legs, and place the other arm behind the patient's back. Swing the patient's legs over the side of the bed while pivoting the patient's body, so that the patient ends up sitting on the edge of the bed with the feet hanging down. This is termed **dangling**.	This uses the patient's body weight to facilitate the movement and lessens back strain for the nurse.
f. Allow the patient to sit for a few minutes. Be sure the patient sees the chair and its position. If the patient is visually impaired, explain the location of the wheelchair, and, if possible, place the patient's hand on it.	Sitting allows circulation to stabilize and prevents light-headedness or **orthostatic hypotension,** which can occur with any sudden change in circulation caused by lowering the legs and raising the head. To promote a feeling of security, support the patient if he or she feels dizzy (Fig. 18-2). If the patient sees the chair, he or she is able to participate in the process more effectively. 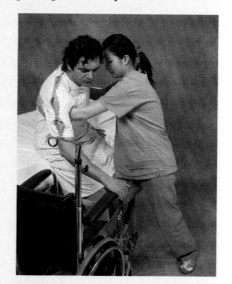 **FIGURE 18-2** Bed to wheelchair: Support the patient who reports feeling dizzy. Allow him to sit and rest momentarily before proceeding to transfer him to the wheelchair.
g. Place a gait or transfer belt around the patient's waist and firm slippers or shoes on the patient's feet.	This belt provides you with something firm to grasp during the transfer. Slippers give the patient a sense of security, prevent slipping and foot injury, and protect against contaminated floors.

(continued)

Action	Rationale
h. Position the patient's feet firmly on the floor and slightly apart, with the patient's hands on the bed. *Note:* This is the time to consider using the transfer disk. This disk would facilitate the patient to pivot into the chair. The patient's feet are placed securely on the disk before standing. The patient will need assistance to balance during the pivot.	To protect yourself from injury, do not let the patient hold on to you. If the patient is holding on to you and begins to fall, you may receive a back injury from the twisting weight applied to your spine.
i. Take a wide stance, bend your knees, and grasp the sides of the belt. You may want to straddle the patient's weaker leg with your own legs, or you may want to stabilize the patient's knees by supporting them with your own knees. *Note:* A mechanical sit-to-stand lift could be used at this time if the patient is very heavy. This device avoids any lifting by staff and ensures the safety of the patient through a safety belt. The entire device is moved to pivot the patient. Follow the directions for the specific lift.	To provide you with a broad base of support. The belt helps you grasp strongly. The mechanical stand lift does the lifting and prevents back injuries for the caregiver.
j. Inform the patient that you will assist him or her to a standing position on a count of "one, two, three, stand" and that he or she should lean slightly forward and push up with the hands on the bed.	To provide the patient with information to facilitate cooperative action.
k. On the count of "three," straighten your knees, assisting the patient to a standing position.	To bring all effort simultaneously to help the patient stand.
l. Stand close to the patient and pivot to the chair.	Pivoting requires less energy than walking.
m. Instruct the patient to place both hands on the arms of the chair.	Using both hands keeps the patient balanced over both legs.
n. Lower the patient to the seat.	Stabilizing the patient prevents the patient from falling backward.
18. Be sure the patient's body is positioned firmly back in the chair seat and upright.	Correct positioning preserves function and promotes comfort.
19. Follow step 19 of the General Procedure: Wash or disinfect your hands.	

EVALUATION

20. Follow step 20 of the General Procedure: Evaluate using the individualized patient outcomes previously identified: safe transfer; correct alignment; comfort; no fatigue; and pulse, respiratory rate, and blood pressure remain stable.

DOCUMENTATION

21-22. Follow steps 21 and 22 of the General Procedure: Document the transfer on the nursing plan of care and on the patient's record as appropriate. Include means of transfer used and any aids or devices needed; number of people needed to help; patient's ability to cooperate; exact nature of the activity; time it was carried out; and the patient's response to the activity (consider pain, fatigue, pulse, respiratory rate, blood pressure changes, and dizziness).

Bed to Chair: Two-Person Maximal Assist

This procedure is appropriate for the patient who cannot bear weight or bears it only minimally and who cannot move without assistance. Using two people provides greater safety for the caregivers and the patient.

ASSESSMENT

1-7. Follow steps 1 to 7 of the General Procedure: Review records, assess ability to move, vital signs, pain, ability to cooperate, need for glasses or hearing aid, and identify available equipment.

ANALYSIS

8-9. Follow steps 8 and 9 of the General Procedure: Critically think through your data, and identify specific problems.

PLANNING

10-11. Follow steps 10 and 11 of the General Procedure: Identify the appropriate individualized patient outcomes of the transfer: safe transfer; correct alignment; comfort; no fatigue; pulse, respiratory rate, and blood pressure remain stable; and devise a plan to transfer the patient. Obtain an assistant for the procedure.

IMPLEMENTATION

Action	Rationale
12-15. Follow steps 12 to 15 of the General Procedure: Wash your hands, obtain needed assistive devices, identify the patient, and explain the transfer technique.	
16. Place the bed in the position so that the patient's feet will be flat on the floor from the bedside.	To allow correct body mechanics, protection from back injury, and ease of patient participation.
17. Transfer the patient from bed to chair, using the following steps:	
a. Angle the wheelchair or armchair at a 45-degree angle to the bed so that the chair is on the patient's stronger side. If the footrests are removable, remove them at this time; otherwise, fold them out of the way.	This arrangement will allow the patient to pivot on the stronger leg and to move the shortest distance.
b. Lock the wheels of the bed and wheelchair.	To prevent them from moving during transfer.

(continued)

Action	Rationale
c. Begin with the patient in a supine position, with the hips placed where the bed will bend as the head of the bed is raised, and close to the edge of the bed.	To allow the bed mechanism to be used to lift the patient.
d. Raise the head of the bed slowly until the patient is in a sitting position.	To decrease the effort for you and the patient. Raising the bed slowly helps prevent dizziness from position change.
e. Slide one arm under the patient's legs, and place the other arm behind the patient's back. Swing the patient's legs over the side of the bed while pivoting the patient's body, so that the patient is sitting on the edge of the bed with the feet hanging down.	This uses the patient's body weight to facilitate the movement and lessens back strain for the nurse.
f. Allow the patient to sit for a few minutes. Support the patient while he or she is sitting to prevent falling. Be sure the patient sees the chair and its position. If the patient is visually impaired, explain the location of the wheelchair, and, if possible, place the patient's hand on it.	Sitting allows circulation to stabilize and prevents light-headedness or orthostatic hypotension, which can occur with any sudden change in circulation caused by lowering the legs and raising the head. If the patient sees the chair, he or she can participate in the process more effectively.
g. Place a gait or transfer belt around the patient's waist.	The belt provides you with something firm to grasp during the transfer.
h. Position the patient's feet firmly on the floor and slightly apart, with the patient's hands on the bed. *Note:* A transfer disk could be used to facilitate the pivot. A sit-to-stand lift with a platform for the feet or a mechanical lift is preferred for use at this time because these eliminate all lifting. Follow manufacturer's instructions for using the device.	The patient's weight is on the bed and then transferred to the feet. However, there is a lift involved in getting the patient up to a standing position. To protect yourself from injury, do not let the patient hold on to you. If the patient is holding on to you and begins to fall, you may receive a back injury from the twisting weight applied to your spine. The disk would facilitate pivoting the patient to the chair. A mechanical lift would eliminate the need for this person to be lifted by caregivers. In this transfer, the patient's entire weight is not lifted.
i. *Nurse 1* stands in front of the patient, taking a wide stance, bending the knees, and grasping the patient at the sides of the belt. *Nurse 1* may want to straddle the patient's weaker leg with his or her own legs or stabilize the patient's knees by supporting them with his or her own knees. *Nurse 2* stands between the wheelchair and the bed with one knee on the bed and grasps the transfer belt at the patient's back and front (Fig 18-3).	This provides the nurse with a broad base of support. The belt facilitates a strong grip. Nurse 2 is in a position to provide strong lifting help.

(continued)

Action	*Rationale*

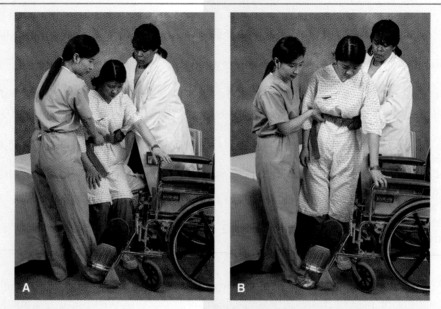

FIGURE 18-3 Bed to chair: two-person maximal assist. (**A**) *Nurse 2* (right) grasps the transfer belt firmly and establishes a firm base of support while (**B**) *Nurse 1* (left) prepares the patient for transfer to the chair on the count of "one, two, three, lift."

j. *Nurse 1* informs the patient that the move will occur on a count of "one, two, three, lift" and then signals "one, two, three, lift." Both nurses lift and pivot the patient on the count of "three" and then transfer the patient into the wheelchair.	Pivoting expends less energy than lifting entirely. The patient's weight and momentum assist in the pivot.
18. Be sure the patient's body is positioned upright and firmly back in the chair seat.	Correct positioning preserves function and promotes comfort.
19. Follow step 19 of the General Procedure: Wash or disinfect your hands.	

EVALUATION

20. Follow step 20 of the General Procedure: Evaluate in relation to the individualized patient outcomes previously identified: safe transfer; correct alignment; comfort; no fatigue; and pulse, respiratory rate, and blood pressure remain stable.

DOCUMENTATION

21-22. Follow steps 21 and 22 of the General Procedure: Document the transfer on the nursing plan of care and on the patient's record if appropriate. Include means of transfer used and any aids or devices needed; number of people needed to help; patient's ability to cooperate; exact nature of the activity; time it was carried out; and the patient's response to the activity (consider pain, fatigue, pulse, and respiratory rate, blood pressure changes, and dizziness).

Bed to Chair: Mechanical Lift

The mechanical lift enables nurses to lift heavy patients or those who are badly incapacitated without relying on physical strength. The use of a lift is always preferable to manual lifts because of the potential injuries to caregivers with manual lifting. All lifts have a sturdy frame that supports the patient's weight; a sling or seat of some type, which is positioned under the patient; and a lifting mechanism. Lifts are useful when providing hygienic care for patients (Fig. 18-4).

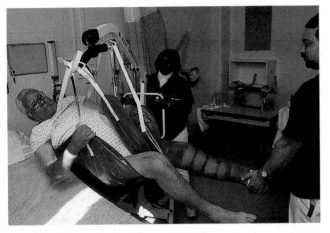

FIGURE 18-4 Mechanized lifts are helpful for moving large or immobile patients. Here, a hydraulic lift with a secure sling device is utilized to move the patient from the bed to a chair.

Consult the lift device directions for specifics about the particular brand and model used in your facility. The following is a general outline of the procedure when using a device with a sling. Two people are usually needed to ensure the patient's safety. Two people are essential for incapacitated patients who cannot support their own heads. The transfer belt is not used for this transfer technique.

ASSESSMENT

1-7. Follow steps 1 to 7 of the General Procedure: Review records, assess ability to move, vital signs, pain, ability to cooperate, need for glasses or hearing aid, and identify available equipment.

ANALYSIS

8-9. Follow steps 8 and 9 of the General Procedure: Critically think through your data, and identify specific problems.

PLANNING

10-11. Follow steps 10 and 11 of the General Procedure: Identify the appropriate individualized patient outcomes of the transfer: safe transfer; correct alignment; comfort; no fatigue; and pulse, respiratory rate, and blood pressure remain stable; and devise a plan to transfer the patient. Obtain an assistant for the procedure.

IMPLEMENTATION

Action	Rationale
12-15. Follow steps 12 to 15 of the General Procedure: Wash your hands, obtain needed assistive devices, identify the patient (two identifiers), and explain the transfer technique.	
16. Place the chair or commode so that it is at a 90-degree angle to the bed so that the nurses will have enough room to work. If the footrests are removable, remove them at this time; otherwise, fold them out of the way. Remove the wheelchair arms if possible. Lock or brace both chairs or the bed and chair.	To allow you to use correct body mechanics and protect yourself from back injury. Locking the chair prevents the chairs or bed from moving and creating the potential for falling.
17. Using the mechanical lift, transfer the patient as indicated below.	
a. Place patient in supine position.	This position provides for the most support in lifting.
b. Position sling under the patient's body by rolling the patient onto the sling. Be sure that the sling is positioned well under the thighs.	To ensure that the patient will not slide out of the sling as it lifts.

(continued)

Action	*Rationale*
c. Drape the patient if necessary.	To maintain modesty.
d. Place the bed in the low position.	To ensure that the sling is as low as possible as the patient is moved, which is safer and less distressing to the patient.
e. Position the lift over the patient.	The lift will raise the patient straight up.
f. Place the patient's arms across the chest.	To ensure that the arms do not get pinched in the fastening devices.
g. Fasten lift's chains securely.	To ensure that the sling does not come loose during the lift.
h. *Nurse 1* stands at patient's head and keeps a hand on the part of the sling nearest the head.	To make sure that the head is supported and the sling does not begin to rotate.
i. *Nurse 2* operates the lift and engages the lifting mechanism slowly.	This provides for constant monitoring of the functioning of the lift. Slow lifting is less likely to cause the sling to begin swinging.
j. *Nurse 1* guides and supports the patient's head while *Nurse 2* moves the lift away from bed.	This ensures that the patient is not bumped or jarred.
k. Double-check draping.	To maintain modesty.
l. Slowly move the lift to the new position.	Move slowly to prevent possible swinging into objects.
m. Position the patient above the next resting place and lower slowly.	Slow movement prevents inadvertent injury.
n. Turn off switch or close valve.	To prevent the lift arm from moving down onto the patient.
o. Detach chains from sling and move the lift away.	To allow the patient to engage in activity.
18. Be sure the patient's body is positioned firmly back in the second chair seat and upright.	Correct positioning preserves function and promotes comfort.
19. Follow step 19 of the General Procedure: Wash or disinfect your hands.	

EVALUATION

20. Follow step 20 of the General Procedure: Evaluate in relation to the individualized patient outcomes previously identified: safe transfer; correct alignment; comfort; no fatigue; pulse, respiratory rate, and blood pressure remain stable.

DOCUMENTATION

21-22. Follow steps 21 and 22 of the General Procedure: Document transfer on the nursing plan of care and on the patient's record as appropriate. Include means of transfer used and any aids or devices needed; number of people needed to help; patient's ability to cooperate; exact nature of the activity;

time it was carried out; and the patient's response to the activity (consider pain, fatigue, pulse, respiratory rate, blood pressure changes, and dizziness).

Chair to Chair: Two-Person "Bucket" Lift

This lift, often called a "bucket lift," has a high potential for back injury for nurses because one nurse must lift from a bent position. Another concern with this technique is that the nurse's arms may place pressure on the brachial plexus under the patient's arms, causing injury. For these reasons, many facilities encourage staff to use the six-point seated transfer (described below) instead of this lift. This lift can be done safely, however, if the patient is small and Nurse 1 is tall, quite strong, and uses good body mechanics. Given the current ANA recommendation of lifting no more than 51 lb, the patient would weigh less than 102 lb. The best option remains the mechanical lift.

ASSESSMENT

1-7. Follow steps 1 to 7 of the General Procedure: Review records, assess ability to move, vital signs, pain, ability to cooperate, need for glasses or hearing aid, and identify available equipment.

ANALYSIS

8-9. Follow steps 8 and 9 of the General Procedure: Critically think through your data, and identify specific problems.

PLANNING

10-11. Follow steps 10 and 11 of the General Procedure: Identify the appropriate individualized patient outcomes of the transfer: safe transfer; correct alignment; comfort; no fatigue; pulse, respiratory rate, and blood pressure remain stable; and devise a plan to transfer the patient. Obtain an assistant for the procedure.

IMPLEMENTATION

Action	Rationale
12-15. Follow steps 12 to 15 of the General Procedure: Wash your hands, obtain needed assistive devices, identify the patient (two identifiers), and explain the transfer technique.	
16. Place the chair or commode so that it is side by side with the wheelchair so that the patient will be lifted horizontally as much as possible. If the footrests are removable, remove them at this time; otherwise, fold them out of the way. Remove the wheelchair arm closest to the chair if possible.	To allow you to use correct body mechanics and protect yourself from back injury.
17. Lock or brace both chairs.	To prevent the chairs from moving and decrease the potential for falling.
18. Transfer the patient from chair to chair using the following steps.	Correct transfer technique and patient positioning preserves function and promotes comfort.
a. The taller nurse *(Nurse 1)* stands behind the chair.	
b. The shorter nurse *(Nurse 2)* stands facing the patient.	
c. *Nurse 1* folds the patient's arms across the patient's chest. The nurse then reaches under the patient's arms from	

(continued)

Action	**Rationale**

behind the patient and grasps the opposite wrist with each hand.

d. *Nurse 2* bends knees and hips, adopting a squatting position, and grasps the patient under the knees to support the legs (Fig. 18-5A).

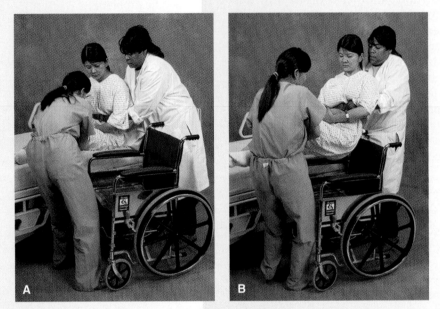

FIGURE 18-5 Bed to chair: Two-person "bucket" lift. (**A**) One nurse lifts from behind the person. The other nurse places an arm under the person's legs to lift. (**B**) On the count of "one, two, three, lift," the nurses raise the patient carefully from the bed and lower her into the chair.

e. *Nurse 1* informs the patient that the move will occur on the count of "one, two, three, lift."

f. *Nurse 1* counts ("one, two, three, lift"), and both lift at the same time. *Nurse 1* controls the timing because that nurse bears the greatest weight.

g. When the word "lift" is said, both nurses lift the patient and move over to the second chair (or commode), lowering the patient immediately, slowly, and smoothly (Fig. 18-5B). Be sure the patient's body is positioned firmly back in the second chair seat and upright.

19. Follow step 19 of the General Procedure: Wash or disinfect your hands.

EVALUATION

20. Follow step 20 of the General Procedure: Evaluate in relation to the individualized patient outcomes previously identified: safe transfer; correct alignment; comfort; no fatigue; and pulse, respiratory rate, and blood pressure remain stable.

DOCUMENTATION

21-22. Follow steps 21 and 22 of the General Procedure: Document transfer on the nursing plan of care and on the patient's record as appropriate. Include means of transfer used and any aids or devices needed; number of people needed to help; patient's ability to cooperate; exact nature of the activity; time it was carried out; and the patient's response to the activity (consider pain, fatigue, pulse, respiratory rate, blood pressure changes, and dizziness).

Bed to Chair or Chair to Chair: Two-Person Six-Point Lift

This procedure can easily be adapted to transfer between any two surfaces on which the patient can sit. Physical therapists state that this transfer provides greater protection from back injury for personnel and eliminates the potential for brachial plexus injury that the traditional two-person lift creates. It is called a six-point transfer

because the patient uses both arms for support, and each of two nurses are using two arms for support. This lift can be done more safely if both nurses are similar in height. This should only be done with a very lightweight patient and strong nurses. Given the current ANA recommendation of lifting no more than 51 lb, we are referring to a patient who weighs less than 102 lb. The best option remains the mechanical lift.

ASSESSMENT

1-7. Follow steps 1 to 7 of the General Procedure: Review records, assess ability to move, vital signs, pain, ability to cooperate, need for glasses or hearing aid, and identify available equipment.

ANALYSIS

8-9. Follow steps 8 and 9 of the General Procedure: Critically think through your data, and identify specific problems.

PLANNING

10-11. Follow steps 10 and 11 of the General Procedure: Identify the appropriate individualized patient outcomes of the transfer: safe transfer; correct alignment; comfort; no fatigue; pulse, respiratory rate, and blood pressure remain stable; and devise a plan to transfer the patient. Obtain an assistant for the procedure.

IMPLEMENTATION

Action	Rationale
12-15. Follow steps 12 to 15 of the General Procedure: Wash your hands, obtain needed assistive devices, identify the patient (two identifiers), and explain the transfer technique.	
16. Place the chair or commode at a 90-degree angle to the bed so that the nurses will have enough room to work. If the footrests are removable, remove them at this time; otherwise, fold them out of the way. Remove the wheelchair arms if possible. Lock or brace both chairs or the bed and chair.	To allow you to use correct body mechanics and protect yourself from back injury. Locking the chair prevents the chairs or bed from moving and decreases the potential for falling.
17. Transfer the patient from bed to chair or chair to chair using the following steps.	
a. Both nurses stand facing the patient, one on each side.	To position the nurses to lift effectively.

(continued)

Action	Rationale
b. Secure a transfer belt around the waist of the patient.	To provide a firm mechanism for holding onto the patient.
c. Both nurses place the forearm nearest the patient under patient's thighs from the inner side, and lean forward alongside the patient. *Note:* A second transfer belt may be secured around both thighs of the patient to facilitate grasping, but this is often more uncomfortable for the patient.	To position the nurse for lifting the legs.
d. Instruct and assist the patient to lean forward with arms resting over the backs of the nurses (Fig. 18-6A).	To facilitate the balance of the patient.

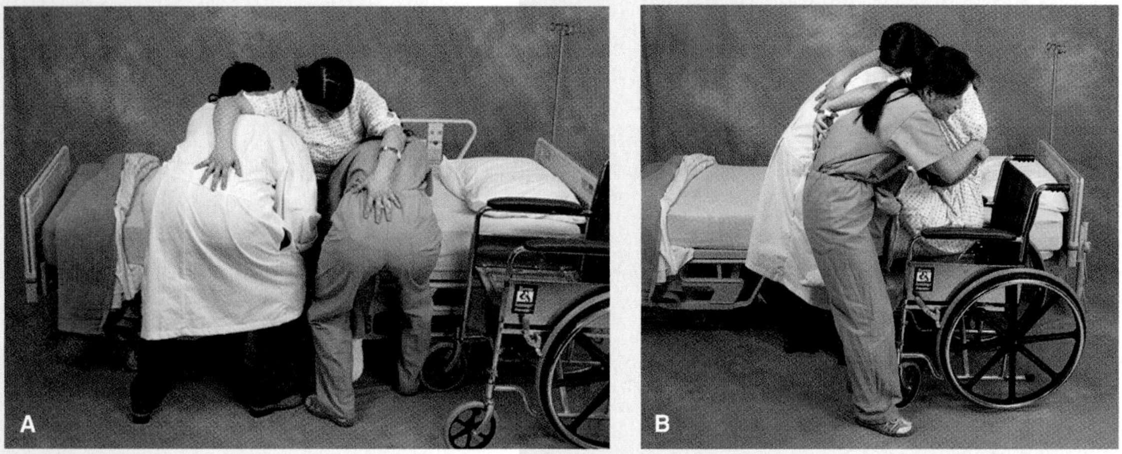

FIGURE 18-6 Six-point transfer, two-person lift. (**A**) The patient leans forward with her arms resting over the backs of the nurses. The nurses lift the patient by coming to a standing position with their shoulders back. (**B**) The patient is lowered to the chair.

Action	Rationale
e. Both nurses grasp the patient's transfer belt around the waist with the outside hand.	To provide a firm grasp on the patient's trunk.
f. Inform the patient of the signal. The count will be "one, two, three," and patient will be lifted on three.	To help ensure patient's cooperation and lessen patient's fear of being lifted.
g. Count. On "three," both nurses lift patient straight up by coming to a complete standing position with shoulders back. Patient flexes forward.	This uses the large leg muscles to lift and coordinates efforts.
h. Nurses turn and place patient onto the chair (Fig 18-6B).	The patient is held firmly during the lift.
18. Be sure the patient's body is positioned firmly back in the second chair seat and upright.	Correct positioning preserves function and promotes comfort.
19. Follow step 19 of the General Procedure: Wash or disinfect your hands.	

EVALUATION

20. Follow step 20 of the General Procedure: Evaluate in relation to the individualized patient outcomes previously identified: safe transfer; correct alignment; comfort; no fatigue; and pulse, respiratory rate, and blood pressure remain stable.

DOCUMENTATION

21-22. Follow steps 21 and 22 of the General Procedure: Document transfer on the nursing plan of care and on the patient's record as appropriate. Include means of transfer used and any aids or devices needed; number of people needed to help; patient's ability to cooperate; exact nature of the activity; time it was carried out; and the patient's response to the activity (consider pain, fatigue, pulse, respiratory rate, blood pressure changes, and dizziness).

Horizontal Slide: Using a Transfer Slider Board

This procedure is appropriate for the patient who must be moved from a bed to a stretcher or from a stretcher to a bed without getting up. A slider board bridges the gap between the bed and the stretcher and reduces friction, thus facilitating sliding the patient between the two surfaces.

ASSESSMENT

1-7. Follow steps 1 to 7 of the General Procedure: Review records, assess ability to move, vital signs, pain, ability to cooperate, need for glasses or hearing aid, and identify available equipment.

ANALYSIS

8-9. Follow steps 8 and 9 of the General Procedure: Critically think through your data, and identify specific problems.

PLANNING

10-11. Follow steps 10 and 11 of the General Procedure: Identify the appropriate individualized patient outcomes of the transfer: safe transfer; correct alignment; comfort; no fatigue; pulse, respiratory rate, and blood pressure remain stable; and devise a plan to transfer the patient. Obtain an assistant for the procedure.

IMPLEMENTATION

Action	Rationale
12-15. Follow steps 12 to 15 of the General Procedure: Wash your hands, obtain slider board, identify the patient (two identifiers), and explain the transfer technique.	
16. Raise the bed to the position that is level with the stretcher and positioned so caregivers do not need to bend over.	To allow caregivers to use correct body mechanics and protect themselves from back injury.
17. Transfer the patient from bed to stretcher, using the following steps.	
a. Move the patient toward one side of the bed, using techniques from Module 6.	To reduce the distance the patient must be moved.
b. *Nurse 1* stands on the side of the bed where the stretcher will be placed (usually closest to the door), and *Nurse 2* stands on the opposite side of the bed.	Positioning in this way safeguards the patient from falls and facilitates cooperation.
c. *Nurse 1* lowers the side rail nearest the door and places the stretcher with the slider board, covered with a sheet, alongside the bed.	To prepare for the move.

(continued)

Action	*Rationale*
d. *Nurse 2* rolls the patient away from the stretcher while *Nurse 1* slides the board across the dividing space between the stretcher and the bed and partially under the patient.	This provides a firm, smooth surface on which to slide the patient to the stretcher (Fig. 18-7). **FIGURE 18-7** Plastic slider board facilitates transfer from the bed to the stretcher.
e. *Nurse 2* rolls the patient back over partially onto the slider board and pulls the cover sheet out on the far side of the bed, rolling the patient as necessary to accomplish this.	The sheet provides a base that can move across the slider board.
f. *Nurse 1* reaches across the stretcher and grasps the sheet firmly at the level of the patient's shoulders and hips.	This allows the nurse to slide the patient's weight using pulling muscles.
g. *Nurse 2* lifts the edge of the sheet, transferring the patient's weight toward the slider board as *Nurse 1* firmly pulls the sheet and the patient across the slider board onto the stretcher. If the patient is incapacitated or very heavy, additional assistance may be needed on the stretcher side to support the head and pull the patient.	By transferring the weight onto the slider board, which reduces friction, the patient will move more easily. *Note:* If the patient is being returned to bed, remove the transfer sheet by turning the patient side to side. The transfer sheet remains under the patient if the patient will soon be transferred again (such as from the stretcher to the x-ray table).
18. Be sure the patient's body is positioned correctly on the stretcher.	Correct positioning preserves function and promotes comfort.
19. Follow step 19 of the General Procedure: Wash or disinfect your hands.	To decrease the transfer of microorganisms that could cause infection.

EVALUATION

20. Follow step 20 of the General Procedure: Evaluate in relation to the individualized patient outcomes previously identified: safe transfer; correct alignment; comfort; no fatigue; and pulse, respiratory rate, and blood pressure remain stable.

DOCUMENTATION

21-22. Follow steps 21 and 22 of the General Procedure: Document transfer on the nursing plan of care and on the patient's record as appropriate. Include means of transfer used and any aids or devices needed; number of people needed to help; patient's ability to cooperate; exact nature of the activity; time it was carried out; and the patient's response to the activity (consider pain, fatigue, pulse, respiratory rate, blood pressure changes, and dizziness).

Horizontal Lift: Two- or Three-Person Assist

This procedure can easily be adapted to transfer between any two surfaces on which the patient is lying, such as bed to stretcher or stretcher to bed. It is described simply as bed to stretcher for clarity. This lift can be done more safely if all three caregivers are similar in height. The better option remains the mechanical lift.

ASSESSMENT

1-7. Follow steps 1 to 7 of the General Procedure: Review records, assess ability to move, vital signs, pain, ability to cooperate, need for glasses or hearing aid, and identify available equipment.

ANALYSIS

8-9. Follow steps 8 and 9 of the General Procedure: Critically think through your data, and identify specific problems.

PLANNING

10-11. Follow steps 10 and 11 of the General Procedure: Identify the appropriate individualized patient outcomes of the transfer: safe transfer; correct alignment; comfort; no fatigue; pulse, respiratory rate, and blood pressure remain stable; and devise a plan to transfer the patient. Obtain an assistant for the procedure.

IMPLEMENTATION

Action	Rationale
12-15. Follow steps 12 to 15 of the General Procedure: Wash your hands, obtain needed assistants, identify the patient (two identifiers), and explain the transfer technique.	
16. Place the stretcher at a 90-degree angle to the bed so that the nurses will have enough room to work. Lock or brace both the bed and the stretcher. Place the far side rail on the stretcher up.	To allow nurses to use correct body mechanics and protect themselves from back injury. Locking or bracing the bed and the stretcher prevents them from moving and decreases the potential for falling.
17. Transfer the patient from bed to stretcher using the following steps.	
a. All three nurses stand facing the patient alongside the bed. One stands at the head and shoulders. One stands at the hips. The third stands at the knees.	This lift is easier to accomplish if the nurses are approximately the same height because the patient remains **horizontal.** If they are not the same height, the tallest one is at the head and the shortest at the legs in order to keep the patient's head higher than the feet.
b. Move the patient to the edge of the bed.	To lessen bending and reaching, which would strain backs.
c. All three nurses slide their arms under the patient, palms up (Fig. 18-8A).	To engage the strongest flexor muscles of the arms.
d. *Nurse 1* informs the patient that they will lift together on the signal of "one, two, three, lift."	Anxiety is lessened when the patient understands what will happen.

(continued)

Action	*Rationale*

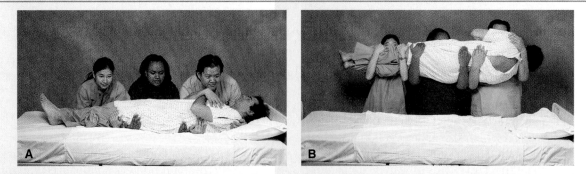

FIGURE 18-8 Horizontal lift: Three-person assist. (**A**) Three nurses slide their arms under the patient with the tallest nurse at the patient's neck and shoulder area. (**B**) Then they roll the patient toward their bodies and lift, standing straight with the patient's body against their bodies in preparation to transfer the patient to the stretcher or bed.

Action	*Rationale*
e. *Nurse 1* counts "one, two, three, lift." Using elbows as levers, all three nurses roll the patient toward their bodies and lift, standing straight with the patient's body against their bodies (Fig 18-8B).	Coordinating effort helps ensure that no individual is lifting too great a load.
f. *Nurse 1* states "Ready, walk." All nurses move back away from the bed and turn toward the stretcher.	To manage the patient's weight; it is essential that movement be coordinated.
g. When the nurses are at the edge of the stretcher, *Nurse 1* states "Ready, down," and at that signal, all nurses lower the patient to the stretcher.	This ensures that the patient is lowered carefully onto the stretcher.
18. Be sure the patient's body is positioned correctly and comfortably on the stretcher.	Correct positioning preserves function and promotes comfort.
19. Follow step 19 of the General Procedure: Wash or disinfect your hands.	

EVALUATION

20. Follow step 20 of the General Procedure: Evaluate in relation to the individualized patient outcomes previously identified: safe transfer; correct alignment; comfort; no fatigue; and pulse, respiratory rate, and blood pressure remain stable.

DOCUMENTATION

21-22. Follow steps 21 and 22 of the General Procedure: Document transfer on the nursing plan of care and on the patient's record as appropriate. Include means of transfer used and any aids or devices needed; number of people needed to help; patient's ability to cooperate; exact nature of the activity; time it was carried out; and the patient's response to the activity (consider pain, fatigue, pulse, respiratory rate, blood pressure changes, and dizziness).

Acute Care

Because lifts are used less frequently in acute care settings, staff sometimes feel uncertain about their use and, therefore, do manual lifts when a mechanical lift would be more appropriate. As a registered nurse on the unit, you can encourage education sessions to instruct staff in the use of lifting devices.

You also can encourage the assistive personnel to care for themselves by avoiding manual lifting. Nurses can also be effective in encouraging facilities to purchase transfer and lift devices that are suited to their particular settings and in storing them in locations that facilitate ease of use.

Long-Term Care

Care providers in long-term care settings have the potential to be involved in more transfers where maximum assistance is needed than those in most acute care settings. A serious concern is the potential for repetitive strain injury to the back. The Occupational Safety and Health Administration is studying the problem and considering ways that workers can be protected from injury. It is critical that these care providers use techniques and mechanical devices designed to reduce the need for their physical exertion. Thus, you may see mechanical lifts used more frequently in long-term care. Many new types of lifting devices are being developed as their value is demonstrated through fewer on-the-job injuries. When a two-person lift is needed, the authors recommend the six-point seated transfer.

Home Care

Those caring for people at home also need to know how to carry out safe and effective transfers. You may be asked to teach family members appropriate procedures for their situation. It may also be useful for you to assess the home environment so that it can be adapted to accommodate the client's needs, including adequate space and special equipment necessary for maximum safety. Home caregivers may be elderly individuals themselves who do not have the strength or balance to effectively transfer a dependent family member. Transfer and lift devices are also available for home use.

LEARNING TOOLS

DEVELOP YOUR BACKGROUND KNOWLEDGE

1. Review the Learning Outcomes.
2. Read the section on transfer in your assigned text.
3. Look up the Key Terms in the glossary.
4. Review this module and mentally practice the techniques described. Study so that you would be able to teach these skills to another person. Use the Performance Checklists on the CD-ROM in the front of this book as a guide.

DEVELOP YOUR SKILLS

1. In the practice setting, select two other students and form a group of three.
2. Alternating so that each has the opportunity to play the role of the patient, perform each of the following procedures. Those who are not participating at a given time can observe and evaluate the performances of the others. As you do each of the following, be sure to communicate effectively with the "patient" as you proceed.
   a. Place a colored tie or scarf around your partner's left arm and another on the left leg (or right arm and right leg). This will be the nonfunctional side.
   b. Transfer your partner from a supine position in bed to an upright position, sitting on the side of the bed. This is called dangling and is often preparatory to any type of transfer.
   c. Transfer your partner from the bed to a chair using a one-person, minimal-assist transfer.
   d. With a third person, transfer your partner from a bed to a chair using a two-person, maximal assist transfer.
   e. Transfer your partner from bed to chair using a mechanical lift device if one is available.
      (1) Obtain the lift.
      (2) Review the specific directions for its use.
      (3) Practice raising and lowering the device without a person in it.
      (4) Using the directions in this module, transfer another student from a bed to a chair and back to the bed using the lift.
      (5) Ask the student who was transferred to describe how it felt.
   f. Transfer your partner from chair to chair and from bed to chair using each of the two-person lift transfer techniques—do this only if your partner is within the weight lift limits—Chair to Chair: Two-Person "Bucket" Lift, Bed to Chair, or Chair to Chair: Two-Person Six-Point Lift.
   g. Transfer your partner from a bed to a stretcher, using a horizontal slide.
   h. Transfer your partner from a bed to a stretcher using a two- or three-person horizontal lift, ensuring that each person is lifting no more than 51 lb.

3. Change roles as patient and nurse, and repeat all of the transfers until each person participating has had an opportunity to be in each role.

DEMONSTRATE YOUR SKILLS

In the clinical setting

1. Consult with your instructor regarding the opportunity to transfer a patient.

2. Evaluate your performance with the instructor.

CRITICAL THINKING EXERCISES

1. Martha Evans, age 77, fractured her hip in a fall at home. The surgeon repaired the fracture 2 days ago and has just ordered that Ms. Evans be up in a chair with no **weight-bearing** on the affected leg. Ms. Evans is alert and oriented and states that she fell when she got dizzy, although she has no idea why that might have happened. She is a thin, slightly frail woman. Based on this information, choose a method of transfer. Explain what additional information you would like to have before transferring the patient into a chair. Describe the specific criteria you will use to evaluate Ms. Evans' transfer.

2. Maude Jefferson is an 84-year-old nursing home resident. She goes to the dining room in a wheelchair for her meals. Although she can walk a few steps to a chair with assistance, she is unsteady and states that she is afraid of falling. You are to plan her care for the day. Evaluate the various types of transfers possible in relation to the abilities and deficits Ms. Jefferson appears to have. Identify the reasons each particular transfer technique would be appropriate or inappropriate for use with this individual. Plan an appropriate transfer technique.

SELF-QUIZ

SHORT-ANSWER QUESTIONS

1. State two reasons for having the patient wear shoes or slippers with firm soles when being transferred.

   a. _____

   b. _____

2. What should you do if a patient begins to fall during a transfer?

   _____

   _____

3. How would right-sided paralysis affect a patient's transfer?

   _____

4. What is the purpose of a transfer belt?

   _____

5. Name two transfer techniques for which a transfer belt is used.

   a. _____

   b. _____

6. Why is a patient changed from a lying-down to a sitting position slowly?

   _____

7. In what situation would you use a plastic transfer slider board?

   _____

MULTIPLE CHOICE

_____ 8. A patient is able to stand once up on her feet, but she has great difficulty rising to a standing position from the bedside chair. Which device would be the best choice to assist her in this process?
   a. Hydraulic sling lift
   b. Sit to stand electrical lift
   c. Transfer disk
   d. Transfer belt with two-person transfer

_____ 9. A patient has expressed fear of being lifted using the hydraulic sling lift. Which action is the most appropriate initial response to this situation?
   a. Explain exactly how the device works.
   b. Ask her what about the device makes her afraid.
   c. Reassure her that the device will not be used and that she will be lifted by staff.
   d. Tell her that there is nothing to be afraid of; it is perfectly safe.

_____ 10. A nurse is assisting a patient to get into a chair for the first time since his hospitalization. After standing up beside the bed and starting to pivot, the patient gets dizzy and weak and begins to collapse. The correct action by the nurse is to
   a. hold the patient up in place while calling for help.
   b. hold the patient, and try to pivot the patient back into the bed.
   c. continue the pivot into the chair, using the patient's weight as momentum.
   d. support the patient while lowering the patient to the floor.

Answers to the Self-Quiz questions appear in the back of the book.

Ambulation: Simple Assisted and Using Cane, Walker, or Crutches

SKILLS INCLUDED IN THIS MODULE

General Procedure for Ambulation
Procedures for Specific Types of Ambulation
  Simple Assisted Ambulation
  Using a Cane
  Using a Walker
  Using Crutches
    Crutchwalking Up Stairs
    Crutchwalking Down Stairs

PREREQUISITE MODULES

Module 1	An Approach to Nursing Skills
Module 2	Documentation
Module 3	Basic Body Mechanics
Module 4	Basic Infection Control
Module 5	Safety in the Healthcare Environment
Module 18	Transfer

The following modules may be needed for assessment of some patients before ambulation:

Module 11	Assessing Temperature, Pulse, and Respiration
Module 12	Measuring Blood Pressure

KEY TERMS

gait
gait belt
loss of balance
partial weight-bearing (PWB)

OVERALL OBJECTIVE

▸ To assist the patient to walk, or to use a walker, cane, or crutches effectively.

LEARNING OUTCOMES

The student will be able to

1. Assess the patient to determine the patient's ability to walk, activity tolerance, and previous use of assistive devices for ambulation.
2. Analyze the data to determine whether the patient needs assistance with ambulation and what assistive devices are needed.
3. Determine appropriate patient outcomes relative to frequency of ambulation and distance or duration of ambulation, and recognize the potential for adverse outcomes.
4. Plan interventions that support ambulation, including assistance and teaching as needed.
5. Effectively assist a patient to ambulate.
6. Teach the patient the correct technique for using a walker, cane, or crutches.
7. Evaluate the patient's ability to ambulate, tolerance of the activity involved, and technique in using assistive devices.
8. Document ambulation and teaching according to the facility policy.
9. Record effective strategies used for ambulation on the patient's plan of care.

Ambulation maintains and restores muscle tone, muscle strength, and joint flexibility. In addition, it helps individuals improve balance. Mobility also improves appetite and stimulates the respiratory and circulatory systems, increasing the effective functioning of each system. It stimulates bowel action, thus facilitating elimination. It also enhances the patient's psychological well-being, which is a move toward optimal health.

NURSING DIAGNOSES

- Activity Intolerance: related to immobility secondary to illness
- Impaired Mobility: related to any of a variety of musculoskeletal and neurologic conditions
- Deficient Knowledge: related to importance of activity/mobility in healing
- Risk for Injury: falls related to unsteady gait or loss of balance

DELEGATION

Ambulation is often delegated to assistive personnel after a physician, physical therapist, or nurse determines the amount and type of assistance necessary for the patient to ambulate safely. If assistive devices are needed, a physical therapist or nurse will do the initial teaching to the patient and family as appropriate. The nurse must then determine whether or not the assistive personnel have been taught the appropriate techniques to enable them to safely ambulate the patient. The nurse must also determine that the assistive personnel know how to appropriately assess the patient before

and after ambulation and recognize symptoms that are important to report.

GENERAL PROCEDURE FOR AMBULATION

ASSESSMENT

1. Identify the patient's capabilities. **R:** This helps you plan for patient participation.
2. Identify the level of activity ordered. **R:** When individuals are ill, the physician orders the level of activity that is appropriate for the medical condition.
3. Check the patient's previous level of activity. **R:** This provides a baseline for assessing later activity.
4. Determine whether assistive devices were previously used. **R:** Again, this provides a baseline.
5. Assess the patient's pulse, respirations, and blood pressure to provide a baseline.

ANALYSIS

6. Critically think through your data, carefully evaluating each aspect and its relation to other data. **R:** This enables you to determine specific problems for this individual in relation to ambulation.
7. Identify specific problems and modifications of the procedure needed for this individual. **R:** Planning for the individual must take into consideration the individual's problems.

PLANNING

8. Determine individualized patient outcomes in relation to ambulation or using a cane, walker, or crutches, including the following. **R:** Identification of outcomes guides planning and evaluation.

a. The patient is able to ambulate safely, correctly using a cane, walker, or crutches if needed.

b. The patient does not experience a drop or rise in blood pressure of more than 10 mm Hg, a rise in respiratory rate to tachypnea, or a change in pulse rate of more than 20 beats per minute while ambulating.

c. The patient is aware of signs and symptoms that indicate his or her need to rest.

d. The patient ambulates the desired distance and/or duration without undue fatigue or discomfort.

9. Plan for pain relief, if indicated, before ambulation. Be sure to allow enough time for the medication to take effect before the patient begins to ambulate. **R:** Pain will interfere with the patient's willingness and ability to move.

10. With the patient, set a tentative goal for how far the patient will ambulate. **R:** Setting goals helps the patient understand what is expected.

11. Decide how much support the patient will need. **R:** This determines the appropriate assistance or special devices to be obtained.

12. Plan to use a specific technique for assisting with ambulation. **R:** The technique used will depend on the individual patient situation. Planning ahead allows you to proceed more safely and effectively.

IMPLEMENTATION

Action	Rationale
13. Wash or disinfect your hands.	To decrease the transfer of microorganisms that could cause infection.
14. Identify the patient, using two identifiers.	Verifying the patient's identity helps ensure that you are performing the right skill for the right patient.
15. Explain to the patient what you are planning to do, and encourage questions.	Explaining the procedure helps relieve anxiety or misperceptions that the patient may have about a procedure or activity and sets the stage for patient participation.
16. Obtain the patient's robe and firm-soled, supportive shoes. If shoes are not available, use nonslip slippers.	The patient must be covered for warmth and modesty. Firm-soled, supportive shoes give the patient stability. Avoid "scuffs," which can easily slip off, and cloth slippers, which tend to slide on smooth floors. The area should be litter-free and spill-free so that the patient does not slip or fall.
17. Adjust the bed to an appropriate low position for the patient to transfer to a standing position, and help the patient to stand, using the techniques and devices discussed in Module 18 and later in this module.	To promote safety and prevent falls.
18. Using the directions given for the specific type of ambulation, assist the patient to ambulate.	Following directions carefully increases the potential for safety.
19. Watch the patient carefully for signs of any adverse responses.	To be able to respond immediately to any problem. Knowledge of the environment will make you aware of where the patient can sit and rest if he or she becomes weak or unsteady.
20. After completing the desired ambulation, return the patient to bed or to a chair, and position for comfort.	To ensure comfort and provide an opportunity to rest.

(continued)

Action	Rationale
21. Recheck pulse, respirations, and blood pressure.	To provide information related to the patient's ability to tolerate the activity.
22. Wash or disinfect your hands.	To decrease the transfer of microorganisms.

EVALUATION

23. Evaluate using the individualized patient outcomes previously identified, including the following. **R:** Evaluation in relation to desired outcomes is essential for planning future care.
    a. The patient was able to ambulate safely, correctly using a cane, walker, or crutches if needed.
    b. The patient did not experience a drop or rise in blood pressure of more than 10 mm Hg, a rise in respiratory rate to tachypnea, or a change in pulse rate of more than 20 beats per minute while ambulating.
    c. The patient was aware of signs and symptoms that indicate his or her need to rest.
    d. The patient ambulated the desired distance and/or duration without undue fatigue or discomfort.

DOCUMENTATION

24. Document the ambulation as appropriate for your facility. Include the time, the distance ambulated, any assistance or assistive devices used, and the patient's response. **R:** Documentation is a legal record of the patient's care and therapy; it also communicates nursing activities to other nurses and caregivers.
25. Document on the nursing care plan any new information about ambulating this patient. Include assistive aids or number of people needed, specific techniques that worked well, and the patient's ability to participate. **R:** To help ensure continuity of care.

■ POTENTIAL ADVERSE OUTCOMES AND RELATED INTERVENTIONS

1. The patient experiences fatigue or faintness.
Intervention: If the patient feels faint, move him or her to the nearest chair to sit with the head down to enhance blood flow to the brain. Ask someone else to get a wheelchair, so you can return the patient to bed.
2. The patient experiences **loss of balance.**
Intervention: If the patient loses balance slightly, help him or her regain it.
3. The patient's knees buckle, and the patient makes no attempt to straighten up.
Intervention: Control the descent to the floor. Do not try to hold the patient up: this is likely to injure you and is often unsuccessful. Simply steady and support the patient, making sure that the patient's head does not strike anything, as you allow him or her to slide slowly to the floor. Ask for help to return the patient to bed.

PROCEDURES FOR SPECIFIC TYPES OF AMBULATION

Simple Assisted Ambulation

This is the most commonly used procedure for ambulation. The person who is ill and may be unsteady, the elderly person with some disability, and the person recovering from recent surgery are examples of people who may need assistance with ambulation.

ASSESSMENT

1-5. Follow steps 1 to 5 of the General Procedure: Assess the patient's capabilities, activity order, previous level of activity, assistive devices previously used, and vital signs.

ANALYSIS

6-7. Follow steps 6 and 7 of the General Procedure: Think through your data, and identify specific problems and modifications.

PLANNING

8. Determine individualized patient outcomes in relation to ambulation. **R:** Identification of outcomes guides planning and evaluation. Include
    a. The patient is able to ambulate safely with assistance.
    b. The patient does not experience a drop or rise in blood pressure of more than 10 mm Hg, a rise in respiratory rate to tachypnea, or a change in pulse rate of more than 20 beats per minute while ambulating.
    c. The patient is aware of signs and symptoms that indicate his or her need to rest.
    d. The patient ambulates the desired distance and/or duration without undue fatigue or discomfort.
9-11. Follow steps 9 to 11 of the General Procedure: Plan for pain relief, set a tentative goal, and decide on support needed.
12. Obtain a **gait belt** (sometimes called a transfer or ambulation belt). **R:** A gait belt provides support and a firm way to hold on to the patient.

IMPLEMENTATION

Action	Rationale
13-17. Follow steps 13 to 17 of the General Procedure: Wash or disinfect your hands, identify the patient (two identifiers), explain what you are planning to do, obtain a robe and shoes or nonslip slippers, put the bed in low position, and help the patient to stand.	
18. Assist the patient to walk in the following way:	
a. In most cases, walk on the patient's weaker or affected side.	If the patient falters, you can give assistance and support. However, if the patient has poor balance and tends to lean toward the person assisting, walk on the patient's strong side, so that the patient's weight is shifted to the strong leg, rather than the weak leg, when he or she leans.
b. Use the gait belt around the patient's waist. A gait belt is made of strong webbing. It has a safety release buckle. When using a gait belt, walk on the patient's weaker side and slightly behind, with one hand grasping the belt in the center back. The other arm may be extended at the patient's side for the patient to grasp.	To provide safety with minimal support (Fig. 19-1). **FIGURE 19-1** Ambulation. The nurse stands on the patient's weaker side and grasps the ambulation belt. The patient may hold a cane on the stronger side.
c. Support the patient as you walk, but do not allow the patient to put an arm around your shoulders. Instead, offer support by extending an arm bent at the elbow with the palm up. The patient can then rest a hand on your arm.	If the patient has an arm around your shoulders and starts to fall, the weight could place a twisting strain on your back and cause severe injury. With an extended arm, you can maintain a firm support, and the patient can determine how much support to use.

(continued)

Action	Rationale
d. Walk slowly and with an even **gait.** Synchronize your steps with the patient's. Also, try to make your steps the same size as the patient's.	Smooth, coordinated movements, a steady gait, and synchronized steps will give the patient consistent support, promote confidence in you, and diminish fear of falling.
19-22. Follow steps 19 to 22 of the General Procedure: Watch the patient for adverse responses, return the patient to the bed or chair, recheck vital signs, and wash or disinfect your hands.	

EVALUATION

23. Follow step 23 of the General Procedure: Evaluate whether the technique used to assist the patient was effective. **R:** Evaluation in relation to desired outcomes is essential for planning future care. Evaluate using the individualized patient outcomes previously identified:
    a. The patient was able to ambulate safely with assistance.
    b. The patient did not experience a drop or rise in blood pressure of more than 10 mm Hg, a rise in respiratory rate to tachypnea, or a change in pulse rate of more than 20 beats per minute while ambulating.
    c. The patient was aware of signs and symptoms that indicate his or her need to rest.
    d. The patient ambulated the desired distance and/ or duration without undue fatigue or discomfort.

DOCUMENTATION

24-25. Follow steps 24 and 25 of the General Procedure: Document activity according to facility policy (time, distance ambulated, assistance used, and patient's response), and record on the nursing care plan any new information (assistive aids or number of people needed, specific techniques that worked well, patient's ability to participate).

USING A CANE

A cane is used by those who need help with balance or who are able to bear weight on both legs but have one leg weaker than the other. All canes should have a rubber tip to prevent slipping. The height of the cane should be that of the waist, allowing for 25% to 30% bend at the elbow when the patient places weight on the cane. If the cane is used to help in balance, encourage the patient to use a normal gait and to go slowly so that the cane is easy to use. This takes time to perfect. A quad cane, which has four tips, is used when maximum support is needed (Fig. 19-2). When a cane is used to augment a weak leg, a special gait is often useful. The gait usually is taught by a physical therapist, who also is responsible for securing and measuring the cane. The nurse supports the therapist's instructions and helps the patient practice.

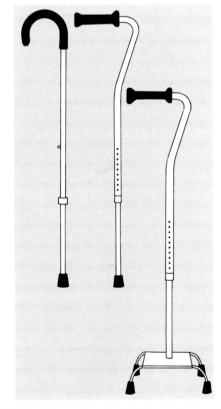

FIGURE 19-2 (**Left**) examples of adjustable aluminum canes. (**Right**) example of an adjustable quad cane, which provides excellent support during ambulation.

Specific Procedure for Using a Cane

ASSESSMENT

1-5. Follow steps 1 to 5 of the General Procedure: Assess the patient's capabilities, activity order, previous level of activity, assistive devices previously used, and vital signs.

ANALYSIS

6-7. Follow steps 6 and 7 of the General Procedure: Think through your data, and identify specific problems and modifications.

PLANNING

8. Determine individualized patient outcomes in relation to using a cane. **R:** Identifying outcomes guides planning and evaluation.

a. The patient is able to ambulate safely with assistance.

b. The patient does not experience a drop or rise in blood pressure of more than 10 mm Hg, a rise in respiratory rate to tachypnea, or a change in pulse rate of more than 20 beats per minute while ambulating.

c. The patient is aware of signs and symptoms that indicate his or her need to rest.

d. The patient ambulates the desired distance and/or duration without undue fatigue or discomfort.

9-11. Follow steps 9 to 11 of the General Procedure: Plan for pain relief, set a tentative goal, and decide on support needed.

12. Obtain a gait belt. **R:** Gait belts provide support and a firm way to hold onto the patient.

IMPLEMENTATION

Action	Rationale
13-17. Follow steps 13 to 17 of the General Procedure: Wash or disinfect your hands, identify the patient (two identifiers), explain what you are planning to do, obtain a robe and shoes or nonslip slippers, and put the bed in the low position.	
18. Teach the patient to stand up from a sitting position and walk with a cane, as follows:	
a. Grasp the cane in the hand opposite the affected leg for support.	This is the hand that will hold the cane while ambulating.
b. Slide the hips forward on the side of the bed or in the chair (if sitting in a chair).	To make standing easier.
c. Place the palm of the free hand down on the bed, or grasp one arm of the chair with the free hand. With the other hand, grasp the cane and the chair arm, if possible. If the patient cannot grasp both, only the cane is grasped.	To provide maximum stability.
d. Push to a standing position, using the mattress or the arms of the chair for support. Encourage this type of independence. If the patient needs help to stand, give only the help that is needed, and encourage maximum independence.	To develop muscle strength and balance and promote psychological well-being.

(continued)

Action	*Rationale*
e. After standing, pause in place. Then, to best maintain balance, have the patient place the cane close to his or her foot so that the patient remains erect, not bent over (Fig. 19-3).	To establish balance, to place the cane initially, and to keep the patient from tripping on the cane.

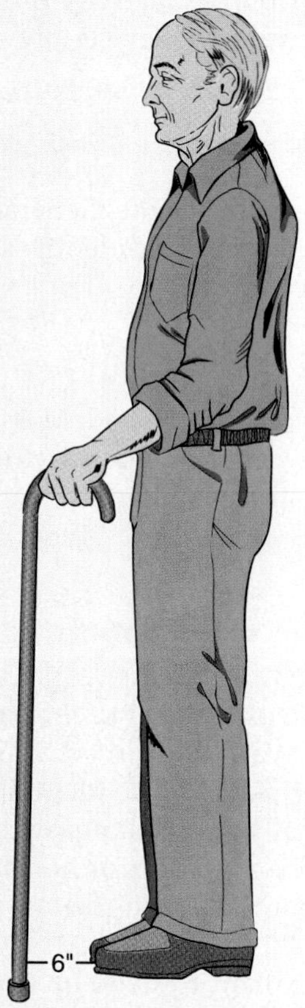

FIGURE 19-3 Proper cane stance. Cane on strong side; elbow slightly flexed. Cane is to the side and 6 inches in front of the foot.

Action	*Rationale*
f. Walk to the side and slightly behind the patient. You may want to use a gait belt until you have determined that the patient is strong enough to walk without the added support.	To position you to provide support if needed.
g. Teach the patient to carry out the gait pattern, as follows: (1) Move the cane ahead approximately 4 to 6 inches. (2) Move the affected leg ahead opposite the cane. (3) Place the weight on the affected leg and the cane.	To promote a normal walking pattern. This pattern provides for support when placing the weight on the weak leg and avoids having the patient lean toward the weak side, which contributes to falls.

(continued)

Action	Rationale
(4) Move the unaffected leg forward. The steps of both legs should remain equal.	
(5) Repeat the sequence.	
h. Teach the patient to sit, as follows:	This pattern promotes balance and independence when sitting and arising from the bed or chair.
(1) Using the cane, approach the chair, turn around, and back up to the bed or chair.	
(2) Reach behind to place the palm of the free hand on the mattress or to grasp one arm of the chair. With the other hand, grasp the cane and the other arm of the chair, if possible. If the patient cannot grasp both, only the cane is grasped.	
(3) The patient lowers himself or herself onto the bed or into the chair, placing the cane beneath the bed or chair so that someone else does not fall over it. If the cane is a quad cane, it is placed to the side of the bed or chair, within easy reach of the patient.	
19-22. Follow steps 19 to 22 of the General Procedure: Watch the patient for adverse responses, return the patient to the bed or chair, recheck vital signs, and wash or disinfect your hands.	

EVALUATION

23. Follow step 23 of the General Procedure: Evaluate using the individualized patient outcomes previously identified, including the following. **R:** Evaluation in relation to desired outcomes is essential for planning future care.

  a. The patient was able to ambulate safely with a cane.

  b. The patient did not experience a drop or rise in blood pressure of more than 10 mm Hg, a rise in respiratory rate to tachypnea, or a change in pulse rate of more than 20 beats per minute while ambulating.

  c. The patient was aware of signs and symptoms that indicate his or her need to rest.

  d. The patient ambulated the desired distance and/or duration without undue fatigue or discomfort.

DOCUMENTATION

24-25. Follow steps 24 and 25 of the General Procedure: Document activity according to facility policy (time, distance ambulated, assistance used, and patient's response), and record on the nursing care plan any new information (assistive aids or number of people needed, specific techniques that worked well, patient's ability to participate).

USING A WALKER

Walkers are assistive devices used by patients who have at least one weight-bearing leg and arms strong enough for **partial weight-bearing (PWB).** They also may be used by patients with generalized weakness and those with balance problems. A walker provides greater support and stability than a cane. Walkers are of two types, pick-up and rolling. The pick-up walker is more stable; it does not slip when the patient leans on it (Fig. 19-4). The rolling walker allows a smooth, normal gait but is less steady. Usually, the physical therapist determines which style of walker will be used. When there is a question, the more stable pick-up walker is generally recommended. Walkers can be adjusted in height. Ideally, they should reach slightly below waist level so that the handgrips can be grasped with comfort and so that the arms are slightly flexed to give strength to the support.

Specific Procedure for Using a Walker

ASSESSMENT

1-5. Follow steps 1 to 5 of the General Procedure: Assess the patient's capabilities, activity order, previous level of activity, assistive devices previously used, and vital signs.

ANALYSIS

6-7. Follow steps 6 and 7 of the General Procedure: Think through your data, and identify specific problems and modifications.

PLANNING

8. Determine individualized patient outcomes in relation to using a walker, including the following. **R:** Identification of outcomes guides planning and evaluation.
   a. The patient can ambulate safely with a walker.
   b. The patient does not experience a drop or rise in blood pressure of more than 10 mm Hg, a rise in

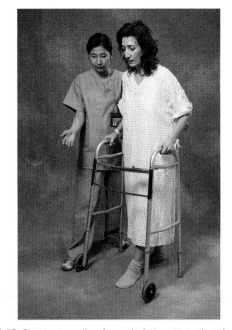

FIGURE 19-4 Using a walker for ambulation. Note that the arms are slightly bent and the walker is placed squarely in front of the person.

respiratory rate to tachypnea, or a change in pulse rate of more than 20 beats per minute while ambulating.
   c. The patient is aware of signs and symptoms that indicate his or her need to rest.
   d. The patient ambulates the desired distance and/or duration without undue fatigue or discomfort.

9-11. Follow steps 9 to 11 of the General Procedure: Plan for pain relief, set a tentative goal, and decide on support needed.

12. Obtain a gait belt to provide support and a firm way to hold on to the patient.

IMPLEMENTATION

Action	Rationale
13-17. Follow steps 13 to 17 of the General Procedure: Wash or disinfect your hands, identify the patient (two identifiers), explain what you are planning to do, obtain a robe and shoes, and put the bed in the low position.	
18. Assist the patient to stand and walk with a walker in the following way:	
a. Place the walker in front of the bed or chair. (You may wish to place a gait belt on the patient's waist until you are certain the patient is stable.)	This positions the walker where the patient can maintain balance while standing to use it. The patient uses the chair or bed instead of the walker when getting up because the lower surface allows him or her to push

(continued)

Action	Rationale
b. Place both hands on the arms of the chair or one hand on the mattress and the other grasping the upper side rail and push up to a standing position. You can grasp the gait belt for safety if needed.	with more force. Pushing or pulling on the walker may cause it to tip as the patient puts weight on it.
c. Move the hands to the handgrips of the walker one at a time to maintain balance during the transfer.	
d. Walk closely behind and slightly to the side of the patient.	To maintain safety for the patient.
e. Teach the patient to carry out the gait pattern, as follows: **(1)** Move the walker and the affected leg simultaneously ahead 4 to 6 inches. **(2)** Place weight on the arms for support. Place partial weight on the affected leg, if permitted. If no weight-bearing is allowed on the affected leg, the arms must support all the weight. **(3)** Move the unaffected leg forward. **(4)** Repeat the pattern.	This pattern helps the patient to maintain balance and stability.
f. Teach the patient to sit, as follows: **(1)** Turn around in front of the bed or chair, and back up until the legs touch the bed or chair. **(2)** Reach behind with one hand and then the other to grasp the arms of the chair or grasp the upper side rail with one hand. **(3)** Using the arms of the chair or the upper side rail, lower onto the bed or into the chair.	To place the patient in the correct position to sit directly onto the chair or bed. The walker is used for support during this maneuver. The arms of the chair or the upper side rail provide a solid and stable support and help the patient with balance.
19-22. Follow steps 19 to 22 of the General Procedure: Watch the patient for adverse responses, return the patient to the bed or chair, recheck vital signs, and wash or disinfect your hands.	

EVALUATION

23. Follow step 23 of the General Procedure: Evaluate using the individualized patient outcomes previously identified, including the following. **R:** Evaluation in relation to desired outcomes is essential for planning future care.

   a. The patient was able to ambulate safely with a walker.

   b. The patient did not experience a drop or rise in blood pressure of more than 10 mm Hg, a rise in respiratory rate to tachypnea, or a change in pulse rate of more than 20 beats per minute while ambulating.

   c. The patient was aware of signs and symptoms that indicate his or her need to rest.

   d. The patient ambulated the desired distance and/or duration without undue fatigue or discomfort.

DOCUMENTATION

24-25. Follow steps 24 and 25 of the General Procedure: Document as appropriate for your facility (time, distance ambulated, assistive devices used, patient's response), and document on the nursing care plan any new information (assistive aids or number of people needed, specific techniques that worked well, patient's ability to participate).

USING CRUTCHES

The physical therapist is usually responsible for initiating crutchwalking. This includes correctly adjusting the length of the crutches, determining the gait appropriate for the patient's condition, and initiating patient teaching. You must be aware of the basis for the therapist's decisions so that you can reinforce the teaching. In addition, in some settings, for example, the emergency department, you may be expected to carry out some of these functions when a physical therapist is not available.

Crutches are adjusted so that when a patient stands upright, the tip of the crutch rests approximately 6 inches in front of the foot and 2 inches to the side of the foot (Fig. 19-5). The top of the crutch rests against the chest wall, with approximately 2 inches between the crutch top and the axilla (Fig. 19-6). The patient should not rest on the crutches in a way that puts pressure on the axillae. Doing so causes pressure on the nerves that control the hand and can lead to numbness, tingling, muscle weakness, and even paralysis from nerve damage (known as crutch palsy).

Specific Procedure for Using Crutches

ASSESSMENT

1-5. Follow steps 1 to 5 of the General Procedure: Assess the patient's capabilities, activity order, previous

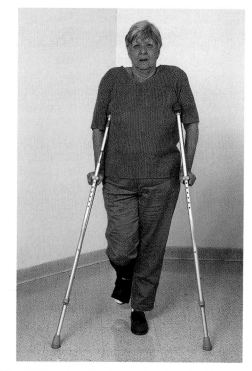

FIGURE 19-5 Tripod position for crutchwalking. Position the crutch tip to the side and 6 inches ahead of the foot.

level of activity, assistive devices previously used, and vital signs.

ANALYSIS

6-7. Follow steps 6 and 7 of the General Procedure: Think through your data, and identify specific problems and modifications.

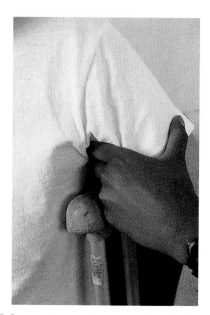

FIGURE 19-6 Measuring crutches for a proper fit. The top of the crutch should fall about 2 inches below the axilla.

PLANNING

8. Determine individualized outcomes in relation to walking with crutches, including the following. **R:** Identification of outcomes guides planning and evaluation.

   a. The patient can ambulate safely using crutches.

   b. The patient does not experience a drop or rise in blood pressure of more than 10 mm Hg, a rise in respiratory rate to tachypnea, or a change in pulse rate of more than 20 beats per minute while ambulating.

   c. The patient is aware of signs and symptoms that indicate his or her need to rest.

   d. The patient ambulates the desired distance and/or duration without undue fatigue or discomfort.

9-11. Follow steps 9 to 11 of the General Procedure: Plan for pain relief, set a tentative goal, and decide on support needed.

12. Obtain a gait belt to provide support and a firm way to hold on to the patient.

IMPLEMENTATION

Action	Rationale
13-17. Follow steps 13 to 17 of the General Procedure: Wash or disinfect your hands, identify the patient (two identifiers), explain what you are planning to do, obtain a robe and shoes, and put the bed in the low position.	
18. Assist the patient to stand, walk with crutches, using one of the gaits provided, and sit down as shown below:	
a. Stand using crutches.	This process promotes balance throughout the procedure.
(1) Place feet securely on the floor.	
(2) Slide hips forward on the bed or chair.	
(3) Hold both crutches in the hand of the unaffected side.	
(4) Grasp upper side rail or arm of chair with hand opposite of crutches.	
(5) Push up from the bed or chair.	
(6) Stabilize the body by standing on the unaffected leg.	
(7) Place crutches under both arms.	
(8) Take a crutch stance, with crutch tips at least 2 inches to the side and 6 inches ahead of the feet.	

(continued)

Action	Rationale
b. Using a gait. Always begin the gait with the patient in the standing crutch stance with weight bearing on the leg or legs as prescribed by the physician. Consistently use the gait prescribed by the physical therapist. Start at the bottom and move forward. Follow the description in the illustration carefully (Fig. 19-7 and Fig. 19-8):	Each gait requires somewhat different abilities and balance. When no gait has been prescribed, the nurse uses the descriptions of the gaits to choose the best option based on the patient's weight-bearing abilities and arm and shoulder strength.

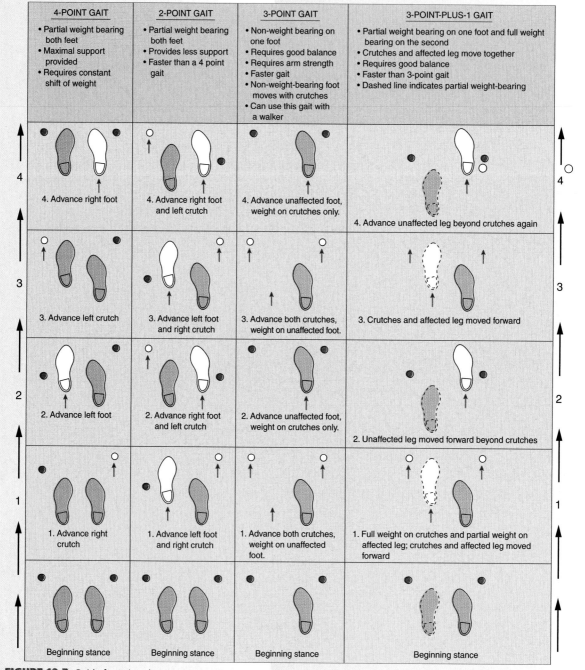

FIGURE 19-7 Guide for using the 4-point, 3-point, 3-point-plus 1, and the 2-point gaits. Start at the bottom and move forward. Note: Shaded areas indicate weight-bearing.

(continued)

Action	Rationale
	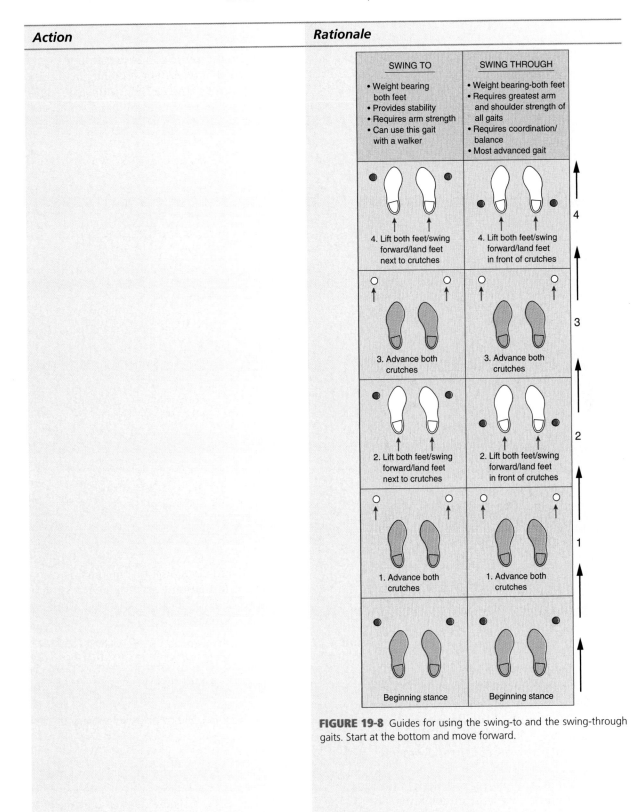

FIGURE 19-8 Guides for using the swing-to and the swing-through gaits. Start at the bottom and move forward.

(continued)

Action	Rationale
c. Sitting down with crutches: Teach patient to do the following: (1) Walk to the bed or chair. (2) Turn around so his or her back is to the bed or chair and the backs of the legs touch the bed or the chair. (3) Grasp both crutches in one hand. (4) Reach back with the free hand, and grasp the upper side rail or the arm of the chair. (5) Lower into the chair, using the support of both crutches and the bed or chair. (6) Sit back on the bed or in the chair using proper body mechanics. *Note:* Do not hyperextend the knees if the patient's legs are elevated.	This places the patient in the correct position to sit directly onto the bed or chair. The crutches are used for support during this maneuver. The upper side rail or the arms of the chair provide a solid and stable support and help the patient with balance.
19-22. Follow steps 19 to 22 of the General Procedure: Watch the patient for adverse responses, return the patient to the bed when appropriate, recheck vital signs, and wash or disinfect your hands.	

EVALUATION

23. Follow step 23 of the General Procedure: Evaluate using the individualized patient outcomes previously identified:
    a. The patient was able to ambulate safely using crutches and the appropriate gait.
    b. The patient did not experience a drop or rise in blood pressure of more than 10 mm Hg, a rise in respiratory rate to tachypnea, or a change in pulse rate of more than 20 beats per minute while ambulating.
    c. The patient was aware of signs and symptoms that indicated his or her need to rest.
    d. The patient ambulated the desired distance and/or duration without undue fatigue or discomfort.

DOCUMENTATION

24-25. Follow steps 24 and 25 of the General Procedure: Document as appropriate for your facility (time, distance ambulated, assistive devices used, patient's response), and document on the nursing care plan any new information (assistive aids or number of people needed, specific techniques that worked well, patient's ability to participate).

Specific Procedure for Crutchwalking Up Stairs

The patient must be able to bear weight on one leg.

ASSESSMENT

1-5. Follow steps 1 to 5 of the General Procedure: Assess the patient's capabilities, activity order, previous level of activity, assistive devices previously used, and vital signs.

ANALYSIS

6-7. Follow steps 6 and 7 of the General Procedure: Think through your data, and identify specific problems and modifications.

PLANNING

8. Determine individualized patient outcomes in relation to crutchwalking up stairs, including the following. **R:** Identification of outcomes guides planning and evaluation.
   a. The patient is able to walk up stairs safely using crutches.
   b. The patient does not experience a drop or rise in blood pressure of more than 10 mm Hg, a rise in respiratory rate to tachypnea, or a change in pulse rate of more than 20 beats per minute while walking up stairs with crutches.
   c. The patient is aware of signs and symptoms that indicate his or her need to rest.
   d. The patient walks up stairs on crutches without undue fatigue or discomfort.
9-11. Follow steps 9 to 11 of the General Procedure: Plan for pain relief, set a tentative goal, and decide on support needed.
12. Obtain a gait belt if the patient is not already wearing one. **R:** The gait belt provides support and a firm way to hold on to the patient.

IMPLEMENTATION

Action	Rationale
13-17. Follow steps 13 to 17 of the General Procedure: Wash or disinfect your hands, identify the patient (two identifiers), explain what you are planning to do, obtain a robe and shoes, put the bed in the low position if the patient is in bed.	
18. Assist the patient to walk upstairs with crutches in the following way:	This pattern provides a constant source of support for the patient at each step.
a. Position the crutches under the arms as if walking.	
b. Put weight on the hands.	
c. Raise the unaffected leg to the first step, and pull up the affected leg (Fig. 19-9).	

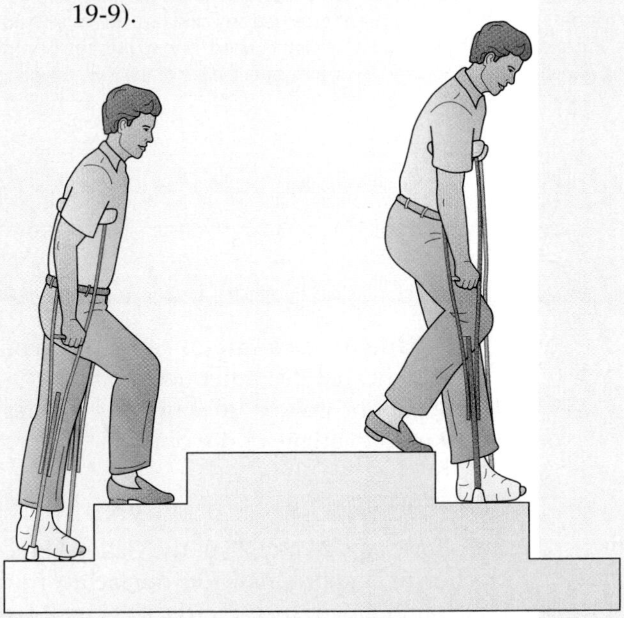

FIGURE 19-9 Using crutches to walk up and down stairs without a railing. The person pulls up the unaffected leg and advances the crutches to the same step. On the way down, the person puts his weight on the unaffected leg and places the crutches on the next lower step. The person also places partial weight on the hands and crutches and moves the affected leg to the lower step.

(continued)

Action	Rationale
d. Advance the crutches to the step on which you are standing.	
e. Again, raise the unaffected leg to the next higher step, and pull up the affected leg, advancing the crutches as before.	
f. If a railing is present, hold both crutches with one hand, and use the other to grasp the railing. R: The railing provides more stability than the two crutches will provide (Fig. 19-10).	

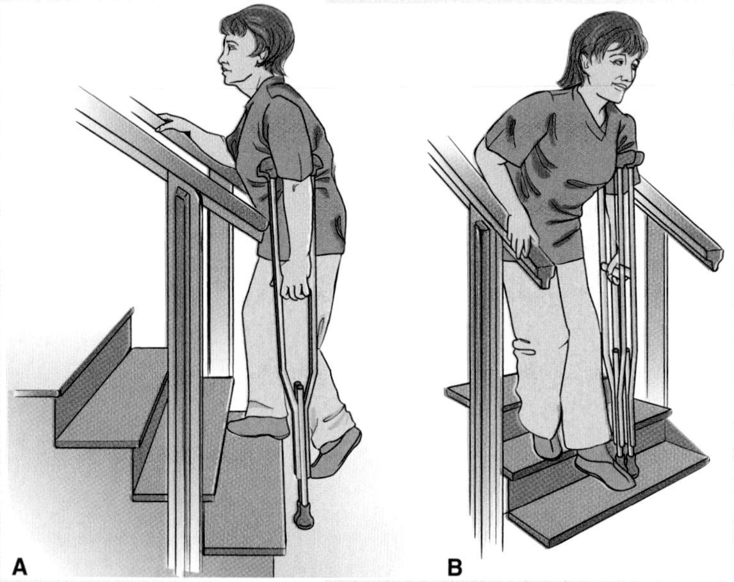

A **B**

FIGURE 19-10 Using crutches to navigate stairs with a railing. (**A**) Both crutches are held under one arm while the patient grasps the railing with the other hand and raises the unaffected leg up to the next step, followed by the affected leg and crutches. (**B**) To descend stairs with a railing, the patient again holds crutches under one arm and grasps the railing with the other hand. Placing the crutches on the next lower step, the patient puts partial weight on the hand, crutches, and railing and moves the affected leg to the lower step.

19-22. Follow steps 19 to 22 of the General Procedure: Watch the patient for adverse responses, return the patient to the bed or chair, recheck vital signs, and wash or disinfect your hands.

EVALUATION

23. Follow step 23 of the General Procedure: Evaluate using the individualized patient outcomes previously identified, including the following.
   a. The patient was able to walk up stairs safely using crutches.
   b. The patient did not experience a drop or rise in blood pressure of more than 10 mm Hg, a rise in respiratory rate to tachypnea, or a change in pulse rate of more than 20 beats per minute while walking up the stairs with crutches.
   c. The patient was aware of signs and symptoms that indicated his or her need to rest.
   d. The patient walked up stairs on crutches without undue fatigue or discomfort.

DOCUMENTATION

24-25. Follow steps 24 and 25 of the General Procedure: Document as appropriate for your facility (time, distance ambulated, assistive devices used, patient's response), and document on the nursing care plan any new information (assistive aids or number of people needed, specific techniques that worked well, patient's ability to participate).

Specific Procedure for Crutchwalking Down Stairs

ASSESSMENT

1-5. Follow steps 1 to 5 of the General Procedure: Assess the patient's capabilities, activity order, previous level of activity, assistive devices previously used, and vital signs.

ANALYSIS

6-7. Follow steps 6 and 7 of the General Procedure: Think through your data, and identify specific problems and modifications.

PLANNING

8. Determine individualized patient outcomes in relation to crutchwalking down stairs, including the following. **R:** Identifying outcomes guides planning and evaluation.

  a. The patient is able to walk down stairs safely using crutches.

  b. The patient does not experience a drop or rise in blood pressure of more than 10 mm Hg, a rise in respiratory rate to tachypnea, or a change in pulse rate of more than 20 beats per minute while walking up stairs with crutches.

  c. The patient is aware of signs and symptoms that indicate his or her need to rest.

  d. The patient walks down stairs on crutches without undue fatigue or discomfort.

9-11. Follow steps 9 to 11 of the General Procedure: Plan for pain relief, set a tentative goal, and decide on support needed.

12. Obtain a gait belt if the patient is not already wearing one to provide support and a firm way to hold on to the patient.

IMPLEMENTATION

Action	Rationale
13-17. Follow steps 13 to 17 of the General Procedure: Wash or disinfect your hands, identify the patient (two identifiers), explain what you are planning to do, obtain a robe and shoes or nonslip slippers, put the bed in the low position if the patient is in bed.	
18. Assist the patient to walk down stairs with crutches in the following way:	This pattern provides a constant source of support for the patient at each step.
a. Position crutches under the arms as if walking.	
b. Place weight on the unaffected leg.	
c. Place crutches on the next lower step.	
d. Put partial weight on the hands and crutches.	
e. Move the affected leg to the lower step.	
f. Put total weight on the crutches and the affected leg (see Fig. 19-9).	

(continued)

Action	Rationale
g. Move the unaffected leg to the same step as the crutches and the affected leg.	
h. If a railing is present, hold both crutches with one hand, and use the other to grasp the railing (see Fig. 19-10). The railing provides more stability than the two crutches will provide.	
19-22. Follow steps 19 to 22 of the General Procedure: Watch the patient for adverse responses, return the patient to the bed or chair, recheck vital signs, and wash or disinfect your hands.	

EVALUATION

23. Follow step 23 of the General Procedure: Evaluate using the individualized patient outcomes previously identified, including the following.
  a. The patient was able to walk down stairs safely using crutches.
  b. The patient did not experience a drop or rise in blood pressure of more than 10 mm Hg, a rise in respiratory rate to tachypnea, or a change in pulse rate of more than 20 beats per minute while walking down stairs with crutches.
  c. The patient was aware of signs and symptoms that indicate his or her need to rest.
  d. The patient walked down stairs on crutches without undue fatigue or discomfort. **R:** Evaluation in relation to desired outcomes is essential for planning future care.

DOCUMENTATION

24-25. Follow steps 24 and 25 of the General Procedure: Document as appropriate for your facility (time, distance ambulated, assistive devices used, patient's response), and document on the nursing care plan any new information (assistive aids or number of people needed, specific techniques that worked well, patient's ability to participate).

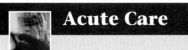

Acute Care

In the acute care environment, the physical therapist is available for the patient who has been admitted and is ordered to begin walking on crutches. The nurse helps the patient to follow the instructions given by the physical therapist. However, the person who comes to the emergency room may be sent home with instructions to rent or purchase crutches and use them for a period of time. These individuals can easily develop problems associated with poorly fitting crutches and an ineffective gait. Written instructions that can be reviewed with the patient before discharge may help them make the adjustment to crutches more effectively.

Long-Term Care

A major focus in all long-term care facilities is assisting the residents to stay as independent as possible. Supporting residents in maintaining their activity is an important component of that independence. Contrary to what many think, residents in long-term care can increase their ability to engage in activity with regular exercise. Assistance when necessary and encouragement to continue efforts help to sustain motivation in this process. Safety is a major concern because those who reside in long-term care facilities are often fragile and susceptible to falls.

Regular exercise programs in long-term care facilities can contribute to a feeling of increased well-being for all residents. Recent research has shown that even people in their eighties can benefit from regular muscle-strengthening exercises.

Home Care

Typically, more barriers to maintaining activity exist for those receiving care at home. Stairs, narrow doors, rugs, furniture placement, and inadequate lighting may all pose problems for the person trying to ambulate. You can assist clients and families to identify safety concerns and barriers to ambulation. When these problems have been identified, you can often be a resource for planning modifications. Handrails and grab bars may be installed in bathrooms and hallways. Area rugs that slip may be removed. Night-lights, brighter lightbulbs, and white lines painted on the edges of steps make it easier for individuals with disabilities to ambulate safely. The goal is to prevent injury and maintain or increase the present level of activity.

Ambulatory Care

Ambulatory care presents a situation similar to an emergency room. The client who has been prescribed crutches needs careful instruction before leaving the setting so that correctly fitting crutches may be chosen, and the person can use them correctly. Nurses in ambulatory care settings may begin to know clients over time and have the opportunity to discuss concerns related to ambulation in the home as part of health promotion activities.

LEARNING TOOLS

DEVELOP YOUR BACKGROUND KNOWLEDGE

1. Review the Learning Outcomes.

2. Read the section on activity in your assigned text.

3. Look up the Key Terms in the glossary.

4. Review this module, and mentally practice the techniques described. Study so that you would be able to teach these skills to another person.

DEVELOP YOUR SKILLS

In the practice setting, select one other student.
1. Practice ambulation with a partner. Take turns being the patient and being the nurse. Use a colored tie or scarf to mark one of the patient's legs as the affected leg.

2. Using the procedures in the module, practice each ambulation technique. Review the teaching and explanations for the patient each time. When you are the patient, evaluate your partner's performance using the Performance Checklist on the CD-ROM in the front of this book as a guide. Practice each of the following techniques:
   a. simple assisted ambulation
   b. using a cane
   c. using a walker
   d. using crutches (including three-point gait, three-point-plus-one gait, four-point gait, sitting down with crutches, and crutches on stairs)

3. When you believe that you have mastered these skills, ask your instructor to evaluate your performance.

4. If there is not enough equipment for each two students, one can be the patient, one the nurse, and a third can be the observer-evaluator. With this larger group, change roles as you did before so that each student has an opportunity for each role.

DEMONSTRATE YOUR SKILLS

In the clinical setting
1. Consult with your instructor regarding the opportunity to ambulate a patient.

2. Evaluate your performance with the instructor.

3. Consult with your instructor regarding the opportunity to visit physical therapy while initial teaching and support for ambulation and using assistive devices is conducted.

CRITICAL THINKING EXERCISES

A frail 84-year-old woman living with her family has balance problems occasionally, but she does not require assistive devices. You are making a home visit and find the situations described below. Analyze each situation, and suggest appropriate interventions or possible alternatives.
1. The living room, dining room, kitchen, two bedrooms (one used as an office), one bathroom, and a powder room are located on the first floor. Three bedrooms, one bathroom, and a sewing room are located on the second floor. The grandmother's room is on the second floor. Two teenagers occupy the other two upstairs bedrooms. The daughter and her husband sleep in the bedroom on the first floor. Suggest alternatives to these arrangements and implications for the family.

2. The grandmother's room on the second floor could use some updating. Furnishings include a double

bed. A small, crowded bedside table has a lamp shaded by a cracked glass globe, a clock radio, seven bottles and blister packs of medications, two books, a stack of letters and other mail, a glass of water, and a box of chocolate chip cookies. The bureau opposite the bed has four crowded drawers with some items of clothing crowding out of the drawers. In front of the bureau is a small rag rug, and beside the bed is another small rag rug. One standup lamp on the far side of the bedside table has only one lightbulb and an extralong cord visible between the grandmother's bed and adjoining bath. There is no overhead light and no telephone. Piled high in front of the closet door is a basket overflowing with sweaters, nightclothes, and blankets. Also on the floor beside the bed are a cat and the cat's bedding. What changes do you think will help increase safety in this room?

3. The older bathroom that adjoins the grandmother's room and that is used by the teenage grandchildren as well is large enough for two people to use at a time. It has a small sink, toilet, supply chest, medicine closet, and enclosed tub with shower. The room has no window. Lighting is supplied by a hanging unshaded bulb. Grandmother is hoping to get a new lighting fixture when she saves enough money to buy the one she wants. The floor is a shiny ceramic tile without carpeting. The shower door has lost its handle, and there are no grab bars and no soap dish inside the shower. Since there is no towel bar, the grandmother piles her towels and robe in the far corner in front of the toilet. The grandchildren leave their towels where they fall. The sink is small, and there is no cabinet space beneath it. There is some room for the grandmother to store her teeth in the glass cup she keeps at the edge of the sink. She can store other supplies in the small medicine chest above the sink.

SELF-QUIZ
SHORT-ANSWER QUESTIONS

1. Name four ways physical activity can improve patient status.

   a. _____

   b. _____

   c. _____

   d. _____

2. What is the major hazard of ambulation for patients?

   _____

3. Why are shoes better than most slippers for ambulation?

   _____

4. What types of assistive devices could be used for a person with one affected leg and one unaffected leg?

   _____

5. How is the crutch length determined?

   _____

   _____

6. Which gait pattern is indicated for the patient with muscular weakness, lack of balance, or lack of coordination?

   _____

7. Describe the safest way to teach a patient to stand up from a chair to use a walker.

   _____

8. On which side does the patient hold a cane?

   _____

9. When a patient using crutches sits down, what should he or she do with the crutches?

   _____

10. Which gait is appropriate for a patient using crutches who cannot bear weight on one leg?

    _____

11. When crutchwalking down stairs without a railing, what is the order of crutches, affected leg, and unaffected leg?

    _____

12. Name three safety precautions related to ambulation you would discuss with a patient recovering at home.

    a. _____

    b. _____

    c. _____

MULTIPLE CHOICE

_____ 13. Your patient is to ambulate today after being on bedrest for 6 days. Which of the following would indicate that the patient is not tolerating this amount of activity?
   a. Patient tends to walk in a bent posture.
   b. Pulse increases from 78 to 120.
   c. Blood pressure increased from 122/60 to 134/84.
   d. Respiratory rate increases from 12 to 22.

_____ **14.** The patient has one weak leg and will have to use a cane. Which method of holding the cane effectively supports the weak leg?
  a. Holding the cane on the unaffected side
  b. Holding the cane on the affected side
  c. Holding the cane where it is most comfortable
  d. Holding the cane on the unaffected side while moving and the affected side while sitting

_____ **15.** You are in an ambulatory clinic and must measure a client for crutches. How much space should there be between the crutch top and the axilla?
  a. No space, the crutch should touch the axilla
  b. One inch
  c. Two inches
  d. Three inches

Answers to the Self-Quiz questions appear in the back of the book.

MODULE 20

Implementing Range-of-Motion Exercises

SKILLS INCLUDED IN THIS MODULE

Procedure for Range-of-Motion Exercises
  Range of Motion for the Neck
  Range of Motion for the Elbow
  Range of Motion for the Wrist
  Range of Motion for the Hip and Knee
  Range of Motion for the Ankle
  Range of Motion for the Toes
  Range of Motion for the Spine

PREREQUISITE MODULES

Module 1	An Approach to Nursing Skills
Module 2	Documentation
Module 3	Basic Body Mechanics
Module 4	Basic Infection Control
Module 5	Safety in the Healthcare Environment
Module 6	Moving the Patient in Bed and Positioning

KEY TERMS

abduction	hyperextension
adduction	internal rotation
ball-and-socket joint	inversion
	opposition
circumduction	pivotal joint
condyloid joint	plantar flexion
contracture	pronation
contraindicated	proximal
distal	radial deviation
dorsiflexion	rotation
eversion	saddle joint
extension	supination
external rotation	synovial fluid
flexion	synovial joint
gliding joint	ulnar deviation
hinge joint	

OVERALL OBJECTIVE

▶ To perform range-of-motion (ROM) exercises on patients' joints, using proper sequence and joint positioning and support.

LEARNING OUTCOMES

The student will be able to
1. Assess a patient to determine the need for planned range-of-motion (ROM) exercises.
2. Analyze assessment data to determine if any specific problems are present that could affect the patient's ability to perform ROM exercises.
3. Determine appropriate patient outcomes for the individual patient's situation in regard to ROM exercises, and recognize the potential for adverse outcomes.
4. Plan an appropriate time to do ROM exercises.
5. Plan for patient teaching in regard to ROM exercises.
6. Implement ROM exercises safely and correctly for the patient.
7. Evaluate the effectiveness of ROM exercises for the individual patient.
8. Document ROM exercises according to the policy of the facility.

A joint that has not been moved sufficiently can begin to stiffen within 24 hours and will eventually become inflexible. With longer periods of joint immobility, the tendons and muscles can be affected as well. The flexor muscles contract strongly, leading to a shortening of flexor tendons and muscles and a permanent position of **flexion.** This fixed joint flexion position is called a **contracture.**

Many people with an illness or injury become unable to move one or more of the body's joints by themselves. The nurse must promptly take over this function to maintain joint and extremity mobility until the patient can move joints independently. With skill in handling the various body parts and knowledge of their movements, the nurse can prevent joint stiffening and contractures. Implementing range-of-motion (ROM) exercises for patients can often save them a lengthy rehabilitation.

When joint function has already been compromised and for patients at very high risk of joint contractures, a physical therapist usually prescribes appropriate exercises and may even use splints to maintain joints in functional positions.

NURSING DIAGNOSES

An appropriate nursing diagnosis for patients who are not able to move one or more of the body's joints independently is Impaired Physical Mobility. The ROM exercises in this module are essential for such patients.

DELEGATION

After the nurse has assessed the patient and planned for ROM exercises, the exercises are frequently delegated to assistive personnel. The nurse must know what the assistive personnel were taught about performing these exercises in order to determine whether teaching will be needed in order to delegate. The nurse will evaluate the effectiveness of the exercises and monitor the performance of the assistive person.

TYPES OF JOINTS

In all joints of the body, the ends of the bones are encased in a capsule and are lubricated with a viscous fluid secreted by the membrane within the capsule. This fluid is called **synovial fluid,** and the membrane that secretes it is called synovial membrane. Supporting cartilage provides a smooth gliding surface that is lubricated by the synovial fluid as the joint is moved. There are several types of joints: **ball-and-socket, hinge, condyloid, saddle, gliding, synovial, pivotal,** and combination. Each type can move only in certain ways. Table 20-1 lists the various types of joints and their movements.

RANGE-OF-MOTION EXERCISES

ROM exercises are exercises in which a person moves each joint through as full a range as possible without causing pain. Most people move and exercise their joints through the normal activities of daily living. When any joint is not moved in this way, the patient or nurse must move the joint to maintain muscle tone and joint mobility.

GOALS OF RANGE-OF-MOTION EXERCISES

The two goals of ROM exercises are to maintain current joint function and restore joint function that has been lost through disease, injury, or lack of use. The restora-

table 20-1. Body Areas, Types of Joints, and Movement

Body Area	Type of Joint	Movement
Neck	Pivotal joint	Flexion
		Extension
		Hyperextension
		Lateral flexion
		Lateral rotation
Shoulder	Ball-and-socket	Flexion
		Extension
		Vertical abduction
		Vertical adduction
		Internal rotation
		External rotation
		Horizontal abduction
		Horizontal adduction
Elbow	Hinge	Flexion
		Extension
Wrist and forearm	Condyloid	Flexion
		Extension
		Radial deviation
		Ulnar deviation
		Circumduction
		Pronation
		Supination
Hands (two types of joints)		
Hand knuckles	Condyloid	Flexion
		Extension
		Abduction
Finger joints	Hinge	Adduction
		Flexion
		Extension
Thumb (two types of joints)		
Joint near wrist	Saddle	Flexion
		Extension
		Abduction
		Adduction
		Opposition
Joint at base of thumb	Condyloid	Flexion
		Extension
		Abduction
		Adduction
Joint at end	Hinge	Flexion
		Extension
Hip	Ball-and-socket	Flexion
		Extension
		Abduction
		Adduction
		Internal rotation
		External rotation
Knee	Hinge	Flexion
		Extension
Ankle	Gliding and hinge	Dorsiflexion
		Plantar flexion
		Inversion
		Eversion
Toe (two types of joints)		
Joint near foot	Condyloid	Flexion
		Extension
		Abduction
		Adduction
Joints on toe	Hinge	Flexion
		Extension
Spine	Gliding	Flexion
		Extension
		Hyperextension
		Lateral flexion
		Rotation

tive process requires the special skills and techniques of a physical therapist. Maintaining current function may be done by the patients, nurses, physical therapists, assistants, and family members.

CONTRAINDICATIONS TO RANGE-OF-MOTION EXERCISES

ROM exercises require energy and tend to increase circulation. Any illness or disorder in which increasing the level of energy expended or increasing the demand for circulation is potentially hazardous is a contraindication to routine ROM exercises. This is seen particularly in patients with heart and respiratory diseases. If these conditions are present, the nurse should consult with the physician to determine whether ROM exercises are appropriate or are **contraindicated** by the patient's condition.

ROM exercises also put stress on the soft tissues of the joint and on the bony structures. These exercises should not be performed if the joints are swollen or inflamed or if the musculoskeletal system in the vicinity of the joint has been injured. Gentle exercises may be appropriate in some of these situations, but this requires consultation with the physician.

JOINTS NEEDING EXERCISE

When an individual is weak or inactive, exercises of all joints may be needed because the ordinary activities of daily living may not provide sufficient exercise of the joints to maintain range of motion. In particular, elderly individuals may need assistance in planning for ROM exercises when a sedentary lifestyle places them at risk for loss of joint function. Daily ROM exercises are usually adequate to maintain full mobility for these individuals.

When extremities or joints are just weak or partially affected, focus your assessment on abilities and disabilities. How far can the patient move the joint independently? This may be indicated in degrees of motion. How far can the joint be moved with assistance? Is there any stiffness or barrier to passive movement?

Any joint that is completely immobile as a result of paralysis is in particular need of ROM exercises. When a patient is completely paralyzed on one side of the body, the joints ideally should be exercised four or five times daily for full maintenance of joint flexibility. In reality, however, you may see exercise limited to only one or two times a day because of inadequate staffing. Limited ROM exercising does not lead to optimum joint mobility.

When a patient receives ROM exercises for the first time, exercise affected and unaffected joints bilaterally to establish a baseline of normal functioning for the patient. With each ROM procedure, move each joint through its range six to eight times. If you also are bathing or ambulating the patient, you will not have to exercise all the joints as many times because several of the bathing movements are ROM movements. As a nurse performing ROM, you must never force a joint to the point of pain because this may injure the joint. However, restorative therapy by a physical therapist may sometimes push a joint to the point of pain.

TYPES OF RANGE-OF-MOTION EXERCISES

ROM exercises may be classified as active, active-assisted, and passive.

ACTIVE RANGE-OF-MOTION EXERCISES

In active ROM, instruct the patient to perform the movements on a nonfunctioning joint. When patients are taught a planned ROM program, they feel more independent because they are participating actively. They also can carry out additional ROM by participating in their own care. Combing the hair exercises joints of the upper extremity; lifting the foot for bathing exercises joints of the lower extremity. Encourage other appropriate activities as well.

ACTIVE-ASSISTIVE RANGE-OF-MOTION EXERCISES

Active-assistive ROM is carried out with both patient and nurse participating. Encourage the patient to carry out as much of each movement as possible, within the limitations of strength and mobility. The nurse supports or completes the desired movement.

PASSIVE RANGE-OF-MOTION EXERCISES

Passive ROM is performed by a nurse or other care provider on a patient's immobilized joints. Your assessment skills are needed to determine which parts or joints must be exercised and with what frequency.

After certain types of major joint surgery (such as a knee replacement or shoulder surgery), restoring the patient's ROM is a significant concern. In such cases, a machine called a continuous passive motion (CPM) device may be used (Fig. 20-1). The CPM device for the knee provides a sling support for the thigh and calf, with a hinged connection at the knee. A footplate maintains the foot at a right angle to prevent footdrop. The CPM device is placed in the bed under the leg; the motor is placed under the bed and plugged into a convenient outlet. The leg is then positioned in correct alignment with the knee at the flex point and secured to the CPM device with Velcro straps. (Usually padding or an artificial sheepskin is placed under the leg for comfort.) A control allows you to set the degree of flexion ordered by the surgeon. When the machine is turned on, it automatically flexes and extends the knee joint at

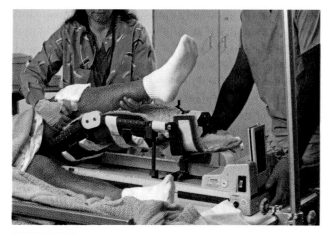

FIGURE 20-1 Continuous passive motion machine.

a slow, continuous rate. There also are CPM machines designed to move the shoulder after surgery. They operate on the same principle as the CPM device for the knee.

When caring for a patient using a CPM device, determine how many hours the device is to be used and what degree of flexion has been ordered. Remove the CPM device for such activities as bathing, skin care, ambulating, or going to the bathroom. Some CPM devices have an on-off switch that allows for patient control, enhancing self-care. The patient using a CPM device will continue to have physical therapy for concentrated exercise.

SEQUENCE OF EXERCISES

Joints are exercised sequentially, starting with the neck and moving downward. Joints move in different ways. The knee and elbow move in just one direction; the neck, wrist, and hip move in several directions. Several movements can be done together. For example, flexion of the knee and external **rotation** of the hip can be done simultaneously, as can **abduction** and **external rotation** of the shoulder. Never grasp joints directly. Instead, grasp the extremities gently but firmly either **distal** or **proximal** to the joint. This is more comfortable for the patient and results in easier movement through the entire ROM. Cup the heel in your hand when exercising the leg. When it is necessary to support the joint itself, gently cup your hand under the joint, and allow the joint to rest on the palm of the hand. This prevents pressure on the joint. Do not grasp the fingernails or toenails; this can be uncomfortable for the patient. When exercising extremities, work from the proximal joints toward the distal joints.

Every joint should receive adequate exercise, but it is crucial that several particular joints remain functional to provide independence. For example, flexion of the thumb must be maintained so that there is **opposition** of the thumb to the other fingers to promote optimum function. Hip and knee **extension** allow the patient to walk successfully when he or she is again mobile. Maintaining ankle flexion helps to prevent footdrop, which interferes with walking.

PROCEDURE FOR RANGE-OF-MOTION EXERCISES

While performing ROM exercises for the patient, keep in mind correct body mechanics for yourself to prevent musculoskeletal strain (see Module 3).

ASSESSMENT

1. Assess the patient's joint mobility and activity status. **R:** This determines the need for ROM exercises.
2. Assess the patient's general health status. **R:** To determine whether any contraindications to ROM exercises are present.
3. Assess the patient's ability and willingness to cooperate in ROM exercises. **R:** This facilitates patient self-care as much as possible.
4. Check for any physician's orders related to activity. **R:** A review of orders ensures that planning for ROM exercises is done within the context of the overall plan of care.

ANALYSIS

5. Critically think through your data, carefully evaluating each aspect and its relation to other data.

R: To determine specific problems for this individual in relation to ROM exercises.

6. Identify specific problems and modifications of the ROM procedure needed for this individual. **R:** Planning for the individual must take into consideration the individual's problems.

PLANNING

7. Identify appropriate individualized patient outcomes of the ROM exercises, including the following. **R:** Individualized outcomes facilitate planning and evaluation.
   a. Joints have flexibility to move through full ROM.
   b. Patient is willing and able to complete ROM exercises independently.
   c. Patient is comfortable throughout the ROM exercises.
8. Plan when ROM exercises should be done. **R:** For example, bath time is an appropriate time to complete ROM exercises. The warm bathwater relaxes the muscles and decreases their potential to spasm. Additionally, during the bath, areas are exposed so that the joints can be moved and observed. Other appropriate times might be when the patient is rested in the morning or before bedtime.
9. Plan whether exercises will be active, active-assistive, or passive, and which joints will be included (see discussion above for choosing). **R:** Maximum patient participation results in the most effective outcome. Planning ahead allows you to proceed more safely and effectively.

IMPLEMENTATION

	Action	Rationale
✳	10. Wash or disinfect your hands.	To decrease the transfer of microorganisms that could cause infection.
	11. Obtain any needed supportive devices or assistance.	To save time and promote efficiency.
▲	12. Identify the patient, using two identifiers.	Verifying the patient's identity helps ensure that you are performing the right skill for the right patient.
	13. Explain the procedure you are about to perform.	Explaining the procedure helps relieve anxiety or misperceptions that the patient may have about a procedure or activity and sets the stage for patient participation.
▲	14. Raise the bed to an appropriate working position based on your height.	To allow you to use correct body mechanics and protect yourself from back injury.

(continued)

Action	Rationale
15. Follow the procedure below to complete ROM on one side of the body. Complete ROM on joints you have determined should be exercised. After each movement, return the part to its correct anatomic position. Each joint movement is described separately here. Remember that it is possible to move two joints, such as the shoulder and the elbow, at the same time. A plan for exercising all joints follows.	
a. Range of motion of the neck (Fig. 20-2) **(1) Hyperextension:** Position the head as if looking up at the ceiling. The elderly person should not perform this movement, which can lead to pain or cervical fractures. **(2)** Extension: Position the head as if looking straight ahead (not shown in Fig. 20-2).	This sequence includes all the movements that are possible for the neck.

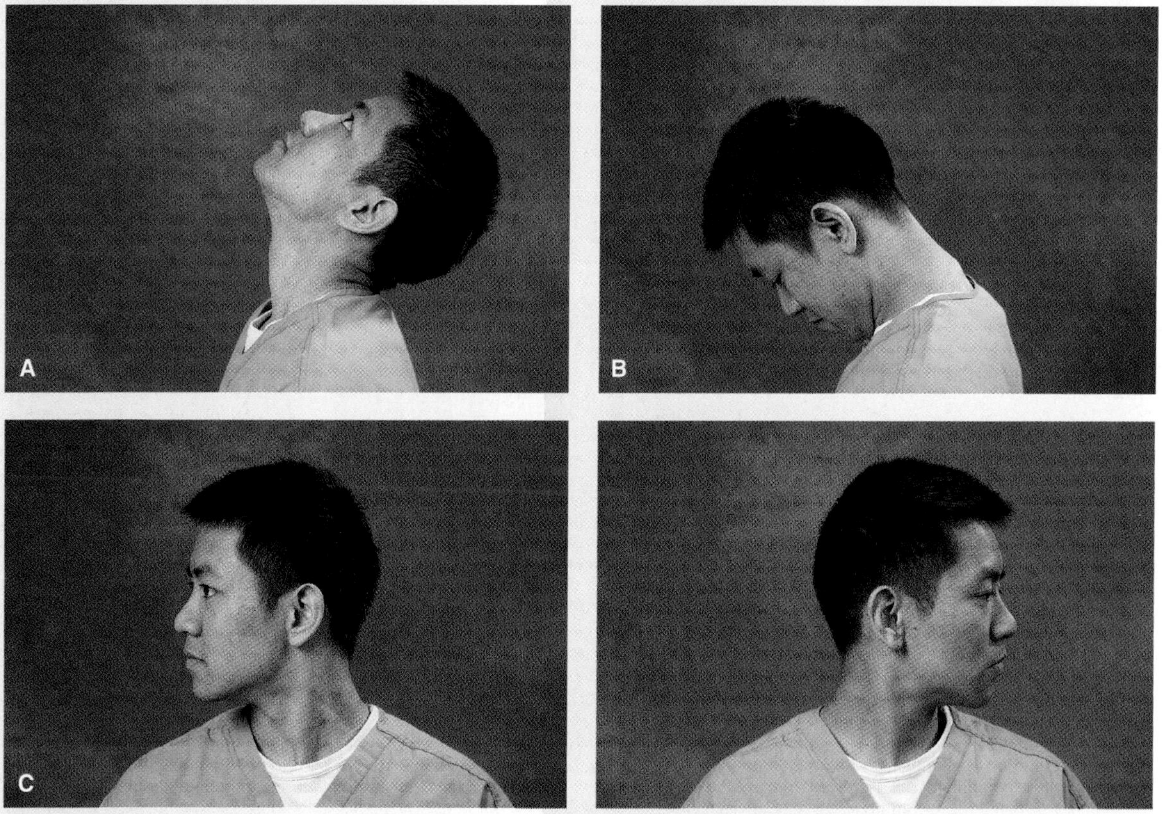

FIGURE 20-2 Exercising the neck. (**A**) Hyperextension: Person lifts head straight backward with eyes toward ceiling. (**B**) Flexion: Person lowers head to chest with eyes toward floor. Lateral flexion: Person moves head toward one shoulder and then the other. (**C**) Lateral rotation: Person moves head in twisting motion from side to side.

(continued)

Action	Rationale
(3) Flexion: Position the head as if looking at the toes.	
(4) Lateral flexion: While the head is positioned looking straight ahead, tilt the head toward the shoulder, first to the left and then to the right (not shown in Fig. 20-2).	
(5) Lateral rotation: Position the head so that the head is looking first toward the right and then toward the left.	
b. Range of motion of the shoulder (Fig. 20-3)	This sequence includes all the movements that are possible for the shoulder.

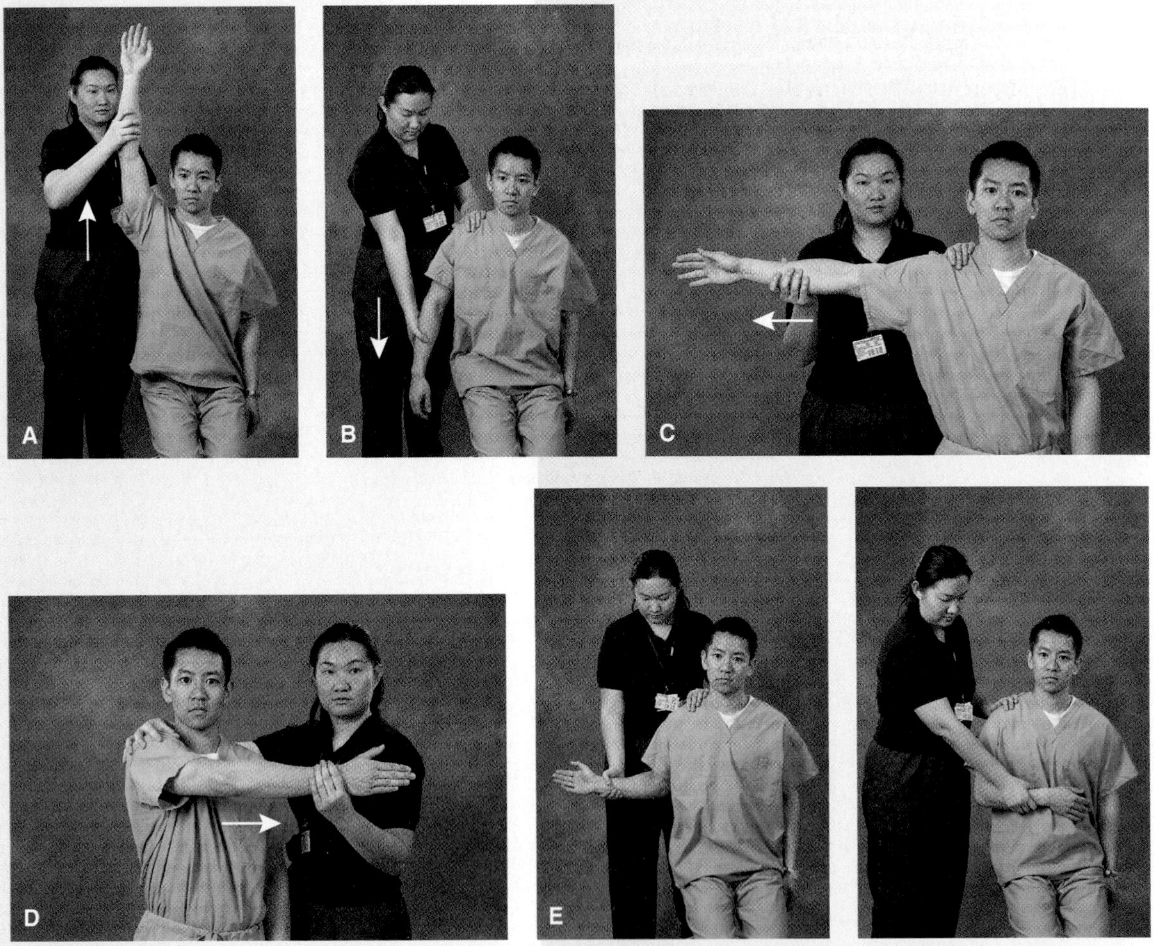

FIGURE 20-3 Exercising the shoulder. (**A**) Flexion: Raise arm forward and overhead. (**B**) Extension: Return arm to side of body. (**C**) Vertical abduction: Swing arm out and up. (**D**) Internal rotation: Swing arm up and across body. (**E**) External rotation: Rotate arm out and back.

(continued)

Action	Rationale
(1) Flexion: Raise the arm forward and overhead. The elbow may be bent to avoid the head of the bed.	
(2) Extension: Return the arm to the side of the body.	
(3) Vertical abduction: Swing the arm out from the side of the body and up.	
(4) Vertical **adduction:** Return the arm to the side of the body (not shown in Fig. 20-3).	
(5) Internal rotation: Swing the arm up and across the body.	
(6) External rotation: Rotate the arm out and back, keeping the elbow at a right angle.	
c. Range of motion of the elbow (Fig. 20-4): These movements can be performed in conjunction with the shoulder movements. When doing these, the caregiver needs to be sure to support the elbow.	This sequence includes all the movements that are possible for the elbow.
(1) Flexion: Bend the elbow.	
(2) Extension: Straighten the elbow.	
d. Range of motion of the wrist (Fig. 20-5)	This includes all the movements possible for the wrist joint.
(1) Flexion: Grasping the palm with one hand and supporting the elbow with the other hand, bend the wrist forward.	
(2) Extension: Straighten the wrist joint and move dorsally.	
(3) Radial deviation: Bend the wrist toward the thumb.	
(4) Ulnar deviation: Bend the wrist toward the little finger.	
(5) Circumduction: Move the wrist in a circular motion.	

(continued)

Action	*Rationale*

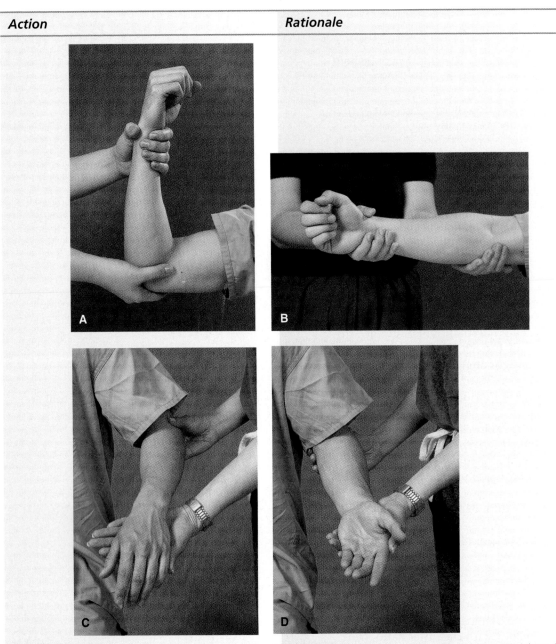

FIGURE 20-4 Exercising the elbow. (**A**) Flexion: Cupping the elbow in the hand, bend the arm. (**B**) Extension: Straighten the arm. (**C**) Pronation. (**D**) Supination. Note that the elbow is always supported.

(6) **Pronation:** Turn the hand so that the palm is downward.

(7) **Supination:** Turn the hand so that the palm is upward.

(continued)

Action	*Rationale*

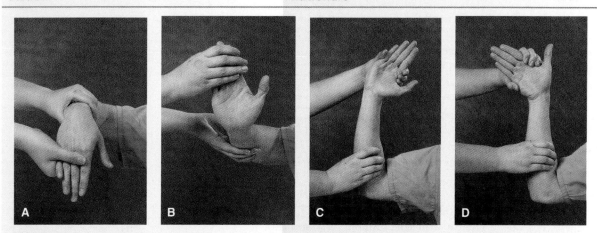

FIGURE 20-5 Exercising the wrist. (**A**) Flexion: Support elbow with one hand; grasp palm and bend wrist forward. (**B**) Extension: Straighten wrist and move dorsally. (**C**) Lateral flexion for radial deviation: Bend the wrist toward the thumb. (**D**) Lateral flexion for ulnar deviation: Bend the wrist toward the little finger.

e. Range of motion of the fingers and thumb (Fig. 20-6). A hand can be partially functional if a patient is able to place the thumb in opposition to the index finger or third finger. Therefore, take special care to exercise these joints as thoroughly as possible. You can move all three joints of each finger and the fingers and thumb through flexion and extension together.

(1) Flexion: Bend the fingers and thumb onto the palm.

(2) Extension: Return them to their original position.

This sequence includes all the movements possible for the fingers and thumb.

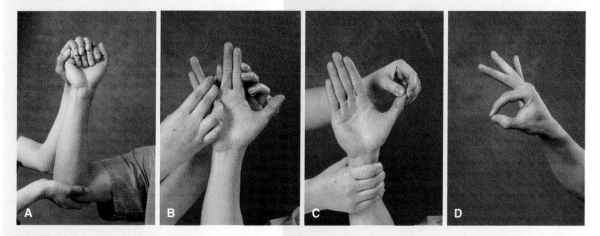

FIGURE 20-6 Exercising the fingers and thumb. (**A**) Flexion: Bend the fingers and thumb onto the palm. (**B**) Abduction: Spread the fingers. (**C**) Circumduction of the thumb: Move thumb in circular motion. (**D**) Opposition: Touch end of thumb to each of fingers in turn.

(continued)

Action	Rationale
(3) Abduction: Spread the fingers. (4) Adduction: Return the fingers to the closed position. (5) Circumduction: Move the thumb in a circular motion. (6) Opposition: Touch the end of the thumb to each of the fingers in turn.	
f. Range of motion of the hip and knee (Fig. 20-7): The hip and knee can be exercised together. Place one hand under the patient's knee, and with the other hand, support the heel. (1) Flexion: Lift the leg, bending the knee as far as possible toward the patient's head. (2) Extension: Return the leg to the surface of the bed, and straighten. (3) Abduction: With the leg flat on the bed, move the entire leg out toward the edge of the bed.	This sequence includes all the movements of the knee and hip.

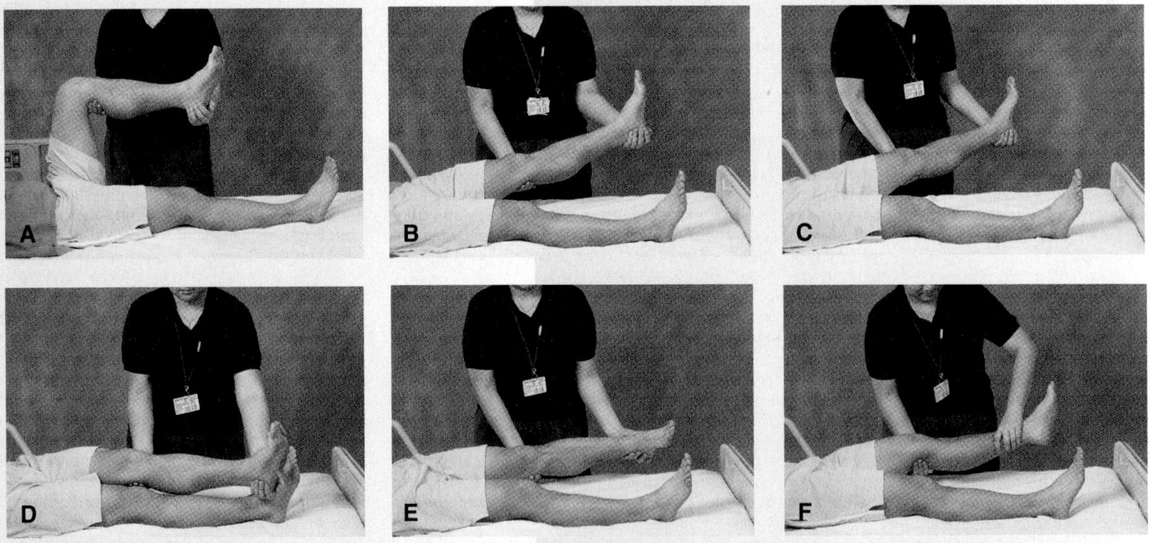

FIGURE 20-7 Exercising the hip and knee. (**A**) Flexion: Cupping the heel in your hand, bend knee toward head. (**B**) Extension: Return leg to bed. (**C**) Abduction: Move leg outward to edge of bed. (**D**) Adduction: Bring leg back to midline. (**E**) Internal rotation: Roll entire leg inward. (**F**) External rotation: Roll entire leg outward.

(continued)

Action	Rationale
(4) Adduction: Bring the leg back toward the midline or center of the bed. *Note:* Steps (3) and (4) can be performed with the knee bent. This allows you to give better support to some patients and affords a greater range of movement. **(5)** Internal rotation: With the leg flat on the bed, roll the entire leg inward so that the toes point in. This will rotate the hip joint internally. **(6)** External rotation: With the leg flat on the bed, roll the entire leg outward so that the toes point out. This will rotate the hip externally.	
g. Range of motion of the ankle (Fig. 20-8) **(1) Dorsiflexion:** Cup the patient's heel with your hand, and rest the sole of the foot against your forearm. Steady the leg just above the ankle with your other hand. Put pressure against the patient's sole	This sequence includes all the movements of the ankle.

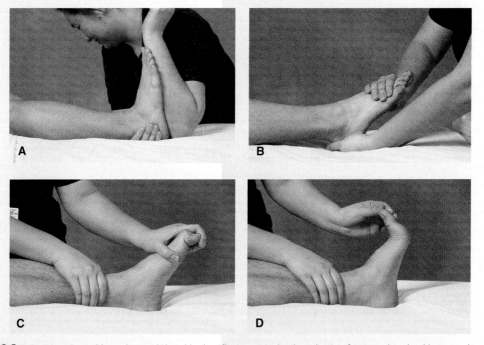

FIGURE 20-8 Exercising the ankle and toes. (**A**) Ankle dorsiflexion: Cup heel, and using forearm, bend ankle toward upper body. (**B**) Ankle plantar flexion: Cup heel and push ankle downward to point toes. (**C**) Flexion of toes: Bend toes downward. (**D**) Extension of toes: Bend toes upward.

(continued)

Action	Rationale
of the foot with your arm to flex the ankle.	
(2) **Plantar flexion:** Change your hand from above the ankle to the ball of the foot. Move the other arm away from the toes, keeping the hand cupped around the heel, and push the foot downward to point the toes.	
(3) **Circumduction:** Rotate the foot on the ankle, moving it first in one direction and then in the other.	
h. Range of motion of the toes (see Fig. 20-8)	This sequence includes all the movements of the toes.
(1) Flexion: Bend the toes down. Avoid grasping the nails because this can be uncomfortable for the patient.	
(2) Extension: Bend the toes up.	
i. Range of motion of the spine (Fig. 20-9): These exercises can be done only by an individual who is able to stand. Direct the elderly person to hold the back of a chair or a railing for balance while doing these exercises. If the person experiences back pain, the exercise should be stopped.	This includes the movements possible for the spine.
(1) Extension: Stand straight.	
(2) Flexion: Bend forward from the waist.	
(3) Hyperextension: Bend backward from the waist.	
(4) Lateral flexion: Bend toward the side, first left, then right.	
(5) Rotation: Twist from the waist to the side, first left, then right.	
16. Return the bed to the lower position for the patient to get in and out.	To facilitate patient activity and provide for safety.
17. Wash or disinfect your hands.	To decrease the transfer of microorganisms that could cause infection.

(continued)

Action	Rationale

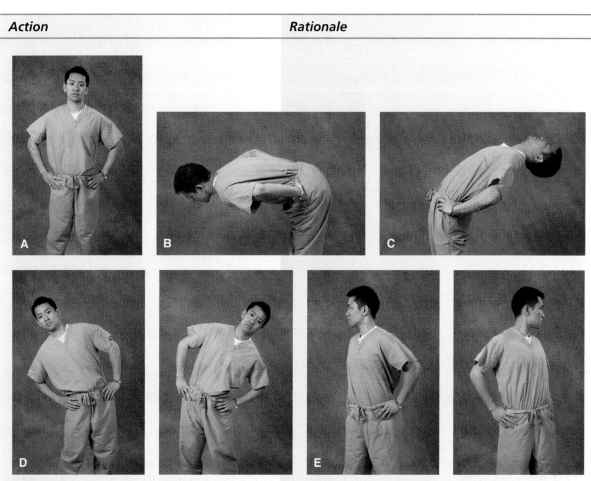

FIGURE 20-9 Exercising the spine. (**A**) Extension: Stand straight. (**B**) Flexion: Bend forward. (**C**) Hyperextension: Bend backward. (**D**) Lateral flexion: Bend toward each side. (**E**) Rotation: Twist from the waist.

EVALUATION

18. Evaluate the effectiveness of the ROM regimen in relation to the individualized outcomes previously identified, including the following. **R:** Evaluation in relation to desired outcomes is essential for planning future care.
   a. Joints have flexibility to move through full range of motion.
   b. Patient was willing and able to complete ROM exercises independently.
   c. Patient remained comfortable throughout the procedure.

DOCUMENTATION

19. Document the ROM exercises as appropriate for your facility. The specific activity carried out, the time, the ability to move the joints, and the patient's response are usually noted on the patient's chart, either on a flow sheet or in the nurse's progress notes. **R:** Documentation is a legal record of the patient's care and therapy and communicates nursing activities to other nurses and caregivers.

20. Document plans for future ROM exercises, such as any new information about times planned for them, the best method, and the patient's ability to participate, on the nursing care plan. **R:** To ensure continuity of care.

POTENTIAL ADVERSE OUTCOMES AND RELATED INTERVENTIONS

1. Patient experiences pain when joints are moved. *Intervention:* Slow the movement initially. Joints may sometimes be moved slowly through movements that cause pain when the movement is rapid. If discomfort continues, encourage maximum movement possible without pain. Give pain medication prn (as needed) if available. Consult with physician about joint pain.

2. Joints are stiff and do not move through full range of motion. *Intervention:* Move the joint as far as possible, and encourage the patient to continue ROM exercises to maintain joint flexibility that is still present.

Acute Care

In hospitals, ROM exercises are most often done by physical therapists based on specific rehabilitation needs. However, nurses may note the need for ROM exercises and consult with the physician and the physical therapist with regard to how this might be incorporated into the plan of care.

Long-Term Care

Many long-term care facilities have an activities coordinator. These staff people frequently lead a daily exercise group for residents, during which active exercises are done. Even those confined to wheelchairs can join in the exercises. Bowling with special equipment and other types of activities may provide excellent range of motion. As a staff nurse, you can encourage residents to participate in activities that provide these important movements. Many elderly residents have the problem of fatigue. In these cases, it is useful to schedule ROM exercises for the morning hours when fatigue may be less of a problem than it is later in the day.

Many residents experience joint inflexibility due to arthritis. Move arthritic joints to maintain function, but avoid stress on the joints. Individuals with arthritis may benefit from a combination of active, active-assistive, and passive exercises. For the staff, scheduling ROM exercises at the same time each morning is most convenient because baths may be given only one to two times per week. If performing ROM exercises becomes routine and is done at the same time, the resident or caregivers are more likely to remember it.

Many of the residents in long-term care facilities have had a stroke or have other neuromuscular impairments. Participating in ROM exercises is essential for these people to maintain joint mobility, strengthen muscles, and enhance the function of affected extremities. An accurate assessment of these individuals is necessary before proceeding with ROM exercises. Usually a physical therapist performs an assessment and determines the specific prescription for exercise. A physical therapy assistant or activity aide may carry out the activity. Restoration of function is an important goal for many individuals in long-term care. When function cannot be restored, maintenance of flexibility may be the goal.

Home Care

As more incapacitated people are receiving care by family members in the home, maintaining the highest degree of mobility becomes a priority. Activities of daily living, such as eating, dressing, and ambulating, are enhanced when joint mobility is improved. If you are the nurse providing home care, you may perform ROM exercises for the client and teach a family member to perform them on the person's joints. The nurse should encourage the disabled client to participate as fully as possible so that the person feels involved in the process. If teaching the procedure, use a chart indicating the sequence of exercises. This chart might also include a place to record completion of exercises each day. Use another chart showing progress to motivate the client and the family member. Progress is usually slow, and improvements on a daily basis may be difficult to see.

Ambulatory Care

When teaching elderly individuals in a primary care office, emphasize the importance of ROM exercises to preserve functional status. Often range of motion is incorporated into activities of daily living, but for those whose lives are very sedentary, a planned ROM program may be very valuable. These may be done at home independently. Senior centers often have exercise groups to help older adults maintain flexibility.

LEARNING TOOLS

DEVELOP YOUR BACKGROUND KNOWLEDGE

1. Review the Learning Outcomes.

2. Read the section on activity in your assigned text.

3. Look up the Key Terms in the glossary.

4. Review this module, and mentally practice the techniques described. Study so that you would be able to teach these skills to another person. Use the Performance Checklists on the CD-ROM in the front of this book as a guide.

5. Standing, move the joints on one side of your body through ROM exercises. Begin with your neck. Consider what your own range of motion is. How does it feel to move each joint deliberately through

its full range? Do you encounter difficulties in doing complete ROM exercises?

DEVELOP YOUR SKILLS

1. In the practice setting, select one other student, and form a pair to work together.

2. Changing so that each has the opportunity to play the role of the patient, perform each of the following procedures. If you need to have more than two people in a group, one person can serve as an evaluator.
   a. Practice ROM exercises with a partner for one side of the body.
   b. Change positions, and have your partner perform the exercises on one side of your body.
   c. Together, evaluate your performances.

DEMONSTRATE YOUR SKILLS

In the clinical setting
1. Consult with your instructor regarding the opportunity to observe a physical therapist perform ROM exercises.
2. Consult with your instructor regarding the opportunity to perform ROM exercises for a patient.
3. Evaluate your performance with the instructor.

CRITICAL THINKING EXERCISES

1. Mildred Ogden was admitted to a long-term care facility from the hospital after a stroke that left her right side paralyzed. She is receiving rehabilitative services that include physical therapy twice a week. Determine what factors you should consider when deciding whether she needs ROM exercises provided by the nursing staff. Specify what joints might be most in need of ROM, and explain why. Who might be the best person to consult for assistance in making decisions regarding this aspect of care?
2. Joseph French, age 75, was admitted with emphysema and pneumonia. His admission data state that he has been housebound due to shortness of breath for the past month. As he tries to turn over in bed, he says, "This old body is pretty stiff!" Consider the problems associated with his medical diagnosis. Is this man a candidate for ROM exercises? If not, why not? If he is, determine what specific precautions are needed.

SELF-QUIZ
SHORT-ANSWER QUESTIONS

1. List two goals of ROM exercises.
   a. _____
   b. _____

2. Identify two contraindications to ROM exercises.
   a. _____
   b. _____

3. Contractures occur when the stronger muscle group of an extremity shortens or pulls. What are these muscles called?

   _____

4. Give an example of a hinge joint, and explain how it moves.

   _____

5. Give an example of a saddle joint, and explain how it moves.

   _____

6. What type of joint is found in the spine?

   _____

7. What is the term used to indicate ROM exercise that is performed by the patient?

   _____

8. What is the term used for when the hand is held in an outward, upward position?

   _____

9. What position is the shoulder in when combing the hair?

   _____

MULTIPLE CHOICE

____ 10. When should ROM exercises be performed?
   a. Every time a patient is repositioned
   b. At bath time
   c. When ordered by the physician
   d. Four to five times a day

____ 11. In what order should the joints of the body be exercised?
   a. Alternately, from one side to the other
   b. From distal to proximal
   c. From proximal to distal

____ 12. "Scissoring" one leg over the other may bring about what movement of the hip joint?
   a. Hip flexion
   b. Hip extension
   c. Adduction
   d. Circumduction

Answers to Self-Quiz questions appear in the back of this book.

SKILLS INCLUDED IN THIS MODULE

Procedure for Initial Care of the Patient in a Cast
Guidelines for Continuing Care of the Patient in a Cast
Procedure for Assisting With the Application of a Cast
Procedure for the Application of a Brace

PREREQUISITE MODULES

Module 1	An Approach to Nursing Skills
Module 2	Documentation
Module 3	Basic Body Mechanics
Module 4	Basic Infection Control
Module 5	Safety in the Healthcare Environment
Module 6	Moving the Patient in Bed and Positioning
Module 11	Assessing Temperature, Pulse, and Respiration
Module 14	Nursing Physical Assessment
Module 18	Transfer
Module 19	Ambulation: Simple Assisted and Using Cane, Walker, or Crutches
Module 20	Implementing Range-of-Motion Exercises
Module 37	Applying Bandages and Binders

KEY TERMS

bivalving
cast padding
cervical collar
circulation, motion, and sensation (CMS)
epigastrium
excoriation
fiberglass
gluteal settings
isometric exercises
kyphosis
neurovascular status
petaling
plaster of Paris
quadricep settings
scoliosis
stockinette
tepid
torso
trapeze
twist support
walking heel
windowing

OVERALL OBJECTIVES

▸ To accurately assess the patient for complications and prevent problems related to the presence of a cast or brace and to assist efficiently with the application of a cast or brace.
▸ To provide psychological support during and after the application of a cast or brace.

LEARNING OUTCOMES

The student will be able to

1. Assess the patient's record for the type of injury and the type of cast to be applied, the reason for the cast, and the condition of the body part to be immobilized in the cast.
2. Analyze assessment data to determine special problems or concerns that must be addressed during cast or brace application and care of the patient with a cast or brace.
3. Determine appropriate patient outcomes for a patient with a cast or brace, and recognize the potential for adverse outcomes.
4. Assist with application and adaptation of the cast (or brace), using appropriate equipment.
5. Position the patient in anatomically correct and effective positions to assist with cast application, to foster cast drying, and to prevent complications.
6. Provide emotional support during and after the cast procedures.
7. Teach the patient how to care for himself or herself while wearing a cast or brace.
8. Intervene to prevent complications after application of a cast or brace.
9. Evaluate patient knowledge of techniques to support self-care.
10. Document the type of cast applied, the patient's tolerance, the patient's neurovascular status, and the instruction provided.

The treatment of fractures by immobilizing a body part with a cast is very old, as is the treatment of sprains, skeletal abnormalities, and minor fractures with braces. To be effective and relatively problem-free, casts and braces must be applied carefully. A specific cast or brace may be applied by the patient's physician or by a specialty technician according to the physician's order. Nurses are responsible for assessment to detect problems and for interventions that prevent the complications that might develop. They must also teach the patient and caregivers how to manage the cast effectively.

NURSING DIAGNOSES

Examples of nursing diagnoses common to patients with casts and braces include

- Impaired Physical Mobility: related to a cast
- Impaired Home Maintenance Management: related to body cast
- Impaired Tissue Perfusion: related to peripheral compression caused by a leg cast or brace
- Risk for Injury: sensory or motor deficits related to pressure from casts, braces, crutches, or canes
- Risk for Impaired Skin Integrity: related to pressure from cast or brace
- Risk for Peripheral Neurovascular Dysfunction: related to pressure from cast or brace

DELEGATION

Assistive personnel routinely assist with the care of patients in casts and braces. Some also assist with the application of casts. While assistive personnel should be aware of appropriate positioning and comfort measures, the nurse remains accountable for assessment and for teaching the patient and family about appropriate home care and observations.

CASTS

Casts immobilize the trunk or a body part so that a fracture of a bone, a dislocation, or an injury to soft tissue can heal. The various casting materials are impregnated with a substance that hardens after being applied to the body part. To be effective, casts must be contoured or molded carefully to the surface being covered. Although padding is used on the skin, pressure from the hard casting material can produce complications in the covered area, including pain, decreased sensation, or skin breakdown.

MATERIALS

Many casting materials have been used over the years, and each has advantages and disadvantages for the patient. The type of cast to be applied and the material to be used are ordered by the physician. The patient may be taken to a special casting room, where all the casting equipment is available. Or, instead, a "cast cart" with the materials needed may be brought to the treatment site.

Casting and splinting materials most often used include **plaster of Paris,** the oldest and still common, or synthetic materials. These are described in greater detail later.

Stockinette and **cast padding** or wrapping are used beneath both types of cast before the material is applied. Soft cotton material is the fabric of choice for the plaster of Paris cast because it absorbs perspiration, thereby decreasing skin irritation. Synthetic material is preferred for the fiberglass cast because cotton can fray under the hardness of the fiberglass surface, causing skin-irritating particles to become embedded beneath the cast (Pifer, 2000).

PLASTER OF PARIS CASTS

When combined with water, plaster of Paris, or calcium sulfate, forms gypsum, which is a hard but fairly light substance. Crinoline (a firmly woven cotton fabric) rolls impregnated with plaster of Paris are first immersed in water and then molded to a body part to form a cast. Plaster casts require 24 to 72 hours to completely dry and weight-bearing should not occur prior to this time. During this time, the extremity should be supported with the palms of the hands and not handled with the fingertips because fingers may produce indentations that will create pressure points under the cast.

After drying, the resulting cast is hard and fits the body part exactly. Plaster of Paris is used to immobilize fractures and damaged soft tissue parts and to protect newly amputated limbs. They are inexpensive and relatively nonallergenic. Disadvantages are that the larger casts are heavy, and the material has a tendency to crumble if worn for long periods or if it becomes damp or wet.

SYNTHETIC CASTS

The synthetic materials used for casting include **fiberglass**, polyester, and thermoplastic. They come in a wide variety of colors (such as purple, bright green, yellow, and white) and are especially popular with children. Synthetic casts are lightweight and can be immersed in water if padded with material that dries quickly. Synthetic casting materials are molded to the body part after being activated by submersion in cool or **tepid** (warm) water. Some brands of fiberglass material require "finishing" the cast with aerosol fiberglass material. Synthetic casts set rapidly in 5 minutes to 15 minutes, depending upon the resin. One type sets even

more rapidly if exposed to ultraviolet light. Synthetics can withstand weight-bearing in 15 to 30 minutes, depending on the specific material used. The specific instructions for the brand in use should be followed in terms of preparation of the product, the setting time, and when weight-bearing is allowed.

Synthetic casts, like those made from plaster of Paris, have advantages and disadvantages. Synthetic casts are easier to apply, more rigid, and more durable than plaster of Paris, making them suitable for active children with minor fractures and injuries. Another advantage is that casts dry in less than 1 hour. Although synthetic casts are more resistant to moisture and water than plaster of Paris casts, they should not be immersed in water unless polypropylene stockinette and polyester padding, which dry easily, were used when the cast was applied.

There are several disadvantages to synthetic casting material. It is more expensive than plaster of Paris. The substance is not as "forgiving" as plaster, so once the cast is molded to the part, the rigidity may cause problems if even minimal swelling occurs. When the cast is dry, this rigidity may continue to cause problems for the underlying tissue.

COMMON TYPES OF CASTS

There are many variations on the types of casts commonly used. Each type carries with it the complications specific to having a particular part of the body enclosed. Figure 21-1 illustrates the various casts.

- Short arm casts extend from below the elbow to the fingers. The elbow can be flexed.
- Short leg casts extend from below the knee to the toes. The knee can be flexed.
- Long arm or hanging arm casts extend from under the axilla to the fingers. The elbow is maintained in flexion so that the arm can be supported by a sling or strap. Module 37 gives directions for tying a sling.
- Long leg casts extend from above the knee to the toes.
- Shoulder spica casts immobilize the upper **torso** and one shoulder and arm. A support bar is used for stability, and a window is cut over the **epigastrium** to promote comfort after eating.
- Hip spica casts can extend over the torso from just under the axilla or from the lower rib cage downward, enclosing both hips. One, one and one-half, or both legs may be casted, depending on need (Clarke & Dowling, 2003). A support bar is used if both legs are enclosed, and a window is again placed at the epigastrium.

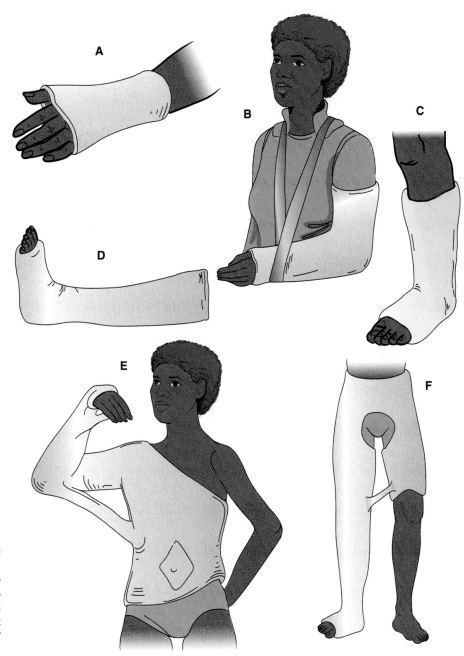

FIGURE 21-1 The various types of casts cover different parts of the body. The greater the surface of the body that is casted, the greater the chance for potential problems. (**A**) Short arm cast. (**B**) Hanging arm cast. (**C**) Short leg cast. (**D**) Long leg cast. (**E**) Shoulder spica cast. (**F**) Hip spica cast.

CAST FINISHING, CAST ADAPTATIONS, AND CAST CHANGES

Casts may be changed or adapted for the needs of the patient.

CAST FINISHING

The rough edges of the cast are smoothed or trimmed with a cast knife or cast cutter and may be covered with stockinette. The stockinette may simply be folded down over the outer surface of the cast and fastened with tape (Fig. 21-2). Edges also may be finished using "petals" (Fig. 21-3) once the cast has dried. This process is discussed later.

TWIST SUPPORTS AND WALKING HEELS

The person applying the cast may wish to incorporate a **twist support** and **walking heel** into the cast. Twist supports and walking heels can be incorporated before the cast has dried, or they can be glued on later. Twists are made by twisting a roll, wrapping the ends around the two sites of attachment, then rolling another roll around the twist. When dry, this appears as a strong bar

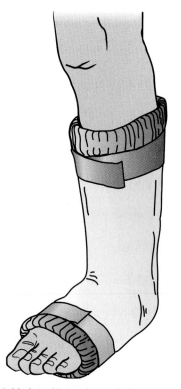

FIGURE 21-2 Folded stockinette beneath the case protects the skin from the sharp edges of the cast.

between two extremities or between an extremity and the patient's body (Fig. 21-4).

BIVALVING

A usable cast can be bivalved instead of being totally removed and discarded. An electric cast saw is used to cut the cast lengthwise in two pieces. **Bivalving** usu-

ally is done because of swelling, infection, or discomfort when a fracture is partially healed, and although support is still needed, an enclosed cast is unnecessary. An elastic bandage wrap can be used when the patient is moving to keep the two parts together. The top half can be lifted off when the patient is resting to relieve constant pressure from the cast (Fig. 21-5).

WINDOWING

Windowing involves cutting a square or diamond-shaped section from the cast to allow for the observation and care of the skin underneath. In some cases, this is done to care for a surgical incision under the cast. In others, pins that have been used to hold bones together must be removed through a window in the cast. Windows also are cut to relieve pressure when the tissue below includes a bony prominence or an area that will expand or swell. The swelling might be due to injury or, more commonly, to gastric enlargement caused by eating. Edges of windows should be "petaled" to prevent skin irritation (see step 2 of "Continuing Care of the Patient in a Cast"). Handle the windowed part of a cast carefully, because it is the weakest point, and cracking can occur.

CAST CHANGES

Casts are changed for a variety of reasons. The cast may become too tight as a result of swelling or weight gain. The cast may no longer immobilize effectively as a result of weight loss, a decrease in swelling, or a decrease in underlying muscle bulk related to disuse. In the infant or child requiring long-term casting, normal growth patterns can cause the original cast to become too snug, and

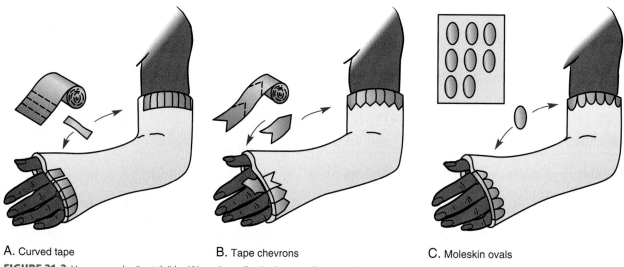

A. Curved tape   B. Tape chevrons   C. Moleskin ovals

FIGURE 21-3 You can make "petals" by (**A**) cutting adhesive into small strips or (**B**) chevrons. You can also make petals from moleskin cut ovals (**C**). Tuck petals smoothly over the edge of the cast to protect the skin from crumbling plaster and rough edges.

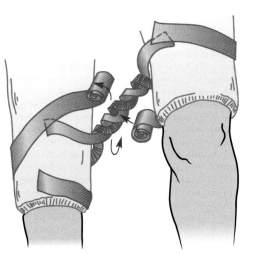

FIGURE 21-4 A "twist" support is made to act as a rigid bridge between the casts of two lower extremities. The wet casting bandage is twisted into a support and anchored into each leg cast.

a new one must be applied. Wrinkling of the padding under the cast can cause extreme discomfort and necessitate a change. The cast also can be changed because of the possibility of infection beneath it. The cast may soften, crumble, or become badly soiled or foul smelling. When this happens, a cast change may be needed.

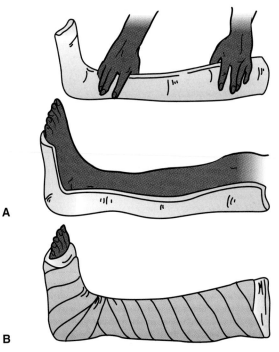

FIGURE 21-5 Bivalving. (**A**) If the patient experiences swelling or infection, the cast may be bivalved (cut horizontally into two pieces). The top section can be removed to relieve pressure. (**B**) The two halves are usually held together by elastic wrap to immobilize the casted area.

PROCEDURE FOR INITIAL CARE OF THE PATIENT IN A CAST

The patient with a newly applied cast is at risk for specific problems. These problems are more likely to occur and to be more severe if a large proportion of the body or extremity is casted. Many important nursing actions can be taken to ensure the patient's comfort and safety. Consider the following carefully, and incorporate these into the plan of care for the patient immediately after casting (Schoen, 2001). The patient and caregiver may carry out this plan of care at home because many orthopedic procedures are done as day surgeries. In such cases, the nurse must teach the patient and caregiver.

ASSESSMENT

1. Identify the type of cast and its purpose. **R:** This helps with determining the assessment and patient education needed.
2. Inspect the bed for the type of mattress support. **R:** A firm surface promotes proper body alignment and supports a heavy cast. In the hospital, beds usually have a flat metal surface supporting the mattress. In long-term care facilities, beds may have a flat spring. In this case, a special bed board is usually available to support the mattress. Placing a board between the mattress and box spring will provide the necessary support in the home.
3. Check to see if a **trapeze** has been placed on the bed. **R:** Such devices can help the patient with a large cast to move more easily in bed. When this is not possible in the home, a rope tied to the foot of the bed and with a large knot where the patient can grasp it will help the patient move about in bed.

ANALYSIS

4. Critically think through your data, carefully evaluating each aspect and its relation to other data. **R:** This enables you to determine specific problems for this individual in relation to traction.
5. Identify specific problems and modifications of the procedure needed for this individual. **R:** Planning for the individual must take into consideration the individual's problems.

PLANNING

6. Determine individualized patient outcomes in relation to the cast, including the following. **R:** Identification of outcomes guides planning and evaluation.
   a. Patient expresses comfort. **R:** Discomfort may indicate injury, trauma, or pressure. Complaints of pain or burning may indicate impaired circulation.

b. The cast is supported. **R:** To prevent strain on muscles and joints.

c. The patient engages in activity. **R:** To prevent complications of the cast and of immobility.

d. **Neurovascular status** in extremity remains stable. **R:** Cast may impair nerve function.

e. Skin at the edges of the cast remains free of breakdown. **R:** Rough cast edges may abrade skin.

f. There are no signs or symptoms of infection or the complications of immobility.

7. Identify any transfer device or assistance that will be needed to move the patient into the bed. **R:** Two care providers may be needed in order for one person to support the cast while the other assists the patient. Supporting the cast well prevents undue strain on muscle groups adjacent to it.

IMPLEMENTATION

Action	*Rationale*
8. Wash or disinfect your hands.	This is to prevent the spread of microorganisms.
9. Identify the patient, using two identifiers.	Verifying the patient's identity helps ensure that you are performing the right skill for the right patient.
10. Transfer the patient to the bed, using care to support the cast with the palms of your hands and to avoid putting point pressure on the cast.	Point pressure can deform the cast, creating a place that rubs.
11. Conduct neurovascular monitoring, also called **circulation, motion, and sensation (CMS)** checks, immediately and then every hour while the cast is in the drying stage. Explain the purpose of these checks to the patient (Box 21-1).	

> **box 21-1** *Neurovascular Monitoring Circulation, Motion, and Sensation (CMS) Checks*
>
> ■ Circulation
>   Skin temperature of extremity
>   Color of nail beds and skin of extremity
>   Comparison of pulse rates and quality of pulses of the two extremities
>   Capillary refill on nail beds and skin of extremity
> ■ Motion
>   Ability of the patient to move fingers and toes
> ■ Sensation
>   Patient's ability to feel pressure
>   Patient's report of pain
>   Patient's report of numbness and tingling

a. *Circulation checks:*	
(1) Check skin temperature of the toes or fingers of the extremity. They should be warm. Do not rely on the patient's report that the fingers or toes do not feel cool. Feel the surface of the skin with your own hand.	Areas with decreased circulation become colder. Restricted circulation reduces sensitivity.

(continued)

Action	Rationale
(2) Check the color of the nails and the color of the extremity.	Any differences could indicate compromised circulation. Nail bed should be pink. Swelling and darkening indicate impaired venous return.
(3) Check for capillary filling by pressing on tissues. This causes blanching (loss of color) by emptying the capillary bed. Release the pressure, and observe for the return of pink. It should return immediately. When capillary filling is delayed, you should time how long it takes to occur.	Delayed capillary filling indicates that arterial circulation is impaired.
b. *Motion checks:*	
(1) Ask the patient to move the fingers or toes.	Decreased ability to do this may indicate pressure on nerves from swelling or decreased circulation.
c. *Sensation checks:*	
(1) Ask whether the patient can feel pressure when you press on the nails of the fingers or toes.	The patient should be able to feel the pressure. Decreased sensation may indicate pressure on nerves.
(2) Ask also about pain.	Pain from the injury is expected, but severe pain may result from decreased circulation or tissue swelling.
(3) Ask about abnormal sensations (paresthesias), such as numbness or tingling.	Paresthesias may indicate pressure on nerves from the cast or from swelling.
12. Monitor the amount, color, and odor of any drainage that appears on the outside of the cast. Mark the boundaries of the drainage area so that increases in size can be identified.	Drainage may reflect an open wound under the cast, and the color and odor of the drainage may indicate infection.
13. Elevate the extremity with the cast if possible. This may be done with several pillows or by elevating the foot of the bed for a lower extremity.	Elevation increases venous return and decreases the potential for swelling.
14. Change the patient's position during the drying process so that pressure on the cast does not remain in one spot.	This is primarily a concern with plaster casts. A plaster cast left lying flat while drying may deform to have a flat side that may put pressure on underlying tissue.
15. Teach the patient how to prevent complications through activity.	

(continued)

Action	Rationale
a. Encourage the patient to turn after the cast is completely dry.	Turning prevents respiratory complications and helps elimination, as does other exercise.
b. Teach the patient to move in one plane.	This is done so that muscle groups are not stretched.
c. Give instructions in performing **isometric exercises** including **gluteal settings** and **quadricep settings** if the patient is on continuous bed rest.	This is to help prevent loss of muscle tone and strength in the muscles required for ambulation. It is also to facilitate venous return in the lower extremity, preventing swelling and venous thrombosis.
16. Ensure that a nurse or physical therapist has given the ambulatory patient in a leg cast safe-walking instructions.	The weight of the cast can affect body balance, leading to unsteadiness and possible falls. Assistive aids, such as canes, crutches, or a walker, may be necessary (see Module 19, Ambulation: Simple Assisted and Using Cane, Walker, or Crutches) for such patients.
17. Wash or disinfect your hands.	To prevent the spread of microorganisms.

EVALUATION

18. Evaluate in relation to the previously identified outcomes. **R:** Evaluation in relation to desired outcomes is essential for planning future care.
  a. The patient expresses comfort.
  b. The cast is supported to prevent strain on muscles and joints.
  c. The patient engages in activity to prevent complications of the cast and of immobility.
  d. Neurovascular status in extremity remains stable.
  e. Skin at the edges of the cast remain free of breakdown.
  f. There are no signs or symptoms of infection or the complications of immobility.

DOCUMENTATION

19. Document evaluation of status including specific findings relating to circulation, motion, and sensation. These observations are most often entered on a flow sheet. Also record any relevant psychological data. **R:** Documentation is a legal record of the patient's care and communicates nursing activities to other nurses and caregivers.

POTENTIAL ADVERSE OUTCOMES AND RELATED INTERVENTIONS

Long-term immobilization of a body part in a cast or brace can lead to a variety of complications. These can, in large part, be prevented through conscientious nursing assessment and intervention. For problems that do arise, early intervention is essential. The nurse needs to provide skillful immediate and ongoing care for the patient with a cast or brace. Any cast or brace, regardless of type or size, forces the patient to make some immediate and long-term adaptations.

  1. The patient experiences edema distal to the cast or the brace.

Intervention: Elevate the extremity above the level of the heart. Apply ice over the area of the injury or surgery. The cold will be transferred through the cast to the tissue. Report the situation to the physician.

  2. The patient experiences a change in neurovascular status and comfort.

Intervention: Notify the physician; the cast may need to be bivalved (cut in half lengthwise along the cast and secured in place with a wrapped bandage) to prevent nerve or tissue damage due to pressure from edema. A brace may need to be adjusted to relieve pressure on specific areas.

  3. Drainage from the cast becomes foul smelling or yellow in color. This may indicate infection.

Intervention: Check the patient's temperature, and report your assessment to the physician.

  4. Skin at the edges of the cast or under pressure points of the brace becomes abraded, creating open wounds.

Intervention for cast: Make sure that all debris from the cast is cleaned out from under the edge. Pad the edge of the cast. Notify the physician. Sometimes, the edge of the cast can be reconfigured to decrease rubbing. *For brace:* Remove the brace, and provide padding over pressure points before reapplying.

GUIDELINES FOR CONTINUING CARE OF THE PATIENT IN A CAST

In 24 to 48 hours after the initial casting, the acute danger of swelling under the cast is gone; however, problems may still occur. The following should be part of the plan of care, whether the person is hospitalized or at home (Schoen, 2001).

1. Conduct ongoing assessment of the following:
   a. *Circulation, motion, and sensation.* These checks (as described previously) are continued to identify any problems. After the initial period, if all is stable, the checks are gradually spaced out to longer and longer intervals until they are done just once a day by the patient. Neurovascular compromise remains a concern when a cast is in place.
   b. *Tightness or looseness.* Either of these conditions can cause complications. You or the patient should be able to slip one finger easily between the cast and the patient's skin. **R:** The cast may become tight if swelling occurs. The cast may become loose if the patient loses weight or the muscles under the cast atrophy from disuse.
   c. *Drainage.* Observe for signs of drainage coming through the cast. Report, record, and describe the size of any area stained with drainage. Most facilities have a policy of outlining the area of drainage with a felt-tipped pen, noting the date and time. This allows increases in drainage to be seen quickly. Because some patients can become anxious over this procedure, reassure the patient that this is a method of assessment so that he or she does not become unduly alarmed. **R:** Drainage may help to identify a wound under the cast that is not healing well or the beginning of an infection.
   d. *Odor.* Check the odor of the cast. **R:** A musty, foul odor can signal infection and should be reported immediately. Unpleasant odors may also be caused by perspiration and bacteria, especially if the cast is extensive. These odors are different from the odor of infection. Commercial cast deodorants, which are sometimes mixed with the casting materials, are largely ineffective. A cast change is sometimes necessary if the odor becomes too unpleasant.
2. Edge the cast. The edge of a cast must be finished in a way that protects the skin from the cast material and the cast material from perspiration, urine, or feces. This may have been done when the cast was applied by folding padding material over the edges and fastening it on the outside of the cast; it also may be done after the cast is dry by petaling or placing plastic around openings.
   a. ***Petaling:*** Make adhesive petals by cutting small strips of adhesive tape into pointed or rounded ends. Place these strips perpendicular to the cast edge and then smooth over the edge and tuck inside the cast. Pointed petals wrinkle more readily than rounded ones. Moleskin cut into round sections provides a smoother and softer surface and has less tendency to wrinkle up than tape (see Fig. 21-3). Commercially made cast-edging petals also are available.
   b. Protect casts that surround the perineal or anal area from soiling by edging or covering them with plastic secured by tape (Fig. 21-6).
3. Protect the exposed toes of a patient in a leg cast against cold with a heavy sock. Also prevent contact with sharp or dangerous objects. **R:** Because of the cast, the extremity cannot be flexed and withdrawn from danger.
4. Discourage the patient from attempting to scratch beneath the cast with sharp objects. **R:** Sharp objects can damage or even puncture the underlying skin surfaces. These abrasions or injuries may remain undetected and become infected. Itching is usually present to some degree and is especially likely when the cast is in place for a long time.
5. Teach strategies to manage itching.
   a. The best intervention for itching is distraction. Keeping the mind focused on something interesting will make other sensations recede.

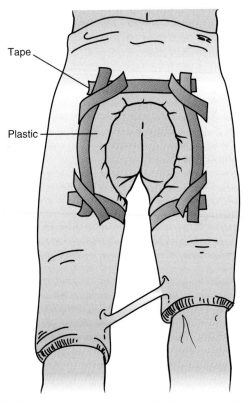

FIGURE 21-6 To protect casts surrounding the anal or perineal area from soiling, cut wide strips of plastic and tuck these smoothly over the soft padding around the cast edges. Tape the plastic in place on the cast. (Note the completed twist support.)

b. A cool environment also helps, because perspiration under the cast increases itching.

c. Blowing cool air from a hairdryer into the cast may also help to alleviate the itching.

d. Sometimes the physician may recommend an over-the-counter analgesic such as acetaminophen to relieve itching at bedtime when it is hard to maintain distraction.

Note: Physically, little can be done about this problem except changing the cast.

6. Listen to the patient! Never ignore the patient's complaints. They could be the first indication of a problem that could develop into serious complications. Offer emotional support to all patients in casts. Being encased within a cast of any size imposes restrictions on activities of daily living that concern and inconvenience the patient.

7. Plan strategies for moving the patient that will not damage the cast or cause muscle strain to either the caregiver or the patient. This may mean additional help or the use of a transfer device (see Module 18).

8. Assist the patient when a cast is removed.

a. During the procedure, the loud whine of the cast saw may be distressing. Also, the patient may fear that skin will be cut by the cast saw. Reassure the patient that the saw is designed to cut cast material and that the soft tissue of the skin will not be cut. Explain the sound in advance so that the patient can be prepared for it.

b. Gently bathe the skin that was under the cast to remove dead skin and encrustations. Do not rub because that may damage the skin.

c. Apply lotion to the skin. This will soften any remaining skin flakes and crusts so that they will eventually be removed with bathing.

d. Reassure the patient, who may feel very vulnerable without the cast. Explain that the cast would not have been removed if the bone were not sufficiently healed to support itself.

PROCEDURE FOR ASSISTING WITH THE APPLICATION OF A CAST

Casts are most frequently applied in the emergency room in a special cast room where all the equipment is located. The physician or an orthopedic technician may apply the cast. The nurse may care for the patient in preparation for the casting and may assist with the casting procedure itself. Nurses also need to gather the appropriate equipment and assist the person applying the cast and to provide the patient with emotional support during and after the casting procedure. Nurses need to recognize and prevent problems and to teach patients and/or caregivers self-care techniques. Because the area or part being treated is covered by the cast, it can be dif-

ficult to discern problems unless the nurse carries out frequent and careful assessments. Nursing interventions also may prevent the occurrence of some problems.

ASSESSMENT

1. Review the patient's record, and read the physician's notes about casting. **R:** To determine the kind of injury and type of cast to be applied.

2. Inspect the skin over which the cast is to be applied for lacerations, abrasions, or interruptions in skin integrity. Look for signs of edema that may intensify pressure caused by the cast. Incisions and wounds may be exposed for inspection through a "window" (a small cutout in the cast) after the cast has been applied. **R:** This promotes wound healing and reduces the incidence of skin breakdown.

3. Assess what the patient knows about the procedure. **R:** To enable you to clarify, if necessary, any information that has been given.

4. Assess the patient for pain or anxiety. **R:** To determine the need for sedation prior to casting.

ANALYSIS

5. Critically think through your data, carefully evaluating each aspect and its relation to other data. **R:** To determine specific problems for this individual in relation to casting.

6. Identify specific problems and modifications of the procedure needed for this individual. **R:** Planning for the individual must take into consideration the individual's problems.

PLANNING

7. Determine individualized patient outcomes in relation to the application of a cast. **R:** Identification of outcomes guides planning and evaluation.

a. Patient understands the purpose of the cast.

b. Patient expresses comfort. **R:** Discomfort may indicate injury, trauma, or pressure. Complaints of pain or burning may indicate impaired circulation.

c. The cast is supported to prevent strain on muscles and joints.

d. Neurovascular (CMS) status in extremity remains stable.

e. Skin at the edges of the cast is intact and without irritation.

8. Gather equipment appropriate to the type of cast being applied if a special cast cart is not available:

a. stockinette—this soft, stretchy, ribbed tubular material comes in different circumferences. When pulled over a body part, it provides a smooth surface and protection from the inner surface of the cast. Choose an appropriate circumference, and cut off a length 6 inches longer than the area to be casted.

b. large, heavy-duty scissors
c. cast padding
d. a cast knife for trimming
e. a cast saw if windowing is needed (see "Windowing," earlier).
f. adhesive cloth tape
g. a plastic apron and gloves; these are used by the physician or technician applying the cast to protect the clothing and hands. It is also prudent practice for you to wear clean gloves to protect your hands from casting materials.
h. materials specific to the type of cast
   Plaster of Paris cast materials
   (1) rolls of plaster of Paris. (Assemble more than you think might be needed, and include various widths.)
   R: The physician may want to reinforce certain areas or add more casting material than originally planned. It is frustrating not to have enough casting rolls on hand. Physicians usually elect to use the larger rolls because they produce a smoother cast with less chance of undue constriction.
   (2) a bucket or deep container
   R: This is for immersing the rolls.

(3) cotton cast padding or "wadding." Gather several rolls of various widths. This padding is "waffled," consisting of soft, thin cotton layers between two outer layers of more closely woven cotton material.
R: This is to decrease pressure on bony prominences. The texture allows for molding to the body part and decreases wrinkling underneath the cast.
Synthetic cast materials
(4) sealed rolls of synthetic casting material
R: Casting materials may be damaged if exposed to air prior to use.
(5) synthetic cast padding
R: This decreases retention of moisture under the cast.
(6) a bucket or deep container
R: This is for immersing the rolls of synthetic casting material.

9. Plan to position and maintain the part to be casted in the anatomical alignment indicated by the physician during the casting procedure. **R:** Planning ahead allows you to proceed more safely and effectively.

IMPLEMENTATION

Action	*Rationale*
10. Wash or disinfect your hands.	To decrease the transfer of microorganisms that could cause infection.
11. Obtain any needed supportive devices or assistance.	To promote efficiency. An additional person may be needed to assist the patient to maintain the needed position.
12. Identify the patient, using two identifiers.	Verifying the patient's identity helps ensure that you are performing the right skill for the right patient.
13. Drape the patient as needed.	To avoid undue exposure and protect other body parts from contact with casting materials.
14. Place a plastic-covered sheet or pillow under the part to be casted.	To protect the linen from moisture and casting materials.
15. Offer the patient emotional support and reassurance.	To help reduce anxiety and facilitate coping.
16. Explain the casting procedure.	Explaining the procedure helps relieve anxiety or misperceptions that the patient may have about a procedure or activity and sets the stage for patient participation.

(continued)

Action	Rationale
17. Raise the bed to an appropriate working position based on your height.	To allow you to use correct body mechanics and protect yourself from back injury.
18. Assist the person applying the cast to	
a. Wash and dry the part to be casted, treat breaks in the skin as prescribed, and apply sterile dressings.	To promote wound healing and reduce the incidence of skin breakdown.
b. Place knitted material (e.g., stockinette) over the part to be casted in a smooth and nonconstrictive manner.	To protect the skin from casting materials and from pressure. Fold the stockinette over the cast edges when finishing the application to create a smooth, padded edge that protects the skin from abrasion.
c. Wrap soft nonwoven roll padding smoothly and evenly around the body part.	To protect the skin from the pressure of the cast.
d. Use additional padding around bony prominences and nerve grooves.	To protect the skin at bony prominences and to protect superficial nerves.
e. Prepare the casting materials, and assist with casting as appropriate for the specific casting material. Check the label for specific directions.	
Plaster of Paris cast	
(1) Fill the bucket with warm water. Put on gloves to protect your skin from the plaster.	Warm water facilitates the drying process.
(2) Stand a plaster roll on its end in the water.	So that absorption of water is more uniform.
(3) As soon as the bubbling stops, remove the roll, and gently squeeze (but do not twist) out the excess water. "Free up" the end of the roll.	When the bubbling stops, the plaster roll has absorbed sufficient water; twisting can cause plaster to be squeezed from the roll.
(4) Hand the roll to the person applying the cast. The casting rolls are wrapped around the body part in an overlapping fashion, adding rolls until the cast is the desired shape and size.	To create a smooth, solid, well-contoured cast.
Synthetic cast materials	
(5) Fill the bucket with cool or tepid water.	The temperature of the water is determined by the specific manufacturer's directions.

(continued)

Action	Rationale
(6) Put on gloves.	To protect your skin from the casting material.
(7) Cut open packages, and immerse each roll in the water for the designated time (8 to 10 seconds are common), and then gently squeeze out excess water, "free up" the end of the roll, and hand the roll to the person casting the patient. The casting rolls are wrapped around the body part in an overlapping fashion, adding rolls until the cast is the desired shape and size. *Note:* If you're utilizing material that does not require immersion in water, simply cut open the package and hold the package so the person applying the cast can lift out the roll.	To create a smooth, solid, well-contoured cast.
19. When the casting is completed, clean excess material from the patient's skin. Water can be used for plaster, and a solvent is used for synthetics.	To prevent particles from sliding beneath the cast.
20. Position the patient so that the cast is supported, and the patient is comfortable.	
a. Handle a cast carefully until it is completely dry. Use the flat palms of the hands so that your fingers do not place indentations in the wet or damp cast.	To prevent weakening the surface and causing uneven pressure on the skin.
b. Place small plastic-covered pillows under and around the cast, leaving some air space at the sides until the cast is dry. Extend the pillows above and below the cast.	To allow the cast to dry more evenly and keep the cast from pulling on muscle groups.
c. Elevate the extremity slightly higher than the heart.	To improve venous return and thereby help prevent swelling of the tissues and excessive tightness of the cast.
d. Leave the cast uncovered during the drying period. A fan or a hair dryer on a cool setting can be used to hasten the drying process of a plaster cast. Never apply heat.	Heat tends to dry the surface of the plaster cast too quickly while interior layers are still wet, causing cracking.

(continued)

Action	Rationale
21. Provide patient teaching, including the following:	Educating patients and caregivers facilitates immediate and ongoing care.
a. monitoring that will be done (observations for pain; circulation, motion, and sensation [often referred to as CMS] of body part distal to the cast; edema)	
b. length of time cast takes to dry (48 to 72 hours for a plaster of Paris cast, depending on the size; 5 to 15 minutes for a synthetic cast)	
c. how the cast feels as it dries (patient will experience a warm sensation)	
d. optimum position for the casted part (and when weight-bearing will be possible, if appropriate)	
e. importance of immediately reporting feelings of pain, pressure, or altered sensation (can indicate pressure that could result in tissue damage)	
f. need to keep the extremity immobile until the cast is dry (cast should not harden in an undesired position)	
22. Care for equipment and supplies and clean the area as needed.	
a. Clean off any casting material on the surfaces by wiping with a moist cloth for plaster or a solvent for synthetic materials.	Dried casting material is difficult to remove and may damage equipment.
b. Dispose of water from a cast application in a special sink with a plaster trap.	Plaster or synthetic casting material will clog a regular sink.
c. Discard opened packages and used materials. (Unopened package, if kept clean, may be returned to a supply location.)	To facilitate the next cast application. (Clean, unopened packages are not contaminated and cost-effective care requires that materials not be wasted.)
d. Remove your gloves while avoiding touching any casting material.	Casting materials are caustic and irritate the skin.
23. Move the patient to a wheelchair or stretcher for transport from the casting room to a hospital room or to a vehicle for transport home.	Weight-bearing will not be allowed on a lower leg cast. The patient is usually very fatigued after a cast application due to the injury as well as the casting and is more susceptible to falls, even with an upper extremity cast.
24. Wash or disinfect your hands.	To prevent the spread of microorganisms.

EVALUATION

25. Evaluate using the individualized patient outcomes previously identified. **R:** Evaluation in relation to desired outcomes is essential for planning future care.
    a. Patient understands the purpose of the cast.
    b. Patient reports comfort.
    c. The cast is supported.
    d. Neurovascular (CMS) status in extremity remains stable.
    e. Skin at the edges of the cast is intact and without irritation.

DOCUMENTATION

26. Document the following on the appropriate form. **R:** Documentation is a legal record of the patient's care and communicates nursing activities to other nurses and caregivers.
    a. Type of cast applied
    b. Neurovascular status
    c. Patient comfort

BRACES

Braces are rigid devices that may be applied for several purposes:

- to provide protection and healing of minor fractures
- to maintain therapeutic alignment for body parts
- to protect soft-tissue injuries
- to provide support after orthopedic surgery
- to correct skeletal malformations

Braces are made of foam, soft or rigid plastic, metal, or a combination of these materials. Because of their many applications, braces are contoured to all parts of the body—cervical spine, lower spine, and extremities. Braces are available with movable joints when this feature is appropriate.

Some braces are named after the place they were developed. For example, the Boston, Milwaukee, and Philadelphia braces were developed in those respective locations. Other braces are named after the designer, such as the Thomas brace. Many commercial companies produce the same brace under their own brand names.

Potential complications are associated with wearing braces. The patient may report initial discomfort and then develop skin problems. All braces should be applied over skin that is protected by clothing so that **excoriation** (abrasion of the skin) does not occur. Some braces have a protective soft inner lining sufficient for this purpose. The patient may have difficulty adjusting to changes in mobility if the brace is a body or leg brace.

Braces for patients in a healthcare facility are ordered from a commercial company that sends a representative to measure the patient to ensure a correct fit. These representatives also may measure patients at home. Braces for children and adolescents may have to be refitted periodically due to growth changes. Older people also may need to have braces changed from time to time due to shortening of the spine and structural changes in other bones.

This module discusses only common types of braces and the appropriate parts of the body to which they are applied. The name "splint" is sometimes used for the term brace.

TYPES OF BRACES

There are many different types of braces. Many are fabricated specifically for the individual patient.

CERVICAL COLLAR

The **cervical collar** is used for a neck strain. Immobilizing the neck so that neither flexion nor extension can occur treats trauma such as whiplash. It is difficult to rotate the head with a cervical collar in place. In addition, the collar supports the weight of the head. Cervical collars may also be used with stable cervical vertebral fractures or following cervical fusion. Cervical collars are available in a soft version made from foam rubber with a cloth cover or a hard plastic collar with a padded cuff (Fig. 21-7). The Aspen collar is an example of a rigid plastic collar.

To apply the cervical collar, encircle the neck as the patient looks straight ahead. Fasten firmly with the

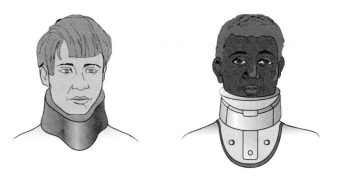

A. Soft collar   B. Plastic collar

FIGURE 21-7 Cervical collar. The cervical collar is available in both padded cotton (**A**) and rigid plastic materials (**B**). It is used for neck sprains and limits flexion and extension. Apply by encircling neck and fastening. Patient should look straight ahead.

Velcro or straps provided with the specific collar being used. Check the patient for any impingement on breathing or swallowing.

THORACIC LUMBOSACRAL SPINE BODY JACKET

This is a multipurpose brace that provides anterior and posterior support. Sometimes called a "clamshell" brace, it is widely used for many types of orthopedic conditions. The brace may be worn to prevent the progression of deformity in **scoliosis** (lateral spinal curvature). It also may be worn after surgery for scoliosis or other orthopedic surgery (Fig. 21-8). Lumbosacral corsets may also be used to provide support following lumbar surgery.

BOSTON SCOLIOSIS BRACE

The Boston scoliosis brace is effective as support for the thoracic-lumbar region. It can be used for a lower back strain or for scoliosis if the curvature is primarily of the lower spine (Fig. 21-9). This brace has now replaced the heavier Milwaukee brace that was designed for the same purpose.

BOSTON BRACE

The Boston brace supports the lumbosacral region. The brace is made of a rigid but flexible plastic material and is molded to the contours of the wearer. It is available with straps or Velcro fastenings (Fig. 21-10).

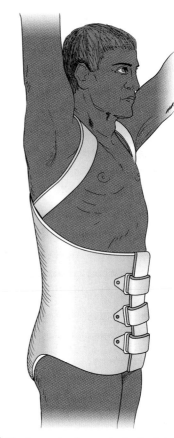

FIGURE 21-8 The thoracolumbosacral spine body jacket provides both anterior and posterior support. It is contoured to the body. Apply by wrapping around trunk and fastening with straps or Velcro. Adjust shoulder straps.

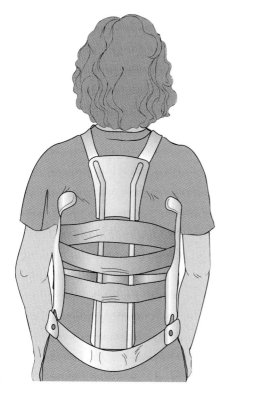

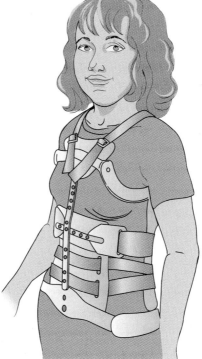

FIGURE 21-9 Boston scoliosis brace (Kosair). This brace has steel supports both anteriorly and posteriorly to correct lateral spinal curvature. It is fitted to the patient and is applied by holding the brace in place and adjusting with the straps provided.

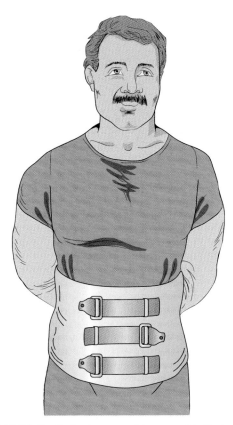

FIGURE 21-10 The Boston brace provides support to the lumbosacral region. Apply it by fitting it snugly around the body so that it is positioned around the lower spine and fasten with Velcro or straps.

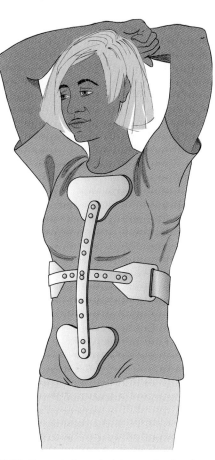

FIGURE 21-11 The anterior spinal hyperextension brace prevents anterior flexion of the thoracic spine. To apply, place in position and secure with straps that fasten at the back.

ANTERIOR SPINAL HYPEREXTENSION BRACE

A brace that prevents anterior flexion of the thoracic spine is the anterior spinal hyperextension brace. It can be used to prevent the progression of **kyphosis** (a "humpback" spinal curvature) in elderly patients. The flexible soft plastic "plates" are comfortable for the patient and can be concealed under ordinary clothing (Fig. 21-11).

CAST/BRACE COMBINATIONS

Braces are applied in combination with casts in certain conditions. Patients undergoing amputation of the lower extremity may have a cast applied during the surgical procedure and a walking brace attached to the cast. These people begin ambulation earlier than they previously would have because of these assistive devices.

The cast/brace also is used with severe fractures, based on the same rationale. The cast material protects the fracture, and the brace provides support for minimal weight-bearing earlier than would be possible without such devices (Fig. 21-12).

KNEE AND LEG BRACES

Many kinds of knee and leg braces are available. Some are rigid so that the patient's knee is immobilized. Others are jointed so that the patient can maintain knee

joint mobility. Because these braces are complicated, to be safe and effective, they require a person who has been instructed in the techniques for their application. The study of sports medicine has greatly added to knowledge in this area (Fig. 21-13).

PROCEDURE FOR THE APPLICATION OF A BRACE

Nurses commonly assist with the application of braces. An understanding of braces used for specific problems and how patients wear them is important for the nurse who must assist an individual to put on and wear a brace correctly. Braces can be complicated devices and difficult for the patient and family to understand without proper instruction. The nurse provides teaching to support effective self-care and patient confidence in these situations.

ASSESSMENT

1. Review the patient's record. **R:** To determine the injury or condition and the type of brace ordered.
2. Read any instructions that accompany the brace. **R:** To familiarize you with the specific brace.

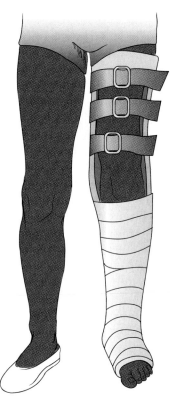

FIGURE 21-12 The combination of the cast and brace allows earlier ambulation for the person who has had a severe leg fracture. It is applied during the surgical procedure.

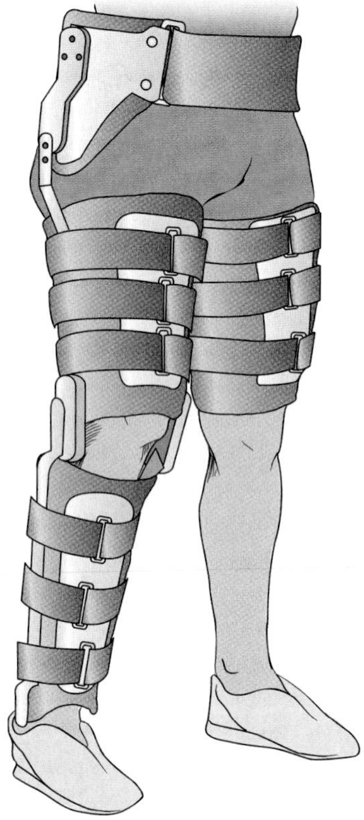

FIGURE 21-13 Knee and leg braces are available as rigid support or with the option of a flexible knee joint. This complex brace is designed for one leg but also has waist and opposite leg stabilizers. Most leg braces are designed to fit onto one leg only.

3. Assess what information the patient has been given. **R:** To clarify, if necessary, any information that has been given.
4. Assess the patient's understanding and how much assistance the patient can give. **R:** To help determine how much assistance the patient will need and how much the patient can participate in the application.

ANALYSIS

5. Critically think through your data, carefully evaluating each aspect and its relation to other data. **R:** To determine specific problems for this individual in relation to brace application.
6. Identify specific problems and modifications of the procedure needed for this individual. **R:** Planning for the individual must take into consideration the individual's problems.

PLANNING

7. Determine individualized patient outcomes in relation to the application of a brace. **R:** Identification of outcomes guides planning and evaluation.
   a. The patient understands the need for the brace.
   b. The patient is able to apply and remove the brace independently or assist when another is doing it.
   c. The patient understands the rationale for observations to make while the brace is in place.
   d. There are no adverse effects of the brace such as skin irritation or breakdown.
8. Inspect the brace, and plan the method for application. **R:** Planning ahead allows you to proceed more safely and effectively.

IMPLEMENTATION

Action	Rationale
9. Wash or disinfect your hands.	To decrease the transfer of microorganisms that could cause infection.

(continued)

Action	Rationale
10. Identify the patient, using two identifiers.	Verifying the patient's identity helps insure that you are performing the right skill for the right patient.
11. Explain how you intend to apply the brace, and explain the various parts and fastening devices.	Explaining the procedure helps relieve anxiety or misperceptions that the patient may have about a procedure or activity and sets the stage for patient participation.
12. Raise the bed to an appropriate working position based on your height.	To allow you to use correct body mechanics and protect yourself from back injury.
13. Have the patient put on clothing or other protection for the skin, if indicated for the specific brace.	This will provide protection from the pressure of the brace, if needed.
14. Help the patient to a position that will facilitate the application of the brace.	To assist with application and provide comfort for the patient.
15. Apply the brace to the body part for which it is intended.	To provide the appropriate support.
16. Position the patient in a comfortable position.	To ensure that comfort is maintained.
17. Provide patient teaching as appropriate to the specific brace (see manufacturer's instructions).	Educating patients and caregivers facilitates immediate and ongoing care.
18. Lower the bed, and wash or disinfect your hands.	For patient safety and to decrease the transfer of microorganisms that could cause infection.

EVALUATION

19. Evaluate using the individualized patient outcomes previously identified. **R:** Identification of outcomes guides planning and evaluation.
    a. The patient understands the need for the brace.
    b. The patient is able to apply and remove the brace independently or assist when another is doing it.
    c. The patient understands the rationale for observations to make while the brace is in place.
    d. There are no adverse effects of the brace such as skin irritation or breakdown.

DOCUMENTATION

20. Document the following on the appropriate form. **R:** Documentation is a legal record of the patient's care and communicates nursing activities to other nurses and caregivers.

    a. Type of brace applied
    b. Neurovascular status
    c. Patient comfort

EMOTIONAL SUPPORT

Casts and braces are long-term treatments. Being in a cast or having to wear a brace places stress on the individual. People in casts realize that they are restricted physically and that they cannot easily perform some of their routine daily tasks. These tasks may be essential, such as bathing, eating, or moving around the setting rapidly. There also are minor inconveniences. In the healthcare facility, the patient may have difficulty finding a comfortable position in which to read in bed. As an outpatient, the person may have limited access to restaurants, theaters, and other social places. In the extreme, the person confined to bed in a body cast may understandably worry about safety in the case of a fire or emergency.

An adult of advanced age who is required to wear a spinal brace on a permanent basis may have feelings of lowered self-esteem related to restrictions on activity. Body image is particularly important to teenagers, and some casts and braces cannot be totally concealed under clothing. To the teenager, this may be embarrassing and may lead to emotional distress. The teenager in a jacket brace cannot participate in sports with companions and may feel excluded.

Whatever the degree of stress, you can offer understanding, and allow the person to talk about the temporary or permanent adjustments that must be made. In the case of temporary adjustments, short-term planning with the patient may help him or her to feel some control over the situation. If the cast or brace will be used over a long period, you can emphasize activities the person can do and minimize attention to activities that must be postponed or eliminated. Planning realistically and positively can greatly reduce stress.

Acute Care

The need for a cast application in the acute care setting is frequently the result of a surgical intervention or following trauma. The patient may be recovering from anesthesia following the cast application, requiring astute nursing care to ensure proper care of the cast and prompt assessment for adequate circulation and normal nerve function. The nurse assesses circulation by observing the color, temperature, and capillary refill of the distal extremity. Nerve function is assessed by observing the patient's ability to move the fingers or toes and by assessing for numbness, tingling, and burning distal to the cast. Elevation and the application of ice may be helpful in managing edema. Prior to discharge, the patient and caregiver need instruction in cast care, transfer and mobility, and recognition of complications.

Long-Term Care

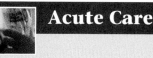

Mobility limitations imposed due to a cast, especially a long leg cast or spica cast, may require an individual to use long-term care. It is essential that the nurse have the knowledge of cast care to provide safe and effective care for these vulnerable individuals. Many residents in long-term care are elderly and have changes brought on by the aging process as

well as other medical conditions that can further compromise skin care, circulation, and mobility.

Home Care

People in the home may have casts or may be fitted with braces. Apply the same principles of assessment and care as those used in the healthcare facility. Casts and braces may interfere with the home maintenance role, causing the person to feel more dependent on others than usual. Some states have laws that prohibit a person with any cast or brace in place that inhibits full movement of the body from driving a motor vehicle. This adds to the person's dependence and may affect the ability to fulfill important responsibilities.

A home care nurse can instruct the client and caregiver in ways to handle such situations and provide continuing assessment. An important part of this assessment includes the knowledge that even when a cast or brace has been in place for an extended time, the potential for skin problems remains. Family members need to become proficient with assessing the cast and the client's skin for any sign of pressure or damage. General concerns surrounding immobilization also must be taken into consideration for the client at home.

Caregiving families and the people with a cast or brace who are cared for in their homes require health teaching to ensure proper healing without complications. The family may be responsible for assisting with transfers and the use of mobility aids. Assisting the caregiver to learn these techniques may require demonstration and feedback on your part and a return demonstration by the caregiver and/or the client.

Ambulatory Care

Many fractures are casted in an emergency department or outpatient setting. These clients often require no hospitalization. Regardless of the type of casting material used, a cast can interfere with circulation and nerve function because of excessive edema after application. Client teaching is an important nursing responsibility to prevent complications. The client or caregiver must be taught about cast care, the potential complications, and the need for frequent neurovascular assessment to prevent long-term problems. The importance of follow-up care should be stressed.

LEARNING TOOLS

DEVELOP YOUR BACKGROUND KNOWLEDGE

1. Review the Learning Outcomes.

2. Read the section on immobilization in your assigned text.

3. Look up the Key Terms in the glossary.

4. Review this module, and mentally practice the techniques described. Study so that you would be able to teach these skills to another person.

DEVELOP YOUR SKILLS

1. In the practice setting, observe any available casts, casting materials, or braces.

2. In the practice setting, select three other students, and form a group of four.

3. Apply each of the following braces, changing so that each has the opportunity to play the role of the patient. Those who are not participating at a given time can observe and evaluate the performances of the others.

   a. cervical collar
   b. lumbosacral brace
   c. leg mobilizer

DEMONSTRATE YOUR SKILLS

In the clinical setting

1. Consult with your instructor regarding the opportunity to observe or assist in the application of a cast or brace. Evaluate your performance with the instructor.

2. Consult with your instructor regarding the opportunity to care for a patient in a cast or brace. Use the Performance Checklists on the CD-ROM in the front of this book as a guide. Evaluate your performance with the instructor.

CRITICAL THINKING EXERCISES

1. Jeff Whitman, age 22, was injured in a motorcycle accident. He has been admitted to your unit with a fractured hip, pelvis, and left femur that have been surgically fixated; a hip spica body cast has been applied. This is his first hospitalization. Synthesize information you know about psychosocial development, the process of bone healing, and cast care, and identify major priorities in nursing care for this young man.

2. Amy Johnson, age 10, fell off her bike while riding and broke her left wrist. You have helped with applying a cast in the emergency room. She is to be discharged for care at home. Plan the teaching that will be necessary for Amy and her parents.

SELF-QUIZ
SHORT-ANSWER QUESTIONS

1. Name two kinds of casts.
   a. _____
   b. _____

2. Name two advantages of a plaster of Paris cast.
   a. _____
   b. _____

3. Name two advantages of a synthetic cast.
   a. _____
   b. _____

4. Why is the skin inspected carefully before casting?
   _____

5. Name two methods for finishing or covering the rough edges of a cast.
   a. _____
   b. _____

6. Name three ways to check neurovascular function when a person is in a cast or wearing a brace.
   a. _____
   b. _____
   c. _____

7. Name three kinds of materials used for constructing braces.
   a. _____
   b. _____
   c. _____

8. Why might patients wearing braces have difficulty ambulating?
   _____

MULTIPLE CHOICE

_____ 9. Spica casts cover basically
   a. an arm or leg only.
   b. the body.
   c. the body and only one arm or leg.
   d. the body and one or more extremities.

_____ 10. Windowing is done to
   a. enlarge the cast.
   b. relieve pressure on underlying tissue.
   c. feel the fracture.
   d. view the fracture.

_____ 11. The toes or fingers of the patient in a cast that is not yet dry should be checked
   a. every 15 minutes.
   b. every hour.
   c. once per shift.
   d. once per day.

_____ 12. The brace on a child may have to be changed periodically due to
   a. increased activity.
   b. noncompliance.
   c. growth changes.
   d. wear and damage of the appliance.

_____ 13. Printed instructions for applying a brace will most likely come from
   a. the physician.
   b. the company supplying the brace.
   c. a nurse clinical specialist.
   d. central supply department.

Answers to Self-Quiz questions appear in the back of this book.

MODULE 22

Caring for the Patient in Traction or With an External Fixation Device

SKILLS INCLUDED IN THIS MODULE

Procedure for Applying Skin Traction
Procedure for Caring for the Patient in Traction or With an External Fixation Device

PREREQUISITE MODULES

Module 1	An Approach to Nursing Skills
Module 2	Documentation
Module 3	Basic Body Mechanics
Module 4	Basic Infection Control
Module 5	Safety in the Healthcare Environment
Module 6	Moving the Patient in Bed and Positioning
Module 14	Nursing Physical Assessment
Module 18	Transfer
Module 20	Range-of-Motion Exercises
Module 21	Caring for Patients With Casts and Braces
Module 24	Basic Sterile Technique: Sterile Field and Sterile Gloves
Module 37	Applying Bandages and Binders

KEY TERMS

anorexia	iliac crest
cervical halter traction	occiput
	popliteal space
countertraction	prism glasses
excoriation	pulleys
external fixation device	reduction
	skull tongs traction
fixation	spreader bar
footboard	thrombophlebitis
footdrop	traction
footrest	trapeze
humerus	

OVERALL OBJECTIVE

▸ To apply skin traction to the patient and to maintain commonly used skin and skeletal traction devices effectively and safely while maximizing comfort and self-care without complications.

LEARNING OUTCOMES

The student will be able to

1. Assess the patient's record for the type of traction or external fixation to be used, the weight to be applied, if appropriate, and the restrictions on the patient's activity.
2. Analyze assessment data to determine possible complications of traction or the presence of an external fixation device and immobilization.
3. Determine appropriate outcomes for a specific patient in traction or with an external fixation device, and recognize the potential for adverse outcomes.
4. Assist with the application and adaptation of traction, using appropriate equipment.
5. Position the patient in anatomically correct and effective alignment, and position to ensure effective traction.
6. Provide emotional support during and after the procedure.
7. Intervene to prevent complications following application of traction or an external fixation device.
8. Evaluate traction for correct, unobstructed placement and patient knowledge of techniques to prevent complications and to support self-care.
9. Document the type of traction or external fixation device applied, the weight applied if any, the patient's tolerance of the procedure, the patient's neurovascular status, and the instructions provided.

Traction relies on the application of force or "pull" in two directions simultaneously to maintain the stability of a body part. Traction is commonly applied by using weights to pull in one direction and the body's own weight to provide pull or "**countertraction**" in the other direction. Traction also may be applied by arranging sets of weights that provide pull in opposing directions. Traction may be applied continuously or intermittently, depending on its purpose. Traction is most commonly applied to the arms, legs, and spine, including the cervical spine, or neck.

Traction devices can be used to treat many injuries and conditions of the musculoskeletal system. Nurses on the unit can safely and effectively apply the simple, commonly used traction devices to keep an injured body part in proper alignment, using the prescribed pull or tension. However, nurses or technicians will need special training to apply some of the more complicated traction devices. If reduction of a fracture requires surgery, the patient may return from the operating room to the unit with traction already in place. The nurse then maintains the traction properly. Traction and the immobility associated with it place the patient at risk for other complications, such as skin breakdown, muscle atrophy, urine retention, hypoventilation, and pneumonia.

The use of traditional traction is not common in contemporary healthcare in the United States. Skin traction as a treatment for lower back and cervical pain (see below) has been largely replaced by different types of physical therapy and medications that treat muscle spasm. Buck's traction (see below) is used as a temporary measure to relieve pain and muscle spasm for the person with a hip fracture. Many types of skeletal tractions that require the patient to remain in bed have been replaced by surgical procedures to fix fractures with pins and plates or by the use of external fixation devices. Skeletal tractions for large bone fractures may be a temporary measure for the person who has experienced multiple traumatic injuries and for whom the correction of fractures is a lower priority. Having said this, traction is still a potential treatment modality, and the nurse must be able to competently care for the patient in traction.

An **external fixation device** consists of a system of pins and wires passing through bone and connected to a rigid external metal frame consisting of circular rings with interconnecting rods that hold the fractured bone in place. The frame rods maintain tension between the skeletal pins or wires and the frame. Some external fixation devices are simple and have only two or three connecting rods. Others are complex, with rods arranged at different angles to maintain the position of fractured bone fragments. External rigid fixation allows fractures to heal by primary bone union. It promotes healing of complex fractured bones of the upper and lower extremities and pelvis (Bailey, 2003).

An external fixation device has two major advantages. First, it is useful when skin wounds are present. A cast would cover these wounds, making infection a greater possibility. With an external fixation device, the skin is uncovered, and wounds can be observed and treated as needed. Also the patient with an external fixation device is more mobile than one with a bed-based skeletal traction system. Therefore, the complications of immobility are decreased (Fig. 22-1).

NURSING DIAGNOSES

Examples of some nursing diagnoses related to traction include the following:

- Impaired Physical Mobility: related to traction or the presence of an external fixation device
- Disturbed Sleep Pattern: related to discomfort and confinement by traction or an external fixation device
- Impaired Skin Integrity: related to immobility secondary to traction
- Risk for Infection: related to presence of skeletal pin sites
- Deficient Diversional Activity: related to confinement imposed by traction

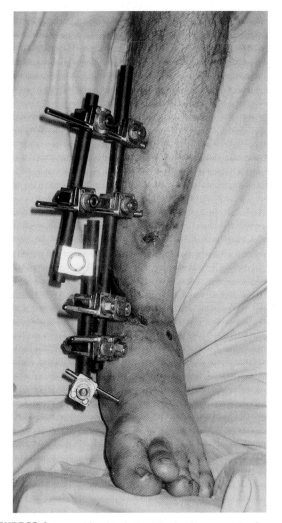

FIGURE 22-1 External fixation device. Metal rods exert traction between two sets of skeletal pins.

DELEGATION

Assistive personnel may be trained (often by a physician or orthopedic physician's assistant) to set up traction devices that are attached to the patient's bed. The traction devices may be applied to the patient by the physician or by the nurse, depending upon the type of traction. The maintenance of appropriate traction is a nursing responsibility. The nurse may delegate checking specific aspects of the traction to the nursing assistant and establish plans for reporting any deviations to the nurse. The care of patients in external fixation devices may also be delegated to assistive personnel, but the nurse must be certain the personnel know what signs and symptoms must be reported.

PURPOSES OF TRACTION

Traction has several uses in treating musculoskeletal conditions and injury. **Reduction** of a fracture is placing the fractured ends in alignment so that bone healing can occur. **Fixation** of a fracture is establishing a mechanism to hold the reduced fracture in its proper alignment throughout the healing process. Traction has been used for both reduction and fixation of fractures. Through the use of pins and rods, which are inserted through the skin, traction can be exerted on bones (skeletal traction), providing pull for the reduction of fractures. Traction can be applied to a fracture that has already been reduced to maintain the position and provide the conditions in which bone healing can occur.

Traction is also applied to create pull on muscles, thereby decreasing pressure on nerves and providing relief from muscle spasm. This is used as a temporary measure for hip fractures prior to surgery and as a treatment for lower back and cervical strain.

EQUIPMENT AND SETUP

The equipment and application methods for traction may vary somewhat from one healthcare setting to another. Essentially, the equipment consists of a traction bed that has a frame to which traction equipment can be attached and that provides correct body alignment for the patient. Traction pull is supplied by various ropes, **pulleys,** and weights. Discussions of each of these follow.

THE TRACTION BED AND FRAME

A regular hospital bed can be easily converted to a traction bed by installing a horizontal overhead bar attached to vertical bars at the head and foot. A **trapeze** device can be added to the overhead bar, so the patient can grasp this to assist in moving (Fig. 22-2).

All traction beds should have a firm, solid base under the mattress. Modern hospital beds have a flat metal base under the mattress. Older beds with a spring base require the use of a bedboard to provide a firm foundation, which helps maintain good body alignment. Many special mattresses and therapeutic beds and frames may be used for patients who have special problems and who also need traction. (See Module 9, Bedmaking and Therapeutic Beds.)

ROPES

Ropes are used to attach weights to traction devices. Use only clean ropes in good condition. Inspect all ropes for kinking or fraying. Ropes must hang freely without interference from bedding or bars. Wrap the ends of ropes with a pull tape to prevent slipping and fraying. You can do this by covering the end of the rope with adhesive tape and folding the two free ends of the tape over on themselves to form two pull tabs that can easily be removed (Fig. 22-3). Ropes that move past hard surfaces need to be wrapped where friction might fray and weaken the rope. When tying ropes, use a traction knot, as shown in Figure 22-4. All knots are taped for safety so that they do not separate.

PULLEYS

Be sure all pulleys move freely and function properly. Most pulleys are prelubricated. If they do not move easily, lubricate them with an oiled cotton sponge or silicone spray.

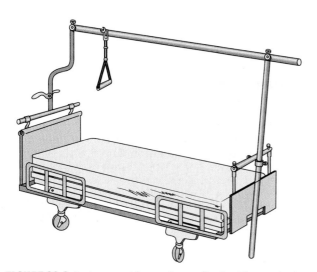

FIGURE 22-2 Bed prepared for traction application. The traction bars and overhead trapeze are in place. (Courtesy Zimmer, Inc., Warsaw, Indiana.)

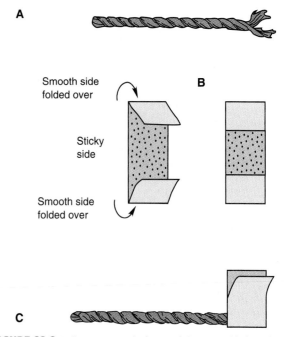

FIGURE 22-3 Pull-tape on end of rope. (**A**) Rope with frayed ends. (**B**) Prepared tape with folded-over ends to make removal easy. (**C**) Tape folded over end of rope to prevent further fraying.

WEIGHTS

The physician orders how many pounds of weight are to be applied. Metal blocks or sand bags, with hooks for attachment to the ropes, are used as weights. Each weight is marked with the number of pounds. Typically, a combination of weights is needed to achieve the desired traction. To avoid jarring the patient when weights are used intermittently or the amount of weight is changed, remove or add them slowly and gently while support is simultaneously given to the affected body part. You may need assistance to do this properly. Weights must hang freely from the pulleys at all times. When not in use, store weights carefully out of the way to avoid injuries.

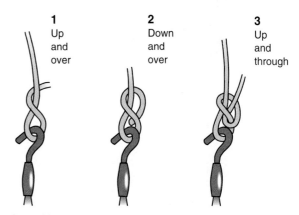

FIGURE 22-4 How to tie a traction knot.

SKIN TRACTION

Skin traction applies traction to muscles or bones by pulling on the skin, using traction tapes, a foam boot, or harnesses with protective padding. Skin traction has some limitations because of the danger of skin irritation and breakdown. It cannot be applied over skin that is broken or has poor blood supply because of the danger of more serious tissue damage. The weights are usually limited to fewer than 10 lb and are left on for fewer than 3 weeks.

Skin traction is generally used to treat fractures in children and minor fractures in adults and to temporarily immobilize fractures in adults before permanent fixation. It also is commonly used for muscle strains or spasms.

Although the physician decides the type of skin traction to be used, the nurse or a specially trained technician can apply it. Whether it can be removed intermittently to facilitate hygiene, elimination, or exercise depends on the physician's order and/or the facility's policy. The decision is usually guided by the purpose of the traction. For example, if the traction is being used to immobilize a fracture, it will generally not be removed. If the patient is being treated for muscle strain or spasm, the traction can usually be taken off for varying periods.

Be sure the skin is clean and dry before traction is applied. Follow the policies of the physician or facility regarding skin preparation. Sometimes, the area to be confined or taped is shaved to reduce pain and irritation when the tape is removed. A skin protectant is commonly applied to the skin to prevent skin damage from the traction.

TYPES OF SKIN TRACTION

There are many variations of skin traction. This module discusses commonly used types: Dunlop's (side-arm), Buck's, Russell's, Bryant's traction, pelvic sling, and cervical halter traction. Dunlop's and Russell's traction are less frequently used and are used for shorter periods because orthopedic surgery is used to establish reduction and fixation of fractures immediately after the injury. The medical management for injuries of the shoulder and femur more frequently involve open reduction and internal fixation or use of an external fixator device. Skin breakdown is a concern with all the following types of traction. See Table 22-1 for an overview of areas of potential skin breakdown related to the various types of traction.

DUNLOP'S (SIDE-ARM) TRACTION

Dunlop's skin traction is used for stabilizing fractures of the upper arm and for shoulder dislocations (Fig. 22-5).

table 22-1. Areas of Potential Skin Breakdown

Type of Traction	Area of Potential Skin Breakdown
Dunlop's	Elbow, scapula, sacrum, ischial tuberosities
Buck's	Medial and lateral malleoli, heel, scapula, sacrum, ischial tuberosities, greater trochanter
Russell's	Medial and lateral malleoli, heel, groin, scapula, sacrum, ischial tuberosities
Bryant's	Medial and lateral malleoli, scapula, sacrum
Pelvic	Iliac crest, scapula, sacrum, ischial tuberosities, greater trochanter
Cervical halter	Chin, ears, cheeks, occiput, scapula, sacrum, ischial tuberosities
Cervical tongs	Shoulder, clavicle, scapula

The patient is in the supine position. The head may be elevated for comfort as long as the forearm is in flexion and is extended 90 degrees from and in the same plane as the body.

Traction is applied in two directions by producing horizontal pull on the abducted **humerus** and vertical pull on the flexed forearm (ulna and radius). Procedures

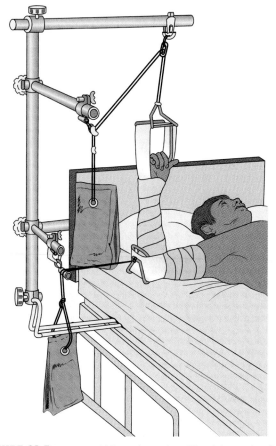

FIGURE 22-5 Humerus (side-arm) traction. The right angle of the elbow and the application of weights maintain alignment. (Courtesy Zimmer, Inc., Warsaw, Indiana.)

vary with the preference of the physician, but generally the following steps are used.

- Thoroughly cleanse the skin.
- Apply skin protectant.
- Attach strips of a special commercial adhesive to the skin, with the ends of the tape protruding above the hand.
- Wrap the part with an elastic bandage. (Refer to Module 37, Applying Bandages and Binders, for directions.) To protect the skin over the bony prominence of the elbow, use moleskin or lamb's wool padding.

Problems associated with this type of traction include skin breakdown, particularly over the elbow, and compromised neurovascular function. Observe the patient's fingers closely for data related to circulation, motion, and sensation (CMS). See Box 21-1 in Module 21 for an outline of neurovascular checks. These are most often caused by wrappings that are too tight and interfere with circulation. If any of these danger signs appear, rewrap the bandage for comfort and safety.

BUCK'S TRACTION

Buck's extension skin traction may be applied to one leg (unilateral) or both legs (bilateral). It is used primarily for temporary immobilization of a hip fracture to reduce muscle spasm and pain while awaiting surgery, for immobilizing fractures of the femur, and for lower spine "hairline" or simple fractures. Muscle spasm of the lower back also can be treated with Buck's traction.

Place the patient in the supine position with the bed flat. Position the head of the bed somewhat lower than the foot (Trendelenburg's position) if the patient's medical condition permits. Most electric beds are designed so that the foot end can be disengaged from the electric control, lowering the head to the desired level. This position allows the weight of the patient's body to provide countertraction.

Traction is applied in one direction on the leg or legs distally and with straight alignment. A foam traction boot with a hook and loop (Velcro) fastener is commonly used to apply the traction and is the most convenient and comfortable means of doing so. An elastic bandage may be used to hold a footplate and traction tapes to the leg instead of using a boot. To do this, apply wide strips of traction tape lengthwise on the inner and outer aspects of the calf. Then pad the calf, place a footplate near the bottom of the foot, and wrap the calf and footplate with the elastic bandage to hold them in place. A **spreader bar** may be attached to the footplate. Position the ropes, pulleys, and weights at the foot of the bed (Fig. 22-6).

Problems include possible skin breakdown at the ankle and over the heel. Wrappings that are too tight may compromise circulation, motion, and sensation.

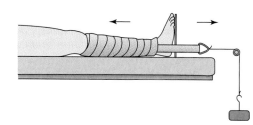

FIGURE 22-6 In unilateral Buck's extension traction, the patient has a foam boot with Velcro straps. The leg is positioned flat and the weight hangs freely. In bilateral Buck's extension traction, both legs are positioned in the same way with the same amount of weight attached for each leg.

The foot should not be in contact with the footplate, but free to perform dorsiflexion and plantar flexion exercises and should be covered only by light bed linen to prevent **footdrop** (permanent plantar flexion of the foot). If the diagnosis permits, remove the boot and wrappings for observation and skin care every 8 hours, and then rewrap. When traction is held in place by elastic bandages only, rewrapping every 8 hours is usually essential.

RUSSELL'S TRACTION

Russell's traction combines, in principle, Buck's and balanced suspension traction (discussed elsewhere in this module). Russell's traction is used for children to reduce or align fractures of the femur or treat knee injuries and is applied as skin traction. With adults, Russell's traction is usually skeletal, with the pull being exerted on a pin or wire that has been surgically inserted through the distal portion of the femur. Skeletal traction is used because the skin of an adult could not tolerate the pull required for the reduction of the fracture of an adult bone.

In general, with this type of traction, the patient lies supine, and the bed is flat. If ordered, elevate the head to a more comfortable level. Russell's traction allows more mobility than Buck's or balanced suspension traction, and the patient can be in high Fowler's position and can move a little from side to side with care.

With this traction, two methods can be used to provide two-directional pull on the leg. In the first, two weights are used—one hangs from an overhead bar to lift the knee, and the second one hangs at the foot of the bed to exert a pull on the lower leg. In the second method, a single weight is added to a system that exerts two-directional pull (Fig. 22-7).

Neurovascular status of the extremity may be compromised by swelling and pressure. Excessive pressure on the **popliteal space** behind the knee can impinge on nerves and constrict circulation. Establish a routine to assess circulation, motion, and sensation for the patient in Russell's traction. (See Box 21-1 in Module 21.) Pressure over the heel can irritate the skin and cause breakdown. Extra padding may be needed. The **footrest** may be used to maintain the foot in flexion to prevent footdrop, however dorsiflexion and plantar flexion exercises

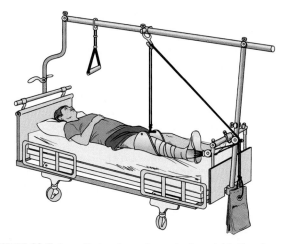

FIGURE 22-7 Russell's traction using a single weight. The sling supports the leg at the knee. (Courtesy Zimmer, Inc., Warsaw, Indiana.)

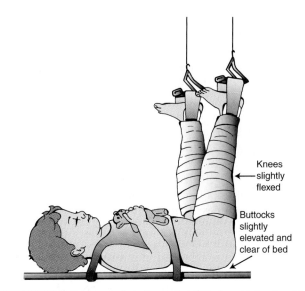

FIGURE 22-8 Representation of a small child in Bryant's traction. The buttocks are lifted slightly off the bed to enable the child's weight to serve as countertraction. (In the clinical setting, side rails would be in place unless someone is at the crib side.)

should be performed frequently for that purpose as well. Put a sock on the foot for warmth.

BRYANT'S TRACTION

Bryant's traction is a variation of bilateral Buck's traction and is used for children younger than 2 years who have an unstable hip joint or a fractured femur. Traction boots are preferable to tape, particularly with children, because the boots are less likely to cause skin breakdown. Place the child supine with the bed flat. Apply traction boots to both lower legs. Thread ropes from the footrests of each boot through pulleys on the overhead bar and onto the foot of the bed, where a weight is hung. Suspend the legs so that the hips are flexed at 90 degrees to the bed surface. The buttocks should be a few inches off the mattress to ensure proper traction on the legs (Fig. 22-8). The traction must be applied to both legs to maintain proper alignment of the affected leg.

Children adjust surprisingly well and quickly to such an apparently uncomfortable position but are at risk for a variety of problems. Assess both feet frequently for circulation, motion, and sensation. Motion and sensation may be decreased. Inspect the skin, including the back, for **excoriation.** When Bryant's traction is first applied, the child may need to have the upper body restrained for a short time until he or she no longer attempts to roll the body or pull on the traction ropes or boots. Give the child in Bryant's traction additional support and comfort, and plan to spend extra time with him or her. The family also can comfort and support the youngster and provide ideas for the amusement and diversion that are so important to the child's contentment.

PELVIC TRACTION

Pelvic traction is used to treat minor fractures of the lower spine, lower back pain, and muscle spasm. A flan-

nel or foam-lined canvas girdle or belt is placed snugly around the patient's pelvic area, often over pajama bottoms. The belt is placed somewhat lower than an abdominal binder; the lower portion ends just below the greater trochanter. It is secured with buckles or hook and loop (Velcro) closures, and traction is applied through attached straps. Traction is applied in the direction of the foot of the bed, either with two weights—one weight pulling to each side of the patient—or with only one weight, which is attached to a connector bar (Fig. 22-9).

Orders on the position of the patient vary. The most common is William's position, in which the patient is supine with the knees elevated. The patient's head is

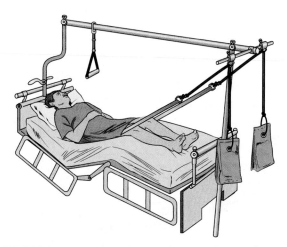

FIGURE 22-9 Pelvic traction. The knees and lower legs are elevated to flatten the lumbosacral curve of the spine, and the head is kept low to provide countertraction in the correct direction. (Courtesy Zimmer, Inc., Warsaw, Indiana.)

usually not elevated higher than the knees except for meals. For greater countertraction, elevate the foot of the bed. In certain cases, usually for patients with muscle spasm or minor disorders such as back strain, the traction is ordered as intermittent, meaning that it may be removed for elimination or hygiene. For more serious conditions, such as minor aligned vertebral fractures, the traction usually is applied continuously so that the pull remains constant. A fracture pan is used for elimination in these cases.

If the pelvic belt becomes soiled, replace it. Inspect skin frequently for irritation from the belt, particularly over the **iliac crest,** and provide any special skin care or padding needed. You also may need to initiate measures to prevent or relieve constipation.

Additionally, a correctly used **footboard** will keep the feet at right angles, thereby preventing footdrop. Foot and leg exercises and position changes help to relieve cramping, maintain muscle tone, and prevent venous stasis, which could lead to **thrombophlebitis.**

PELVIC SLING TRACTION

Pelvic sling traction is used to treat a fracture of the pelvis that has separated the pelvic bones. A flannel-lined sling provides compression on the pelvic region by suspending it slightly. Ropes are threaded through pulleys to a free-swinging weight at the foot of the bed. The patient lies supine with the bed flat. Continuous traction is usually ordered, so problems of hygiene and elimination may arise. As in pelvic traction, a footboard is needed. Breathing exercises and exercises of the lower legs can help prevent the complications of immobility (Fig. 22-10).

CERVICAL HALTER TRACTION

Cervical halter traction is used to treat a variety of conditions of the cervical spine (neck), including arthritis, whiplash injuries, spasms, and minor fractures. A

flannel-lined chin-head halter exerts pull on the cervical spine from the chin and **occiput** through a series of ropes and pulleys leading to a weight hanging freely over the head of the bed. Countertraction, if ordered, can be accomplished either by raising the head of the bed to a low Fowler's position or by placing the head of the bed on blocks. Place a rolled piece of flannel or a small, flat pillow under the neck to increase extension and add to the patient's comfort. Use a footboard to help prevent footdrop (Fig. 22-11).

Inspect the occipital area (back of the head) routinely because a pressure ulcer may develop. Be aware that the chin, cheeks, and ears also are susceptible to skin breakdown. The patient's diet may have to be modified if chewing becomes a problem. Provide **prism glasses** that direct vision upward and then horizontally so that the patient can watch television and read books while in the supine position and thus relieve boredom.

PROCEDURE FOR APPLYING SKIN TRACTION

ASSESSMENT

1. Review the patient's record, and read the physician's notes about the type of traction to be used. **R:** To determine the kind of injury and type of traction to be applied, the weight to be applied, and allowances for or restrictions on the activity of the patient.
2. Inspect the skin over which the traction apparatus is to be applied for interruptions in skin integrity and circulatory impairment. Problems of this type

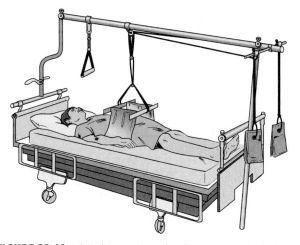

FIGURE 22-10 Pelvic sling traction. The sling supports the body and allows the pelvis to move as a unit without pull on the fracture site. (Courtesy Zimmer, Inc., Warsaw, Indiana.)

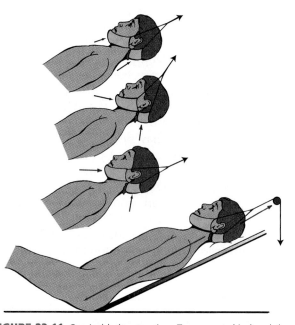

FIGURE 22-11 Cervical halter traction. To prevent skin breakdown, the ears must not be under the halter. The head of the bed is elevated for the body to provide countertraction.

may preclude the use of skin traction. **R:** To reduce the incidence of skin breakdown and circulatory impairment.

3. Assess what the patient knows about the procedure. **R:** To clarify, if necessary, any information that has been given.

ANALYSIS

4. Critically think through your data, carefully evaluating each aspect and its relation to other data. **R:** To determine specific problems for this individual in relation to traction.

5. Identify specific problems and modifications of the procedure needed for this individual. **R:** Planning for the individual must take into consideration the individual's problems.

PLANNING

6. Determine individualized patient outcomes in relation to traction, including the following. **R:** Identification of outcomes guides planning and evaluation.

a. Patient expresses comfort. **R:** Discomfort may indicate injury, trauma, or pressure. Complaints of pain or burning may indicate impaired circulation.

b. Ropes, pulleys, and weights are correctly placed. **R:** To ensure that proper traction is being applied.

c. There are no signs or symptoms of adverse outcomes, such complications of immobility, skin breakdown, or changes in circulation, motion, and sensation of the affected body part. **R:** Complications that continue can result in permanent disability.

7. Plan the correct patient position indicated for the traction. **R:** Planning ahead allows you to proceed more safely and effectively.

8. Gather equipment appropriate to the type of traction. Skin traction may require several of the following: skin protectant, traction tapes, traction boots, bandages, harnesses, halters, ropes, pulleys, weights, padding, trapeze, spreader bars, footrests, or footboard. **R:** Planning ahead allows you to proceed more safely and effectively.

IMPLEMENTATION

Action	Rationale
9. Wash or disinfect your hands.	To decrease the transfer of microorganisms that could cause infection.
10. Identify the patient, using two identifiers.	Verifying the patient's identity helps ensure that you are performing the right skill for the right patient.
11. Provide for privacy, and drape the patient as appropriate.	To avoid undue exposure.
12. Explain the procedure you are about to perform. Explain the purpose of the traction, whether weights are to be used intermittently or continuously, and how much the patient will be allowed to turn or move.	Explaining the procedure helps relieve anxiety or misperceptions that the patient may have about a procedure or activity and sets the stage for patient participation.
13. Raise the bed to an appropriate working position based on your height.	To allow you to use correct body mechanics and protect yourself from back injury.
14. Place the bed in the proper position for the specific type of traction being applied. With some types of skin traction, the patient's body weight serves as a counterbalance, necessitating the elevation of the foot or the head of the bed.	The degree of pull or tension required for effective traction often depends on the level of the bed and the relative position of the patient.

(continued)

Action	*Rationale*
15. Cleanse and prepare the skin according to the procedure of the facility. If tape is to be applied, the skin is often shaved beforehand. A skin protectant may be applied.	Skin may be shaved to reduce pain and irritation when the tape is removed. The skin protectant is used to protect the skin from abrasion by the traction appliance.
16. Secure the traction to the patient by applying the tape, boots, slings, or halters appropriate to the specific procedure. Make sure all appliances are the right size for the patient.	To ensure proper traction pull and lessen the risk of skin breakdown.
17. Thread and knot the ropes through lubricated pulleys. Check that both are aligned properly for the traction you are applying.	To ensure proper traction pull.
18. Using the hooks provided, attach the ropes to the patient's appliance. Then tug gently on the attached rope.	To check for the security of the tapes, boot, or wrappings.
19. If more than one weight is to be applied, gently add one at a time, lowering the weights slowly until the ordered weight is attained.	To avoid jerking the body part.
20. Tape the end of the rope.	To prevent fraying.
21. Carefully check that all appliances are functioning effectively, with weights hanging freely and not resting on the bed or floor.	To ensure that traction is applying correct direction and magnitude of pull to obtain therapeutic effect.
22. Check circulation, motion, and sensation (CMS) of the affected extremity as a baseline. a. Assess *circulation* by checking peripheral pulses, color, capillary refill, and temperature of the extremity. b. Assess *motion* by having the patient move fingers or toes on the affected extremity. c. Assess *sensation* by asking the patient about pain, tingling, numbness, or other sensations in the extremity.	CMS checks done regularly will provide early warning of potential complications. See Box 21-1 in Module 21.
23. Place the call signal, all personal possessions, and items needed for self-care within easy reach of the patient.	To prevent the patient's having to reach for objects or call signals that could misalign the traction or cause a fall.
24. Lower the bed as far as possible without allowing the weights to touch the floor.	If the patient should fall from the bed, there is less potential for injury if the bed is lower.
25. Wash or disinfect your hands.	To decrease the transfer of microorganisms that could cause infection.

EVALUATION

26. Evaluate based on the individualized patient outcomes in relation to traction. **R:** Evaluation in relation to desired outcomes is essential for planning future care. Include
    a. Patient expresses comfort.
    b. Ropes, pulleys, and weights are correctly placed (Box 22-1).
    c. There are no signs or symptoms of adverse outcomes, such as complications of immobility, skin breakdown, or changes in circulation, motion, and sensation (often referred to as CMS) of the affected body part.

DOCUMENTATION

27. Document on the appropriate form. **R:** Documentation is a legal record of the patient's care and communicates nursing activities to other nurses and caregivers.
    a. patient comfort and tolerance of the procedure
    b. type of traction and weight applied
    c. neurovascular status (circulation, motion, and sensation) and any observations or concerns.

◼ POTENTIAL ADVERSE OUTCOMES AND RELATED INTERVENTIONS

Many of the adverse outcomes of traction are related to immobility. Others are related to the pressure of the traction device. To combat immobility, encourage as much movement as possible within the confines of the traction, including active range of motion and passive range of motion when that is not possible (see Table 22-1).

1. Impaired skin integrity related to the pressure of the traction apparatus or from prolonged bedrest.
Intervention: Closely monitor skin in contact with traction tape and foam devices as well as pressure points on the back. Remove skin traction, and inspect skin three times a day. Place patient on a pressure ulcer prevention protocol if your facility has one. Include back care every 2 hours and special mattress overlays to minimize development of pressure ulcers. For both skin and skeletal

---

box 22-1 *Checking a Traction Set-Up*

- Patient's body in correct anatomic alignment
- All points where traction apparatus touches body padded to protect skin
- Ropes intact and not frayed, knots secure, and running through pulleys without restriction
- Pulleys moving freely
- Weights are the correct weight ordered, hanging freely, not touching floor

---

traction, you may need to adjust devices or place extra padding over bony prominences to relieve pressure.

2. Circulatory impairment in the affected extremity that may include edema from impaired venous return, decreased arterial flow, and/or thrombophlebitis.
Intervention: Assess for swelling by documenting appearance of fingers and toes and measuring the circumference of the extremity. Elevate the extremity when possible to increase venous return. Report edema that causes constriction from bandages or traction equipment. Assess arterial *circulation* by checking peripheral pulses, color, capillary refill, and temperature of the extremity. Have patient carry out active foot or hand exercises, as appropriate, every hour. Reapply skin traction to relieve excess constriction on circulation. Report calf tenderness, swelling, and positive Homans' sign, which may be signs of thrombophlebitis. Report dusky or pale color of extremity.

3. Peripheral nerve pressure that may interfere with function.
Intervention: Assess *motion and sensation* regularly. Immediately investigate complaint of burning sensation under the traction bandage or boot. Promptly notify physician of alterations in sensation and motor function.

4. Pulmonary complications, such as atelectasis and/or pneumonia related to immobility, slow respiratory rate, and shallow breathing.
Intervention: Assess breath sounds. Have patient perform deep-breathing exercises or utilize incentive spirometer every 2 hours. Assist patient to cough effectively to remove any secretions in the lungs. Reposition the patient within the confines of the traction requirements.

5. Gastrointestinal disturbances such as **anorexia** and constipation related to immobility.
Intervention: Provide an appealing diet that is rich in fiber. Adjust amounts served to the patient's appetite, and provide small, frequent meals. Encourage adequate fluid intake to aid bowel function. An intake of at least 3,000 mL fluid daily helps to prevent constipation and prevents urinary stasis (see number 6 below). Initiate any protocol for giving a stool softener, or if no protocol exists, consult with the physician about prescribing a stool softener.

6. Urinary stasis leading to urinary tract infection related to immobility.
Intervention: Encourage fluid intake up to 3,000 mL per day. Place in sitting position for urination if traction permits. Provide catheter care if patient requires Foley catheter.

7. Pain related to the underlying orthopedic problem or the traction itself.
Intervention: Provide adequate pain management through comfort measures and administering prescribed pain medication.

8. Disorientation and/or delirium related to underlying health problem (such as trauma) and sensory deprivation.

Intervention: Give frequent explanations and reassurance. Keep low light in the room during the night to avoid disorientation when awakening. Encourage family or significant others to stay with the patient. Avoid restraints because they often increase agitation and result in skin damage under the restraints and disruption of the traction.

9. Boredom related to lack of meaningful activities.

Intervention: Make the room as colorful and attractive as possible. Plan diversional activities for the patient. These might include music, television, crafts, or other activities suggested by the patient or family. These measures greatly alleviate irritability, restlessness, and boredom.

10. Fear and anxiety related to feelings of powerlessness secondary to the immobility. Patients may have secret fears of being trapped or abandoned.

Intervention: Provide opportunity for the patient to reveal fears and concerns, and explain the strategies in place to ensure that the patient will be able to express needs and be cared for regardless of what happens.

SKELETAL TRACTION

Skeletal traction is accomplished by applying traction to wires, pins, or rods that have been surgically attached to or placed through bones. This type of traction, which exerts direct pull on the bones, allows up to 30 lb of weight to be applied for continuous periods of traction of up to 4 months. Although the skin is not covered or pulled, it is still at risk for breakdown, particularly in the elderly. Pulleys and ropes may abrade adjacent skin, and the traction pull may exert shearing force on skin in contact with the bed.

Skeletal traction is used for more serious fractures of the bones and more often in adults than in children. This is because with adults, more weight must be applied to align and reduce fractures effectively.

Although the principles of care for the patient in skin and skeletal traction are similar, the nurse who cares for the patient in skeletal traction has added responsibilities. Skeletal traction is constant and must never be discontinued or interrupted without a specific order. The state of immobility is more complete, thus frequent and conscientious assessment for potential problems is required. Circulation, motor function, and sensation may be impaired in an extremity being treated with skeletal traction just as in skin traction. One additional potential problem is that of infection, because the skin barrier is broken. Bone infections are very difficult to treat successfully.

Understandably, patients in skeletal traction may fear that they cannot be moved or transferred quickly or easily in the event of a fire or natural disaster. It is sometimes advisable to explore these feelings and reassure the patient that in such an event, they would be given special attention. Having the call signal constantly within reach of these patients greatly allays fears. Answer any questions the patient may have. Because skeletal traction devices are usually applied in surgery, the nurse's responsibilities center on maintenance and safety.

TYPES OF SKELETAL TRACTION AND EXTERNAL FIXATION DEVICES

In this module, two of the more common types of skeletal traction are discussed: balanced suspension traction and **skull tongs traction.** Halo traction and other external fixation devices are also explained.

BALANCED SUSPENSION TRACTION

Balanced suspension traction is used to stabilize fractures of the femur. For this type of skeletal traction, a pin or wire is surgically placed through the distal end of the femur. (Skin traction may be used for balanced traction on rare occasions. If skin traction is used, tape and wrapping or a traction boot of the kind described under Buck's traction is applied.)

The patient is in the supine position, with the head of the bed elevated for comfort. As the name suggests, the affected leg is suspended by ropes, pulleys, and weights in such a way that traction remains constant, even when the patient moves the upper body.

Two important components of balanced suspension traction are the Thomas splint and the Pearson attachment. The Thomas splint consists of a ring, often lined with foam, that circles and supports the thigh. Two parallel rods are attached to the splint and extend beyond the foot. A Pearson attachment consists of a canvas sling that supports the calf. A footrest completes the setup (Fig. 22-12).

Parallel rods lead from the pin sites on the distal end of the femur to the attachment for the rope. Traction to the femur is applied through a series of ropes, pulleys, and weights. These weights hang freely at the foot of the bed.

The skin should be inspected frequently to identify problems early. The ring of the Thomas splint can excoriate the skin of the groin. Special padding may have to be used. Again, the foot should always be at a right angle on the footrest to prevent footdrop.

SKULL TONGS TRACTION

Skull tongs are used to immobilize the cervical spine in treating unstable fractures or dislocation of the cervical

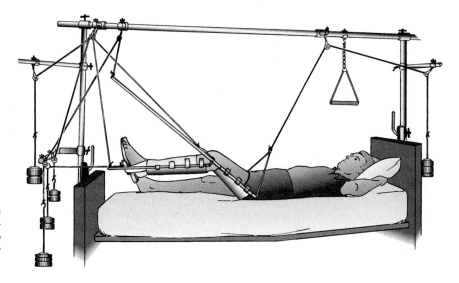

FIGURE 22-12 Balanced suspension traction with Thomas leg splint. Pulleys provide directional pull to enable weights to support the extremity in correct alignment, while other weights exert traction on skeletal pins.

spine. Although Crutchfield tongs were used almost exclusively in the past, Gardner-Wells skull tongs are in wide use currently. Some think these are less likely to pull out than the Crutchfield tongs. The patient is prepared for either type with a local anesthetic to the scalp. The tongs are surgically inserted into the bony cranium, and a connector half-halo bar is attached to a hook from which traction can be applied (Fig. 22-13).

The patient is supine and is usually on a special frame instead of the regular hospital bed. If a hospital bed is used, two or more people are required to assist the patient with any turning movements (logrolling). The head of the bed may be elevated to provide countertraction.

Because patients may remain in this type of traction for an extended period, observe the precautions taken for the patient in other types of skeletal traction. Difficulties with the performance of activities of daily living, infection at the tong sites, and restlessness and boredom are common. It is useful to teach the patient range-of-motion exercises, provide good nutrition, and suggest recreational or occupational activities.

HALO TRACTION

Halo traction is a type of external fixation device. Halo traction provides stabilization and support for fractured cervical vertebrae. The surgeon inserts pins into the skull. A half circle of metal frame connects the pins around the front of the head. Vertical frame pieces extend from the halo section to a frame brace that rests on the patient's shoulders. The vertical frame exerts traction by maintaining tension between the halo and the shoulder frame. The halo traction allows the patient to be out of bed and mobile while stabilizing the cervical vertebrae until they heal. The frame cannot be removed because any movement of the vertebrae could injure the spinal cord (Fig. 22-14).

PIN SITE CARE

When pins are used for fixation, pin sites must be cared for to remove any secretions or crusts and to prevent

FIGURE 22-13 Skull tongs traction. Weights attached to the tongs provide traction to cervical vertebrae. The body weight provides countertraction.

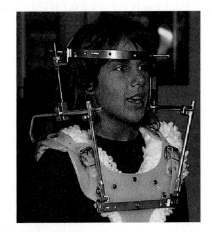

FIGURE 22-14 Halo traction. The external frame of the halo is attached to pins embedded in the skull.

infection. There has historically been a lack of consistency and some controversy regarding the appropriate clinical guidelines for pin site care. The National Association of Orthopedic Nurses is in the process of developing Evidence-Based Practice guidelines on skeletal pin care (Krassner, 2003). Consult the physician, and review your facility's policy for the specific procedure for pin site care to be used where you practice.

A common approach to pin site care is cleaning each pin site separately three times a day. Use sterile cotton-tipped applicators soaked with sterile saline solution to clean away all crusts and drainage. The skin around the pin may be massaged gently to bring any drainage to the surface, where it can be cleaned away. A dressing may be applied while drainage continues. When there is no drainage, the dressings are usually omitted. After healing occurs, the pin sites are cleansed carefully with soap and water and rinsed thoroughly. Some facilities use an ointment around the pin. There is concern as to whether the use of ointment decreases or actually increases the incidence of pin site infection.

Whatever the type of pin site care used, you should constantly assess for infection at the pin sites. Indications of infection at the sites include redness, heat, drainage, swelling, and pain. Fever is a non-specific indicator of infection that may not be present for a localized tissue infection.

EXTERNAL FIXATION DEVICE CARE

Any external fixation device must also be kept clean. The device may become soiled in the process of daily living. A cloth with soap and water may be used to clean the device. Be sure to rinse off any soap. Do not allow water to run from the device into pin sites because it may carry bacteria into the pin sites.

PROCEDURE FOR CARING FOR THE PATIENT IN SKELETAL TRACTION OR WITH AN EXTERNAL FIXATION DEVICE

ASSESSMENT

1. Review the physician's order. The patient has usually returned to the unit from the operating room, and the order will be listed in the postoperative orders. **R:** To determine the type of traction or external fixation device, the weight to be used for traction, allowances for or restrictions on activity, and perhaps the position of the head or foot of the bed.
2. Assess patients returning to the unit from surgery for signs of general discomfort or pain. (See Module 42, Providing Postoperative Care, for more details.) For other patients being maintained in skeletal traction or with an external fixation device, carry out a complete systems assessment, with particular attention to skin, respiratory, gastrointestinal, musculoskeletal, and psychosocial systems. Especially assess circulation, motion, and sensation in the extremities affected by the traction. **R:** This will help determine adverse effects from anesthesia, from the injury, or from immobility.
3. Assess what the patient knows about the procedure. **R:** To clarify, if necessary, any information that has been given.

ANALYSIS

4. Critically think through your data, carefully evaluating each aspect and its relation to other data. **R:** To determine specific problems for this individual in relation to traction.
5. Identify specific problems and modifications of the procedure needed for this individual. **R:** Planning for the individual must take into consideration the individual's problems.

PLANNING

6. Determine individualized patient outcomes in relation to the specific skeletal traction or external fixation device. Include
   a. Patient expresses comfort. **R:** Discomfort may indicate injury, trauma, or pressure. Complaints of pain or burning may indicate impaired circulation.
   b. For traction: Ropes, pulleys, and weights are correctly placed. For external fixation: All components must be in place without pressure. **R:** If not appropriately placed, the traction will not be applied correctly. Pressure on components of an external fixation device may change the direction of force on the bone.
   c. Pin sites are clean without signs of infection. **R:** Pin site infection has the potential to create a bone infection.
   d. There are no signs or symptoms of adverse outcomes, such as pain, burning, complications of immobility, skin breakdown, pin site infection, or changes in circulation, motion, and sensation of the affected body part. **R:** Complications may result in long-term or even permanent disability.
7. Identify the correct position for the patient. **R:** The correct position is needed to maintain the traction or external fixation device and the patient in anatomic alignment.
8. Gather equipment needed for the traction or external fixation device and to maintain comfort and alignment, such as pillows or padding. Obtain assistance if needed. **R:** Planning ahead allows you to proceed more safely and effectively. Assistance may be needed to move the patient without risk to either patient or caregivers.

IMPLEMENTATION

Action	Rationale
9. Wash or disinfect your hands.	To decrease the transfer of microorganisms that could cause infection.
10. Identify the patient, using two identifiers.	Verifying the patient's identity helps ensure that you are performing the right skill for the right patient.
11. Raise the bed to an appropriate working position based on your height.	To allow you to use correct body mechanics and protect yourself from back injury.
12. Inspect the devices: **a.** For traction, all ropes and pulleys should be in proper alignment, correct weights should be attached, and ropes should be hanging freely. **b.** For an external fixation device, all components should be free of pressure and the extremity supported.	To be sure that the device is applied correctly and effectively.
13. Inspect all operative sites including pin or tong insertions for excessive bleeding or drainage, and provide pin site care according to facility policy.	To identify complications early and prevent infection.
14. Carry out nursing interventions appropriate to the problems identified in assessment. Give pain medication as needed.	To ensure patient safety and to alleviate any anxiety or discomfort.
15. Check circulation, motion, and sensation (CMS) of the affected extremity as a baseline. **a.** Assess *circulation* by checking peripheral pulses, color, capillary refill, and temperature of the extremity. **b.** Assess *motion* by having the patient move the fingers or toes on the affected extremity. **c.** Assess *sensation* by asking the patient about pain, tingling, numbness, or other sensations in the extremity.	CMS checks done regularly will provide early warning of potential complications.
16. Place the call signal, all personal possessions, and items needed for self-care within easy reach of the patient.	To prevent the patient's having to reach for objects that could misalign the traction or cause a fall.
17. Teach the patient methods for moving in bed and any appropriate exercises.	To ensure patient involvement in self-care.

(continued)

Action	Rationale
18. Lower the bed as far as possible while keeping the weights off the floor.	If a fall should occur, there is less likely to be injury if the bed is low.
19. Wash or disinfect your hands.	To decrease the transfer of microorganisms that could cause infection.

EVALUATION

20. Evaluate using the individualized patient outcomes previously identified. **R:** Evaluation in relation to desired outcomes is essential for planning future care.
    a. Patient expresses comfort.
    b. For traction: Ropes, pulleys, and weights are correctly placed. For external fixation: All components are in place without pressure.
    c. Pin sites are clean without signs of infection.
    d. There are no signs or symptoms of adverse outcomes, such as pain, burning, complications of immobility, skin breakdown, pin site infection, or changes in circulation, motion, and sensation of the affected body part.

DOCUMENTATION

21. Document the following on the appropriate form. **R:** Documentation is a legal record of the patient's care and communicates nursing activities to other nurses and caregivers.
    a. Patient comfort and tolerance of the procedure
    b. Type of traction and weight applied
    c. Neurovascular status (circulation, motion, and sensation) and any observations or concerns

Acute Care

Most patients requiring skin or skeletal traction will be cared for in the acute care setting initially. Frequent reinforcement of information regarding the traction therapy will increase understanding of the therapy and promote the patient's participation in his or her healthcare. Immobility and confinement pose continuing challenges for the patient in traction. Immobility-related problems may include pressure ulcers, stasis pneumonia, constipation, loss of appetite, urinary stasis, urinary tract infection, and venous stasis. Astute assessment and nursing interventions directed toward these problems are essential. The neurovascular and circulatory status of the body part in traction should be assessed on a regular basis. The nurse should encourage the patient to exercise muscles and joints not in traction to guard against their deterioration. Frequent visits by the nurse and family as well as diversional activities are helpful in allaying apprehension and in fostering coping.

Physical therapy will usually be started sometime during the acute phase. The nurse must work with the physical therapist to ensure a consistent approach to activity and movement and reinforcement of desired behaviors. Prior to discharge, the patient with an external fixation device and the caregiver need instruction in pin care, transfer, and mobility, and recognition of complications.

Long-Term Care

Mobility limitations imposed by traction, particularly skeletal traction, may require a resident to utilize long-term care. It is essential that the nurse have the knowledge of traction management to provide safe and effective care for these vulnerable residents. Many residents in long-term care are elderly and have changes brought on by the aging process as well as other medical conditions that can further compromise skin care, circulation, and mobility.

Home Care

Clients with external fixators or halo traction frequently return home for continuing treatment. Use the same principles of assessment and care as you would for those in the healthcare facility. These traction devices may interfere with mobility and affect family and home maintenance roles, causing the client to feel more dependent on others than usual. The client or caregiver must be proficient in providing pin site care and in recognizing signs of infection at the sites.

A home care nurse can instruct the client and caregiver in ways to handle such situations and provide continuing assessment. An important part of this assessment includes the knowledge that the potential for skin problems remains. Family members will need to become proficient with assessing the client's skin for any sign of pressure or damage. General concerns surrounding immobilization also must be considered for the client at home.

Caregiving families and the people with skeletal traction devices who are cared for in their homes require health teaching to ensure proper healing without complications. The family may be responsible for assisting with transfers and the use of mobility aids. Assisting the caregiver to learn these techniques may require demonstration and feedback on your part and a return demonstration by the caregiver and/or the client.

Ambulatory Care

Most clients requiring traction are treated in an inpatient setting, however some clients with muscle strain requiring pelvic or cervical halter traction may be treated in the outpatient setting. Client teaching is an important nursing responsibility to ensure proper use of traction and to prevent complications. The importance of follow-up care should be stressed.

LEARNING TOOLS

DEVELOP YOUR BACKGROUND KNOWLEDGE

1. Review the Learning Outcomes.
2. Read the section on immobility in your assigned text.
3. Look up the Key Terms in the glossary.
4. Review the information on CMS checks in Module 21.
5. Review this module, and mentally practice the techniques described. Study so that you would be able to teach these skills to another person.

DEVELOP YOUR SKILLS

In the practice setting
1. Observe any available traction equipment or devices.
2. With a partner, practice applying one type of skin traction to experience the pulling sensation. Use both tape and a boot if possible.

3. Together, evaluate the traction experience with attention to the feeling of immobility and psychosocial concerns.
4. Apply each of the following traction devices, changing so that each has the opportunity to play the role of the patient.
   a. Buck's traction boot
   b. cervical traction halter

DEMONSTRATE YOUR SKILLS

In the clinical setting
1. Consult with your instructor regarding the opportunity to observe or assist in the application of skin or skeletal traction. Use the Performance Checklist on the CD-ROM in the front of this book as a guide. Evaluate your performance with the instructor.
2. Consult with your instructor regarding the opportunity to care for a patient in skin or skeletal traction. Review the nursing care plan for this patient, paying particular attention to the parts of the plan relating to traction or problems with immobilization. Evaluate your performance with the instructor.

CRITICAL THINKING EXERCISES

1. Zachary, an active 19-month-old boy, has had an unstable left hip since birth. The physician has ordered him placed in Bryant's traction to correct this problem. How does his age affect his nursing plan of care? Evaluate the physical and psychosocial concerns you should consider when developing his care plan. Describe how you will involve the parents in planning and providing care. Identify the outcomes that you anticipate.
2. Imagine that you are assigned to care for two patients: the 65-year-old male is in humerus side-arm traction, and the 35-year-old female is in halo traction. You may make up personal data related to the two patients. Design complete care plans for the two patients. Then compare and contrast the plans, providing rationale for differences and similarities.

SELF-QUIZ
SHORT-ANSWER QUESTIONS

1. Name two types of skin traction.

   a. _____

   b. _____

2. List materials commonly used when performing pin site care.

   _____

3. List two methods for preventing footdrop in patients in traction who must remain immobilized.

a. _____

b. _____

4. List four common patient problems that may result from the immobilization associated with traction.

a. _____

b. _____

c. _____

d. _____

MATCHING EXERCISES

5. Match the most likely area for potential skin breakdown with the type of traction listed below. (More than once choice may be used.)

_____ **1.** Dunlop's elbow   **a.** ankle

_____ **2.** Buck's   **b.** back

_____ **3.** Russell's   **c.** chin

_____ **4.** Bryant's   **d.** elbow

_____ **5.** pelvic   **e.** groin

_____ **6.** cervical halter   **f.** heel

_____ **7.** cervical tongs   **g.** iliac crest

                             h. occipital

MULTIPLE CHOICE

_____ **6.** A major advantage of a halo traction for a person with a cervical spine injury is that the
   a. vertebrae will heal more quickly.
   b. vertebrae are more stable than with any other type of fixation.
   c. person experiences less pain with a halo traction.
   d. person can be mobile.

_____ **7.** An external fixation device can be
   a. adjusted in tension by the nurse.
   b. removed for bathing and hygiene.
   c. applied when skin wounds are present.
   d. attached to a frame of weights and pulleys.

Answers to the Self-Quiz questions appear in the back of this book.

REFERENCES AND SUGGESTED RESOURCES: UNIT 4

American Nurses Association. (2002). *Preventing back injuries: Safe patient handling and movement.* Washington, DC: Author.

Bailey, J. (2003). Getting a fix on orthopedic care. *Nursing 2003, 33*(6), 58–63.

Clarke, S., & Dowling, M. (2003). Spica cast guidelines for parents and health professionals. *Journal of Orthopaedic Nursing, 7*(4), 184–191.

Krassner, H. (2003). Call for panelists: NAON develops pin care guidelines. *Orthopedic Nursing, 22*(5), 378.

Pifer, G. (2000). Casting and splinting: Prevention of complications. *Topics in Emergency Medicine, 22*(3), 1, 7.

Schoen, D. C. (2001). *NAON core curriculum for orthopaedic nursing* (4th ed.). Philadelphia: W. B. Saunders.

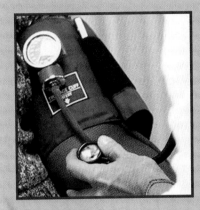

5

Implementing Complex Infection Control

MODULES

MODULE
23

Isolation Procedures

SKILLS INCLUDED IN THIS MODULE

Specific Isolation Techniques
    Preparing the Room
    Entering the Room
    Removing Items From an Isolation Room
    Leaving the Room
General Procedure for Isolation Technique

PREREQUISITE MODULES

Module 1	An Approach to Nursing Skills
Module 2	Documentation
Module 3	Basic Body Mechanics
Module 4	Basic Infection Control

KEY TERMS

Airborne
    Precautions
category-specific
    precautions
common vehicle
    transmission
compromised host
Contact
    Precautions
disease-specific
    precautions
droplet nuclei
Droplet
    Precautions
isolation
methicillin-
    resistant
    *staphylococcus
    aureus* (MRSA)

microorganisms
protective isolation
reverse isolation
sensory deprivation
Standard
    Precautions
Transmission-Based
    Precautions
vancomycin-
    resistant
    *staphylococcus
    aureus* (VRSA)
vectorborne
    transmission

OVERALL OBJECTIVE

▶ To carry out correct isolation technique, emphasizing safety from infectious agents for patients, visitors, staff, and self while maintaining high-quality patient care.

LEARNING OUTCOMES

The student will be able to

1. Assess an individual patient to identify signs and symptoms of an infection.
2. Analyze assessment data regarding the infection to determine the means of transmission.
3. Determine appropriate outcomes for both the patient and others in the setting, and recognize the potential for adverse outcomes.
4. Plan specific isolation procedures to be used, taking into consideration the means of transmission as well as facility policies.
5. Carry out isolation procedures correctly.
6. Evaluate the effectiveness of the infection control measures used.
7. Document infection control measures appropriately.

The **isolation** of an institutionalized patient is used for patients "known or suspected to be infected or colonized with epidemiologically important pathogens that can be transmitted by airborne or droplet transmission or by contact with dry skin or contaminated surfaces" (Centers for Disease Control and Prevention, http://www.cdc.gov/ncidod/hip/ISOLAT/Isolat.htm). The nurse must understand the rationale for isolation procedures and be able to carry out the procedures correctly. This is true not only to maintain safety for the patient and others but also to provide explanations regarding the procedures to the patient, the patient's visitors and family, and the assistive personnel.

Historically, two main systems have been used for isolation: **disease-specific precautions** and **category-specific precautions.** Both approaches were accepted by the Centers for Disease Control and Prevention (CDC), and facilities chose to implement either type. In 1994, the CDC published draft guidelines for a new approach to isolation called **Transmission-Based Precautions.** In 1996, the CDC published its guidelines for "Transmission-Based Precautions" as an approach to isolation and recommended their use (Garner, 1996). These CDC Guidelines have been used since that time. Although CDC recommendations do not have the force of law, most regulatory and accrediting groups (such as state health departments and JCAHO, 2005) require that healthcare agencies comply with these recommendations or justify any differences. Each facility will have infection control policies to guide you in determining the appropriate precautions to use in an individual situation. The CDC Web site provides the complete reference on these Guidelines and the detailed evidence upon which these precautions are based (http://www.cdc.gov/ncidod/hip/ISOLAT/Isolat.htm).

In this module, the types of Transmission-Based Precautions and guidelines for their use are discussed briefly. Specific techniques that can be used for any system, including the preparation of the room for isolation and the correct method for entering and leaving the room, are outlined.

NURSING DIAGNOSES

The following nursing diagnoses relate to problems commonly experienced by patients in isolation. Assessment for these problems is an important part of caring for the patient in isolation.

- Social Isolation: related to confinement imposed by isolation regimen. This occurs when individuals become cut off from their support systems, causing them to feel alone and in distress. A patient may experience this either as a result of the effects of the isolation procedures or as a result of concerns about safety for family and friends.
- Deficient Knowledge: related to lack of experience with infection control measures. Isolation procedures are better tolerated when the individual understands them.
- Deficient Diversional Activity: related to confinement imposed by isolation. This is a particular concern when an individual has a chronic infectious condition. As the individual reaches a convalescent state, the lack of diversional activities may be very distressing.
- Disturbed Sensory Perception: related to lack of stimuli in environment. Certain conditions restrict stimuli. For instance, persons entering an isolation room may be unrecognizable, and the room may have been stripped of amenities to prevent contamination.

■ Risk for Infection: related to suppressed immune system or to the overgrowth of resistant organisms. The individual whose original infection is related to a suppressed immune system may lack the physical resources to fight off additional infections. When severe infections are treated, **microorganisms** not susceptible to the anti-infective drug may have the opportunity to proliferate, creating secondary infections.

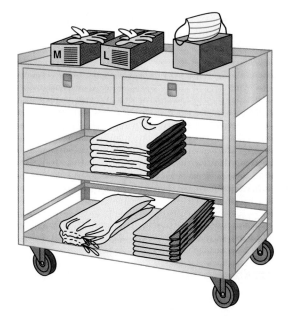

FIGURE 23-1 Example of a stand outside of the room. The stand contains all supplies needed to carry out isolation precautions. The supplies are fairly standard in accord with CDC guidelines that call for specific items to be worn going into the room and containers for things that are removed from the room. The usual supplies are gloves and disposable masks (usually in boxes on the top of the stand); paper bags to put things in that need to be disinfected or sterilized before handling; plastic bags for refuse (usually in an upper drawer of the stand); gowns on a shelf; and laundry bags (some facilities use a red laundry bag; others use a standard bag).

INSTITUTIONAL RESOURCES FOR ISOLATION PROCEDURES

To meet the healthcare agency accreditation standards, each facility must have an infection control officer. This officer is commonly a nurse with specific expertise in infection control or someone on the laboratory staff with such expertise. In large medical centers, the infection control officer is sometimes a physician epidemiologist. The infection control officer monitors infections and helps establish policy regarding all infection control procedures and training within the facility.

A facility's procedure manual outlines the specific isolation methods staff members are required to use. Review this resource for clarification regarding isolation if you are unsure how to proceed in an individual situation. If written materials do not provide the information you need, contact the infection control officer for direction. A supply cart or stand is placed outside of the door of an isolation room for all the supplies needed to carry out the appropriate Transmission-Based Precautions (Fig. 23-1). An isolation sign is posted as well.

CREATING BARRIERS TO MICROORGANISMS

The underlying principle of isolation technique is the creation of a physical barrier that prevents the transfer of infectious agents. The key to this is knowing how the organisms are transmitted and taking measures to prevent that transmission. For example, if an organism is airborne, it is reasonable to wear masks and keep the door of the patient's room closed. If, however, the organisms are transferred only by contact with drainage or secretions on linen and items used in care, masks are unnecessary, and only direct contact with the patient is hazardous. The barriers created for effective isolation should be appropriate to the goal—preventing the spread of select microorganisms from the patient to the environment or from the environment to the patient.

TYPES OF ISOLATION PROCEDURES

With the widespread use of **Standard Precautions,** many facilities use a specific isolation designation only rarely because *all patients* are being treated as if they have infections that can be transferred by blood, body fluids, or any other body substance. (See Module 4, Basic Infection Control.) A specific isolation designation may be used only for those whose infections are not contained by these measures.

The transmission precautions in the guidelines from the CDC recognize this fact and are based on the use of Standard Precautions for all individuals (considered level 1 precautions). Thus, the only situations requiring any additional isolation procedures (considered level 2 precautions) are those in which disease transmission occurs in ways other than through contact with moist body substances. All descriptions below are from the CDC Guidelines (Garner, 1996 and http://www.cdc.gov/ncidod/hip/ISOLAT/Isolat.htm). See Box 23-1 for an overview of types of precautions and selected diseases requiring those precautions.

AIRBORNE PRECAUTIONS

Airborne precautions are used for patients known or suspected to have serious illnesses in which infectious agents are transferred on **droplet nuclei** or dust particles that may remain suspended in the air and that spread easily on air currents. Examples of these diseases are measles, varicella (chickenpox), and tuberculosis. The following precautions are needed in addition to Standard Precautions.

1. Place the individual in an isolation room that has negative air pressure (ensuring that air from the room does not exit to the rest of the institution when the door opens).
2. Ensure that the isolation room has six or more exchanges of air per hour and that air be exhausted to the outside or be recirculated through HEPA (high-efficiency particulate air) filters. This type of filter can remove very small microbes from the air.
3. Keep the door to the room closed at all times except when entering and exiting.
4. Masks must be worn by all caregivers.

The CDC recommends that everyone entering the room should wear special respirators that are certified to exclude particles of 5 microns or less and are fitted to prevent air from entering around the mask (designated as N95 masks). For caregivers or others

---

box 23-1 *Types of Precautions and Selected Conditions Requiring the Precaution**

Standard Precautions

Use Standard Precautions for the care of all patients (see Appendix A).

Airborne Precautions

In addition to Standard Precautions, use Airborne Precautions for patients known or suspected to have serious illnesses transmitted by airborne droplet nuclei. Examples of such illnesses include

- Measles
- Varicella (including disseminated zoster)†
- Tuberculosis‡

Droplet Precautions

In addition to Standard Precautions, use Droplet Precautions for patients known or suspected to have serious illnesses transmitted by large particle droplets. Examples of such illnesses include

- Invasive *Haemophilus influenzae* type b disease, including meningitis, pneumonia, epiglottitis, and sepsis
- Invasive *Neisseria meningitidis* disease, including meningitis, pneumonia, and sepsis
- Other serious bacterial respiratory infections spread by droplet transmission, including
  Diphtheria (pharyngeal)
  Mycoplasma pneumonia
  Pertussis
  Pneumonic plague
  Streptococcal (group A) pharyngitis, pneumonia, or scarlet
    fever in infants and young children
- Serious viral infections spread by droplet transmission, including
  Adenovirus†
  Influenza

Mumps
Parvovirus B19
Rubella

Contact Precautions

In addition to Standard Precautions, use Contact Precautions for patients known or suspected to have serious illnesses easily transmitted by direct patient contact or by contact with items in the patient's environment. Examples of such illnesses include

- Gastrointestinal, respiratory, skin, or wound infections or colonization with multidrug-resistant bacteria judged by the infection control program, based on current state, regional, or national recommendations, to be of special clinical and epidemiologic significance
- Enteric infections with a low infectious dose or prolonged environmental survival, including *Clostridium difficile*
- For diapered or incontinent patients: enterohemorrhagic *Escherichia coli* O157:H7, *Shigella,* hepatitis A, or rotavirus
- Respiratory syncytial virus, parainfluenza virus, or enteroviral infections in infants and young children
- Skin infections that are highly contagious or that may occur on dry skin, including
  Diphtheria (cutaneous)
  Herpes simplex virus (neonatal or mucocutaneous)
  Impetigo
  Major (noncontained) abscesses, cellulitis, or decubiti
  Pediculosis
  Scabies
  Staphylococcal furunculosis in infants and young children
  Herpes zoster (disseminated or in the immunocompromised host)†
  Viral/hemorrhagic conjunctivitis
  Viral hemorrhagic infections (Ebola, Lassa, or Marburg)*

---

*See Appendix A of the CDC Guidelines for a complete listing of infections requiring precautions, including appropriate guidelines.
†Certain infections require more than one type of precaution.
‡See CDC Guidelines for Preventing the Transmission of Tuberculosis in Healthcare Facilities.
Source: Centers for Disease Control and Prevention. (Updated February 18, 1997). (Online). http://www.cdc.gov/ncidod/hip/ISOLAT/isotab_1.htm. Accessed April 3, 2005.

with documented immunity to the specific disease (such as measles or chicken pox), this mask may be omitted. Because individuals do not develop immunity to tuberculosis, the CDC recommends that all individuals entering the room of a patient with either suspected or diagnosed tuberculosis wear this type of mask.

Wearing the specific type of mask that meets a standard for blocking 95% of airborne pathogens (N95) continues to be a challenge. Although HEPA respirators are effective barriers, the masks are hot and somewhat uncomfortable, and they muffle voices, making oral communication more difficult. The masks are difficult to fit and pose particular problems to some individuals, thus rendering them ineffective for those individuals.

In 1993, the Occupational Safety and Health Administration (OSHA) took the position that HEPA filtration was essential to protect healthcare personnel. OSHA has regulatory authority and therefore, facilities were required to conform to this standard (OSHA, 1997). In 2003, OSHA revoked this rule because the overall incidence of tuberculosis in the community is low, and healthcare workers are more likely to be exposed by the person who has not been diagnosed than by the patient in isolation. The agency determined that the institution of these procedures would not significantly alter the incidence of tuberculosis among healthcare workers (OSHA, 2003). Many facilities responded to this regulation by adopting the use of standard surgical masks instead of N95 masks for those with known or suspected airborne infections. The CDC recommendation is still that the N95 masks be used. Therefore, some institutions require them. This is especially true in institutions where drug-resistant tuberculosis is found in the population being treated. Be sure to check the policies of your facility.

5. Discard, clean, or bag and send for processing any articles used by the patient on removal from the room.

6. Transport the patient only if necessary. If transport is essential, the patient wears a surgical mask and is covered by a sheet. If the patient cannot wear a mask, the healthcare worker transporting the patient should wear a HEPA respirator and keep the patient at a distance from others. This may require calling ahead or using a separate elevator.

For all airborne illnesses, a major factor in transmission lies in droplet nuclei deposited in tissues and the hands of the infected individual. Hand hygiene by patients and all others in the environment is most effective against this transmission. Coughing into the air by patients is responsible for most airborne transmission of tuberculosis. Patients can be taught to cover coughs with a disposable tissue, to dispose of tissues correctly into a biohazard bag, and to wash or disinfect their hands every time they use a tissue. Healthcare workers can also maintain distance from patients with tuberculosis as much as possible even while wearing masks. The greatest danger of tuberculosis transmission is often during the period before the tuberculosis is suspected or diagnosed.

DROPLET PRECAUTIONS

Droplet Precautions are used when infectious agents are transferred on large particle droplets directly from the source patient to the oronasal surfaces of the recipient. These large particle droplets tend to settle out of the air rapidly. Examples of diseases for which Droplet Precautions are used are pertussis (whooping cough), influenza, mumps, and rubella.

In addition to Standard Precautions, for Droplet Precautions, the following are included:
1. The patient should be in a private room if at all possible.
2. Those working within 3 feet of the patient must wear a mask. This can be a standard surgical mask. The CDC Guidelines note that some facilities may prefer to have individuals wear a mask upon entry into the room.
3. Patient transport should be minimized, and the patient should wear a mask during transport.

CONTACT PRECAUTIONS

Contact Precautions are used when the infectious agent can be spread by contact with the patient's skin or by surfaces within the room. Examples of diseases for which Contact Precautions are used include acute diarrhea, rash of unknown etiology, respiratory infections in infants and children, wound infections, and infection with a drug-resistant organism, such as **methicillin-resistant *staphylococcus aureus* (MRSA)** or **vancomycin-resistant *staphylococcus aureus* (VRSA).**

In addition to Standard Precautions, the following precautions are added:
1. The patient should be in a private room if possible.
2. In addition to wearing gloves when required by Standard Precautions, gloves are worn while providing direct care to the patient or touching any surface in the room. Gloves are removed before exiting the room, hands are washed or disinfected thoroughly, and nothing is touched before exiting the room. The door handle may be opened with a paper towel that is then discarded.
3. In addition to wearing a gown when required by Standard Precautions, a gown is worn when entering the room if there will be contact with the patient, with environmental surfaces (such as sheets),

or with objects used in care. Remove the gown carefully before leaving the room. Be sure that your clothing does not touch any surface as you leave.

4. When possible, all patient care items should be restricted to the single patient or else adequately cleaned and disinfected after use.

OTHER MODES OF PATHOGEN TRANSMISSION

CDC Guidelines also discuss diseases spread by **common vehicle transmission.** These are diseases borne by food or water. CDC Guidelines also address **vector-borne transmission,** which refers to diseases transmitted by an intermediate host (or vector) such as an insect. This includes diseases such as malaria and West Nile virus that are transmitted by mosquitoes. In general, these modes of transmission are not a concern in hospitalized individuals but rather the preventive actions needed are part of public health actions. In developing countries, these modes of transmission do become a concern for healthcare facilities.

PROTECTING THE INFECTION-SUSCEPTIBLE PATIENT

Additional categories of isolation are used to protect patients who have a suppressed immune system and are therefore highly susceptible to contracting an infection. One category is called compromised-host precautions, and the other is termed **protective isolation,** which is sometimes referred to as **reverse isolation.** Although it has been proved that the most effective measure for infection control is hand hygiene, additional precautions are added to increase safety for these individuals.

PROTECTIVE ISOLATION

Some facilities have eliminated the use of this most restrictive category because infection rates may not be different when this is instituted. However, some institutions find differences in infection rates when protective isolation is used. The following guidelines apply to protective isolation:

1. A private room with positive air pressure (when the door opens, outside air is prevented from coming in) and the door closed is required.
2. Gowns and masks must be worn by all who enter the room.
3. Gloves must be worn by those having direct contact with the patient.
4. All persons, including visitors, must wash hands on entering and leaving the room.
5. People with infections should not enter the room.

6. All items taken into the room should be individually evaluated for their potential to carry pathogens and harm the patient. Usually plants are not permitted because of the microorganisms in the soil. Flowers are not permitted because the standing water becomes a reservoir for microbial growth.
7. Because the room and its contents are considered clean, no special measures are taken when removing articles and linens.

COMPROMISED HOST PRECAUTIONS

The designation **compromised host** usually means that the patient has a suppressed immune system and is therefore less capable of self-protection against pathogens. Many facilities are now using the procedure for compromised host more often than that for protective isolation, because it appears to be as effective and is less restrictive to the person involved. The procedure is more acceptable to patients because it usually does not require use of mask and gown. It includes

1. meticulous hand hygiene by both staff and visitors
2. excluding persons with a cold or other infection from the room or from coming close to the patient
3. instructing patients in careful hand hygiene to protect them from what others may bring in and the microorganisms they carry in their own intestinal tract
4. prohibiting (in some facilities) live plants and flowers in the environment just as in protective isolation
5. limiting visitors to immediate family and special friends, and attempting to have consistent caregivers in order to decrease the number of different organisms to which the person is exposed

PATIENT, FAMILY, AND STAFF COOPERATION

A responsibility inherent in carrying out isolation procedures is making sure the patient and the patient's family understand the reasons for isolation and that they respond to this knowledge with appropriate actions. This responsibility extends to the hospital staff and the physician as well. No one likes isolation procedures, perhaps the patient least of all. For this reason, emphasize the do's rather than the don'ts. A positive approach encourages cooperation.

COMBATING SENSORY DEPRIVATION

Closely related to the idea that isolation procedure is extra work that no one really likes to do is the idea that patients in isolation feel that the staff is reluctant to take care of them. This feeling may be prompted by the sense that they are always the last to be cared for, by careless remarks made outside doors but within hearing of the patient, and by countless nonverbal exchanges. In addition, those who visit isolated patients (family, friends, staff) are often covered from head to toe, making normal communication impossible. Isolation rooms are usually stripped of pictures, plants, and other decorative items, making the total setting rather dreary. The variety of stimulation isolated patients receive is less, and it can be less meaningful as well. Often these patients experience **sensory deprivation** from limited interaction with others. As a result, patients in isolation may become less alert and less motivated, and complaints may increase along with loneliness, depression, and anger.

You can intervene positively by giving care to an isolated patient first, by answering the call signal promptly, and by stopping in the doorway to wave. Provide the patient with puzzles, paperback books, and other paper items that can be disposed of when no longer needed. For patients on protective isolation or compromised host precautions, such items should be new in order to avoid bringing in organisms. These items can be freely removed from the room of the patient on protective isolation. Typically, the family or friends can provide such items.

SPECIFIC TECHNIQUES USED IN ISOLATION PROCEDURES

Each isolation situation should be considered in terms of which specific techniques are needed. Choose those appropriate to the precautions in use for the individual patient. Use only those techniques prescribed by your facility. Using techniques that are not needed adds time and cost to the patient's care.

PROCEDURE FOR PREPARING THE ROOM

This procedure is appropriate for patients in droplet or Airborne Precautions. For the patient in Contact Precautions, a private room is not required but may be desirable. Two patients with the same infectious agent needing Contact Precautions may be placed in the same room.

1. Be sure the patient in droplet or Airborne Precautions is in a private room. **R:** There is potential for spreading infection to a roommate especially if either patient moves about in the room.
2. Post a sign outside indicating the type of isolation precautions in use or giving instructions for all visitors to report to the nursing station before entering the room. **R:** To communicate to all healthcare workers the need to take special precautions and indicate to visitors that they should check with the nursing staff for instructions for their own protection.

3. Be sure a stand is outside the room with appropriate supplies (disposal bags, gowns, masks, gloves as needed). **R:** To provide caregivers and visitors with the supplies needed for appropriate personal protection.
4. Place a laundry hamper inside the room. **R:** To keep the laundry contained and prevent infectious material from being spread around the room. A laundry bag in the room also facilitates removing soiled laundry from the room with ease.
5. Be sure a wastebasket with a plastic liner is inside the room. **R:** While a plastic-lined wastebasket is standard in most institutional settings, its lack is a particular problem within an isolation room because it is more difficult for the caregiver to dispose of gloves and wash hands before exiting the room.
6. If nondisposable equipment, such as a thermometer, blood pressure cuff, and stethoscope, is to be used for the patient's care, make certain those supplies have been obtained and placed in the room. **R:** Items used for caring for a patient in any type of isolation should be not be moved to another patient's bedside. Once you take the equipment into isolation, it is no longer available for use in other patient situations.

PROCEDURE FOR ENTERING THE ROOM

This procedure is used when a gown, gloves, and a mask have been prescribed for the isolation procedure. If one is not needed, simply move to the next procedure.

1. Obtain all needed equipment. **R:** To minimize time demands and help with organization.
2. Wash or disinfect your hands. **R:** For infection control.
3. Put your watch in a plastic bag. **R:** So that the watch face is visible and remains clean.
4. Put on a gown, if indicated by the mode of transmission.
   a. Put on the gown, making sure your uniform is covered.
   b. Fasten the ties securely. **R:** A gown is always needed when entering the room of the patient on Airborne Precautions because microorganisms are in the air. For the patient in Droplet Precautions, a gown is only needed when you are working within 3 feet (the distance droplets travel) of the patient. Some facilities, however, require a gown at all times because once you are in the room, you may need to do something you had not anticipated. A gown is needed during direct care activities for the patient in Contact Precautions to protect the uniform from contact with the patient's linen and the patient. This also protects other patients from infectious agents you might transfer to them from your uniform.

5. Put on a mask, if indicated by the mode of transmission.
   a. Place the mask over your nose and mouth.
   b. If the mask has ties, fasten both sets of ties securely. If the mask has an elastic strap, place it around your head where it will not slip off.
   c. Tuck the bottom edge of the mask under your chin, and fit the top edge snugly across the bridge of your nose. **R:** To be sure that air passes through and not around the mask, thereby protecting yourself from microorganisms in the air.
6. Put on clean gloves if needed.
   a. Put on both gloves.
   b. Pull the wrists of the gloves over the ends of the sleeves. **R:** To protect yourself from infectious agents that are transmitted on room surfaces and to protect other patients from infectious agents you might transfer from one room to another.

PROCEDURE FOR REMOVING ITEMS FROM AN ISOLATION ROOM

This procedure is used to remove contaminated items from inside an isolation room in a way that creates a clean outer surface for those who handle the materials after the materials are outside the patient room. It is often referred to as "bagging out" the room. This procedure may be used for soiled linens, for medical equipment, and for trash. The bag is usually marked so that others will know that it contains infectious material. In some facilities, a red biohazard outer bag is used. In others, a simple label is added.

1. *Inside nurse:* Place used items in appropriate containers or bags. Carefully close and secure each bag. Some items do not need to be double-bagged but may be placed directly into the single bag that the outside nurse holds. **R:** The inside nurse is responsible for evaluating the potential for contamination of those outside the room and providing a means of safeguarding other healthcare workers.
2. *Outside nurse:* Form a cuff on a bag, and hold with your hands underneath the cuff. This may be a linen bag, a paper bag for equipment to be disinfected, or a plastic bag for trash. **R:** The cuff protects your hands from accidental contact with the material from inside the room.
3. *Inside nurse:* Place the bag holding contaminated items directly into the bag being held by the outside nurse, being careful to touch only the inside of that bag. If an item does not need to be double-bagged, simply place the item into the bag held by the outside nurse (Fig. 23-2). **R:** To protect the outside of the bag from contamination so that it can be safely handled for disposal or processing.
4. *Outside nurse:* Fold over the cuffed edge, and carefully secure the top of the bag. **R:** To ensure that the contaminated items do not accidentally fall

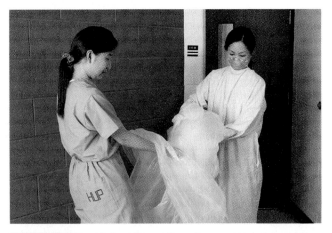

FIGURE 23-2 Double-bagging wet linens from an Airborne Precautions isolation room.

out of the bag and thereby contaminate people or surfaces.
5. Mark the bag in the manner prescribed by the facility. **R:** Marking the bag alerts others to handle the bag with appropriate technique.
6. Dispose of the bag in the proper place, or send it to the appropriate department for processing. **R:** Contaminated materials left in hallways continue to have the potential to spread infectious agents.

PROCEDURE FOR LEAVING THE ROOM

1. Review your tasks to ensure that you have completed what you had planned to do, and also check with the patient regarding any further needs the patient has. **R:** Entering and exiting an isolation room is time consuming. Careful planning will minimize the number of trips in and out.
2. Remove soiled gloves by turning the gloves inside out as you pull them off.
   a. Peel first glove off, touching only the outside with other gloved hand.
   b. Hold first glove in second hand.
   c. Slide ungloved fingers inside of second glove, and turn glove inside out over first glove while removing it. **R:** To ensure that the contaminated surface is inside where it is unlikely to touch a clean surface.
3. Untie waist ties. **R:** These are at your back and should be relatively cleaner than other surfaces.
4. Wash or disinfect your hands. **R:** To remove soil and pathogens. The waist ties have the potential to be contaminated.
5. Untie ties at the neck of the gown, and pull out and forward, dropping gown off the shoulders (Fig. 23-3). **R:** Ties near the head should have remained clean, and you have not recontaminated your hands.
6. Pull off the gown, touching only the inside. Carefully place the gown in a laundry hamper or waste-

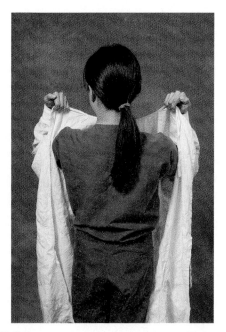

FIGURE 23-3 Removing an isolation gown by touching only the neck and inside surfaces.

basket. **R:** The inside should have remained clean, so it will not contaminate your hands.

7. Untie the mask ties, or grasp the rubber band holder, and discard the mask carefully, touching ties or rubber band only. **R:** The mask itself may have infectious agents on the exterior surface.
8. Wash or disinfect your hands. **R:** To prevent any inadvertent contamination.
9. Open the door, using a paper towel to grasp the door handle. **R:** The door handle is potentially contaminated.
10. Wash or disinfect your hands outside of the room. **R:** This final hand hygiene is an extra safeguard both for you and others in the environment.

CARING FOR LINEN

Inside the room, handle the linen carefully to avoid creating currents of air on which microorganisms can move. Use gloves for handling linens, and take care to keep the outside of the linen bag clean. If the patient is in Droplet or Airborne Precautions, the linen bag in the room will be removed by placing in a clean bag that is outside the door as described above.

CARING FOR DISHES AND FOOD TRAYS

Disposable dishes and tableware are used in some settings. However, the strong detergents and high temperatures used in washing dishes in a healthcare institution will remove any infectious agents on the dishes. Trays and dishes may be placed in a clean bag as described above for transport to the kitchen.

TRANSPORTING THE PATIENT IN ISOLATION

Sometimes, a patient in isolation must be transported to another area. This should be done only when absolutely necessary. Precautions vary according to the type of isolation in use. Generally, it is essential to consider the person that you are protecting and from what type of infection you are protecting others. A patient in protective isolation must be protected from all those with whom he or she comes in contact. This patient may wear a mask during transport; all who care for the patient in another department must wear gowns and masks. During transport, a patient in airborne or droplet isolation must wear a mask to protect others and is usually covered with a sheet so that contaminated clothing is not exposed. A patient in contact isolation should wear a gown, but a mask is not necessary. All items that are touched by the patient must be disinfected. Consult your facility procedure book for specific instructions.

GENERAL PROCEDURE FOR ISOLATION TECHNIQUE

ASSESSMENT

1. Check the type of isolation ordered. **R:** The isolation type should be clearly documented so that all healthcare personnel can carry out correct technique.
2. Identify the reason for isolation. **R:** The reason for isolation informs appropriate actions to take as barriers to transmission.
3. Check equipment outside and inside the patient's room. **R:** By doing this, you will make sure you have everything you need.

ANALYSIS

4. Critically think through your data, carefully evaluating each aspect and its relation to other data. **R:** To determine specific problems for this individual in relation to isolation precautions.
5. Identify specific problems and modifications of the procedure needed for this individual. **R:** Planning for the individual must take into consideration the individual's problems.

PLANNING

6. Determine individualized patient outcomes in relation to isolation. **R:** Identification of outcomes guides planning and evaluation.
   a. Patient understands the need for isolation and the rationale for specific precautions.
   b. Isolation precautions are carried out appropriately by patient, visitors, and staff.
7. Gather necessary equipment that is not found outside or inside the patient's room. **R:** To save time and promote efficiency.

IMPLEMENTATION

Action	Rationale
8. Wash or disinfect your hands.	To decrease the transfer of organisms that could cause infection.
9. Identify the patient, using one identifier.	One identifier is all that is usually available outside the room and permits you to use the correct precautions when entering. If you are doing procedures for the patient inside the room, you will need to check two identifiers there as JCAHO (2005) requires before performing procedures.
10. Open the door so that the patient can see your face, explain what you are doing and that you are entering, and ask the patient about any specific needs.	When the patient has seen your face, you are more of a person and seem less intimidating to the patient. This also reduces feelings of isolation. Patients in isolation often feel neglected because people do not come and go freely. Asking about needs in time to meet them provides the patient with a feeling of being cared for. At the doorway, you are far enough away to protect yourself from infectious agents.
11. Carry out techniques needed to enter the room based on the type of precautions in place.	Each type of transmission requires its own set of safeguards to prevent transmission of infectious agents.
12. Give care as planned.	Your planning should have provided you with everything you need to carry out appropriate patient care.
13. Carry out techniques necessary to leave the room.	Each type of transmission requires its own set of safeguards to prevent transmission of infectious agents.

EVALUATION

14. Evaluate using the individualized patient outcomes previously identified. **R:** Identification of outcomes guides planning and evaluation.
    a. Patient understands the need for isolation and the rationale for specific precautions.
    b. Isolation precautions are carried out appropriately by patient, visitors, and staff.

DOCUMENTATION

15. Document according to facility policy. In most instances, a simple notation that the patient remains in isolation using specified precautions is made. **R:** To provide the legal record of care.

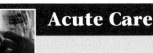

Acute Care

The multidrug-resistant organisms present in acute care hospitals have created a serious concern in regard to nosocomial infections. Standard Precautions are essential to preventing the spread of infections among patients. Nurses need to be alert to early symptoms of infections in order that patients can be assessed and isolation precautions instituted where appropriate. Nurses may need to be role models for others on the healthcare team in terms of carrying out the precautions that are needed for the individual patient.

Long-Term Care

Isolation requirements for Airborne Precautions include engineering standards regarding negative pressure in the room and air circulation and exchange. Long-term care facilities do not usually meet these standards. As a result, these facilities usually elect to transfer any resident thought to have any type of airborne infection to an acute care hospital that has these structural elements in place.

Contact precautions are perhaps the most common type of isolation used in long-term care. This is very challenging in an environment where the residents may not have the cognitive abilities to cooperate in the processes needed. Caregivers must be alert to resident behaviors that could endanger others.

Home Care

Many individuals with infectious diseases are cared for at home, and family members must be taught how to protect themselves as they provide care. Because family members are less likely to be susceptible individuals (as would be found in any health-care institution), instances of communicating most infections in home environments are rare. Airborne infections, which are highly contagious, are the exception. With infections such as tuberculosis, small children and the elderly who are most susceptible may be advised not to live in the same house with the client until the client's treatment regimen decreases the potential for transmission.

Ambulatory Care

Ambulatory care settings are challenged by clients coming into the facility with communicable diseases using no precautions at all. Pediatrician's offices and clinics may have a particular problem as children who are ill and communicable arrive and leave. Many of these settings have established procedures to move individuals with potentially communicable diseases directly into private examination rooms where other clients will not be exposed. Planning ahead for these problems is an important responsibility in ambulatory care.

LEARNING TOOLS

DEVELOP YOUR BACKGROUND KNOWLEDGE

1. Review the Learning Outcomes.

2. Read the section on isolation in your assigned text.

3. Look up the Key Terms in the glossary.

4. Review this module, and mentally practice the techniques described. Read about all three systems

for planning isolation to be sure you understand the underlying principles, and then focus your study on the system in use where you currently have clinical practice. Study so that you will be able to teach these skills to another person.

DEVELOP YOUR SKILLS

1. In the practice setting, select at least one other student with whom to work. You may also form a group of three so that someone is available to observe and critique your performance.

2. With your partner, practice preparing to enter and leave the various types of isolation rooms based on the technique needed. Changing so that each has the opportunity to play the role of the patient as well as the nurse, perform each of the following procedures. Those who are not participating at a given time can observe and evaluate the performances of the others. As a patient, consider how these procedures would make you feel.

   Airborne Precautions
   Droplet Precautions
   Protective Isolation
   Contact Precautions

3. With a partner, practice removing items from an isolation room, alternating so that each of you has a turn being inside the room and outside the room. After you have done the procedure the first time, evaluate yourselves, using the Performance Checklist on the CD-ROM in the front of this book. Then switch roles, and repeat the procedure. Again, evaluate yourselves, and repeat the procedure as necessary.

4. When you are satisfied that you can carry out the procedure, have your instructor evaluate your performances.

DEMONSTRATE YOUR SKILLS

In the clinical setting
1. Consult with your instructor regarding the opportunity to carry out isolation precautions.

2. Evaluate your performance with the instructor.

CRITICAL THINKING EXERCISES

1. Mrs. Mendoza has been in isolation for 10 days. She seems irritable and shows no interest in eating or in the physical therapy ordered by the physician. What could be the source of her problem? Plan at least three nursing actions that might help Mrs. Mendoza.

2. A patient is being admitted. On the telephone, the physician states, "Mrs. Jones has a foot ulcer that appears to be infected. Please culture the wound

as soon as she arrives." What is the nurse's responsibility in regard to infection control for this patient? What is the most appropriate type of transmission-based precaution to use?

SELF-QUIZ

SHORT-ANSWER QUESTIONS

1. What are the two major purposes of isolation?

   a. _____

   b. _____

2. The organism that is causing Mr. P.'s infection can be transmitted either by droplets or by contact. What type of isolation would be appropriate for him?

   _____

3. Mrs. R. is a postoperative patient whose care has been complicated by a pathogen transmitted by direct contact, the mode of transmission being the gastrointestinal system. What type of isolation would be appropriate for her?

   _____

4. List three items required in preparing a room for isolation when the organism is airborne.

   a. _____

   b. _____

   c. _____

5. How are items removed from a protective isolation room?

   _____

6. If you are the outside nurse removing items from an isolation room, and the inside bag touches your hand, what should you do?

   _____

   _____

   _____

7. A patient with severe leukemia has been placed in protective isolation. What is the purpose of isolation for this patient?

   _____

MULTIPLE CHOICE

_____ 8. The patient is diagnosed with a wound infection caused by MRSA. Which type of precautions is needed?
   a. Standard Precautions only
   b. Contact Precautions
   c. Droplet Precautions
   d. Airborne Precautions

_____ 9. The patient is admitted with a diagnosis that includes a notation to R/O (rule out) tuberculosis. Which type(s) of precautions are needed?
   a. Standard Precautions only
   b. Contact Precautions
   c. Droplet Precautions
   d. Airborne Precautions

_____ 10. The patient is on Droplet Precautions. You need to take the patient's medications into the room to administer them. Which of the following precautions would you include?
   a. Standard Precautions only
   b. Gown and mask
   c. Gown, mask, and gloves
   d. Mask only

_____ 11. The patient is on Contact Precautions, and you are to give the patient a bath. Which of the following precautions would you include?
   a. Standard Precautions only
   b. Gown and gloves
   c. Gown, mask, and gloves
   d. Mask only

Answers to the Self-Quiz questions appear in the back of this book.

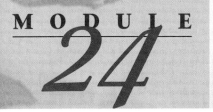

MODULE 24

Basic Sterile Technique: Sterile Field and Sterile Gloves

SKILLS INCLUDED IN THIS MODULE

General Approaches and Principles of Surgical Asepsis
Setting Up for Sterile Technique
   Opening a Sterile Pack
   Adding Items to a Sterile Field
   Adding Liquids to a Sterile Field
   Putting on Sterile Gloves Using Open Technique

PREREQUISITE MODULES

Module 1	An Approach to Nursing Skills
Module 4	Basic Infection Control
Module 14	Nursing Physical Assessment

KEY TERMS

contamination	spores
disinfectant	sterile
disinfection	sterile conscience
medical asepsis	sterile technique
microorganisms	sterilization
pathogen	surgical asepsis

OVERALL OBJECTIVES

▸ To identify situations in which sterile technique is needed and to recognize breaks in technique when they occur.
▸ To open a sterile pack, set up a sterile field, add sterile items or fluid to a sterile area, and put on sterile gloves using open technique.
▸ To implement sterile procedures without contamination and without increased risks for nosocomial infections.

LEARNING OUTCOMES

The student will be able to

1. Assess the need for surgical asepsis, and explain the rationale for the decision.
2. Analyze assessment data to determine special patient problems in relation to maintaining surgical asepsis.
3. Describe criteria that would be used to support the use of surgical asepsis and the equipment necessary for implementation.
4. Determine appropriate outcomes related to surgical asepsis, and recognize the potential for adverse outcomes.
5. Implement surgical asepsis, maintaining all principles and identifying behaviors that lead to contamination.
6. Evaluate the effectiveness of the sterile technique procedure(s) used for the specific patient.
7. Document the appropriate information related to the sterile procedure and the patient response.

Strict sterile technique, or **surgical asepsis,** is frequently necessary in nursing. It is used most extensively in operating rooms, delivery rooms, and for invasive procedures. Surgical asepsis is also essential when performing such nursing procedures as injections, catheterizations, some dressing changes, and intravenous therapy. Surgical asepsis differs from **medical asepsis** in that surgical asepsis eliminates all **microorganisms.** Medical asepsis is also known as clean technique, which is used to reduce the number of microorganisms, usually through handwashing and barrier methods.

Sterile technique is used to protect patients from possible infection when normal body defenses are not intact. Sterile technique consists of practices and principles to initiate and maintain sterility. Nurses are responsible for identifying clinical data and situations in which sterile technique is necessary for preventing patient infection. It is important to review your institution's policies and procedures and current wound and skin care guidelines to determine the procedure appropriate to the specific situation: either medical or surgical asepsis. Critical thinking must be applied to clinical situations to determine the correct procedure for a specific patient. The nurse must practice the psychomotor skills related to surgical asepsis to competently perform them in the clinical setting.

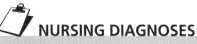

NURSING DIAGNOSES

The most common nursing diagnosis related to the need for surgical asepsis or sterile technique is Risk for Infection related to impaired skin integrity secondary to surgical or traumatic wound. Risk for Infection may also be related to invasive procedures that bypass the body's normal defense mechanisms.

DELEGATION

Assistive personnel usually are not taught sterile technique. Therefore, sterile procedures are not delegated to assistive personnel. There are some settings where assistive personnel are delegated tasks, such as measuring blood glucose levels, which require sterile technique. In those settings, sterile technique must be taught to enable assistive personnel to carry out assigned responsibilities.

SITUATIONS REQUIRING STERILE TECHNIQUE

Healthy, intact skin and mucous membranes provide an effective barrier to microorganisms; however, underlying tissue provides an excellent medium for bacterial growth. Therefore, when most underlying tissue is exposed due to a wound or surgical incision, it must be protected against the entry of a **pathogen** by sterile technique. Pathogens are disease-causing microorganisms. The nurse must assess the extent to which the normal defenses are being breached and the related potential for infection. The classic classification system for surgical wound includes: I, clean; II, clean-contaminated; III, contaminated; and IV, dirty (Mangrem, et al., 1999). This classification system (Table 24-1) provides the nurse

table 24-1. Classification of Wounds	
Wound Classification	**Description**
I—Clean	A clean surgical wound in which no inflammation or contamination is encountered
II—Clean contaminated	A surgical wound originating from the respiratory, alimentary, genital, or urinary tracts, which are likely to have normal flora
III—Contaminated	Fresh traumatic wounds or a wound that encounters gross spillage from the gastrointestinal tract
IV—Dirty	Old traumatic wounds that have current infection, purulence, or perforated viscera

table 24-2. Sterilization Methods	
Sterilization Category	**Method**
Thermal	Moist heat—steam under pressure
	Hot air—dry heat
	Microwaves
Chemical	Ethylene oxide gas
	Hydrogen peroxide plasma/vapor
	Ozone gas
	Liquid chemical sterilant—peracetic acid
Ionizing radiation	Radiation source to which items can be exposed

with insight to decide if medical asepsis or surgical asepsis is indicated. Further, it enables the nurse to identify the risk for postsurgical infection.

Some internal body areas, such as the urinary bladder and the lungs, are normally free of pathogenic microorganisms. To maintain this status, sterile technique is used whenever these areas are entered. Although the eyes are not normally sterile, sterile technique is used in many procedures relating to them, because the eyes are susceptible to infection, and the consequences of even a minor infection in the eye can be serious. Common situations in which sterile technique is used include inserting urinary catheters, changing some surgical dressings, preparing and administering injections, and performing venipunctures.

The nurse must also identify patients at increased risk for infection. Diseases such as diabetes, peripheral vascular disease, renal or liver failure as well as immunosuppression may also be factors when deciding whether to use sterile technique rather than clean technique to reduce the potential for infection. The nurse must examine the white blood cell (WBC) count and other laboratory data and the patient's history and physical examination results to determine an individual patient's risk for infection.

UNDERSTANDING CONCEPTS OF STERILIZATION

Sterilization is "the complete elimination of all forms of microbial life" (AORN 2004, p. 413). The ideal method of sterilization should render an item free of all microorganisms (including **spores** and vegetative forms). It also should not damage the item being sterilized and be relatively simple to use, inexpensive, and safe for those in the workplace. Unfortunately, no single method of sterilization meets all these criteria for all items that must be sterilized. Table 24-2 identifies the major types of sterilization in use. Many items used in modern healthcare

facilities arrive from manufacturers in presterilized packages, and it is imperative that the nurse identifies indications on the manufacturer's wrapper that the item is sterile (Fig. 24-1).

INDICATORS OF STERILITY

Indicators that react to steam under pressure or gas when exposed to it for a prolonged period are used to demonstrate an item's sterility. These indicators are commonly seen on packs in the form of special tape. Dark lines appear on the tape after a package has been exposed to a temperature for sufficient time to sterilize the item. Some sterile indicators are placed inside large packs to indicate sterilization has penetrated and occurred within a bulky package.

Every commercial product has some indicator of sterility. It is the nurse's responsibility to check the manufacturer's literature for this information, so that sterility of an item is confirmed before its use. Wrapped packages retain their sterility for various lengths of time, depending on the type of wrapping material, the condi-

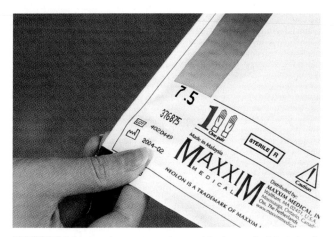

FIGURE 24-1 Manufacturer's package with the sterile label clearly visible.

tions of storage, and the integrity of the package. If an event renders a package contaminated (no longer sterile), such as getting wet or being dropped on the floor, then the package must be taken out of circulation to prevent usage. An expiration date often appears on a sterile package. Do not use the contents after that date, and take the package out of circulation, so others will not use it (Fig. 24-2).

Many items may be sterilized in a department of your workplace. General staff nurses are involved in using sterile materials for patient care activities and in sending items to an appropriate processing department for sterilization. Familiarity with sterilization and **disinfection** methods available in the healthcare setting as well as with the care and handling of sterile materials is important to the safe care of patients, healthcare personnel, and equipment.

If you are employed at a facility where you are required to carry out sterilization procedures, you will need more extensive education. In addition, some sterilization and **disinfectant** chemicals are toxic and hazardous to health. Read all directions, and wear protective equipment, such as eyewear, gloves, masks, and splash-proof skin protection, when indicated.

Any items to be sterilized must first be completely clean, no matter which method of sterilization is used, because, among other reasons, protein, which is a part of all body secretions and excrement, often coagulates, providing a protective barrier for microorganisms that helps them survive even the most careful sterilization procedure (see Table 24-2 for a description of sterilization techniques).

Disinfection is used when items cannot be sterilized or in situations where no method of sterilization is available. Disinfection is done to eliminate as many microorganisms (minute life forms) from an item or from the environment as possible, although it does not eliminate spores. Low-level disinfectants are used for housekeeping purposes and for noncritical items that either do not touch the patient or that only contact intact skin. Intermediate-level disinfectants are used for semicritical items that come in contact with intact skin or mucous membranes but do not enter body tissues. High-level disinfectants are used for critical items that will come in contact with body tissues below the skin or mucous membranes but will not be introduced into the intravascular system. When possible, critical items should be sterilized (AORN, 2004). It is important to eliminate as many pathogens as possible to prevent illness-causing microorganisms from infecting the patient.

According to the Environmental Protection Agency (EPA), a disinfectant is an agent that kills growing or vegetative forms of bacteria. Agents are labeled "virucidal" if effective against viruses, "fungicidal" if effective against fungi, and "sporicidal" if effective against spores. Only agents labeled as "tuberculocidal" are effective against the tubercle bacillus. Disinfectants labeled "tuberculocidal" are also effective against the human immunodeficiency virus (HIV). The hepatitis B virus can survive exposure to many disinfectants. Disinfectants are evaluated based on both their efficacy in destroying microorganisms and their safety for those who must use them and for the environment. Each healthcare facility will have a list of disinfectants to be used for specific purposes.

Items should be disinfected to eliminate as many microorganisms as possible immediately before and after use. The nature of the **contamination,** the composition of the items to be disinfected, and the chemical agent to be used affect the method of application chosen. Read the label on the container, and follow the policies in your healthcare setting. Wear protective equipment to protect your eyes, hands, and skin when handling disinfectants, because most are harsh to skin and potentially toxic. Alcohol, chlorine compounds (such as household bleach in water), and iodophors (such as Betadine) are examples of chemical disinfectants.

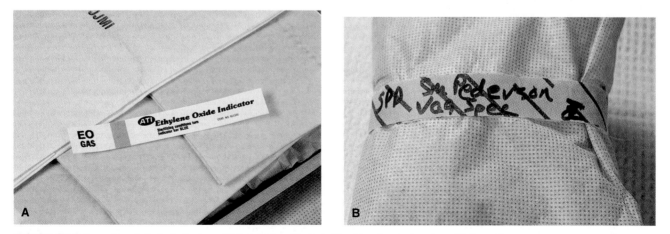

FIGURE 24-2 Examples of sterile indicators: (**A**) Label of product sterilized by chemical means. (**B**) Example of color indicator strips that change color to indicate that sterilization has occurred.

GENERAL APPROACHES AND PRINCIPLES OF SURGICAL ASEPSIS

1. Check sterility indicators, expiration dates, and package integrity prior to placing supplies on a sterile field. **R:** All items used in a sterile procedure must be sterile.
2. Assess the patient for latex allergy. **R:** Some sterile products and many sterile gloves contain latex, and the patient must be assessed for latex allergy. If the patient has a latex allergy, nonlatex gloves and equipment must be used.
3. Minimize air movement or control its direction through special ventilation to limit the movement of microorganisms. When a sterile field is open, keep doors closed, and do not shake drapes and gowns, even if they are sterile. **R:** Microorganisms move through space on air currents. Thus, items that are exposed to the air for a prolonged period are considered to be contaminated.
4. In a setting where sterility is critical (for example, the operating room), personnel wear masks. In some settings, a mask may be omitted, but avoid talking across a sterile field, turn your head away when speaking, and speak only when necessary around a sterile environment. If a healthcare provider has an upper respiratory infection, it is best not to be involved with sterile procedures. **R:** Microorganisms are released into the air on droplet nuclei whenever a person breathes or speaks. Masks provide a barrier to these droplet nuclei.
5. Keep sterile objects at a distance from unsterile ones to prevent the transfer of microorganisms. Pick up or handle sterile items with sterile gloves on. **R:** Microorganisms are transferred from one surface to another whenever an unsterile object touches another object. Any contact, no matter how brief, renders sterile items unsterile.
6. Keep unsterile objects, among them your own arm, from being placed over a sterile field. **R:** Microorganisms move from one object to another as a result of gravity when an unsterile object is held above another item.
7. If moisture connects an unsterile surface to a sterile one, the sterile surface is considered contaminated. **R:** Microorganisms travel rapidly along moisture by a wicking action. Some draping and packaging materials contain a moisture-resistant barrier to prevent wicking. Then, if a moisture-resistant barrier exists, a sterile field is maintained in the presence of liquid.
8. Keep sterile objects away from the edge of the field. **R:** Microorganisms moving in from unsterile items and surfaces can potentially contaminate the edge of any sterile field. Because microorganisms are in constant motion in a variety of ways, providing wide margins for safety must protect sterile areas. One inch is considered a minimum safety margin.
9. Consider anything that is out of sight to be contaminated. Keep gloved hands in front of you above your waist and below your shoulders, in your line of vision. Once a sterile field is created, it should be visually monitored to ensure the maintenance of sterility. **R:** Because you cannot guarantee what you cannot see, it is common practice to consider anything that is out of sight to be unsterile. A person's back is considered unsterile. Remember that all items below your waist or below table level are considered unsterile because they are out of full view.
10. When an item becomes contaminated or when in doubt about the sterility of any item, consider it unsterile, and take corrective action. **R:** The nurse must possess an ethical perspective of **sterile conscience,** which provides the moral mandate to monitor and correct one's behavior in the absence of others. Whenever a break in technique is identified, the procedure must be stopped and actions taken to correct the situation. Failing to take corrective action places the patient at higher risk of infection.

SETTING UP FOR STERILE TECHNIQUE

ASSESSMENT

1. Assess the patient's status and risk for infection. **R:** To determine whether sterile technique is needed.
2. Assess the situation. **R:** To determine the supplies that you will need.

ANALYSIS

3. Think about how the patient's status may determine whether surgical or medical asepsis is necessary. **R:** This enables you to determine specific problems for this individual in relation to infection control.
4. Identify potential problems or areas for contamination. **R:** Planning for the individual must take into consideration the individual's problems.

PLANNING

5. Identify individualized patient outcomes related to the specific procedure. **R:** Identifying outcomes guides planning and evaluation. Include
   a. Sterile technique is maintained for patient safety.
   b. Patient expresses understanding of the process (if the patient is competent).
6. Gather the sterile supplies you will need for the procedure. **R:** Planning ahead allows you to proceed more safely and effectively.

IMPLEMENTATION

Action	Rationale
7. Wash or disinfect your hands. *Note:* The following are various specific techniques that will be used for implementation of sterile technique, although not all techniques are used at each time.	To decrease the transfer of microorganisms that could cause infection.
8. Identify the patient, using two identifiers.	Verifying the patient's identity helps ensure that you are performing the right skill for the right patient.
9. Explain the forthcoming procedure to the patient.	Explaining the procedure helps relieve anxiety or misperceptions that the patient may have about a procedure or activity and sets the stage for patient participation.
10. Open a sterile pack, and create a sterile field as follows:	
a. Choose a flat, hard, dry surface on which to prepare a sterile field, and remove clutter from the working space. As a beginner, you will find you need at least a 12-inch-square field.	The area must be dry to prevent contamination from wicking of fluid. You will need a large amount of space to prevent contamination from nearby unsterile items. Clutter increases the potential for inadvertently contaminating the sterile field.
b. Open a wrapper from a sterile item to be used, or use a separate moisture-resistant drape to spread out on the surface at waist level to create a sterile field.	The wrapper or drape, when opened and placed on a table, provides a barrier from the table. The inside of the wrapper remains sterile if it is not touched while opening the package.
c. When opening a sterile package, do not reach over a sterile object or area. Grasp only the outside edge of the wrapper. To accomplish this, open the far flap first, then the side flaps, and finally the flap closest to you. The item can also be turned, or you can walk around it. In some instances, you may	Touching sterile items with anything nonsterile contaminates them.

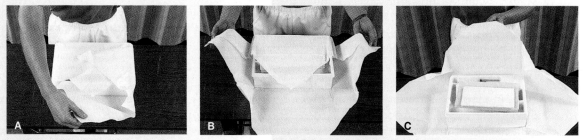

FIGURE 24-3 Opening a sterile package. (**A**) The nurse folds the topmost wrapper part away from her body. (**B**) She unfolds the next layer outward to the side. (**C**) She then unfolds the last layer toward her to avoid reaching over the sterile field.

(continued)

Action	Rationale
reach around the object, but it is difficult to do this without contaminating the item. Figure 24-3 shows the proper sequence for opening a wrapped sterile package.	
11. Add items to a sterile field as follows.	
a. Determine that the package is sterile.	Sterility indicators provide assurance that the package is sterile.
b. As you add additional sterile items, place them well within the edge of the sterile field, using a drop or slight toss method. Keep your unsterile hands or packaging away and 6 inches above the sterile field.	Touching sterile items with anything nonsterile contaminates them. A margin from the edge provides greater protection. Microorganisms could fall onto the sterile field from your arm if you reach over the field.
c. Unwrap the item as for any sterile package as noted above, and then pick it up by sliding your hand underneath the sterile covering. Gather the ends of the covering back around your wrist, forming a sterile cover for your hand, and keep the ends from dragging.	The sterile covering over your hand prevents microorganisms on your hand from falling onto the sterile field.
d. Place items well within the sterile field, keeping your hands as far away from the field as possible. Small items, such as gauze dressings, may be dropped from 6 to 8 inches above the sterile field. Large items should be put down carefully (Fig. 24-4).	Placing items well within the sterile field prevents them from contacting the potentially unsterile edge.

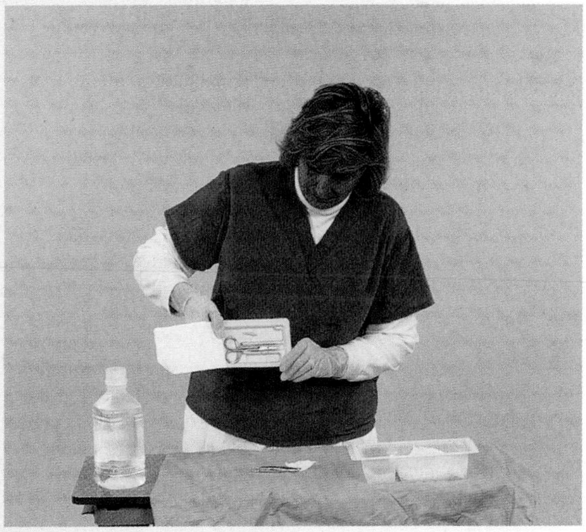

FIGURE 24-4 The nurse holds the package, touching only the outside, and drops the sterile contents onto the sterile field.

(continued)

Action	Rationale
e. Some commercially packaged products come in packages that peel open. Use your thumbs to peel edges away from one another exposing the sterile item (Fig. 24-5). Hold the item securely, and gently toss the item on the field carefully, avoiding the package edges.	The ends you have grasped to peel back are contaminated and should not touch the sterile item, nor should they be held over the sterile field. The edges of a peel package are not considered sterile, and the objects must be removed without sliding them off the side of the package. 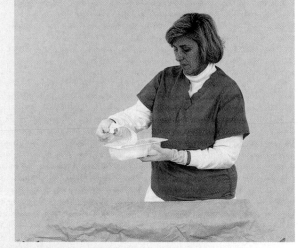 **FIGURE 24-5** In opening a peel pack, the nurse avoids contaminating the contents by touching only the outside of the package.
12. Add liquids to a sterile field as follows:	
a. To pour a liquid into a container in the sterile field, pour the liquid slowly from 6 to 8 inches above the receiving container. Keep your arm as far as possible from the sterile field. Avoid reaching over the sterile field if possible.	This avoids the possibility of the two containers touching (Fig. 24-6). 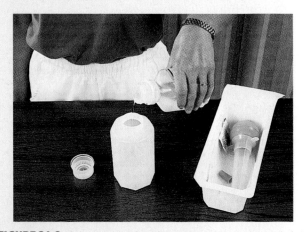 **FIGURE 24-6** The nurse pours liquid into a container on the sterile field by not reaching over the field and not pouring from a height that could cause splashing. (Photo © B. Proud.)

(continued)

Action	Rationale
b. Pour slowly to prevent splashing.	If liquid spills onto the sterile field, the spot is considered contaminated if the moisture can soak through to the unsterile surface beneath. Remember that microorganisms move rapidly through moisture. If the drape is waterproof (many disposable drapes have a plastic layer), and the sterile liquid pools up on the surface, the area is still sterile. Ideally, you should use a moisture-resistant barrier to prevent contamination from liquid.

13. Put on sterile gloves as follows (Fig. 24-7).

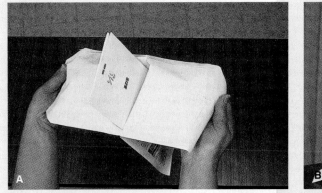

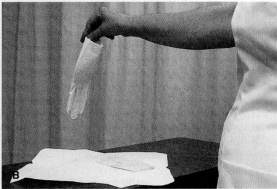

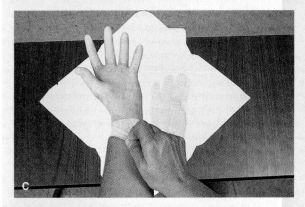

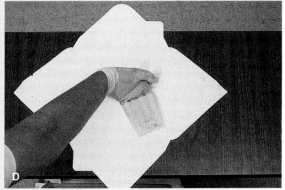

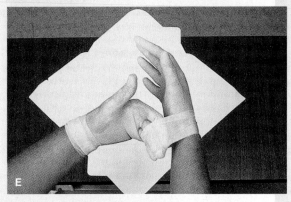

FIGURE 24-7 To put on sterile gloves, obtain a sealed package of gloves. (**A**) Open the outer wrapper, following the directions on the package; then open the inner folder at the corner without touching the gloves. (**B**) Lift up the left glove, touching only the folded cuff, and (**C**) put it on with the cuff still folded. (**D**) Put on the right glove by sliding your fingers under the cuff and (**E**) inserting your hand with the glove's cuff still folded.

(continued)

Action	Rationale
a. Remove all rings. Also, acrylic finger-nails and nail tips are known to harbor microorganisms and should not be worn. Some facilities have a policy prohibiting them.	Jewelry may harbor microorganisms around decorative elements. A ring can also make gloving more difficult and tear the glove. Acrylic nails harbor microorganisms and fungus in the microscopic spaces between the fingernail and the acrylic nail (Boyce & Pittet, 2002).
b. Determine your correct glove size (Table 24-3).	The correct size will be easier to get on and less likely to break through if fingertips of gloves are in touch with wearer's fingertips.

table 24-3. Choosing Glove Sizes

Glove Size	Female Hand	Male Hand
5	Extra small	—
$5\frac{1}{2}$	Extra small	—
6	Small	Extra small
$6\frac{1}{2}$	Medium	Small
7	Large	Medium
$7\frac{1}{2}$	Extra large	Medium large
8	—	Large
$8\frac{1}{2}$ +	—	Extra large

Action	Rationale
c. Open the sterile sealed package in the same way you would open any other sterile package. Inside the sterile pack-age is a folder containing the gloves. You may handle the exterior of the wrapper that contains the gloves, and dispose of the outer packaging.	The outer surface of the glove folder does not need to remain sterile. The outer wrapper may hit the sterile gloves if left under or near the inner packaging.
d. Lay the folder open and flat on the table. The gloves themselves will still be par-tially covered by folds of paper. Inside the folder, the gloves are arranged palm upward, with the left glove on the left side and the right glove on the right side. Each glove has a cuff of 2 to 4 inches.	The folded-back margin of the inner package protects the sterile glove from your fingers.
e. Put on the first sterile glove without touching the outside of the glove, so contamination does not occur. Gloves are packaged uniformly to facilitate this procedure. Open one side of the folder, either left or right, touching only the folded-back edge of the pack-age. Pick up the exposed glove with your opposite hand (the left glove with the right hand or the right glove with the left hand) by the folded cuff that will touch your skin. Watch your hands, making sure they do not touch the outside of the sterile gloves.	You are touching the surface of the glove that will touch your skin.

(continued)

Action	Rationale
f. Insert your free hand into the glove without touching skin to the outside of the glove. (The rhyme "skin side to inside" may help you remember this.) Be sure you hold the glove well away from your body and from the table or package as you work.	A common error is to brush the tips of the glove fingers against an unsterile surface (table top, forearms or edges of glove wrapper) while maneuvering, thus contaminating the gloves.
g. Open the second side of the folder with your ungloved hand, exposing the second glove. Pick up the second glove with your gloved hand from under the cuff, which is the outside surface. Be sure to keep the thumb of the gloved hand rigidly extended outward or folded against the palm, so you are not tempted to use it to grasp the other glove. Hold the glove under its cuff by your four gloved fingers.	The cuff on the second glove protects the gloved hand from contamination by touching and also from microorganisms moving by gravity. By only touching the outer portion of the second glove, you keep sterile glove touching sterile glove surface.
h. Carefully maneuver the second hand into the second glove.	A slow, deliberate movement will help prevent contamination and enable you to visualize any potential sources for contamination.
i. When both gloves are on, turn the cuffs up by flipping them, taking care not to roll the outside of the gloves onto your skin.	Rolling the gloves causes the outside of the glove to touch your skin.
j. You may then make any necessary adjustments to the fingertips so the gloves fit smoothly. Do not touch above the wrist after the gloves are donned.	Smoothly fitting gloves will promote dexterity. Touching the skin above the wrist will contaminate the gloves.

EVALUATION

14. Evaluate using the individualized patient outcomes previously identified. **R:** Evaluation in relation to desired outcomes is essential for planning future care. Include
   a. Sterile technique is maintained for patient safety.
   b. Patient expresses understanding of the process (if the patient is competent).

DOCUMENTATION

15. Document the procedure, time of procedure, and the patient response to the procedure. Complete charge forms if these are required by the agency. **R:** Documentation is a legal record of the patient's care and communicates nursing activities to other nurses and caregivers.

Acute Care

Most sterile supplies in hospitals are disposable and come in sterile packages from the manufacturer. However, there are many types of equipment in hospitals that are reused and must be sterilized between uses. These include surgical instruments, endoscopes, and other diagnostic instruments. To ensure sterility, hospitals use a wide variety of sterilization methods. Those who work with reusable equipment must have a thorough understanding of the cleaning and sterilization process and carry out all checks to make sure that there is no contamination spreading from one patient to another.

Home Care

Some procedures carried out using sterile technique in the hospital or nursing home are commonly done using clean technique in the home setting. For example, urinary catheterization in the acute care setting is routinely done using surgical asepsis. However, in a home care setting, clients needing chronic self-catheterization may use medical asepsis or clean technique.

A common disinfectant in the home may be a simple household bleach solution. This solution can kill weak viruses such as the HIV virus and bacteria but not all microorganisms. It must be made clear that this agent merely disinfects and does not sterilize items or surfaces the solution contacts. Another disinfectant not used in acute care but used in the home is boiling water. Boiling water is an old method of disinfection but is still valuable in some situations, such as in the home and in circumstances where other methods of disinfection or sterilization are not available. This method is most often used for items, such as bedpans and emesis basins, when disinfection is needed between uses. To use boiling water for disinfection, completely cover the items so that all surface areas are exposed to the water. Start timing only after the water comes to a rolling boil. Boil for a minimum of 30 minutes. If sodium carbonate is added to the water to make a 2% solution, the recommended boiling time is 15 minutes. Caution: Boiling water does not destroy some spore forms.

LEARNING TOOLS

DEVELOP YOUR BACKGROUND KNOWLEDGE

1. Review the Learning Outcomes.

2. Read the chapter related to performing sterile nursing procedures and the chapter on infection control in your assigned text.

3. Look up the Key Terms in the glossary.

4. Review the module as though you were preparing to teach this information to another person.

5. Mentally practice specific procedures.

6. Review the Performance Checklist on the CD-ROM in the front of this book.

DEVELOP YOUR SKILLS

In the practice setting
1. Open sterile packs.

2. Add items to a sterile field.

3. Pour liquids into sterile containers.

4. Put on sterile gloves. Use the Performance Checklist as a guide.

5. When you can perform these tasks correctly, select a partner.
   a. Have your partner observe your performance and evaluate you, using the Performance Checklist.
   b. Observe and evaluate your partner, using the checklist.
   c. Repeat this exercise until you have mastered the skills.

6. Arrange with your instructor for a time to have your technique checked.

DEMONSTRATE YOUR SKILLS

In the clinical setting
1. Arrange a visit to the central supply department of a hospital. Examine supply packaging for sterility indicators. Observe the methods of sterilization used in the facility.

2. Identify situations in which sterile technique is needed.

3. With other students, discuss situations that require sterile technique and how to proceed when technique is broken.

CRITICAL THINKING EXERCISES

1. You are changing a surgical dressing when you inadvertently contaminate your left glove (you are right-handed). There is no other staff member in the room who can get another pair of gloves for you. Propose several ways you could handle this situation.

2. You are in a hurry to a patient's room to change a dressing prior to the patient's discharge. You drop some of the supplies. What will you do?

3. Research the disinfectants in use in the facility where you have clinical practice. Identify the purpose of each one that is used and the active ingredient in the disinfectant.

SELF-QUIZ
SHORT-ANSWER QUESTIONS

1. Compare and contrast sterilization and disinfection.

_____

_____

_____

2. What is sterile conscience?

_____

3. How does liquid or moisture contribute to contamination?

_____

4. If a disinfectant kills fungi, how will it be labeled?

_____

5. Why should acrylic fingernails be avoided by healthcare workers?

_____

MULTIPLE CHOICE

_____ 6. The best definition of sterile is
   a. absence of all fungi.
   b. absence of disease-producing microorganisms.
   c. absence of disease-producing microorganisms and their spores.
   d. absence of all forms of life.

_____ 7. Upon handwashing, a healthcare worker's hands are rendered
   a. sterile.
   b. contaminated.
   c. disinfected.
   d. clean.

_____ 8. You are taking a Foley catheter kit to a patient's room, and you accidentally drop it on the floor. You should
   a. use it, since the floor was just mopped.
   b. discard the kit and remove it from circulation.
   c. put the kit back in the storeroom.
   d. wipe the package off with alcohol, and then use it.

_____ 9. Which of the following is the most common sterilization process used in homes?
   a. Boiling water
   b. Steam under pressure
   c. Bleach solution
   d. Sporicidal chemicals

_____ 10. You are watching a staff nurse insert a Foley catheter and see the catheter touch an unprepped leg before the catheter is about to enter the meatus. You should
   a. tell the nurse later that she contaminated the catheter.
   b. tell the nurse quietly that she contaminated the catheter, and get her a new one.
   c. tell the patient the catheter is about to enter her bladder and to bear down.
   d. report the incident to a supervisor.

_____ 11. Sterile technique is needed for which of the following?
   a. Changing a dressing over a surgical wound of the hip
   b. Changing a warm pack over an inflamed joint
   c. Measuring a blood pressure
   d. Changing a colostomy bag

Answers to the Self-Quiz questions appear in the back of this book.

MODULE 25

Surgical Asepsis: Scrubbing, Gowning, and Closed Gloving

SKILLS INCLUDED IN THIS MODULE

Procedure for Surgical Hand Scrubbing, Gowning, and Closed Gloving

Guidelines for Working in Sterile Attire

PREREQUISITE MODULES

Module 1	An Approach to Nursing Skills
Module 2	Documentation
Module 4	Basic Infection Control
Module 24	Basic Sterile Technique: Sterile Field and Sterile Gloves

KEY TERMS

alcohol-based hand rub	personal protective equipment (PPE)
antimicrobial	sterile
antiseptic	subungual
microorganisms	surgical asepsis
normal flora	

OVERALL OBJECTIVE

▸ To put on and function appropriately in sterile attire, identifying breaks in technique if they occur and taking corrective action.

LEARNING OUTCOMES

The student will be able to

1. Assess the need for a surgical scrub, gowning, and closed gloving.
2. Analyze patient assessment data to determine special patient problems indicating the need for surgical asepsis. Analyze institutional procedures to ensure safety of patient and healthcare personnel.
3. Determine appropriate patient outcomes related to surgical asepsis and recognize the potential for adverse outcomes.
4. Gather the supplies and plan the three-part process of surgical hand scrub, gowning, and closed gloving.
5. Implement a surgical hand scrub, gowning, and closed gloving, maintaining all principles and identifying all behaviors that lead to contamination.
6. Carry out recommended guidelines for nursing behaviors and actions to maintain sterility while practicing in a sterile field and to readily identify behaviors leading to contamination.
7. Evaluate the effectiveness of the procedures.
8. Document the name and role of personnel performing in the sterile procedure as well as relevant patient responses.

Handwashing alone does not eliminate **normal flora** (natural body **microorganisms**) on the hands. Even what we consider to be normal flora can produce infection when introduced into an open wound. During surgical procedures, infant deliveries, and invasive procedures, sterile gloves are worn. However, because gloves can tear in the course of a procedure, it is important that the hands be rendered as nearly free of microorganisms as possible. A gown, too, can become moist or tear, allowing microorganisms to move from the arms to the surface of the gown or from the patient's blood to the healthcare provider. Surgical gloves and gowns protect the patient from contamination by the healthcare provider, but they also serve as **personal protective equipment (PPE),** so the healthcare provider is not exposed to bloodborne pathogens.

Surgical scrubbing lowers the total count of microorganisms on the hands and arms. It also removes dirt and oil from the skin, decreasing the ability of remaining microorganisms to multiply. The agent to decontaminate the hands should be an **alcohol-based hand rub** or long-acting **antimicrobial** soap. After scrubbing, a residue of antimicrobial cleansing agent remains on the skin, which further reduces the growth of microorganisms.

Gowns and gloves worn for **sterile** procedures must be put on in a way that ensures that nothing unsterile touches the outer surfaces. To maintain the highest standard of sterility, proper scrubbing, gowning, and closed gloving technique is essential. These procedures are complex psychomotor skills and require demonstration and practice prior to implementing them in a patient care situation.

Every facility has its own routine for performing a surgical scrub. These routines should be based on current recommendations and standards and used to ensure that all individuals maintain the same standard of care. The Association of periOperative Nurses (AORN) recommends that consultation with the infection control committee should take place in each practice setting regarding scrub policies and procedures (AORN, 2004). Always follow the procedure established by your facility or, if none exists, work to establish an appropriate procedure. Policies and procedures for the surgical scrub should be standardized and reviewed annually in individual facilities. The approved procedure should be available to healthcare personnel in areas requiring these procedures.

NURSING DIAGNOSES

The most common nursing diagnosis related to the need for **surgical asepsis** or sterile technique is Risk for Infection related to impaired skin integrity due to surgical or traumatic wound.

DELEGATION

Surgical asepsis is not taught to nursing assistive personnel. These techniques are a part of the educational program for roles such as operating room technician.

OVERVIEW OF SURGICAL SCRUBBING, GOWNING, AND CLOSED GLOVING

The surgical scrub, gowning, and closed gloving procedure may be used in an operating room, certain special procedure rooms, and in the obstetrical delivery room. General guidelines apply to the surgical scrub, gowning, and gloving procedures. They include the following:

- *Preparation:* Before scrubbing, the nurse puts on surgical attire and personal protective equipment (Fig. 25-1). All jewelry should be removed prior to this procedure because rings, watches, and bracelets harbor bacterial growth (Boyce & Pittet, 2002). Fingernails should be well groomed, and natural nail tips should be less than ¼ in long (Boyce & Pittet, 2002). Acrylic fingernails should be avoided. In addition, hands and forearms should be free of open lesions or breaks in skin (Boyce & Pittet, 2002).
- *Preventing moisture on attire:* The scrub sink should be deep and wide enough so you can hold both arms over it and water cannot splash out onto your scrub attire. Moisture can contaminate the sterile gown donned over wet scrub attire. Therefore, disposable surgical attire is moisture resistant. Foot- or knee-operated faucets (rather than hand-operated ones) are preferred to prevent contamination of the hands after you have scrubbed them.
- *Cleaning the nails and scrubbing the hands:* Surgical scrub procedures necessitate an initial cleaning of the **subungual** area followed by a systematic washing of fingers, hands, and forearms to just

above the elbow. The specific procedure for scrubbing may differ from one facility to another, but certain principles of aseptic technique are common. One must ensure sufficient exposure of *all* skin surfaces to light friction during a traditional scrub using an antimicrobial soap or an alcohol-based rub.

Because the hands are in the most direct contact with the sterile field, begin the steps of any scrub procedure with the hands and finish with the elbows. Also, keep the hands higher than the elbows during the scrub procedure to allow water to flow from the cleanest area (the hands) to the less clean area (the elbows) (AORN, 2004). The recommended duration of a surgical scrub is 2 to 6 minutes. Facilities are encouraged to use the scrub agent manufacturer's recommendations when instituting policies and procedures for scrub times. The hands are dried with a sterile towel.

- *Putting on the sterile gown:* After you have scrubbed and dried your hands, you are ready to put on a sterile gown. Gowning is a two-person procedure. Surgical gowns are disposable and moisture resistant. You will need an assistant to put on a sterile gown without contamination.
- *Closed glove technique:* A closed glove technique is used to put on sterile gloves with a sterile gown. This special technique maintains the sterility of the gown and the entire outside surface of the gloves. Sterile gloves are put on prior to entering a sterile field.

PROCEDURE FOR SURGICAL HAND SCRUBBING, GOWNING, AND CLOSED GLOVING

A surgical hand scrub is followed by donning a surgical gown and then a closed gloving procedure. This is a three-step process.

Preprocedure Preparation

ASSESSMENT

1. Determine which surgical attire used in your facility is to be worn. These are called "scrub" garments. All personnel should wear scrub attire consisting of a two-piece pantsuit, cap or hood, and shoe covers when entering the surgical or scrub area. **R:** Surgical attire must be worn in the entire area where scrubbing, gowning, and gloving will take place. Wearing surgical attire prevents bringing outside organisms into the area.

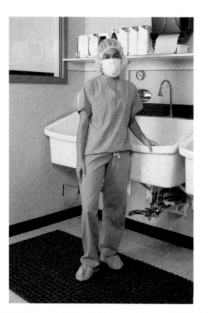

FIGURE 25-1 Before scrubbing, the nurse puts on surgical attire (scrub garments) and proceeds to cleanse hands. Note that the sink is knee operated.

The cap or hood should be put on first to prevent hair and dander from collecting on the scrub attire. All facial and head hair must be completely covered to prevent microorganisms from moving from hair to the environment. If pierced-ear studs are worn, they must be completely covered by the cap or hood. The scrub shirt should be tucked into the scrub pants or fit close to the body so that loose garments do not come into contact with scrubbed hands and arms or with the sterile drying towel. Shoe covers prevent the introduction of outside microorganisms into the clean environment and protect personnel from exposure to blood and body fluids that might contain infectious agents.

2. Determine patient allergies and the procedural implications if the patient or healthcare personnel have a latex allergy. **R:** If latex allergy is present in either staff or patient, nonlatex gloves and other equipment must be obtained.

3. Check that a table set up with a sterile gown, sterile gloves in your size (Box 25-1), and a sterile towel to dry your hands has been set up for your use and that someone will be available to assist you to put on the gown. **R:** Planning ahead prevents delay.

ANALYSIS

4. Critically determine how the patient's status determines the necessary supplies and need for surgical asepsis. **R:** Each situation is different and adjustments may be required.

5. Identify specific potential problems and modifications of the procedure. Gloves and gowns are often standardized, and a healthcare provider with extremely large or small hands or body size may have difficulty locating supplies. **R:** Planning for the individual must take into consideration the individual's uniqueness.

PLANNING

6. Identify the desired outcomes of the procedure. **R:** Identification of outcomes guides planning and evaluation.
   a. Hands are prepared in accord with the policies of the facility.
   b. The sterile gown is donned without contamination of the outside of the gown.
   c. Sterile gloves are donned so that the outside remains sterile and the cuffs cover the cuffs of the gown with no skin showing.

7. Identify where supplies are located, including the following. **R:** To be effectively organized for your tasks.
   a. Hand-scrubbing sponge impregnated with antimicrobial soap or alcohol-based hand rub
   b. Nail-cleaning implement (this may be in the package with the hand-scrubbing sponge)

---

box 25-1 *Guidelines for Working in Sterile Attire*

1. Everything below the waist or table height is considered nonsterile. Therefore, keep your hands above your waist and keep sterile equipment on top of the tables. When you are waiting, it is often convenient to clasp your gloved hands together in front of you to protect them.
2. Your back is considered potentially contaminated because you cannot see if it touches anything unsterile. Do not turn your back on any sterile area. Always pass with your face toward the sterile area.
3. For the same reason, when passing another person in sterile attire, pass back to back with your sterile hands in front of you.
4. Sterility is a matter of certainty, not conjecture. If you even suspect that a part of your attire has been contaminated, notify the appropriate person (eg, circulating nurse) for assistance in changing.
5. Moisture allows microorganisms to wick quickly and easily from one area to another. If your attire becomes wet, consider it contaminated and change, or cover the wet area with a sterile towel.
6. Contamination commonly occurs accidentally. To prevent this, whenever you move close to anyone, warn them verbally. Do not assume that you will be seen.

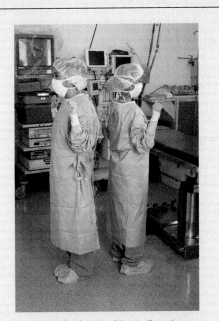

Passing back to back in sterile attire.

IMPLEMENTATION

Action	Rationale
PREPARATION	
8. Remove all watches, rings, and bracelets.	Jewelry and watches harbor microorganisms beneath them (Boyce & Pittet, 2002).
9. Examine your hands and forearms for cuts or blemishes. Do not scrub if there are any open lesions or breaks in skin integrity.	Breaks in the skin can cause contamination in the surgical wound and increase the potential for exposure of healthcare personnel to bloodborne pathogens.
10. Ensure that fingernails are in good condition with no nail polish or artificial nails and no longer than the tips of the fingers.	Chipped nail polish tends to harbor microorganisms. Artificial fingernails or tips should not be worn because studies show that a higher number of microorganisms have been cultured from the fingertips of nurses wearing artificial nails than from the fingertips of nurses with natural nails. Additionally, because of moisture being trapped between the natural and artificial nails, fungal growth often occurs under artificial nails. Long nails may puncture gloves.
11. Put on a mask and protective eyewear. a. Mask: The mask should cover both nose and mouth. Fit it to your face by molding the nosepiece to the bridge of your nose so that air moves through, not around, the mask. It is generally accepted policy for masks to be worn in sterile settings and for individuals to don a fresh mask between procedures. (Handle only the ties of a used mask when discarding a mask after use to prevent contamination of the hands by a soiled mask.) b. Eyewear: Protective eye gear must be worn to protect the eyes and mucous membranes from accidental splashes of blood or other body fluid. Side shield attachments that protect against side splashes are available for eyeglasses. Individuals who wear glasses should clean them before scrubbing. Surgical masks are available with an integral eye shield/splash guard.	The mask protects the vulnerable patient from exposure to microorganisms that might be in the respiratory tract of the caregiver. The mask and eye protection also serve as personal protective equipment to protect the caregiver from exposure to blood or body fluids. Each facility should have clear policies and procedures established for proper personal protective equipment to be worn in that setting. All personnel must conform to the established policy.
PREWASH AND NAIL CLEANING	
12. Turn on the water and adjust the temperature so that it is comfortably warm.	Warm water emulsifies fats more effectively than cold water does, and hot water is harsh on the skin.
13. Moisten your hands and arms, keeping your hands higher than your elbows so that water will drain off your elbows.	The water will flow from the cleanest area (hands) to the less clean area (elbows).

(continued)

Action	Rationale
14. Using one of the surgical hand scrub agents provided, lather your hands and arms for 1 minute.	This prewash reduces bioburden (skin oils that support microorganisms) and prepares the skin for either a traditional scrub or an alcohol-based rub.
15. Remove a prepackaged, disposable nail cleaner, and clean under each fingernail and around each cuticle (Fig. 25-2). If a traditional scrub is being done, the nail cleaner may be included with the scrub sponge. Dispose of the nail cleaner after cleaning underneath each fingernail.	Subungual areas harbor microorganisms and should be cleansed at the time of the first scrub of the day or when visibly soiled. 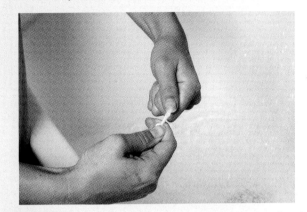 **FIGURE 25-2** The nurse cleanses under the nailtip (subungual) at the first scrub of the day.

TRADITIONAL SCRUB

Note: Use steps 16a to 16i when the facility requires the traditional scrub.

16. Perform hand scrub.

Action	Rationale
a. Wet hands and arms thoroughly and dispense scrub agent according to manufacturer's recommendation, or use an impregnated brush or sponge that you wet thoroughly.	To ensure the ability to lather the scrub agent.
b. Begin the first hand by scrubbing the nails, being sure to scrub the corners of each nail.	This procedure ensures that all surfaces are mechanically scrubbed to remove microorganisms and that the **antiseptic** agent has optimum contact with all surfaces for disinfection.
c. Next, scrub the fingers. Envision each finger as having four surfaces. Scrub all four surfaces of the thumb and then of each finger in turn, moving from the thumb to the fifth finger.	
d. Then scrub the dorsal surface of the hand and then the palmar surface of the hand.	
e. Next scrub around the wrist and continue around the forearm, proceeding up the arm to 2 inches above the elbow (Fig. 25-3).	

(continued)

Action	Rationale

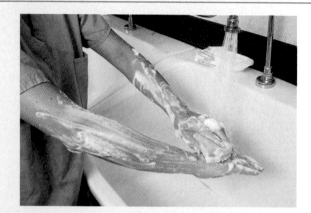

FIGURE 25-3 After the nails are cleansed, the nurse scrubs with a sterile brush or sponge.

Action	Rationale
f. Transfer the scrub sponge to other hand and repeat the scrub on the second hand in the same way, using steps b to e. This process should take a total of 2 to 6 minutes.	
g. Rinse the scrub agent from your skin by passing each hand and arm through the water in one direction from fingertips to elbow (Fig. 25-4) with hands higher than the elbow. The movement should be from distal (hands) to proximal over the elbows.	Rinsing moves microorganisms from the skin surface in the lather. The position prevents water from running over the unscrubbed area beyond the elbows back onto the hands.

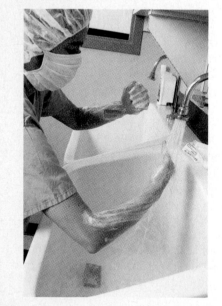

FIGURE 25-4 The nurse rinses the arms, keeping the hands higher than the elbows.

Action	Rationale
h. Keep hands extended in front of you and above the height of your waist to avoid contamination. Walk to the table where the towels are kept. If you	To protect your hands from touching any nonsterile surface.

(continued)

Action	Rationale
must go through closed doors, back through. Allow water to drip from your elbows (Fig. 25-5).	

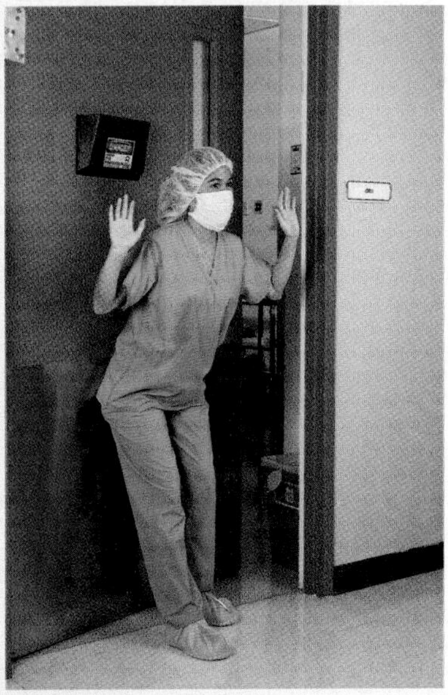

FIGURE 25-5 The nurse backs through a closed door with arms raised to prevent contamination.

Action	Rationale
i. Dry your hands, making sure that each hand and arm are dried by a separate sterile section of the towel.	The sterile towel maintains antisepsis of the hands. Blotting is less harsh on the hands than rubbing.

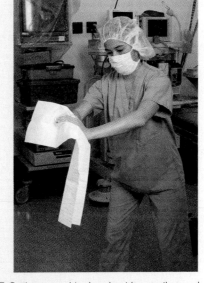

(1) Pick up the sterile towel by one end.

(2) Allow the towel to unfold.

(3) Holding one hand under half of the towel, use that half to blot the opposite hand dry (Fig. 25-6). Start drying the fingers, and move gradually up the arm.

(4) Place the dry hand under the other half of the towel and use that half of the towel to blot the second arm dry. Again, start at the fingers, and move up the arm.

FIGURE 25-6 The nurse dries hands with a sterile towel.

ALCOHOL-BASED RUB

Note: Use steps 17a to 17d when the facility policy requires an alcohol-based hand rub.

17. Perform the hand rub.

Action	Rationale
a. After the prewash and nail cleansing, dry your hands.	If hands remain wet, the effectiveness of the alcohol-based rub is diminished.

(continued)

Action	Rationale
b. Dispense the manufacturer-recommended amount of the alcohol-based product, and apply it to your hands and forearms.	For maximum effectiveness, the correct amount is necessary.
c. Rub the agent onto all skin surfaces, being sure to cover all areas between fingers and around nails and arms up to 2 inches above the elbows, continuing to rub until skin surface feels dry. Repeat if recommended.	Antimicrobial action occurs when alcohol is in direct contact with skin. Skin must be dry to apply gloves.
d. Holding your hands in front of you and above your waist, leave the scrub sink area, and proceed to surgical gown and gloves, backing through the door if necessary.	To protect your hands from touching any nonsterile surface.

GOWNING

18. Pick up the sterile gown carefully by the neck edge.	The area touched is no longer sterile. The neck edge will not be close to sterile objects.
19. Facing the sterile field, hold the gown by the inside, top neckline in front of you, and allow it to unfold, letting gravity assist you (Fig. 25-7).	To maintain the sterility of the gown.

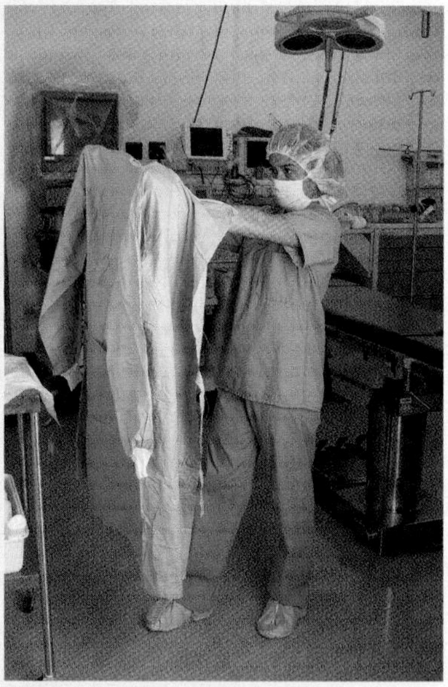

FIGURE 25-7 To put on a sterile gown, face the sterile field and hold the gown by the inside neckline. Allow it to fall open, and work your hands and arms carefully into the gown.

20. Position the gown so that the back opening is facing you.	To enable you to access the opening with your hands and arms.
21. Work your hands and arms carefully into the gown and into the sleeves, as far as the seam between the sleeve and the cuff.	To maintain the sterility of the exterior of the gown.

(continued)

Action	Rationale
Take your time and proceed slowly. Do not push your hands out through the ends of the sleeves.	
22. Turn your back to your assistant, who will now grasp the inside of the back, pull it securely onto your shoulders, and tie the neck and back waistline ties.	The assistant will touch the inside, which is not sterile.
23. Leave the front waistline tie tied in front of you.	To prevent contaminating the outside of your gown.

CLOSED GLOVING

24. Using the closed glove technique, put on the sterile gloves.	This closed glove procedure ensures that only the inside of the gown and gloves are touched, maintaining the outside of the gown as sterile, and that the gloves are over the cuffs of the gown so that no skin is exposed.

  a. Use your left hand still inside the gown to pick up the folded edge of the right glove (Fig. 25-8).

  b. Hold your right hand out, with the palm up, still inside the sleeve.

  c. Lay the right glove on the right palm (which is still inside the sleeve). Position it with the glove fingers pointing toward the elbow and the cuff end pointing toward the fingertips. The thumb of the glove should be over the thumb of your right hand.

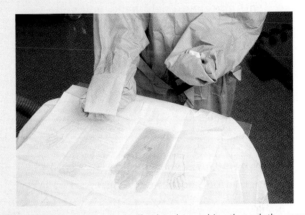

FIGURE 25-8 Position the sterile glove by reaching through the gown with your opposite hand. Lay the right glove on the right palm (which is still inside the sleeve). Position it with the glove fingers pointing toward the elbow and the cuff end pointing toward the fingertips. The thumb of the glove should be over the thumb of your right hand.

  d. Use your right hand (which is still inside the gown sleeve) to grasp the bottom fold of the cuff end of the right glove. You are touching sterile gown to sterile glove.

  e. With your left hand (which is still inside the gown sleeve), grasp the right glove cuff by the top fold of the cuff end, and pull the right glove cuff up and over the right gown cuff (Fig. 25-9).

  f. Adjust the right glove cuff over the right gown cuff as necessary, keeping the left hand inside the gown.

  g. Work your right hand down into the glove. If the fingers are not in place, do not be concerned. You can correct them when both gloves are on.

(continued)

Action	Rationale
h. Pick up the left glove with the gloved right hand. **i.** Hold your left hand, palm up, inside the gown sleeve. **j.** Place the left glove on the left palm (which is still inside the gown), with the glove fingers pointing toward the elbow and the cuff end pointing toward your fingertips. Position the glove thumb over the left thumb of your hand. **k.** Use your left hand (which is still inside the sleeve) to grasp the bottom fold of the cuff end of the left glove. **l.** Grasp the top fold of the cuff edge with the gloved right hand, and pull the glove cuff up and over the gown cuff (Fig. 25-10). **m.** Work your left hand down into the left glove. **n.** Turn up and adjust the cuffs of both gloves (Fig. 25-11). **o.** Pull the glove fingers out at the ends to reposition your fingers if necessary.	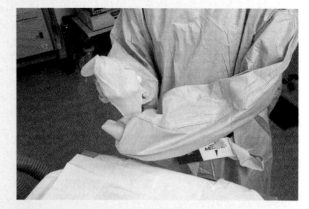 **FIGURE 25-9** Pull up the first glove with your opposite hand still inside the gown. With your left hand (which is still inside the gown sleeve), grasp the right glove cuff by the top fold of the cuff end, and pull the right glove cuff up and over the right gown cuff. 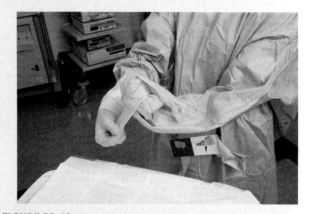 **FIGURE 25-10** The second glove can be pulled up by the hand wearing the sterile glove. Grasp the top fold of the cuff edge with the gloved right hand, and pull the glove cuff up and over the gown cuff. 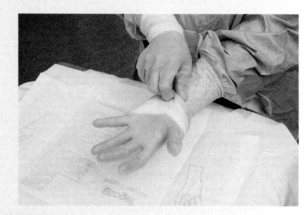 **FIGURE 25-11** When sterile gloves are on both hands, the cuffs may be safely adjusted. Turn up and adjust the cuffs of both gloves.

(continued)

Action	Rationale
FASTEN THE GOWN	
25. With your gloved hands, untie the front waist tie of your gown.	With sterile gloves on your hands, you will not contaminate your gown.
26. Hold the ends of the ties carefully, keeping them above your waist.	To prevent the ties from inadvertently touching something else.
27. Hold the shorter tie in one hand.	To keep it sterile.
28. With the other hand, hold the longer tie, which is attached to a brightly colored cardboard tag, out for your assistant (Fig. 25-12).	The assistant can touch the tag without contaminating the tie.

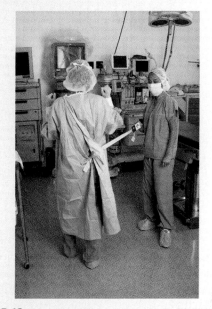

FIGURE 25-12 Take the cardboard tie holder and have an assistant hold it while you turn. Your assistant should dispose of the cardboard holder after this process. With the other hand, hold the longer tie, which is attached to a brightly colored cardboard tag, out for your assistant.

Action	Rationale
29. While your assistant is holding the tag, turn around carefully, wrapping the gown around you as you turn. Be sure you are well away from all equipment when you turn.	This completely covers your back with the sterile gown.
30. Retrieve the tie from your assistant (who will retain the tag) and tie the two ties together in the front. You are now in scrub attire (Fig. 25-13). You are now prepared to handle sterile equipment and to assist the physician performing a surgical procedure.	To maintain the sterility of the ties and the gown front.

(continued)

Action	Rationale
	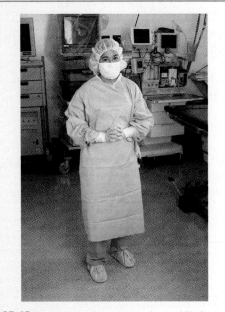 **FIGURE 25-13** The nurse is now properly scrubbed, gowned, and gloved. The nurse clasps gloved hands above the waist to protect them.
31. Clasp your hands together in front of your waist.	To protect your gloved hands from contact with the environment.

EVALUATION

32. Evaluate based on the desired outcomes previously identified.
   a. Hands were prepared in accord with the policies of the facility.
   b. The sterile gown was donned without contamination of the outside of the gown.
   c. Sterile gloves were donned so that the outside remains sterile and the cuffs cover the cuffs of the gown with no skin showing.

DOCUMENTATION

33. Documenting the scrubbing, gowning, and gloving procedures is not standard.

LEARNING TOOLS

DEVELOP YOUR BACKGROUND KNOWLEDGE

1. Review the Learning Outcomes.

2. Read the section on medical and surgical asepsis in your assigned text.

3. Look up the Key Terms in the glossary.

4. Review this module and mentally practice the techniques described. Study so that you would be able to teach these skills to another person.

DEVELOP YOUR SKILLS

1. Select a partner. Together, set up the equipment for donning sterile attire. Use the Performance Checklist on the CD-ROM in the front of this book as a guide.

2. Practice surgical scrubbing, gowning, and closed gloving. Evaluate each other's performance.

DEMONSTRATE YOUR SKILLS

In the clinical setting
1. Consult with your instructor regarding the opportunity to observe personnel scrubbing, gloving, and gowning.

2. Consult with your instructor regarding the opportunity to practice these skills in a surgical setting.

3. Evaluate your performance with the instructor.

CRITICAL THINKING EXERCISES

1. You are in a facility that requires a surgical hand scrub. You are sensitive to the antibacterial soap used in the facility. How might you research the options that would be available to you that might enable you to work in the surgical setting?

2. Do a literature search on surgical hand preparation, and identify what specific antiseptic agents are recommended by authoritative sources. Compare the recommendations for the surgical scrub procedure in at least two literature resources.

SELF-QUIZ
SHORT-ANSWER QUESTIONS

1. Name three items that are considered personal protective equipment, and explain the purpose of each.

   a. _____

   b. _____

   c. _____

2. How long is it recommended to perform a traditional hand scrub?

   _____

3. What parts of your hands require special attention before performing a surgical hand scrub?

   _____

4. How should arms and hands be held when waiting to begin a sterile procedure? Why?

   _____

MULTIPLE CHOICE

_____ 5. Identify the correct sequence of events.
   a. Clean nail beds, open gown, put on hair cover, use alcohol-based rub.
   b. Dress in surgical attire, scrub hands, don gown, don gloves.
   c. Dress in surgical attire, apply PPE, open gown, open gloves.
   d. Apply PPE, dress in surgical attire, open gown, open gloves.

_____ 6. Which statement is correct?
   a. Wedding bands may be worn when doing a surgical scrub.
   b. Acrylic fingernails may not be worn when doing a surgical scrub.
   c. Scrub or rub forearms 1 inch below the elbows.
   d. Keep hands lower than elbows when proceeding to gown and gloves.

_____ 7. You are observing a patient in labor and delivery and have appropriately scrubbed, gowned, and closed gloved. Which statement is true?
   a. Protective eyewear is optional.
   b. It is fine to hold the patient's hand when she is having contractions.
   c. Your arms must remain above your waist.
   d. No one else should be in the sterile field with you.

Answers to the Self-Quiz questions appear in the back of the book.

REFERENCES AND SUGGESTED RESOURCES: UNIT 5

AORN, Inc. (2004). *Standards, Recommended Practices, and Guidelines.* Denver, CO: AORN.

Centers for Disease Control and Prevention. (1996). (Online). Available at http://www.cdc.gov/ncidod/hip/ISOLAT/Isolat.htm. Retrieved October 31, 2005.

Boyce, J. & Pittet, D. (2002). Guidelines for hand hygiene in health-care settings: Recommendations of the Healthcare Infection Control Practices Advisory Committee and the HICPAC/SHEA/APIC/IDSA Hand Hygiene Task Force. (Online). Available at http://www.cdc.gov/mmwr/PDF/RR/RR5116. Retrieved May 1, 2005.

Garner, J. S., & Hospital Infection Control Practices Advisory Committee. (1996). Guideline for isolation precautions in hospitals. *Infection Control Hospital Epidemiology* (1996). 17, 53–80, and *American Journal of Infection Control.* (1996). 24, 24–52. (Online). Available at www.cdc.gov/ncidod/hip/ISOLAT/isolat.htm. Retrieved April 3, 2005.

JCAHO. (2005). National Patient Safety Goals 2005. (Online). Available at http://www.jcaho.org/accredited+organizations/patient+safety/05+npsg/05_npsg_hap.htm. Retrieved April 8, 2005.

Mangrem, A., Horan, T., Pearson, M., et al. (1999). Guideline for prevention of surgical site infection. *Infection Control and Hospital Epidemiology, 27*(2), 97–132.

Occupational Safety and Health Agency. (1993). OSHA enforcement policy and procedures for occupational exposure to tuberculosis. *Infection Control and Hospital Epidemiology, 14*(12), 694–699.

Occupational Safety and Health Agency. (2003). Occupational exposure to tuberculosis; proposed rule; termination of rulemaking respiratory protection for M. tuberculosis; final rule; revocation Federal Register #68: 75767–75775. (Online). Available at http://www.osha.gov/pls/oshaweb/owadisp.show_document?p_table=FEDERAL_REGISTER&p_id=18050. Retrieved April 3, 2005.

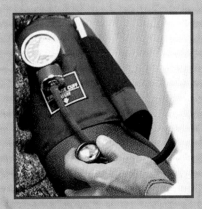

UNIT 6

Managing Special Elimination and Nutrition Needs

MODULES

MODULE 26

Administering Enemas

SKILLS INCLUDED IN THIS MODULE

General Procedure for Administering a Cleansing Enema
Specific Procedure for Administering a Return-Flow Enema
Specific Procedure for Administering a Premixed Disposable Enema

PREREQUISITE MODULES

Module 1	An Approach to Nursing Skills
Module 2	Documentation
Module 3	Basic Body Mechanics
Module 4	Basic Infection Control
Module 5	Safety in the Healthcare Environment
Module 6	Moving the Patient in Bed and Positioning
Module 14	Nursing Physical Assessment
Module 18	Transfer

KEY TERMS

anal sphincter	hypotonic
anorectal	instillation
bowel impaction	isotonic
descending colon	left lateral position
distention	normal saline
electrolytes	peristalsis
enema	reflex contraction
feces	sigmoid flexure
flatus	Sims' position
hypertonic	

OVERALL OBJECTIVE

▸ To safely and effectively administer enemas to adult patients.

LEARNING OUTCOMES

The student will be able to

1. Assess the patient for last bowel movement, presence of abdominal **distention** (swollen and firm), sphincter control, and ability to use the toilet, bedside commode, or bedpan.
2. Analyze assessment data to determine special problems or concerns that must be addressed to safely administer an enema to the individual patient.
3. Determine appropriate patient outcomes for a patient receiving an enema, and recognize the potential for adverse outcomes.
4. Plan to administer an enema by verifying the physician's order, selecting appropriate solutions, gathering appropriate equipment, and verifying the integrity of the equipment.
5. Implement safe and effective enema administration, including explaining the procedure to the patient and choosing an anatomically correct position.
6. Evaluate the effectiveness of the enema.
7. Document patient's response (presence of stool, ability to retain enema, abdominal discomfort), amount and characteristics of stool, and any adverse effects.

ADMINISTERING ENEMAS

An **enema** is a solution that is instilled directly into the rectum and large intestine. The solution dilates the intestine and irritates the intestinal mucosa. This action increases **peristalsis,** thereby promoting evacuation of **feces** and **flatus.** There are several types of enema solutions and purposes to be accomplished by their administration (Table 26-1). The most common use is for temporary relief of constipation. Other uses include cleansing bowels prior to diagnostic or surgical procedures and prior to the onset of bowel programs. Nurses must be familiar with varying solutions, their purpose, and how to properly administer them.

NURSING DIAGNOSES

These nursing diagnoses are appropriate for patients who may need an enema:

- Constipation: related to lack of fiber in diet, lack of fluids, or inactivity
- Altered Comfort: related to abdominal distention or passing hard feces
- Risk for Ineffective Therapeutic Regimen: related to lack of knowledge
- Deficient Knowledge: related to managing personal bowel care
- Nausea: related to disruption in bowel function

DELEGATION

Administration of enemas may be delegated to assistive personnel after they have received proper instruction and supervision. The nurse should inform the assistive personnel of any special positioning or other needs of the patient as well as what signs and symptoms to report and when to stop the procedure, if necessary.

CLEANSING ENEMAS

There are two types of cleansing enemas: the large-volume enema and the small-volume or prefilled, disposable enema. Both encourage full evacuation of stool from the colon. Each has a specific purpose and is appropriate for certain patients. Tap water and **normal saline** are commonly used solutions for large-volume enemas. Soapsuds enemas are occasionally ordered but these are very irritating to the bowel. For this reason, some facilities have a policy prohibiting the use of soap in an enema solution. Tap water is **hypotonic** and will therefore draw electrolytes from the body into the fluid. Normal saline solution is **isotonic** and does not cause a movement of electrolytes.

table 26-1. Types of Enemas

Type	Indication	Examples
Cleansing (used to remove feces from colon)	Preparation for diagnostic tests	Large-volume tap water or soap suds enema
	Prevents escape of feces during surgical procedures	Prefilled disposable enema
	Relief of constipation	
Return flow	Abdominal distention	Tap water or normal saline solution
Retention		
Oil	Introduction of oil to soften feces	Mineral oil enema
Medicated	Introduction of medications	Kayexelate enema, dexamethasone enema

Because it does not create electrolyte disturbances as readily as does tap water, normal saline solution is preferred for patients who are vulnerable to electrolyte imbalances, such as the elderly, the very young, and the severely debilitated. When several enemas are ordered for an individual, normal saline enemas should be administered to prevent alterations in electrolyte balance. Although a commercially prepared irrigating solution is preferred, an acceptable substitute mixture can be made by adding 1 teaspoon salt to each 500 mL water.

A commercial enema set includes a container for the fluid, attached tubing with a rectal tip, lubricant for the rectal tip (if the tip is not prelubricated), a drape for the bed, and a pair of clean gloves. A packet of Castile soap is found in some commercial enema equipment sets but is seldom used. Enema sets can be washed at the sink, dried, and reused for the same patient. When this is done, you will need to obtain gloves and lubricant separately (Fig. 26-1).

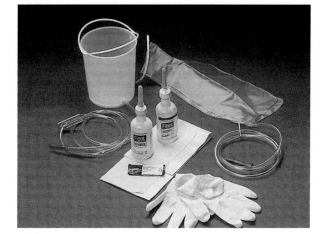

FIGURE 26-1 Types of enema equipment. A bucket or bag to fill with fluid or a small-volume medicated solution may be used for a cleansing enema. A premixed, prefilled oil retention enema may be used to soften stools.

GENERAL PROCEDURE FOR ADMINISTERING A CLEANSING ENEMA

ASSESSMENT

1. Verify the physician's orders. **R:** The nurse is responsible for verifying orders to ensure that an enema has been ordered and that the type of enema is appropriate for the specific patient.
2. Assess for abdominal distention. **R:** Abdominal distention and firmness could be a symptom of constipation, supporting the need for an enema.
3. Assess the patient's ability to tolerate and retain fluid and his or her ability to use the toilet, bedside commode, or bedpan. **R:** To determine whether the patient requires assistance.
4. Assess vital signs to establish a baseline prior to administering an enema. **R:** These baseline data can be utilized to evaluate the patient's response or tolerance of procedure.

ANALYSIS

5. Critically think through your data, carefully evaluating each aspect and its relation to other data.

R: To determine specific problems for this individual in relation to medical problems, ability to tolerate enemas, and ability to ambulate to the toilet or commode.
6. Identify specific problems and modifications of the procedure needed for this individual. **R:** Planning for the individual must take into consideration the individual's problems.

PLANNING

7. Determine individualized patient outcomes in relation to the enema administration. **R:** Identification of outcomes guides planning and evaluation.
   a. The patient understands the need for the enema.
   b. The patient experiences minimal discomfort during the procedure.
   c. Stool and fluid are completely evacuated from the bowel.
   d. The patient is clean and comfortable.
8. Assemble appropriate equipment: enema container, water-soluble lubricant, protective pad for bed, ordered fluid, and clean gloves (see Fig. 26-1). **R:** Gathering equipment ahead of time allows you to proceed more safely and effectively. Equipment includes enema supplies as well as toileting materials, such as a bedside commode or a bedpan.

IMPLEMENTATION

Action	Rationale
9. Wash or disinfect your hands.	To reduce transmission of microorganisms that could cause infection.

(continued)

Action	Rationale
10. Verify patient's identity, using two identifiers.	To ensure that the enema is being administered to the correct patient.
11. Explain the procedure you are about to perform.	Explaining the procedure helps relieve anxiety or misperceptions that the patient may have about a procedure or activity and sets the stage for patient cooperation.
12. Lubricate approximately 5 cm (2 inches) of the enema tip.	Lubrication enables the rectal tube to be inserted comfortably and without trauma.
13. Clamp the tubing.	Clamping prevents the solution from flowing, thereby allowing the container to fill properly.
14. Fill the bag or bucket with approximately 500 to 1,000 mL of the appropriate solution at slightly warmer than body temperature (100° to 105°F; 39.7° to 40.5°C). (*Note:* Some facilities recommend starting with 1,000 mL; you can always stop instilling fluid before the container is empty.) Check the temperature of the solution using a bath thermometer, or estimate the temperature by testing it on the inner aspect of your forearm. It should feel comfortably warm but not hot.	If the solution is slightly warmer than body temperature, by the time it is instilled through the tubing, it will be approximately at body temperature. Fluid at body temperature helps to maintain homeostasis.
15. Prime the tubing by allowing a small amount of solution to flow from the bucket or bag to the end of the tubing.	Priming prevents **instillation** of air, which could contribute to unnecessary abdominal pain or distention.
16. Close the door, and pull the curtain completely around the bed.	To provide privacy.
17. Raise the bed to an appropriate working position based on your height.	To allow correct use of body mechanics to prevent back injuries.
18. Put on clean gloves.	Gloves act as a barrier, preventing the transfer of microorganisms that could cause infection.
19. Assist the patient to a **left lateral position** with right leg flexed (**Sims' position**), and place a moisture-proof pad under the hips.	This position allows solution to flow by gravity into the sigmoid colon and **descending colon;** both are located on the left side. Flexing the right leg provides adequate exposure of anus. The moisture-proof pad protects the bed.
20. Directing the enema tip toward the umbilicus, slowly insert approximately 7 to 10 cm (3 to 4 inches), just beyond the internal sphincter. Have the patient breathe through the mouth to relax the **anal sphincter.** Another technique for	This angle follows the normal contour of the rectum. Slow, smooth insertion prevents sphincter spasms, and inserting the tube 7 to 10 cm (3 to 4 inches) places the tube beyond the sphincter and into the rectum. This prevents fluid from placing pressure against the sphincter and decreases the potential for trauma

(continued)

Action	Rationale
relaxing the sphincter is to touch the enema tip to the sphincter, wait for the **reflex contraction** to subside, and then insert the tip. If you encounter an obstruction, stop the procedure immediately, and report your findings to the physician.	to the intestinal wall, as would farther insertion. It is possible to traumatize the intestinal mucosa severely, especially if the tubing is inserted into the **sigmoid flexure** or the descending colon. Mouth breathing will relax the anal sphincter to ease insertion.
21. Slowly administer enema solution according to orders at a low pressure. If the patient complains of fullness, stop the flow for about 30 seconds, and resume at a slower rate (Fig. 26-2).	The flow rate is controlled by the height of the solution. The top of the fluid in the container should be no higher than 30 to 45 cm (12 to 18 inches) above the rectum for low pressure. Higher pressure may damage the colon mucosa. 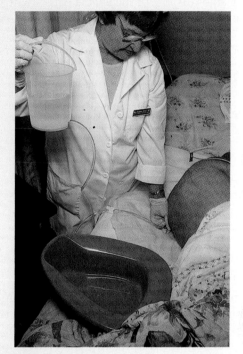 **FIGURE 26-2** Flow rate and fluid pressure are regulated by the height of the container. For low pressure, the fluid container may be held 12 to 18 inches above the rectum. Higher pressure may injure the colon. Negative pressure, used for siphoning, is achieved by positioning the container below the rectum.
22. Encourage the patient to retain the enema solution.	Retaining the fluid for a period of time increases stool softening and makes the enema more successful. Sometimes, a patient cannot retain the fluid because of weakness or lack of control of the anal sphincter. In such a case, hold the buttocks firmly together around the tubing to help the patient retain the fluid. If small amounts of fluid drain back constantly, place the curved side of an emesis basin against the buttocks to catch the fluid as it drains out. In some instances, the patient must be placed on a bedpan to avoid extreme soiling of the bed, which would be upsetting to the patient.

(continued)

Action	Rationale
23. Assist the patient to a sitting position on the bedpan, commode, or toilet, and instruct the patient not to flush the toilet.	A sitting position assists with defecation. Not flushing ensures that the nurse can observe the stool to evaluate the effectiveness of the procedure.
24. Promote patient comfort by helping the patient with cleaning the **anorectal** area if needed. If the patient can clean the area independently, provide an opportunity for handwashing and then assist him or her to return to bed or a chair.	Cleansing and handwashing provide comfort and protection from infectious agents.
25. Clean or dispose of the enema equipment appropriately.	Some disposable equipment may be cleaned and reused for the same patient. If this is so, dry the equipment thoroughly to prevent the growth of microorganisms, and label it with the date and the patient's name. If nondisposable equipment is used, send it to the appropriate area to be disinfected.
26. Remove gloves and discard.	Removing gloves prevents cross-contamination. This should be done prior to implementing additional interventions and prior to contact with other patients.
27. Wash or disinfect your hands.	To reduce transmission of microorganisms that could cause nosocomial infections.

EVALUATION

28. Evaluate using the individualized patient outcomes previously identified: The patient understands the need for the enema; the patient experiences only minimal discomfort during the procedure; stool and fluid are completely evacuated from the bowel; the patient is clean and comfortable. **R:** Evaluation in relation to desired outcomes is essential for planning future care.

DOCUMENTATION

29. Document the amount and type of enema, the amount and characteristics of the stool, and the response of the patient. Adverse reactions should be documented as well. **R:** Documentation is a legal record of the patient's care, and it communicates nursing interventions to other nurses and other disciplines.

◼ POTENTIAL ADVERSE OUTCOMES AND RELATED INTERVENTIONS

1. The bowel does not empty, and only fecal-colored solution returns.

Intervention: Notify the physician. A different type of enema may be needed to soften the stool.

2. All the fluid is not expelled.

Intervention: Note the amount retained, and notify the physician.

RETURN-FLOW ENEMAS

A return-flow enema is used to remove intestinal gas and stimulate peristalsis. It may be referred to as a Harris flush. A large volume of fluid is used, as in a cleansing enema, but the fluid is instilled in small increments (100 to 200 mL). Then the fluid is siphoned out by lowering the container below the level of the bowel. This action carries the flatus (gas) out with the fluid. The procedure may be repeated three to five times or until no flatus returns. Be careful not to tire the patient unduly.

If tap water solution is used, the patient's **electrolytes** may be depleted, especially if several return-flow enemas are given in a day. Normal saline solution will lessen electrolyte depletion. You should first determine whether the absorption of sodium will be detrimental to the patient by checking the patient's diagnosis.

SPECIFIC PROCEDURE FOR ADMINISTERING A RETURN-FLOW ENEMA

ASSESSMENT

1-4. Follow steps 1 to 4 of the General Procedure. Verify the physician's orders, assess presence of abdominal distention, assess the patient's ability to tolerate and retain fluid, and his or her ability to use the toilet, bedside commode, or bedpan. Also assess vital signs.

ANALYSIS

5-6. Follow steps 5 and 6 of the General Procedure. Critically think through your data, carefully evaluating each aspect and its relation to other data, identifying specific problems and modifications of the procedure needed for this individual.

PLANNING

7. Determine individualized patient outcomes in relation to the return-flow enema administration. **R:** Identification of outcomes guides planning and evaluation.

   a. The patient understands the need for the return-flow enema.

   b. The patient experiences only minimal discomfort during the procedure.

   c. Gas is completely evacuated from the bowel, and the abdomen is soft.

   d. The patient is clean and comfortable.

8. Follow step 8 of the General Procedure. Assemble appropriate equipment: enema container, water-soluble lubricant, protective pad for bed, ordered fluid, and clean gloves.

IMPLEMENTATION

Action	Rationale
9-20. Follow steps 9 to 20 of the General Procedure: Wash hands or disinfect hands, verify patient's identity (two identifiers), and explain the procedure you are about to perform. Lubricate approximately 5 cm (2 inches) of the enema tip, clamp tubing, fill bag or bucket with appropriate solution, and prime tubing by allowing a small amount of solution to flow from bucket or bag to end of tubing. Close the door and curtains around bed. Raise the bed to an appropriate working position based on your height, put on clean gloves, assist the patient to a left lateral position with the patient's right leg flexed, direct the enema tip toward the umbilicus, and slowly insert the tip of the tubing approximately 7–10 cm (3–4 inches).	
21. Administer enema solution as follows.	
a. Instill 200 mL of fluid.	The fluid will move into the bowel where flatus can dissolve into the fluid.
b. Lower the enema container below the level of the patient's bowel, and siphon the fluid and gas from the bowel.	This action creates negative pressure that draws the fluid and gas out. If the fluid does not return, you may have to move the tip of the tubing slightly so that it is in contact with the fluid in the bowel.

(continued)

Action	Rationale
c. Repeat steps 21a and 21b only until no more gas returns.	Continuing after the gas is removed will increase electrolyte depletion and patient fatigue.
22. Clamp the tubing before removing it from the patient's rectum.	To avoid soiling the bed.
23-27. Follow steps 23 to 27 of the General Procedure: Assist the patient to a sitting position (bedpan, toilet, or commode), help the patient with cleaning the rectal area if needed, provide an opportunity for handwashing, and assist with the patient's return to bed or a chair. Clean or dispose of the enema equipment, remove gloves and discard, wash or disinfect your hands.	

EVALUATION

28. Evaluate using the individualized patient outcomes previously identified: The patient understands the need for the enema; the patient experiences only minimal discomfort during the procedure; gas is completely evacuated from the bowel, and the abdomen is soft; the patient is clean and comfortable. **R:** Evaluation in relation to desired outcomes is essential for planning future care.

DOCUMENTATION

29. Follow step 29 of the General Procedure. Document amount and type of enema administered, amount of flatus returned, patient's subjective feelings of comfort, and any adverse reaction.

POTENTIAL ADVERSE OUTCOMES AND RELATED INTERVENTIONS

1. Patient experiences severe abdominal cramping and discomfort as peristalsis is stimulated.
Intervention: Stop the procedure, maintain patient in side-lying position, and notify the physician.
2. No flatus returns, but the patient continues to express discomfort, and the abdomen continues to be distended.
Intervention: Flatus may be higher in the colon than the enema was able to reach. Encourage the patient to walk to restore peristalsis and move gas down in the colon.

PREMIXED DISPOSABLE ENEMAS

Premixed disposable enemas come in a variety of formulations based on the purpose of the enema.

SMALL-VOLUME CLEANSING ENEMA

The most common disposable product is the small-volume cleansing enema, such as the Fleet's Phosphosoda enema. These small-volume enemas can be used for treating constipation and also for cleansing the bowel in preparation for tests. The enema solutions may contain either bisocodyl or sodium phosphate, which are both rectal stimulants. These solutions are **hypertonic** and thus draw fluid into the bowel, softening and loosening the fecal mass. Because hypertonic enemas use the body's own fluid supply to moisten and loosen the feces, they are inappropriate for patients who are dehydrated or in a situation in which immediate evacuation is desired. These solutions are also irritants, causing strong peristalsis and subsequent evacuation. These enemas are available in two sizes: 150 mL and 37 mL. Because both are of small volume, patients should be able to retain the enema solution for at least 20 minutes to allow fluid from the body to enter the colon.

Prepackaged disposable enemas are being used in place of large-volume enemas more frequently because they are adequate for treating uncomplicated constipation (Fig. 26-3). People can easily be taught to administer them at home. They also have other advantages. They do not have the potential to create electrolyte depletion as does tap water. In addition, they can be given more rapidly than the large-volume enema, they cause less abdominal distention and discomfort for the patient, and they are more convenient for the person administering the enema. When using a commercially prepared enema, read and follow the package directions. The general directions for the procedure still apply.

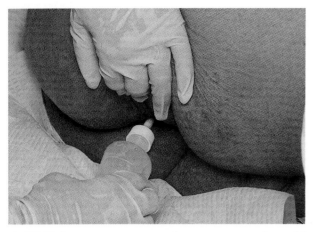

FIGURE 26-3 Small-volume premixed enemas are typically used for relieving constipation or for bowel preparation before tests. Their contents are instilled by slowly squeezing the container.

RETENTION ENEMAS

Retention enemas also come as premixed disposable enemas. They contain a therapeutic agent that has its effect when it is retained in the bowel for 30 minutes to 1 hour. If fecal material has hardened or cannot be expelled (a **bowel impaction**), an oil-retention enema may be ordered to soften the feces. Commercially packaged oil-retention enemas contain 90 to 120 mL solution (see Fig. 26-1). Approximately 90 to 120 mL is instilled into the patient's colon. The patient should retain the solution as long as possible—30 minutes to 1 hour—for the enema to be effective. This enema is usually followed by a cleansing enema. If a commercially prepared oil enema is not available, mineral oil may be used. It is instilled by using a 30 mL bulb syringe barrel attached to a rectal tube. Oil is poured into the open barrel and allowed to flow into the bowel by gravity.

MEDICATED ENEMAS

Medicated enemas contain various drugs that may be administered as an enema. These include steroid preparations for their effect in the bowel, antibiotics used to reduce infection during colon surgeries, electrolyte preparations to treat electrolyte imbalances, and preparations that absorb certain chemicals (such as ammonia) in the bowel. To safely administer medicated enemas, you will need to follow the procedures to administer medications as well as procedures for administering enemas.

SPECIFIC PROCEDURE FOR ADMINISTERING A PREMIXED DISPOSABLE ENEMA

ASSESSMENT

1-4. Follow steps 1 to 4 of the General Procedure. Verify the physician's orders, assess for abdominal distention, assess the patient's ability to tolerate and retain fluid, and his or her ability to use the toilet, bedside commode, or bedpan. Also assess vital signs.

ANALYSIS

5-6. Follow steps 5 and 6 of the General Procedure. Critically think through your data, carefully evaluating each aspect and its relation to other data, and identify specific problems and modifications of the procedure needed for this individual.

PLANNING

7. Determine individualized patient outcomes in relation to the specific packaged enema being administered. **R:** Identification of outcomes guides planning and evaluation.
    a. The patient understands the need for the specific enema.
    b. The patient experiences only minimal discomfort during the procedure.
    c. The patient retains the enema for the appropriate length of time.
    d. The purpose of the enema is met:
        (1) Bowel evacuation occurs when being given for bowel cleansing.
        (2) The specific purpose of the medicated enema must be identified for evaluation.
    e. The patient is clean and comfortable.
8. Follow step 8 of the General Procedure. Assemble appropriate equipment: enema container, water-soluble lubricant, protective pad for bed, ordered fluid, and clean gloves.

IMPLEMENTATION

Action	Rationale
9-11. Follow steps 9 to 11 of the General Procedure. Wash or disinfect your hands, verify the patient's identity (two identifiers), and explain the procedure you are about to perform.	

(continued)

Action	Rationale
12. Warm the enema by immersing the plastic container in a basin of warm water.	The warming solution enhances the comfort and effectiveness of the enema.
13. Close the door, and draw the curtain completely around the bed.	To provide privacy.
14. Raise the bed to an appropriate working position based on your height.	To allow correct use of body mechanics to prevent back injuries.
15. Put on clean gloves.	Gloves act as a barrier, preventing the transfer of microorganisms that could cause infection.
16. Assist the patient to a left lateral position with the right leg flexed, and place a moisture-proof pad under the hips.	This position allows solution to flow by gravity into the sigmoid and descending colons; both are located on the left side. Flexing the right leg provides adequate exposure of the anus. The moisture-proof pad protects the bed.
17. Directing the enema tip toward the umbilicus, slowly insert until the tip is beyond the internal sphincter. (Premixed enemas usually have a prelubricated tip.)	This angle follows the normal contour of the rectum. Slow, smooth insertion prevents sphincter spasms, and inserting the tube beyond the sphincter prevents fluid from flowing out while being instilled.
18. Slowly administer the enema based on the type.	
a. Squeeze the plastic container from the bottom to instill fluid while maintaining steady pressure.	To prevent the suction of instilled fluid back into the container and allow complete administration of the enema.
b. Instruct the patient to retain the fluid in accord with the therapeutic intent.	Cleansing enemas are held until there is a strong urge to defecate. Oil-retention enemas are held for 30 to 90 minutes to soften the stool. Medicated enemas are held for the prescribed amount of time, which varies from drug to drug.
19. Hold the rolled container tightly while removing it from the patient's rectum, and discard the container and your gloves into the waste container.	To avoid soiling the bed.
20. Assist the patient to a sitting position on the bedpan, toilet, or commode. Instruct the patient not to flush the toilet.	Sitting promotes effective bowel evacuation, and not flushing allows the nurse to evaluate the effectiveness of the enema.
21. If necessary to assist with cleansing the anorectal area, put on clean gloves, and cleanse the patient's anorectal area, or assist the patient with handwashing.	To make the patient comfortable and remove fecal material.

(continued)

Action	Rationale
22. Remove your gloves and discard, and assist the patient to wash his or her hands and return to a position of comfort.	Removing gloves prevents cross-contamination. This should be done prior to implementing additional interventions and prior to contact with other patients. The patient is helped to a comfortable position before the nurse leaves the bedside.
23. Wash or disinfect your hands.	To prevent transmission of infectious agents.

EVALUATION

24. Evaluate the patient's response based on the individualized patient outcomes previously identified: The patient understands the need for the specific enema, the patient experiences only minimal discomfort during the procedure, the patient retains the enema for the appropriate length of time, the purpose of the enema is met, and the patient is clean and comfortable. **R:** Evaluation in relation to desired outcomes is essential for planning future care.

DOCUMENTATION

25. Document the amount and type of enema, amount and characteristics of the stool returned, the patient's subjective feelings of comfort, and any adverse reaction. **R:** Documentation provides a legal record of care and communicates care to the rest of the healthcare team.

Acute Care

Hospitalized patients may require enema administration for various reasons. Diagnostic examinations in which unrestricted direct visualization (an invasive form of visualizing internal organs) of the bowel is necessary often require enemas as a part of the bowel cleansing protocol. The following are examples of the above-mentioned examinations: colonoscopy, sigmoidoscopy, and proctoscopy. Barium enemas are utilized when indirect visualization (noninvasive form of visualizing the shape or function of internal organs) of the bowels is necessary. These enemas are administered fluoroscopically, which allows continuous visualization of the barium's progression throughout the bowels by projecting X-ray films onto a screen. Last, patients may require enemas to relieve constipation that often occurs in conjunction with surgery, use of narcotic medications, and immobility.

Long-Term Care

Developing intolerance to certain foods along with decreased activity may place elderly residents in long-term care settings at risk for alterations in bowel function. Because of the physiologic changes that occur, these foods and limited mobility may cause abdominal discomfort, distention, flatus, and more commonly, constipation. Bowel programs are often a part the resident's plan of care. Typically, these programs schedule daily dosing of stool softeners with the use of laxatives as needed. Enemas are considered when routine medications are no longer effective.

When an enema is a part of the care of an elderly resident, several considerations are important. First, the nurse should be aware of any medical conditions that could affect the resident's response to the enema (e.g., cardiac disorders and/or fluid volume disturbances). Second, enemas should be administered very slowly because elderly persons often experience a reduction in sphincter control, resulting in an inability to hold large volumes of fluid. Nurses may also be responsible for teaching other staff members to administer enemas.

Home Care

Enemas may be administered at home in preparation for gastrointestinal studies performed in ambulatory care settings or for occasional episodes of constipation. Nurses have the responsibility to instruct clients on the use of enemas to avoid injury and to ensure that stool has been properly evacuated prior to gastrointestinal studies. Clients should be encouraged to administer enemas as directed and advised to report any adverse effects immediately.

LEARNING TOOLS

DEVELOP YOUR BACKGROUND KNOWLEDGE

1. Review the Learning Outcomes.

2. Read the section on enemas in your assigned text.

3. Look up the Key Terms in the glossary.

4. Review this module, and mentally practice the techniques described. Study so that you would be able to teach these skills to another person.

5. Note the different types of enemas discussed in the module. Which would be more appropriate for a patient undergoing gastrointestinal studies?

DEVELOP YOUR SKILLS

In the practice setting

1. Review the procedure for administering enemas.

2. Select two other students, and form a group.
   a. Role-play communicating with a patient about receiving an enema, with one student playing the role of the patient, another playing the role of the nurse, and the third serving as the evaluator.
   b. Role-play teaching a patient how to self-administer an enema.
   c. Role-play should continue until each student has had the opportunity to play each role.

3. Using the equipment available in the skills laboratory and a mannequin, complete the entire procedure for giving a tap water enema using the Performance Checklist on the CD-ROM in the front of this book to evaluate one another's technique.

4. Inspect examples of medicated enemas if they are available in your practice setting.

DEMONSTRATE YOUR SKILLS

In the clinical setting

1. Identify your facility's policy regarding bowel care intervention that may be initiated by the nurse.

2. Consult with your instructor regarding the opportunity to administer an enema to a patient or resident.

3. Ask your instructor to supervise and evaluate your performance.

CRITICAL THINKING EXERCISES

1. Mr. C. is a 70-year-old male who complains of constipation. He takes Fibercon tablets (an over-the-counter fiber tablet) daily but states that he hasn't had a bowel movement in 2 weeks. He complains of passing small amounts of brown liquid but no formed stool. Upon assessment, you discover Mr. C.'s abdomen to be firm and distended. What observations are most important? How would you respond to this patient? List appropriate interventions.

2. Mrs. H. is a 23-year-old female. She is to receive a large-volume enema. During administration, she complains of abdominal pain and distention. She has received 100 mL of the enema solution. What should you do next? Explain your reasoning.

SELF-QUIZ
SHORT-ANSWER QUESTIONS

1. List three types of enemas.

   a. _____

   b. _____

   c. _____

2. List four observations to be made of the patient while administering an enema.

   a. _____

   b. _____

   c. _____

   d. _____

3. List two types of premixed enemas.

   a. _____

   b. _____

4. How far should an enema tip be inserted?

   _____

5. How much volume is given in cleansing enemas?

   _____

6. Give two instances in which patients might administer their own enemas.

   a. _____

   b. _____

MULTIPLE CHOICE

_____ 7. Which type of enema should not be used for the dehydrated patient?
   a. Tap water
   b. Return-flow
   c. Small-volume irritant such as Fleet's Phosphosoda
   d. Small-volume containing a prescribed medication

_____ 8. Two days after having a right knee replacement, a 64 year old states that she feels the urge to defecate but cannot pass any stool. She is taking narcotic medications to control her pain and hasn't had a bowel movement in 3 days. Upon assessment, you find abdominal distention and decreased bowel sounds. Which of the following is the most appropriate nursing diagnosis for this patient?

a. Constipation related to anxiety
b. Constipation related to immobility and decreased peristalsis secondary to opioid medication
c. Constipation related to postoperative knee pain
d. Perceived constipation related to inaccurate information about bowel patterns

_____ 9. The nurse should observe for changes in electrolyte levels after administering which type of enema?
a. Large-volume tap water enemas
b. Normal saline enemas
c. Soap suds enemas
d. Steroid enemas

_____ 10. Return-flow enemas are used to
a. administer medications.
b. evacuate stool.
c. expel flatus.
d. soften stool.

Answers to the Self-Quiz questions appear in the back of this book.

MODULE 27

Assisting the Patient Who Requires Urinary Catheterization

SKILLS INCLUDED IN THIS MODULE

Procedure for Catheterization
Caring for a Patient With an Indwelling Catheter
Procedure for Removing an Indwelling Catheter
Teaching the Procedure for Intermittent
   Self-Catheterization
Procedure for Bladder Irrigation

PREREQUISITE MODULES

Module 1	An Approach to Nursing Skills
Module 2	Documentation
Module 3	Basic Body Mechanics
Module 4	Basic Infection Control
Module 5	Safety in the Healthcare Environment
Module 6	Moving the Patient in Bed and Positioning
Module 7	Providing Hygiene
Module 8	Assisting With Elimination and Perineal Care
Module 13	Monitoring Intake and Output
Module 14	Nursing Physical Assessment
Module 24	Basic Sterile Technique: Sterile Field and Sterile Gloves

KEY TERMS

bladder scan	meatus
catheter	penis
catheterization	perineum
continuous bladder irrigation (CBI)	retention catheter
Foley catheter	straight catheter
foreskin	three-way catheter
hemostasis	urethra
indwelling catheter	void

OVERALL OBJECTIVES

▸ To insert a urinary catheter utilizing sterile technique
▸ To maintain and properly discontinue a urinary catheter
▸ To irrigate a bladder safely and effectively

LEARNING OUTCOMES

The student will be able to

1. Assess the patient to determine the need for catheterization and whether a straight or indwelling catheter is needed.
2. Analyze assessment data to prepare for problems or concerns that should be addressed prior to inserting a urinary catheter.
3. Identify desired outcomes for the patient who requires urinary catheterization or whose catheter is to be irrigated or removed and any potential adverse outcomes.
4. Plan catheter insertion, care, or removal by verifying the physician's order and selecting appropriate equipment.
5. Implement safe catheter insertion, care, and removal.
6. Evaluate effectiveness of catheterization and comfort and safety of patient.
7. Document size of catheter and patient response (characteristics of urine, level of comfort before and after, and any adverse effects).

Urinary **catheterization** introduces tubing (rubber, plastic, latex, silicone, or polyvinyl), called a **catheter,** into the **meatus.** The tubing is then advanced until it reaches the bladder. Catheterization is usually performed to drain urine from the bladder or to instill solution into the bladder. Because the risk exists for introducing microorganisms into the bladder, catheterization is performed only when necessary, and strict sterile technique is utilized to limit contamination of the bladder and kidneys. Although sterile technique is used, the risk for infection continues to exist because the catheter is a foreign body, and the natural defense mechanism of voiding, which flushes microorganisms from the **urethra,** is altered. Urinary catheters are the most common cause of hospital-acquired (nosocomial) infections (Tambyah, Knasinski, & Maki, 2002).

The nurse is responsible for understanding the anatomy of the male and female urinary systems to avoid injury due to improper catheter insertion. A review of these systems may be helpful. Catheters should be inserted slowly, following the natural contours of the urethra. Once catheterization has been performed, the nurse is responsible for maintaining the catheter. Maintenance includes—but is not limited to—proper drainage position, daily catheter care, assessing for trauma or signs of infection, and patient education.

NURSING DIAGNOSES

- Risk for Infection: related to indwelling catheter that provides a pathway for microorganisms to ascend to the bladder. The presence of an indwelling catheter is a frequent causative factor in urinary tract infections.
- Impaired Urinary Elimination: related to decreased bladder capacity, or irritation secondary to infection, or interference with the function of the urinary sphincter. This nursing diagnosis may be present before the catheter is inserted and be the reason for the use of the catheter. When the catheter is used for another purpose, it may create these conditions, which then may cause ongoing problems with urinary elimination.
- Risk for Impaired Skin Integrity: related to mechanical irritants or pressure secondary to indwelling catheter. The tissue at the meatus is sensitive to the pressure exerted by the catheter and may break down from catheter pressure or movement.

DELEGATION

Insertion of urinary catheters is not usually delegated to assistive personnel nor are bladder irrigations. However, care of the patient with a catheter and removal of a catheter may be delegated to those who have been taught these skills.

ASSESSING THE PATIENT FOR URINARY RETENTION

A common reason for catheterization is urinary retention. This may be a problem after surgery or illness or after a catheter has been removed. While the bladder can be palpated to detect a full bladder, this is not an exact process. In many facilities, the bladder is assessed using a portable ultrasound bladder scanning machine. The **bladder scan** provides a readout of the volume of urine that is being retained in the bladder. This precise knowledge guides nursing actions. The specific directions of the bladder ultrasound scanning machine should be followed for an accurate assessment.

PREPARING THE PATIENT

Many patients are anxious about catheterization, fearing pain and discomfort. They react emotionally to any procedure related to the genitourinary system—one that involves penetration of the body. Some facilities protect privacy by establishing a policy for male patients to be catheterized by male nurses and female patients to be catheterized by female nurses, unless the catheterization is an emergency. If an emergency occurs, and because there are fewer male nurses than female nurses, some facilities have specially trained male technicians or nursing assistants who can catheterize male patients. Other institutions permit both male and female nurses to perform catheterizations on a patient of either sex.

Always assess the patient's feelings about the procedure, and review the policy of your facility to cause the patient as little embarrassment as possible. In preparing the patient, use a calm, straightforward, professional manner to relieve his or her anxiety. Explain the procedure completely, and tell the patient what to expect. Then, give the patient an opportunity to ask questions and express concerns. Pay careful attention to privacy by closing doors, draping the patient, and exposing only the area involved in the procedure. These actions show your concern for the patient's privacy and should alleviate some distress.

EQUIPMENT FOR CATHETERIZATION

A catheterization kit contains the basic equipment needed for the procedure. Some variation from one brand to another may exist, but usually the kit includes the following items in this order.

- Sterile wrapper: When opened, the inside of the wrapper provides a sterile field. The outside is usually impervious to moisture. Therefore, it must be opened to preserve the sterility of the inside of the wrapper.
- Sterile gloves: These are usually on top, so all other items can be set up using sterile technique. As a beginner, you may want to have an extra pair of gloves in the room in case of inadvertent contamination.
- Sterile drapes: Two drapes are usually provided. One is a plain drape to slide under the female

patient or to spread out under the **penis** of the male patient. The other drape is typically fenestrated (has a hole in it). The fenestrated drape is placed over the **perineum,** with the opening over the meatus for a female patient or around the penis of a male patient.

- Sterile cleansing wipes: These may be cotton balls for use with a separate cleansing solution or a packet of premoistened wipes with a short handle attached.
- Thumb forceps or "pickups" if the cleansing wipes are not on a stick. You will need these to handle the cotton balls without contaminating your gloves.
- Cleansing solution for use with cotton balls: The solution container is opened, and solution poured into a space in the tray. Most sets contain a water-soluble iodine solution, which is an excellent antibacterial agent.
- Water-soluble lubricant for lubricating the catheter
- Sterile catheter: The catheter may be in the set, or it may be packaged separately and need to be added to the sterile field during the procedure. Either a plain (straight) catheter or an indwelling catheter can be used. (See Figure 27-1 for an illustration of catheter types.) Catheters are available in sizes 8 to 20 French (French is a method of sizing). Size 8 French is used for infants and young children. Size 16 French is commonly used for adults. For patients who drain urine around an indwelling catheter, size 18 or 20 French is used. Selecting the smallest size that will be effective decreases the likelihood of infection. Larger catheters irritate the wall of the urethra, causing it to be prone to invasion by microorganisms. This is more significant when an indwelling catheter is to be inserted because it remains in contact with the urethra for a longer time. The composition of the catheter also makes a difference in infection rates. Silicone catheters that are softer and cause less irritation than latex rubber catheters can be left in place longer with a lower risk for infection. Silicone catheters are essential for the patient who is sensitive to latex. Additional materials in the kit differ, depending upon whether an indwelling or straight (intermittent) catheter is being inserted.

Safety Alert

Note: *An important step in choosing a catheter involves assessing and/or monitoring the patient for latex sensitivity or allergy, which if present, may lead to serious complications.*

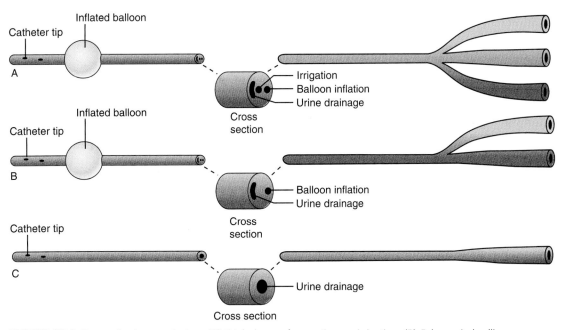

FIGURE 27-1 Types of urinary catheters. (**A**) Triple lumen for continuous irrigation. (**B**) Foley or indwelling catheter. (**C**) Straight catheter.

An **indwelling catheter** is also referred to as a **retention catheter** or a **Foley catheter,** named after its originator. The indwelling catheter has a balloon at the end that is inflated to hold the catheter in the bladder (Fig. 27-2). The inflated balloon holds the catheter in the bladder. Balloons are available in several sizes. Nurses most commonly insert catheters with balloons that hold 5 or 6 mL sterile water, depending on the manufacturer. Catheters with larger balloons are available and can be used for patients who have difficulty retaining the indwelling catheter. The larger balloon secures it within the bladder. During surgery, physicians sometimes insert catheters with balloons as large as 30 mL, which they secure with traction to promote **hemostasis** at a urologic surgical site.

- Drainage tubing and a collection bag may be attached to the indwelling catheter or be separate within the set. If the indwelling catheter set does not contain drainage tubing and a collection bag, this must be obtained in a separate package.
- Sterile syringe filled with sterile water is used to fill the balloon of an indwelling catheter. (Note: Saline is *not* used because it can crystallize in the balloon, making it difficult to extract.)
- A plastic clamp used to secure the indwelling catheter tubing to the bed may be included. In many settings, it was the practice to use a safety pin and rubber band for this purpose. Because of concern for injury to the hands from a sharp stick, these are being eliminated.
- A specimen container and label may be found in the set for the **straight catheter.**

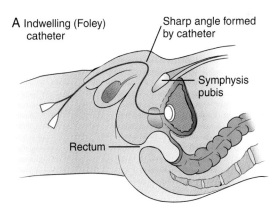

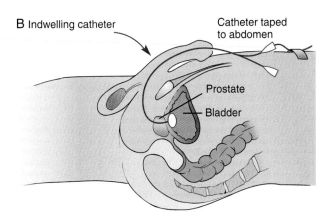

FIGURE 27-2 The inflated balloon holds the catheter in the bladder. (**A**) Note the sharp angle formed at the penile-scrotal junction when the penis is directed toward the thigh. (**B**) Note how correct taping of the catheter in the male patient eliminates the potential for abrasion and erosion of the penile-scrotal angle.

PROCEDURE FOR CATHETERIZATION

ASSESSMENT

1. Verify physician's orders. **R:** The nurse is responsible for verifying orders to ensure that catheterization has been ordered for the patient.
2. Determine appropriate method of catheterization (straight or indwelling). **R:** Straight catheters are used only in specimen collections, assessment of postvoid residual urine, or for intermittent emptying of the bladder. Indwelling catheters are used when continuous bladder emptying is needed.

ANALYSIS

3. Critically think through your data, carefully evaluating each aspect and its relation to other data. **R:** This enables you to determine specific problems for this individual in relation to catheterization.
4. Identify specific problems and modifications of the procedure needed for this individual. In particular, determine whether the patient will be able to maintain the proper position for catheterization or whether assistance will be needed. **R:** Planning for the individual must take into consideration the individual's problems.

PLANNING

5. Determine individualized patient outcomes in relation to the urinary catheterization. **R:** Identification of outcomes guides planning and evaluation.

   a. The patient understands the need for the catheter.
   b. The patient experiences only minimal discomfort during the procedure.
   c. Sterile technique was maintained to prevent infection.
   d. Urine is completely drained from the bladder.
   e. If an indwelling catheter was inserted, both catheter and drainage bag are positioned correctly.
   f. The patient is clean and comfortable.
6. Collect the appropriate equipment. **R:** Gathering equipment ahead of time allows you to proceed more safely and effectively.

   a. Correct catheterization kit with the specific type (indwelling or straight) and size of catheter to be used. (*Note:* You may wish to have extra equipment, such as extra sterile gloves available in case an item is contaminated.)
   b. Additional lighting if the room does not have adequate lighting to enable you to see the perineum clearly. (A portable gooseneck lamp or a flashlight may be used to improve existing lighting.)
   c. A bath blanket or sheet to drape the patient
   d. Tape or special device for securing the indwelling catheter to the patient: Cath-Secure is a disposable cloth patch with an adhesive backing and a hook and loop fastener (Velcro) that fastens the catheter to the patch. There are also a variety of leg straps that can be used.

IMPLEMENTATION

Action	Rationale
7. Wash or disinfect your hands.	To reduce the transfer of microorganisms that could cause infection.
8. Identify the patient, using two patient identifiers.	To be sure you are performing the procedure on the correct patient.
9. Explain the procedure to the patient, and answer his or her questions.	Explanations relieve anxiety and provide the patient with information regarding the procedure.
10. Close the door of the room, or draw the bed curtains.	To provide privacy.
11. Raise the bed to an appropriate working position based on your height.	This allows you to use correct body mechanics and protect yourself from back injury.
12. Position and drape the patient.	To provide good visualization and convenience and preserve patient privacy.

(continued)

Action	Rationale
a. Place a female patient in the dorsal recumbent position (Fig. 27-3), with knees flexed and legs spread. Sometimes, it is more comfortable for the patient to have her knees supported with pillows. Drape the bath blanket so that both legs are covered, and only the perineum is exposed. If the patient cannot assume the dorsal recumbent position, the Sims' position can be used. For a pediatric patient or one who is disoriented or confused, you may need another person (sometimes two others) to assist the patient to maintain the proper position. **b.** Place a male patient in a dorsal recumbent position. Expose only the penis and a small surrounding area.	 **FIGURE 27-3** Female in dorsal recumbent position.
13. Arrange the lighting so that you can see the perineum easily. (If the perineal area is soiled, you will have to pause at this point to provide perineal care, wearing clean gloves and using soap and water, before you begin catheterization. You may be able to identify the meatus while providing perineal care.)	Adequate lighting is essential for viewing the meatus well. Any soiling of the perineum increases the potential for contamination and infection.
14. If the drainage bag is in a separate package, open the package, and attach it to the bed with the end of the tubing covered and conveniently available for later use.	To maintain sterility of the end of the tubing and to ensure that it is conveniently accessible when needed.
15. Place the catheterization kit on an overbed table at the foot of the bed or on the bed between the patient's legs, and set up the equipment.	Equipment should be set up prior to insertion to avoid cross-contamination and to facilitate its utilization.
a. Remove the plastic bag containing the kit, and prop it open away from where you will prepare your sterile field. (A bedside bag or several paper towels may also be used.)	This can be used as a receptacle for soiled cleansing wipes and to dispose of used materials away from the sterile field as you work.
b. Open the catheterization kit wrapper carefully, touching only the outside to maintain sterility, and place this drape with the kit in the middle of it in a convenient location as a sterile field.	This creates your initial working sterile field.
c. Put on gloves, and place the first sterile drape. The process differs based on what is found on the top layer of the kit.	To maintain sterility of contents and set up sterile field while protecting your gloves from contamination. *(continued)*

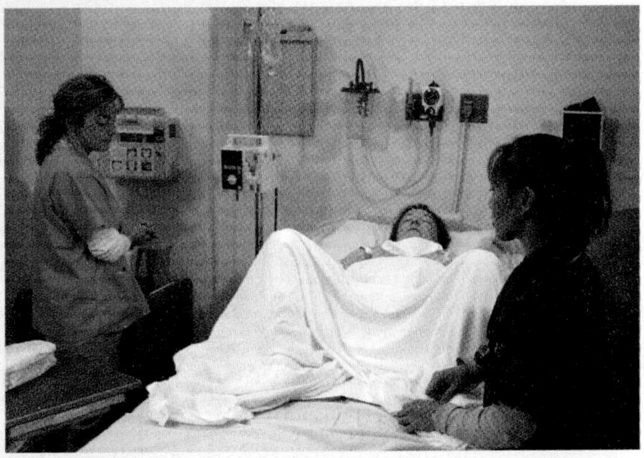

Action	Rationale
(1) *If a sterile drape is on top of the set,* you will need to place the sterile drape under your patient with ungloved hands, and put on sterile gloves later. To do this, grasp the drape by one corner, and then open it with care, touching only the under, shiny side and ½ to 1 inch of surrounding edges.	This keeps your hands away from the sterile top surface. Using the sterile supplies as they occur in the kit enables you to handle them in a way that ensures that the ones still in the container remain sterile.
(a) *For the female patient:* Ask the female patient to lift her hips. Next, keeping the top sterile and keeping your ungloved hands underneath the drape, carefully slide the drape under the buttocks. The soft side should be up against the patient, and the shiny waterproof side should be down. Then carefully slide your hands out, and put on sterile gloves.	These techniques keep the top side of the drape sterile and you are left ready to put on gloves.
(b) *For the male patient:* Hold the drape with your hands under it. Next, slide the drape under the penis and across the groin. Then slide your hands out, and put on sterile gloves.	
(2) *If sterile gloves are on top of the set,* put the gloves on first; then place the first sterile drape as follows: Carefully take the first drape by one corner and unfold it, keeping your gloved hands at the top of the drape. Grasp two adjacent corners of the drape with the soft side toward you and the shiny plastic side away from you, and turn your hands so that the drape covers the gloves.	
(a) *For the female patient:* Ask the female patient to lift her hips. Next, keeping the top sterile and keeping your gloved hands on top and covered by the corners of the drape, carefully slide the drape under the buttocks. The soft side should be up against the patient, and the shiny waterproof side should be down. Then carefully slide your hands out (Fig. 27-4).	This keeps the top soft side sterile and provides a sterile field next to the patient. You are left wearing sterile gloves, and you are ready to handle the rest of the equipment.

(continued)

Action	Rationale
	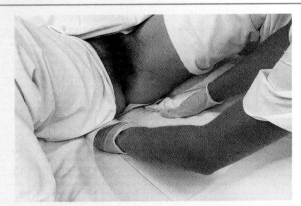 **FIGURE 27-4** Placing a sterile drape under the female patient without contaminating sterile gloves.
(b) *For the male patient:* Hold the drape with gloved hands on top of the drape with the corners wrapped around them. Next, slide the drape under the penis and across the groin. Then, slide your hands out.	
d. Place the second drape to secure and enlarge the sterile field. If it is fenestrated, place the opening over the penis of the male patient. The drape can be placed over the meatus of the female patient, but many nurses find that it tends to fall forward, obscuring their vision and potentially contaminating the catheter. An alternative is to fold the drape in half, and place it over the pubic area.	This enlarges the sterile field.
e. If the cleansing solution is separate, open the cleansing solution, and pour it over the swabs. If there are moist wipes for cleansing, open that package.	The cleansing materials will be used first. Packages must be opened when two hands are available.
f. Open the lubricant, and place a small amount onto the tray in your sterile field. Place the tip of the catheter into lubricant, and leave it in place until ready for insertion.	Lubricant minimizes trauma and discomfort to the urethra when the catheter is inserted. A catheter that remains on the sterile field is less likely to become contaminated.
g. Prepare for either an indwelling catheterization or a straight catheterization.	

(continued)

Action	Rationale
(1) If an indwelling catheter is being inserted, attach the prefilled syringe to the balloon port. Test the balloon by instilling all of the sterile water and then deflating it by withdrawing the water.	This allows you to assess for defects. If the catheter is defective, ask someone to get another catheter kit, or remove your gloves and get another catheter kit and pair of sterile gloves. If the catheter is without defects, leave the syringe attached. (This can simplify later work because you will want to hold the catheter in place with one hand, which leaves you only one hand to manipulate the syringe.)
(2) If the drainage bag is in the set, connect the distal end of the catheter to the drainage tube. If a specimen is needed, you can either not connect the catheter to the drainage tube at this time, and use the specimen container as a collection device, or obtain a specimen from the sterile drainage bag after you have finished.	This prevents urine spilling from a collecting container while you are performing the procedure.
(3) If this is a straight catheterization, and a sterile urine specimen is needed, remove the top from the specimen container included in the set, and place it upside down.	This is so that the container remains convenient and sterile.
16. Use your nondominant hand to expose the meatus. Remember that this hand is now contaminated and cannot be used to handle sterile equipment again.	
a. *For a male:* Raise the penis at a 45-degree angle from the scrotum, and retract the **foreskin,** if necessary, to expose the meatus.	Clear visualization of the meatus is essential to maintaining sterility during the catheterization.
b. *For a female:* Separate both the labia majora and the labia minora. Place the thumb and forefinger or first and second fingers on the two labia just anterior to the vagina. By separating these two fingers, retract the labia in an upward and outward direction. A common error is to place the fingers too high to expose the meatus. If the meatus is not identifiable, move your hand position for better exposure. Always identify the meatus before any other equipment is contaminated (Fig. 27-5). If the perineum is clearly exposed, and you cannot identify the meatal opening, you may ask the patient to cough because coughing usually causes the meatus to open slightly and aids in identification. Cleansing, the next step, will help you positively identify the meatus.	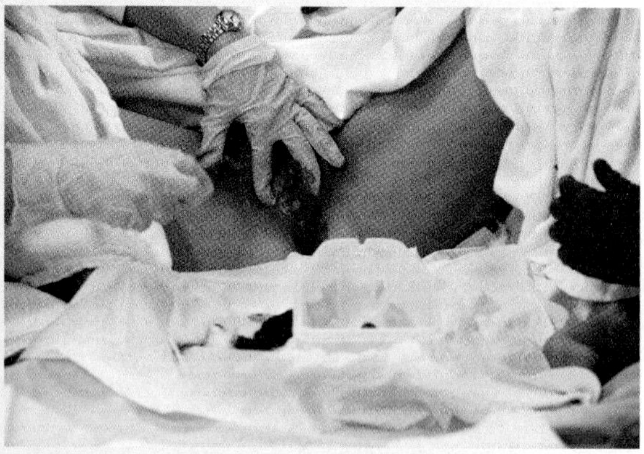 **FIGURE 27-5** Locating the female meatus for catheterization.

(continued)

Action	Rationale
17. Cleanse the meatus. Use forceps to handle the cleansing wipes to maintain sterility of your dominant gloved hand for handling the catheter, or hold by the end of the swab stick (Fig. 27-6). Use each wipe only once, and then discard in the prepared location, where it will not contaminate your field. To prevent bacteria from falling onto the sterile field, do not pass the used cleaning wipes over the sterile field.	The principle governing this pattern is to cleanse from the area of lesser accumulation of secretions and organisms (labia) to the area of greater concentration (meatus). Some persons recommend that the first cleansing strokes be down the center, across the meatus, and that subsequent strokes move outward. The principle governing this pattern is to move from the area you want to be the cleanest area (meatus) to the area that is less critical (labia). Research has not identified which of these procedures is better. The most critical point seems to be that each swab be used only once and that the path of the swab be from anterior to posterior to avoid moving microorganisms from the rectal area to the meatus. For this step, follow your facility's policy or procedure. If the labia close over the meatus, the site will become contaminated and will need to be cleaned again.

a. *For a male:* Clean in a circular motion, starting at the meatus, without retracing any area to move bacteria away from the meatus (Fig. 27-7).

b. *For a female:* After the meatus is exposed and identified, continue to hold the labia separate, and begin cleaning. Cleanse the labia and meatus using separate moistened wipes for each stroke. Each stroke should begin at the anterior and move toward the anus. Start with the outside labia on one side and then the other, and with each separate swab move closer to the meatus (see Fig. 27-6). The final stroke should be vertical to clean the meatus itself. The last stroke, if done slowly, may open the meatus slightly, thereby ensuring identification. Continue holding the labia apart with the non-dominant hand after cleaning until the catheter is inserted.

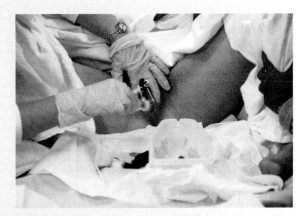

FIGURE 27-6 Cleansing the female meatal area before catheterization. Wipe from anterior to posterior, outside to inside.

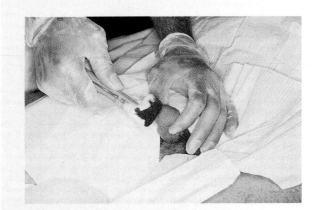

FIGURE 27-7 Cleansing the male meatal area using a circular motion.

(continued)

Action	Rationale
18. Use the sterile-gloved dominant hand (clean hand) to move the tray containing the catheter close to the patient (between the legs of the female patient and beside the male patient). Touch only the inside of the tray. Pick up the catheter several inches back from the tip to keep the tip sterile. If a collecting bag is not attached, be sure to keep the end of the catheter in the tray.	This is to maintain the sterility of the catheter and prevent urine from spilling onto the area.
19. Insert the lubricated catheter smoothly, approximately 2 to 3 inches (5 to 8 cm) into the female and 10 to 12 inches (25 to 30 cm) into the male (Fig. 27-8). This distance places the end of the catheter beyond the urethra into the bladder. Do not use force. If you encounter resistance, ask the patient to breathe deeply (to relax the muscles), and gently rotate the catheter to see if it will advance. If it still will not enter, consult a physician before trying again. It is possible to damage the urethra and the urinary sphincters by pushing against resistant tissue. Once urine returns in the tubing, insert the catheter 1 inch (2 to 3 cm) farther. (Note length of insertion for male in Figure 27-8.)	The catheter must be inserted far enough to be inside the bladder, not in the urethra. The return of urine indicates that the catheter is in the bladder, and the extra inch ensures that the balloon does not inflate in the urethra.

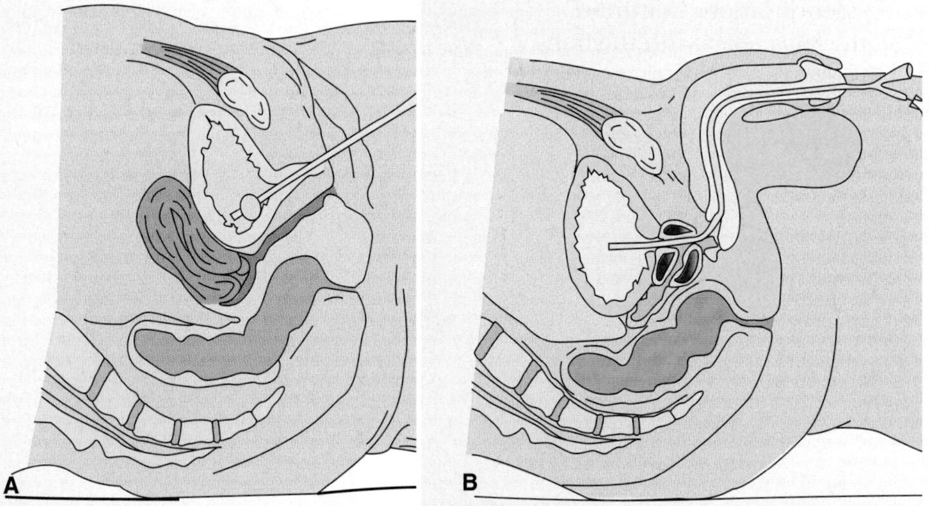

FIGURE 27-8 (**A**) The lubricated catheter is inserted approximately 2 to 3 inches (5 to 8 cm) into the female and (**B**) 10 to 12 inches (25 to 30 cm) into the male. These distances place the end of the catheter beyond the urethra into the bladder.

(continued)

Action	Rationale
20. If you are using a straight catheter, hold the catheter in place with the nondominant hand while you allow urine to fill the specimen container, then drain the bladder fully into the basin that is in the set, pinch the catheter closed to prevent further dripping, and remove the catheter. Some facilities have a policy that no more than 1,000 mL is drained at one time.	Urine left in the bladder is a reservoir for microbial growth. If the patient is having difficulty voiding, leaving stagnant urine in the bladder contributes to urinary tract infection. If the bladder has been stretched by more than 1,000 mL, there may be discomfort and even bladder spasm with rapid removal.
21. If you are inserting an indwelling catheter, release the labia, and hold the catheter in place with your nondominant hand. Then pick up the syringe with the dominant hand, and fill the balloon. The catheter can continue to drain into the receptacle while this is being done. Use the amount of fluid indicated on the catheter itself plus 4 or 5 mL.	Because the fluid must fill the tube leading to the balloon as well as the balloon itself, you will need this extra amount. Manufacturers indicate that balloons will not overinflate or rupture from using this amount. If you use too little fluid, the catheter may slip out. Check the security of the catheter by gently pulling it until you feel resistance.
22. In most indwelling catheter sets, the bag is attached to the catheter. If it is not, connect the bag at this time. Be sure to maintain the sterility of the ends of the tubing at the connecting point.	This is to establish the closed sterile drainage system.
23. Place the tubing over the top of the patient's thigh, so the leg does not occlude the tubing; then tape the catheter to the patient, or use a catheter-securing device to hold the catheter in place. *For a male,* tape the catheter without tension to the side of the lower abdomen or upper thigh. *For a female,* tape the catheter to the inner thigh. A commercial catheter-securing device is also available (Fig. 27-9).	Taping prevents pulling on the neck of the bladder as the patient moves and secures the catheter where it will drain. The position for the male patient prevents the formation of a fistula at the penile-scrotal angle.

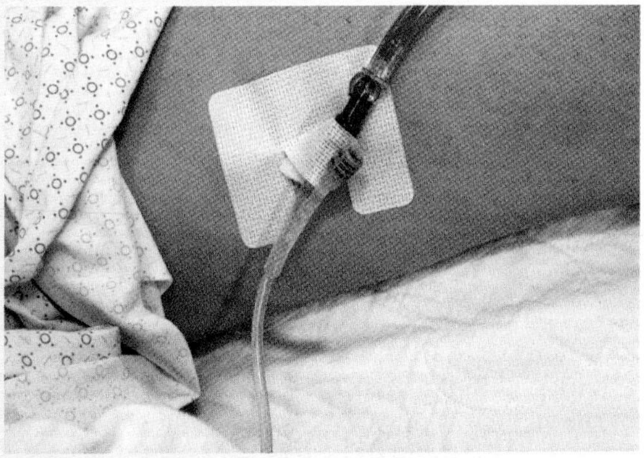

FIGURE 27-9 Securing a catheter. To decrease the chance of a tape strip pulling loose, the catheter is secured in a loop of tape, leg straps, or a peel-off patch of interlocking mesh fastener. Alternately, the catheter may be attached by using a combination of tape and rubber band.

(continued)

Action	*Rationale*
24. Coil excess tubing flatly on the bed, and attach the tubing to the side of the bed with a plastic catheter clamp (which may be included in the set) or with a rubber band and safety pin. Wrap the rubber band around the tubing, pin the rubber band to the sheet, and hang the bag on the bed frame below the level of the bladder. Make sure the bag does not touch the floor (Fig. 27-10). Be very careful if using a safety pin, to guard against a puncture wound.	To promote unimpeded drainage. Urine collecting in the tube provides a medium for bacteria to multiply and ascend into the urinary tract. Microbes from the floor could ascend the outside of the catheter. 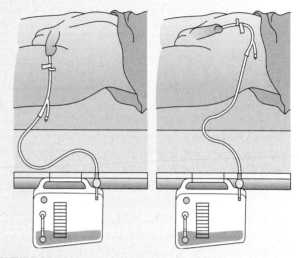 **FIGURE 27-10** The catheter bag needs to hang below bladder level with the catheter secured in two different ways and the bag attached to the bed frame. Ideally, excess tubing is coiled on the bed next to the patient.
25. Remove your gloves, and assist the patient to a comfortable position, straighten and lower the bed, and open the bed curtains.	To ensure patient comfort and safety.
26. Teach the patient about the catheter and its appropriate care. The patient may have further questions or concerns. Tell the patient that the balloon will hold the catheter in place and that it is all right to move. Stress the need for fluids (if the patient's medical condition permits) to maintain adequate kidney function. Because of the pressure of the balloon, the patient with an indwelling catheter usually feels as though he or she needs to **void**. Explain that this feeling will pass as the tissue becomes less sensitive to the constant stimulation.	Knowledge of the catheter and how it works facilitates the patient's participation in care. Understanding the cause of discomfort helps the patient to tolerate it.
27. Discard gloves and disposable equipment properly outside of the patient's room.	For infection control as well as aesthetics.
28. Wash or disinfect your hands.	To decrease the transfer of microorganisms that could cause infection.

EVALUATION

29. Evaluate using individualized patient outcomes previously identified. Include
    a. The patient understands the need for the catheter.
    b. The patient experienced only minimal discomfort during the procedure.
    c. Sterile technique was maintained to prevent infection.
    d. Urine is completely drained from the bladder.
    e. If an indwelling catheter was inserted, both catheter and drainage bag are positioned correctly.
    f. The patient is clean and comfortable.

DOCUMENTATION

30. Document the following. **R:** Documentation is a legal record of the patient's care and communicates nursing interventions to other healthcare team members.
    a. date and time of catheterization
    b. type and size of catheter inserted and volume of water instilled into balloon if relevant
    c. whether a specimen was obtained and sent to the laboratory
    d. amount of urine drained (add to the output record if appropriate)
    e. description of the urine
    f. patient's response to the procedure

▮ POTENTIAL ADVERSE OUTCOMES AND NURSING INTERVENTIONS

1. Urinary tract infection as evidenced by elevated temperature, discomfort over bladder area, and cloudy urine.
Intervention: Increase fluid intake. Ensure that perineal hygiene is being provided. Notify physician.
2. Rupture of the urethra as evidenced by sudden severe pain when the water is instilled into the balloon. If the balloon is in the urethra when inflated, the balloon pressure can rupture the urethral wall.
Intervention: Immediately remove the catheter, and notify the physician.
3. Loss of bladder tone and ongoing urinary retention from prolonged use of an indwelling catheter.
Intervention: Consult with the physician. Often a program of clamping the catheter and draining it intermittently can restore the normal fill and empty cycle and begin to increase bladder tone.
4. Catheter cannot be advanced into the bladder.
Intervention: Do not use force. If you encounter resistance, ask the patient to breathe deeply (to relax the muscles), and gently rotate the catheter to see if it will advance. If it still will not enter, consult a physician before trying again. It is possible to damage the urethra and the urinary sphincters by pushing against resistant tissue.

CARING FOR A PATIENT WITH AN INDWELLING CATHETER

The urinary tract is normally sterile. The introduction of organisms through the catheter is a common cause of urinary tract infection. Various measures are used to decrease the risk of infection.

1. Place the patient on intake and output measurement. **R:** Measurement assesses the functioning of the catheter.
2. Encourage the patient to increase fluid intake. **R:** Large intake causes a constant flow of urine out of the kidneys and bladder, which tends to inhibit the upward movement of microbes. By increasing fluid intake, the system is being irrigated internally. Up to 3,000 mL fluid daily (for the patient without circulatory problems and with no fluid restriction) is best. This quantity may be unrealistic for an elderly patient or child, but encourage any increase.
3. Maintain the closed system. **R:** Every time the system is opened, microorganisms can enter. Carry out all procedures so that the system is uninterrupted if possible (see Module 15 for a method of obtaining urine specimens without interrupting the system).
4. Maintain external cleanliness around the catheter. Catheter and perineum should be washed with warm soap and water daily along with perianal care. **R:** Secretions that build up are an optimum location for bacterial growth, which could ascend the outside of the catheter.
5. Keep the catheter drainage bag below the level of the bladder at all times. **R:** This prevents potentially contaminated urine from draining back into the bladder. Some brands of collection bags have one-way valves to prevent backflow.
6. Keep the tubing coiled by the patient's side, allowing urine to drain properly. **R:** Tubing that hangs off the bed in loops allows urine to collect in the tubing, creating a possible reservoir for microbes, which could then ascend.
7. Keep the drainage bag off the floor by attaching it to the bed frame. **R:** If the bag touches the floor, the outside picks up microorganisms that can then move up the outside of the bag and the catheter. If attached to a side rail, moving the side rail will pull on the catheter.
8. Tape or coil the catheter in a way that prevents pulling. **R:** Pulling irritates the patient's urethra and can actually dislodge the catheter and inflated balloon. In addition to causing the patient trauma and discomfort, irritation and inflammation predispose the tissue to infection.
9. Take extra care when moving or ambulating a patient. Watch the position of the tubing and bag at all times. **R:** Pulling on the catheter can damage

the meatus and cause discomfort. It may even pull the catheter out with the balloon intact.

10. Observe the skin around the meatus for irritation. If any is evident, provide catheter care to the area more frequently. **R:** This will help to prevent skin breakdown. Report your findings to the physician.

11. Empty the bag at regular intervals (usually every 8 hours). Empty more frequently if large amounts of urine are being excreted. **R:** This ensures that the bag does not overfill and cause urine to back up in the tubing.

PROCEDURE FOR REMOVING AN INDWELLING CATHETER

ASSESSMENT

1. Verify the order to discontinue the indwelling catheter, and find out if a single dose of antibiotic has been ordered to prevent urinary tract infection. **R:** Verifying orders ensures that the procedure has been ordered for this patient. Some facilities are encouraging the use of a single dose of antibiotic that is effective for urinary tract infections at the time of catheter removal to decrease the incidence of nosocomial infections. If this is the case, consult Module 44 for the Procedure for Administering Oral Medications.

2. Determine whether a urine specimen is needed. **R:** Doing so helps you plan to have the equipment needed to secure a specimen.

ANALYSIS

3. Critically think through your assessment data, carefully evaluating each aspect and its relation to other data. **R:** This enables you to determine specific problems for this individual in relation to catheterization.

4. Identify specific problems and modifications of the procedure needed for this individual. **R:** Planning for the individual must consider the individual's problems.

PLANNING

5. Determine individualized patient outcomes related to removal of the urinary catheter, including the following. **R:** Identification of outcomes guides planning and evaluation.
   a. Catheter is removed without trauma to the urethra.
   b. Patient's perineum is clean, and the patient is comfortable.
   c. Patient understands how to participate in self-care by maintaining high fluid intake and measuring output.
   d. Patient is able to void within 8 hours and at regular intervals (a minimum of 250 mL each time).

6. Obtain the necessary equipment to allow for an easy uninterrupted catheter removal. You will need
   a. several paper towels for wrapping the soiled catheter after removal
   b. a 10-mL syringe
   c. padding and a small container to catch the fluid
   d. clean gloves

IMPLEMENTATION

Action	Rationale
7. Wash or disinfect your hands.	This is to decrease the transfer of microorganisms that could cause infection.
8. Identify the patient, using two identifiers.	This is to be sure you are performing the procedure for the correct patient.

9. Teach the patient about removal of the catheter and appropriate care after removal. Teaching should include the following points:
 	
  a. Removal will be felt but should not hurt.
 	
  b. A mild burning sensation may accompany urination for a short time because of the irritation caused by the catheter. If this persists, it should be reported to the nurse.
	Explanation helps to reduce anxiety, provides the patient with information about the procedure, and maximizes patient participation and cooperation.

(continued)

Action	Rationale
c. Voiding may be more frequent and in smaller amounts than normal at first because the bladder has been kept empty and may have to relearn how to respond to a sensation of fullness. Again, if this persists, it should be reported to the nurse because it may indicate infection.	
d. For the first 24 hours after the catheter is removed, the nurse should be called to measure each voiding to facilitate assessment. If the patient can go to the bathroom, explain how measurement is carried out. Catheters should be removed during the day when adequate assessment of voiding can be implemented.	
e. It is essential to continue increased fluid intake to maintain proper kidney and bladder function.	
10. Close the door, and/or draw curtains.	To provide privacy before exposing the patient.
11. Raise the bed to an appropriate working position based on your height.	To allow you to use correct body mechanics and protect yourself from back injury.
12. Position the patient in a dorsal recumbent position, and fold the bedding back.	To expose the catheter.
13. Put on clean gloves.	To protect you from body substances that may transmit microorganisms.
14. Empty the drainage bag into a graduated cylinder.	To measure urine output.
15. Remove the catheter as follows.	
a. Place paper towels under the catheter.	To keep the soiled catheter off the bedding as it is removed.
b. Use the syringe to slowly remove sterile water from the balloon.	Aspirating the balloon too rapidly may collapse the inflation lumen and prevent deflation. Some nurses cut the balloon-filling tube of the catheter with scissors to remove the sterile water. This is unwise, because there is always a chance that the balloon has become encrusted with sediment and will not deflate with this method. If this occurs, the physician will have to introduce a special instrument to deflate the balloon so that the catheter can be removed.

(continued)

Action	Rationale
c. Pull gently on the catheter to ensure that the balloon is deflated.	Damage may occur to the urethra if the catheter is removed when the balloon is not deflated.
d. Pinch the catheter, and pull it out slowly. If there is resistance, try again to remove water from the balloon. With your free hand, wrap the end of the catheter in the paper towel as you pull it out. This action should not cause discomfort but will be felt. Ask the patient to breathe in and out through the mouth to relax while you withdraw the catheter.	Keeping it pinched closed prevents leakage and soiled bedding. Relaxation techniques prevent the patient from contracting the sphincter and increasing the discomfort of catheter removal.
e. Hold the end of the catheter up to allow urine to drain from the tubing into the collection bag.	This prevents urine from dripping onto the bedding.
16. Make the patient comfortable.	
a. Wash perineum with soap and water, and dry thoroughly.	To provide cleanliness.
b. Assist the patient to a comfortable position, and lower the bed.	To maintain comfort and safety.
17. Empty the drainage bag into a graduated cylinder, measure urine output, and dispose of the equipment into the proper waste receptacle outside the patient's room.	For both aesthetics and infection control. Urine is measured for assessment.
18. Remove your gloves, and wash or disinfect your hands.	To decrease the transfer of microorganisms that could cause infection.

EVALUATION

19. Evaluate using the individualized patient outcomes previously identified:
   a. Catheter is removed without trauma to the urethra.
   b. Patient's perineum is clean, and the patient is comfortable.
   c. Patient understands how to participate in self-care by maintaining high fluid intake and measuring output.
   d. Patient is able to void within 8 hours and at regular intervals (approximately 250 mL each time) without discomfort.

DOCUMENTATION

20. On the patient's record, document the time the catheter was removed, the volume of water withdrawn from the balloon, the amount of urine output, and the patient's response to the procedure. Also, document the amount and appearance of the first voiding and whether the patient experienced discomfort when voiding. **R:** Documentation is a legal record of the patient's care and communicates nursing activities to other nurses and caregivers.

TEACHING THE PROCEDURE FOR INTERMITTENT SELF-CATHETERIZATION

Individuals with bladders that do not empty may be able to avoid an indwelling catheter by performing self-catheterization at intervals throughout the day. This intermittent self-catheterization is performed using clean rather than sterile technique. Because the patient is not exposed to outside microorganisms on an ongoing basis, the body can defend against the few microorganisms introduced with the catheter each time. Additionally, patients in their home and working environments are rarely exposed to the antibiotic-resistant microorganisms found in the healthcare environment. Conscientious handwashing is essential to prevent infection. Regular emptying of the bladder is another factor involved in avoiding urinary tract infections. The procedure is performed every 2 to 3 hours during the day and once during the sleeping hours, if necessary.

PROCEDURE FOR INTERMITTENT SELF-CATHETERIZATION

ASSESSMENT

1. Check the order. **R:** This ensures that self-catheterization has been ordered for the patient.
2. Identify the medical diagnosis and whether the patient is learning the procedure for purposes of temporary or permanent urinary drainage. **R:** This enables you to plan an appropriate teaching session.
3. Assess the patient's knowledge of anatomy and any feelings of anxiety that may interfere with learning. **R:** This assessment provides baseline information about the patient's level of knowledge and the factors that must be included in teaching.

ANALYSIS

4. Critically think through your assessment data, carefully evaluating each aspect and its relation to the other. **R:** This enables you to develop appropriate outcomes criteria as well as preparing for problems that are associated with catheterizations.
5. Identify specific problems and modifications of the procedure that will be needed for this individual. **R:** Planning for the individual must take into consideration the individual's problems.

PLANNING

6. Determine individualized patient outcomes for self-catheterization. Include
   a. Patient understands the procedure and carries out the skill.
   b. Patient empties bladder completely.
   c. Patient maintains clean technique.
7. Collect the following equipment. **R:** Organizing equipment ahead of time saves time and decreases patient distress.
   a. A 14- or 16-French straight catheter (two or more)
   b. Water-soluble lubricant
   c. Small hand mirror (for the female patient)
   d. Small clean pan, container, or leakproof plastic bag
   e. Additional clean plastic bag for storing catheter

IMPLEMENTATION

Action	Rationale
8. Wash your hands.	To decrease the transfer of microorganisms that could cause infection.
9. Identify the patient, using two identifiers.	To ensure that you are teaching the procedure to the correct patient.
10. Review the equipment you have selected with the patient, identifying each item, explaining its use, and answering the patient's questions.	Reviewing equipment with the patient allows him or her to participate in the process and learn to plan for personal actions.
11. Review the steps of the procedure in detail.	To help the patient visualize the whole process as a step in learning.
12. Have the patient wash or disinfect hands and clean the perineal area with soap and water.	For infection control.
13. Position the patient.	

(continued)

Action	Rationale
a. *If the patient is female,* have her assume the dorsal recumbent position with her legs spread, and use a mirror to view the perineum. Elevate her head, and position the mirror so that she can see the perineum. Spread the labia. You can point to the meatus with a sterile cotton-tipped applicator to help the patient identify the structure. Later, when she has learned to self-catheterize without using a mirror, she can sit on a chair or on the toilet.	This position allows the female patient to visualize the meatus with the mirror.
b. *If the patient is male,* he can sit on a chair, toilet, or commode. He is then taught to use one hand to retract the foreskin, if appropriate, and the other hand to elevate the penis so that it is at a right angle to the body.	From this position, the male can clearly see the meatus.
14. Lubricate the catheter with water-soluble lubricant or clean water.	Water-soluble lubricant allows the catheter to glide smoothly into the meatus. After the patient becomes familiar with the process, using water may allow catheterization in settings where the lubricant is more difficult to use.
15. The lubricated catheter is introduced through the meatus, 2 to 3 inches (5 to 8 cm) for the female, 9 to 12 inches (25 to 30 cm) for the male, or until urine begins to flow into the clean pan or a leak-proof plastic bag.	This prevents the catheter from going in too far and damaging the bladder wall.
16. When the flow stops, teach the patient to pinch and withdraw the catheter.	To prevent further drainage.
17. The patient can wipe away any urine that is on the perineum with a tissue. Then he or she can stand up and redress.	To enable the patient to return to activities.
18. The urine collected in the bag can be discarded in the toilet.	For disposal. Measurement is not commonly required for the patient using intermittent catheterization.
19. Instruct the patient to wash the catheter in warm water with soap, rinse it thoroughly, and then dry it and store it in a clean leak-proof plastic bag until its next use.	The catheter is maintained as a clean item.

EVALUATION

20. Evaluate according to the following criteria. **R:** This helps determine whether desired outcomes have been met and whether the patient needs additional practice.
    a. Patient understands the procedure and carries out the skill.
    b. Patient empties bladder completely.
    c. Patient maintains clean technique.

DOCUMENTATION

21. Document the following. **R:** Documentation provides a legal record of the patient's care and communicates nursing activities to other healthcare team members.
    a. performed self-catheterization
    b. patient's degree of understanding and proficiency
    c. any problems with performing the procedure

PROCEDURE FOR BLADDER IRRIGATION

The terms *bladder irrigation* and *catheter irrigation* are often used interchangeably. Sterile technique is essential because the inside of the bladder is sterile. An open or closed technique can be used for bladder irrigations.

The closed technique is used most frequently. This ensures that the system is not interrupted, which could allow microorganisms to enter the sterile environment of the urinary tract. To use closed technique, a **three-way catheter** is inserted (Fig. 27-11). The catheter then can be connected to irrigation fluid (irrigant) by one channel and to the drainage bag by another. In patients who have had prostate or bladder surgery, a **continuous bladder irrigation (CBI)** is typically used to maintain patency of the catheter.

Open irrigation is used when a standard (not three-way) catheter is in place. It may be used when the catheter becomes obstructed by clots or mucous plugs or when medications have been ordered to be instilled. Because the system is being opened, special care must be taken to maintain sterility. Open irrigation is also referred to as "manual" irrigation because the pressure is from the hand.

ASSESSMENT

1. Verify the physician's orders. **R:** This lets you be sure that bladder irrigation has been ordered for this patient.
2. Assess for discomfort, bladder spasms, or bladder distention (palpating just above the pubis symphysis). **R:** This provides information on any underlying problem that might affect irrigation.

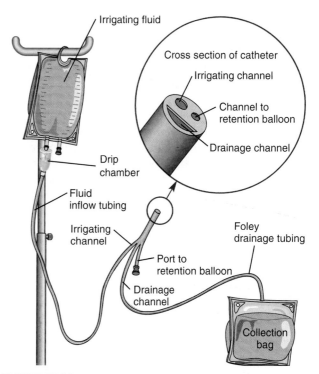

FIGURE 27-11 Three-way irrigation setup.

3. Assess the patient's current urinary drainage system. **R:** This determines whether a closed irrigation system is in place or whether an open irrigation will be needed.

ANALYSIS

4. Critically think through your data, carefully evaluating each aspect and its relation to other data. **R:** This enables you to determine specific problems for this individual in relation to the disease process. Consider the patient's diagnosis: Manual irrigation should not be performed on transurethral resection of a bladder tumor due to risk of rupture of a bladder that has just undergone surgery.
5. Identify specific problems and modifications of the procedure that will be needed for this individual. **R:** Planning for the individual must take into consideration the individual's problems.

PLANNING

6. Determine individualized patient outcomes for the irrigation. Include
    a. Catheter is patent and draining freely.
    b. Fluid returned equals fluid instilled.
    c. Patient expresses comfort.
    d. Patient remains free of urinary tract infection
7. Gather equipment first. **R:** Planning ahead allows you to proceed more safely and effectively.
    a. *For a closed irrigation with a three-way catheter in place:*

(1) irrigant in a bag suitable for hanging on a pole; bladder irrigant commonly comes in bags that are similar to intravenous (IV) fluid bags but are much larger. The correct solution is essential. Normal saline is the most commonly used solution because it does not pose the risk of electrolyte imbalance.

(2) tubing designed for connection to a fluid bag and for connection to the inflow channel of the three-way catheter (large lumen tubing with a graduated end to enable it to seal into the catheter end)

(3) clean gloves

(4) alcohol wipe

b. *For an open irrigation with a standard catheter in place:*

(1) irrigation set that contains a 30-mL or larger irrigating syringe: This might be a bulb syringe or a large plunger syringe with a tip that will fit into a catheter. This is often referred to as a Toomey syringe.

(2) container of sterile irrigant: Normal saline is the most commonly used solution.

IMPLEMENTATION

Action	*Rationale*
8. Wash or disinfect your hands.	To decrease the transfer of microorganisms that could cause infection.
9. Identify the patient, using two identifiers.	Verifying the patient's identity helps ensure that you are performing the right skill for the right patient.
10. Explain the procedure you are about to perform. Reassure the patient that irrigation should not be painful or uncomfortable. However, premedicate the patient if indicated. Bladder spasms may occur secondary to manual irrigation.	Explaining the procedure helps relieve anxiety or misperceptions that the patient may have about a procedure or activity and sets the stage for patient participation.
11. Close the door, and/or draw the curtains around the bed.	To provide privacy.
12. Apply clean gloves.	To protect you from body substances.
13. Empty the contents of the drainage bag, making sure to record the amount and appearance.	To allow for a more accurate record of output during irrigation.
14. Remove your gloves, and rewash or disinfect your hands.	To prevent the spread of microorganisms.
15. Irrigate the catheter:	
a. *For closed system with a three-way catheter:*	
(1) Close the clamp on the tubing, remove the covering on the spike of the irrigation tubing, and insert it into the solution bag.	This sets up the fluid without allowing leaking while you are working with it.
(2) Hang the bag on an IV pole, and open the clamp, allowing the solution to prime the tubing.	This removes air, preventing it from being introduced into the bladder.

(continued)

Action	Rationale
(3) Put on clean gloves.	To protect you from body substances that may contain infectious agents.
(4) Cleanse the catheter inflow port with alcohol wipe.	To decrease the potential for microorganisms moving to the inside of the catheter.
(5) Connect irrigation tubing to the input port on the three-way catheter.	To allow the fluid to flow into the bladder.
(6) Check that the outflow on the catheter is open, connected to a drainage bag, and functioning.	To ensure that fluid entering the bladder will be able to flow out and will not distend the bladder.
(7) Open the clamp, and begin the flow at the rate prescribed or at a steady rate of drip if the order simply reads "continuous irrigation."	
b. *For an open system using an irrigating syringe:*	
(1) Open the sterile irrigation set, avoiding touching the tip of the syringe.	To maintain the sterility of the portion that touches the inside of the catheter.
(2) Open the sterile fluid, and pour approximately 250 mL into the solution container in the set, and recap the container. This container should be marked with the date and time it was opened.	This amount will usually allow adequate irrigation. A sterile solution that has been opened is usually discarded after 24 hours due to potential for contamination.
(3) Put on clean gloves.	To protect you from body substances that may contain infectious agents.
(4) Use an alcohol wipe to cleanse the connection between the catheter and the tubing.	To decrease the potential for microorganisms moving to the inside of the catheter.
(5) Take the catheter drainage tubing out of the catheter. Be sure to keep this tip sterile. It may be covered with a sterile cap or placed inside the impervious wrapper of the alcohol swab.	To maintain sterility for reinsertion of the drainage tubing into the catheter.
(6) Place the drainage basin of the irrigating set on the bed, and put the catheter end into it.	To keep the catheter end clean and protect the bedding from urine drainage.

(continued)

Action	Rationale
(7) Fill the irrigating syringe with fluid, connect it to the catheter, and instill the fluid into the catheter. Use slow, steady pressure, but do not use excessive force. Allow the fluid to drain into the drainage basin. Repeat this until you have instilled and returned approximately 250 mL of fluid or until any thick mucus or clots no longer return.	Excessive force may irritate the bladder and create bladder spasms. It may also disrupt clots at a surgical site (if there is one in the bladder) and increase bleeding. The purpose of the irrigation is to ensure effective catheter drainage.
(8) Reconnect the catheter to the drainage tubing, and check that it is draining freely.	This prevents bladder distention from inadvertent blockage of the catheter.
16. Remove your gloves, and wash or disinfect your hands.	To prevent the spread of microorganisms.

EVALUATION

17. Evaluate using the individualized patient outcomes previously identified. **R:** Evaluation of outcomes is essential for planning future care. Include
    a. Catheter is patent and draining freely.
    b. Fluid returned equals fluid instilled.
    c. Patient expresses comfort.
    d. Patient remains free of urinary tract infection.

DOCUMENTATION

18. Document the following. **R:** Documentation is a legal record of the patient's care and communicates nursing activities to other nurses and caregivers.
    a. Time at which procedure was initiated
    b. Type and amount of irrigating solution
    c. Patient's response
    d. Intake and output
    e. Appearance of the drainage

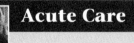

Acute Care

In the acute care environment, catheters are often inserted before specific procedures, with the expectation that they will be removed as quickly as possible. However, sometimes urinary catheters are inserted as a mechanism to manage urinary incontinence. This is especially true when an elderly cognitively impaired individual develops incontinence in the stress of major illness and hospitalization. A urinary tract infection is always a potential problem and can lead to an increased length of stay in the hospital. Additionally, the elderly person whose bladder becomes deconditioned from the presence of a catheter may not be able to regain continence after discharge. While incontinence creates the potential for skin breakdown and increases the workload of the nursing staff, the expert nurse recognizes the serious consequences of an indwelling catheter and seeks alternatives to catheterization for management of incontinence.

Long-Term Care

Some of the residents in long-term care facilities have problems with a flaccid bladder that does not empty. This necessitates a permanent indwelling catheter. In long-term care, indwelling catheters are rarely used to manage incontinence because of the adverse effects of long-term catheter placement.

Adaptations may have to be made when catheterizing women of advanced age because many have difficulty maintaining the dorsal recumbent position for an extended period. Additionally, arthritis may make it very difficult to abduct the legs from the midline. The Sims' position may be more effective for visualizing the meatus and preventing discomfort of the resident's joints. Certainly, providing privacy is always essential for any resident being catheterized, but for the elderly, this issue is particularly sensitive because many were reared with strong attitudes about not exposing their bodies.

An additional problem for older residents who have an indwelling catheter inserted is the increased potential for urinary tract infections. This increased risk may be caused by a less active immune system, poor hygiene, and enlargement of the prostate in the male, which partially obstructs drainage of the bladder. Many institutionalized elderly people develop urinary tract infections at some time; this is particularly true in those with indwelling catheters.

To decrease the chance of urinary tract infection, the nurse in long-term care settings can see that perineal hygiene is performed properly, that fluid intake is adequate, and that assessment for infection is done routinely.

Home Care

Because more chronically ill persons are being cared for in the home, it is more common for individuals receiving home care to have an indwelling urinary catheter. The person may be discharged with a catheter in place, or the home health nurse may insert one. In either case, meticulous care should be provided to prevent complications. Showering rather than tub bathing decreases the risk of ascending infection on the outside of the catheter. Home care policies indicate that the catheter should be changed once a month or more often if there is evidence of infection.

If the client can be up in a chair or ambulate, the drainage system should be appropriate to the specific client. The drainage system for the person who is not bedridden should be one that does not use rubber straps which irritate the skin, is leakproof, eliminates lengthy tubing, maintains correct positioning of the drainage bag, and is suited to the domestic environment. For reasons of client safety and comfort, the home healthcare nurse should provide ongoing assessment and education.

LEARNING TOOLS

DEVELOP YOUR BACKGROUND KNOWLEDGE

1. Review the Learning Outcomes.

2. Read the section on urinary elimination in your assigned text.

3. Look up the Key Terms in the glossary.

4. Review this module, and mentally practice the techniques described. Study so that you would be able to teach these skills to another person.

5. List the differences between a straight and an indwelling catheter, noting the uses for each.

DEVELOP YOUR SKILLS

In the practice setting
1. Arrange for a practice partner.

2. Together view the equipment for urinary catheterization.

3. If a nonsterile catheterization set is available, go through it carefully, to visualize how it is organized and to handle the equipment without gloves. This will help with your later manual dexterity.

4. One partner should catheterize a female mannequin. Go slowly to be sure that you do not contaminate the equipment. The person catheterizing should verbalize each step to help fix it in his or her mind. The partner should watch carefully for breaks in sterile technique, and make sure that all steps are completed, giving cues when needed.

5. Change roles with your partner so that you both have done a complete catheterization. Practice additional times as possible to help you become more proficient with the equipment.

6. Together with your partner, set up a continuous bladder irrigation set (CBI), and connect it to a three-way catheter.

7. Obtain the appropriate supplies, and perform an open catheter irrigation using a mannequin.

8. Change roles with your partner so that both have performed an open irrigation. Practice additional times, as possible, to help you become proficient with the equipment.

DEMONSTRATE YOUR SKILLS

In the clinical setting
1. Consult with your instructor regarding the opportunity to care for a patient with an indwelling catheter and one who needs bladder irrigation.

2. Consult with your instructor regarding the opportunity to catheterize a patient.

3. Evaluate your performance with the instructor.

CRITICAL THINKING EXERCISES

1. Your elderly male patient has an indwelling catheter. During shift report, the nurse states that the patient has had no urinary output on her shift (night shift). She further states that the patient has

been irritable and had an elevated pulse. In reviewing the nurses' notes, you discover that the patient pulled the catheter out yesterday afternoon. Compose a list of appropriate nursing assessment activities for this patient and the rationale for each.

2. Your elderly, confused, female patient has an order for catheterization. As you enter her room to make an assessment, she is shouting and flailing her arms. Specify four to five nursing actions that could be taken to ensure her safety, and identify at what step in the procedure these actions should be taken.

3. An 18-year-old woman who has had surgery has not been able to void for 9 hours. On assessment, you find that her bladder is very distended. She has an order for catheterization, but she adamantly states she does not want to be catheterized. The responses listed below might be given to persuade her that the procedure is necessary. Evaluate each response, explaining why it is appropriate or inappropriate. Then, compose two responses that would be appropriate to give this patient.
   "Your doctor has written the order for the procedure."
   "It won't hurt at all and will only take a minute."
   "I had this procedure once, and it went fine."
   "We catheterize patients all the time after surgery."
   "If you're worried about privacy, we will close the door."
   "Your bladder can only hold so much urine, and it is dangerous not to drain it."

SELF-QUIZ

SHORT-ANSWER QUESTIONS

1. List three common concerns of patients being catheterized.

   a. _____

   b. _____

   c. _____

2. Mrs. Tigerson was to have a catheter inserted preoperatively. The nurse explained to Mrs. Tigerson what the procedure was, why it was being done, and what she should expect. The nurse then carried out the catheterization. What step in dealing with the patient's concerns did the nurse omit?

   _____

3. List the four important points to include when teaching the patient whose indwelling catheter is to be removed.

   a. _____

   b. _____

c. _____

d. _____

4. List two important evaluation activities that should be noted when removing a catheter.

   a. _____

   b. _____

5. List two purposes of bladder irrigation.

   a. _____

   b. _____

MULTIPLE CHOICE

_____ 6. How far should the catheter be inserted for the adult male patient?
   a. 6 to 9 inches
   b. 7 to 8 inches
   c. 8 to 10 inches
   d. 10 to 12 inches

_____ 7. How far should the catheter be inserted for the adult female patient?
   a. ½ to 1 inch
   b. 1 to 2 inches
   c. 2 to 3 inches
   d. 3 to 4 inches

_____ 8. When you are catheterizing a female patient, the catheter touches the meatus but then slides downward on the perineum and does not enter the urethra. Your next action should be to
   a. get better lighting.
   b. clean the area again.
   c. obtain a sterile catheter.
   d. clean the catheter with the remaining cleansing solution.

_____ 9. The most essential point of cleaning the female perineum for catheterization is to
   a. clean in a circular motion.
   b. clean from inner to outer areas.
   c. clean toward the anus.
   d. clean in any manner so long as you do it thoroughly.

_____ 10. Which of the following items is usually part of a catheterization set? Choose all that apply.
   a. Drapes
   b. Gloves
   c. Catheter
   d. Safety pin
   e. Lubricant

_____ 11. A drape with a hole in it is called
   a. fenestrated.
   b. sequestered.
   c. windowed.
   d. no special name.

_____ 12. Which of the following must you chart after performing a catheterization?
   a. Only the name of the procedure and the time done
   b. Only those aspects that differed from a routine catheterization procedure
   c. Type and size of catheter, amount and description of urine, patient's response, and time of procedure

_____ 13. The catheter used for self-catheterization should be stored between uses in
   a. a sterile pan in solution.
   b. the paper package it came in.
   c. a paper towel.
   d. a clean leakproof plastic bag.

Answers to the Self-Quiz questions appear in the back of this book.

Caring for the Patient With an Ostomy

SKILLS INCLUDED IN THIS MODULE

Procedure for Changing an Ostomy Pouch
Procedure for Irrigating a Colostomy
Procedure for Catheterization of a Urinary Diversion

PREREQUISITE MODULES

Module 1	An Approach to Nursing Skills
Module 2	Documentation
Module 3	Basic Body Mechanics
Module 4	Basic Infection Control
Module 5	Safety in the Healthcare Environment
Module 6	Moving the Patient in Bed and Positioning
Module 7	Providing Hygiene
Module 13	Monitoring Intake and Output
Module 14	Nursing Physical Assessment
Module 15	Collecting Specimens and Performing Common Laboratory Tests
Module 18	Transfer
Module 26	Administering Enemas
Module 27	Assisting the Patient Who Requires Urinary Catheterization

KEY TERMS

adhesive	effluent
anastomosis	ileobladder
Asepto syringe	ileoconduit
cecostomy	ileoloop
colostomy	ileostomy
continent urinary reservoir (CUR)	ostomate
	ostomy
descending colostomy	skin barrier
	stoma
double-barreled colostomy	transverse colostomy
	ureterostomy

OVERALL OBJECTIVE

▶ To care for patients with an ostomy, using safe and appropriate technique while maintaining cleanliness and an environment conducive to the patient's dignity and self-respect.

LEARNING OUTCOMES

The student will be able to

1. Assess the patient with an ostomy to determine the purpose of the ostomy and the condition of the stoma.

2. Analyze assessment data to determine specific problems of the individual patient.

3. Determine appropriate patient outcomes for the person with an ostomy, and recognize the potential for adverse outcomes.

4. Plan effective care for the patient with an ostomy that maintains stoma and skin integrity, hygiene, and comfort.

5. Implement planned care of an ostomy and teaching relative to the ostomy in a manner respectful of the patient's psychological response to the ostomy.

6. Change ostomy pouches and care for skin around the stoma effectively.

7. Irrigate a colostomy safely.

8. Catheterize a urinary diversion in a safe and effective manner.

9. Evaluate the effectiveness of the pouching system, the functioning of the ostomy, the ability of the patient to perform self-care, and the response of the patient to the ostomy.

10. Document ostomy care according to facility policies.

Advanced surgical techniques have led to increasing numbers of patients with surgical diversions of fecal and urinary elimination pathways. Comprehensive care requires that the nurse understand the different types of diversions and the reasons for them. Cleanliness, skin care, and odor control are other concerns. Because a surgical diversion is a profound change in body structure and function, the nurse must also provide supportive care, helping patients to make the necessary psychosocial adjustments.

Ostomies drain either fecal material or urine through a surgically altered passage. Rarely does the same **ostomy** drain both. Bowel diversion ostomies and urinary diversion ostomies, although similar in appearance and in appliances used, differ in one important element: fecal matter drains from the bowel, and urine drains from the sterile ureters. Any opening into the urinary system offers a pathway for infection directly to the kidneys.

The nurse must also constantly assess the condition of the skin surrounding the ostomy for problems that can be caused by constant moisture on the skin as well as by urine or fecal material.

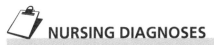

NURSING DIAGNOSES

Examples of some nursing diagnoses that may be appropriate for the patient with an ostomy include the following:

- Risk for Impaired Skin Integrity: related to skin around stoma being exposed to urine or fecal material

- Disturbed Body Image: related to presence of stoma and surgical alteration of elimination
- Deficient Knowledge: management of the ostomy and performance of procedures for care

DELEGATION

Care of the patient with a new ostomy must be done by the nurse, who can assess the stoma and plan for the type of pouching system to be used. The nurse must provide the teaching in self-care for the patient. When an ostomy has been established and is functioning well, the basic care may be delegated to assistive personnel if they receive appropriate teaching. In many settings, assistive personnel are not taught these skills, and the care of the ostomy patient remains a nursing responsibility.

TYPES OF BOWEL DIVERSION OSTOMIES

Bowel diversion ostomies may be temporary or permanent. Persons with a chronic disease of the bowel may have an ostomy so that the diseased bowel can rest for a time to heal. Others who have severe bowel injury that requires reconstructive surgery may also have a temporary diversion so that healing can take place. More commonly, a permanent bowel diversion is performed for the person who has a malignancy of the rectum or lower bowel.

All bowel diversion ostomies drain fecal material. The consistency of the material depends on the portion of the bowel that remains, the length of time the ostomy has been in place, and the location chosen for the placement of the **stoma** (the opening to the external environment).

An **ileostomy** empties from the end of the small intestine. Because a large part of the water in the stool in the ileum is normally absorbed in the large intestine, the fecal material may be very liquid. After the ileostomy has been in place for a time, the ileum often assumes a degree of this water-absorbing function, which results in a less liquid stool, although not one that is truly formed. The discharge from the stoma also contains digestive enzymes, which increase the risk for impaired skin integrity. Odor is not usually a major problem.

A surgical ileostomy technique, called the continent ileostomy or Kock pouch (named for Dr. Nils Kock of Sweden), is created by forming a pouch of small intestine to serve as a reservoir for feces for the person whose entire large bowel has been removed. A "nipple" valve is formed where the pouch is attached to the skin. A catheter is introduced at regular intervals to drain the liquid fecal material. When not accessed, the valve closes so that stool does not drain, and therefore the patient does not need to wear an appliance. Sometimes, a small amount of leakage occurs. In that case, the person wears a light dressing for absorption.

A **cecostomy** empties from the first part of the large intestine. Some digestive enzymes are usually present, and the stool may be liquid. The unformed stool moves through the intestinal tract without stimulation. A person with an ileostomy or a cecostomy wears a drainage pouch, formerly referred to as a bag.

A **colostomy** can be located anywhere along the entire length of the large intestine. The farther along the bowel it is located, the more solid the stool, because the large intestine reabsorbs water, and the colon is less active than more proximal portions of the intestine. The larger the portion of intestine that remains, the less frequent the bowel movements, because there is more space for fecal material to accumulate.

There are several types of colostomies. In a **descending colostomy** (or sigmoid colostomy), the diseased portion of the colon is removed, and a permanent colostomy is formed. In a **transverse colostomy,** a portion of the diseased transverse colon is removed, and a loop of bowel is formed, which is either cauterized in the operating room (a current procedure) or brought through the abdominal wall with a glass rod beneath the loop to be cauterized later (an older procedure).

After the diseased portions of the colon are surgically removed, both ends of the intestine may be brought to the surface. This is known as a **double-barreled colostomy.** Two stomas are formed: the proximal delivers stool, and the distal, which connects to the rec-

tum, produces mucus. The latter is sometimes referred to as a mucus fistula. Both loop and double-barreled colostomies may be temporary in cases in which the distal bowel primarily needs a period in which to heal from severe infection or surgery. The ends of the severed bowel are rejoined later by **anastomosis,** a surgical procedure that reconnects the bowel and preserves patency.

As with the ileostomy and cecostomy, the longer a colostomy has been in place, the more normal the consistency of the stool, because remaining portions of the intestine increase water reabsorption to compensate for the excised bowel. The general location of a planned ostomy, which depends on the underlying pathology, is determined by the surgeon. However, in many large medical centers, the enterostomal therapist (ET), usually a nurse, is consulted. Several factors regarding the placement of the stoma are taken into consideration. Patients should be able to see the stoma easily, so that if they are caring for themselves, they can see what they are doing. The stoma should never be placed in areas such as a body crease, near scar tissue, or by bony prominences, because any of these could interfere with the appliance's secure fit (Fig. 28-1).

TYPES OF URINARY DIVERSION OSTOMIES

All urinary diversions provide for drainage of urine that bypasses the bladder. A **ureterostomy** is an opening of a ureter directly onto the abdominal surface. Uretero-

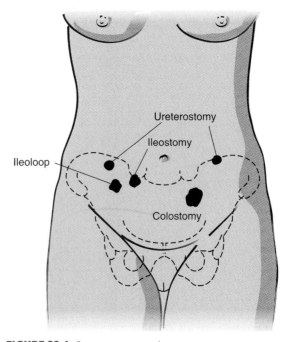

FIGURE 28-1 Common ostomy sites.

stomies can be right, left, or bilateral. In the bilateral ureterostomy, each opening is covered by a separate appliance. Another variation is to suture one ureter into the other and bring that ureter to the skin, forming only one stoma. The opening is small—about as large in diameter as a pencil—and drains urine continuously so that an appliance must be worn.

Another type of urinary diversion is called **ileoloop, ileobladder,** or **ileoconduit.** (The prefix *ileal* is also used.) In this procedure, a section of the ileum (small intestine) or some other part of the intestine, such as the cecum, is dissected from the rest of the intestine, and the intestinal ends are reattached. (Although some surgeons use sections other than the ileum, the term ileo is still used.) Both ureters are attached to this separate segment of intestine and drain into it. One end of the intestinal segment is closed, forming a substitute bladder, and the other passage opens onto the abdomen as a stoma (Fig. 28-2). The stoma is the size of an ileostomy (about 1½ inches wide) and drains urine continuously. The advantage of this type of urinary diversion is having one stoma that is larger and more easily fitted with an appliance. This procedure reduces the risk of ascending kidney infection because the mucous membrane of the intestinal segment serves as a barrier to microorganisms.

A procedure being done with increasing frequency is known as the **continent urinary reservoir (CUR).** The advantage for the patient of having this procedure is that no appliance needs to be worn. It is similar to the bowel diversion technique known as the continent ileostomy or Kock pouch. A portion of the ileum is dissected and folded back on itself to form a structure for urine storage. A nipple valve is constructed onto the skin so that a stoma is formed, and a catheter can be introduced at intervals to drain the urine.

APPEARANCE OF A NORMAL STOMA

The patient with an ostomy and the nurse, as well, must understand the appearance of a normal stoma so that changes can be identified, problems prevented, and interventions planned if necessary. Because there are no nerve endings in this tissue, the stoma can be irritated and even necrotic without causing the patient pain. This fact mandates careful and continual assessment. To avoid early complications, assess the appearance of the stoma every 2 hours for the first 24 hours and then every 4 hours for the next 48 to 72 hours after surgery. Thereafter, assessment of the stoma is a part of all stoma care procedures.

The normal stoma is highly vascular, appears red and smooth, and the surface resembles other mucous membranes of the body (Fig. 28-3). The color is sometimes described as "beefy red." During the first few days after surgery, the stoma may appear shiny and swollen. This is normal postoperative edema but should be observed to make sure that it begins to subside. The swelling usually subsides in 5 to 10 days. Meanwhile, there may be a small amount of bleeding from the suture line around the stoma in the immediate postoperative period. This is normal.

HEALTH TEACHING ABOUT SELF-CARE

Unless the patient is very debilitated or seriously ill, an important nursing goal is to teach the patient to perform

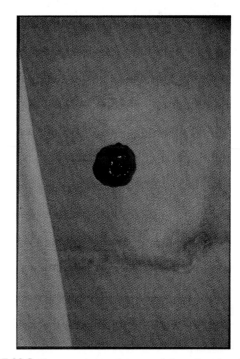

FIGURE 28-3 The appearance of a normal stoma is red and smooth with a mucous membrane surface.

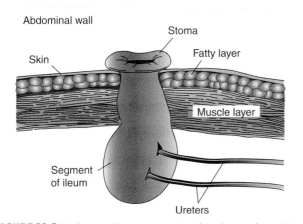

FIGURE 28-2 To form an ileoloop, a portion of the ileum is formed into a pouch for storing urine.

personal ostomy care. The nurse needs to be totally accepting of the stoma's appearance and competent and knowledgeable about caring for ostomies.

At first, the patient may be reluctant to actively enter a teaching program because of fear and depression related to the realization that such a basic function as elimination has been surgically altered. This may be particularly true if the surgery has been done as an emergency, and the patient had little time to prepare. Many patients with ostomies are not sufficiently skilled in self-care at the time of discharge and need to continue to improve their performance after leaving the hospital. Community resources may need to be contacted. Your approach in the healthcare setting should be one that is straightforward and supportive of the patient who will quickly understand the goal as one of regaining independence.

Some hospitals have a health teaching outline for educating the patient with a new ostomy. If the facility has a nurse ostomy specialist on the staff, he or she may help to design the teaching plan. Some specialty nurses are prepared exclusively in enterostomal therapy. Others are specialists in wound, ostomy, and continence nursing (WOCN). A specialty nurse is especially helpful for the person with a new ostomy because this nurse has detailed knowledge of the products available for care and is skilled in assessment of the stoma. This nurse may give instructions to the patient or be a useful resource to others on the staff to facilitate teaching the patient. An ostomy specialty nurse is the best resource person to consult when selecting pouching systems and supplies. If no specialist is available, the staff nurse must choose between the types of pouching equipment the facility stocks. After the nurse has determined the appropriate pouching system to be used, a teaching plan for using that system should be set up and shared with the healthcare team.

Before discharge, the patient should be made aware that there are a variety of care supplies and options so that he or she can make personal choices for ongoing care. After discharge, the patient may consult a representative from the surgical supply store regarding available options. Manufacturers will sometimes provide sample products to facilitate choices by the patient. Ostomy appliances and accessories can be ordered at most local pharmacies. There also are many online equipment distributors.

OSTOMY MANAGEMENT SUPPLIES

A variety of supplies are used to effectively manage the drainage from an ostomy and to care for the skin surrounding the stoma.

OSTOMY POUCHES

Ostomy pouches are the "bags" applied over the stoma to collect the elimination product. Ostomy pouches are manufactured by a number of companies, and no one type of appliance is best for all patients. A variety of different configurations for pouches are available, although for economic reasons, a healthcare facility may choose to use a single brand with limited variations. Use a clear plastic pouch while the patient is in the hospital with a new stoma so that staff can easily see the stoma and assess its condition.

ONE-PIECE AND TWO-PIECE POUCHES

While in the hospital, a one-piece disposable pouch with a type of **skin barrier** that also serves as the **adhesive** material to adhere the pouch to the skin (Fig. 28-4) is the most common one available. An opening approximately the same size as the stoma is cut into the square skin barrier. The pouches come with a measuring template that can be used to accurately measure the stoma so that the pouch opening can be cut precisely. Patients who have had a colostomy for some time may use a pouch with an opening that is preformed to the size of the stoma. Only the mucous membrane of the stoma is permitted to project through the hole because the skin surrounding the stoma can be irritated easily if there is contact with urine or stool. The mucus on the membrane protects the stoma itself from irritation. After the opening is cut, the protective film is peeled from the adhesive backing (like contact paper), and the pouch is applied to the skin.

If the stoma is irregular or if it is difficult to create a close fit, a paste barrier or a moldable barrier material may be placed around the stoma to fill irregularities and ensure that all skin is protectively covered before the pouch is applied. This also ensures that the pouch seals well across irregularities. Some pouch brands have a tape edge around the adhesive barrier for additional support to the pouch.

After discharge, patients have the option of using a two-part pouching system. Two-part systems have a solid plastic faceplate that fits around the stoma (see Fig. 28-4B). Faceplates come in various sizes, and the size needed by an individual patient may change over time as the stoma tissue shrinks. The faceplate is held in place by a skin barrier that is adhesive: a karaya gum ring, a solid-pectin adhesive (such as Stomahesive), or a liquid adhesive. The pouch has a plastic rim that fastens onto the faceplate. A belt is available that the patient may attach to the faceplate and wear around the waist (see Fig. 28-4C). The belt is designed to support the weight of the pouch as it fills, preventing it from pulling the adhesive loose and causing leakage. Belts are more commonly worn by people who are heavy or who have a soft abdomen. There are also belts for children who are

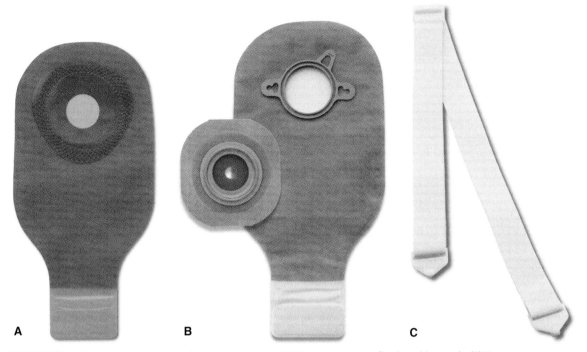

FIGURE 28-4 Examples of common colostomy equipment. (**A**) One-piece, cut-to-fit, drainable pouch. (**B**) Two-piece drainable pouch with faceplate. The pouch latches onto the faceplate. (**C**) An ostomy belt which is worn to keep the pouch securely in place.

very active and need the security of the belt to keep the pouch from pulling loose.

OPEN-ENDED AND SEALED POUCHES

Both one- and two-piece pouches are manufactured in styles with open bottoms and with closed bottoms. Most hospitals choose open-ended pouches for use while the patient is hospitalized.

An open-ended pouch is sealed closed with a special clamp. If the pouch is partially full, it can be opened and drained from the bottom. It can then be rinsed with an **Asepto** (bulb) **syringe** and warm water while in place. The pouch is left in place as long it remains secure because removing and reapplying pouches can irritate the skin. Although the clamp on the bottom of an open-ended pouch may create a "lump" under clothing, some clamps are designed to have a curved, low profile that does not show through clothing. The pouch clamp is reused even when the pouch is removed and discarded.

Sealed pouches are closed at the bottom and tend to lie flatter under clothing than those with a clamp at the bottom. One-piece sealed pouches are removed from the skin and discarded each time the pouch fills. The skin is then cleansed and a new pouch applied. With two-piece sealed pouches, the pouch may be removed from the faceplate and emptied from the top or simply discarded and a new one placed on the faceplate without having to change the seal against the skin. An individual with

an ostomy (**ostomate**) may prefer not to have to empty a pouch and would rather simply change the pouch and discard the one that contains fecal material. This may also be done during the day in a public restroom where emptying a pouch is more difficult.

URINARY OSTOMY POUCHES

Pouches used for urinary drainage ostomies that are not continent urinary reservoirs (CURs) are similar to those already described. They are usually one-piece pouches that are replaced every 2 to 3 days to prevent urinary infection. Special adhesives that cannot be broken down by urine are used. All urinary pouches are designed to drain from the bottom.

OSTOMY SKIN MANAGEMENT SUPPLIES

A variety of supplies are available to assist in managing the potential for skin problems around ostomies (Table 28-1). A paste or moldable barrier can be used to fill in skin creases or irregular stoma borders so that a seal is possible. Special nonirritating cleaning solutions may be used to clean the skin around the stoma. Also, there are adhesive removal products that reduce the irritation resulting from pulling the adhesive off the skin when changing the pouch. A variety of materials that create a film of skin protection can be used. These are not compatible with all types of adhesive barriers; some

table 28-1. Commonly Used Ostomy Products

Product	Description	Purpose
Moldable barrier	A soft, pliable material that can be molded to fit skin irregularities around a stoma. Available in strips, in ovals or circles, and in flat sheets	To ensure a tight seal and protect the skin from contact with ostomy effluent
Paste barrier	A soft paste in a tube that can be extruded into skin irregularities around a stoma	To ensure a tight seal and protect the skin from contact with ostomy effluent
Deodorant	Liquid that can be placed inside of a colostomy pouch	To decrease odor from stool
Moisturizing cream	A soft cream that is rubbed into the skin around a stoma	To lubricate dry skin around the stoma. Moisturizing creams must be absorbed into the skin and not remain on the surface where they will impede pouch adhesion.
Powders	Some skin barriers are available in a powder form to put under the main adhesive barrier.	To facilitate adhesion over a moist or weeping skin surface
	There are also antifungal powders prescribed for fungal infections of the skin.	To treat fungal infections
	Note: Body and bath powders and cornstarch should not be used.	
Skin protectant liquid	This may come on wipes or in a spray bottle.	Dries to form a protective film on the skin under the adhesive. Care must be taken to check compatibility with the adhesive product in use.
Skin barrier/adhesives	A flat layer of material that may be a colloidal product, a karaya gum product, or other material that is attached to the back of the faceplate or to the pouch.	To adhere the pouch or faceplate to the skin. These materials can be removed with minimal irritation to the skin. *Note:* Individuals may develop sensitivity to a product.

adhesive barriers will not adhere tightly with these films on the skin. Therefore, the directions on the products need to be read carefully. Hospitals do not routinely stock all these products, but they usually can be ordered for specific needs. Nurses need to be alert to the need to adapt product use to the individual's needs.

COLOSTOMY DRESSINGS

Colostomy dressings are uncommon except in the case of a newly created colostomy that is nonfunctioning. Because most colostomies are functioning, the patient returns from the operating room with a pouch in place. If a dressing is used, a sterile 4- × 4-inch gauze pad, held in place with paper tape, is usually sufficient. After healing, a person whose colostomy control is well-established may wear only a flat dressing over the stoma after having a daily stool.

FREQUENCY OF EMPTYING AND CHANGING POUCHES

Most pouches are designed to remain in place for several days and are not replaced until they begin to pull loose or leak. The more often the pouch is changed, the more the skin is irritated.

A pouch that fills completely is heavy and more likely to pull loose from the skin. Therefore, the pouch should be emptied when it is one-third to one-half full. This makes it easier to manage, lessens the potential for spilling during the process, and protects the integrity of the pouch seal against the skin.

OBTAINING SPECIMENS FROM OSTOMIES

At times, a stool or urine specimen is needed from the patient with a fecal or urinary diversion to monitor for blood, glucose, bacteria, or parasites. Even if the pouch has just been changed, it is preferable to secure the specimen directly from the stoma, because it will not have had time to deteriorate in the pouch or to become contaminated if the pouch is not new. Use a tongue blade to gently collect a specimen of stool from an intestinal stoma and a syringe without a needle to aspirate a small amount of urine from a urinary diversion. Review these procedures in Module 15, Collecting Specimens and Performing Common Laboratory Tests.

PROCEDURE FOR CHANGING AN OSTOMY POUCH

ASSESSMENT

1. Identify the type of ostomy the patient has and its location.
2. Determine whether the patient is being taught self-care at this time. **R:** This will help you to continue the teaching plan.
3. Review the plan of care. **R:** This cues you to the types of pouching system and care products being used.

ANALYSIS

4. Critically think through your data, carefully evaluating each aspect and its relation to other data. **R:** This enables you to determine specific problems for this individual in relation to ostomy care.

5. Identify specific problems and modifications of the procedure needed for this individual. **R:** Planning for the individual must take into consideration the individual's problems.

PLANNING

6. Determine the desired patient outcomes for the individual patient in relation to the ostomy. **R:** Identification of outcomes guides planning and evaluation.
   a. Ostomy pouching system is satisfactory.
      (1) Previous pouch is secure before being changed, with no leakage.
      (2) Skin is intact without indications of adverse responses to products used or to **effluent** (waste material).
      (3) The area around the stoma is clean.
      (4) Patient is odor-free.
      (5) Patient is comfortable.
   b. Patient is making a satisfactory adjustment to the ostomy.
      (1) Patient accepts changes in body image.
      (2) Patient demonstrates ability to care for self.

7. Gather the equipment needed to change a pouch or dressing, including the following. **R:** Planning ahead allows you to proceed more safely and effectively.
   a. Cleansing supplies, including tissues, warm water, a soft cloth, and a towel; in some facilities, clean disposable cloths are used for cleaning colostomies. **R:** These supplies promote cleansing around the stoma without causing irritation.
   b. Clean pouch of the type currently being used. **R:** Using consistent supplies results in faster learning for the patient.
   c. Seal or tape if needed. **R:** To prevent leakage; the tape may be attached to the pouch.
   d. Skin management materials, such as paste or moldable barrier for creases, skin protectant spray or liquid. **R:** To prevent skin breakdown around the stoma.
   e. Adhesive solvent. **R:** If needed to remove the existing pouch.
   f. Receptacle for the soiled pouch or dressing; a bedpan can be used initially. For both aseptic and aesthetic reasons, place the soiled pouch or dressing in a disposal bag, or wrap it in newspaper or paper towels for disposal outside the room when you leave. **R:** To keep the linen clean and help prevent odor in the room.
   g. Clean gloves. **R:** To protect against microorganisms.
   h. Waterproof pad. **R:** To protect the bedding from soiling.

8. Plan for teaching and patient participation as indicated by the plan of care. **R:** To move toward patient self-care.

9. Choose the appropriate location for carrying out the procedure. The bathroom offers the patient more privacy and is more like the setting the patient will use at home. The bedside can also be used and is usually more convenient for the nurse because the stoma can be clearly seen, and there is a place to put needed equipment. The new postoperative patient may not have the strength to be out of bed for the procedure. **R:** Always plan based on the patient's needs.

IMPLEMENTATION

Action	Rationale
10. Wash or disinfect your hands.	This is to decrease the transfer of microorganisms that could cause infection.
11. Identify the patient, using two identifiers.	Verifying the patient's identity helps ensure that you are performing the right skill for the right patient.
12. Explain the procedure you are about to perform.	Explaining the procedure helps relieve anxiety or misperceptions that the patient may have about a procedure or activity and sets the stage for patient participation.

(continued)

Action	Rationale
13. Raise the bed to an appropriate working position based on your height, and draw the curtains; *or* help the patient to the bathroom.	To allow you use correct body mechanics and protect yourself from back injury and to provide privacy for the patient.
14. Put on clean gloves. Wear gloves when handling any soiled material.	To protect yourself from microorganisms (or from contact with feces and urine).
15. Fold back the linen, and place a waterproof pad along the side of the patient over the bedding.	To expose the site and protect the bedding from soiling.
16. Remove the pouch that is in place by gently pulling the skin away from the adhesive barrier. A solvent for the adhesive may be needed.	Seals must be detached from the skin in a way that does not irritate or abrade the skin.
17. Note the amount and characteristics of any fecal material or urine in the pouch. Using the measuring device kept in the bathroom, measure any liquid for the intake and output record before discarding stool into the toilet. Remove any clamp for use on the new pouch before discarding the old pouch.	To evaluate the patient's elimination pattern.
18. Assess stoma condition, skin integrity around the stoma, and the effectiveness of the current pouch.	To determine if you need to make any modifications in the plan of care.
19. Cleanse the skin around the stoma thoroughly, using warm water with a soft cloth or with special cleansing wipes if they are being used for the patient.	To remove feces or urine.
20. Cover the stoma with a tissue, and change tissues as necessary during the procedure.	To prevent feces or urine from contact with the clean skin.
21. Dry the skin around the stoma carefully, patting gently. Do not rub.	To avoid irritating the skin. The skin must be dry for the new pouch to adhere.
22. Apply a skin protective liquid film if needed and appropriate to the type of adhesive barrier. Use sparingly, because a thin coating is sufficient for protection and will not interfere with pouch attachment.	The adhesives themselves and the need to remove adhesives from the skin increase the potential for skin irritation and breakdown. Some adhesive barriers will not adhere over the surface of skin protectants.
23. Prepare the new pouch for application.	

(continued)

Action	Rationale
a. *One-piece pouches:* The pouch has an adhesive surface with a peel-off covering. An opening that matches the shape and size of the stoma must be cut into the surface. A measuring guide is usually found in the stoma supplies. Often a template is created by an ostomy nurse so that each pouch is cut correctly. The opening should be just a bit larger than the stoma. Any space between the edge of the pouch opening and stoma must be filled with a skin barrier. If the pouch is open-ended, check to be sure that the clamp to close the bottom is included or was removed from the previous pouch.	If the opening is too large, the skin is exposed to stool. If the opening is too small, the pouch does not seal around the stoma and the stoma is irritated. If the edges of the pouch rub against the stoma, they will create irritation, which may lead to ulceration. The clamp is reusable.
b. *Two-piece pouches:* Make sure that you have a matching faceplate and pouch.	Two-piece pouches are manufactured to fit precisely. A pouch will not fit on the wrong size faceplate.
24. Remove the tissue from the stoma, and apply the clean pouch or dressing.	
a. If the fit is not exact, put a ring of paste or moldable barrier around the stoma, and smooth it into place with a finger, or place the barrier around the opening of the pouch.	If skin is exposed to effluent, it will become irritated and eventually will break down.
b. Carefully place the barrier adhesive opening over the stoma. Starting at the stoma, smooth it down so that all parts are in contact with the skin, and there are no wrinkles.	Any wrinkle or place where contact is not firm allows for leakage onto the skin.
c. Place tape around the edges of the adhesive barrier, or fasten down the tape that is part of the pouch if tape is needed.	Tape around the edges helps to support the weight of the pouch as it fills and prevents it pulling loose. Tape may irritate the skin of some individuals.
d. If this is a two-part pouch, fasten the pouch to the faceplate by gently pushing it onto the ring. Do not push too hard.	The pouch and faceplate must be securely sealed, but pushing hard may cause pain in incisional areas around the new stoma.
25. Remove your gloves, and wash or disinfect your hands.	This is to decrease the transfer of microorganisms that could cause infection.

EVALUATION

26. Evaluate using the individualized patient outcomes previously identified. **R:** Evaluation in relation to desired outcomes is essential for planning future care.
    a. Ostomy pouching system is satisfactory.
       (1) Previous pouch is secure before being changed, with no leakage.
       (2) Skin is intact without indications of adverse responses to products used or to effluent (waste material).
       (3) Area around the stoma is clean.
       (4) Patient is odor-free.
       (5) Patient is comfortable.
    b. Patient is making a satisfactory adjustment to the ostomy.
       (1) Patient accepts changes in body image.
       (2) Patient demonstrates ability to care for self.

DOCUMENTATION

27. Record the following information:
    a. the amount, color, and consistency of the fecal material or urine in the pouch
    b. the condition of the skin
    c. the application of the clean pouch and dressing change
    d. the patient's psychological response
    e. the knowledge and ability of the patient to participate in the procedure or ability to change the pouch independently

◼ POTENTIAL ADVERSE OUTCOMES AND RELATED INTERVENTIONS

1. Peristomal skin problems develop such as a chemical burn, producing redness and/or excoriation from contact with urine or feces.
Intervention: Contact the physician for a topical medication to treat the problem. Review the type of pouch and the material used for an adhesive barrier. A different material may need to be used.
2. Bacterial infections develop in hair follicles.
Intervention: Contact the physician for a topical antibacterial medication to treat the problem.
3. Fungal infections of the skin cause what appears to be "pimples" surrounding the stoma.
Intervention: Contact the physician for a topical antifungal medication. Review the pouching process, and make sure that the skin is thoroughly dried before a pouch is applied.
4. Patient develops contact dermatitis (rash and/or itching) from the products being used.
Intervention: Communicate with the prescriber, and change to a different type of product that has a different basic compound.

5. Stoma appears bluish or dark and dusky.
Intervention: These discolorations indicate deterioration from impaired blood supply. Notify the physician. Surgical intervention may be needed.
6. Stoma ulcerates.
Intervention: Consult with the prescriber regarding treatment. Change the pouch frequently to avoid contact of ulcerated area with effluent.

IRRIGATING A COLOSTOMY

Only colostomies that are in the sigmoid or descending colon are irrigated. If there is a colostomy higher in the gastrointestinal (GI) tract, there is not enough space to hold the fluid from an irrigation. The physician determines when a colostomy should be irrigated. For example, irrigation may be done if constipation develops or before certain diagnostic procedures. The enema-type irrigation loosens stool and stimulates the bowel to evacuate.

Routine irrigations are sometimes used to manage colostomies. However, frequent irrigation distends the bowel, decreases normal bowel evacuation responses, and depletes electrolytes. Therefore, most ostomy nurses recommend use of colostomy irrigation only for a specific purpose in the same way that an enema is only used for a specific purpose and not for routine bowel management. You will use the General Procedure for Cleansing Enema (see Module 26) as the basis for this procedure.

PROCEDURE FOR IRRIGATING A COLOSTOMY

ASSESSMENT

1-4. Follow steps 1 to 4 of the General Procedure for a Cleansing Enema (Module 26): Verify prescriber's orders; assess presence of abdominal distention; assess the patient's ability to tolerate and retain fluid and ability to use the toilet, bedside commode, or bedpan; assess vital signs.

ANALYSIS

5-6. Follow steps 5 and 6 of the General Procedure for a Cleansing Enema: Critically think through your data, carefully evaluating each aspect and its relation to other data, and identify specific problems and modifications of the procedure needed for this individual.

PLANNING

7. Determine desired outcomes for the individual patient in relation to the irrigation:
   a. Total amount of fluid instilled returns.
   b. Stool is evacuated.
   c. If patient participates, the patient understands and can carry out the procedure.
8. Follow step 8 of the General Procedure for a Cleansing Enema: Assemble appropriate equipment. The equipment needed for a colostomy irrigation includes
   a. colostomy irrigating bag with cone tip. **R:** The cone tip fits securely into the stoma, blocking fluid from returning as it is instilled. The cone does not penetrate deeply enough to injure the bowel wall (Fig. 28-5).
   b. ordered fluid, e.g., tap water or normal saline solution. **R:** Tap water may be absorbed more easily and contribute to fluid excess. It may also cause electrolytes to move from the bowel into the fluid, thereby depleting electrolytes. Normal saline solution prevents electrolyte depletion, but in the person on a low-sodium diet, this solution may increase serum sodium through absorption.
   c. waterproof pad. **R:** To protect the patient and bedding if irrigation is done in the bed
   d. irrigation pouch with long-tailed open end at the bottom for drainage and an opening in the top into which to fit the tubing and cone tip.

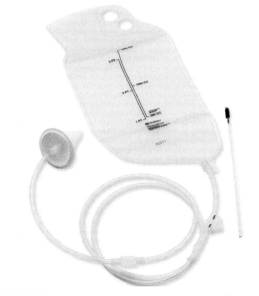

FIGURE 28-5 Equipment for a colostomy irrigation with cone tip.

   R: This bag prevents irrigation fluid and feces from flowing onto the patient's skin and the surroundings.
   e. water-soluble lubricant to lubricate the cone tip. **R:** Water-soluble lubricant is used because it is easily cleansed from the tissue by the mucus that flows.
   f. clean gloves. **R:** For infection control
   g. bedpan or commode if the patient cannot use the bathroom for the procedure

IMPLEMENTATION

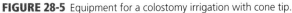

Action	Rationale
9-11. Follow steps 9 to 11 of the General Procedure for a Cleansing Enema: Wash or disinfect your hands, verify patient's identity (two identifiers), and explain the procedure you are about to perform.	
12. Pull the curtains and raise the bed, or move the patient to the bathroom. The patient may sit on the toilet or on a chair in the bathroom facing the toilet.	To provide privacy.
13. Position the patient so that the stoma is exposed. Spread the waterproof pad so that any drainage will be absorbed by the pad.	To facilitate visualization of the stoma and to keep the patient comfortable.
14. Put on clean gloves.	To protect your hands from exposure to feces.
15. Remove and discard the soiled pouch as described above.	To expose the stoma.

(continued)

Action	Rationale
16. Wash around the stoma with warm water and mild soap. Dry well.	This is so the irrigation bag will fit securely.
17. Place the irrigation bag or sleeve over the colostomy, and position it for drainage.	
a. In bed, place the bedpan on a disposable protective pad on the bed. Then place the end of the irrigation sleeve in the bedpan. Use another disposable pad to cover the bedpan as the colostomy empties, to help contain odor and prevent splashing. *Note:* Sometimes, a patient who cannot sit on a commode but who can sit in bed is placed in high Fowler's position. The bedpan is then placed beside the patient's hips. If the patient is lying on the side, the tail should be positioned down on that side into a bedpan.	
b. If the patient is sitting by or on the toilet, the irrigating bag is positioned with the tail down into the toilet (Fig. 28-6).	This is to facilitate drainage of irrigating fluid and feces. 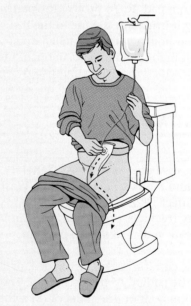 **FIGURE 28-6** Patients can sit on a toilet and perform self-irrigation of the colostomy.
18. Drape a towel or bath blanket over the patient's lap.	This provides for warmth and preserves modesty.
19. Irrigate the colostomy.	

(continued)

Action	Rationale
a. Hang the irrigation container on the IV pole, with the fluid level approximately 12 to 18 inches above the stoma. This positions the bottom of the container at the patient's shoulder for appropriate pressure.	Hanging the container allows you to have both hands free to manage the cone tip and the irrigation bag.
b. Expel all air from the tubing.	Air will cause discomfort and interfere with fluid movement in and out of the bowel.
c. Lubricate the tip of the cone.	To facilitate its sliding into the stoma.
d. Gently insert the cone tip into the stoma. The cone tip fits into the stoma only far enough to dam the flow of water. If the colostomy is double-barreled (has two stomas), you will be irrigating the proximal loop.	The cone tip is designed to prevent injury to the bowel wall. The proximal end of a double-barreled colostomy is the one connected to the GI system, and that has fecal material in it.
e. Press the cone firmly against the stoma.	The cone occludes the opening around the catheter, so the fluid does not flow out.
f. Unclamp the tubing to allow the fluid to flow into the bowel. If cramping occurs, stop the flow and wait, as you would with a conventional enema.	Rapid bowel distention may cause cramping. This is uncomfortable and will interfere with instilling the fluid.
g. When all the fluid has been instilled, remove the cone to allow the bowel to empty, and close the top of the irrigation bag with a clamp.	This allows the fluid to flow into the toilet or receptacle and not to overflow from the top of the irrigating bag.
20. Instruct the patient to sit for approximately 15 minutes. Massage the abdomen if needed.	To allow the bowel to empty. Gently massaging the abdomen encourages bowel emptying.
21. Drain the irrigation sleeve, and then rinse it by pouring fluid in the top and allowing it to empty out the bottom.	Rinsing the irrigating sleeve lessens the potential for dripping fecal material on the patient or surroundings.
22. Turn up the bottom of the irrigating sleeve, and fasten it closed. Leave this in place for approximately 30 to 45 minutes. The patient may get up and move about during this time.	To ensure that all the irrigant has been expelled.
23. Remove the irrigating bag, clean and dry the skin, and apply a clean pouch, using the Procedure for Changing an Ostomy Pouch (above).	

(continued)

Action	Rationale
24. Clean all the equipment, dry it, and put it away for future use.	Irrigating equipment, such as enema equipment, is used only for the individual patient but may be washed and reused if needed.
25. Remove gloves, and wash or disinfect your hands.	To decrease the transfer of microorganisms.

EVALUATION

26. Evaluate using the desired patient outcomes previously identified. **R:** Evaluation in relation to desired outcomes is essential for planning future care.
    a. The total amount of fluid instilled returns.
    b. Stool is evacuated.
    c. If the patient participated, the patient understood and was able to carry out the procedure.

DOCUMENTATION

27. Record the irrigation procedure, including the amount of fluid instilled and returned, a description of stool returned, and the patient's reaction. **R:** The patient's record is the legal record of all care provided.
28. Document the patient's level of knowledge and ability to carry out the procedure. **R:** This will facilitate further teaching by other members of the healthcare team.

▪ POTENTIAL ADVERSE OUTCOMES AND RELATED INTERVENTIONS

1. The fluid does not return.
Intervention: First, try to siphon fluid back. Do not instill additional fluid. Watch the patient carefully for later fluid return.
2. No stool returns.
Intervention: Consult with the physician. A large-volume irrigation is not usually repeated without specific consultation with the physician because of electrolyte depletion.
3. The fluid flows out as fast as you put it in, which will not promote adequate emptying of the bowel.
Intervention: Stop the irrigation, and devise a better way to occlude the stoma opening before you begin again.
4. A patient with an old colostomy tells you he or she uses a lot more fluid than you are planning to use. (Some patients increase the amount of fluid instilled on their own at home, and some have been known to instill 4,000 to 5,000 mL and to take 2 hours for an irrigation.)
Intervention: Explain the rationale for the procedure as you are going to do it. Then consult with the physician. You may have to increase the amount of fluid to obtain any results.

5. The patient states that he or she always inserts a traditional enema catheter 8 or 10 inches into the colostomy.
Intervention: Explain the rationale for the short distance, and do not insert the catheter any further. The patient should be provided with information on obtaining an appropriate colostomy irrigation set with a cone tip if he or she will need an irrigation while at home.

PROCEDURE FOR CATHETERIZATION OF A URINARY DIVERSION

The procedure for catheterizing the stoma of a urinary diversion is similar to that used for the Procedure for Intermittent Self-Catheterization but with some modifications. A clean technique is used for this procedure. The mucous membrane of the ileal pouch is fairly resistant to infection caused by microorganisms that may be introduced to the urinary tract. Also, the time between catheterizations allows the patient's immune system to remain active in fighting off infection. It must be remembered that resistance to pathogens is not as active in persons who are ill or debilitated.

ASSESSMENT

1. Check the physician's order. **R:** You need to be sure that catheterization of the urinary drainage ostomy has been ordered for the patient.
2. Identify the medical diagnosis and whether the patient is learning the procedure for purposes of temporary or permanent urinary drainage. **R:** This enables you to plan teaching appropriately.
3. Assess the patient's knowledge of own anatomy and any feelings of anxiety that may interfere with learning. This provides baseline information about the patient's level of knowledge and the factors that must be included in teaching.

ANALYSIS

4. Critically think through your assessment data, carefully evaluating each aspect and its relation to the other. **R:** This enables you to develop appropriate

outcomes as well as preparing for problems that are associated with catheterizations.

5. Identify specific problems and modifications of the procedure needed for this individual. **R:** Planning for the individual must take into consideration the individual's problems.

PLANNING

6. Determine individualized patient outcomes in relation to catheterization of the urinary diversion.

R: Identification of outcomes guides planning and evaluation.
   a. Urine is effectively drained.
   b. The patient understands and can complete the process independently.
7. Collect appropriate equipment:
   a. straight catheter that is 12 French or smaller
   b. lubricant
   c. clean, small basin
   d. moisture-proof pad

IMPLEMENTATION

Action	Rationale
8. Wash your hands.	To decrease the transfer of microorganisms that could cause infection.
9. Identify the patient, using two identifiers.	To ensure that you are teaching the procedure to the correct patient.
10. Review the equipment you have selected with the patient, identifying each item, explaining its use, and answering the patient's questions.	Reviewing equipment with the patient allows him or her to participate in the process and learn how to plan for personal actions.
11. Review the steps of the procedure in detail.	This helps the patient visualize the whole process as a step in learning.
12. Have the patient wash or disinfect hands and the peristomal area.	For infection control.
13. Have the patient sit in a comfortable position; this could be on a straight-backed chair or on the toilet or commode with the protective drape under the stoma across the lap.	To avoid soiling the patient's clothing or surroundings with urine.
14. Lubricate the catheter with either lubricating jelly or clean water.	To facilitate insertion of the catheter.
15. Have the patient introduce the catheter through the urinary diversion stoma 2 to 3 inches or until the urine begins to flow into a small pan or a leak-proof plastic bag.	Inserting the catheter too far could cause injury to the mucosa.
16. When the flow stops, instruct the patient to pinch and withdraw the catheter.	To prevent drainage of urine onto the skin.
17. The patient can wipe away any urine that is on the skin with a tissue.	For cleanliness and comfort.

(continued)

Action	Rationale
18. The urine collected may be measured and then be discarded in the toilet.	To dispose of the urine. Measurement is not commonly required for the patient catheterizing a well-established urinary diversion but is required for a new urinary diversion.
19. The patient washes the catheter in warm water with soap and rinses it thoroughly.	This is a clean procedure and does not need sterile equipment.

EVALUATION

20. Evaluate using the individualized patient outcomes previously identified. **R:** Evaluation in relation to desired outcomes is essential for planning future care.
    a. Urine is effectively drained.
    b. The patient understands and can complete the process independently.

DOCUMENTATION

21. Document the following. **R:** Documentation is a legal record of the patient's care and communicates nursing activities to other nurses and caregivers.
    a. patient-performed self-catheterization of the urinary diversion and the amount drained if measured
    b. patient's degree of understanding and proficiency
    c. any problems with performing the procedure

Acute Care

In the acute care environment, the nurse often supports the individual with a new ostomy. In addition to recovering from surgery and adjusting to the major physical change, the patient is also faced with the psychological adjustments of body image and overall self-concept. Nursing care that addresses all of the aspects of adjustment will start the patient on the path toward overall health. Recognition that this adjustment is not accomplished quickly requires that the astute nurse plan for referrals to facilitate continuing care after discharge from the hospital.

Long-Term Care

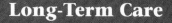

The nurse in the long-term care setting has an added responsibility when caring for the older resident who has had an ostomy for some time and may be living in the facility because of impairments other than elimination. Some of these people have been doing their own ostomy care for years but find they have gradually lost the ability to manage ostomy care. It is important for you to understand the type of ostomy and the procedure needed for a specific resident so that you can offer what has been usual and satisfactory to the resident. It also becomes vital to maintain proper exercise and diet to maintain adequate fecal elimination through an ostomy.

For those with a urinary diversion, it is essential to provide sufficient oral fluids to ensure adequate urinary elimination and decrease the risk of urinary tract infection. With adaptations for the individual resident, you can modify certain procedures in this module for use in the long-term care setting.

Home Care

After an ostomate is discharged from the hospital, visits from the home health nurse make the transition much easier. The nurse can promote self-care as the client faces what may be a new and frightening experience.

In some cases, the pouch that worked well for the client in the hospital may be unsatisfactory when used at home because of the resumption of normal activity. If this is the case, the home health nurse can consult with the enterostomal therapist to identify a pouch that may be more effective. Again, it is important to emphasize exercise and adequate diet and fluid intake so that elimination, both bowel and urinary, is facilitated. To avoid excessive intestinal gas formation, advise clients to avoid gas-producing foods, such as beans and cabbage. The home health nurse can also act as a resource. Self-help groups in many communities meet regularly to talk about the physical and psychological impacts of living with an ostomy. These groups offer ways of overcoming any disruptions in life caused by having an ostomy and have proven invaluable for many people with a temporary or permanent elimination diversion.

Ambulatory Care

People who have had a colostomy for years often continue with management techniques that are cumbersome and difficult because they do not know of other options. When a person with a long-standing ostomy comes into an ambulatory care setting for care, the nurse needs to assess the person's strategies for managing the ostomy. The nurse needs to inquire about the current equipment used, the individual's satisfaction with that equipment, and the individual's knowledge about resources available. Often a discussion of options and a referral to resources may help the client to have a more satisfactory lifestyle.

LEARNING TOOLS

DEVELOP YOUR BACKGROUND KNOWLEDGE

1. Review the Learning Outcomes.

2. Read the section on ostomy care in your assigned text.

3. Look up the Key Terms in the glossary.

4. Review this module, and mentally practice the techniques described. Study so that you would be able to teach these skills to another person. Use the Performance Checklist on the CD-ROM in the front of this book as a guideline.

DEVELOP YOUR SKILLS

In the practice setting, with a partner

1. Examine the various types of equipment/pouches available, and discuss their uses.
2. Read the instructions on any pouches and adhesives available.
3. Examine colostomy irrigation equipment.
4. Using a simulated ostomy on a mannequin, take turns doing the following procedures and checking one another:
   a. Change the ostomy pouch using the Performance Checklist on the CD-ROM in the front of this book as a guide. Have your partner check your performance.
   b. Set up a colostomy irrigation using the equipment available. Do a mock irrigation if possible, using the mannequin.
5. When you have mastered these skills, ask your instructor to check your performance.

DEMONSTRATE YOUR SKILLS

In the clinical setting

1. Arrange with an instructor to make rounds with an ostomy specialty nurse.
2. Arrange with your instructor to perform any of the following procedures for a patient with an ostomy:
   a. changing an ostomy pouch
   b. teaching the procedure for changing an ostomy pouch
   c. performing a colostomy irrigation
   d. teaching the irrigation of a colostomy
3. Ask your instructor to evaluate your performance.

CRITICAL THINKING EXERCISES

1. You are preparing to change the colostomy pouch for an 80-year-old resident who has just transferred to your long-term care facility for recuperation after surgery. When you checked the pouch, you noted a strong odor in the room and leakage on the patient's clothing. What might be contributing factors for these problems? What changes might you consider in the pouching system to alleviate these problems?
2. You are to teach two patients to change their own colostomy pouches. The first patient is a 72-year-old male gas station owner who had his colon and rectum removed because of cancer. The second patient is a 23-year-old female college student who had a portion of her colon resected because of a chronic inflammation of the bowel. Analyze how and why your teaching methods might be similar or different for these two patients. Contrast both physical and psychosocial concerns.

SELF-QUIZ
SHORT-ANSWER QUESTIONS

1. What is an ileostomy?

   _____

2. What special problems does a patient with an ileostomy have?

   _____

3. Describe the appearance of a normal stoma.

   _____

4. Describe a continent urinary reservoir (CUR) and the major advantage it provides for the patient.

   _____

   _____

5. What is the best position for the patient having a colostomy irrigation?

   _____

6. How many milliliters of fluid are used for a colostomy irrigation?

_____

7. How long should the patient remain on the toilet after the irrigation fluid is instilled?

_____

8. After the initial draining, how long should the irrigation pouch be left in place before the clean appliance is applied?

_____

9. Why is special attention to cleanliness necessary when changing a urinary drainage appliance?

_____

10. What are two important services provided by the home health nurse to the person with an ostomy who has been recently discharged from the hospital?

a. _____

b. _____

MULTIPLE CHOICE

_____ **11.** What product is best to manage an indented scar on the abdomen near an ostomy?

a. A skin protectant liquid
b. A barrier paste
c. A two-piece ostomy system
d. A protectant powder on the skin

_____ **12.** When assessing a new stoma immediately after surgery, what is the expected appearance?
a. Red, swollen, smooth surface
b. Red and beefy in appearance
c. Raw and weeping
d. Pale pink and dry

_____ **13.** How often should the patient plan to change the ostomy pouch?
a. Daily
b. Every time stool is in the bag
c. Every other day
d. When the pouch loosens and may leak

_____ **14.** The patient refuses to look at the ostomy and does not want to participate in self-care. What is the most likely underlying cause of this behavior?
a. Body image disturbance
b. Regression
c. Major depression
d. Rejection

Answers to Self-Quiz questions appear in the back of this book.

Inserting and Maintaining a Nasogastric Tube

SKILLS INCLUDED IN THIS MODULE

Procedure for Inserting a Nasogastric Tube
Procedure for Irrigating a Nasogastric Tube
Procedure for Removing a Nasogastric Tube

PREREQUISITE MODULES

Module 1	An Approach to Nursing Skills
Module 2	Documentation
Module 3	Basic Body Mechanics
Module 4	Basic Infection Control
Module 7	Providing Hygiene
Module 13	Monitoring Intake and Output
Module 14	Nursing Physical Assessment

KEY TERMS

aspirate	nasogastric tube
bulb syringe	patent
dyspnea	peristalsis
enteral	pharynx
gag reflex	silicone
gastric sump tube	sternum
intubation	stylet
lavage	trachea
Levin tube	xyphoid process
lumen	

OVERALL OBJECTIVES

▸ To insert different types of nasogastric tubes to enable gastric suctioning, irrigation of the stomach, or the instillation of enteral feedings and/or medications.
▸ To irrigate nasogastric tubes to maintain patency.
▸ To remove nasogastric tubes safely.

LEARNING OUTCOMES

The student will be able to

1. Assess the patient effectively to determine the need for a nasogastric (NG) tube and the purpose of the tube.

2. Analyze assessment data to determine any special problems or concerns that must be addressed before inserting an NG tube.

3. Determine appropriate patient outcomes of nasogastric **intubation** and/or irrigation or removal and the potential adverse outcomes that may occur.

4. Choose the appropriate equipment based on the purpose of the tube, and identify assistance that will be needed.

5. Insert and maintain an NG tube, ensuring comfort and safety for the patient and maintaining safety for the nurse.

6. Evaluate correct placement of the NG tube, patency of the tube, and the comfort of the patient.

7. Remove an NG tube that is in place.

8. Evaluate the patient's response to the various procedure(s).

9. Document the nasogastric intubation, irrigation, or tube removal in the patient's plan of care and in the patient's record as appropriate.

A **nasogastric** (NG) **tube** is inserted to decompress and drain the stomach before or after surgery, or to **lavage** (wash out) the stomach. When suction is applied to the tube, gastric secretions and any accumulated gas are removed, preventing nausea and vomiting and making the patient more comfortable. After abdominal surgeries and other major stressors to the body, the gastrointestinal (GI) system may cease **peristalsis,** allowing secretions and gas to accumulate. Distention from these accumulated secretions and gas is not only uncomfortable but can also place tension on an abdominal suture line, increasing the risk for disrupting the wound and for nausea and vomiting as well. To prevent these conditions, the physician may order an NG tube inserted immediately before surgery or to be inserted during the surgical procedure.

A large-bore NG tube may also be used on a short-term basis to instill liquid nourishment and medications for the patient who cannot swallow without aspirating or who cannot eat by mouth. Because many patients cannot take food orally after surgery or during a chronic illness, continuous **enteral** nutrition provided via a tube is sometimes necessary. For these patients, a smaller bore feeding tube or a gastrostomy tube may be used. In some instances, these feedings may be continued in a long-term care facility or in the home. Physical and muscular debilitation caused by stroke is a common condition that may necessitate tube feeding for an extended time.

Most healthcare professionals consider the use of an NG tube a routine procedure, but it can be frightening and unfamiliar to patients and their families. It is the nurse's responsibility to help patients overcome their anxieties about the tube's insertion and removal and to make these procedures as comfortable as possible. All patients with NG tubes in place for treatment should have their intake and output monitored.

NURSING DIAGNOSES

Patients may need an NG tube for a variety of nursing diagnoses.

- Impaired Swallowing: related to decreased neuromuscular control of the mouth and throat. The person with a stroke, one with a brain tumor, or other disorder that disturbs neuromuscular control may have difficulty swallowing. The nurse is often the individual who identifies that the patient is choking on food or food is being pocketed in the cheek and not swallowed.

- Risk for Aspiration: related to impaired swallowing. The patient with impaired swallowing always is at risk for aspiration. Aspiration may be noticed with coughing and choking, but the severely impaired person may **aspirate** silently.

- Impaired Comfort: related to presence of an NG tube. Once an NG tube is in place, the patient may experience discomfort of the nose and throat and also of the nares (nostrils), where the tube may cause irritation. This is a more pronounced problem with larger tubes made of a harder plastic material.

The insertion of NG tubes is not delegated to assistive personnel because they lack the background education in anatomy and physiology to insert the tube and to understand all the potential complications. Assistive personnel may care for the patient with an NG tube in place, but the insertion, irrigation, and removal of the tube are the responsibility of the nurse.

TYPES OF NASOGASTRIC TUBES

There are different types of NG tubes based on their differing purposes. They may be made of rubber, plastic, or **silicone.** The tube diameter, or **lumen,** also varies; lumen sizes range from small (5 French) to quite large (18 French).

NASOGASTRIC TUBES FOR SUCTION OR IRRIGATION

For gastric suction and irrigation, a firm plastic tube, size 12 French, is often used for adult patients. A very-large-bore NG tube, such as an Ewald tube, between size 29 and 36 French, is used for emergency treatment if a patient has ingested toxic substances and the stomach must be emptied through lavage. This is most frequently seen in the emergency department, where the emergency physician may insert the tube and begin the procedure with the nurse continuing the process once the physician determines that the patient does not need further medical intervention immediately.

The **Levin tube** is a commonly used single-lumen NG tube (Fig. 29-1). A double-lumen tube, the **gastric sump tube** (also called a Salem sump tube), has one smaller lumen that is used as an air vent and another larger lumen used to drain gastric contents or ingested air. Its advantage is that the smaller lumen (color-coded blue) is left open to room air, allowing equalization of pressure and therefore continuous, steady suction without pull on the tissues. Suction pull above the level of capillary fragility, which can damage tissues, is prevented (see Fig. 29-1). An antireflux valve may be put in this lumen to prevent gastric contents from siphoning out.

SMALL-BORE, SILICONE FEEDING TUBES

A variety of small-bore, silicone tubes are available to use for **enteral** feeding. Their soft material and small size are less irritating to the nose and throat. In addition, the cardiac sphincter closes more tightly around them, lessening the possibility of regurgitation and aspiration. Their softness and small size make them more comfortable for the patient. They usually come with a firm metal **stylet** threaded through the lumen, which facilitates insertion. Final positioning is verified by x-ray film with the stylet in place. Then the stylet is removed. The stylet should be saved because the tube might be removed or pulled out and need to be reinserted. A weighted tube

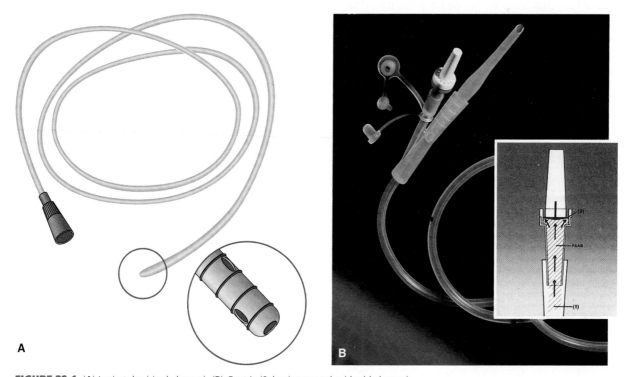

FIGURE 29-1 (**A**) Levin tube (single lumen). (**B**) Gastric (Salem) sump tube (double lumen).

will move with peristalsis into the small intestine if the tube is not taped with tension to the patient's nose. This feature makes it especially suitable for delivering enteral feedings. See Table 29-1 for a summary of tube types and uses.

PROCEDURE FOR INSERTING A NASOGASTRIC TUBE

ASSESSMENT

1. Validate the medical orders in the patient's record. **R:** This determines the type of tube to be inserted and the reason for insertion of the tube, such as decompression, suctioning, or instillation of nutrition or medication.
2. Assess the patient's mental and physical status. **R:** Assessment helps determine if there are problems that may need to be considered prior to NG intubation. There may be facial injuries or abnormalities that need to be considered. Mental status will determine whether the patient can assist in the procedure.

ANALYSIS

3. Critically think through your assessment data, carefully evaluating each aspect and its relation to other data. **R:** This enables you to determine specific problems for this individual in relation to NG intubation.
4. Identify specific problems and modifications of the procedure that may be needed for the individual. **R:** Planning for the individual must take into consideration the individual's problems.

PLANNING

5. Determine desired outcomes for the individual patient in relation to the insertion of an NG tube:

table 29-1. Types of Nasogastric Tubes

Type	Purpose	Sizes	Composition
Levin	Decompression Medication administration	5–18 French (diameter)	Flexible plastic or rubber Single lumen
Salem sump	Decompression	5–18 French (diameter)	Flexible plastic Double lumen
Small-bore silicone	Enteral nutrition Medication administration	5–12 French (diameter) 22–60 inches (length)	Soft silicone Metal stylet Weighted/nonweighted

Note: Special purpose tubes include the Ewald, Cantor, and Miller-Abbott tubes. They are used infrequently on nursing units and are commonly inserted by the physician when needed as part of the medical plan of care.

a. The tube is accurately positioned.
b. The rate and rhythm of breathing are normal.
c. The patient is comfortable.
d. There is no irritation at the nostrils.
e. There is no indication of nausea or regurgitation.

6. Locate the equipment. **R:** Some items may not be kept on the unit and will need to be ordered from the central supply department.
7. Gather the equipment, including suction equipment or equipment related to providing nutrition as indicated prior to beginning the procedure. In addition to the tube, you will need the following:

Safety Alert

Note: *If inserting a small-bore feeding tube, be sure that the internal stylet is not protruding through the holes in the tube.* R: *This could cause tissue irritation or damage.*

---

a. clean gloves to protect yourself from body secretions
b. water-soluble lubricant, which, if aspirated, will not cause aspiration pneumonia
c. emesis basin in case the patient vomits
d. tape or adhesive bandage (such as a Coverlet) to secure the tube to the patient's nose
e. tissues for patient's secretions
f. bath towel to protect the patient and linen from gastric secretions
g. a glass of water and straw to help the patient swallow the tube
h. large syringe with an adapter or a **bulb syringe** for aspiration if necessary
i. stethoscope
j. rubber band and safety pin to attach the tube to the patient's gown
k. To set up suction, you will need the following:
   (1) a source of negative pressure (either wall suction or a portable suction machine)
   (2) a connecting tube with adapter
   (3) a suction container (to receive gastric contents)

8. Plan for any assistance you will need to perform the procedure. **R:** Extra support and encouragement during the procedure may be appreciated by the patient. A confused or disoriented patient may need to have assistance to remain still and follow directions.
9. If a special weighted tube is to be used, review the manufacturer's directions for insertion. **R:** Reviewing prior to insertion of tube makes the procedure go more smoothly.

IMPLEMENTATION

Action	Rationale
10. Wash or disinfect your hands.	To decrease the transfer of microorganisms that could cause infection.
11. Identify the patient, using two identifiers.	To ensure that you are performing the procedure for the correct patient.
12. Close the door to the room, and pull the curtain around the patient's bed.	To provide for the patient's privacy.
13. Explain the procedure and why it is needed.	Knowledge of the procedure, the reason for the procedure, and the equipment to be used help relieve anxiety in the patient and set the stage for patient participation.
14. Raise the bed to the appropriate working position based on your height.	This allows you to use correct body mechanics, to work with maximum comfort, and to protect yourself from back injury.
15. Assess the patient's nostrils. **a.** Ask the patient if either nostril is obstructed (history of broken nose, deviated septum, or nasal surgery). **b.** Using a flashlight, assess the patient's nostrils for intactness, irritations, and/or abrasions. **c.** Ask the patient to breathe through one nostril while occluding the other.	To select the nostril that has the greater airflow and will cause the least discomfort to the patient during the insertion of the tube.
16. Place the patient in high Fowler's position, if possible.	Gravity will aid in the insertion of the tube.
17. Place a towel over the patient's chest.	This protects bed linens and makes it easier to clean up any spills quickly.
18. Stand to the patient's right, if you are right-handed, and measure the portion of the tube to be inserted by extending it from the tip of the patient's nose to the earlobe and from the earlobe to the **xyphoid process.** Mark the tube with tape at this point (Fig. 29-2). *If inserting a nasoduodenal tube, mark the tubing again 4 to 10 inches farther along.*	To ensure that the tube will rest in the stomach. In an especially tall person, you may need to add 2 inches to the portion of the tube to be inserted to ensure entrance into the stomach.
19. If the patient's skin is oily, use an alcohol wipe to cleanse the nose.	This prepares the skin for later tape application.

(continued)

Action	Rationale
	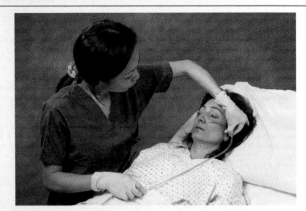 FIGURE 29-2 Measuring the portion of the tube to be inserted.
20. Put on gloves.	This is to protect you from possible contact with body secretions.
21. Lubricate the first 4 inches of the tube with water-soluble lubricant. *Note:* Some small-bore tubes self-lubricate when dipped in water.	Water-soluble lubricant will not cause aspiration pneumonia if aspirated and will prevent damage to the nasopharyngeal mucosa when you insert the tube.
22. Ask the patient to flex the head slightly back against the pillow.	This facilitates the insertion of the initial part of the tube.
23. Grasp the tube with your right hand, about 3 inches from the end, and gently insert it into the nostril, guiding it straight back along the floor of the nose. Have an emesis basin and tissues in the patient's lap.	Guiding the tube along the floor of the nose avoids the turbinate folds at the top of the nasal passage. An emesis basin and tissue may be needed in case the patient experiences temporary gagging and watery eyes.
24. Next, ask the patient to tilt the head slightly forward.	This is to facilitate passage of the tube into the GI tract. The tube is less likely to pass into the **trachea** because the glottis closes the trachea in this position.
25. Have the patient sip water and swallow while you gently but steadily advance the tube.	To assist the patient to swallow the tube. A smooth, steady advance of the tube will decrease discomfort caused by the **gag reflex.**
26. If the tube will not progress, ask the patient to open the mouth, and use a flashlight to check if the tube is curled in the back of the throat. If it is, withdraw it until it is straight, and try again. If you still cannot advance the tube, remove it, relubricate it, and try the other nostril.	This is to prevent injury and discomfort to the patient.
27. If coughing persists, or if **dyspnea** (shortness of breath) occurs, remove the tube.	The tube may have entered the trachea.

(continued)

Action	Rationale
28. When the tube has been advanced as far as the tape marker, secure the tube to the patient's nose using tape or the adhesive bandage if the tube is to remain in the stomach. If the tube is to be allowed to move by peristalsis into the duodenum, then it is not taped down at this time (see below).	
a. If you are using tape	
(1) Place a vertical strip down the bridge of the nose.	This method is comfortable for the patient and prevents irritating the side of the nostril while firmly holding the tube in place to prevent it slipping out.
(2) Cut the lower end of the tape into two "tails," and wrap them around the tube. *Note:* If you are using an hourglass-shaped Coverlet adhesive bandage, the wide end may be placed on the nose and the other around the tubing (Fig. 29-3).	

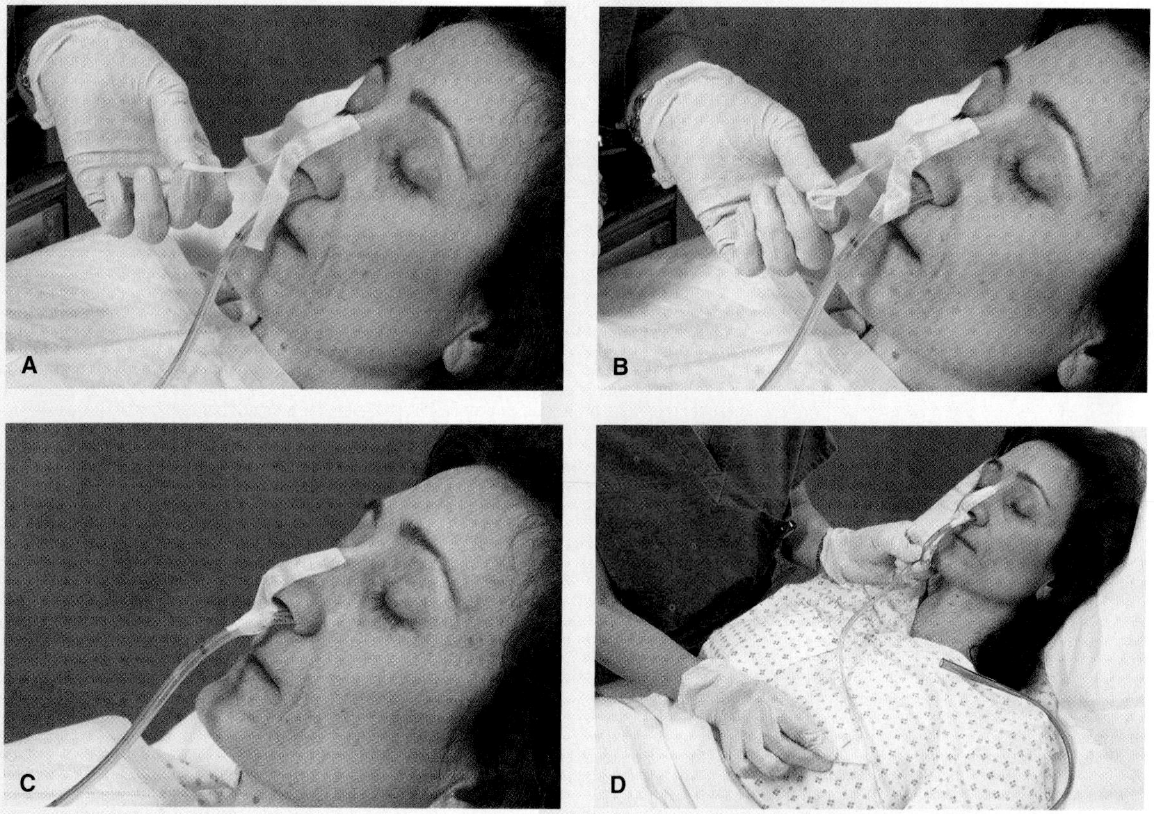

FIGURE 29-3 Securing the NG tube. (**A**) Tape torn lengthwise for several inches is placed lengthwise on the nose, with tails extending beyond the end of the nose. (**B**) The first tape tail is spiraled around the tube, which in this case is a Levin tube. (**C**) Second tail spirals around tube in opposite direction. Another tape strip (not shown) may be placed crosswise over the bridge of the nose for additional security. (**D**) The tubing is held to provide pull while the tubing is secured to the gown.

(continued)

Action	Rationale
29. Check to see if the end of the tube is in the stomach. Visualize the back of the throat with a flashlight to determine if the tube is curled in the throat.	If the tube is curled in the back of the throat, it is uncomfortable and ineffective.
30. Check for proper placement of the NG tube. See Table 29-2 for techniques. Follow the protocol for the techniques required at your facility.	Insufflating air into the tubing while listening for "swooshing" sounds with a stethoscope just below the **sternum** is usually used for initial determination of tube placement. Aspiration of secretions may indicate gastric placement. Gastric contents usually appear cloudy and green, tan, off-white, bloody, or brown (Lord, 2001). Gastric pH can be checked with a test strip. A pH between 1 and 5 (very acidic) indicates gastric rather than respiratory placement (Metheney & Titler, 2001). If feeding formula will be instilled into the tubing, the patient is usually sent to the radiology department for an x-ray determination of placement. If the tubing will be used only for suction, the x-ray image is not usually required.
31. Attach the end of the tube to a suction device, or clamp/plug the end of the tubing. *Note:* If the tube is to be placed in the duodenum or jejunum, it will be advanced by peristalsis. Leave 4 to 10 inches of the tube free before taping it. Then position	This is to prevent leakage. If the patient is having tube placement confirmed by x-ray, clamp the tube.

table 29-2. Verifying Placement of a Nasogastric Tube

Method	Accuracy and Recommendations
1. Aspirate and test secretions	When gastric secretions are aspirated and can be identified visually, the placement of the tube in the stomach is confirmed. This alone is often used for large-lumen nasogastric (NG) tubes that are to be used for suction only. Determining the pH value of the aspirate provides greater certainty of stomach placement. A pH strip is used for testing. Gastric secretions are acidic with a pH of 1–5. A pH of 6 or greater may reflect either secretions from the lungs or from the small intestine. Therefore, pH testing can confirm placement in the stomach but cannot confirm where the end of the tubing is located if an alkaline pH is detected.
2. x-ray visualization of tube placement	This is the standard for accurate verification of small-bore tubes because it provides assurance that the end of the tube is in the stomach or duodenum. Small-bore tubes may be in the lungs without causing coughing or respiratory distress. In general, no feedings should be instilled into a small-bore tube until after a tube's placement has been verified by an x-ray image.
3. Insufflation of air into the tube with auscultation over the stomach for the sound	The swooshing or gurgling sound of air moving through secretions is heard via the stethoscope. This has long been used for verification of NG tube placement, but research indicates that when there are secretions in the lungs, air moving through those secretions can be mistaken for air moving in stomach secretions. Because x-ray confirmation is time-consuming and costly, this method may be used as a general guide for correct tube placement, which may then be verified by x-ray. This prevents ordering an x-ray image when the tube is clearly incorrectly placed.
4. Placing the end of the tubing in water to watch for bubbling	This method was used for many years under the mistaken belief that if the tube were in the lungs, air would exit forcefully enough to bubble in the water. This is very unreliable. Eructation of gas in the stomach may bubble in water. A tube that is in the lungs but against tissue may not create bubbles in water. The patient with weak, shallow respirations may not breathe with enough force for air to bubble out of the tubing.

(continued)

Action	Rationale
the patient on the right side to aid peristalsis. Do not remove the internal stylet until placement is confirmed by x-ray.	
32. To suction, proceed as follows:	
a. If you are using wall suction, insert the suction regulator into the suction port. If you are using a portable suction machine, plug the machine into a power source.	This prepares the suction source.
b. Attach the suction tubing to the suction container and to the suction device (wall suction or portable suction). Turn the suction on, and check to see if the equipment is functioning. Turn the suction off.	To be sure the equipment is functioning properly.
c. Wash or disinfect your hands, and put on clean gloves.	To decrease the transfer of microorganisms that could cause infection and to protect you from body secretions.
d. Remove the plug or syringe from the end of the NG tube. Connect the NG tube to the suction tubing. Set the suction device to the type of suction (intermittent or continuous) and pressure ordered.	To provide suction.
33. To provide enteral nutrition, see Module 30, Administering Tube Feedings.	
34. Lower the bed.	To promote patient safety.
35. Wash or disinfect your hands.	To decrease the transfer of microorganisms that could cause infection.

EVALUATION

36. Evaluate using the individualized patient outcomes previously identified. **R:** Evaluation in relation to desired outcomes is essential for planning future care.
  a. Tube is properly placed.
  b. Rate and rhythm of breathing are normal.
  c. The patient is comfortable.
  d. There is no irritation at the nostrils.
  e. There is no indication of nausea or regurgitation.

DOCUMENTATION

37. Document the procedure on the patient's record, and add to the care plan. Include type and size of tube inserted, amount and characteristics of any drainage, suction pressure applied, and the patient's response to the procedure. **R:** Documentation is a legal record of the patient's care and therapy and communicates nursing activities to other nurses and caregivers.

POTENTIAL ADVERSE OUTCOMES AND RELATED INTERVENTIONS

1. The patient begins to choke, gag, or cough during the insertion of the tube.
Intervention: Withdraw the tube slightly, and pause. Have the patient take sips of water as you continue to advance the tube.

2. The patient vomits during the insertion of the tube. *Intervention:* Place the patient in high Fowler's position. Suction if necessary. Have the patient rest before proceeding.

INSERTING A NASOGASTRIC TUBE WHEN THE PATIENT IS UNCONSCIOUS

An unconscious patient may require insertion of an NG tube to relieve gastric distention or to receive enteral nutrition.

Observe all the principles described in the previous procedure, with the following important adaptations. Place the patient in low to mid-Fowler's position, again with the head flexed forward slightly to facilitate passage of the tube past the trachea. The main danger is the possible insertion of the tube through the bronchus into the lung. The unconscious patient may have lost gag and cough reflexes, so you may not accurately know the position of the tube because the patient will not cough if the tube is positioned incorrectly. An easy but effective way to avoid this problem is to insert an oropharyngeal airway into the patient's mouth. The distal end of the airway acts as a guide, moving the tube smoothly down into the esophagus (Fig. 29-4). Even if you have used an airway, carefully check tube placement. When you are sure the location is correct, remove the airway.

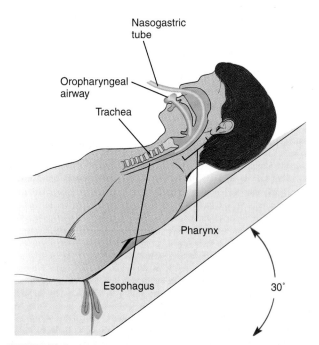

FIGURE 29-4 Insertion of an NG tube into an unconscious patient. The oropharyngeal airway prevents the NG tube from coiling forward, so the tube passes easily into the esophagus.

PROCEDURE FOR IRRIGATING A NASOGASTRIC TUBE

An NG tube is irrigated to keep it **patent** and functioning well.

ASSESSMENT

1. Check the physician's order or agency policies to verify the following:
   a. amount and type of irrigating fluid (irrigant) to be used. **R:** This promotes safety and maximum therapeutic effect.
   b. how often the irrigations are to be done. **R:** Irrigating too frequently could damage the stomach mucosa and deplete electrolytes.
2. Check the patient's record to determine whether an irrigation has been performed previously. Note any specifics about how the procedure was carried out and the patient's response to it. **R:** This facilitates continuity of care.
3. Assess what the patient knows about the procedure. **R:** Understanding what to expect will allow the patient to participate in his or her own care to the fullest extent.

ANALYSIS

4. Critically think through your assessment data, carefully evaluating each aspect and its relation to other data. **R:** This enables you to determine specific problems for this individual in relation to NG tube irrigation.
5. Identify specific problems and modifications of the procedure needed for this individual. **R:** Planning for the individual must take into consideration the individual's problems.

PLANNING

6. Determine individualized patient outcomes in relation to the irrigation of an NG tube.
   a. The NG tube is patent.
   b. The patient's abdomen is not distended.
   c. The patient is comfortable.
7. Decide whether the irrigation is to be clean or sterile. **R:** You will usually use clean technique because the acid environment of the stomach is resistant to bacteria. However, if a surgical incision has been made in the area to be irrigated, sterile technique may be used to prevent infection.
8. Identify and gather the equipment needed, including
   a. solution. Normal saline is usually used. **R:** Normal saline solution reduces electrolyte depletion. It is essential that the correct solution in the correct concentration and amount be used.

b. prepackaged irrigation set *or* 60-mL syringe with an adapter, an Asepto (bulb) syringe, or a catheter-tip syringe along with a fluid container
c. emesis basin for returned irrigating fluid
d. protective padding (towel or disposable water-proof pad) to keep the patient and the environment dry

e. clean gloves to protect you from contact with body secretions. It is also important to protect the patient from microorganisms that you may harbor in small cracks in your skin or on a minor abrasion. Sterile gloves are worn when sterile equipment must be touched.

IMPLEMENTATION

Action	*Rationale*
9. Wash or disinfect your hands.	To decrease the transfer of microorganisms that could cause infection.
10. Identify the patient, using two identifiers.	Verifying the patient's identity helps ensure that you are performing the right skill for the right patient.
11. Close the door to the room, and draw the curtain around the patient's bed.	To provide for patient privacy.
12. Explain the procedure you are about to perform.	Explaining the procedure helps relieve anxiety or mis-perceptions that the patient may have about a procedure or activity and sets the stage for patient participation.
13. Raise the bed to an appropriate working position based on your height.	To allow you to use correct body mechanics and pro-tect yourself from back injury.
14. Position the patient so that the connec-tion between the NG tube and the suction tubing is accessible.	To promote efficiency.
15. Place the protective covering over the patient's chest, under the connection.	To protect the patient's gown and environment.
16. Put on clean gloves.	To protect you from body secretions.
17. Irrigate the NG tube.	
a. Turn off suction, and disconnect the NG tube from the connecting tubing.	To access the appropriate site for irrigation.
b. Determine that the NG tube is properly placed by checking the pH of stomach aspirate, if possible.	Checking the pH of the aspirate is one of the most reliable methods to determine that the tube is in the stomach. Gastric secretions will have a pH between 1 and 5 (Metheney & Titler, 2001).
c. Draw up 30 mL of irrigant into the syringe.	This is the usual amount, but up to 60 mL may be used if ordered.
d. Insert the tip of the syringe catheter into the end of the NG tube, and slowly instill the irrigant.	Instilling solution slowly is more comfortable for the patient and is more effective than a rapid infusion.
e. If you're unable to instill fluid, reposi-tion patient, and try again.	Repositioning may move the end of the tube away from the stomach wall.

(continued)

Action	Rationale
f. When irrigating solution has been instilled, aspirate the fluid back, and discard it into the basin. If the fluid does not return after several attempts at aspiration, instill another 30 mL fluid. Do not continue to instill fluid if the first 60 mL does not return. Report the situation to the physician.	Instillation of fluid without its return may cause excessive distention.
g. In some facilities, the fluid is not aspirated. After instillation, the tubing is reconnected, and the suction machine aspirates the fluid. The fluid must then be added to the intake record or to a separate record of the irrigant. Follow the policy of your facility.	It is important to keep an accurate record of intake and output in order to evaluate fluid balance accurately.
h. Repeat the procedure if needed, instilling and aspirating fluid.	To clear the tubing of clotted material or thick mucus.
i. Reconnect the tubing to the suction machine, attach clamp, or insert plug.	To prevent spillage.
18. Remove and discard your gloves; wash or disinfect your hands.	To prevent the transfer of microorganisms that could cause infection.
19. Make sure the patient is dry and comfortable.	To leave the patient relaxed and able to rest.
20. Lower the bed.	To protect the patient from potential falls.
21. Care for the used equipment, following the policy of your facility.	If the equipment is reusable, you may need to wash it thoroughly and return it to the appropriate department for processing. If it is disposable, you may need to discard it in a specific place.

EVALUATION

22. Evaluate using individualized patient outcomes previously identified.
   a. The NG tube is patent.
   b. The patient's abdomen is not distended.
   c. The patient is comfortable.

DOCUMENTATION

23. Document the details of the procedure on a flow sheet, in the nursing care record, and/or on the nursing care plan. **R:** Documentation is a legal record of the patient's care and communicates nursing activities to other nurses and caregivers.
   a. Type of irrigation done
   b. Amount, color, consistency, and odor of secretions washed out with the irrigant
   c. Response of the patient

PROCEDURE FOR REMOVING A NASOGASTRIC TUBE

ASSESSMENT

1. Verify that the physician has ordered removal of the NG tube. **R:** Reinserting a tube that was not supposed to be removed is distressing for the patient.
2. Assess the patient to determine whether the patient's condition still supports the removal of the tube or whether the physician should be notified of the changed condition.

ANALYSIS

3. Critically think through your data, carefully evaluating each aspect and its relation to other data. **R:** This enables you to determine specific problems for this individual in relation to removal of the NG tube.

4. Identify specific problems and modifications of the procedure needed for this individual. **R:** Planning for the individual must take into consideration the individual's problems.

PLANNING

5. Determine individualized patient outcomes in relation to the removal of an NG tube.
   a. The NG tube is removed with minimal discomfort for the patient.

b. The patient experiences no nausea, vomiting, or distention after the tube is removed.

6. Gather the equipment you will need, including the following. **R:** Planning ahead allows you to proceed more safely and effectively.
   a. Clean gloves to protect you from body secretions
   b. Bath towel or waterproof pad for handling and covering the soiled tube
   c. Protective padding (towel or disposable waterproof pad) to protect the patient from secretions
   d. Tissues and emesis basin for patient secretions or emesis
   e. Disposable plastic bag to hold the soiled tube

IMPLEMENTATION

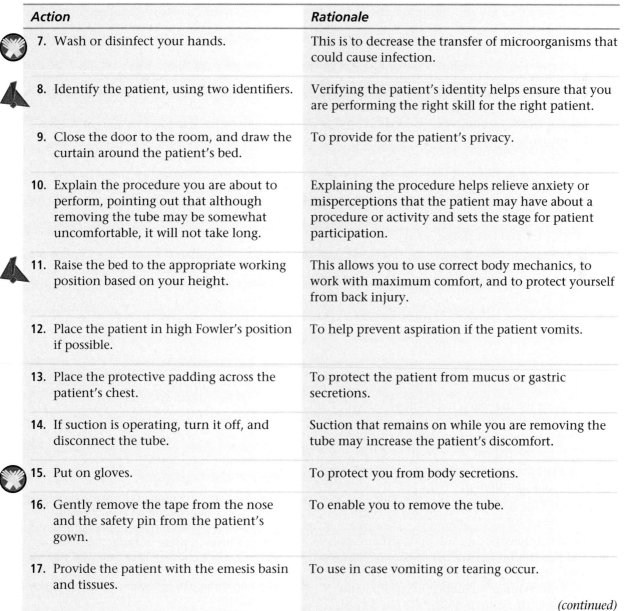

Action	Rationale
7. Wash or disinfect your hands.	This is to decrease the transfer of microorganisms that could cause infection.
8. Identify the patient, using two identifiers.	Verifying the patient's identity helps ensure that you are performing the right skill for the right patient.
9. Close the door to the room, and draw the curtain around the patient's bed.	To provide for the patient's privacy.
10. Explain the procedure you are about to perform, pointing out that although removing the tube may be somewhat uncomfortable, it will not take long.	Explaining the procedure helps relieve anxiety or misperceptions that the patient may have about a procedure or activity and sets the stage for patient participation.
11. Raise the bed to the appropriate working position based on your height.	This allows you to use correct body mechanics, to work with maximum comfort, and to protect yourself from back injury.
12. Place the patient in high Fowler's position if possible.	To help prevent aspiration if the patient vomits.
13. Place the protective padding across the patient's chest.	To protect the patient from mucus or gastric secretions.
14. If suction is operating, turn it off, and disconnect the tube.	Suction that remains on while you are removing the tube may increase the patient's discomfort.
15. Put on gloves.	To protect you from body secretions.
16. Gently remove the tape from the nose and the safety pin from the patient's gown.	To enable you to remove the tube.
17. Provide the patient with the emesis basin and tissues.	To use in case vomiting or tearing occur.

(continued)

Action	Rationale
18. Pinch the tube closed by doubling it over, or plug it.	This is to prevent secretions from leaking into the esophagus and **pharynx.** The secretions in the tube are stomach acids and therefore are irritating.
19. Pull the tube down from the nose, pulling smoothly in a continuous motion, coiling it in the towel as you go.	Any nausea and gagging that occur are increased by pulling the tube too slowly, which stimulates the posterior pharynx. Coiling the tube in the towel confines spillage of gastric secretions and gets it out of sight.
20. Provide a tissue for the patient to wipe the nostrils to remove any secretions that are present or do this for the patient.	To promote patient comfort.
21. Place the soiled tube in the disposable plastic bag, and place it out of the patient's view.	The soiled tube is aesthetically unpleasant.
22. Measure the secretions in the collection container, and note their appearance.	For accurate intake and output records.
23. Dispose of the equipment appropriately. Follow biohazard procedure for your facility.	This limits the transfer of organisms and provides a pleasant environment for the patient.
24. Remove your soiled gloves, and wash or disinfect your hands.	To decrease the transfer of microorganisms.
25. Provide for oral care if desired by the patient.	For patient comfort.
26. Lower the bed, and leave the patient in a position of comfort.	For patient safety and comfort.

EVALUATION

27. Evaluate using the individualized patient outcomes previously identified.
   a. The NG tube was removed with minimal discomfort for the patient.
   b. The patient experienced no nausea, vomiting, or abdominal distention.

DOCUMENTATION

28. Document the time the tube was removed, the volume and description of material in the collection container, and the patient's response to the procedure in the manner prescribed by your facility. Be sure to add the volume to the output record.
   R: Documentation is a legal record of the patient's care and therapy and communicates nursing activities to other nurses and caregivers.

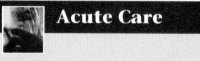

Acute Care

Nasogastric tubes are used in the acute care facility primarily for patients undergoing abdominal surgery and for those who need short-term enteral nutrition. Nurses in these settings may need to teach the patient and family or caregiver how to manage the enteral feedings and keep the tube functioning if the patient is sent home with such a tube in place.

Long-Term Care

Inserting and removing a small-bore NG feeding tube is a skill that may be used by the nurse in the long-term care setting. The purpose is to introduce nutrients (enteral feedings) on a temporary or permanent basis for residents who are unable to eat a diet normally. On occasion, a resident may have suffered a stroke or is not conscious for other reasons; therefore, the directions for inserting a feeding tube in the unconscious person are useful. Maintaining safety while performing these skills is an extremely important consideration for the nurse practicing in any setting. The same precautions must be taken so that the tube is positioned correctly and does not become dislodged. Most long-term care settings must have an outside agency bring portable x-ray equipment for use in validating proper tube placement.

The nurse may also be responsible for teaching assessment techniques regarding the presence of an NG tube to other staff members and for acting as a resource person. In addition, nurses working in long-term care who interact with families are responsible for answering questions regarding the potential risks and benefits of using a feeding tube.

Home Care

People who at one time would have remained in the acute or chronic care setting for convalescence are now receiving care in the home. The insertion of a small-bore NG tube may be ordered for introducing enteral nutrition.

This procedure may be frightening for the client or the care providers and family. By demonstrating expertise and following all safety precautions, the home care nurse can reassure everyone. Depending on the agency, an x-ray image may be required for checking placement. It is therefore important that the home health nurse review the policies and procedures of the agency.

Clear explanations of all steps of the procedure to the client and others giving care also are important. Teaching the client and caregivers about which data are needed for continual assessment aids the nurse in responding to concerns that arise. Ongoing evaluation is a process that can be shared with the client and care providers in the home.

LEARNING TOOLS

DEVELOP YOUR BACKGROUND KNOWLEDGE

1. Review the Learning Outcomes.

2. Read the section on enteral nutrition and care following abdominal surgery in your assigned text.

3. Look up the Key Terms in the glossary.

4. Review the anatomy of the upper gastrointestinal tract.

5. Review this module and mentally practice the techniques described. Study so that you would be able to teach these skills to another person.

DEVELOP YOUR SKILLS

1. In the practice setting, do the following:
   a. Inspect the various NG tubes available. Note the differences in diameter, size of lumen, length, and composition.
   b. Carefully read over the procedure and the Performance Checklist on the CD-ROM in the front of this book.

2. Working with two other students
   a. Simulate the insertion, irrigation, and removal of an NG tube, using a mannequin. Give instructions and support to the mannequin as if it were an actual patient.
   b. Change roles so that each student has the opportunity to play the role of the nurse, the support person, and the evaluator.

3. Within your group of three or with the rest of the class, discuss the experience, focusing especially on what you learned from watching the other students.

DEMONSTRATE YOUR SKILLS

1. In the clinical setting, do the following:
   a. Examine the equipment available in the clinical facility to which you are assigned. Also familiarize yourself with the suction equipment used in the facility. Access the facility's procedure(s) for the insertion, irrigation, and removal of NG tubes.
   b. Consult with your instructor regarding the opportunity to observe the insertion, irrigation, and removal of an NG tube if possible by either your instructor or a staff nurse.
   c. Consult with your instructor regarding the opportunity to assist with the care of a patient with an NG tube with suction applied.

2. Consult with your instructor regarding the opportunity to insert an NG tube, verify proper placement,

irrigate the tube, and if possible, remove the tube. Evaluate your performance with the instructor.

CRITICAL THINKING EXERCISES

1. An 82-year-old, alert woman in long-term care has refused to eat for the past 5 days. Her physician ordered the insertion of an NG tube for the purpose of tube feeding. The resident pulled out the tube, stating that it made her nose and throat uncomfortable. Identify additional assessment data that are important for you to collect. Describe what steps you might take to determine whether or not the tube is to be reinserted. Depending on what you determine, relate how you would interact with the resident.

2. A 48-year-old man has had an NG tube in place since his abdominal surgery 2 days ago. Today, his abdomen is distended and tight, and he is complaining of feeling "full" and uncomfortable. He is frightened and wants to know what is going on. What should you tell him? What should your next action be? Give rationale for your responses.

SELF-QUIZ
SHORT-ANSWER QUESTIONS

1. List three reasons why an NG tube might be inserted.

   a. _____

   b. _____

   c. _____

2. Why is the NG tube lubricated?

   _____

3. What is accomplished by removing an NG tube smoothly but swiftly?

   _____

MULTIPLE CHOICE

_____ 4. To determine the proper distance to insert the NG tube for the adult patient, measure
   a. from the tip of the earlobe to the cricoid.
   b. from the nose to the umbilicus.
   c. from the tip of the nose to the earlobe and then to the xyphoid process.
   d. from the tip of the earlobe to the nose and then to the umbilicus.

_____ 5. When advancing the tube, have the patient's head
   a. in extension initially and then flexed slightly forward.
   b. in flexion initially and then in extension.
   c. in extension through the procedure.
   d. in flexion throughout the procedure.

_____ 6. The NG tube is advanced more easily if the patient is
   a. in low Fowler's position.
   b. flat in bed.
   c. in high Fowler's position.
   d. positioned on the left side.

_____ 7. When checking the position of the tube, which of the following methods is most reliable?
   a. Introduce a small amount of air into the tube, and listen with a stethoscope over the gastric region for the entrance of air into the stomach.
   b. Aspirate the gastric contents gently with a syringe, and observe.
   c. Obtain an x-ray image.
   d. Measure gastric pH.

_____ 8. A primary safety factor to remember when applying suction to a patient's NG tube is to
   a. turn the equipment on to the low position always.
   b. test the functioning of the equipment before attaching it to the patient's tube.
   c. be sure the seals on the collection bottle are tight.
   d. never use extension cords.

Answers to the Self-Quiz questions appear in the back of this book.

Administering Tube Feedings

SKILLS INCLUDED IN THIS MODULE

General Procedure for Administering a Tube Feeding
Specific Procedure for Administering a Gastrostomy or
Jejunostomy Feeding

PREREQUISITE MODULES

Module 1	An Approach to Nursing Skills
Module 2	Documentation
Module 4	Basic Infection Control
Module 5	Safety in the Healthcare Environment
Module 6	Moving the Patient in Bed and Positioning
Module 7	Providing Hygiene
Module 13	Monitoring Intake and Output
Module 14	Nursing Physical Assessment

KEY TERMS

aspiration	nasal mucosa
comatose	nasogastric tube
distention	osmolarity
elemental feeding	patent
enteral feeding	percutaneous
esophagus	endoscopic
gag reflex	gastrostomy
gastric gavage	(PEG) tube
gastrostomy	regurgitation
jejunum	reservoir
lumen	

OVERALL OBJECTIVE

▸ To safely administer continuous and intermittent tube feedings, to recognize complications that might occur, and to intervene appropriately.

LEARNING OUTCOMES

The student will be able to

1. Assess the patient effectively to determine the need for tube feedings.
2. Analyze assessment data to determine any special problems or concerns that must be addressed prior to initiating tube feedings.
3. Determine appropriate patient outcomes of tube feeding, and recognize the potential for adverse outcomes.
4. Plan to administer tube feeding, including gathering the equipment, the proper formula, and any assistance needed.
5. Implement tube feeding safely.
6. Evaluate the patient's response to the procedure and tolerance of the tube feeding.
7. Document the tube feeding in the patient's plan of care and in the patient's record as appropriate.

The purpose of tube feeding is to enhance the nutritional status of patients who are unable to take adequate amounts of food orally. For example, patients with chronic conditions, such as cancer or acquired immune deficiency syndrome (AIDS), may experience wasting from inadequate nutrition and may need supplements that they are unable to take orally. Unconscious patients need nutrients supplied for them until they regain consciousness. Tube feeding formulas can supply them with a well-balanced and complete diet. It is one of the nurse's primary functions to carefully and efficiently provide feedings through the feeding tube until patients can take meals orally.

NURSING DIAGNOSES

Patients who require tube feeding may be assessed with problems that would reveal the following nursing diagnoses:

- Imbalanced Nutrition: Less Than Body Requirements: related to inability to ingest food and fluids orally
- Impaired Swallowing: related to stroke or reduced level of consciousness
- Risk for Aspiration: related to reduced level of consciousness or depressed cough/gag reflexes
- Impaired Skin Integrity: related to inadequate nutrition and hydration, or to irritation from a tube in the nares (nostrils), or to skin irritation or breakdown at the gastrostomy/jejunostomy site
- Diarrhea: related to tube feedings

DELEGATION

Tube feedings usually are not delegated to assistive personnel. However, licensing regulations vary from state to state. In some states, assistive personnel who have specific training may administer gastrostomy and jejunostomy feedings for the stable patient. If that is the case where you practice, you must be aware of exactly what the regulations permit and what the assistive personnel are taught. The registered nurse remains responsible for assessing the patient, ensuring that the patient is stable, and making sure that this is a well-established procedure. The nurse will check tube placement on a regular schedule and also make sure that the tube is **patent.** Assistive personnel should be instructed to have the patient sitting upright in a chair or in bed, to run the feeding slowly, and to report any discomfort reported by the patient or difficulties encountered.

TYPES OF FEEDING TUBES

Tube feeding, or **gastric gavage,** is done by introducing the feeding or formula through a tube directly into the gastrointestinal (GI) tract. Tube feedings may also be referred to as **enteral feeding.** The tube most commonly used is a **nasogastric tube,** which is advanced through the nose, down the **esophagus,** and into the stomach (Fig. 30-1).

Standard nasogastric (NG) tubes are made of firm, clear plastic and come in three general sizes: adult, pediatric (for small children), and infant. Another type of tube used is the small-diameter (small-bore) silicone

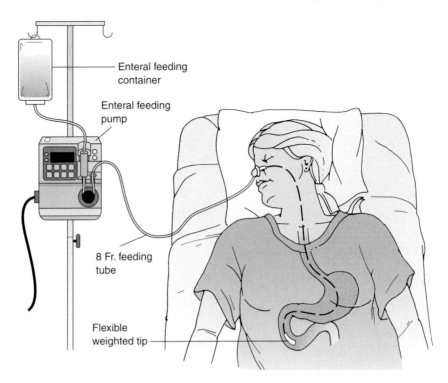

Enteral feeding
container

Enteral feeding
pump

8 Fr. feeding
tube

Flexible
weighted tip

FIGURE 30-1 Nasoenteric tube in place.

tube. These tubes are made of a white, very soft, non-irritating silicone. They are used because they cause less irritation and because the cardiac sphincter at the top of the stomach closes more tightly around them, thus decreasing the potential for **regurgitation** of stomach contents around the feeding tube. One disadvantage of the small-bore tubes is difficulty in aspirating GI contents to validate proper placement.

In adults and children, the tube is usually advanced through the nostril into the stomach and remains in place for intermittent or continuous feedings. A clean tube should be inserted into the other nostril when the current tube is no longer patent, irritating the **nasal mucosa,** or possibly harboring microorganisms. Because there are no clearly defined times, the decision to change the tube often rests with the nurse. Some facilities have a policy specifying the interval between tube changes.

For infants, such as those who are premature and who must be fed by an NG tube, introduce the tube through the mouth each time a feeding is needed, administer the formula, and remove the tube. Use a clean tube each time.

You will also be caring for patients who are being fed through a tube that has been surgically placed directly through the abdominal wall into the stomach. This surgical procedure is called a **gastrostomy.** The tube used has a much larger **lumen** than the NG tube, may be sutured into place until healing is complete, and is protected by a light dressing.

A **percutaneous endoscopic gastrostomy (PEG) tube** is a gastrostomy tube that has been placed through the skin into the stomach using an endoscope to ensure correct placement rather than using an open surgical procedure to place the tube (Fig. 30-2). These tubes may be used for those with long-term feeding needs, such as the chronically ill, the **comatose** patient, or the child with burns of the esophagus.

A jejunostomy tube is used for feedings for some patients. This tube may be inserted in the same way a gastrostomy tube is inserted, but its end is positioned in the **jejunum** (see Fig. 30-2). Because the feeding goes directly into the jejunum, the possibility of regurgitation and **aspiration** of feedings is almost eliminated, although vomiting may still occur with resultant aspiration.

TUBE FEEDING CONTENTS

Many types of formula are used for tube feeding, some offering a more balanced diet than others. Most commercially prepared formulas contain approximately 1 Kcal/mL. Some companies also make a high-calorie formula that provides 1.5 or 2 Kcal/mL. This high-nutrient content is valuable for those whose caloric needs are so great that too large a volume of the standard formula would have to be administered to provide the desired calories. The high-calorie formula is more likely to cause adverse responses, such as diarrhea and vomiting.

The standard formulas contain all the required basic nutrients. They contain proteins that provide all the essential amino acids, and they are enriched with a wide array of vitamins and minerals. Essential fatty acids are included, and most have polyunsaturated fats

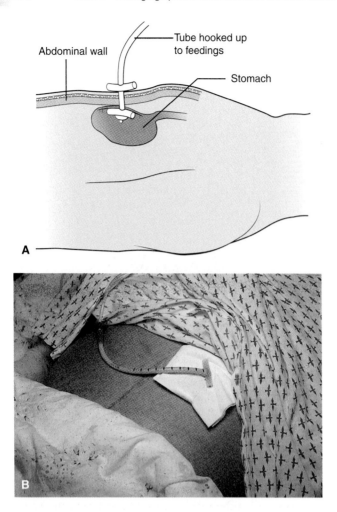

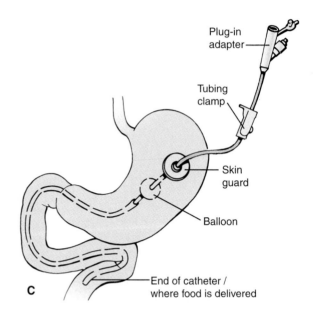

FIGURE 30-2 (**A**) Percutaneous endoscopic gastrostomy (PEG) tube in place. (**B**) A dressing over the PEG tube protects the site. (**C**) A jejunostomy tube is placed similarly to the PEG tube but is positioned in the jejunum.

as opposed to saturated fats. Carbohydrates provide the needed calories. The standard formulas are designed to provide a complete nutritional balance when all dietary calories are derived from the formula.

A variety of specialized formulas are also available. Some contain soluble fiber to assist with bowel function. Some have a specific low lipid content for those whose dietary intake of fat needs to be restricted. Lactose-free formula is available for the lactose-intolerant person who develops diarrhea and bloating from ingesting foods containing lactose.

Formulas with various concentrations are also available. Concentration of formula is usually measured in terms of **osmolarity**, which is the number of particles (measured in milliosmoles) per kilogram of water. Most formulas are isotonic to blood, which has a concentration of approximately 300 mOsm/kg. High-calorie formulas are hypertonic with a high osmolarity. Some individuals develop diarrhea from high-osmolarity formula or even from isotonic formula. These individuals may be given a special low-osmolarity formula or formula is administered at half strength to decrease osmo-

larity. The individual may then have a gradually increasing concentration administered and thus develop tolerance to the formula.

Formulas are also available that contain only substances that require little or no digestion and that do not leave residue in the intestine. These are known as **elemental feedings**. They can be administered into the stomach or directly into the small intestine. They may be used when digestion is impaired or when the bowel must be rested.

Commercially canned formulas need not be refrigerated until they are opened. They are then promptly stored in the refrigerator to prevent growth of microorganisms. If the opened refrigerated can is not used within 24 hours, it is discarded. Check the can of formula for an expiration date, and do not administer if outdated.

Additional water is usually needed by the person receiving tube feedings. The amount may be ordered by the physician or may be adjusted by the nurse based on observation of the urine. If the urine remains pale and dilute (of a low specific gravity), then the patient is usually receiving enough water. Dark or concentrated urine usually indicates that the patient needs more water. The water may be given after intermittent feedings to rinse out the tube, before and after medications are administered, and at prescribed times.

When tube feedings are first initiated, the formula may be used in a dilute form, and an amount less than the expected caloric needs may be given—for example, equal parts of formula and water. Then, gradually, the feedings may be increased in strength and amount. This practice helps to prevent diarrhea, which can result from the sudden change in consistency and content of the diet.

IDENTIFYING ASPIRATION OF TUBE FEEDINGS

Identifying aspiration of tube feedings is a continuing concern because individuals receiving tube feedings often have an inadequate **gag reflex.** When individuals cough or choke during feedings, this clearly points to aspiration, but this response cannot be relied upon. A chest x-ray is required to accurately diagnose aspiration.

In the past, a blue food coloring was added to tube feedings to make it easier to identify formula-contaminated respiratory secretions. In a health advisory, the Food and Drug Administration (U.S. Food & Drug Administration, 2003) warned against this practice because exposure to food dye has been shown to be dangerous for some individuals and can lead to potentially fatal liver toxicity. In these individuals, Blue I dye is absorbed systemically, resulting in a bluish coloring of the skin, mucous membranes, and body fluids. For this reason, nurses are encouraged to avoid this practice (Kohn-Keeth & Frankel, 2004).

Checking respiratory secretions for glucose has been recommended to verify aspiration. The research by Metheney and colleagues (1998) provided evidence that suctioning respiratory secretions and testing them for glucose was not an accurate measure of aspiration. While glucose is not usually present in respiratory secretions in amounts sufficient to be measured, glucose did appear in measurable quantities even when no aspiration had occurred. Additionally, the absence of glucose does not clearly show that no aspiration has taken place. If small amounts are aspirated, and there are large amounts of secretions, the presence of glucose may be masked.

SCHEDULING TUBE FEEDINGS

The physician, often in consultation with the dietitian, will determine the type and amount of tube feeding and the intervals at which it is to be administered. The most common method is continuous infusion over a 24-hour period. When tube feedings are initiated, it is common practice to begin with a slow administration rate (20 mL/hr) and gradually increase the rate as the patient exhibits the ability to tolerate the feeding without adverse effects.

Bolus feedings usually are used for the patient who needs a supplemental feeding in addition to regular oral intake or for the patient who is ambulatory. A prescribed volume is given four to six times a day. *Cycled* feedings are scheduled to accommodate the patient's schedule. The tube feeding may be given over a prescribed period of time (for example, during the night) freeing the patient for other activities during the day. Intermittent feedings, whether bolus feedings or cycled feedings, are delivered using a pump for consistent rate of administration.

ADMINISTERING MEDICATIONS THROUGH AN ENTERAL TUBE

When patients are receiving tube feedings, oral medications may also be delivered via the feeding tube. Ideally, medications administered by tube should be in liquid form. Consult with the pharmacist and the physician to facilitate obtaining medications that are available in liquid form. However, some medications are not available in liquid form, or the liquid form may contain sweeteners or other additives that are contraindicated.

For medications not in liquid form, the following guidelines apply. Gelatin-like medications such as stool softeners can be briefly microwaved in a paper cup on a low setting to liquefy the product. They are cooled and then administered by tube. Products containing psyllium are dissolved in large quantities of water because they tend to solidify and obstruct the feeding tube. When psyllium is used for treating diarrhea, the product should be mixed with formula at room temperature. Tablets that are not enteric coated must be finely crushed and dissolved in at least 30 mL of water to be administered. Capsules are opened, and the contents dissolved in water. Sometimes, the contents do not dissolve well but may be suspended in the water long enough for administration. Thorough flushing with water after administering medications is essential.

Enteric-coated tablets and time-release capsules or tablets should not be crushed for administration because the time of absorption will be changed, resulting in too much drug at one time and not enough at another. Whenever possible, it is desirable to administer medications through a medication port on the tube. Stop the feeding, use an alcohol wipe to disinfect the port, and flush the tube with 30 mL of water before and after administering the medication(s). Then restart the feeding (Padula, et al, 2004). If there is no port on the tubing, disconnect the feeding tube from the administration set while the medications and flushing solution are given. Be sure to protect the ends of the tubing to avoid contamination.

It is best to give medication at the beginning of a feeding so that if, for any reason, the full amount of formula is not given, the medication will have been administered. Medications should never be dissolved in the formula because you cannot ensure that the patient receives the whole dose in a timely manner.

PREVENTING CONTAMINATION OF THE FORMULA

Use clean technique when you administer a tube feeding, and handle both the formula and the administration set carefully because careless handling of the formula and administration set can lead to contamination, which in turn can be the cause of nosocomial (hospital-acquired) infections. The formula should be at room temperature. Do not warm formula because milk products with added nutrients are an ideal medium for the growth of bacteria, and warmth increases the ability of bacteria to grow. Providing tube feedings at refrigerator temperature can cause cramping. Additionally, cold formula has been found to increase diarrhea. Commercial formulas have been heat sterilized and are considered safe for administration if they do not remain at room temperature longer than 12 hours with open systems and 24 to 48 hours with closed systems (Padula, et al., 2004). Be sure to check the manufacturer's guidelines.

RESIDUAL FORMULA IN THE STOMACH

"Checking for residual" refers to determining whether residual formula from the previous feeding remains in the stomach. Gastric contents are aspirated, measured, and usually returned to the stomach in order to not disturb the body's electrolyte balance. However, some suggest that removing and returning gastric residual volumes can lead to a higher incidence of tube clogging and bacterial contamination of feedings (Powell, et al, 1993). Because there is no definitive research supporting either practice, follow your facility policy or the medical orders for the individual patient.

In the past, it was believed that when feedings are given on a continuous basis, the formula should be consistently moving into the small intestine so that the residual amount is less than 50 mL. It was further believed that when there was a large residual volume, the patient was more likely to regurgitate formula through the gas-

tric sphincter into the esophagus. From there, the formula could be aspirated into the lungs, thereby increasing the incidence of aspiration pneumonia. In many settings, feedings were withheld if the residual volume was more than 100 to 150 mL. According to research (McClave, et al, 1999), stopping feedings until residual formula in the stomach is less than 150 mL can contribute to malnutrition from the reduction in calories administered.

McClave & Snider (2002) found that in most instances, gastric tube feedings can safely be given if the residual volume is less than 400 to 500 mL. Exceptions to this practice include patients at high risk for aspiration, such as those who are sedated or obtunded or who have impaired GI function. In these instances, the patient has a greater chance of regurgitation and aspiration. However, you must follow the physician's order or facility policy if they indicate that the feeding should be withheld when a specified amount of residual is obtained.

DETERMINING TUBE LOCATION

Check the feeding tube for position and patency before beginning each feeding and at regular intervals, typically every 8 hours, when continuous feedings are given. Research indicates that the most reliable bedside method for determining tube position is the aspiration method that includes observing gastric contents and checking their pH level (Metheney & Titler, 2001). Use a minimum amount of pressure when aspirating a small-bore tube to keep it from collapsing. Rinse the tubing with water after checking for correct position. This helps to prevent clogging of the tubing and lessens the risk of the growth of microorganisms in the tubing.

Observing the contents of the aspirated material is most useful when differentiating between gastric and intestinal placement. Gastric contents are usually brown to greenish-brown and may contain shreds of mucus or sediment. When mixed with formula in the stomach, they appear tan, while intestinal aspirate is usually more transparent, varying in color from yellow to brownish-green. Observation is less useful when the tube might be in the lung because the appearance of the aspirate (off-white to tan mucus) could have originated in either the respiratory or gastric tract.

The pH of the aspirated contents can also be tested to check for placement. If measured to be acidic (5 or below), the feeding tube is most likely placed correctly in the stomach. The pH of material aspirated from the intestinal or respiratory tract is usually 7 or above. This method must be used cautiously because medications and some medical conditions as well as the tube feeding itself can alter the gastric pH (Metheney & Titler, 2001).

Auscultation is another method often used to verify tube placement. A small amount of air is introduced through the tube while auscultating over the stomach through a stethoscope for gurgling sounds. Metheney and Titler (2001) consider the aspiration method as more reliable to verify feeding tube placement than the auscultatory method. The use of both methods together is recommended.

Because placement is so critical, and bedside methods are uncertain, when a small-bore feeding tube is initially placed, it is standard practice to check for placement with an x-ray image. The observation and auscultatory methods often are used at tube placement as an initial guide before sending the patient for an x-ray image. Once it has been established that the tube is not in the respiratory tract, a pH of 6 or greater is usually considered adequate to ensure that a small-bore tube is located in the duodenum (Metheney & Titler, 2001).

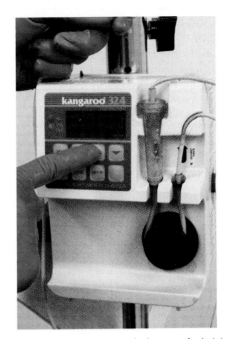

FIGURE 30-3 A feeding pump controls the rate of administration for the tube feeding. (Photo by Rick Brady.)

SYSTEMS FOR ADMINISTERING TUBE FEEDINGS

Tube feedings may be administered either by open or closed systems. A pump may be attached to the feeding apparatus, or the force of gravity may be used.

OPEN VERSUS CLOSED FEEDING SYSTEMS

Tube feedings may be delivered via a closed system in which the tubing connects directly to the bottle or bag containing the formula. The closed system lessens the potential for outside contamination of the feeding and requires less time for setup and preparation. If the feeding is intermittent rather than continuous, the tubing can be clamped, the pump turned off, and the setup remain connected until the next feeding.

Open systems consist of an open bag attached to the tubing for the feeding. The desired amount of formula is poured into the open bag and then administered. The bag and tubing are changed every 24 hours. There are more opportunities for contamination because the original container must be opened and the formula poured into the open bag. If the feeding is to be intermittent, the bag should be thoroughly rinsed after it empties. This decreases the potential for microbial growth while the bag remains hanging until the next feeding.

USE OF A PUMP FOR TUBE FEEDINGS

A rate-controlled pump is used to deliver tube feedings at a precise rate or through very small-diameter tubes (Fig. 30-3). These pumps apply constant positive pressure to the feeding tube. A tubing compatible with the particular pump is used with a closed-system (spike set or prefilled bag) or an open system (**reservoir** or bag set). The procedure is identical to the procedure when a closed or open system without a pump is used, except that when the entire setup is complete, the tubing is threaded through the pump according to the directions provided by the manufacturer, and the flow rate is set on the machine. The machine is equipped with a warning signal that is activated if the flow is interrupted or if the tubing runs dry.

Even when feedings are provided continuously, the position of the tube should be rechecked each time additional formula is added to the reservoir. Simple observation of the location of the tubing at the nostril may reveal a tube that has become dislodged. Then use auscultation and the aspiration techniques to determine tube placement. This prevents unsafe administration of tube feeding in the event that the tubing has moved out of correct position.

PROCEDURE FOR ADMINISTERING A TUBE FEEDING

ASSESSMENT

1. Validate the order for the type and specific amount of formula and water to be given as well as the rate at which they are to be administered and the method of formula delivery to be used. Specific times may also be indicated if the formula is not to be administered on a continuous basis. **R:** Proceeding in this way verifies the accuracy of the feeding to be administered.

2. Check the patient's record for any notes regarding tolerance of previous feedings and any complications. **R:** Doing this helps determine if any adjustments need to be made with regard to the type, amount, and flow rate of formula ordered.

ANALYSIS

3. Critically think through your assessment data, carefully evaluating each aspect and its relation to other data. **R:** This enables you to determine specific problems for this individual in relation to tube feeding.
4. Identify specific problems and modifications of the procedure that may be needed for the individual. **R:** Planning for the individual must take into consideration the individual's problems.

PLANNING

5. Determine individualized patient outcomes for the individual patient related to the tube feeding.

R: Identification of outcomes guides planning and evaluation.
   a. The patient receives the correct formula in the correct amount at the correct rate.
   b. The patient experiences no complications during or after the tube feeding is administered.
6. Identify and select the specific equipment you will need. **R:** Planning ahead allows you to proceed efficiently.
   a. A stethoscope for checking for bowel sounds and for checking the position of the feeding tube if the auscultation method will be used
   b. The ordered formula
   c. Clean gloves
   d. A 60-mL syringe with adapter
   e. pH test strips
   f. A pump (if one is being used) and IV pole
   g. Warm irrigant (water or normal saline solution)
   h. Closed system (spike set) or open system (bag set)

IMPLEMENTATION

Action	Rationale
7. Wash or disinfect your hands.	To decrease the transfer of microorganisms that could cause infection.
8. Identify the patient, using two identifiers.	Verifying the patient's identity helps ensure that you are performing the right skill for the right patient.
9. Explain the procedure you are about to perform.	Explaining the procedure helps relieve anxiety or misperceptions that the patient may have about a procedure or activity and sets the stage for patient participation.
10. Elevate the head of the bed between 30 and 45 degrees unless contraindicated. The patient should be left with head elevated throughout the feeding and for at least 30 minutes afterward. The unconscious patient should have the head turned to the side.	The elevated position assists gravity to empty the stomach and prevents regurgitation and aspiration (Keithley & Swanson, 2004; Opilla, 2003). With the head turned to the side, the unconscious patient is less likely to aspirate if regurgitation occurs.
11. Check bowel sounds.	Active bowel sounds indicate a functioning bowel, which is necessary to avoid gastric **distention.**
12. Put on clean gloves.	Gloves protect you from contact with GI secretions.
13. Validate correct placement of the tube.	To ensure that the tube is in the stomach and has not dislodged.
a. Place your stethoscope over the stomach, and auscultate while injecting 30 mL of air into the tube.	

(continued)

Action	Rationale
b. Aspirate the stomach contents, examine and test the pH of the contents, and return the contents to the stomach.	
14. Check for residual formula.	Residual formula in the stomach may indicate that the stomach is not emptying. Follow the medical orders or facility policy regarding the action to take based on the residual volume.
15. Flush the tubing.	To ensure that the tube remains patent.
16. Proceed with the feeding, using one of the following approaches for *continuous feeding with a feeding pump:*	
a. *Closed system (spike set):*	
(1) Prepare the formula (see Figure 30-4 for an example of a prefilled bag of formula). Turn the container containing the formula upside down, and shake it vigorously.	To mix the components of the formula thoroughly.

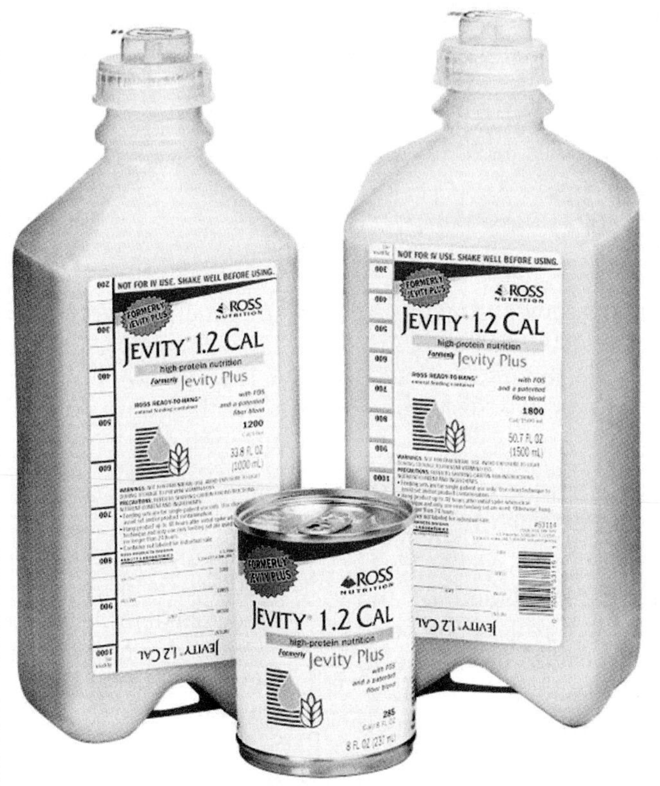

FIGURE 30-4 A prefilled tube feeding set provides convenience for the patient on continuous infusion. (Courtesy Ross Laboratories, Columbus, Ohio.)

(continued)

Action	Rationale
(2) Remove the protective cap, and insert the piercing pin into the port on the cap.	To connect the formula to the administration set.
(3) Close the clamp on the administration set, invert the container, and hang it on the IV pole.	To prevent the formula from spilling and to ready it for administration.
b. *Open system (bag or reservoir set):*	
(1) Obtain the ordered formula. If it is canned, use alcohol wipes to clean both the can opener and the top of the can.	To prevent the spread of microorganisms.
(2) Open the can, and pour formula into the container (never pour more formula than enough for 4 hours), and label the container with the date and time it is to be changed.	To be certain that the formula is discarded after 24 hours.
17. Prime the tubing, and place it in the pump according to the package instructions.	The tubing is filled with formula to ensure that air is not instilled into the stomach. Air will cause abdominal distention and increase the potential for regurgitation. Each pump has specific tube placement requirements in order to function effectively.
18. Attach the formula administration set to the patient's feeding tube. Secure all connections.	To prevent spillage.
19. Open the clamp.	To allow the formula to flow.
20. If a pump is being used, follow the manufacturer's operating instructions.	To ensure timely delivery of the formula.
21. Remove your gloves, and wash or disinfect your hands.	To decrease the transfer of microorganisms that could cause infection.

EVALUATION

22. Return to check on the patient in 30 minutes, and evaluate using the individualized patient outcomes previously identified. **R:** Evaluation in relation to desired outcome is essential for planning future care.
  a. The patient is receiving the correct formula at the correct rate.
  b. The patient is experiencing no complications.

DOCUMENTATION

23. Document the specific patient outcomes in relation to the tube feeding according to the policies of the facility.

24. Document the volume of tube feeding formula and water or normal saline flush and the amount of any residual (if measured) on the appropriate flow sheet. **R:** Documentation is a legal record of the patient's care and therapy and communicates nursing activities to other nurses and caregivers.

POTENTIAL ADVERSE OUTCOMES AND RELATED INTERVENTIONS

1. The patient experiences diarrhea.
Intervention: Check medications to determine whether any are associated with diarrhea, and consult with the physician for a change if indicated. Check also to be

sure that feedings are being administered at room temperature, and check with the dietitian to determine if a change of formula is indicated. Remember to maintain cleanliness, and act to prevent skin breakdown and dehydration.

2. The patient appears to have aspirated.

Intervention: Follow institutional protocol regarding the use of reagent strips to test for glucose. There is glucose in tube feedings, and this may be evident on testing, however, glucose may be found in the absence of aspiration (Metheney, et al, 1998). Contact the physician for an order to obtain a chest x-ray. Keep the head of the bed elevated between 30 and 45 degrees during and after tube feedings to prevent aspiration (Keithley & Swanson, 2004).

3. The tube becomes occluded.

Intervention: Pancreatic enzymes may be used to restore patency to clogged tubes. In some cases, pancreatic enzyme solution may be used prophylactically to prevent clogging in addition to routine flushing with water (Bourgault, et al., 2003). The use of enzymes is based on specific medical orders or facility protocol.

4. The patient experiences dry mouth.

Intervention: Provide frequent mouth care (at least every 8 hours).

5. The skin around the nostrils or the gastrostomy/jejunostomy tube becomes red, sore, or eroded.

Intervention: Provide wound care as described in Module 40.

ADMINISTERING A GASTROSTOMY OR JEJUNOSTOMY FEEDING

ASSESSMENT

1. Validate the order for the type and specific amount of formula and water to be given as well as the rate at which they are to be administered and the method of formula delivery to be used. Specific times may also be indicated if the formula is not to be administered on a continuous basis. **R:** This ensures the accuracy of the feeding to be administered.

2. Check the patient's record for information regarding tolerance of previous feedings and any complications. **R:** This helps determine if any adjustments need to be made with regard to the type and amount of formula ordered or to the flow rate.

ANALYSIS

3. Critically think through your assessment data, carefully evaluating each aspect and its relation to other data. **R:** This enables you to determine specific problems for this individual in relation to tube feeding.

4. Identify specific problems and modifications of the procedure that may be needed for the individual. **R:** Planning for the individual must take into consideration the individual's problems.

PLANNING

5. Determine desired patient outcomes for the individual patient related to the tube feeding. **R:** Identification of outcomes guides planning and evaluation.
   a. The patient receives the correct formula in the correct amount at the correct rate.
   b. The patient experiences no complications during or after the tube feeding is administered.
   c. The skin at the tube or stoma site is dry and intact.

6. Identify and select the specific equipment you will need:
   a. stethoscope for checking for bowel sounds
   b. the ordered formula
   c. clean gloves
   d. 30- to 60-mL syringe with adapter
   e. pH test strips
   f. pump and IV pole
   g. warm irrigant (water or normal saline solution)
   h. closed system (spike set) or open system (bag set)

IMPLEMENTATION

Action	Rationale
7. Wash or disinfect your hands.	This is to decrease the transfer of microorganisms that could cause infection.
8. Identify the patient, using two identifiers.	Verifying the patient's identity helps ensure that you are performing the right procedure for the right patient.
9. Close the door, and draw the curtains around the bed.	To provide privacy.

(continued)

Action	*Rationale*
10. Explain the procedure you are about to perform.	Explaining the procedure helps relieve anxiety and sets the stage for patient participation.
11. Elevate the head of the bed between 30 and 45 degrees unless contraindicated.	This position assists gravity to empty the stomach and prevents regurgitation and aspiration (Keithley & Swanson, 2004; Opilla, 2003).
12. Check bowel sounds.	Active bowel sounds indicate a functioning bowel, which is necessary to avoid gastric distention.
13. Put on clean gloves.	Gloves protect you from direct contact with GI secretions.
14. Check the gastrostomy or jejunostomy site for drainage and skin irritation or breakdown.	Pressure from the tube or drainage can cause skin breakdown, which can lead to infection.
15. Validate correct placement of the tube.	To ensure that the feeding is administered into the correct site.
a. Gastrostomy tube: Aspirate stomach contents, examine contents, and test pH, and return contents to stomach.	
b. Jejunostomy tube: Aspirate intestinal secretions, examine, and test pH.	
16. For gastrostomy tube, measure residual formula. (The measurement of residual formula on jejunostomy tubes is not necessary.)	Residual formula in the stomach may indicate that the stomach is not emptying. Follow the orders or facility policy regarding the action to take based on the residual volume.
17. Flush the tubing.	To ensure that the tube remains patent.
18. Proceed with the feeding, using one of the following approaches for *continuous feeding with a feeding pump:*	
a. *Closed system (spike set):*	
(1) Prepare the formula: Turn the container of formula upside down, and shake it vigorously.	To mix the components of the formula thoroughly.
(2) Remove the protective cap, and insert the piercing pin into the port on the cap.	To connect the formula to the administration set.
(3) Close the clamp on the administration set, invert the container, and hang it on the IV pole.	To prevent the formula from spilling and to ready it for administration.

(continued)

Action	Rationale
b. *Open system (bag or reservoir set):*	
(1) Obtain the ordered formula. If it is canned, use alcohol wipes to clean both the can opener and the top of the can.	To prevent the spread of microorganisms.
(2) Open the can, and pour the formula into the container (never more than enough for 4 hours), and label the container with the date and time it is to be changed.	To be certain that the formula is discarded after 24 hours.
19. Prime the tubing, and place it in the pump according to the package instructions.	To ensure that the formula is delivered without difficulty.
20. Attach the formula administration set to the patient's feeding tube. Secure all connections.	To prevent spillage.
21. Open the clamp.	To allow the formula to flow.
22. If a pump is being used, follow the manufacturer's operating instructions.	To ensure timely delivery of the formula.
23. Remove your gloves, and wash or disinfect your hands.	To decrease the transfer of organisms that could cause infection.

EVALUATION

24. Return to check on the patient in 30 minutes, and evaluate using the individualized patient outcomes previously identified. **R:** Evaluation in relation to desired outcomes is essential for planning future care.
  a. The patient is receiving the correct formula in the correct amount at the correct rate.
  b. The patient is experiencing no complications.
  c. The skin at the tube or stoma site is dry and intact.

DOCUMENTATION

25. Document the specific patient outcomes in relation to the tube feeding according to the policies of the facility.
26. Document the volume of tube feeding formula and water or normal saline flush solution on the appropriate flow sheet. **R:** Documentation is a legal record of the patient's care and therapy and communicates nursing activities to other nurses and caregivers.

Acute Care

Some hospitalized patients cannot swallow or may need their oral intake supplemented by enteral feedings to facilitate healing or to sustain or regain optimal weight. These patients are often seen in critical care units although they may be on acute care and rehabilitation units as well. Benefits of enteral feedings in these situations include decreased infection, improved wound healing, and shorter hospital stays. Nurses in acute care settings must be aware of both the rationale for enteral feedings as well as recent changes in practice recommendations.

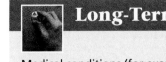

Long-Term Care

Medical conditions (for example, dysphagia or problems with dentition) as well as ethical considerations and personal wishes play a part in the decision to consider enteral feedings for those who reside in long-term care settings. Thorough nutritional, physical, and psychological assessments should be done before making this decision. It is possible that consideration of medication changes, resident preferences, and environmental issues could improve food intake. The resident and family should be informed of the potential risks and benefits of tube feeding as well as realistic expectations for favorable outcomes. Nurses in long-term care settings must be aware of the technical aspects of administering tube feedings as well as of the psychological impact on the resident of receiving nourishment in this way.

Home Care

Tube feedings may be administered at home for relatively short periods or over a long term. The person(s) responsible for providing this aspect of care must be assisted to appreciate both the technical aspects of the procedure as well as the need the client may have for social interactions such as the ones traditionally associated with meals, family or holiday celebrations, and religious events. The nurse will need to assess the administration of the tube feeding, the care and storage of equipment and formula, and of course, the well-being of the client.

LEARNING TOOLS

DEVELOP YOUR BACKGROUND KNOWLEDGE

1. Review the Learning Outcomes.

2. Read the section on tube feeding in your assigned text.

3. Look up the Key Terms in the glossary.

4. Review the module and mentally practice the techniques described. Study so that you would be able to teach these skills to another person. Use the Performance Checklist on the CD-ROM in the front of this book.

5. Review the anatomy of the gastrointestinal and respiratory tracts.

DEVELOP YOUR SKILLS

In the practice setting

1. If tube feeding equipment is available, arrange for time to become familiar with the equipment you will need to carry out the tube feeding procedure.

2. If a mannequin is available, simulate the procedure using both closed and open system sets.

3. Evaluate your performance with a partner or your instructor.

DEMONSTRATE YOUR SKILLS

In the clinical setting

1. Consult with your instructor regarding the opportunity to observe a staff nurse or your instructor prepare for and begin tube feeding.

2. Consult with your instructor regarding the opportunity for you to administer a tube feeding under the supervision of your instructor. Evaluate your performance with the instructor.

3. Document the procedure according to facility policies.

4. Share your documentation with your instructor.

CRITICAL THINKING EXERCISES

1. Your 62-year-old male patient had a stroke (CVA) 2 weeks ago and has been in a coma. For the past 3 days, he has been on continuous tube feeding and has had copious diarrhea. Identify three possible causes of the diarrhea that relate to tube feeding. What assessment might you carry out to determine the cause(s) of the diarrhea? For each possible cause, identify the nursing actions you might take.

2. Your patient has a small-diameter feeding tube in place. The medical order is "Begin tube feeding. One can of complete nutritional formula (Compleat) every 8 hours." You observe that the patient has a low-grade fever and is very diaphoretic. Devise an individualized care plan for this patient that addresses the problems described.

SELF-QUIZ
SHORT-ANSWER QUESTIONS

1. When is plain water given to a patient through a feeding tube?

2. How can you check respiratory secretions to determine if the patient has aspirated formula?

3. If there is 150 mL of residual volume aspirated after tube feeding, what should be your next step?

4. What is one of the most common causes of diarrhea for the person who is receiving tube feedings?

5. How might an occluded feeding tube be opened?

MULTIPLE CHOICE

_____ 6. Each milliliter of standard tube feeding formula yields approximately
   a. 1 kcal.
   b. 2 kcal.
   c. 5 kcal.
   d. 10 kcal.

_____ 7. For administration, the formula temperature should be
   a. hot.
   b. cold.
   c. room temperature.
   d. at whatever temperature is convenient.

_____ 8. To prevent gastric distention, you should
   a. feed the patient only every 4 hours.
   b. allow as little air as possible to enter the tube.
   c. rinse the tube well with water after the feeding.
   d. feed rapidly.

_____ 9. The head of a comatose patient should be turned to the side after feeding to prevent
   a. vomiting.
   b. aspiration.
   c. distention.
   d. indigestion.

_____ 10. The patient should be checked approximately 30 minutes after feeding for
   a. vomiting.
   b. drowsiness.
   c. anorexia.
   d. diarrhea.

_____ 11. If the tubing does not appear to be in the stomach when you check it, your first action should be to
   a. give the feeding slowly.
   b. remove the tube immediately.
   c. not give the feeding.
   d. call the physician for a decision.

_____ 12. If the patient begins to gag while you are tube feeding, you should
   a. stop the feeding for a time.
   b. continue with the feeding as planned.
   c. give additional feeding.
   d. give medication for nausea.

Answers to the Self-Quiz questions appear in the back of the book.

REFERENCES AND SUGGESTED RESOURCES: UNIT 6

Bourgault, A., Heyland, D., Drover, J., et al. (2003). Prophylactic pancreatic enzymes to reduce feeding tube occlusions. *Nutrition in Clinical Practice, 18* (5), 398–401.

Collins, N. (2001). What's in that feeding formula anyway? *Nursing 31,* 12.

Keithley, J., & Swanson, B. (2004). Enteral nutrition: An update on practice recommendations. *Medsurg Nursing, 13* (2), 131–134.

Kohn-Keeth, C., & Frankel, E. (2004). Taking the blue dye out of tube feedings. *Nursing 2004, 34,* 14.

Lord, L. (2001). How to insert a large-bore nasogastric tube. *Nursing 2001, 31* (9), 46–48.

McClave, S., Sexton, L., Spain, D., et al. (1999). Enteral tube feeding in the intensive care unit: Factors impeding adequate delivery. *Critical Care Medicine, 27* (7), 1252–1256.

McClave, S., & Snider. (2002). Clinical use of gastric residual volumes as a monitor for patients on enteral tube feeding. *Journal of Parenteral and Enteral Nutrition, 26* (Supplement 6), S43–S50.

Metheney, N. A., St. John, R. E., Clouse, R. E. (1998). Measurement of glucose in tracheobronchial secretions to detect aspiration of enteral feedings. *Heart and Lung, 27,* 285–292.

Metheney, N., & Titler, M. (2001). Assessing the placement of feeding tubes. *American Journal of Nursing, 101* (5), 36–45.

Opilla, M. (2003). Aspiration risk and enteral feeding: A clinical approach. Nutrition Issues in Gastroenterology Series #4. *Practical Gastroenterology,* 89–96. (Online). Available at http://www.healthsystem.virginia.edu/internet/ digestive-health/apr03opillaarticle.pdf. Retrieved April 11, 2005.

Padula, C., Kenny, A., Planchon, C., et al. (2004). Enteral feeding: What the evidence says. *American Journal of Nursing, 104* (7) 62–69.

Powell, K., Marcuard, S., Farrier, E., et al. (1993). Aspirating gastric residuals causes occlusion of small-bore feeding tubes. *Journal of Parenteral and Enteral Nutrition, 17* (3), 243–246.

Tambyah, P. A., Knasinski, V., & Maki, D. G. (2002). The direct cost of nosocomial catheter-associated urinary tract infections in the era of managed care. *Infection Control and Hospital Epidemiology, 23,* 27–31.

U.S. Food and Drug Administration. (2003). *Reports of blue discoloration and death in patients receiving enteral feedings tinted with the dye, FD&C Blue No. 1.* (Online). Available at http://vm.cfsan.fda.gov/~dms/col-ltr2.html. Retrieved January 3, 2004.

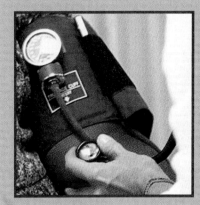

UNIT 7

Supporting Oxygenation and Circulation

MODULES

Administering Oxygen

SKILLS INCLUDED IN THIS MODULE

General Procedure for Administering Oxygen
Specific Procedures for Administering Oxygen
   Procedure for Administering Oxygen by Nasal Cannula
   Procedure for Administering Oxygen by Nasal Catheter
   Procedure for Administering Oxygen by Mask
Using Oximetry to Measure Oxygen Saturation
Self-Inflating Breathing Bag and Mask

PREREQUISITE MODULES

Module 1	An Approach to Nursing Skills
Module 2	Documentation
Module 4	Basic Infection Control
Module 7	Providing Hygiene
Module 11	Assessing Temperature, Pulse, and Respiration
Module 12	Measuring Blood Pressure
Module 14	Nursing Physical Assessment

KEY TERMS

ambient	dyspnea
apnea	flowmeter
cannula	hypoxemia
capnogram	oronasal
capnography	oximetry
carbon dioxide	pulse oximetry
catheter	tracheostomy
claustrophobia	transtracheal
combustion	

OVERALL OBJECTIVE

▸ To administer oxygen to patients, using equipment appropriately in a safe and effective manner.

LEARNING OUTCOMES

The student will be able to

1. List general conditions that necessitate oxygen administration.
2. Assess the patient for indicators of oxygen need including **dyspnea,** feelings of breathlessness, dusky nail beds or mucous membranes, oxygen saturation level, anxiety or cognitive changes, and other factors that may be affecting oxygenation.
3. Identify the benefits and hazards of oxygen administration.
4. Plan for oxygen administration, including identifying the desired outcomes and the most effective method for the patient situation.
5. Implement oxygen therapy effectively.
6. Evaluate the patient's oxygenation after therapy as well as the patient's response to the method of administration.
7. Document oxygen administration, including amount of oxygen administered, method of administration, and the patient's responses to oxygenation.

Oxygen is essential to life. An optimum level of oxygen must be maintained in the blood to sustain cellular functioning. **Hypoxemia** is the state in which the level of oxygen in the blood is lowered. The term *hypoxia* may also be used to refer to a generalized oxygen deficiency. When hypoxemia is present, the administration of oxygen may be essential to increase its concentration in the blood. However, pure oxygen is a therapeutic agent that can have adverse effects when given improperly. Therefore, the nurse must be familiar with the indications for oxygen use and the various types of equipment for oxygen delivery. The nurse must also be skilled in administering oxygen.

NURSING DIAGNOSES

- Impaired Gas Exchange: Oxygen therapy is used most often for the patient with the nursing diagnosis of "Impaired Gas Exchange," which may be related to a variety of factors, including excessive secretions in the lungs; hypoventilation; a disease process that decreases the gas exchange surfaces in the lungs; or a condition that decreases circulation of blood through the lungs. Not all conditions producing hypoxemia are alleviated by oxygen administration alone. For oxygen to be effective, unoxygenated blood must be circulated through the lungs, alveolar membranes must be capable of gas exchange, and the oxygen delivery method must succeed in increasing the percentage of oxygen in the alveolar air.
- Ineffective Breathing Pattern: A breathing pattern may become ineffective with shallow ventilations and slow respiratory rate due to pain, sedation, surgery, or head injury. The underlying problem causing the ineffective breathing pattern must be addressed. However, the administration of oxygen may assist in maintaining blood oxygen levels in the face of hypoventilation while other measures are being instituted.

DELEGATION

Assessments in relation to oxygenation and the decision about using oxygen or the type of oxygen delivery system to be used are not delegated to assistive personnel. However, assistive personnel are taught how to put on and remove oxygen delivery devices, as necessary, to promote activities of daily living. Assistive personnel also may be taught to check the flow rate and the fluid level in a humidification bottle.

SAFETY CONCERNS RELATED TO ADMINISTERING OXYGEN

A variety of safety concerns are related to the use of oxygen. The physical dangers include fire, pressure hazards, and equipment malfunctions.

FIRE HAZARDS

Although oxygen itself is not explosive, it supports **combustion.** This means that extremely rapid burning takes place in the presence of high oxygen concentration, almost as if the oxygen itself were explosive. Thus, it is essential to prevent sparks or fire in an environment where oxygen is being used. Observe the precautions listed in Box 31-1.

PRESSURE HAZARDS

Oxygen can be stored in several ways. Most acute care facilities have a piped-in system, with outlets on the wall beside the bed; gas flow is adjusted by means of a flowmeter that attaches to the wall outlet. This oxygen comes from a large holding tank that is usually located outside the building. When oxygen is not piped in, facilities may use tanks that hold oxygen as a compressed gas at more than 2,000 lb pressure per square inch (psi). Because of the extreme pressure, these tanks should be handled with great care. Large tanks are chained to stands to prevent falling and possible rupture of the valve. Smaller, portable tanks of liquid oxygen are available and are largely replacing the older compressed air tanks in homes and long-term care settings that do not have piped-in oxygen. Oxygen in this form is safe because of its low pressure. Storage and transport savings have made liquid oxygen an economical method of oxygen delivery. These tanks are light and can be easily moved by caregivers. Small containers are portable and can be transported by the patient using either a small wheeled cart or a shoulder or backpack.

MALFUNCTIONING EQUIPMENT

Regardless of the method or appliance used, oxygen should always be turned on and checked before being administered to a patient. Regulators and flowmeters do malfunction, so each time oxygen is to be started on a patient, check all equipment first.

OXYGEN EQUIPMENT

Various pieces of equipment are needed for administering oxygen.

FLOWMETER

A **flowmeter** is a device that attaches to the oxygen outlet to adjust the amount of oxygen being delivered (Fig. 31-1). Two types of flowmeters are available: ball and gauge. Both types register the number of liters of oxygen delivered per minute (L/min). Orders for oxygen typically are stated in liters, although the meaning is liters per minute.

Safety Alert

A note of caution: *Many hospitals have outlets for air as well as oxygen. They are usually color-coded, with yellow outlets reserved for air and green outlets for oxygen. Be sure to place the oxygen flowmeter into the oxygen outlet, not the air outlet.*

HUMIDIFIER

Humidification, if indicated, is provided by containers of sterile water, which may be prefilled and are disposable. They are attached to the oxygen delivery equipment. Oxygen bubbles through the water and picks up moisture, which prevents drying of the mucous membranes.

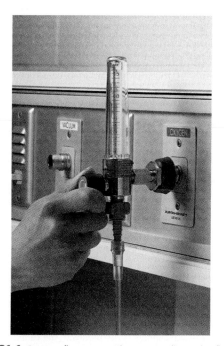

FIGURE 31-1 Oxygen flowmeter. The nurse adjusts the flowmeter, which registers the number of liters of oxygen delivered per minute.

The water must be sterile to prevent infection. Sterile water is used because stagnant water is a medium in which the microorganisms present in tap water may begin to multiply. These organisms can then pose a significant infection hazard to the ill person. Each facility has a policy on how frequently the container is changed. It is usually changed every 24 hours or when the water level becomes low.

OXYGEN ADMINISTRATION SYSTEMS

Oxygen administration systems can be classified in two ways: low flow and high flow. Low-flow oxygen systems provide only part of the patient's total inspired air. Generally, these systems are more comfortable for the patient, but oxygen delivery varies with the patient's breathing pattern. High-flow oxygen systems provide the total inspired atmosphere to the patient. There is consistent oxygen delivery, which can be regulated precisely and which does not vary with the patient's breathing pattern.

NASAL CANNULA

The nasal **cannula** (also called nasal prongs) is composed of plastic tubing that has two small open prongs to be positioned over the patient's face under the nose (Fig. 31-2). It is the most common method of administering oxygen, because it is effective, easy to apply, and comfortable for the patient. The patient receiving oxygen through a nasal cannula can communicate easily, eat, and engage in activities of daily living. These are all important factors in choosing this method of administration. The nasal cannula is a low-flow system.

Although patients commonly mouth-breathe and appear as if they are not receiving the oxygen, they do receive a consistent supply. The oxygen flows into the nose, and the entire upper airway (nose, **oronasal** pharynx, and mouth) becomes a reservoir for oxygen. In addi-

tion, some of the oxygen tends to flow down over the mouth, because it is heavier than air. Thus, when the patient breathes in, the inspired air provides a significant oxygen concentration, even if the patient breathes through the mouth.

Oxygen by nasal cannula is given at 1 to 6 L/min and provides 22% to 50% oxygen in the inspired air, with lower rates of oxygen administration resulting in lower percentages of oxygen in the inspired air. The exact concentration inspired is determined by the interaction of the liter flow of oxygen (volume of oxygen delivered each minute), the respiratory rate and pattern, and the volume of each inspired breath. Therefore, the patient's degree of oxygenation must be assessed to determine the adequacy of the oxygen delivery. Oxygen by nasal cannula is most commonly delivered in low flow rates of 2 or 3 L/min. An excess of 6 L/min does not increase the oxygen delivery. It does, however, increase the drying of mucous membranes and air swallowing.

NASAL CATHETER

The nasal **catheter** is a plastic tube with perforations through which oxygen can flow. It is inserted into the nasopharynx through the nostril. It operates as a low-flow oxygen system. The nasal catheter is rarely used because it can irritate a patient's nostrils, is unpleasant to have inserted, and must be changed every 8 hours.

OXYGEN MASKS

Oxygen masks cover the nose and mouth, are sealed around the edges, and provide the most consistent, effective method of oxygen delivery. Masks are the only method to reliably deliver a high level of oxygen and thus are preferred in critical care situations. There are, however, several disadvantages to their use. The mask interferes with the patient's ability to communicate. It must be removed when eating, drinking, and taking

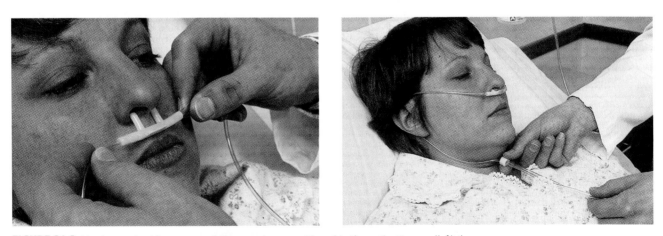

FIGURE 31-2 Nasal cannula. After prongs of the cannula are positioned in the patient's nose (*left*) the oxygen delivering tubing is adjusted for comfort. The patient can communicate easily, eat, and engage in activities of daily living while receiving oxygen.

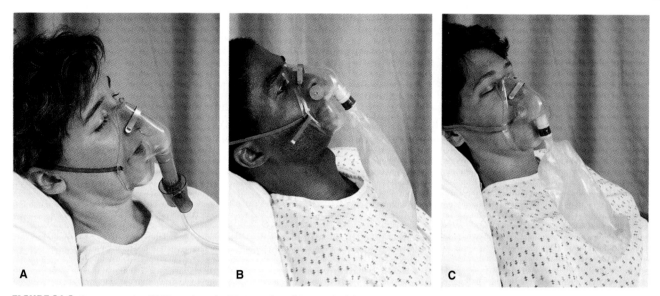

FIGURE 31-3 Oxygen masks. (**A**) Venturi mask. (**B**) Non-rebreathing mask. (**C**) Partial rebreather mask. Photos © Ken Kaspar.

medications, and it makes some individuals experience **claustrophobia.** In addition, because masks are uncomfortable for many patients, they are not consistently left in place, thereby making it impossible to guarantee the percentage of oxygen actually received by the patient (Fig. 31-3).

The *simple mask* (or *rebreathing mask*) is a low-flow system. It has side vents and a reservoir over the face into which oxygen flows, so the patient breathes in air with a higher concentration of oxygen. It is usually used on a short-term basis when an oxygen concentration of 30% to 60% is desired. (Oxygen dose is often abbreviated as FIO_2, which means fraction of inspired oxygen.) Guidelines for estimating FIO_2 with simple masks are shown in Table 31-1. Use of this device requires a flow rate of 6 to 8 L/min. The actual percentage of oxygen received by the patient depends on the patient's tidal volume, respiratory rate, and the fit of the mask as well as the liter flow rate. Because the patient breathes out into the same reservoir, the **carbon dioxide** (CO_2) content of the inspired air tends to increase. The flow rate of 6 to 8 L/min assists in flushing CO_2 from the mask, so for most patients, this is not a concern. The slightly higher CO_2 may actually stimulate respirations.

However, if the patient retains excess CO_2, this type of mask is contraindicated.

The *non-rebreathing mask,* a high-flow system, has a bag attached to the bottom and can deliver 50% to 100% oxygen. The oxygen flows into the bag and accumulates there as a reservoir. When the patient breathes out, a special valve between the bag and the mask closes, and exhaled air exits through the vents in the side of the mask. When the person breathes in, the valve opens so that the inspired air comes from the bag and has a high oxygen concentration. This overcomes the problem of excess CO_2 in the inspired air and prevents room air from diluting the oxygen. A flow rate of 12 to 15 L/min may be needed to keep the bag inflated (see Fig. 31-3).

The *Venturi,* or *air-entraining, mask,* another high-flow system, is designed to deliver oxygen at a specific percentage between 24% and 50%. Pure oxygen delivered at a high rate flows past special vents, and the "Venturi effect" causes this oxygen to mix with the room air at a predictable level. The patient, therefore, receives a constant oxygen concentration, regardless of the rate or depth of respiration. Color-coded adapters are included to set the oxygen flowmeter correctly for the amount of oxygen prescribed. For example, a green adapter indicates that the flowmeter needs to be set at 12 L/min for the patient to receive 35% oxygen. A Venturi mask can be used with or without humidification. It is the most common type of mask used for the critically ill person (see Fig. 31-3).

An additional type of mask is the *tracheostomy mask.* It is designed for the patient who has a **tracheostomy.** It is a small mask, which simply fits over the site of the tracheostomy to deliver oxygen. The oxygen is humidified to keep pulmonary secretions thin and prevent

table 31-1. Guidelines for Estimating FIO_2 With Oxygen Masks	
Oxygen Flow Rate in Liters	**FIO_2**
5–6	40%
6–7	50%
7–8	60%

drying of the mucosa. This type of oxygen delivery may be referred to as flow-by, since it flows by the tracheostomy.

TRANSTRACHEAL OXYGEN CATHETERS

A **transtracheal** catheter is a small-diameter plastic tube with several openings near the tip. It is surgically inserted into the trachea after the patient receives a local anesthetic. When individuals need oxygen on a long-term basis, the problems associated with having a facial mask or nasal cannula become a greater concern. The transtracheal oxygen catheter provides an alternative means of oxygen delivery. This device has advantages over the use of nasal prongs or masks. Because the oxygen runs directly into the trachea, a low flow rate is satisfactory, so the therapy is less costly. In addition, there is no oxygen flow into the **ambient** air, making safety issues less of a problem. The catheter can be completely or partially covered by clothing, so the therapy is more socially acceptable and aesthetically pleasing.

The catheter does need to be irrigated on a daily basis with normal saline solution. This removes any secretions on the inside of the tubing. It is then flushed with air to dry it. The small insertion site is routinely cleaned in the bath or shower. Any secretions can be removed with a cotton-tipped applicator moistened with hydrogen peroxide.

OXYGEN EXTENSION TUBING

Tubing that may be used to connect the delivery device to the oxygen source is usually long enough to accommodate the patient in bed or in a chair near the oxygen source. When a patient needs to move about the room, extension tubing provides for oxygen delivery at longer distances. A small plastic connector is used to join the main oxygen delivery device to the extension tubing. Some homebound patients use tubing that allows them to go around a bedroom and into the bathroom without moving the oxygen tank. In an acute care facility, a patient may be able to ambulate around the room and into a bathroom while receiving oxygen from the piped-in wall source near the bed.

COMPRESSED OXYGEN TANK WITH REGULATOR

Oxygen tanks are not used in hospitals because of the high pressure and their potential for serious injuries if the pressure valve is broken. They are sometimes used in home care or in the nursing home. An additional device, called a regulator, must be attached to the valve of the tank of compressed gas (oxygen or air) to reduce the pressure to a safe, functional working level. The amount of gas registers on the gauge in pounds per square inch (*psi*). When the tank is almost empty, the needle points to a red area, warning that the tank must be replaced soon. The pressure in the tank delivers the oxygen so that no power is needed to use it.

LIQUID OXYGEN TANK

Small tanks that hold liquefied oxygen are used for those who must use oxygen as they go about their daily lives. A large container is kept in the home. A small, light-weight portable tank that can be worn over a shoulder is refilled as needed. This type of oxygen delivery system encourages an individual to be up and active. It can deliver oxygen at a high flow rate. Because it requires no electricity, it is not affected by power outages. It operates quietly with only the low sound of air moving. This type of oxygen may also be used in long-term care facilities.

OXYGEN CONCENTRATOR

The oxygen concentrator is a device operated on ordinary electrical current that selectively removes the nitrogen from the ambient air, producing concentrated oxygen. The units can provide up to 5 liters a minute of air with an oxygen concentration of 95%. These are primarily used for individuals in home care or in nursing homes. The device is a large stationary machine and thus is most suited for the person who remains in one room. There is a continuous sound from the machine that most people do not find objectionable. The oxygen concentrator eliminates the need for oxygen tanks or other oxygen supplies but is dependent on a reliable electrical supply. The device has a filter, which should be changed on a regular basis.

OXYGEN CONSERVERS

Oxygen-conserving devices can be used by patients receiving oxygen at home to reduce the number of refills needed to replenish their supply. This can reduce costs. The equipment is used with either liquid oxygen or compressed oxygen supplies. These devices can decrease oxygen requirements by 50% and can be used with either compressed or liquid oxygen. The most common are known as "demand flow" systems: Oxygen flow begins as the patient inhales and stops when the patient exhales (Pruitt & Jacobs, 2003). A demand nasal cannula and a reservoir nasal cannula are other types of demand systems.

GENERAL PROCEDURE FOR ADMINISTERING OXYGEN

ASSESSMENT

1. Assess the patient for dyspnea, difficulty in breathing, feelings of shortness of breath, dusky color in

nail beds or mucous membranes, hypoventilation and oxygen saturation level (see Pulse Oximetry below), anxiety and/or cognitive changes. **R:** Assessment determines whether oxygen administration is indicated.

2. Check the physician's order to verify that there is an order for oxygen. If so, check the concentration and equipment ordered. If at any time, you assess that a patient is experiencing acute hypoxemia, you can administer oxygen without a doctor's order, and notify the physician as soon as possible. Such a decision requires skilled nursing judgment, and there may be a specific protocol to follow for this type of situation. If a patient's condition makes this a possibility, a physician may order oxygen prn (as needed) so that the nurse can start or discontinue administration according to the patient's needs. This order may be written to give a variable amount of oxygen (e.g., up to 5 L) to maintain hemoglobin oxygen saturation at a specific level (e.g., 92%). In this instance, the nurse would measure hemoglobin saturation using pulse oximetry (see below). Then the oxygen would be started, increasing the flow rate at intervals until the desired hemoglobin oxygen saturation is reached.

   If the patient's respiratory status is such that he or she is in danger, proceed with administering oxygen, and obtain an order as soon as possible. Be cautious in administering oxygen to a patient with chronic obstructive pulmonary disease. A flow rate of greater than 2 L/min may cause the patient to stop breathing.

3. Assess the patient's immediate respiratory status. If the patient is anxious, have someone stay with him or her while you determine equipment availability.

4. Identify the types of oxygen equipment and oxygen source(s) in your facility.

ANALYSIS

5. Critically think through your data, carefully evaluating each aspect and its relation to other data. **R:** This enables you to determine specific problems for this individual in relation to administering oxygen.

6. Identify specific problems and modifications of the procedure needed for this individual. **R:** Planning for the individual must take into consideration the individual's problems.

PLANNING

7. Determine individualized patient outcomes in relation to oxygen administration, including the following. **R:** Identifying outcomes guides planning and evaluation.
   a. Breathing pattern regular and at normal rate
   b. Pink color in nail beds, lips, conjunctiva of eyes
   c. No disorientation, confusion, or difficulty with cognition
   d. Laboratory measurement of arterial oxygen concentration (PaO_2) within normal limits (80 to 100 mm Hg) or hemoglobin oxygen saturation (HgSat) within normal limits (95% to 100%).
   e. Patient resting comfortably with no irritation on the face or over the ears where oxygen device lies

8. Plan for any assistance needed to ensure the patient's safety. **R:** Typically, patients who are "oxygen hungry" become extremely restless and even disoriented. In such cases, you may need assistance.

9. Choose the appropriate equipment for the method of oxygen administration ordered. In an emergency, choose the method that best meets the patient's needs. For example, in some situations, a breathing mask is necessary, whereas in others, when the patient is alert and in mild distress, a nasal cannula is sufficient and more comfortable. Obtain a flowmeter if one is not already attached to the wall outlet or tank and a humidification device if indicated. Long extension tubing may be needed. **R:** Selecting the equipment based on the patient's needs facilitates achieving desired outcomes.

10. Check the immediate environment carefully for any potential source of fire or sparks. **R:** Eliminate any possible risk or, if necessary, move the patient to an area that is safer for oxygen administration.

IMPLEMENTATION

Action	Rationale
11. Wash or disinfect your hands.	To decrease the transfer of microorganisms that could cause infection.
12. Identify the patient, using two identifiers.	To be sure you are performing the procedure for the correct patient.

(continued)

Action	Rationale
13. Carefully and calmly explain what you are going to do. Reassure the patient that your actions will provide more comfort and that trying to relax and breathe more slowly and deeply helps.	Knowledge of the procedure, the reason for the procedure, and the equipment to be used helps relieve anxiety in the patient and sets the stage for patient participation.
14. Attach the oxygen supply tube to the cannula, catheter, or mask and the humidification device to the flow system if indicated. Then turn on the oxygen and test the flow.	To be sure the equipment is functioning properly.
15. Follow the specific procedure for the equipment you are using.	To ensure correct administration of oxygen.
16. Assess the effectiveness of the oxygen delivery. Assess both the patient's breathing and the functioning of the equipment. Check the position of the cannula, catheter, or mask, and make any necessary adjustments.	To determine if any adjustments are needed in the amount of oxygen or mode of delivery.
17. Explain safety precautions to the patient and any family or visitors present.	To prevent injury due to oxygen administration.
18. Assess the patient's nose and mouth, and provide oronasal care.	Because oxygen dries the mucous membranes, it is good nursing practice to administer frequent oronasal care to any patient receiving oxygen therapy. You can do this before you initiate oxygen therapy, if the patient's respiratory status allows.
19. Stay with the patient until you are sure the proper flow rate is maintained and the patient is calm enough to be left alone safely. Holding the patient's hand is often very useful and comforting.	Patient anxiety and restlessness will increase oxygen needs. Calming the patient will help decrease the oxygen demand as well as offer comfort.
20. Post an "oxygen in use" sign on the patient's door.	To ensure safety.
21. Wash or disinfect your hands.	To prevent the transfer of microorganisms that could cause infection.

EVALUATION

22. Evaluate using the individualized patient outcomes previously identified: breathing pattern regular and at normal rate; pink color in nail beds, lips, conjunctiva of eyes; no disorientation, confusion, or difficulty with cognition; laboratory measurement of arterial oxygen concentration (PaO_2) or hemoglobin oxygen saturation (HgSat) within normal limits; patient resting comfortably with no irritation on the face or over the ears where oxygen device lies. **R:** Evaluation in relation to desired outcomes is essential for planning future care.

DOCUMENTATION

23. Document the following in a narrative progress note or on a flow sheet. **R:** Documentation is a legal

record of the patient's care, and it communicates nursing interventions to other nurses and other disciplines.

   a. Date and time oxygen started

   b. Method of delivery

   c. Specific oxygen concentration or flow rate in liters per minute

   d. Subjective and objective observations of patient

   e. Notification of the physician, if appropriate

   f. Oronasal care given and added to nursing care plan if necessary

POTENTIAL ADVERSE OUTCOMES AND NURSING INTERVENTIONS

1. Loss of breathing stimulus: When individuals with chronic obstructive pulmonary disease have experienced impaired gas exchange for a long time, they often have increased blood levels of CO_2. Their respiratory mechanisms may adapt to this abnormal state. The normal stimulus to breathing that changing CO_2 levels creates is lost. In these individuals, the low oxygen level becomes the major stimulus for breathing. This is called hypoxic drive. Abruptly changing the oxygen level without altering the CO_2 level may result in the loss of the stimulus for breathing. The patient's respiratory rate will decrease and may even progress to **apnea.**

Intervention: Oxygen is initially administered at low levels: often 2 L/min for those who have chronic pulmonary disease. The patient's respiratory rate and depth is observed. Usually the oxygen is maintained at this low rate. If a higher oxygen administration rate is ordered by the physician, the rate is gradually increased while the caregiver watches carefully for the patient's response.

2. Drying of respiratory membranes: The nasal mucosa is well designed to moisten air that moves through the nose to the lungs. Anytime that oxygen is administered through a tracheostomy or through an endotracheal tube, bypassing the normal moistening mechanism, humidification of the inspired air and oxygen is essential. For the patient receiving oxygen through the nose, drying of mucous membranes may be a problem if the patient does not have adequate fluid intake.

Intervention: The question of when additional moistening of inspired air or oxygen is necessary is an important one. Some experts believe that when oxygen is administered through the normal breathing route, such as by nasal cannula or mask, humidification is unnecessary. Others believe that humidification is always important as a precautionary measure to decrease the drying effect on the **oronasal** mucosa. Follow the policy in your facility when planning initial administration. If humidification is not routinely used, be sure to assess the patient for dry mucous membranes. Do not apply petroleum-based moisturizers to the patient's lips when oxygen is in use. This is because petroleum can degrade the plastic of the oxygen administration equipment and may cause pulmonary complications if aspirated. Use a water-based product.

3. Anxiety or fear: Oxygen administration, although a common procedure, may make some patients anxious, which may increase difficulty in breathing. Some perceive oxygen administration as a life-saving measure and are reassured by the therapy. Others perceive it as an indication that they are seriously ill and are made anxious. Still others find a mask oppressive and experience claustrophobia when a mask is in place.

Intervention: By explaining the procedure (in simple terms) to the patient and the patient's family as well as by maintaining a calm attitude, you can help to allay many unnecessary fears. For this reason, even semi-comatose patients should be given explanations.

SPECIFIC PROCEDURES FOR ADMINISTERING OXYGEN

For each specific procedure discussed, some steps of the General Procedure may be modified. The text includes the modified steps as well as references to the steps of the General Procedure that remain the same.

Administering Oxygen by Nasal Cannula

ASSESSMENT

  1-4. Follow steps 1 to 4 of the General Procedure: Assess the patient's need for oxygen, check the physician's order, assess the patient's respiratory status, and identify oxygen equipment and source.

ANALYSIS

  5-6. Follows steps 5 and 6 of the General Procedure: Critically think through your data, carefully evaluating each aspect and its relation to other data, and identify specific problems and modifications of the procedure needed for this individual.

PLANNING

  7. Determine individualized patient outcomes in relation to administering oxygen by nasal cannula, including the following. **R:** Identifying outcomes guides planning and evaluation.

   a. Breathing pattern regular and at normal rate

   b. Pink color in nail beds, lips, conjunctiva of eyes

   c. No disorientation, confusion, or difficulty with cognition

   d. Laboratory measurement of arterial oxygen concentration (PaO_2) within normal limits (80 to

100 mm Hg) or hemoglobin oxygen saturation (HgSat) within normal limits (95% to 100%)

e. Patient resting comfortably with no irritation on the face or over the ears from the elastic, or of the nostrils from the cannula

8-10. Follow steps 8 to 10 of the General Procedure: Plan for any assistance needed, choose the appropriate equipment for the method of oxygen administration ordered, and check the immediate environment.

IMPLEMENTATION

Action	Rationale
11-14. Follow steps 11 to 14 of the General Procedure: Wash your hands, identify the patient (two identifiers), explain what you are going to do, and attach the oxygen supply tube to the cannula.	
15. After attaching the oxygen supply tube to the distal end of the nasal cannula, proceed as follows.	
a. Allow 3 to 5 L oxygen to flow through the tubing. Use a humidifier with flow rates greater than 4 L/min.	This makes certain that the equipment is working properly and that the patient's oronasal mucosa is protected.
b. Hold the cannula to the patient's face and gently insert the prongs into the nostrils.	To ensure that the prongs are providing oxygen directly into the nostrils and that the prongs are not rubbing against tissue.
c. Adjust straps either behind the head or around the ears and under the chin, tighten to comfort (see Fig. 31-2), and pad if needed.	The strap holds the nasal cannula in place but may cause skin irritation where it exerts pressure.
d. Adjust the flow rate to the ordered level.	To ensure that the patient is receiving the desired oxygen rate.
16-21. Follow steps 16 to 21 of the General Procedure: Evaluate the effectiveness of the oxygen delivery; explain safety precautions; assess the patient's nose and mouth, and provide oronasal care; stay with the patient until it is safe to leave; post an "oxygen in use" sign; and wash or disinfect your hands.	

EVALUATION

22. Follow step 22 of the General Procedure: Evaluate using the individualized patient outcomes previously identified: breathing pattern regular and at normal rate; pink color in nail beds, lips, conjunctiva of eyes; no disorientation, confusion, or difficulty with cognition; laboratory measurement of arterial oxygen concentration (PaO_2) or hemoglobin oxygen saturation (HgSat) within normal limits; and patient resting comfortably with no irritation on the face or over the ears from the elastic or of the nostrils from the cannula.

DOCUMENTATION

23. Follow step 23 of the General Procedure: Document date and time oxygen started; method of delivery; specific oxygen concentration or flow rate in liters per minute; subjective and objective observations of patient; notification of physician, if appropriate; oronasal care, and add oronasal care to the nursing care plan, if indicated.

Administering Oxygen by Nasal Catheter

ASSESSMENT

1-4. Follow steps 1 to 4 of the General Procedure: Assess the patient's need for oxygen, check the physician's order, assess the patient's respiratory status, and identify oxygen equipment and source.

ANALYSIS

5-6. Follows steps 5 and 6 of the General Procedure: Critically think through your data, carefully evaluating each aspect and its relation to other data, and identify specific problems and modifications of the procedure needed for this individual.

PLANNING

7. Determine individualized patient outcomes in relation to administering oxygen by nasal catheter, including the following:
   a. Breathing pattern at regular and normal rate
   b. Pink color in nail beds, lips, conjunctiva of eyes
   c. No disorientation, confusion, or difficulty with cognition
   d. Laboratory measurement of arterial oxygen concentration (PaO_2) within normal limits (80 to 100 mm Hg) or hemoglobin oxygen saturation (HgSat) within normal limits (95% to 100%)
   e. Patient rests comfortably with no irritation on the face or over the ears from the elastic or of the nostrils from the cannula

8-10. Follow steps 8 to 10 of the General Procedure: Plan for any assistance needed, choose the appropriate equipment for the method of oxygen administration, and check the immediate environment.

IMPLEMENTATION

Action	Rationale
11-14. Follow steps 11 to 14 of the General Procedure: Wash your hands, identify the patient (two identifiers), explain what you are going to do, and attach the oxygen supply tube to the catheter.	
15. After attaching the oxygen supply tube to the distal end of the nasal catheter, proceed as follows.	
a. Allow 3 to 5 L of oxygen to flow through the tubing to make certain the equipment is working properly. Use a humidifier with flow rates more than 4 L/min.	This makes certain that the equipment is working properly and that the patient's oronasal mucosa is protected.
b. Ensure that the tip of the nasal catheter rests in the nasopharynx. Measure from the tip of the patient's nose to the earlobe to determine how far to insert the tube. Lubricate the catheter with water-soluble lubricant, and gently insert it along the floor of the nasal passage.	The external landmarks reflect the distance to the oropharynx. Inserting on the floor of the nasal passages avoids the turbinate bones.
c. Tape the nasal catheter to the nose.	To hold the catheter in place.
d. Adjust the flow rate to the ordered level.	To ensure that the patient is receiving the desired oxygen rate.

(continued)

Action	Rationale
16-21. Follow steps 16 to 21 of the General Procedure: Assess the effectiveness of the oxygen; explain safety precautions; assess the patient's nose and mouth, and provide oronasal care; stay with the patient until safe to leave; post an "oxygen in use" sign; and wash or disinfect your hands.	

EVALUATION

22. Follow step 22 of the General Procedure: Evaluate using the individualized patient outcomes previously identified: breathing pattern regular and at normal rate; pink color in nail beds, lips, conjunctiva of eyes; no disorientation, confusion, or difficulty with cognition; laboratory measurement of arterial oxygen concentration (PaO_2) or hemoglobin oxygen saturation (HgSat) within normal limits; and patient resting comfortably with no irritation on the face or over the ears from the elastic or of the nostrils from the catheter.

DOCUMENTATION

23. Follow step 23 of the General Procedure: Document date and time oxygen started; method of delivery; specific oxygen concentration or flow rate in liters per minute; subjective and objective observations of patient; notification of physician, if appropriate; oronasal care, and add oronasal care to the nursing care plan if indicated.

Administering Oxygen by Mask

ASSESSMENT

1-4. Follow steps 1 to 4 of the General Procedure: Assess the patient's need for oxygen, check the physician's

order, assess the patient's respiratory status, and identify oxygen equipment and source.

ANALYSIS

5-6. Follow steps 5 and 6 of the General Procedure: Critically think through your data, carefully evaluating each aspect and its relation to other data, and identify specific problems and modifications of the procedure needed for this individual.

PLANNING

7. Determine individualized patient outcomes in relation to administering oxygen by mask, including the following.
   a. Breathing pattern regular and at normal rate
   b. Pink color in nail beds, lips, conjunctiva of eyes
   c. No disorientation, confusion, or difficulty with cognition
   d. Laboratory measurement of arterial oxygen concentration (PaO_2) within normal limits (80 to 100 mm Hg) or hemoglobin oxygen saturation (HgSat) within normal limits (95% to 100%).
   e. Patient rests comfortably with no irritation on the face or over the ears where oxygen mask and elastic rest

8-10. Follow steps 8 to 10 of the General Procedure: Plan for any assistance needed, choose the appropriate equipment for the method of oxygen administration ordered, and check the immediate environment.

IMPLEMENTATION

Action	Rationale
11-14. Follow steps 11 to 14 of the General Procedure: Wash your hands, identify the patient (two identifiers), explain what you are going to do, and attach the oxygen supply tube to the mask.	

(continued)

Action	Rationale
15. After attaching the oxygen supply tube to the mask, proceed as follows:	
a. Regulate the oxygen flow. With the non-rebreathing mask, be sure the bag is inflated before placing the mask over the patient's mouth and nose.	To make certain the equipment is working properly.
b. Place the mask against the face, over the mouth and nose, and fit it securely, shaping the metal band on the mask to the bridge of the nose. Adjust the elastic band around the patient's head and tighten.	To prevent leakage. If the mask is not snug against the face, you may need to place gauze pads over the cheek area to ensure a tight fit.
c. Adjust the flow rate to the ordered level.	To ensure that the patient is receiving the ordered oxygen rate.
16-21. Follow steps 16 to 21 of the General Procedure: Evaluate the effectiveness of the oxygen delivery; explain safety precautions; assess the patient's nose and mouth, and provide oronasal care; stay with the patient until it is safe to leave; post an "oxygen in use" sign; and wash or disinfect your hands.	

EVALUATION

22. Follow step 22 of the General Procedure: Evaluate using the individualized patient outcomes previously identified: breathing pattern regular and at normal rate; pink color in nail beds, lips, conjunctiva of eyes; no disorientation, confusion, or difficulty with cognition; laboratory measurement of arterial oxygen concentration (PaO_2) or hemoglobin oxygen saturation (HgSat) within normal limits; patient resting comfortably with no irritation on the face or over the ears where the oxygen mask and elastic rest.

DOCUMENTATION

23. Follow step 23 of the General Procedure: Document date and time oxygen started; method of delivery; specific oxygen concentration or flow rate in liters per minute; subjective and objective observations of patient; notification of physician, if appropriate; oronasal care, and add oronasal care to the nursing care plan, if indicated.

ASSESSING OXYGENATION WITH PULSE OXIMETRY

Pulse oximetry, sometimes referred to simply as **oximetry,** is a noninvasive means of measuring the oxygen saturation of hemoglobin (Fig. 31-4). Oxygen saturation is the percentage of oxygen attached to the hemoglobin that the molecule is capable of holding. Normal hemoglobin is 95% to 98% saturated. The color of the hemoglobin changes, depending on the amount of oxygen versus the amount of carbon dioxide (CO_2) it contains. A very sensitive meter can register the differences in color of the hemoglobin and translate that into the percentage of oxygen saturation. The oximetry device, through the use of diodes, measures the reflectance of light off the hemoglobin molecules in the capillaries close to the surface in the earlobe or fingertip, translates that into an oxygen saturation value, and displays the reading digitally on a monitor screen. The meter will only measure saturation correctly in the finger if the patient is not wearing nail polish on the fingernails. In situations where the finger cannot be used, an earlobe

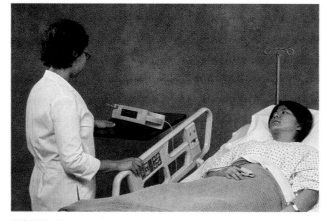

FIGURE 31-4 Oxygen saturation may be checked with the pulse oximeter.

probe may be used. Oximetry is widely used in healthcare facilities to monitor patients at risk for hypoxemia.

Although a laboratory measurement of the actual level of dissolved oxygen in the arterial blood (PaO_2) is more exact, that laboratory test requires a sample of arterial blood to be drawn and immediately analyzed by an appropriate technician. This is painful, requires a high level of skill, and is expensive. The oxygen saturation can be used as a general indicator of oxygenation when exact measurement of blood oxygen is not required. A further explanation of these relationships can be found in a physiology or medical/surgical nursing text.

The physician may order oximetry as a separate order or as a part of oxygen therapy, or the procedure may be done at the discretion of the nurse to monitor the patient's response to care. The saturation (often abbreviated "sat.") may be used as the determining factor in the amount of oxygen to be given. The order may read "Oxygen per nasal prongs up to 6 L/min to maintain saturation at 92%." This means that the nurse makes sure the oxygen saturation is measured and oxygen delivery adjusted appropriately. In some facilities, the oxygen saturation is measured by the respiratory therapist.

EQUIPMENT

A pulse oximeter is a small battery-operated device that can be handheld or placed on the bedside table. There is

an on-and-off switch, a screen where the oxygen saturation reading appears, and a clip-on finger or ear probe attached to the device by a cord (see Fig. 31-4).

USING OXIMETRY TO MEASURE OXYGEN SATURATION

ASSESSMENT

1. Check the patient's record for orders relative to oxygen therapy, oximetry, and respiratory status. **R:** Do this to identify the context and need for this assessment.
2. Review the procedure and the directions for the equipment used in the facility. **R:** Each brand of instrument has unique controls that must be used correctly.
3. Assess the patient, focusing especially on factors that might affect the patient's ability to cooperate or to undergo the procedure, special needs, and knowledge base regarding the test. **R:** This will enable effective planning.

ANALYSIS

4. Critically think through your data, carefully evaluating each aspect and its relation to other data. **R:** This enables you to determine specific problems for this individual in relation to measuring oxygen saturation.
5. Identify specific problems and modifications of the procedure needed for this individual. **R:** Planning for the individual must take into consideration the individual's problems.

PLANNING

6. Determine individualized patient outcome in relation to pulse oximetry: oxygen saturation of 95% or above. **R:** Identification of outcomes guides planning and evaluation.
7. Obtain the oximetry device, and review the directions for the specific brand. **R:** While oximetry devices are similar, making sure that the device is used correctly will ensure an accurate measurement.

IMPLEMENTATION

Action	Rationale
8. Wash or disinfect your hands.	To decrease the transfer of microorganisms that could cause infection.
9. Identify the patient, using two identifiers.	To be sure you are carrying out the correct procedure for the correct patient.

(continued)

Action	Rationale
10. Explain to the patient what you will be doing.	Explaining the procedure helps relieve anxiety or misperceptions that the patient may have about a procedure or activity and sets the stage for patient participation.
11. Carry out the procedure as follows:	
a. Attach the meter's probe to the patient as directed, either to the finger or the earlobe. Be sure the light-emitting diode is directly opposite the light-receiving diode. If the light does not have a direct path, an inaccurate reading will result. Do not fasten the probe so tightly that it impedes blood circulation.	A probe applied too tightly can produce inaccurate readings, and it can interfere with arterial blood flow (Ault & Stock, 2004).
b. Turn on the meter and read the scale when the numbers have stabilized. Ask the patient to remain still while you are taking the reading.	Excessive movement of the body, electrical noise, and low arterial blood pressure can affect readings (Ault & Stock, 2004).
c. Note the oximetry reading, and write it down.	To ensure that you will accurately record the results.
d. Remove the probe from the finger or earlobe.	To relieve pressure and discomfort.
12. Clean the equipment according to the facility procedure.	To prevent the spread of microorganisms.
13. Wash or disinfect your hands.	To prevent the spread of microorganisms that could cause infection.
14. Return equipment to appropriate storage place.	This is so that it is conveniently available for reuse.

EVALUATION

15. Evaluate using the individualized patient outcome previously identified: oxygen saturation of 95% or above. Also compare results with patient's previous readings. **R:** Evaluation in relation to desired outcomes is essential for planning future care. Comparing results determines whether oxygen administration needs to be adjusted.

DOCUMENTATION

16. Document the oximetry reading on the patient's record, either on the appropriate flow sheet or in a narrative note. Also describe patient's activity or signs and symptoms occurring at the same time that may reflect oxygenation. **R:** Documentation is a legal record of the patient's care and therapy and communicates nursing activities to other nurses and caregivers.

SELF-INFLATING BREATHING BAG AND MASK

The self-inflating breathing bag and mask (also referred to as the bag-valve mask or the Ambu bag) can be used for rescue breathing as part of cardiopulmonary resuscitation or to provide deep breaths of high oxygen concentration before suctioning. This device may also provide temporary artificial ventilation (for example, during transport) to a person who is in respiratory arrest or who depends on a ventilator for breathing.

The device is composed of a face mask that covers the mouth and nose and has a soft rim to make an airtight seal. The mask is attached to a firm rubber or plastic bag that has a connector that may be attached to an oxygen source if a high concentration of oxygen is needed. Manual compression of the bag forces air into the patient's nose and mouth. There is a valve that ensures one-way pressure into the mask and that then reinflates from the ambient air (unless attached to an oxygen source). Humidification is not provided with this method.

The bag-valve mask may also have an adapter that fits onto an endotracheal tube in the event that it needs to be used for an intubated patient (Fig. 31-5). Many bag-valve masks are designed with a tube reservoir, which looks like an accordion. This accordion-like reservoir must be stretched open to the expanded position to administer the maximal amount of oxygen to the patient.

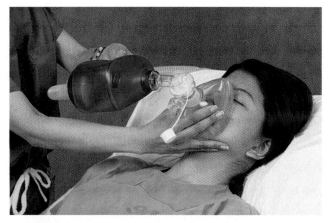

FIGURE 31-5 The self-inflating breathing bag can be used for rescue breathing, as part of CPR, or to provide deep breaths of high oxygen concentration before suctioning.

PROCEDURE FOR VENTILATING A PATIENT WITH A SELF-INFLATING BREATHING BAG AND MASK

ASSESSMENT

1. Assess the patient's need for breathing assistance or for hyperoxygenation before suctioning to determine the need for ventilating the patient with a self-inflating breathing bag and mask.

ANALYSIS

2. Critically think through your data, carefully evaluating each aspect and its relation to other data. **R:** This enables you to determine specific problems for this individual in relation to being ventilated with a self-inflating breathing bag and mask.
3. Identify specific problems and modifications of the procedure needed for this individual. **R:** Planning for the individual must take into consideration the individual's problems.

PLANNING

4. Determine individualized patient outcomes in relation to the ventilation process, including the following. **R:** Identifying outcomes guides planning and evaluation.
   a. Chest rises and falls as the bag is pressed and released.
   b. Skin color shows pink nail beds and conjunctiva.
   c. Oxygen saturation (based on pulse oximetry) is within normal limits (95% to 100%).
5. Obtain the bag-valve mask and an oxygen connector tubing if oxygen will be used to hyperoxygenate the patient. **R:** Obtaining all needed equipment facilitates organization.
6. Obtain assistance if needed. **R:** It is much easier to hyperoxygenate a patient before suctioning if there are two nurses: one nurse to use the breathing bag and one nurse to suction. In the restless patient, one nurse may be needed to hold the patient's head still, while another nurse operates the breathing bag.

IMPLEMENTATION

Action	Rationale
7. Wash or disinfect your hands.	To decrease the transfer of microorganisms that could cause infection.
8. Identify the patient, using two identifiers.	To be sure you are carrying out the procedure for the correct patient.
9. Explain to the patient what you are doing.	Even in an emergency, a patient may feel panic if something is placed over the mouth and nose.
10. Connect the mask to the oxygen supply and turn on to highest flow rate that does not cause the device to stick or jam.	This will more effectively hyperoxygenate the patient before a procedure. In emergencies, the highest concentration possible is needed.

(continued)

Action	Rationale
11. Apply the mask snugly over the patient's nose and mouth to form an occlusive seal. Either hold the mask in place manually or fasten straps behind the patient's head.	Creating a seal ensures that the patient is receiving the correct amount of oxygen.
12. Compress the bag as completely as possible to force air into the patient's nose and mouth.	This gives the patient the maximum amount of oxygen.
13. Release the bag to allow expiration. Count "1, 2, 3, 4" to allow adequate time for expiration and for the bag to reinflate.	The bag needs to be fully reinflated to deliver maximum oxygen.
14. Repeat steps 12 and 13 in a rhythmic pattern.	To provide ventilation at a rate of 12 breaths/min or for the desired number of deep breaths.

EVALUATION

15. Evaluate in relation to the individualized patient outcomes previously identified: Chest rises and falls as the bag is pressed and released; skin color shows pink nail beds and conjunctiva; and oxygen saturation is within normal limits. **R:** Evaluation in relation to desired outcomes is essential for planning future care.

DOCUMENTATION

16. Document the following. **R:** Documentation is a legal record of the patient's care and therapy and communicates nursing interventions to other nurses and other disciplines.
    a. Assessment indicating need for artificial ventilation
    b. Outcomes specific to the therapy that have been met

(See Module 36, Emergency Resuscitation Procedures, for complete directions for emergency resuscitation.)

ASSESSING VENTILATION THROUGH CAPNOGRAPHY

Capnography is often used in critical care settings or during a respiratory arrest to evaluate the effectiveness of ventilation being provided. The amount of carbon dioxide exhaled can reveal whether ventilation is effective. Carbon dioxide is measured using a mechanical device that can be attached to a ventilator or by an adapter attached to an endotracheal tube. Most provide a **capnogram,** a computerized graphic readout of CO_2 during the various phases of ventilation. The results provide an indirect mechanism to assess CO_2 production, pulmonary perfusion, alveolar ventilation, respiratory

patterns, and elimination of CO_2 from the anesthesia circuit and ventilator (Kodali, 2005). Capnography is also used in emergency situations or critical care units with a device that provides a "pH sensitive indicator that changes color when exposed to CO_2. The color varies between expiration and inspiration as the CO_2 level increases or decreases. The color changes from purple (when exposed to room air or oxygen) to yellow (when exposed to 4% CO_2)" (Kodali, 2005, p. 44). The use of either device is beyond the scope of this text and may be found in critical care manuals.

Acute Care

Oxygen use is common in the acute care setting. However, this should not make it so routine that healthcare providers fail to carefully assess the patient and evaluate its use. Oxygen delivered at high levels can have adverse effects on the lungs, oxygen delivery systems are uncomfortable for the patient, and oxygen use contributes to the cost of healthcare. Appropriate monitoring will ensure that oxygen is used when needed and discontinued when no longer needed.

Long-Term Care

Residents in long-term care facilities may also require oxygen therapy—some continuously and some intermittently. Nursing homes rarely have piped-in oxygen sources. Therefore, the oxygen source is provided for each resident who needs supplemental oxygen. A variety of types of equipment may be found in the same facility. The nurse will need to learn about each new type of equipment when it arrives in the setting. Portable oxygen units can be attached to wheelchairs for residents who are not ambulatory and who require constant oxygen. The nurse needs to exercise care to prevent fatigue and maintain mobility for the resident. Techniques to decrease exertion may include the use of a bedside commode, small meals, assistance with feeding, and a calm, low-stress environment. The same safety considerations apply in long-term care as in acute care.

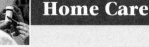

Home Care

Many persons require oxygen therapy at home. These persons or a family member must be taught how to administer oxygen as well as how to care for the equipment. A "no smoking" sign should be posted on the outside door. However, it may be more difficult to get people to cooperate with this restriction in the home than in a healthcare facility. Safety concerns involve not using oxygen in the kitchen if gas flames are used for cooking, avoiding the use of candles in the home, and planning for management of power outages if a concentrator is used. Setting up a plan for refilling oxygen containers is essential in order to not run out of oxygen. Most people receiving oxygen at home use nasal prongs, but some will have had the option to choose transtracheal oxygen therapy.

Ambulatory Care

Clients move quickly through ambulatory care centers. It is vital for the nurse to assess clients' oxygenation status after surgical procedures. If complications in respiratory status develop, the nurse must be able to assess such complications and respond accordingly. The client who develops complications postoperatively may need to be admitted to the hospital as an inpatient.

LEARNING TOOLS

DEVELOP YOUR BACKGROUND KNOWLEDGE

1. Review the Learning Outcomes.

2. Read the section on aeration in your fundamentals text.

3. Look up the Key Terms in the glossary.

4. Review this module and mentally practice the techniques described. Study so that you would be able to teach these skills to another person.

DEVELOP YOUR SKILLS

In the practice setting

1. Inspect and handle the oxygen administration equipment available.

2. Choose a partner and practice applying a mask and a nasal cannula to him or her.

3. Have your partner apply the mask and nasal cannula for you.

4. If a pulse oximeter is available, measure the oxygen saturation of your partner, and then have your partner measure your oxygen saturation.

5. Practice ventilating the mannequin using a self-inflating breathing mask and bag if available. Have your partner evaluate your performance. Then evaluate your partner's performance.

DEMONSTRATE YOUR SKILLS

In the clinical setting

1. Become familiar with the oxygen equipment used in your clinical facility.

2. Locate the pulse oximeter, and read the directions for the particular brand.

3. Talk with a patient who is receiving oxygen, and assess what he or she has been taught regarding oxygen therapy if it is not uncomfortable for the patient to talk.

4. Review the records of patients who are receiving oxygen. Note the medical diagnosis, the orders, the therapy, and any laboratory or diagnostic tests. In a small group, compare the situations of different patients.

5. Observe the administration of oxygen and the measurement of oxygen saturation for a specific patient. Were all safety precautions observed?

6. Consult with your instructor regarding the opportunity to administer oxygen to patients.

7. Under supervision, plan and initiate oxygen therapy, pulse oximetry, or both, as ordered for a patient. Use the Performance Checklists on the CD-ROM in the front of this book as a guide.

8. Document the procedure properly, and share your notes with your instructor.

CRITICAL THINKING EXERCISES

1. You are caring for a patient who has a physician's order that states: "Oxygen per nasal prongs to maintain saturation at 87%. Call me if more than 6 L/min needed." The night nurse informs you that the patient was comfortable all night, and the oxygen saturation remained at 88% with oxygen given at 4 L/min. As you plan for care during the day, identify the times when it is most important to measure oxygen saturation. When would you expect to need to increase the oxygen? What events might increase the need for oxygen?

2. Mr. Singh, who is on long-term oxygen therapy at home, uses compressed oxygen in a tank. He states that he cannot go anywhere without his oxygen on, so he stays in the bedroom, uses a commode, and bathes at the bedside. Considering the various ways to deliver oxygen, identify at least two alternative plans for oxygen therapy that might allow Mr. Singh to leave his bedroom. Determine what other considerations—besides the method of oxygen delivery—may need to be addressed in relation to this client's situation. Explain how the nurse might manage these concerns.

SELF-QUIZ
SHORT-ANSWER QUESTIONS

1. List four methods of delivering oxygen.

   a. _____

   b. _____

   c. _____

   d. _____

MULTIPLE-CHOICE

_____ 2. Oxygen is potentially dangerous because it
   a. burns rapidly.
   b. is explosive.
   c. supports combustion.
   d. combines with nitrogen.

_____ 3. Regardless of the method used, it is important to test and regulate oxygen flow before administering oxygen to the patient because
   a. it is easier to observe the flow rates.
   b. it protects the patient from the danger of a malfunction.
   c. it protects the patient from an explosion.
   d. it limits the amount of oxygen intake.

_____ 4. Oxygen flow (liters per minute)
   a. should never exceed 3 L/min.
   b. should remain below 8 L/min.
   c. should be changed every 8 hours.
   d. is determined by the delivery method and the physician's order.

_____ 5. The self-inflating breathing bag is most likely to be used
   a. for routine oxygen administration.
   b. for rescue breathing.
   c. instead of transtracheal oxygen.
   d. instead of a non-rebreathing mask.

_____ 6. Frequent oronasal care should be given to the patient receiving oxygen primarily because
   a. of the patient's high anxiety level.
   b. oxygen dries mucous membranes.
   c. oxygen is irritating to the skin.
   d. secretions are increased.

_____ 7. Patients who receive oxygen therapy need explanations and reassurance because (Choose all that apply.)
   a. the patient or family may think the patient is seriously ill when this is not true.
   b. the patient may feel claustrophobic.
   c. the patient has had no previous experience with it.
   d. some oxygen appliances are uncomfortable to wear.

_____ 8. What is a disadvantage to the patient of the use of transtracheal oxygen?
   a. It is less safe.
   b. It is more expensive.
   c. It is less socially acceptable.
   d. It requires a surgical procedure to place.

Answers to the Self-Quiz questions appear in the back of the book.

Respiratory Care Procedures

SKILLS INCLUDED IN THIS MODULE

General Procedure for Giving Respiratory Care
Specific Procedures for Giving Respiratory Care
  Assisting the Patient With Deep Breathing
  Teaching the Patient to Cough Productively
  Performing Postural Drainage
  Performing Percussion
  Performing Vibration

PREREQUISITE MODULES

Module 1	An Approach to Nursing Skills
Module 2	Documentation
Module 3	Basic Body Mechanics
Module 4	Basic Infection Control
Module 5	Safety in the Healthcare Environment
Module 6	Moving the Patient in Bed and Positioning
Module 14	Nursing Physical Assessment

KEY TERMS

abdominal (diaphragmatic) breathing	lobes
	lung
	mucus
alveoli	nebulizer
atelectasis	percussion
auscultation	postural drainage
bronchioles	postural
cough	hypotension
diaphragm	segment
expectorate	splinting
expiration	sputum
gatched	Trendelenburg
hyperventilation	position
inspiration	vibration
lingula	

OVERALL OBJECTIVE

▸ To assist patients effectively with deep breathing, coughing, postural drainage, percussion, and vibration as necessary in their individual situations.

LEARNING OUTCOMES

The student will be able to

1. Assess the patient effectively to determine the need for a respiratory care procedure.
2. Analyze assessment data to determine the patient's specific respiratory problem and the type of procedure to be utilized for that problem.
3. Analyze assessment data to determine other special problems or concerns that must be addressed before proceeding with a specific procedure.
4. Determine appropriate patient outcomes based on the purpose of each respiratory care procedure, and recognize the potential for adverse outcomes.
5. Plan the respiratory care procedure, taking into consideration the special needs of the patient and whether a physician's order is needed for the procedure.
6. Implement deep breathing, coughing, postural drainage, percussion, and vibration, using appropriate techniques.
7. Evaluate the effectiveness of the respiratory care procedure implemented in relation to the desired outcomes.
8. Document respiratory care procedures appropriately according to facility policy.

Respiratory care procedures are used to prevent and treat respiratory complications that may occur as a result of bed rest, immobility, and various illnesses. These procedures are effective because they assist in inflating the **alveoli** and in removing secretions that can host microbial growth and interfere with gas exchange. Respiratory care personnel may be responsible for some of this care, but the nurse is always responsible for assessing, monitoring, and evaluating the patient's respiratory status and may be responsible for all respiratory care, including teaching these measures. These measures are often referred to as chest physiotherapy or bronchial hygiene therapy.

NURSING DIAGNOSES

- Risk for Impaired Respiratory Function. This reflects a general category rather than a specific nursing diagnosis within the NANDA framework, but it may be appropriate to use for the individual who does not yet have a specific nursing diagnosis, but who is at risk for developing one of the respiratory-related nursing diagnoses below.
- Ineffective Airway Clearance is appropriate for the person who has secretions in the airway that are not being coughed up.
- Impaired Gas Exchange reflects the condition of the patient who is unable to obtain the oxygen needed or expel the carbon dioxide that has accumulated. Secretions accumulated in the lungs may obstruct respiratory passages and

block air from entering alveoli, resulting in a lack of oxygen.
- Ineffective Breathing Pattern may be evidenced by the patient who is taking very shallow breaths. Shallow breathing may fail to expand alveoli, leading to alveolar collapse and eventually to impaired gas exchange. Shallow breathing may occur because of pain or sedation.
- Risk for Infection Transmission is appropriate for the patient who has a respiratory infection. Coughing up secretions can spread infectious material. Nurses need to be aware of this problem and set up the appropriate measures to protect themselves and others in the environment.

DELEGATION

Respiratory care procedures require assessment of respiratory status as well as teaching as part of each procedure. Therefore, many of these procedures should not be delegated to assistive personnel. In some instances, for patients who need to learn how to deep breathe, cough, and use the incentive spirometer, the nurse may initially teach the patient. Regular oversight of the patient performing the procedure may be delegated to the nursing assistant. In these cases, the assistants must first be taught the correct procedures. The nurse also may need to teach assistive personnel how to protect themselves from infection when working with patients who are coughing.

GENERAL PROCEDURE FOR GIVING RESPIRATORY CARE

ASSESSMENT

1. Count the individual's respiratory rate and assess for depth and chest expansion. **R:** This provides a baseline measure of the patient's respiratory status.
2. Auscultate each **lung,** especially noting areas with diminished breath sounds and areas where moisture is present. **R:** This allows you to note any changes after the respiratory procedure.
3. Assess the patient's activity pattern. **R:** The activity pattern helps you determine the patient's tolerance for the procedure.
4. Identify whether the patient is at risk for respiratory problems because of bed rest, inactivity, or surgical treatment. **R:** Recognizing problems helps you to determine which procedures may benefit the patient.
5. Check the patient for pain or other factors that may limit respiratory effort. **R:** This will help the patient get the maximal benefit from the respiratory procedure.

ANALYSIS

6. Critically think through your data, carefully evaluating each aspect and its relation to other data to determine the specific respiratory problem and the type of respiratory procedure appropriate to that problem. **R:** The procedure must be one that has the potential for resolving the problem. While some procedures require a physician's order, deep breathing and coughing may be initiated by the nurse.
7. Identify specific problems and modifications of the procedure needed for this individual. **R:** Planning for the individual must take into consideration the individual's problems.

PLANNING

8. Determine individualized patient outcomes in relation to the specific respiratory care procedure, include the following, as appropriate. **R:** Identification of outcomes guides planning and evaluation.

---

box 32-1 *Splinting for Safety and Comfort*

A patient who has a surgical wound feels pain when moving the muscles that were cut during surgery. The pain can be minimized by splinting; that is, by holding the incisional area firmly to decrease movement. Splinting can be accomplished by spreading your hands or the patient's hands and holding them firmly over the incision. Also, a pillow can be held firmly over the incisional area to splint it. If pain medication is needed, make sure that you allow enough time for the medication to take effect before you begin the procedure.

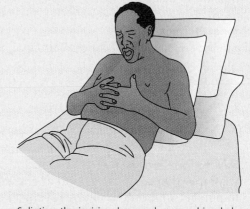

Splinting the incisional area when coughing helps relieve some pain.

---

a. The patient coughs out all secretions present.
b. The lungs are clear to **auscultation.**
c. The respiratory rate is within normal limits.
d. The patient takes deep breaths at intervals.
e. The patient is resting comfortably.

9. Plan for pain relief, if necessary, before performing any respiratory care procedure. Plan also for **splinting** during the procedure if needed. Doing so ensures that the patient gets the maximal benefit from the procedure while remaining as comfortable as possible (Box 32-1).
10. Plan an appropriate time for performing the procedure. Also plan how often the procedure should be repeated. The times should be spaced throughout the day. **R:** The frequency is determined by the desired outcome of the procedure. It is preferable to choose times when the patient is rested.

IMPLEMENTATION

Action	Rationale
11. Wash or disinfect your hands. You may need gloves if there is a chance you will be exposed to respiratory secretions.	To prevent the transfer of microorganisms that may cause infection.

(continued)

Action	Rationale
12. Identify the patient, using two identifiers.	To be sure you are performing the procedure for the correct patient.
13. Explain to the patient why you are concerned about his or her respiratory status in a way that does not increase anxiety. Tell the patient which measures are necessary to prevent or alleviate problems.	To help the patient remain calm and set the stage for maximum patient cooperation and participation.
14. Carry out planned pain relief measures.	To allow maximal benefit from the respiratory procedure.
15. Carry out the specific procedure as outlined below.	To assist the patient in achieving optimal respiratory function.
16. Remove gloves if used, and wash or disinfect your hands.	To decrease the number of microorganisms that could cause infection.

EVALUATION

17. Evaluate using the individualized patient outcomes previously identified: The patient coughs out all secretions present, the lungs are clear to auscultation, the respiratory rate is within normal limits, the patient takes deep breaths at intervals, and the patient is resting comfortably. **R:** Evaluation in relation to desired outcomes is essential for planning future care.

DOCUMENTATION

18. Document the respiratory care procedure performed on a flow sheet, nurses' progress notes, or using computerized charting. **R:** This provides important information for other caregivers.

SPECIFIC PROCEDURES FOR GIVING RESPIRATORY CARE

Note: For each respiratory care procedure discussed, some steps of the General Procedure may be modified. The modified steps have been included completely as have references to the steps of the General Procedure that remain the same.

Assisting the Patient With Deep Breathing

All alveoli are not equally expanded during each breath taken. Normal respiration includes occasional deep breaths that serve to fully expand all alveoli and encourage the movement of secretions. Whenever a person is bedridden or otherwise immobile, continuous shallow respirations are common. This tends to encourage the retention of secretions and **atelectasis** (the collapse of the alveoli).

Deep breathing is a planned part of the nursing care of every immobilized patient, especially those who have increased secretions (persons who have inhaled respiratory anesthetics or who have respiratory disease). For patients who have undergone abdominal or chest surgery, deep breathing may be difficult and even painful. These patients may require a great deal of assistance and support when you help them to deep breathe.

ASSESSMENT

1-5. Follow steps 1 to 5 of the General Procedure: Count respiratory rate and assess depth and chest expansion, auscultate lungs, assess activity pattern, identify whether the patient is at risk for respiratory problems, and check for pain or other factors that may limit respiratory effort.

ANALYSIS

6-7. Follow steps 6 and 7 of the General Procedure: Critically think through your data, and identify specific problems and modifications of the procedure needed.

PLANNING

8. Determine individualized patient outcomes in relation to deep breathing. **R:** Identifying outcomes guides planning and evaluation.

a. Respiratory rate and chest expansion equal to or greater than before the procedure
b. Lungs clear to auscultation
c. Patient resting comfortably

9-10. Follow steps 9 and 10 of the General Procedure: Plan for pain relief and for an appropriate time and frequency for the procedure.

IMPLEMENTATION

Action	Rationale
11-14. Follow steps 11 to 14 of the General Procedure: Wash or disinfect your hands, identify the patient (two identifiers), explain the deep breathing exercises and why they are indicated, and provide pain relief, if indicated.	
15. Assist the patient with deep breathing as follows:	
a. Instruct the patient both by explaining and by demonstrating proper deep breathing. Remember to use the principles of health teaching as you plan for the patient's instruction.	Because the patient must carry out the procedure, he or she must understand what should be done and why. A person who understands and accepts the importance of deep breathing is more likely to cooperate and participate in the exercises.
b. Position the patient for maximum expansion of the lungs. To accomplish this, the chest should not be constricted. Having the patient sit on the edge of the bed or in a chair is ideal, but deep breathing can be done in any position necessitated by the patient's condition.	To provide maximal benefit from the procedure.
c. Have the patient inspire slowly. It is helpful if you count slowly to 2 during **inspiration.**	To allow for more comfortable alveolar expansion. Slow movement usually creates less discomfort than rapid movement.
d. Because normal **expiration** is twice as long as inspiration, have the patient exhale slowly while you count to 4.	This preserves the normal inspiratory–expiratory ratio and encourages maximum filling and emptying of the alveoli.
e. Watch the patient for chest and abdominal expansion.	Maximum expansion of the lungs occurs when both abdomen and chest expand during inspiration. This is called **abdominal (diaphragmatic) breathing.** The expansion of the abdomen is caused by the **diaphragm** moving downward, displacing abdominal contents to allow complete lung expansion.
f. Correct the patient's breathing technique as necessary.	To encourage complete lung expansion.
g. Repeat the procedure for a total of 10 deep breaths.	This provides enough repetitions for the patient to benefit from the procedure.

(continued)

Action	Rationale
16. Follow step 16 of the General Procedure: Wash or disinfect your hands.	

EVALUATION

17. Follow step 17 of the General Procedure: Evaluate using the individualized patient outcomes previously identified: respiratory rate and chest expansion equal to or greater than before procedure, lungs clear to auscultation, and patient resting comfortably.

DOCUMENTATION

18-19. Follow steps 18 and 19 of the General Procedure: Document the deep breathing procedure performed and the patient's response. Include the patient's understanding and ability to do deep breathing independently.

DEVICES THAT ENCOURAGE DEEP BREATHING

A variety of devices are used to encourage deep breathing. These include several types of incentive spirometers and the intermittent positive pressure breathing (IPPB) device.

INCENTIVE SPIROMETERS

Physicians often order an incentive spirometer to encourage the patient to breathe deeply. The incentive spirometer provides immediate objective feedback about performance, thereby increasing motivation to learn and resulting in quicker learning. The achievement signal often is set low at first, allowing the patient to master that level before moving higher. This also allows the patient to progress gradually. Spirometers are quite effective in that many patients breathe far more deeply when using them. Several models of incentive spirometers are available, and all have been developed to encourage the patient to perform deep breathing.

VOLUME-ORIENTED SPIROMETER

The volume-oriented, or electronic, device is set so that a signal is activated when the patient achieves a prescribed inspiratory volume. The patient is instructed in deep breathing, with particular emphasis on the long inspiratory effort. The patient expires normally, and then places the mouthpiece in the mouth and inspires only through the machine. If the inspiratory volume meets the preset amount, the signal is activated. Most incentive spirometers have counters to indicate the number of deep breaths taken.

FLOW-ORIENTED SPIROMETER

The flow-oriented, or mechanical, incentive spirometer has plastic chambers with movable balls similar to ping-pong balls. The patient inhales through the nose, exhales through the mouth, and then inhales through the mouthpiece, attempting to keep the balls at the top of the chambers for 3 seconds (Fig. 32-1). The patient is usually encouraged to do this exercise 10 times every 1 or 2 hours.

INTERMITTENT POSITIVE PRESSURE BREATHING MACHINE

The IPPB machine uses positive pressure to increase inspiration and a **nebulizer** device to deliver moisture (with or without medication) deep into the lungs. Most often, IPPB is used for the patient with respiratory disease who needs to have a medication delivered to the lungs using pressure. According to the AARC clinical practice guideline (Sorenson & Shelledy, 2003), IPPB is not a first-line choice for respiratory treatments. Standard nebulizers and metered-dose inhalers can deliver medication more effectively. When ordered, this treatment is usually performed by the respiratory therapist. A treatment usually lasts 5 to 10 minutes or as long as

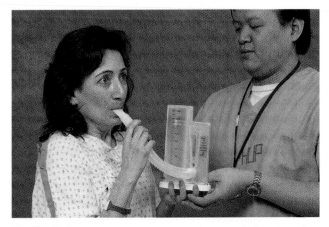

FIGURE 32-1 A mechanical incentive spirometer. By inhaling, the patient attempts to keep the balls at the top of the chambers for 3 seconds.

it takes to get all of the ordered medication delivered. In some cases, a short rest period may be needed during the treatment. The actual procedure is specific to the brand of machine. The manufacturer provides a manual with directions for use.

PRODUCTIVE COUGHING

A **cough** is always combined with deep breathing, but deep breathing may be done without coughing. Deep breathing fully expands the alveoli and enhances the normal respiratory function. Coughing raises respiratory secretions so they do not plug the **bronchioles** (causing atelectasis) or provide a medium for bacterial growth.

Teaching the Patient to Cough Productively

ASSESSMENT

1-5. Follow steps 1 to 5 of the General Procedure: Count respiratory rate and assess depth and chest expan-sion, auscultate lungs, assess activity pattern, identify whether the patient is at risk for respiratory problems, and check for pain or other factors that may limit respiratory effort.

ANALYSIS

6-7. Follow steps 6 and 7 of the General Procedure: Critically think through your data, and identify specific problems and modifications of the procedure needed.

PLANNING

8. Determine individualized patient outcomes in relation to teaching the patient to cough productively:
  a. Any secretions present are coughed out.
  b. Lungs are clear to auscultation.
  c. Respiratory rate is within normal limits.
  d. Patient takes deep breaths at intervals.
  e. Patient is resting comfortably.

9-10. Follow steps 9 and 10 of the General Procedure: Plan for pain relief and for an appropriate time and frequency for the procedure.

IMPLEMENTATION

Action	Rationale
11-14. Follow steps 11 to 14 of the General Procedure: Wash or disinfect your hands, identify the patient (two identifiers), explain that you will be teaching the patient to cough productively and why, and provide pain relief.	
15. Teach the patient to cough productively as follows.	
a. Explain the reasons for coughing.	A patient who understands and accepts the reason for an activity is more cooperative in performing that activity.
b. Assist the patient to a sitting position if possible.	This is normally the most effective position for coughing. Other positions can be used, depending on the patient's needs.
c. Splint, as described above in the General Procedure, step 8, if necessary.	This will allow greater lung expansion by decreasing pain.
d. Provide the patient with tissues if needed for expectorating sputum. (Put on gloves if the patient cannot manage own secretions.)	Respiratory secretions should be coughed into a tissue and discarded into a bedside bag to avoid transferring microorganisms. If the nurse must handle the tissues, gloves protect the nurse from microorganisms.

(continued)

Action	Rationale
e. Have the patient deep breathe, following steps 15c (inspire slowly) and 15d (exhale slowly while you count to 4) as in the Procedure for Assisting With Deep Breathing.	This allows for more comfortable alveolar expansion. Slow movement usually creates less discomfort than rapid movement does. Expiring slowly preserves the normal inspiratory–expiratory ratio and encourages maximum filling and emptying of the alveoli.
f. After the third deep breath, have the patient inspire and hold the breath 3 seconds.	To allow for full expansion of the lungs.
g. Have the patient expire forcefully against the closed glottis, and then release the air abruptly while flexing forward. Use simpler language when explaining this to the patient. For example, instead of "Exhale against the closed glottis," say, "Hold your breath, and then try to breathe out when your throat is closed."	Exhaling against the closed glottis builds up pressure, which tends to create a force that raises secretions. Flexing forward exerts abdominal pressure against the diaphragm, which increases the force of the expired air sufficiently to carry secretions.
h. Repeat for three deep coughs if possible, or repeat until the patient can **expectorate mucus.** Watch for dizziness and tingling of the extremities, the most common symptoms of **hyperventilation.**	Repetition may be needed to raise secretions. Prolonging deep breathing and coughing can cause hyperventilation.
i. Check the lungs by auscultation.	To determine the patient's response to the procedure.
j. Offer oral hygiene.	**Sputum** (expectorated mucus) often leaves a disagreeable taste in the mouth.
k. Repeat deep breathing and coughing hourly as needed or as ordered.	To clear the lungs of secretions.
16. Follow step 16 of the General Procedure: Discard gloves if used, and wash or disinfect your hands.	

EVALUATION

17. Follow step 17 of the General Procedure: Evaluate using the individualized patient outcomes previously identified: Any secretions present are coughed out, lungs are clear to auscultation, respiratory rate is within normal limits, deep breaths are taken at intervals, and the patient is resting comfortably.

DOCUMENTATION

18-19. Follow steps 18 and 19 of the General Procedure: Document the productive coughing exercises and the patient's response. Include the amount and character of sputum coughed up.

POTENTIAL ADVERSE OUTCOMES AND RELATED INTERVENTIONS

1. Atelectasis: Coughing when the patient has no secretions to expectorate may lead to alveolar collapse (atelectasis) and decreased oxygenation.
Intervention: Carefully assess the patient. Do not encourage vigorous coughing when the patient does not have secretions to expectorate.

POSTURAL DRAINAGE

When a large volume of secretions is present in the lungs, raising all of them by deep breathing and coughing may be impossible. **Postural drainage**—positioning the patient so that the force of gravity helps drain the lung secretions—may be required. For most individuals, moderately slanted positions are successful in draining lungs. Because of the branching structure of the lungs, however, a variety of positions must be used to drain each lung **segment** adequately.

Each position is generally held from 3 to 15 minutes (Goodfellow & Jones, 2002). When you have determined the position in which most of the secretions are raised, you can shorten the time the patient spends in some positions and lengthen the time in others. Not all positions are necessary for every patient—only those that drain specific affected areas.

Postural drainage is best tolerated if done between meals, at least 2 hours after the patient has eaten, to decrease the possibility of vomiting. This will also allow the patient time to rest before the next meal. Even if you are not responsible for carrying out the postural drainage because it is done by a respiratory therapist, you are responsible for coordinating all aspects of care in the patient's best interests. The positions in the following procedures (Postural Drainage, Percussion, and Vibration) are moderate. Certain lung segments do not drain in these positions, but if the entire sequence is used, most do.

Performing Postural Drainage

ASSESSMENT

1. Check the chart for a physician's order. **R:** An order is needed to perform postural drainage.
2. Identify the specific segments of the lung to be drained. This may be part of the physician's order, or the areas with excessive secretions may be identified by the physician in the progress notes. The areas with excessive secretions may also be identified through auscultation or by checking the chest x-ray report. **R:** You need to know the segments to be drained to determine in which positions to place the patient.

   Note: Most often, the lower **lobes** are drained. It is assumed that most of the upper lobes drain in normal daily activity, but this would not be true for a severely immobilized patient. The complete postural drainage, or chest physiotherapy, sequence is tiring and can be done with rest periods between positions. Pay particular attention to elderly patients with heart disease who may experience difficulty with the procedure.

ANALYSIS

3. Critically think through your data, carefully evaluating each aspect and its relation to other data. **R:** This enables you to determine specific problems for this individual in relation to postural drainage.
4. Identify specific problems and modifications of the procedure needed for this patient. **R:** The patient may not need to be placed in all positions because he or she may only need certain areas of the lungs drained. Or the patient may not tolerate certain positions well. For instance, patients with respiratory problems do not like to lie flat, because they feel short of breath.

PLANNING

5. Determine the individualized patient outcomes in relation to postural drainage, including the following. **R:** Identification of outcomes guides planning and evaluation.
   a. Secretions coughed up
   b. Lungs clear to auscultation
   c. Respiratory rate within normal limits
   d. Patient resting comfortably
6. Plan how you will place the patient in the various positions. Some beds can be raised in the middle **(gatched)** to provide the correct position for postural drainage. Some beds that cannot be gatched do have a foot section that can be lowered, in which case, you can position the patient with his or her head at the foot of the bed and use the footdrop to achieve the desired position. Most electric beds can be placed in the **Trendelenburg** (head down) **position.** You can use this position for postural drainage, but raising the patient's feet may increase fatigue and is not essential to the procedure's effectiveness. If the bed cannot be positioned properly, you will need one large or two small pillows to place under the patient's hips to provide the correct position. You will also need another pillow to support the patient in the side-lying position. **R:** Planning allows you to be prepared to provide postural drainage with proper positioning.
7. Obtain pillows and a sputum cup and tissues. Also obtain clean gloves if the patient cannot manage his or her own secretions. **R:** The pillows are used to position the patient, and the cup and tissues are for the patient to use for expectorated secretions. Wearing gloves protects you from possible contact with the sputum.

IMPLEMENTATION

Action	Rationale
 **8-9.** Follow steps 8 and 9 of the General Procedure: Wash or disinfect your hands, and identify the patient (two identifiers).	

(continued)

Action	Rationale
10. Explain to the patient the purpose and method of postural drainage, using the basic principles of health teaching.	The informed patient will be less tense and more able to participate.
11. Position the patient.	To drain the proper lobes.
12. Drain the upper lobes.	
a. Have the patient sit up if possible. (Sitting in a straight chair is ideal.) You can also raise the head of the bed to its maximum height.	To facilitate drainage of the upper lobes.
b. Have the patient lean to the right side (45-degree angle) for 5 minutes.	This will drain the left aspect of both upper lobes. Support the patient with pillows if necessary.
c. Then have the patient lean to the left side (45-degree angle) for 5 minutes.	This will drain the upper right lobes. Again, support the patient with pillows if necessary.
d. Have the patient lean forward at a 30- to 45-degree angle, and stay in this position for 5 minutes.	This position drains the posterior segments of the upper lobes. Let the patient brace the elbows on the knees to maintain this position. Or you can pad an overbed table and place it in front of the patient to lean on.
e. Have the patient lean backward at a 30- to 45-degree angle for 5 minutes.	This position drains the anterior segments of the upper lobes. Help the patient maintain the position by having him or her lean back in bed with the headrest at the proper height.
f. Have the patient lie on the abdomen, back, and both sides while horizontal (prone, supine, left and right side-lying).	This will drain the remaining segments of the upper lobes.
13. Drain the lower lobes. *Note:* There are six positions described below. Each can be achieved if the patient starts out lying on one side and gradually turns like a rotisserie.	Each position drains a different lung segment. To identify which lung segments are drained with each position, refer to the drawings in an anatomy text that outline various lung segments. The patient should remain in each position for 5 minutes. Use the same sequence of positions each time to help you remember them easily.
a. Place the patient in the left side-lying position in bed. Use pillows, or adjust the bed so that the patient's head and thorax are 30 to 45 degrees down from the horizontal position.	The 30-degree position is less tiring and creates fewer adverse circulatory effects than the 45-degree position.
(1) Next, have the patient lie on the left side, with the shoulders perpendicular to the bed (Fig. 32-2). Use pillows to support the patient, and place a small pillow under the head, if necessary for comfort.	This position drains the lateral basal segment of the right lower lobe.

(continued)

Action	Rationale
	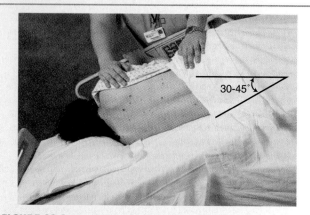 **FIGURE 32-2** To drain the lateral basal segment of the right lower lobe, the patient lies on the left side with the head and thorax 30 to 45 degrees lower than the horizontal position (as shown). To drain the right middle lobe, the shoulders should be raised to a 45-degree angle from the horizontal position.
(2) Turn the patient halfway onto the back, so the shoulders are at a 45-degree angle to the bed. Again, use pillows to support this position.	This position drains the right middle lobe.
(3) Turn the patient to the supine position, flat on the back (Fig. 32-3).	This position drains the anterior basal segments of the right and left lower lobes.
	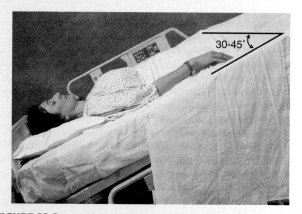 **FIGURE 32-3** To drain the anterior basal segments of both lungs, the patient lies flat on the back (supine) with thorax 30 to 45 degrees down from the horizontal position.
(4) Turn the patient halfway to the right side, so the shoulders are at a 45-degree angle to the bed (Fig. 32-4).	This position drains the **lingula** of the left lower lobe.
(5) Turn the patient completely onto the right side, so the shoulders are again at a 90-degree angle to the bed (Fig. 32-5).	This position drains the lateral basal segments of the left lower lobe.

(continued)

Action	Rationale
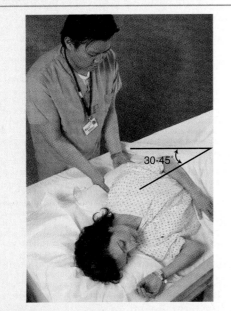

FIGURE 32-4 To drain the lingula of the left lower lobe, the nurse places pillows to support the shoulders at a 30- to 45-degree angle to the bed. |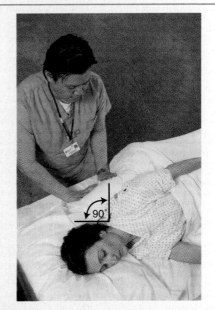

FIGURE 32-5 To drain the lateral basal segments of the left lower lobe, the nurse positions the shoulders at a 90-degree angle to the bed and places pillows to support the position. |
| **(6)** Have the patient turn onto the abdomen (prone), with the head turned to the side (Fig. 32-6). | This position drains the posterior basal segments of the lower lobes. It is usually used last, because secretions are often easier to cough out when the patient is on the abdomen.

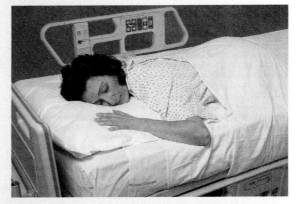

FIGURE 32-6 Draining the posterior basal segments of the lower lobes. This position is also used for coughing out secretions. |
14. Have the patient cough forcefully (lying on the abdomen).	To expel secretions.
15. Return the patient to a comfortable position, offer mouth care, and allow for a rest period.	Secretions often leave a bad taste in the mouth. Positioning, mouth care, and rest provide for comfort of the patient.
16. Follow step 16 of the General Procedure: Remove gloves, if used, and wash or disinfect your hands.	

EVALUATION

17. Follow step 17 of the General Procedure: Evaluate using the individualized patient outcomes previously identified: secretions coughed up, lungs clear to auscultation, respiratory rate within normal limits, and patient resting comfortably.

DOCUMENTATION

18-19. Follow steps 18 and 19 of the General Procedure: Document the postural drainage and the patient's response. Include the positions used for postural drainage and amount and character of any secretions produced.

POTENTIAL ADVERSE OUTCOMES AND RELATED INTERVENTIONS

1. Falling because of dizziness or fainting is a common concern when the patient undergoes postural drainage. Although this problem can occur when the patient is in the head-down position, it is more likely to occur when the patient is returning to the normal position, because of **postural hypotension.**
Intervention: By changing the patient's position slowly, you can help alleviate this problem. To protect the patient, raise the side rails and make frequent observations during the procedure. Some patients cannot be left alone during the procedure, so use careful nursing judgment.

2. Severe respiratory distress: If a large volume of secretions is mobilized from the alveoli and small bronchioles at one time, a larger airway may be temporarily blocked, causing severe respiratory distress, anxiety, and fear. This experience may be so upsetting that the patient may resist future attempts at postural drainage.
Intervention: Explain what is happening, and help the patient cough out the secretions. Support the patient with your continued presence and reassurance. Sometimes, it is necessary to use **percussion** (or clapping) and **vibration** (see below) to remove secretions. If the blockage is severe, suctioning may be required.

Performing Percussion

Percussion is the manual application of light blows to the chest wall. These blows are transmitted through the tissue and help loosen secretions in the lung segment immediately below the area struck. Percussion is done over areas that need to be drained. To decrease friction, percuss over the patient's gown or other light clothing, not against the bare skin.

ASSESSMENT

1. Check the chart for a physician's order. **R:** A physician's order is needed to perform percussion.

2. Identify the specific segments of the lung to be percussed. This may be part of the physician's order, or the areas with excessive secretions may be identified by the physician in the progress notes. The areas with excessive secretions may also be identified through auscultation or by checking the chest x-ray report. **R:** It is necessary to know the segments to be percussed to determine which positions are appropriate for the patient.

ANALYSIS

3. Critically think through your data, carefully evaluating each aspect and its relation to other data. **R:** This enables you to determine specific problems for this individual in relation to percussion.

4. Identify specific problems and modifications of the procedure needed for this individual. **R:** Some patients may tolerate percussion for only brief periods. Patients may have difficulty expectorating secretions that are loosened, and suctioning may be required.

PLANNING

5. Determine individualized patient outcomes in relation to the postural drainage, including the following. **R:** Identifying outcomes guides planning and evaluation.
   a. Secretions coughed up
   b. Lungs clear to auscultation
   c. Respiratory rate within normal limits
   d. Patient resting comfortably

6. Obtain pillows and a sputum cup and tissues. Also obtain clean gloves if the patient cannot manage his or her own secretions. **R:** The pillows are used to position the patient, and the cup and tissues are for the patient to use for expectorated secretions. During percussion, secretions may be expectorated. Wearing gloves protects you from possible contact with the sputum.

7. Plan for any assistance you may need. **R:** You may need to have another person assist you if the patient needs to be held in a position he or she is unable to maintain independently.

IMPLEMENTATION

Action	Rationale
8. Wash or disinfect your hands.	To prevent the transfer of microorganisms that could cause infection.

(continued)

Action	Rationale
9. Identify the patient, using two identifiers.	To be sure you are performing the procedure on the correct patient.
10. Place the patient in the appropriate postural drainage position.	This is so that the proper lobes are percussed and drained.
11. Cup your hands.	The cupped hands form a pocket of air that cushions the blows to the chest.
12. Clap cupped hands over the chest wall (Fig. 32-7). Correctly done, this action should produce a hollow sound and should not be painful for the patient. Instruct the patient to take slow deep breaths during percussion to prevent tensing of the chest and to assist with the mobilization of secretions. *Note:* Mechanical percussion devices that deliver percussion at a set force and rate are used by respiratory therapists. These devices are not commonly available in nursing departments.	To loosen secretions in the chest. **FIGURE 32-7** Performing percussion.
13. Wash or disinfect your hands.	To decrease the transfer of microorganisms that could cause infection.

EVALUATION

14. Evaluate using the individualized patient outcomes previously identified: secretions coughed up, lungs clear to auscultation, respiratory rate within normal limits, and patient resting comfortably.

DOCUMENTATION

15. On a flow sheet, nurses' progress notes, or computerized charting, document the percussion performed. A simple flow sheet is most often used to document respiratory care procedures themselves. Include the areas percussed and the amount and character of the secretions produced. **R:** This provides a legal record of the procedure that was performed.
16. Document the patient's response as evaluated on the appropriate assessment form in the chart. If there is no specific form, complete a narrative progress note or computerized note providing the pertinent information. **R:** This provides valuable information to other caregivers regarding the effectiveness of the procedure and how the patient tolerated it.

Performing Vibration

Vibration is performed for the same purpose as percussion and is as effective as percussion if done correctly. Ask the patient to exhale after a deep inspiration and perform vibration as the patient exhales.

ASSESSMENT

1. Check the chart for a physician's order. **R:** A physician's order is needed to perform vibration.
2. Identify the specific segments of the lung to be vibrated. This may be part of the physician's order, or the areas with excessive secretions may be identified by the physician in the progress notes. The areas with excessive secretions may also be identified through auscultation or by checking the chest x-ray report. **R:** It is necessary to know the segments to be vibrated to determine which positions are appropriate for the patient.

ANALYSIS

3. Critically think through your data, carefully evaluating each aspect and its relation to other data. **R:** This enables you to determine specific problems for this individual in relation to vibration.

4. Identify specific problems and modifications of the procedure needed for this individual. Some patients may tolerate vibration for only brief periods. **R:** Patients may have difficulty expectorating secretions that are loosened; suctioning may be required.

PLANNING

5. Determine the individualized patient outcomes in relation to vibration, including the following. **R:** Identification of outcomes guides planning and evaluation.

   a. Secretions coughed up
   b. Lungs clear to auscultation
   c. Respiratory rate within normal limits
   d. Patient resting comfortably

6. Obtain pillows and a sputum cup and tissues. Obtain clean gloves if the patient is unable to manage his or her own secretions. **R:** The pillows are used to position the patient, and the cup and tissues are for the patient to use for expectorated secretions. Because secretions may be expectorated during vibration, wearing gloves protects you from possible contact with the sputum.

7. Plan for any assistance you may need. **R:** You may need to have another person assist you if the patient needs to be held in a position he or she is unable to maintain independently.

IMPLEMENTATION

Action	Rationale
8. Wash or disinfect your hands.	To prevent the transfer of microorganisms that could cause infection.
9. Identify the patient, using two identifiers.	To be sure you are performing the procedure on the correct patient.
10. Place the patient in the postural drainage position of choice for vibration.	This is so that the proper lobes are percussed and drained.
11. Using flat hands, place your hands firmly against the chest wall, one over the other.	This provides a firm medium for conducting vibration.
12. Keeping your arms and shoulders straight, vibrate your hands back and forth rapidly while the patient exhales (Fig. 32-8).	The vibration is transferred through the tissues and loosens mucus. Mechanical vibrators also loosen secretions by transferring vibrations though the chest wall. Read the directions for the particular brand and model of vibrator available (generally you place the vibrating head firmly against the chest wall over the area where secretions are retained). 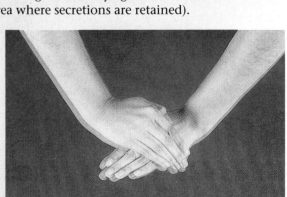 **FIGURE 32-8** Hands positioned to perform vibration.
13. Wash or disinfect your hands.	To decrease the transfer of microorganisms that could cause infection.

EVALUATION

14. Evaluate using the individualized patient outcomes previously identified: secretions coughed up, lungs clear to auscultation, respiratory rate within normal limits, and patient resting comfortably.

DOCUMENTATION

15. On a flow sheet, nurses' progress notes, or computerized charting, document the vibration performed. A simple flow sheet is most often used to document respiratory care procedures themselves. Include the area treated and the amount and character of the secretions produced. **R:** This provides a legal record of the procedure that was performed.

16. Document the patient's response as evaluated on the appropriate assessment form in the chart. If there is no specific form, complete a narrative progress note or computerized note providing the pertinent information. **R:** This provides important information to other caregivers regarding the effectiveness of the procedure and how the patient tolerated it.

NEW FORMS OF BRONCHIAL HYGIENE THERAPY

There are new forms of bronchial hygiene therapy for patients with pulmonary disorders (Table 32-1). Many of these therapies are still being investigated for their effectiveness. As such, they will likely be encountered more often in large metropolitan areas. It is useful to know about such therapies in the event you encounter them.

Acute Care

Percussion, vibration, and positioning for postural drainage can now be done by the patient's bed. Special therapeutic beds can be programmed via their inner computer to perform percussion, vibration, and positioning. It is best to wait to program the bed to perform these functions for respiratory care when the nurse can remain at the bedside to monitor the patient's response.

table 32-1. New Forms of Bronchial Hygiene Therapy

Therapy	Method	Nursing Implications
Manually assisted cough	External application of pressure to thoracic cage or epigastric area coordinated with forced exhalation Helpful for patients, such as those with neuromuscular problems or who have difficulty coughing Involves application of positive pressure with a self-inflating bag	Contraindicated in patients with flail chest, pregnancy, unprotected airway, abdominal aortic aneurysm, or osteoporosis
Autogenic drainage (also called self-drainage)	Method of controlled breathing that requires no equipment Involves timed coughing that mobilizes secretions by varying air flow. The patient is trained to loosen the mucus, collect it in higher airways, and then expel it.	Teaching focuses on the three-step technique to help patients achieve maximal expiratory air flow without airway collapse
Active cycle of breathing (formerly known as forced expiratory technique)	Couples breathing exercises with the "huff cough," which consists of one or two forced expirations without closure of the glottis. This provides less chance of airway collapse.	Teaching focuses on instructing the patient to phonate or huff during exhalation, which keeps the glottis open
Positive expiratory pressure (PEP)	Requires the patient to breathe in and out 5 to 20 times through a flow resistor. This creates positive pressure in the airways during exhalation, which stabilizes smaller airways, preventing collapse.	Most clinical studies of PEP are with cystic fibrosis patients, but its use with patients who have chronic obstructive airway diseases has also been studied.
Flutter valve	Combines PEP with high-frequency oscillations at the airway opening. The flutter valve looks like a fat pipe covered by a perforated cap. It has an inner cone that leads to a loosely supported steel ball. The patient exhales into the pipe. The physiologic changes are equivalent to PEP.	Studies comparing it with PEP show no differences.
High-frequency chest wall oscillation	Consists of an air-pulse generator and an inflatable vest. Volumes of gas are alternately injected and withdrawn from the vest, creating oscillation.	Procedure is usually performed for 30-min sessions, one to six times daily. In studies, it performed no better than PEP, but cost significantly more.
Intrapulmonary percussive ventilation (IPV)	Uses a pneumatic device to deliver bursts of gas, usually through a mouthpiece Positive airway pressure is maintained. Nebulized aerosol treatments may be given through the device.	Recommended treatment time is 20 minutes. Two studies show IPV as effective as standard aerosol and chest physiotherapy with postural drainage.

Compiled from Goodfellow, L. T., & Jones, M. (2002). Bronchial hygiene therapy: From traditional hands-on techniques to modern technological approaches. *American Journal of Nursing, 102* (1), 37–43.

Long-Term Care

Respiratory care procedures may be needed by those in long-term care facilities as well as by those in acute care. Treatments are the same, but may need to be modified for the older adult. For example, the resident may not be able to stay in a position for postural drainage as long, and you may need to use a gentler touch with percussion and vibration techniques.

Home Care

Clients may need to continue respiratory care procedures at home after discharge from the hospital, or those with chronic respiratory problems may need to carry them out on a long-term basis. In any event, you will need to assess the home setting to facilitate teaching the client as well as the family or other caregivers, to supervise the treatments, and to evaluate their effectiveness.

Ambulatory Care

Since many surgeries are performed in the ambulatory care setting, it is vital to be proficient in teaching respiratory care procedures. This is particularly true for coughing and deep breathing techniques. The client needs to attain adequate respiratory status before being discharged to home from the ambulatory care setting.

LEARNING TOOLS

DEVELOP YOUR BACKGROUND KNOWLEDGE

1. Review the Learning Outcomes.

2. Read the material on oxygenation and health teaching in your assigned text.

3. Look up the Key Terms in the glossary.

4. Review the module and mentally practice the techniques described. Study so that you would be able to teach these skills to another person.

5. Using the module directions as a guide

a. Practice deep breathing until you can do deep abdominal breathing easily.

b. Practice coughing until you can create an effective cough.

c. Practice postural drainage at home on your own bed.

   (1) Use pillows to position yourself in a moderately slanted position.

   (2) Consider the fatigue and discomfort caused by various positions.

DEVELOP YOUR SKILLS

1. In the practice setting, obtain a partner. Each of you, in turn, will be the patient while your partner is the nurse. Practice each skill as though you were instructing a patient with no previous knowledge or skill. The person representing the patient should do exactly as told, not what he or she knows to be correct.

a. Teach one another deep breathing.

b. Evaluate one another, using the Performance Checklist on the CD-ROM in the front of this book.

c. Teach one another to cough effectively.

d. Evaluate one another, using the Performance Checklist.

e. Assist one another with postural drainage.

f. While the "patient" is in each position, use percussion and vibration over the area being drained.

g. When you can perform all skills correctly, ask your instructor to evaluate your performance.

DEMONSTRATE YOUR SKILLS

1. In the clinical setting

a. Seek an opportunity to observe respiratory care being given.

b. Seek opportunities to use these skills.

CRITICAL THINKING EXERCISES

1. Mrs. T., age 73, is being seen in the outpatient clinic for a respiratory infection that has been causing a severe cough. The coughing has interfered with her sleep, but it has not been productive. How will you determine what teaching Mrs. T. needs in regard to deep breathing and coughing? Identify the special concerns that might exist for her.

2. J.J., age 8, has cystic fibrosis. He was hospitalized for a respiratory infection. He will be returning home with a regular regimen of postural drainage, vibration, and percussion to remove secretions. His parents will be performing these procedures at home. Identify the nursing role in relation to dis-

charge planning and teaching. Determine the specific actions the nurse should take in this situation.

SELF-QUIZ

SHORT-ANSWER QUESTIONS

1. Why is deep breathing necessary for the inactive or immobile patient?

   _____

2. What is the correct ratio of length of inspiration to length of exhalation?

   _____

3. What is the purpose of postural drainage?

   _____

4. What main position and then five variations are used to drain the upper lobes?

   a. _____

   b. _____

   c. _____

   d. _____

   e. _____

   f. _____

5. What main position and four variations are used to drain the left lower lobe?

   a. _____

   b. _____

   c. _____

   d. _____

   e. _____

6. What is the purpose of percussion? Of vibration?

   _____

7. What is the purpose of the incentive spirometer?

   _____

MULTIPLE-CHOICE QUESTIONS

_____ 8. Which of the following assessments of a patient will help to identify the specific positions needed for postural drainage?
   a. Auscultation of the lungs
   b. Patient's activity pattern
   c. Pain assessment
   d. Patient's respiratory rate and depth

_____ 9. What is the primary purpose of deep breathing?
   a. Increase oxygenation and the movement of secretions
   b. Lessen the risk for pulmonary embolus
   c. Prevent pneumonia
   d. Decrease pain perception

_____ 10. What is the purpose of a mechanical vibrator used on the chest?
   a. To increase the delivery of oxygen
   b. To measure ventilatory capacity
   c. To promote deep breathing
   d. To mobilize secretions

Answers to the Self-Quiz questions appear in the back of the book.

MODULE 33

Oral and Nasopharyngeal Suctioning

SKILLS INCLUDED IN THIS MODULE

Procedure for Oral and Nasopharyngeal Suctioning

PREREQUISITE MODULES

Module 1   An Approach to Nursing Skills
Module 2   Documentation
Module 4   Basic Infection Control
Module 14   Nursing Physical Assessment
Module 24   Basic Sterile Technique: Sterile Field and Sterile Gloves
Module 31   Administering Oxygen
Module 32   Respiratory Care Procedures

For tracheostomy suctioning, see Module 34, Tracheostomy Care and Suctioning.

KEY TERMS

aspirate	nasopharynx
bronchial	oropharynx
bronchoscopy	pharynx
cough reflex	secretions
cyanotic	trachea
hypoxia	Yankauer suction-
mucous	tip catheter
mucus	

OVERALL OBJECTIVE

▸ To suction patients safely and effectively using the oral or nasopharyngeal route.

LEARNING OUTCOMES

The student will be able to

1. Assess patients for signs and symptoms indicating a need for suctioning.
2. Analyze factors that may influence a patient's tolerance for suctioning.
3. Determine appropriate patient outcomes in terms of suctioning, and recognize the potential for adverse outcomes.
4. Plan the best route of suctioning for the individual patient.
5. Implement oral and nasopharyngeal suctioning techniques in the clinical setting.
6. Evaluate the patient's response to suctioning techniques.
7. Document the suctioning technique used and the patient's response.

An abnormal increase in respiratory **secretions** can result from a variety of conditions. Among the more common are lung and **bronchial** infections, central nervous system depression, and exposure to anesthetic gases. In such situations, respiratory secretions must be removed mechanically to facilitate breathing. In the conscious, alert adult, the **cough reflex** is activated when respirations are compromised and secretions are then expectorated. Unconscious or very ill patients are incapable of coughing and must rely on the nurse and the nurse's familiarity with the equipment and various techniques for suctioning to carry out this function for them.

NURSING DIAGNOSES

- Ineffective Airway Clearance: This diagnosis may be related to the patient's inability to cough effectively when copious secretions are present.
- Anxiety: The suctioning procedure itself can produce an anxious state because normal breathing may be temporarily compromised.

DELEGATION

Oral and/or oropharyngeal suctioning with a Yankauer suction device may be delegated to assistive personnel and to the client, family, or caregiver. The nurse is responsible for teaching appropriate suctioning, cleaning, and storage techniques. Nasopharyngeal suctioning may require the use of sterile equipment and sterile technique and is therefore not usually delegated to assistive personnel.

TYPE OF ASEPTIC TECHNIQUE REQUIRED

Because the respiratory tract is continuous and moist, pathogens can readily move downward from the area being suctioned. The bronchi and lungs of an ill person are particularly susceptible to infection, so sterile equipment should be used for suctioning, whether performed orally or nasopharyngeally. If the suctioning route is changed for any reason (such as an obstruction), you must obtain a new sterile catheter.

Wear sterile gloves to perform suctioning. One gloved hand holds the sterile portion of the catheter, which is in contact with the patient, while the other hand operates the machine or clean pieces of equipment. This hand is considered contaminated and is not used to touch sterile equipment.

Sterile water or saline solution is used to flush the catheter and tubing. Tap water contains microorganisms that are not harmful to the well person but may cause infection of the respiratory tract in the ill person.

In some acute care environments, the policy is to begin with new sterile equipment each day or each shift, but to clean, dry, and reuse the equipment for the specified period. These facilities usually monitor infection rates carefully and have determined that this practice does not increase their infection rate. Be sure to check the policy of the facility in regard to the use of sterile equipment for each time suction is needed. The procedure in this module is based on the use of sterile equipment and may be modified if that is not required in the facility.

In the home environment, or the long-term care environment, clean technique may be used for the person who needs suctioning on an ongoing basis. In those environments, the patient may not be exposed to the number of different and potentially drug-resistant microorganisms found in the acute care environment. Therefore, the same cleanliness that is used with food is adequate for suctioning the oropharynx. The catheter is washed and dried carefully after each use and placed in a clean, dry basin. Clean gloves are worn by the nurse to protect against microorganisms.

SUCTION CATHETERS

Suction catheters are available with two types of tips (Fig. 33-1). Each has special advantages. The open-ended catheter has a large opening at the end of the catheter and two openings on the sides of the catheter. This type is effective when the **mucus** is very thick and tenacious, but it does have a tendency to pull at tissue unless it is used carefully. The whistle-tip catheter has a large oblique opening in the end, which has a lesser tendency to grab or pull tissue.

With any catheter, the system must be closed to obtain suction, or pull. Suctioning is easily controlled with a button-type connector by placing the thumb over the opening in the protruding button (Fig. 33-2).

SUCTION SOURCE

In many healthcare facilities, each room has a suction outlet on the wall. A length of clean tubing, a wall outlet control, and a reservoir are needed to connect to the outlet (Fig. 33-3). Most reservoirs are either disposable or have disposable liners to prevent transfer of microorganisms. If wall suction is not available, a portable suction machine (Fig. 33-4) may be obtained.

The equipment should be tested before the procedure. To be effective, suction tubing must be tightly fastened to the outlet to maintain a closed system. The nurse should inspect all plugs and cords on portable units to make sure they are in good repair to prevent

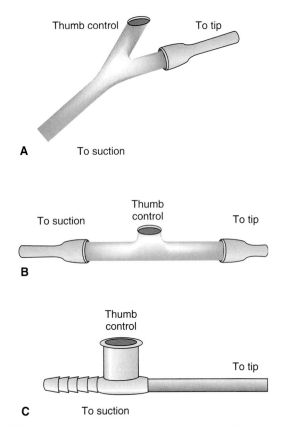

FIGURE 33-2 Suction controls. (**A**) Y-tube connector. (**B**) Button-type connector attached to catheter. (**C**) Button-type connector as part of suction catheter.

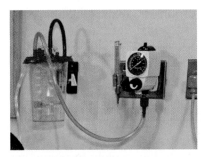

FIGURE 33-3 Wall outlet suction device.

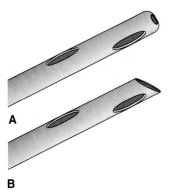

FIGURE 33-1 Suction catheters. (**A**) Open-ended catheter. (**B**) Whistle-tip catheter.

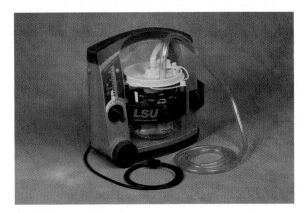

FIGURE 33-4 Portable suction machine. When wall suction is not available, a portable suction machine may be used.

sparks. Remember that sparks can be hazardous when oxygen is in use, and often the patient who is ill enough to require suctioning is receiving oxygen. If the portable unit is battery charged, be sure the charge is adequate before suctioning.

The suction pressure needs to be adjusted properly. Recommended pressure is 80 to 100 mm Hg. Pressures lower than that will not remove secretions well. Pressures higher than that can damage the mucosa and lead to atelectasis (Day, Farnell, & Haynes, et al., 2002).

ROUTES FOR SUCTIONING

The suction catheter may be inserted orally (through the mouth to the back of the throat) or nasopharyngeally (through one of the nostrils). Nasopharyngeal suctioning, particularly if done frequently, can irritate the nasal passages and cause bleeding. For an infant, suctioning must be done orally, because the nostrils are too small to introduce a suction catheter.

With oral suctioning, you can easily assess the length of catheter needed to **aspirate** the back of the throat (Fig. 33-5). When using the nasopharyngeal route, the depth of insertion for the catheter is generally determined by measuring the distance from the tip of the nose to the tip of one ear lobe, or about 5 inches (approximately 12.5 cm) for an adult.

Tracheal or deep suctioning is done by a respiratory therapist or a nurse. In tracheal suctioning, the catheter is introduced past the glottis, deep into the **trachea.** For this procedure, sterile technique is essential. This route is used when the secretions are deep in the respiratory tract, are interfering with ventilation, and cannot be suctioned by another route.

The cough reflex can be stimulated using either route. Although unpleasant for the conscious patient, coughing raises deeper secretions, which can then be removed by suctioning.

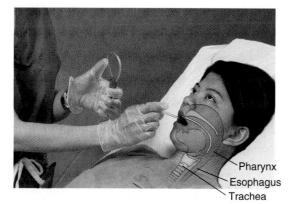

FIGURE 33-5 To measure the length of catheter needed to suction matter orally from the throat, you can place the suction catheter in the pharynx before initiating suctioning.

PROCEDURE FOR ORAL AND NASOPHARYNGEAL SUCTIONING

ASSESSMENT

1. Check for a physician's order for suctioning, if this is your facility's policy. Keep in mind that most facilities do not require a physician's order for suctioning. When it is written, it is usually done as a prn (whenever needed) order. **R:** Suctioning can be performed at the discretion of the nurse who assesses the need for suctioning the patient. If the patency of the patient's airway is threatened, an emergency exists, and you should promptly proceed with suctioning to prevent respiratory obstruction.

2. Carefully assess the patient before you proceed with suctioning unless the patency of the patient's airway is threatened. In such a situation, proceed without delay. Assess by listening to chest sounds and to sounds of the higher respiratory tract. You can sometimes hear gurgling sounds from the **pharynx** (back of the throat). A patient with severely compromised respirations resulting from copious secretions may appear **cyanotic** and have labored breathing. Determine whether the patient needs a short period of hyperventilation with a high concentration of oxygen. **R:** You must be thoughtful about the decision to suction a patient, because the irritation of the catheter may intensify the buildup of secretions. During suctioning, the patient cannot breathe in oxygen. Suctioning performed too frequently can increase the accumulation of secretions and cause a degree of **hypoxia.**

3. Familiarize yourself with the suctioning equipment available and the details of the procedure prescribed by the facility. **R:** This helps the nurse to perform the procedure promptly and skillfully.

ANALYSIS

4. Critically think through your data, carefully evaluating each aspect and its relation to other data. **R:** These measures help determine the specific respiratory problem present and the type of suctioning to be utilized for that problem. The procedure must be the one that can most effectively resolve the problem.

5. Identify specific problems and modifications of the procedure needed for the individual. **R:** Planning for the patient must take into consideration his or her individual problems.

PLANNING

6. Determine individualized patient outcomes for the suctioning procedure, including the following. **R:** Identification of outcomes guides planning and evaluation.
   a. Breath sounds clear
   b. Vital signs stable

c. Patient comfortable and calm

d. Pulse oximetry indicates adequate blood oxygen level and stability. (This outcome may not be necessary for the specific patient if there has already been a determination that oxygenation is not compromised.)

7. Plan for any needed assistance from another staff person. **R:** You may need someone to hold the patient's hands in place or to comfort the patient, because suctioning can cause agitation in patients who feel that breathing is impeded. An assistant may help the patient stay calm and cooperative.

8. Choose the appropriate equipment for the planned route of suctioning. If you are not sure which route will be used, select two catheters for possible change of route (see Module 24, Basic Sterile Technique: Sterile Field and Sterile Gloves). Most healthcare facilities have preassembled suction kits (Fig. 33-6) available that contain the following equipment:

   a. sterile catheter (sizes vary) to enter the airway to remove secretions

    b. sterile gloves to protect the patient and nurse from transfer of microorganisms

   c. sterile container, basin, or cup to hold the solution for flushing the catheter

   d. water-soluble lubricant (for nasopharyngeal suctioning)

   e. clean towel or paper drape for protecting the patient's gown and bedding

9. Add the following:

   a. sterile water or sterile saline solution (if not in set) to flush the catheter

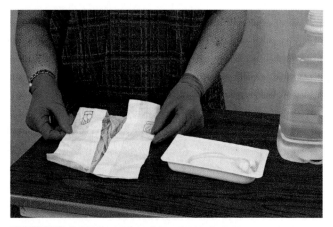

FIGURE 33-6 Commercial sterile suction catheter set.

b. wall suction connector or portable suction machine (if wall suction is not available) to remove the secretions

c. face shield or eye protection, such as eyeglasses or goggles, which provide front and side protection, to protect the nurse from secretions if the patient coughs

d. plastic apron to protect clothing from contamination with secretions and to avoid transferring microorganisms to yourself, the patient, and others if you anticipate that the patient may cough out copious secretions; in some facilities, this is done for all suctioning. **R:** Obtaining equipment ahead of time fosters organization.

IMPLEMENTATION

Action	Rationale
10. Wash or disinfect your hands.	To prevent the transfer of microorganisms that may cause infection.
11. Identify the patient, using two identifiers.	To be sure you are performing the procedure for the correct patient.
12. Explain what you are going to do. Tell the patient that you will insert the catheter gently and that you will stop the procedure if the patient wishes. Ask the patient to relax as much as possible. Inform the patient that coughing may be induced, but explain that this may help to raise the secretions to a level where they can be suctioned.	Suctioning can be threatening to any patient. It is natural to resist foreign objects that enter the respiratory tract. This is, in fact, the basis for the protective cough reflex. You can alleviate the patient's fear and gain increased cooperation by adequately explaining the procedure and the reasons for it.
13. Be sure to have or obtain adequate lighting if the room lighting is inadequate.	To promote adequate visualization.

(continued)

Action	Rationale
14. Position the patient appropriately:	
a. For oropharyngeal suctioning, place the patient in semi-Fowler's position with the head turned slightly toward you.	This allows for maximal visualization of the oral cavity and facilitates access to the oropharynx.
b. For nasopharyngeal suctioning, place the patient in semi-Fowler's position with the neck hyperextended.	To promote smooth insertion of the suction catheter.
c. Place the unconscious patient in the lateral position facing toward you.	To promote drainage of secretions and prevent aspiration.
15. Place the drape (from a suction catheter kit) or a clean towel across the patient's chest.	The drape protects the gown from secretions and general soiling.
16. Preoxygenate the patient. Follow the procedure for using the self-inflating breathing bag and mask in Module 31, Administering Oxygen.	Preoxygenation prevents the patient from becoming hypoxic. Current research advocates preoxygenation for all patients who will receive suctioning (Day, Farnell, & Haynes, et al., 2002).
17. Open the suction kit, maintaining sterile technique. Use the wrapper as a sterile field. If you are not using a kit, use the inner surface of the sterile glove package to provide a sterile field.	To prevent transfer of microorganisms to the patient's respiratory tract.
18. If the sterile solution and container are not in the suction kit, set up the sterile container, and open and pour the sterile solution into it at this time.	The sterile solution is needed to flush the suction catheter.
19. Connect the tubing to the wall or portable suction source.	This allows the suction to be transmitted to the patient.
20. Turn on the wall suction mechanism or the portable suction machine, and test by placing your thumb over the end of the suction tubing (Fig. 33-7).	Testing the suction allows you to determine if connections need to be tightened and if your suction apparatus is functioning properly.

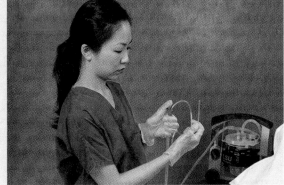

FIGURE 33-7 Testing the suction pressure by turning on the equipment and placing the thumb over the open end of the tubing.

(continued)

Action	Rationale
21. Put on sterile gloves. Kits contain two sterile gloves so that both hands are protected from contact with respiratory secretions and the patient is protected from microorganisms. Reserve the sterile glove on your dominant hand for contact with the suction catheter and use the other hand for any other needs. Fill the container in the kit with sterile solution.	This action protects the patient from contact with microorganisms.
22. Pick up the catheter with your gloved dominant hand and attach the connector end to the suction tubing, which is held in your nondominant hand. Do not touch the tubing with the nondominant hand.	To prevent contamination.
23. Suction a small amount of saline solution or water once through the tubing and catheter.	To test the function of the suction apparatus. The liquid serves to lubricate the catheter.
24. Insert the catheter through the mouth or the nostrils:	
a. *Through the mouth:* Slide the catheter along the side of the mouth to the **oropharynx.** Do not apply suction at this time.	The catheter tip may adhere to the tissues so that secretions cannot be suctioned, or the tissue may be damaged.
b. *Through the nostrils.* (*Note:* If you detect an obstruction in one nostril, try the other side.) Slide the catheter gently along the floor of the unobstructed nostril to the **nasopharynx.** No suction should be applied during this step. Use one catheter only for a single route. If you must change the route, obtain a new sterile catheter. For example, if you have attempted to suction a patient orally, met with resistance and then decided to proceed with the nasopharyngeal approach, discard the first catheter and obtain a second. If you are not using a kit, open separate sterile packs and proceed. Some facilities allow using the same catheter for oral and nasopharyngeal suctioning if the oral suctioning is done last, but this practice should be discouraged.	Precautions are necessary to prevent transmitting microorganisms from the patient's nose to the throat.
25. Holding your thumb over the opening in the catheter, apply suction for 10 to 15 seconds. As a beginner, practice	Keeping suctioning time under 15 seconds prevents hypoxia (Day, Farnell, & Haynes, et al., 2002).

(continued)

Action	Rationale
holding your breath during the suctioning period to help you remember that the patient is not receiving oxygen or inhaling while you suction. When suctioning orally, suction carefully in the cheeks, where secretions tend to pool.	
26. Withdraw the catheter under suction with a continuous, smooth motion. Do not move laterally or rotate the catheter.	Moving the catheter laterally or rotating it causes damage to the mucosa (Day, Farnell, & Haynes, et al., 2002).
27. Flush the catheter.	To remove secretions from the lumen.
28. Using the nondominant hand, turn off the suction to listen to the patient's breath sounds, and assess the need for repeated suctioning. If the patient's breathing is not clear, repeat steps 24 through 27, allowing the patient to rest 20 to 30 seconds between suctioning periods. Also encourage the patient to deep breathe and cough between suctioning periods to get the secretions to a place where they can be reached by suctioning. If you suction the patient more than once, hyperoxygenate between suctionings. When the patient's breathing sounds clear, stop suctioning. Never apply suction more than three times. Sometimes, you will stop because you have not been successful in reaching the secretions. At other times, you may be forced to stop because the patient is actively resisting the procedure. Knowing when to stop suctioning requires good nursing judgment.	Suction no longer than 15 seconds for a maximum of three times, to avoid producing hypoxia, mucosal trauma, exhaustion, and anxiety in the patient.
29. Hyperoxygenate the patient to conclude the procedure.	This postoxygenation prevents hypoxia (Day, Farnell, & Haynes, et al., 2002).
30. Detach the catheter from the tubing.	This is so that you can dispose of the contaminated catheter.
31. With your nondominant hand, grasp the cuff of the sterile glove, and pull it downward over the used catheter in your gloved hand. Dispose of catheter and glove safely in a receptacle.	This method neatly encloses the used catheter in the glove, making disposal more sanitary (Fig. 33-8).
32. Reposition the patient.	To provide comfort.

(continued)

Action	Rationale
	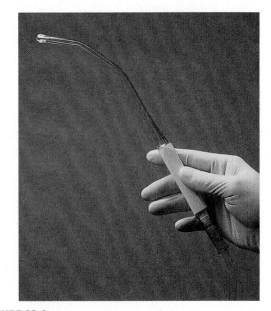 *Note: the image shown here is the disposal figure*
	FIGURE 33-8 Disposing of the suction catheter. The nurse grasps the cuff of the glove and pulls it downward over the used catheter.
33. Provide oral hygiene.	Suctioning can leave a disagreeable taste in the mouth as well as microorganisms. Oral hygiene can help prevent proliferation of microorganisms (Sole, Byers, & Ludy, et al., 2003).
34. Wash or disinfect your hands.	To prevent the transfer of microorganisms that can cause infection.

EVALUATION

35. Evaluate using the individualized patient outcomes previously identified:
  a. Breath sounds clear
  b. Vital signs stable
  c. Patient comfortable and calm
  d. Pulse oximetry indicates adequate blood oxygen level and stability (if appropriate)

DOCUMENTATION

36. Record the procedure on the patient's chart. Include date, time, and the amount and character of secretions removed. Also note the patient's tolerance of the procedure. **R:** Documentation is a legal record of the patient's care and therapy and communicates nursing activities to other nurses and caregivers.

POTENTIAL ADVERSE OUTCOMES AND RELATED INTERVENTIONS

1. The patient may become hypoxic while suctioning is being performed.
Intervention: Monitor the patient's oxygenation by pulse oximetry. If monitoring indicates hypoxia, stop suctioning and hyperoxygenate the patient.

2. The patient may become agitated and anxious.
Intervention: Continually reassure the patient and explain what you are doing. You may need an assistant to help hold the patient's hands for safety and comfort.

3. The patient remains in respiratory distress despite suctioning, and the suctioning does not seem to remove all of the patient's secretions.
Intervention: Sometimes **mucous** plugs form deep in the bronchi, out of reach of a suction catheter. If a patient remains in respiratory distress despite suctioning, notify the physician immediately. An emergency **bronchoscopy** may need to be performed by the physician to visualize and remove the mucous plugs.

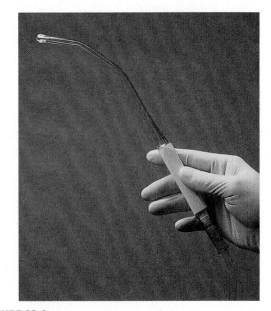

FIGURE 33-9 Yankauer suction-tip catheter.

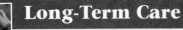
Acute Care

Current research shows that instilling normal saline solution before suctioning causes an increased risk of ventilator-associated pneumonia. In the past, nurses instilled saline solution before suctioning, believing that it would thin secretions and ease suctioning. On the contrary, patients who received saline instillations reported feelings of drowning, and oxygen levels were diminished. Based on this research evidence, the practice of instilling saline solution before suctioning is inappropriate (Sole, Byers, & Ludy, et al., 2003). For thick secretions, use a catheter with a larger lumen (Day, Farnell, & Haynes, et al., 2002).

Long-Term Care

Sometimes the resident in the long-term care facility is able to cough secretions into his or her mouth, but then is unable to expel them. In such cases, oral suctioning is useful. The **Yankauer suction-tip catheter** has a very large lumen designed for oral suctioning of thick secretions (Fig. 33-9). This is a clean technique, which some residents are able to perform themselves.

Home Care

When a client is taught how to perform self-suctioning at home, clean technique instead of sterile technique is sometimes used. This is because the home does not contain the antibiotic-resistant microorganisms found in healthcare facilities. Microorganisms encountered in the home are more likely to be susceptible to the client's own immune system defenses. However, the client is carefully monitored for signs of infection, and maintenance antibiotics are sometimes prescribed.

Ambulatory Care

Since many ambulatory care centers offer surgical services, it is vital for the nurse to know suctioning techniques. Sometimes the effects of anesthetics lead to pooling of respiratory secretions, and the sedated client just arousing from surgery may be unable to cough them out successfully. The nurse will then need to use suction to remove the respiratory secretions until the client is alert enough to resume such activity. Postoperative suctioning may also be needed to remove vomitus from the mouth and pharynx of the client who is still sedated. For this purpose, a very large diameter suction catheter is used.

LEARNING TOOLS

DEVELOP YOUR BACKGROUND KNOWLEDGE

1. Review the specific Learning Outcomes.
2. Read the material on respiration in your assigned text.
3. Look up the Key Terms in the glossary.
4. Review the module as though you were preparing to teach the contents to another person. Mentally practice the skills.

DEVELOP YOUR SKILLS

1. Review the Performance Checklist on the CD-ROM in the front of this book.
2. In the practice setting
   a. Familiarize yourself with the available suctioning equipment.
   b. Work with a partner. Using the available equipment and a mannequin, simulate oral and nasopharyngeal suctioning, taking turns completing the procedures.
   c. Have your partner evaluate your performance, using the Performance Checklist.
   d. Compare your own evaluation with that of your partner.
   e. Reverse roles, and repeat steps b through d.
   f. Practice assessing and recording the suctioning procedure.
   g. When you feel you have practiced the procedure adequately, have your instructor evaluate your performance.

DEMONSTRATE YOUR SKILLS

1. In the clinical setting, consult with your clinical instructor regarding an opportunity to suction an alert adult and a comatose adult.

CRITICAL THINKING EXERCISES

When assessing a semicomatose patient, you determine that the patient needs suctioning. You attempt to provide nasopharyngeal suctioning through the left nostril, but find you are unable to pass the catheter. You change to the oral route, but the agitated patient bites the suction catheter. Analyze this situation. What other assessment data could you have used before you began? What data should you collect at this time? What nursing actions might effectively assist in clearing this patient's airway? Explain how you might involve others in your planning.

SELF-QUIZ

SHORT-ANSWER QUESTIONS

1. List two reasons why the patient must be given an adequate explanation of the suctioning procedure.

   a. _____

   b. _____

2. When using a suction catheter, why must you maintain sterility?

   _____

3. When you are operating the suctioning equipment, why must the system be closed?

   _____

4. In what position should you place the unconscious patient for suctioning?

   _____

5. What are two reasons for placing the unconscious patient in this position?

   a. _____

   b. _____

6. What is the maximum length of time you should suction on each insertion of the catheter?

   _____

7. Ideally, what is the maximum number of times you should suction a patient?

   _____

MULTIPLE CHOICE

_____ 8. The postoperative patient is somewhat somnolent but can be aroused. When you listen to his lungs, you hear gurgles. What is the first intervention you should try to resolve this?
   a. Wake the patient, and encourage the patient to deep breathe and cough.
   b. Obtain an order for an incentive spirometer.
   c. Initiate intermittent positive pressure breathing.
   d. Suction the patient.

_____ 9. The nurse is performing oropharyngeal suctioning, and the patient begins to cough violently. This indicates
   a. the nurse has suctioned too deeply and should refrain from suctioning that deep again.
   b. the nurse should stop all suctioning.
   c. the coughing will bring secretions from deeper in the respiratory tract and is therefore desirable.
   d. the coughing will cause the patient undue distress and should be avoided if possible.

_____ 10. When suctioning the unconscious patient, the nurse identifies that the secretions are very thick and tenacious, and he or she is having difficulty getting the suction catheter to remove the secretions. The appropriate nursing response is
   a. keep trying, and rotate the catheter more as it is removed.
   b. get a larger diameter suction catheter, and try again.
   c. encourage the patient to cough out the secretions.
   d. instill saline solution into the respiratory tract to liquefy the secretions.

Answers to the Self-Quiz questions appear in the back of the book.

Tracheostomy Care and Suctioning

SKILLS INCLUDED IN THIS MODULE

Procedure for Suctioning the Tracheostomy
  Open Suctioning of a Tracheostomy
  Closed (In-Line) Suctioning of a Tracheostomy
Procedure for Administering Tracheostomy Care
Procedure for Changing the Tracheostomy Dressing

PREREQUISITE MODULES

Module 1	An Approach to Nursing Skills
Module 2	Documentation
Module 4	Basic Infection Control
Module 5	Safety in the Healthcare Environment
Module 7	Providing Hygiene
Module 14	Nursing Physical Assessment
Module 24	Basic Sterile Technique: Sterile Field and Sterile Gloves
Module 31	Administering Oxygen
Module 33	Oral and Nasopharyngeal Suctioning

KEY TERMS

Ambu bag	nasotracheal tube
bronchi	necrosis
button	obturator
cannula	open suctioning
catheter	percutaneous
clockwise	tracheostomy
closed suctioning	introducer
counterclockwise	sordes
endotracheal tube	speaking valve
fenestrated tra-	trachea
cheostomy tubes	tracheal ring
hydrogen peroxide	tracheostomy
inflatable cuff	ventilator
lumen	

OVERALL OBJECTIVES

▸ To care for patients with tracheostomies appropriately.
▸ To perform suctioning through the tracheostomy safely and effectively.

LEARNING OUTCOMES

The student will be able to

1. Assess the patient effectively to determine the need for tracheostomy suctioning or tracheostomy care.
2. Analyze assessment data to determine other special problems or concerns that must be addressed before proceeding with tracheostomy suctioning or tracheostomy care.
3. Determine appropriate patient outcomes for tracheostomy suctioning and care procedures, and recognize the potential for adverse outcomes.
4. Plan the tracheostomy suctioning and tracheostomy care, taking into consideration the special needs of the patient.
5. Implement open and closed tracheostomy suctioning and tracheostomy care.
6. Evaluate the effectiveness of the tracheostomy suctioning and tracheostomy care in relation to the desired outcomes.
7. Document tracheostomy suctioning and tracheostomy care, along with patient response.

A **tracheostomy** is a surgical incision into the **trachea** to insert a tube through which the patient can breathe more easily and through which secretions can be removed. At one time, the procedure was performed only as an emergency measure to allow a critically ill patient to breathe when life was imminently threatened by respiratory obstruction. In current practice, tracheostomies are performed initially when it is expected that a **ventilator** will be needed for a prolonged period of time or when swelling is expected, such as after surgery on the neck. A tracheostomy may be performed to decrease dead air space in the respiratory system, therefore decreasing the work of breathing and improving ventilation. A long-term tracheostomy is sometimes performed for the patient who has had the larynx removed. In some situations, a **nasotracheal** or **endotracheal tube** is initially inserted in order to place patients on a ventilator. If left in place for a prolonged period of time, a nasotracheal or endotracheal tube can cause tissue necrosis. Therefore, if the patient must remain on a ventilator, a tracheostomy may then be performed.

The surgeon usually performs the tracheostomy in the operating room. In emergencies, it may be performed in the Emergency Department or even on a patient care unit. A small, horizontal incision is made just below the first **tracheal ring,** and a tracheostomy tube is inserted. There is now a special device that can be used to insert a tracheostomy tube through the patient's endotracheal tube, called a **percutaneous tracheostomy introducer.** This procedure can be done in the critical care unit and is called a percutaneous tracheostomy insertion. In most cases, a tracheostomy is a temporary measure. Once the patient can tolerate temporary closure (sometimes referred to as "buttoning"), starting with short periods and gradually moving to longer ones, the tracheostomy tube is removed, and the incision heals.

Because patients with tracheostomies are cared for in a variety of healthcare settings, the nurse must be familiar with the special care required and the variations needed for suctioning such patients. Normally, the upper respiratory passages protect the trachea, filtering out foreign material and providing some protection from microorganisms. Because the tracheostomy opens directly into the trachea, which is highly susceptible to infection, the nurse must have a thorough knowledge of sterile technique to care for and suction a tracheostomy. In addition, a patent airway must be maintained at all times.

NURSING DIAGNOSES

- Risk for Infection: The risk for infection is always present in the patient with a tracheostomy because the protection of the upper respiratory tract has been disrupted. Much of the care described in this module is directed toward preventing infection by using correct technique when caring for a tracheostomy.
- Ineffective Airway Clearance: Suctioning is needed for an individual with a nursing diagnosis of Ineffective Airway Clearance. The tracheostomy tube irritates the respiratory tract and causes an increase in secretions. If the patient is not able to cough these secretions out effectively, this nursing diagnosis is present, and you will need to suction the patient to remove these secretions.
- Impaired Verbal Communication: The patient with a tracheostomy tube in place is unable to speak, except when a fenestrated tube is used or when the tracheostomy tube is "buttoned"

or occluded. There is also a special valve, called a **speaking valve,** which can be placed on the tracheostomy to allow the patient to speak. Without such special devices, the patient with a tracheostomy cannot speak, because the vocal cords are above the tracheostomy opening. For this reason, the nursing diagnosis of Impaired Verbal Communication is often appropriate.

■ Disturbed Body Image: Any alteration in what is considered normal appearance and function by the patient and others can produce distress. For the person who must have a long-term tracheostomy, both the presence of the tracheostomy and the differences it makes in daily living may contribute to body image disturbance.

DELEGATION

Because tracheostomy care is critical to oxygenation, these procedures are not delegated to assistive personnel. When an assistive person is providing care for the person with a tracheostomy, the individual should be taught what specifically should be reported to the nurse immediately to ensure safety.

TRACHEOSTOMY TUBES

Tracheostomy tubes may be composed of three parts: an outer **cannula,** an inner cannula, and an **obturator.** The outer cannula fits through the tracheostomy opening, is curved, and has a flange near the upper opening. The flange should rest comfortably on the surrounding tissue but not so tightly that it causes tissue irritation or **necrosis.** Ties attached to this flange secure the cannula to the patient's neck.

Inside the outer cannula is an inner cannula, which has a slightly smaller diameter. A latch usually holds this cannula securely and allows it to be removed for cleaning. Some companies now make tracheostomies with disposable inner cannulas. Rather than cleaning an inner cannula, the old one is disposed of and a new one inserted. Some companies make tracheostomy tubes without inner cannulas. These are more often used for short-term problems because they cannot be cleaned as thoroughly and completely as the multipart tracheostomy tube.

An obturator with a smooth, oval end fits inside the outer cannula and protrudes from the end. This makes it easier for the physician or nurse to insert the tracheostomy tube through the opening in the trachea

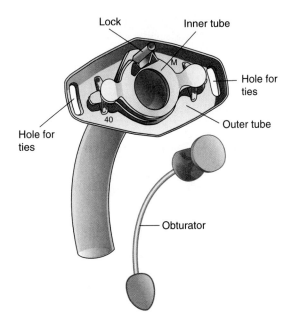

FIGURE 34-1 The parts of a tracheostomy tube.

(Fig. 34-1). The obturator is removed once the tube is in place, and the inner cannula is inserted.

The size of the tube used is the choice of the physician and is usually based on the patient's airway size. Usually, a size 8 is used for men and a size 6 for women. The optimal size is one that is large enough to decrease airway resistance, yet small enough to prevent tracheal stenosis (Tamburri, 2000).

Tracheostomy tubes are commonly made of plastic, but may also be made of metal. The plastic tube is soft and pliable, unlike the metal tube, which is rigid. The plastic tube molds more easily to the trachea, so it causes less irritation and is more comfortable for the patient. Plastic tracheostomy tubes are disposable. Metal tubes may be cleaned, sterilized, and reused by that patient.

There are many specialized types of tracheostomy tubes on the market today. The type of tube is chosen based on a variety of factors, including age of the patient, expected length of time for tracheostomy to remain in place, healthcare setting, physician preference, length of time it will be needed, patient anatomy, and whether the patient needs to be able to speak.

TYPES OF TUBES AND BUTTONING

There are four major types of tracheostomy tubes: cuffed, cuffless, nonfenestrated, and **fenestrated tracheostomy tubes.** See Table 34-1 for a description of these types of tubes with their associated benefits and drawbacks. See also Figures 34-2 and 34-3.

A tracheostomy tube is cuffed to provide an air seal around the tube. If the patient has a tube with an **inflatable cuff,** the nurse and/or respiratory therapist

table 34-1. Types of Tracheostomy Tubes

Type	Benefits	Drawbacks
Cuffed	Inflated, the cuff seals the space between the tube and trachea. This type of tube must be used for a ventilated patient.	The cuff may erode the trachea if the pressure is not checked regularly or if the cuffed tube is left in for a long period. The patient cannot talk unless cuff is deflated.
Cuffless	Allows the patient to eat and talk without having to deflate a cuff	This type of cuff cannot be used in the patient needing ventilation, because oxygen can travel around the tracheostomy tube.
Fenestrated (tube with hole or holes in it)	Allows the patient to breathe through the tube and the fenestrations; may come with fenestrated or nonfenestrated inner cannula Allows the patient to talk	If the patient has a fenestrated inner cannula, a nonfenestrated inner cannula needs to be inserted during suctioning to prevent the suction catheter from going through the fenestrations and injuring the tracheal mucosa. Tracheal tissue can eventually grow into the fenestrations and occlude the tube, so it needs to be changed frequently if in long-term use.
Nonfenestrated	Allows suctioning without having to change a fenestrated inner cannula	The patient will lack the ability to talk if the tube is nonfenestrated and cuffed.

Compiled from Tamburri, L. M. (2000). Care of the patient with a tracheostomy. *Orthopaedic Nursing, 19* (2), 49–60.

needs to check the cuff pressure at intervals dictated by agency policy and additional times if needed based on patient assessment. A pressure gauge is attached to a port on the cuff and provides a reading. By turning a stopcock mechanism on the gauge, the nurse can see the reading on the gauge, indicating the amount of pressure in the cuff. The nurse can then increase or decrease the cuff pressure accordingly.

Normal tracheostomy cuff pressure is 18 to 22 mm Hg (25 to 30 cm H_2O), with 20 mm Hg commonly used. It is best to keep the cuff pressure as low as possible to prevent tracheal tissue breakdown. However, the cuff pressure needs to be high enough to prevent oxygenated air from escaping around the tracheostomy tube. Monitoring the patient's oxygen saturation and listening for cuff leaks can help the nurse make such a determination. When the cuff leaks, the nurse may hear air rushing around the tracheostomy, and if the patient is conscious, he or she will be able to vocalize around the flaccid tracheostomy cuff.

One approach to determining whether an individual can function without a tracheostomy tube in place is to close the tube, usually with a "**button,**" which requires air to move around the sides of the tracheostomy tube (or through the fenestration) as it passes from the upper airway to the lungs and then exits (Fig. 34-4). The patient is closely monitored when the tube is "buttoned" to assess oxygenation. The time during which the tracheostomy is buttoned may be increased gradually until it is clear that the tracheostomy is no longer needed.

SAFETY MEASURES

There are a number of vital safety measures to consider when caring for the patient with a tracheostomy. See Box 34-1 for a listing of these measures.

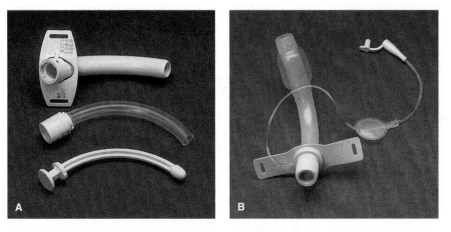

FIGURE 34-2 (**A**) Cuffless nonfenestrated tracheostomy tube. (**B**) Plastic cuffed tracheostomy tube.

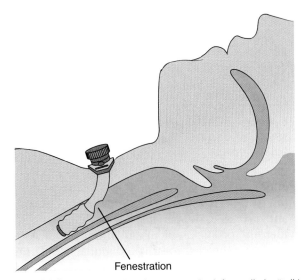

FIGURE 34-3 A fenestrated tracheostomy tube (often called a "talking trach").

SUCTIONING THE TRACHEOSTOMY

A tracheostomy is suctioned to improve oxygenation. This is done by removing secretions that may obstruct the airway, stimulating the cough reflex to raise deep secretions from the lungs, and reducing the work of breathing by providing a clear airway. Two different approaches to tracheostomy suctioning are the open procedure and the closed or in-line procedure. The latter is most often used in intensive care units and settings where the patient needs frequent suctioning. The open approach is more commonly used for the person with a long-term tracheostomy. The procedure for open tracheostomy suctioning is similar to that described for nasopharyngeal suctioning in Module 33, Oral and Nasopharyngeal Suctioning.

Suctioning the trachea and **bronchi** decreases the oxygen available to the lungs and causes collapse of alveoli. The result is hypoxemia (lowered blood oxygen level). To prevent hypoxemia, you must hyperox-

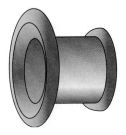

FIGURE 34-4 Tracheostomy button. When a "button" is in place, air passes from the upper airway to the lungs and back out, moving around the sides of the tracheostomy tube.

> **box 34-1** *Safety Measures for the Patient With a Tracheostomy*
>
> - Prevent infection of the wound, bronchi, and lungs when caring for a patient with a tracheostomy. If a patient has a new or recent tracheostomy, use sterile technique when cleaning the tracheostomy or changing the dressing.
> - Keep an extra tracheostomy set at the bedside of the patient with a new tracheostomy. During the acute period, if the tube becomes accidentally dislodged, the opening may close, occluding breathing. In this case, the nurse can open the extra tracheostomy set and insert a new sterile tracheostomy, using the obturator to ease insertion of the outer cannula. If a tube is dislodged or coughed out by a person with a well-established tracheostomy, the opening usually remains patent because the tissue has healed.
> - Use only lint-free cloth material or gauze in tracheostomy care in order to avoid possible aspiration of particles into the respiratory tract. Do not use cut cloth or cut gauze for tracheostomy care.
> - Observe the patient with a tracheostomy carefully, especially if the patient cannot communicate.
> - Place the call signal within reach at all times. An alert patient can summon help by using a call signal if it is within reach.

ygenate the patient with 100% oxygen immediately before and after suctioning. Hyperventilating the patient requires that a volume greater than tidal volume be instilled into the lungs. This prevents and reverses atelectasis, making maximum use of all alveolar surfaces for oxygen exchange. If you suction the patient more than one time, you also need to hyperoxygenate and hyperventilate between suctioning insertions.

Some patients have a tracheostomy in order to be placed on a mechanical ventilator. Many ventilators can be set to provide hyperoxygenation and hyperventilation when it is needed.

You also can use a breathing bag, commonly referred to as an **Ambu bag,** attached to oxygen to hyperoxygenate and hyperventilate the patient. Some equipment is structured so that the breathing bag can be attached directly to the tracheostomy, endotracheal, or nasotracheal tube. In other cases, the breathing bag is attached to a T-shaped piece on the tracheostomy tube. For patients who are not on ventilators, but have tracheostomies, you will need to use an Ambu bag.

In the past, it was common to instill saline into the trachea in an attempt to liquefy secretions. Research (Kinloch, 1999; Ackerman & Mick, 1998) demonstrated that this was not effective and contributed to decreased oxygen saturation and increased nosocomial infections. This practice is no longer recommended.

Procedure for Open Suctioning of a Tracheostomy

Open suctioning requires the use of a new sterile suction **catheter** each time the patient is suctioned. When using the open procedure, the Ambu bag for oxygenation must be used while maintaining sterility of the suction catheter. This is easiest if two people work together. An experienced, skillful individual may do this procedure effectively alone by operating the Ambu bag with one hand; however, this may not result in effective hyperventilation. The procedure presented here is for two people working together performing suctioning and using the Ambu bag for hyperventilation. As you become more proficient, you may be able to do this independently.

The individual handling the suction equipment is designated Person 1, and the individual handling the Ambu bag is designated Person 2. All steps are done by Person 1 except for those that specify Person 2.

ASSESSMENT

1. Assess the patient's respiratory status and need for tracheostomy suctioning and cleaning. **R:** This assessment is especially critical because many of these patients are comatose, and most conscious patients cannot talk because of the tracheal opening.
   a. Listen to the breath sounds. These should be quiet, not labored. **R:** If the respirations are labored, and you hear the movement of secretions (gurgling sounds), the patient's secretions need suctioning. Fine crackles represent moisture in small airways, and this will not be removed by suctioning.
   b. Check oxygen saturation level to determine adequacy of respirations. **R:** An oxygen saturation of 95% or greater is desired.
   c. Observe the condition of the cannula to determine if it is patent or if there are secretions built up within the **lumen. R:** The inner cannula is cleaned on a regular basis according to protocol and whenever inspection reveals that there are secretions built up there.
   d. Inspect the dressing. **R:** Dressings are changed on a regular basis according to protocol and whenever they are soiled with secretions. If suctioning, cleaning, and a dressing change are all

needed, suction first so that the tube and dressing will remain clean after changing.
   e. Check pulse and respiratory rate. **R:** These data will serve as a baseline.

ANALYSIS

2. Critically think through your data, carefully evaluating each aspect and its relation to other data to determine the patient's need for suctioning and the best approach for conducting suctioning. **R:** The approach must be the one that succeeds in removing secretions with the least amount of discomfort and distress to the patient.
3. Identify specific problems and modifications of the procedure needed for this individual. **R:** Planning for the individual must take into consideration the individual's problems.

PLANNING

4. Determine the individualized patient outcomes for the suctioning procedure. **R:** Identification of desired outcomes guides planning and evaluation.
   a. Tracheostomy tube is securely in place.
   b. Respiratory rate and depth are normal. **R:** This provides the ability to maintain oxygenation.
   c. Breath sounds are clear to auscultation. **R:** This indicates that secretions have been adequately removed.
   d. Oxygen saturation is 95% to 100%.
   e. Patient is resting comfortably. **R:** This indicates that the patient has recovered adequately from the procedure.
5. Obtain the necessary equipment. Commercial suctioning kits, which contain the essential items you will need, are available. Check the kit to identify whether any item must be obtained separately or if all items are in the kit, including the following. **R:** To allow you to be fully prepared to conduct the procedure.
   a. Sterile gloves—usually in the kit
   b. Sterile suction catheter—usually in the kit
   c. Sterile basin—in a kit, it is usually a folded cardboard box lined with plastic
   d. Sterile water or sterile normal saline solution—in a kit, it is usually in a foil packet. If not in a kit, it will be in a small bottle that can be opened before beginning the process.
   e. Moisture-proof drape—if not in the kit, a towel may be used.
   f. Suction regulator (if wall suction is available) or a portable suction machine (if no wall suction is available) with connector tubing
   g. Self-inflating breathing bag (Ambu bag) or ventilator with a setting for hyperoxygenating and hyperventilating

box 34-2 *Obtaining a Sputum Specimen Through a Tracheostomy*

A sputum specimen may be obtained when you are suctioning a tracheostomy. Use a special suction trap with two outlets. One outlet is attached to the suction catheter, and the other is attached to the tubing from the suction source. In closed suction techniques, you would need to disconnect the catheter from the suction tubing to attach the suction trap. As the sputum is suctioned, a specimen is collected in the container. The entire container is then sent to the laboratory. This protects the specimen from the possibility of outside contamination, and it protects healthcare workers from contact with the sputum.

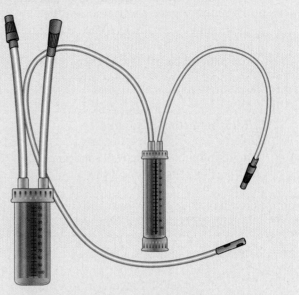

A suction trap for obtaining a sputum specimen.

 h. Mask
i. Eye protection (a shield attached to the mask, goggles, or eyeglasses)

j. Plastic apron or other clothing protector if copious secretions are expected
k. Suction trap if a sputum specimen is needed (Box 34-2)

IMPLEMENTATION

Action	Rationale
6. Wash or disinfect your hands.	To prevent the transfer of microorganisms that may cause infection.
7. Identify the patient, using two identifiers.	To be sure you are performing the procedure for the correct patient.
8. Close the door, and pull the curtain around the bed.	To provide privacy. Suctioning can be a distressing procedure to the patient, so it is essential to maintain privacy. Others may be disturbed by the sight of sputum and the suction equipment.
9. Explain the procedure carefully to the patient whether he or she is responsive or not.	Even though the unresponsive patient cannot respond to you, everything you say may be heard and understood. Without proper psychological preparation, the responsive patient may fear choking, asphyxiation, or hemorrhage. The responsive patient may be asked to cough to raise secretions so that they are more easily suctioned.
10. Establish a way of communicating because the patient with a tracheostomy usually cannot speak. Provide a slate,	Being able to communicate relieves the patient's feelings of helplessness and anxiety.

(continued)

Action	Rationale
paper and pencil, keyboard, or a handout of commonly requested tasks for the alert patient to point at so he or she can respond to you during the procedure. If the patient is unable to use any of these methods, establish a yes or no signal system.	
11. Test the suction apparatus.	
a. Turn on either the wall suction or the portable suction machine.	To determine if the suction power functions.
b. Place your thumb over the end of the unsterile connector tubing that is attached to the suction equipment and test for "pull."	To determine if the suction is functioning adequately.
c. Keep the suction regulated to a range of efficiency at 80 to 100 mm Hg.	Suction pressure less than this will not remove secretions adequately. Suction pressure higher than this may damage tracheal mucosa.
12. Place the patient supine in mid-Fowler's position, with the head slightly toward you or in lateral position facing you.	This allows you to access the tracheostomy.
13. Put on eye protection, mask, and apron.	To protect you from contact with secretions.
14. Open the sterile suction kit and prepare the equipment.	
a. Place the drape from the kit or a clean towel over the patient's chest.	To protect the gown or clothing.
b. Put on the sterile gloves.	To enable you to handle the sterile items in the kit.
c. Open the basin.	Most commercial kits have folded basins that require you to open them.
d. Pour the saline solution into the basin. If the kit does not contain a packet of saline solution, have a bottle open, and use your nondominant hand to pour the solution into the basin.	To maintain the sterility of your dominant hand.
e. Pick up the catheter in your dominant hand, and use the nondominant hand to grasp the suction tubing to attach the catheter.	The nondominant hand is now contaminated and cannot touch the catheter. This contaminated hand will now be used to control the suction and to handle any other nonsterile object. The gloves will protect you from contact with secretions, and the sterile glove in contact with the catheter protects the patient from microorganisms.

(continued)

Action	Rationale
15. Hyperoxygenate and hyperventilate the patient. This may be done in two ways.	
a. *When the patient is on a ventilator:* With the nondominant hand, press the control on the ventilator that delivers 100% oxygen as a sigh to the patient. Allow for three breaths.	Most ventilators have a setting that provides for hyperoxygenation when needed by the patient.
b. *When the patient is not on a ventilator:* Person 2 attaches the breathing bag to the oxygen source, attaches the breathing bag to the tracheostomy tube, and provides three deep breaths coordinated with the patient's breathing pattern.	Having a second person assist with the procedure adds to its ease, and preoxygenating prevents hypoxia during suctioning. Coordinating with the patient's breathing pattern minimizes distress to the patient.
16. Suction as follows by using your unsterile gloved hand placed over the opening in the catheter to start and stop the suction and managing the suction catheter with your sterile hand.	
a. Suction a small amount of sterile water into the catheter.	To ensure that the suction is working properly. The water also lubricates the tip of the catheter.
b. Insert the catheter into the tracheostomy until the patient coughs or resistance is felt (usually about 5 inches [12.5 cm]). Withdraw the catheter about ½ inch (1 to 2 cm) before beginning suctioning. If there is persistent coughing, you should stop the procedure. Do not suction while inserting the catheter.	Resistance indicates that the carina has been touched. Going farther than this can traumatize the tracheal mucosa. Coughing helps raise secretions. Persistent coughing, however, may indicate tracheal spasm. Suctioning while inserting the catheter would deprive the patient of oxygen as well as potentially traumatize the tracheal mucosa.
c. Apply suction for no longer than 10 seconds while withdrawing the catheter. (You can hold your own breath while suctioning to help you time the procedure.) Some recommend that you hold continuous suction and do not rotate the catheter while you withdraw it. Others recommend that the catheter be rotated and suction applied intermittently.	The patient cannot breathe while the catheter is in place. Longer suctioning removes oxygen, causes tissue irritation, and increases secretions. No research data is available that clearly demonstrates the best practice. Follow the policy of your facility.
d. Rinse the catheter with sterile water or normal saline solution.	To remove secretions from the catheter and suction tubing, thereby reducing contamination. It also lubricates the catheter tip in the event that you will be suctioning the secretions again.
17. Hyperoxygenate the patient with the ventilator or by having Person 2 hyperoxygenate the patient with three large breaths.	To restore oxygen levels and to prevent atelectasis by reinflating small airways.

(continued)

Action	Rationale
18. Observe the patient for dyspnea or skin color changes.	To determine if the patient is in respiratory distress.
19. If symptoms of hypoxia occur, Person 2 immediately provides additional deep breaths of oxygen or use ventilator to provide deep breaths.	To reverse the hypoxia.
20. Turn off the suction, and listen for clear breath sounds.	To determine whether the patient's secretions need to be suctioned again.
21. If breath sounds are not clear, repeat steps 16 through 18 up to three times, waiting 30 seconds between attempts.	To achieve the desired outcomes without compromising oxygenation.
22. If breath sounds are clear, Person 2 uses the breathing bag to provide three deep breaths of oxygen or use ventilator to provide three deep breaths.	To restore oxygen levels.
23. Disconnect the catheter from the suction tubing and discard the catheter.	The catheter is used for only one episode of suctioning.
24. Grasp the cuff of the sterile glove and pull the glove down over the used catheter to enclose any secretions, and discard all disposable equipment according to facility policy.	Covering the discarded catheter lessens the opportunity for microorganisms to be spread. Proper disposal of used equipment decreases the potential for spreading nosocomial infections.
25. If a dressing change or fastening of tube ties is needed, refer to the Specific Procedure below.	A clean dressing helps to prevent infection around the tube. Securely fastened tube ties prevent the tracheostomy tube from accidentally dislodging.
26. Remove eye protection, mask, and apron, and dispose of them appropriately. If the eye protection is goggles, these are usually cleaned for future use.	Personal protective items are disposed of to prevent spread of microorganisms.
27. Check the patient's need for oral hygiene. If oral hygiene is needed, refer to Module 7.	The patient who is NPO may accumulate **sordes** (dark crusty material) in the mouth that can lead to stomatitis.
28. Wash or disinfect your hands.	To prevent the transfer of microorganisms.

EVALUATION

29. Evaluate using the individualized outcomes previously identified. **R:** Evaluation in relation to desired outcomes is essential for planning future care.
   a. Tracheostomy tube is securely in place.
   b. Respiratory rate and depth are normal (provides ability to maintain oxygenation).
   c. Breath sounds are clear (indicates that secretions have been adequately removed).
   d. Oxygen saturation is 95% to 100%.
   e. Patient is resting comfortably (indicates that the patient has recovered adequately from the procedure).

DOCUMENTATION

30. Document the procedure and your observations in the patient's record. Some facilities have a flow sheet for this purpose. The entry should include the amount and character of secretions and the patient's response to the procedure. **R:** Documentation is a legal record of the patient's care and communicates nursing activities to other nurses and caregivers.

Procedure for Closed (In-Line) Suctioning of a Tracheostomy

There are now suction catheter systems that are used for **closed suctioning** (Fig. 34-5). In this type of suctioning, the suction catheter is continuously attached to the patient's tracheostomy tube. Depending on the manufacturer's recommendations and agency policy, the closed systems are changed every 24 to 72 hours. The closed suctioning method poses less risk of contamination and infection. The procedure for closed suctioning of a tracheostomy is similar to that of open suctioning. The major difference is that the sterile catheter is already in place with a protective cover, so the nurse does not need to wear sterile gloves or prepare a special suction kit.

ASSESSMENT

1. Follow step 1 of the Procedure for Open Suctioning: Assess the patient's respiratory status and need for tracheostomy suctioning and cleaning.

ANALYSIS

2-3. Follow steps 2 and 3 of the Procedure for Open Suctioning: Critically think through your data, carefully evaluating each aspect and its relation to other data to determine the patient's need for suctioning and the best approach for conducting suctioning. Identify specific problems and modifications of the procedure needed for this individual.

PLANNING

4. Follow step 4 of the Procedure for Open Suctioning: Determine the individualized patient outcomes for the suctioning procedure. **R:** Identification of outcomes guides planning and evaluation.
   a. Tracheostomy tube is securely in place.
   b. Respiratory rate and depth are normal.

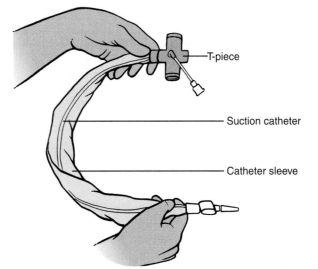

FIGURE 34-5 Closed suction catheter system.

   c. Breath sounds are clear.
   d. Oxygen saturation is 95% to 100%.
   e. Patient is resting comfortably.
5. Obtain the necessary equipment. **R:** Obtaining supplies in advance facilitates effective organization.
   a. Clean gloves
   b. Prepackaged plastic vial of 10 to 15 mL sterile normal saline solution
   c. Wall suction regulator or portable suction machine (if wall suction is not available) with tubing
   d. Self-inflating breathing bag (Ambu bag) or ventilator with a setting for hyperoxygenating and hyperventilating
   e. Mask
   f. Eye protection (a shield attached to the mask, goggles, or eyeglasses)
   g. Plastic apron or other clothing protector if needed
   h. Suction trap (if a sputum specimen is needed)
   i. The in-line suction tubing is changed based on the facility policy. If it is time to change the in-line suction, obtain a new set.

IMPLEMENTATION

Action	Rationale
6-12. Follow steps 6 to 12 of the Open Suctioning Procedure: Wash or disinfect your hands; identify the patient (two identifiers); close the door, and pull the curtain around the bed; explain the procedure; establish a way of communicating;	

(continued)

Action	Rationale
test the suction apparatus; place the patient supine in mid-Fowler's position, with the head slightly toward you, or in lateral position facing you; and put on eye protection, mask, and apron.	
13. Put on clean gloves.	The system is closed; therefore, it is not necessary to wear sterile gloves. Clean gloves will protect you from contact with secretions in case the system disconnects or the patient coughs up secretions around the tracheostomy.
14. Hyperoxygenate and hyperventilate the patient. a. *When the patient is on a ventilator:* Press the control on the ventilator that delivers 100% oxygen as a sigh to the patient. b. *When a breathing bag must be used:* Remove the closed system from the tracheostomy, attach the breathing bag, and give three big breaths. After hyperoxygenation, replace the closed system.	With a closed system, one person is able to manage the procedure with ease because sterility of a glove is not necessary. Hyperoxygenation and hyperventilation prevent hypoxia.
15. If the suction tubing is to be changed a. Detach the old tubing and discard. b. Carefully open the package of new tubing, keeping the connector sterile and the catheter enclosed in the plastic sheath. c. Attach the in-line suction catheter to the connector port of the tracheostomy tube. d. Attach the other end of the suction catheter to the suction tubing.	The in-line suction catheter is not exposed to the environment or in danger of touch from the clean gloves because it is fully enclosed.
16. Suction as follows:	
a. Open suction control and elbow access valves (if present) on the closed suctioning system by turning **counter-clockwise.**	This will make suction available and open the access valve to allow the catheter to enter the tracheostomy.
b. Insert the catheter into the tracheostomy by threading it through the tracheostomy port, using the clear plastic covering over the catheter to guide your movements. You will note that there is a black mark at the distal tip of the	Resistance indicates that the carina has been touched. Going farther than this can traumatize the tracheal mucosa. Coughing helps raise secretions. Persistent coughing, however, may indicate tracheal spasm.

(continued)

Action	Rationale
catheter that enters the port first. Insert until the patient coughs or resistance is felt (usually about 5 inches [12.5 cm]). Withdraw the catheter about ½ inch (1 to 2 cm) before beginning suctioning. If there is persistent coughing, you should stop the procedure. Do not suction while inserting the catheter.	Suctioning while inserting the catheter would deprive the patient of oxygen as well as potentially traumatize the tracheal mucosa.
c. Apply suction for no more than 10 seconds while withdrawing the catheter until you see the black mark at the end of the closed suction apparatus, which shows you have fully withdrawn the catheter from the trachea. (You can hold your own breath while suctioning to help you time the procedure.) Some recommend that you hold continuous suction and do not rotate the catheter while you withdraw it. Others recommend that the catheter be rotated and suction applied intermittently.	The patient cannot breathe while the catheter is in place. Suctioning for longer than 10 seconds removes oxygen, causes tissue irritation, and increases secretions. No research data is available that clearly demonstrates the best practice. Follow the policy of your facility.
17. Hyperoxygenate and hyperventilate.	To prevent hypoxia.
a. *When the patient is on a ventilator:* Press the control on the ventilator that delivers 100% oxygen as a sigh to the patient.	Most ventilators have a setting that provides for hyperoxygenation when needed by the patient.
b. Attach the breathing bag to the oxygen source and to the tracheostomy tube, and provide three deep breaths coordinated with the patient's breathing pattern.	Coordinating with the patient's breathing pattern minimizes distress to the patient.
18. Turn off the suction, and listen for clear breath sounds.	To determine whether the patient needs to be suctioned again.
19. If suction needs to be done again, repeat steps 16 to 18.	To ensure that the secretions are adequately removed.
20. When suctioning is complete, close the elbow access valve (if present) by turning **clockwise.**	To maintain a closed system and prevent migration of the catheter into the tracheostomy, where it would block the trachea.
21. Flush the catheter by twisting and pulling off the end of the vial containing saline solution. Open the irrigation port, attach saline solution to the port, squeeze the solution to dispense, and apply suction.	The purpose of the saline solution is to clear the suction catheter, *not* to go into the patient's trachea. Flushing the catheter with saline solution prevents the growth of microorganisms in the closed system. Instilling saline solution into the patient's trachea increases the risk of infection.

(continued)

Action	Rationale
22. Cap the irrigation port.	Capping the port protects the catheter from contamination.
23. Disconnect the suction tubing, and cap the suction control valve by turning clockwise.	To prevent accidental activation of the suction, which can cause loss of oxygen.
24. Remove eye protection, mask, apron, and gloves, and discard.	Personal protective items are disposed of to prevent spread of microorganisms.
25. Check the patient's need for oral hygiene. If oral hygiene is needed, refer to Module 7.	The patient who is NPO may accumulate sordes in the mouth that can lead to stomatitis.
26. Wash or disinfect your hands.	To prevent the transfer of microorganisms.

EVALUATION

27. Evaluate using the individualized patient outcomes previously identified: tracheostomy tube securely in place, respiratory rate and depth normal, breath sounds clear, oxygen saturation at 95% to 100%, patient resting comfortably. **R:** Evaluation in relation to desired outcomes is essential for planning future care.

DOCUMENTATION

28. Document the procedure and your observations in the patient's record. Include the amount and character of secretions and the patient's response to the procedure. **R:** Documentation is a legal record of the patient's care and communicates nursing activities to other nurses and caregivers.

PROCEDURE FOR ADMINISTERING TRACHEOSTOMY CARE

The tracheostomy tube is cleaned to remove secretions that accumulate and might block ventilation and become a reservoir for infectious agents. Clean by necessity, not by a definite schedule, because some patients have more secretions than others. For example, agency policy may be to clean and dress the tracheostomy once per shift. This may be adequate for some patients, but more frequent care (two or three times per shift) may be necessary for those with copious secretions or drainage. Usually in the first 24 to 48 hours after surgical placement of a tracheostomy, agency policy is to clean and dress the tracheostomy every 4 hours. Never allow the patient to reach the point of labored breathing due to accumulated secretions because this can lead to hypoxia and anxiety for the patient.

ASSESSMENT

1. Inspect the tracheostomy for visible secretions in the tube. **R:** The opening can become obstructed by secretions.

ANALYSIS

2. Critically think through your data, carefully evaluating each aspect and its relation to other data to determine the patient's need for tracheostomy care and the best approach for conducting such care. **R:** The approach must be the one that succeeds in cleaning the tracheostomy with enough regularity to maintain patency and prevent infection.
3. Identify specific problems and modifications of the procedure needed for this individual. **R:** Planning for the individual must take into consideration the individual's problems.

PLANNING

4. Determine individualized patient outcomes in relation to administering tracheostomy care, including the following. **R:** Identification of outcomes guides planning and evaluation.
   a. Tracheostomy tube is completely free of accumulated secretions.
   b. The patient's respirations are quiet and unlabored.
5. Gather the equipment you will need. Commercial tracheostomy kits contain the necessary items (Fig. 34-6). If your facility does not use such kits, obtain the following equipment. **R:** Obtaining supplies in advance facilitates effective organization.

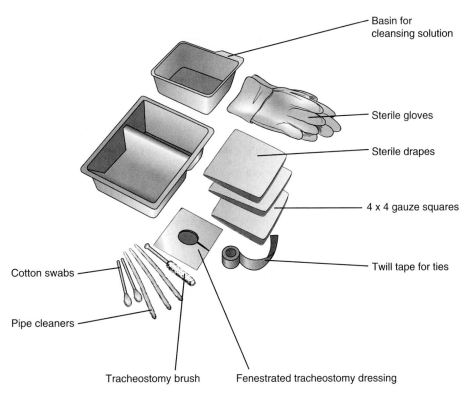

Basin for cleansing solution

Sterile gloves

Sterile drapes

4 x 4 gauze squares

Twill tape for ties

Cotton swabs

Pipe cleaners

Tracheostomy brush

Fenestrated tracheostomy dressing

FIGURE 34-6 A commercially prepared tracheostomy care kit. (Courtesy Sherwood Medical, St. Louis, Missouri.)

a. Sterile gloves if the tracheostomy has been recently performed; nonsterile gloves may be used for a long-term tracheostomy.
b. Eye protection, mask, and apron to prevent transfer of microorganisms to the patient and to prevent contact with secretions for the nurse
c. Four 4- × 4-inch gauze squares for cleansing and drying
d. Cleansing solution (often **hydrogen peroxide** mixed with normal saline)
e. Basin to place inner cannula in for cleansing

f. Tracheostomy brush, pipe cleaners, or swabs to clean the inner cannula surfaces
g. Sterile normal saline solution for cleaning and/or rinsing
  If you plan to change the tracheostomy dressing at this time, obtain the equipment for that procedure to avoid making another trip out of the room for supplies. Add the equipment listed in step 4 of the Procedure for Changing the Tracheostomy Dressing (below).

IMPLEMENTATION

Action	Rationale
6. Wash or disinfect your hands.	To prevent the spread of microorganisms.
7. Identify the patient, using two identifiers.	To be sure you are performing the procedure for the correct patient.
8. Close the door, and pull the curtain around the bed.	To provide privacy.

(continued)

Action	*Rationale*
9. Explain what you are going to do.	Many patients are afraid the tube may become dislodged during care. A clear, step-by-step explanation will reassure the patient.
10. Provide a means for communication for the patient.	The patient feels more secure when able to communicate needs.
11. Put on sterile or clean gloves as necessary as well as a mask, eye protection, and apron.	If the patient coughs, secretions may be blown out into your face or onto your clothes. This is to prevent the spread of microorganisms and to protect you from secretions. Sterile gloves are used for new tracheostomies that have not healed. Clean gloves may be used when tracheostomies have healed.
12. To clean a cannula-type tracheostomy tube	
a. If the inner cannula is to be cleaned, open the catheter care kit, and pour saline or cleansing solution into the basin.	The solution can be used to soften the secretions in the inner cannula.
b. Hold the outer tube carefully in place with one hand as you turn the lock clockwise with your other hand.	To unfasten the inner cannula.
c. Slide out the inner cannula by curving it toward you.	Removing it with the slant of the curve provides the least resistance and trauma.
d. If it is a disposable cannula, discard it. Then proceed to step 12i. If it is not a disposable inner cannula, place it in a basin of cleansing or saline solution.	To soften dried secretions.
e. Apply friction to the cannula with brush, pipe cleaners, or swabs.	To remove any residue.
f. Rinse the cannula well in saline solution.	To remove cleansing solution.
g. Dry the cannula well with a 4- × 4-inch gauze square.	To prevent instillation of fluids into the trachea.
h. If the patient's secretions are copious, or if the patient coughs while you are cleaning the inner cannula (so that the secretions come into contact with the inside surface of the outer cannula), remove the secretions with a gauze square and thoroughly dry the inner surfaces as described in step 12g.	To prevent the surfaces of the two cannulas from adhering.

(continued)

Action	Rationale
i. Hold the outer cannula and replace the clean inner cannula. If you have discarded a disposable inner cannula, now is the time to insert a new, sterile inner cannula, using sterile technique.	To provide an interior surface that can be removed for cleaning.
j. Turn the lock clockwise.	To secure the inner cannula.
k. Test to make sure the inner cannula is firmly in place by gently pulling with the fingers.	To prevent the inner cannula from being accidentally dislodged.
13. If a plastic tube with no inner cannula is being used, carefully clean the inner surfaces with swabs that are dampened, but not saturated, with normal saline solution.	To provide cleaning without risking aspiration.
14. If you are planning to change the tracheostomy dressing, move on to step 10 of the Procedure for Changing the Tracheostomy Dressing. If not, complete this procedure.	After providing tracheostomy cleaning, secretions may be expectorated by the patient, requiring a dressing change.
15. Remove your gloves, apron, mask, and eye protection, and discard them.	To prevent spread of microorganisms to others in the environment.
16. Dispose of the equipment as prescribed by your facility.	To prevent the transfer of microorganisms.
17. Wash or disinfect your hands.	To prevent the transfer of microorganisms.

EVALUATION

18. Evaluate using the individualized patient outcomes previously identified. **R:** Evaluation in relation to desired outcomes is essential for planning future care.
    a. Tracheostomy tube is completely free of accumulated secretions.
    b. The patient's respirations are quiet and unlabored.

DOCUMENTATION

19. Document the procedure in the progress notes or using computerized charting. **R:** Documentation is a legal record of the patient's care and therapy and communicates nursing activities to other nurses and caregivers. Include the amount and character of secretions removed and the patient's response. The procedure is usually documented in conjunction with the dressing change that follows (see Procedure for Changing the Tracheostomy Dressing below).

PROCEDURE FOR CHANGING THE TRACHEOSTOMY DRESSING

ASSESSMENT

1. Assess the patient for any appreciable amount of drainage or soiling of the dressing and ties, which indicates the need for a clean dressing. **R:** Dressings should always be clean and intact, because a tracheostomy is prone to infection. The dressing is often changed after giving tracheostomy care, because the patient may expel secretions during the procedure.
2. Assess the skin integrity around the tracheostomy. **R:** Secretions from the tracheostomy can cause irritation and skin breakdown around the tracheostomy.

ANALYSIS

3. Critically think through your data, carefully evaluating each aspect and its relation to other data to deter-

mine the need for changing the patient's tracheostomy dressing. **R:** The approach must be the one that succeeds in changing the dressing with the least amount of discomfort and distress to the patient.

4. Identify specific problems and modifications of the procedure needed for this individual. **R:** Planning for the individual must take into consideration the individual's problems. For instance, a patient who is coughing up copious secretions onto the dressing will need more frequent dressing changes.

PLANNING

5. Determine individualized patient outcomes in relation to the dressing change, including the following. **R:** Obtaining supplies in advance facilitates effective organization.
    a. Tracheostomy tube is securely in place to prevent it from becoming accidentally dislodged.

b. Tracheostomy dressing and ties are clean, dry, and intact.
c. Skin around tracheostomy is intact without redness or swelling.

6. Obtain a tracheostomy care kit, or gather the following items:
    a. 4- × 4-inch gauze squares and/or special tracheostomy or drain dressings
    b. twill tape ties or tracheostomy tube holder
    c. scissors (if you are removing twill tape ties)
    d. swabs
    e. cleansing solution
    f. oral care equipment
    g. one pair of clean gloves and one pair of sterile gloves, eye protection, mask, and apron
    h. bag for soiled items

IMPLEMENTATION

Action	Rationale
7. Wash or disinfect your hands.	To prevent the transfer of microorganisms.
8. Identify the patient, using two identifiers.	To be sure you are performing the procedure on the correct patient.
9. Close the door, and pull the curtains.	To provide privacy.
10. Explain what you are going to do.	The patient will be more calm and cooperative if you explain what you will be doing.
11. Provide a means of communication, such as paper and pen or eye signals.	Patients feel more secure when they can communicate their needs.
12. Put on clean gloves, mask, eye protection, and apron.	To prevent the transfer of microorganisms to the patient as well as to protect the nurse from contact with secretions. Patients receiving a tracheostomy dressing change may be stimulated to cough, thereby expelling secretions.
13. Remove the old dressing, and discard in bag for soiled items.	This will prevent the spread of microorganisms.
14. Wash or disinfect your hands, and put on sterile gloves.	To prevent the transfer of microorganisms as well as protect the nurse from contact with secretions.
15. With sterile swabs moistened in saline solution, clean around the edges of the tracheostomy opening. If there is copious drainage, you may need to use 4- × 4-inch gauze squares moistened in solution to clean the area; then dry with 4- × 4-inch	Saline will loosen any crusts and will not irritate the tissue. Using hydrogen peroxide may irritate the tissue surrounding the tracheostomy.

(continued)

Action	Rationale
gauze squares. Some facilities use a mixture of 50% hydrogen peroxide and 50% saline solution. If a peroxide mixture is used, then rinse the area with saline solution.	
16. Note any redness or swelling of the wound margins.	Such signs indicate infection, which needs to be reported to the physician.
17. Prepare the dressing. Use a precut tracheostomy dressing (also called a drain dressing or drain sponge), or you can use a 4- × 4-inch gauze square. **a.** *If using a gauze square:* Open the first fold of a 4- × 4-inch gauze square if you are using plain gauze squares. Fold it in half lengthwise. Fold each end toward the center (Fig. 34-7). Slide ends under the tracheostomy flange. **b.** *If using a precut dressing:* Open the dressing package and slide the slit area under the tracheostomy flange.	Having the dressing ready will allow you to move more quickly when replacing the dressing and ties. Either of these types of dressing eliminates the need to cut the material, which could expose the patient to lint, which could be inhaled. 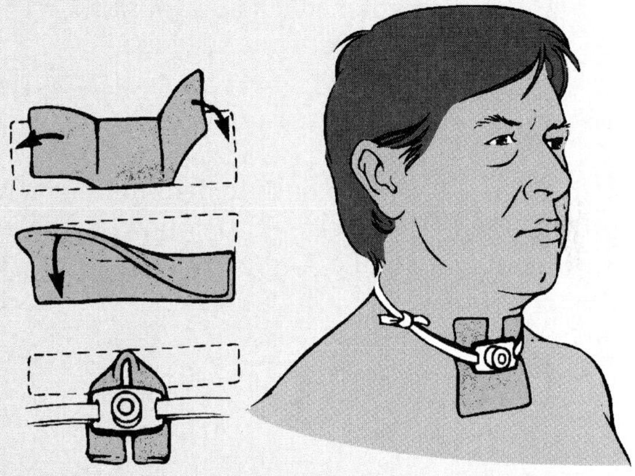 **FIGURE 34-7** Tracheostomy dressing. Open a 4- × 4-inch gauze square, fold it in half lengthwise, and place it around the tube with the ends up. If using a commercially prepared dressing, follow manufacturer's instructions.
18. Remove old tracheostomy ties while carefully holding the tracheostomy tube in place. Tape ties may be cut. A commercial holder can be unfastened and removed. In some situations, it is useful to have another person assist you with this. If you are working alone, you may wish to tie the new tapes into place before cutting the old ones off the tracheostomy flange.	To prevent the tube from becoming accidentally dislodged. In many cases, patients with tracheostomies are unresponsive and unable to move their head. It helps to have another nurse assist with repositioning of the patient's head so that the tube ties or tube holder can be secured in place.
19. Apply dressing and tapes with the tube held in place. **a.** Carefully slip the prepared dressing, ends extending up, around the tube. **b.** Thread the tape through the flange on one side of the neck.	This prevents the tracheostomy tube from becoming accidentally dislodged. Tying the knot on the side prevents discomfort and potential skin breakdown when the patient lies supine.

(continued)

Action	Rationale
c. Bring the tape around the back of the patient's neck. **d.** Thread the loose end through the remaining flange (Fig. 34-8). It is possible to develop the dexterity to hold the tracheostomy tube with the nondominant hand and use the dominant hand to remove the old tape and fasten the new. **e.** After you have attached both new tapes, hold the ties firmly while you tie them around the neck. The knot should be to the side. It is helpful for you or the patient to hold a finger under the tape as it is tightened to allow for slack. Avoid undue pressure on the tissue.	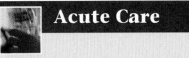 **FIGURE 34-8** Thread the tracheostomy tapes through the flange. Tie tapes toward the side to eliminate pressure on the back of the neck when the patient is supine.
20. Ensure that the tube is securely in place.	To be sure that the airway will remain open.
21. Check the patient's mouth to determine the need for mouth care. If so, follow the procedure in Module 7.	The patient with a tracheostomy has a changed breathing pattern (without air moving freely through the mouth). Also the patient is NPO so that the oral cavity becomes dry and sordes and bacteria build up, causing odor and stomatitis. This is distressing to the patient, family, and to those providing care. Because the patient needs frequent meticulous oral care, make this procedure part of the general tracheostomy care so that it is neither forgotten nor neglected.
22. Remove and dispose of gloves, mask, eye protection, and apron. Goggles may be cleaned for future use.	This is for infection control.
23. Wash or disinfect your hands.	To prevent the transfer of microorganisms.

EVALUATION

24. Evaluate using the individualized patient outcomes previously identified. **R:** Evaluation in relation to desired outcomes is essential for planning future care.
   a. Tracheostomy tube is securely in place to prevent it from becoming accidentally dislodged.
   b. Tracheostomy dressing and ties are clean, dry, and intact.
   c. Skin around tracheostomy is intact without redness or swelling.

DOCUMENTATION

25. Document in the progress notes or using computerized charting the procedure and any observations, such as status of the surrounding skin and the amount and character of drainage. **R:** Documentation is a legal record of the patient's care and therapy and communicates nursing activities to other nurses and caregivers.

Acute Care

When a patient with a new tracheostomy arrives on an acute care unit postoperatively, the nurse is responsible for several aspects of care. The following steps will ensure adequate patient care and safety in relation to the new tracheostomy.

The nurse's responsibilities include the following:

1. ensuring that the airway remains patent, and checking to see if the patient needs suctioning
2. identifying the size and type of tracheostomy that is being used; if it is one with an inner cannula, extra inner cannulas are ordered for the unit.
3. ordering an extra tracheostomy tube immediately, if the surgery staff did not send one with the patient, so that one is at the bedside in case the tube is accidentally dislodged
4. checking that the tracheostomy tube is either tied or strapped on securely and is tight enough to remain in place but not so tight as to cause skin erosion or impair circulation
5. monitoring vital signs as well as pulse oximetry readings
6. checking lung sounds frequently

At a later time, the nurse may prepare a patient to be discharged home with a tracheostomy in place. Teaching both patient and caregivers will be essential to ensure adequate self-care.

Long-Term Care

The same general procedures for suctioning, caring for, and changing a tracheostomy dressing are used in long-term care settings as are used in acute care settings. Clean technique may be used when cleaning or changing a tracheostomy that has been in place for a long time. Sterile technique is always used for suctioning.

Home Care

Caring for the person who returns home with a tracheostomy requires that the client and family members be taught not only how to perform the various aspects of care, but also how to recognize reportable signs and symptoms and how to respond in an emergency. Initially, the client and family members may feel inadequate to the task. However, with complete written instructions and opportunities to observe the nurse and practice the skills, competent and knowledgeable care can be provided by the client and caregivers at home.

Ambulatory Care

There may be times when you will encounter outpatients who have tracheostomies. These clients may be seen postoperatively in ambulatory care settings. It is important for the nurse to know how to properly assess and care for the client with a tracheostomy in the postoperative period, since the client may still be under sedation and unable to care for the tracheostomy independently. Often after surgery, the client may have increased secretions, which cannot be expectorated because of the effects of the anesthetic. In such cases, the nurse needs to suction the client so that the airway remains patent.

LEARNING TOOLS

DEVELOP YOUR BACKGROUND KNOWLEDGE

1. Review the Learning Outcomes.
2. Read material on aeration and the respiratory system in your assigned text.
3. Look up the Key Terms in the glossary.
4. Review the module as though you were preparing to teach the contents to another person. Mentally practice the skills.
5. Review the Performance Checklist on the CD-ROM in the front of this book.

DEVELOP YOUR SKILLS

1. In the practice setting, do the following:
   a. Examine the various tracheostomy tubes available.
   b. Select and gather the equipment for suctioning a tracheostomy.
   c. If a tube can be attached to the mannequin, practice suctioning the tracheostomy, using the Performance Checklist as a guide.
   d. Gather the equipment for cleaning a tube and changing the dressing.
   e. Following the steps in the Performance Checklist, practice cleaning the tube and changing the dressing.
   f. When you think you are prepared to demonstrate the skills, ask your instructor to evaluate your performance.

DEMONSTRATE YOUR SKILLS

1. In the clinical setting, consult with your instructor for an opportunity to care for and suction a patient with a tracheostomy.

CRITICAL THINKING EXERCISES

1. An alert, 61-year-old patient has been transferred from the critical care unit with a tracheostomy. Identify the risks and concerns for care that are present because of the tracheostomy. With each risk or concern identified, describe the nursing actions that may prevent the patient from being placed at risk or actions that are appropriate for alleviating patient concerns.

2. Your patient who has a tracheostomy is to return home. Imagine you are a staff nurse teaching the caregiver how to care for and dress the tracheostomy. Identify which specific teaching instructions you should give. Use this scenario as a health-teaching exercise.

SELF-QUIZ
MULTIPLE CHOICE

_____ 1. Which of the following are purposes of a tracheostomy? (Choose all that apply.)
   a. It allows a critically ill patient to breathe when threatened by respiratory obstruction.
   b. It provides an avenue for nutrition when the patient cannot take food or fluids orally.
   c. It may be done to remove secretions before a patient's breathing is severely compromised.
   d. It may be done so that a ventilator can be used.

_____ 2. The patient with a tracheostomy cannot talk because
   a. he or she is too ill.
   b. air does not reach the vocal cords.
   c. there is swelling of the trachea.
   d. of the presence of secretions.

_____ 3. Which of the following statements explains the reason why an extra tracheostomy set is kept at the bedside of the patient with a tracheostomy?
   a. The set is used in an emergency if the original tube becomes dislodged.
   b. The set is used to change the tracheostomy every 24 hours.
   c. The set is used for routine tracheostomy cleaning.
   d. The set is used when there are no extra supplies available.

_____ 4. The primary reason for periodically deflating a cuffed tracheostomy tube is to
   a. promote the patient's comfort.
   b. adjust the position of the tube.
   c. remove and clean the tube.
   d. prevent tissue necrosis.

_____ 5. Suctioning the trachea and bronchi can improve the patient's respiration through which of the following?
   a. It may cause the patient to cough.
   b. The oxygen available to the lungs is decreased.
   c. It causes collapse of the alveoli.
   d. It increases secretions.

_____ 6. The greatest threat to the patient with a tracheostomy is the danger of
   a. hemorrhaging.
   b. pneumonia.
   c. infection.
   d. airway obstruction.

Answers to the Self-Quiz questions appear in the back of the book.

Caring for Patients With Chest Drainage

SKILLS INCLUDED IN THIS MODULE

Procedure for Assisting With the Insertion of Chest Tubes
Procedure for Caring for the Patient With Chest Tubes
Procedure for Assisting With the Removal of Chest Tubes

PREREQUISITE MODULES

Module 1	An Approach to Nursing Skills
Module 2	Documentation
Module 4	Basic Infection Control
Module 5	Safety in the Healthcare Environment
Module 11	Assessing Temperature, Pulse, and Respiration
Module 12	Measuring Blood Pressure
Module 13	Monitoring Intake and Output
Module 14	Nursing Physical Assessment
Module 17	Assisting with Diagnostic and Therapeutic Procedures
Module 24	Basic Sterile Technique: Sterile Field and Sterile Gloves
Module 40	Providing Wound Care

KEY TERMS

atelectasis
fibrin
hemopneumothorax
hemothorax
mediastinal shift
mediastinal tube
mediastinum
parietal pleura
pleural space
pleural tube
pneumothorax
rubber-shod
  hemostats

serosanguineous
stab wound
subcutaneous
  emphysema
tension
  pneumothorax
thoracentesis
tidaling
trocar
visceral pleura
waterseal drainage

OVERALL OBJECTIVES

▶ To assist in the placement and removal of chest tubes.
▶ To care for patients with chest drainage safely and appropriately, thereby ensuring proper functioning of the chest drainage system.

LEARNING OUTCOMES

The student will be able to

1. Assess the patient having a chest tube inserted or who has a chest tube in place to determine current respiratory status and the functioning of any chest tube system.
2. Analyze assessment data to determine special problems or concerns that must be addressed before proceeding with chest tube placement or removal or with care of the patient with a chest tube.
3. Determine appropriate patient outcomes in terms of the care of a patient with a chest tube, and recognize the potential for adverse outcomes.
4. Recognize complications of chest tube placement occurring in the patient.
5. Plan for ways to resolve complications of chest tube placement.
6. Implement procedures for assisting with insertion and removal of chest tubes and for caring for the patient with a chest tube(s) in place.
7. Evaluate the patient's response to chest tube placement, care, and removal.
8. Document chest tube care according to facility policy.

The most common type of chest tube, the **pleural tube,** is used to drain air or fluid from the pleural cavity and to restore the normal negative intrapleural pressure, making lung expansion possible after surgery or injury to the chest cavity. Another type of chest tube, the **mediastinal tube,** is used to drain fluid from the mediastinal space after cardiac surgery or other surgery in the **mediastinum.** The nurse must anticipate the needs of the patient and physician during the insertion and removal of chest tubes and care safely for the patient with any type of chest drainage system.

NURSING DIAGNOSES

- Risk for Infection: The risk for infection is always present in the patient with a chest tube because the protection of the skin has been disrupted. Part of the care described in this module is directed toward preventing infection by using correct technique when caring for a chest tube.
- Impaired Comfort: Acute Pain is another diagnosis that is commonly encountered in the patient with a chest tube. This is due to pain at

the insertion site of the chest tube. It is important for the nurse to medicate the patient and use alternative modalities for pain reduction (such as imagery and distraction) in order to maximize the patient's comfort.
- Ineffective Breathing Pattern and Impaired Gas Exchange: Patients with chest tubes often have these nursing diagnoses; this is usually due to the underlying disease process requiring the insertion of the chest tube or to complications from chest tube placement.

DELEGATION

The care of chest tubes is not delegated to assistive personnel. If the assistive person is helping to care for the patient, the nurse should teach how to turn and manage basic care without disturbing the chest drainage system. The nurse should also teach what signs and symptoms require immediate notification of the nurse. This would include any indication of respiratory distress or disruption in the chest drainage system.

OVERVIEW

The **pleural space** is a potential space formed by the **visceral pleura** and **parietal pleura.** It contains only enough lubricating fluid to allow the two surfaces to slide smoothly over each other during inspiration and exhalation. On inspiration, the negative pressure is approximately 28 cm water and remains negative on exhalation but somewhat less so, at about 24 cm water. The pleural space does not normally contain air or fluid except for the small amount of lubricating fluid.

When the chest has been opened, there will be some drainage from the wound (the amount will depend on the extent of surgery or trauma). There will also be air in the pleural space that causes collapse of the lung. An accumulation of air in the pleural space is called a **pneumothorax.** Blood in the pleural space is known as a **hemothorax.** The collection of blood and air together is a **hemopneumothorax.** The air and fluid must be removed for the lung to re-expand and for healing to occur.

If additional air enters the space or any fluid accumulates, breathing is compromised because the space normally occupied by the expanded lung is filled with the air or fluid. If too much space is occupied by fluid or air, and the pressure exerted is great enough, the lung may collapse completely.

In an open pneumothorax, breathing is compromised by the air entering the pleural space from outside of the chest. This most commonly occurs because of surgery on the chest or trauma to the chest wall, either of which may allow air to enter the chest, thereby collapsing the lung.

In a closed, or **tension, pneumothorax,** air enters the pleural space from the lung (usually because an alveolus has ruptured) and cannot escape. Pressure builds up in the pleural space with each inspiration as air moves out of the rupture into the pleural space. Because the air is unable to re-enter this opening on exhalation, it accumulates in the pleural space and collapses the lung. The pressure in the pleural space may continue to build until it pushes the structures in the mediastinum toward the opposite side of the chest. This condition, known as **mediastinal shift,** can result in the collapse of the other lung and can rapidly compromise respiratory function. The increased pressure in the pleural space may also interfere with the filling of the ventricles of the heart and lead to circulatory problems.

TYPES OF CHEST TUBES

The insertion of a chest tube or tubes permits removal of air or bloody fluid and allows for re-expansion of the lung and restoration of the normal negative pressure in the pleural space.

PLEURAL TUBES

Because air rises, a chest tube inserted to remove air is usually placed anteriorly through the second intercostal space. A chest tube inserted to remove fluid is placed posteriorly in the eighth or ninth intercostal space because fluid tends to flow to the bottom of the pleural space. If both air and fluid are in the pleural space, two chest tubes may be inserted. Sometimes both tubes are inserted low on the chest through a **stab wound**—a small surgical cut made in the chest after the skin has been anesthetized. The end of one tube is threaded high within the pleural cavity to remove air.

A chest tube inserted at surgery may be brought out of the chest through the surgical incision or through a separate stab wound near the incision. Although two chest tubes can be connected to each other with a Y connector and drain to the same **waterseal drainage** collection device, it is preferable to leave the chest tubes separate for two reasons: fluid or air and drainage returning through each tube may be observed and measured individually, and one tube can be removed without disturbing the other tube or the rest of the setup.

MEDIASTINAL TUBES

The mediastinal space surrounds the heart. After cardiac surgery, there is some **serosanguineous** drainage. Mediastinal tubes are placed to ensure that fluid does not accumulate in the mediastinal space, put pressure on the heart, and interfere with cardiac filling, thereby decreasing cardiac output. Instead, the fluid drains to facilitate cardiac function and healing. Maintaining appropriate drainage is critical to the patient's well-being.

CHEST DRAINAGE CONTAINERS

The chest tube (or tubes) is connected to plastic or rubber tubing, which is attached to a plastic drainage container that has several compartments. Although commercial plastic chest drainage sets are usually used, you may occasionally see glass or plastic bottles used as containers for chest drainage systems. All drainage containers function on the same principles. Therefore, this module explains the principles and provides drawings of bottles as well as pictures of plastic drainage systems.

PRINCIPLES UNDERLYING CHEST DRAINAGE

- The first principle is that air must not be allowed to enter the pleural space from the exterior because that would cause further collapse of the lung and deterioration of oxygenation. Therefore, the drainage system must have a mechanism to allow fluid and air to exit the pleural space but none to enter.

This is usually accomplished by placing the end of the drainage tubing under a waterseal. Air can bubble out through the water, but the water blocks air from entering the drainage tubing. Drainage can flow into the water, and there will not be pressure to push any fluid back into the tubing. An alternative is to have a one-way valve on the system that will not allow air or fluid to enter.

- A second principle is that accurate assessment of the status of the lung is essential. This requires the ability to measure the drainage and determine whether air is exiting the pleural space. The various types of drainage systems each have a mechanism to contain the drainage so that it can be observed and measured. They also allow for observations that indicate whether air is still exiting the pleural space.

- A third principle is that for air to exit the pleural space, the pressure in the lung must be greater than the pressure in the drainage tubing. The pressure of lung expansion by itself can push air out through a drainage tube. Some systems rely on this pressure to remove air and drainage and re-expand the lung. This pressure is low and may not be fast enough to restore effective ventilation to the patient in a timely manner. Therefore, most systems have a mechanism to add suction to pull air and drainage from the pleural space. The tissues of the pleural space and of the exterior of the lung are quite fragile. Any negative pressure applied must be controlled to remain at a low enough level to avoid damage to sensitive lung tissue.

BOTTLE SYSTEM

The original chest systems were composed of glass bottles. Although rarely used now, a bottle system will be described first because the system more clearly demonstrates the principles involved.

Bottle systems may be set up with one or two bottles. The most commonly seen setup of the bottle system is the two-bottle system (Fig. 35-1). The first bottle (or the only bottle in a one-bottle system) is for drainage and waterseal. Drainage moves by gravity down the tubing and accumulates in the bottle. Air moves out with each breath the patient takes. A waterseal at the end of a chest tube is essential to allow air and drainage to escape through the tube but prevent air from traveling back up the tube and into the pleural space. The waterseal drainage system is placed below the level of the patient's chest, taking advantage of gravity to promote drainage and prevent backflow of bottle contents into the pleural space.

To create a waterseal in a bottle, a long glass or plastic tube is inserted through a rubber stopper in the bottle and submerged about 2 cm in the sterile water. Air from

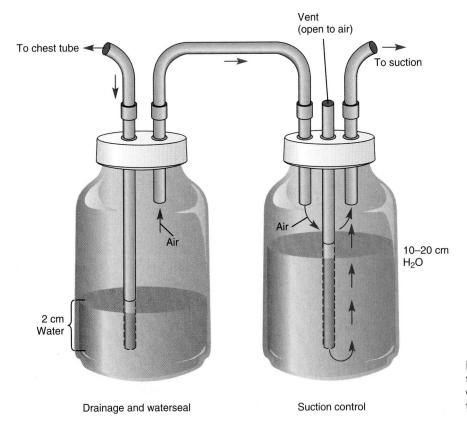

Vent
(open to air)

To chest tube

To suction

Air

Air

2 cm
Water

10–20 cm
H₂O

Drainage and waterseal

Suction control

FIGURE 35-1 Two-bottle system. This system uses one bottle for drainage and a waterseal. The second bottle provides suction control.

the chest passes through the chest tube and bubbles out through the water into the bottle. A short tube is inserted through the second opening in the rubber stopper. This tube acts as an escape valve or vent and allows air to escape from the waterseal bottle, thus preventing pressure build-up in the bottle. Increased pressure in the bottle could cause the water in the bottle to back up toward the chest.

Because the single bottle serves a dual purpose of collecting drainage and providing the waterseal, it must be marked at the original (2 cm) fluid level and again at the end of each shift to keep track of the amount of drainage. A long strip of tape can be attached vertically to the bottle for this purpose. When the amount of fluid in the bottle is increased by drainage, more of the tube is submerged, creating more resistance to drainage.

In an emergency, such as a cracked chest drainage system, you may be able to create a waterseal chest bottle quickly by immersing the end of a chest tube approximately 2 cm into a bottle of sterile water or saline solution at the bedside. Some facilities routinely keep a sealed bottle of sterile water at the bedside of an individual who has a chest tube in place to be used if an emergency occurs.

Suction may also be used on a bottle system. If suction is used, the air vent tube on a waterseal bottle is attached to a suction source. The suction level is regulated by a wall gauge or a gauge attached to the suction machine. Even though the suction is set to a certain level, it is possible for a higher level of suction to be reached at the end of the attached tubing if the tubing is blocked. To prevent this, a second bottle may be added to the system.

This second bottle is a suction control container that limits the amount of suction that can be applied to the chest tube by the suction source. Sterile saline solution is also added to the second bottle. The amount of suction that may be applied is determined by the depth to which the long tube from the suction source is submerged in the sterile water or saline solution. Mechanical suction is responsible for the negative pressure. This pressure is limited to the amount of suction (usually 10 to 20 cm) necessary to pull air in through the vent tube, down through the water, and into the suction tube. When this suction pressure is reached, then air will be pulled into the system, and there will be no increased buildup of suction that could damage the lung. The first bottle continues to provide the waterseal and collect the drainage.

COMMERCIAL CHEST DRAINAGE UNITS

Commercial chest drainage units are more common than bottle systems, but they serve the same purpose. Two of several plastic, disposable chest drainage units

available commercially are the Pleur-Evac and the Atrium units (Fig. 35-2).

The Pleur-Evac is essentially a three-container system: one chamber for drainage, one chamber for the waterseal, and a third chamber for suction control. The drainage compartment is divided into three narrow sections. As one section fills, it spills over into the second section, which then fills. This provides for a more exact measurement of drainage. This chamber has markings to indicate the amount of drainage that has been collected. There is a separate compartment in the center that is labeled as the waterseal chamber. Water is instilled to the marked depth. The container has a molded plastic tube that opens under the water of the waterseal compartment. The system is also equipped with a suction control chamber, which is dry suction control that does not require a waterseal. The system has a positive pressure release valve to prevent the build-up of excessive pressure in the system. The Atrium unit is similar to the Pleur-Evac but does not have the same type of pressure release valve.

Settings for suction level and for measuring drainage are clearly marked. Some systems have an access port to allow for removal of specimens from the unit for examination. With the advent of needleless systems in healthcare settings, some companies are now making such access ports using a needleless design. The units are lightweight, not easily broken, and can hang from the bed frame or be placed in a stand for convenience.

CHEST CATHETER WITH ONE-WAY VALVE

An alternative to standard large-bore chest tubes for treating pneumothorax is a chest catheter, which can be inserted to withdraw air. This process can provide immediate relief of symptoms and correction of the

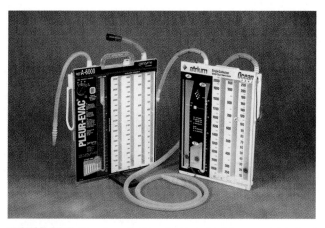

FIGURE 35-2 Pleur-Evac (*left*) and Atrium (*right*) commercial chest drainage systems. Molded into these plastic systems are suction control, waterseal, and drainage containers.

underlying problem. The first 3 inches of the internal end of the catheter have multiple perforations to allow air to flow into the tubing. A Luer-Lok connector at the proximal end allows staff to connect a three-way stopcock after the chest catheter is inserted and to remove the air from the pleural space with a 50-mL syringe.

After as much air as possible has been withdrawn, the Luer-Lok end of the catheter is connected to a Heimlich drainage valve, which permits a one-way flow of air away from the pleural cavity (Fig. 35-3) and does not allow air to reenter the pleural space. This type of chest tube can be connected to waterseal drainage or suction if necessary. The pneumothorax catheter is not recommended for patients who have large amounts of fluid or blood from hemorrhage because its small internal diameter may easily be occluded.

PROCEDURE FOR ASSISTING WITH THE INSERTION OF CHEST TUBES

In hemothorax, pneumothorax, or hemopneumothorax, the chest tube is inserted through a stab wound. Before assisting the physician with the insertion of a chest tube, review Module 17, Assisting With Diagnostic and Therapeutic Procedures, especially noting the procedure for **thoracentesis.**

ASSESSMENT

1. Check the physician's order. **R:** Checking the order ensures that you are preparing the procedure for the correct patient.
2. Check to see if the patient has signed a consent form. If not, notify the physician who is to perform the procedure. **R:** The patient or person responsible for the patient must give written consent for this invasive procedure. Obtaining consent for a medical procedure is the responsibility of the physician.
3. Assess the patient's status and abilities with emphasis on vital signs and respiratory status. **R:** To help you determine what assistance the patient may need during the procedure, such as supplemental oxygenation or assistance with positioning.

ANALYSIS

4. Critically think through your data, carefully evaluating each aspect and its relation to other data to determine the patient's need for chest tube insertion and the observations you will need to make. **R:** Knowing the patient's problem will help you to identify expected findings for that patient. For

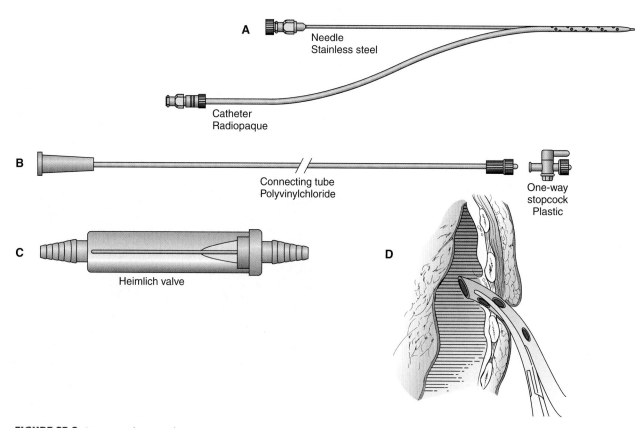

FIGURE 35-3 A pneumothorax catheter set contains (**A**) a trocar with a catheter for insertion, (**B**) a connecting tube to attach the catheter and valve, and (**C**) a Heimlich valve. (**D**) Chest tube inserted.

instance, in a patient with a pneumothorax, you will likely have minimal drainage. A patient with a large hemothorax would be expected to have a large amount of bloody drainage.

5. Identify specific problems and modifications of the procedure needed for this individual. **R:** Planning for the individual must take into consideration the individual's problems.

PLANNING

6. Determine the individualized patient outcomes of the chest tube insertion procedure, including the following. **R:** Identification of outcomes guides planning and evaluation.
   a. Vital signs are stable. **R:** To provide reassurance that the patient is physiologically stable.
   b. Patient states he or she is comfortable. **R:** To allow the patient to rest after the procedure.
   c. Chest tube system is functioning properly: draining, waterseal in place, suction at correct level, and system positioned below the level of the chest. **R:** To allow the lung to begin to expand.
   d. Patient states understanding of situation. **R:** To facilitate compliance with care required while the chest tube is in place.

7. Obtain equipment, including the following:
   a. Chest tube tray: this usually contains the **trocar** (a short, sharply pointed, steel rod used for piercing the chest), sterile drapes, antiseptic solution, syringes, gauze dressing materials, and chest tubes. After you have determined which items are included on the tray in your clinical setting, you can add other needed items.
   b. Chest drainage set: if two drainage tubes will be maintained separately, you will need to prepare two drainage sets. Set up the chest drainage systems. You will need sterile water to fill the waterseal section. Review the directions on the specific set to determine how to fill it. **R:** To ensure proper functioning of the system. Sterile covers should remain over the connectors until they are ready to be connected to the chest tube to maintain sterility of the system.
   c. Other supplies may include sterile water, local anesthetic, antiseptic preparation, suture materials, clean gloves, mask, apron, eye protection, and sterile gloves. **R:** Knowing the specific preferences of the physician inserting the tube is useful and will help the procedure go more smoothly.

IMPLEMENTATION

Action	Rationale
8. Wash or disinfect your hands.	To prevent the transfer of microorganisms that may cause infection.
9. Identify the patient, using two identifiers.	To be sure you are performing the right procedure for the right patient.
10. Explain the procedure to the patient in general terms.	The patient will be less anxious if he or she knows what to expect.
11. Close the door, pull the curtain around the bed, and set up the equipment on a sterile field.	To ensure privacy and readiness for the procedure.
12. Prepare the patient.	
a. Administer pain medication or sedative as prescribed.	Chest tube insertion causes discomfort. Premedication for pain relief will make the patient as comfortable as possible.
b. Assist the patient to the upright position. This positioning may be accomplished in any of the following ways: (1) Pad the back of a straight chair for comfort and have the patient straddle the chair, leaning the arms on the padded back.	The upright position is used so that the pull of gravity consolidates the fluid in the lower portion of the affected side of the chest.

(continued)

Action	Rationale
(2) Have the patient sit upright in bed and lean forward, resting on the overbed table.	
(3) Have the patient sit at the edge of the bed, leaning on the overbed table. The physician will work from the opposite side of the bed.	
13. Put on apron, mask, eye protection, and clean gloves.	To protect yourself from exposure to bloody secretions. This is especially important if the patient has a hemothorax.
14. Reassure the patient, and carefully assess for skin color, diaphoresis, respiratory status, chest pain, and severe anxiety throughout the procedure.	The procedure may cause an adverse response in the patient.
15. Assist with the procedure. You may be asked to assist in any of the following ways:	
a. Pour antiseptic solution over cotton balls or gauze.	The antiseptic will be used to clean the skin. This allows the physician to maintain sterile gloves while handling the antiseptic swabs.
b. Hold the vial of local anesthetic as the physician withdraws the proper dosage. Be sure to state the name of the drug and have the label visible so that the physician can verify the drug she or he will be administering.	Holding the vial allows the physician's gloves to remain sterile. Stating the name of the drug and showing the label supports the safe administration of the right drug.
c. Attach the requested drainage system after the tube has been inserted.	The drainage system allows air and fluid to exit the chest without air entering.
d. Apply an occlusive dressing or dry sterile gauze and tape (Fig. 35-4) to the tube insertion site(s). Wear sterile gloves if you will be handling sterile dressing materials.	The site must be dressed to prevent infection.

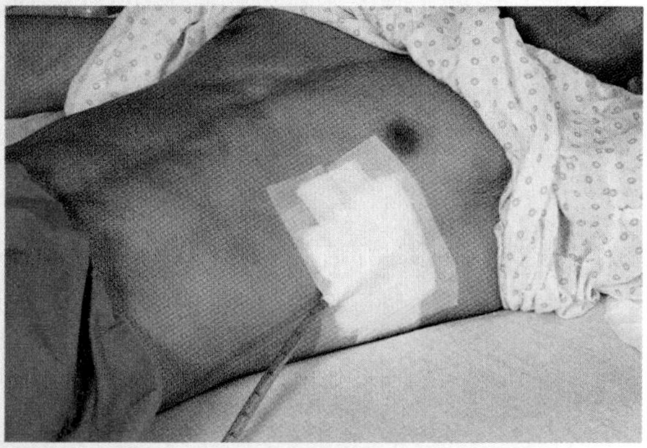

FIGURE 35-4 The chest tube insertion site is protected by a gauze-and-tape dressing.

(continued)

Action	Rationale
e. Make sure a chest x-ray film is ordered following the procedure.	To verify proper placement of the chest tube.
16. Conclude the procedure.	
a. Return the patient to a comfortable position.	So that the patient can rest.
b. If a specimen of fluid is obtained, label it and send it to the laboratory.	For laboratory analysis.
c. Care for the equipment appropriately, including your mask, eyewear, and apron; discard your gloves. Most of the equipment is disposable.	Discard bloody materials and gloves into a biohazard waste container to prevent the spread of infection. Make sure all sharps are placed in a sharps container to avoid accidental sticks.
17. Wash or disinfect your hands.	To prevent the transfer of microorganisms that may cause infection.
18. Recheck the patient's pulse, respirations, and blood pressure, and notify the physician of significant changes.	The procedure may cause physiologic and psychologic stress to the patient, which may require intervention by the physician.

EVALUATION

19. Evaluate using the individualized patient outcomes previously identified. **R:** Evaluation in relation to desired outcomes is essential for planning future care.
   a. Vital signs are stable.
   b. Patient states he or she is comfortable.
   c. Chest tube system is functioning properly: draining, waterseal in place, suction at correct level, and system positioned below the level of the chest.
   d. Patient states understanding of situation.

DOCUMENTATION

20. Document appropriate data. Include the physician's name, vital signs before and after the procedure, type of drainage system in use, amount of suction, and the response of the patient. **R:** Documentation is a legal record of the patient's care and therapy and communicates nursing activities to other nurses and caregivers.

PROCEDURE FOR CARING FOR THE PATIENT WITH CHEST TUBES

To provide safe care for the patient with a chest tube or tubes in place, follow this procedure.

ASSESSMENT

1. Check the patient's record. **R:** To help determine the type of chest tube(s) in place, the suction ordered, and any specific assessment plans.
2. Review appropriate procedures and protocols for your facility. **R:** To ensure that you are performing the procedure within agency guidelines.

ANALYSIS

3. Critically think through your data, carefully evaluating each aspect and its relation to other data to determine the best approach to providing chest tube care. **R:** The approach must be the one that gives the patient maximal benefit while minimizing discomfort.
4. Identify specific problems and modifications of the procedure needed for this individual. **R:** Planning for the individual must take into consideration the individual's problems.

PLANNING

5. Determine the individualized patient outcomes in relation to care of the patient with a chest tube, including the following. **R:** Identification of outcomes guides planning and evaluation.
   a. Respiratory rate is within normal limits, and lung sounds are clear.

b. Patient does not report pain or exhibit anxiety.

c. Integrity of the system is maintained: waterseal intact, no leaks, and correct suction pressure.

d. Drainage type and amount is within expected range for the type of procedure.

e. Wound is healing without signs of infection.

 6. Obtain supplies, including clean gloves, sterile water as needed for containers, and sterile gloves and dressing materials if needed. Having all needed supplies at the bedside in advance will facilitate the procedure, while minimally disturbing the patient.

IMPLEMENTATION

Action	Rationale
7. Wash or disinfect your hands.	To prevent the transfer of microorganisms that can cause infection.
8. Identify the patient, using two identifiers.	To be sure you are performing the procedure for the correct patient.
9. Assess and adjust the drainage system. To protect yourself, put on gloves before manipulating any part of the system in a way that could expose you to body secretions.	
a. Check the entire length of the tubing from the patient to the container. The tubing between the patient and the waterseal bottle should be long enough to allow the patient to move and turn. In addition, it should be coiled on the bed and fastened to the bed so that it will not be kinked or obstructed because the patient is lying on it. If the patient is up in a chair, it must be fastened to the chair in a manner to facilitate drainage.	Dependent loops hanging below the level of the bed allow drainage to accumulate in the tubing, and the pressure of the lung expanding may not be able to push air through the accumulated drainage. Kinks in the tubing will inhibit free drainage.
b. Check the chest tube container to be sure that the waterseal is intact. Also observe whether it is fluctuating **(tidaling)** or if there are bubbles in the waterseal bottle.	The system should be airtight to prevent air from entering the pleural space. Fluctuation of the water level will occur in a waterseal container that is not connected to suction. The water level rises when the patient inhales and falls when the patient exhales. Shallow breathing results in slight fluctuation. When the patient must work harder to breathe, for example, when secretions are retained, negative pressure in the chest is higher, and, therefore, fluctuation is greater. Continuous bubbling in the waterseal bottle can mean either persistent leakage of air from the lung or a leak in the system. When a chest tube is connected to suction, the suction obscures the tidaling in the waterseal container.
c. Position the chest tube container between 2 and 3 feet below the patient's chest. If the drainage container is accidentally raised above the level of the patient's chest, lower it	The container is placed below the level of the patient's chest to provide for gravity to facilitate drainage in the tubing and to prevent any backflow of fluid from the container into the pleural space.

(continued)

Action	Rationale
immediately, encourage the patient to breathe deeply, and observe the patient for signs of further lung collapse and mediastinal shift. If indications of these are seen (see "Potential Adverse Outcomes and Related Interventions"), notify the physician. If the drainage container is on or near the floor, be careful not to lower a bed or side rail onto it because this could break the container and disrupt the entire drainage system.	
d. Secure connections, and retape them with adhesive or plastic tape if needed. In many facilities, the policy is to tape all connections and to check the system on a routine basis to be sure that all connections remain intact.	Taping the connections provides protection against accidental disconnection. Adhesive or plastic tape is used because it is impervious to air. Paper tape is not suitable for this purpose because it will admit air.
e. Observe the amount and character of the drainage and the rate at which it accumulates. This observation is usually made hourly immediately after chest tube insertion and less often thereafter—at least every 8 hours.	To identify excessive bleeding, beginning infection, or tube blockage.
f. If suction is ordered, check the suction level on the suction device. The level must be kept at the amount ordered at all times. The water in the suction control section (unless it is a dry suction system) protects the lung from excess suction.	An inadequate amount of suction may delay lung re-expansion.

Safety Alert *Note: Suction should not be applied to chest drainage without a suction control chamber to protect the lung. A piece of tape placed at the level of solution in the suction control bottle or at the ordered levels on a gauge can be a helpful reminder. If suction control is used, check for gentle, continuous bubbling. Gentle bubbling indicates that suction is constantly reaching the desired level but cannot go higher. If the bubbling is vigorous, the fluid will evaporate more rapidly. The fluid level in the container should be checked periodically to be sure it is the proper depth to provide the amount of suction ordered. If it is not the proper depth, sterile water must be added (unless it is a dry suction system).*

(continued)

Action	Rationale
g. Observe and monitor the patient, check the system, and correct any difficulties.	To decrease the risk of complications of chest tube placement.
h. Keep two large **rubber-shod hemostats** or Kelley clamps at the bedside. Many of the plastic pleural drainage systems are now manufactured with plastic slide clamps that can be closed, rather than using a hemostat for chest tube closure. Use the clamping device only when essential and for only a few minutes. When clamps are used, be careful not to cover them with the sheet or blanket.	The rubber covering over metal clamps prevents damage to the chest tubes. A chest tube is clamped to determine the cause of an air leak when there is bubbling in the waterseal bottle and the chest tube is connected to suction. It is also necessary to clamp a chest tube to empty the collection bottle or replace a broken or cracked container in the system. If the lung is leaking air into the pleural space, air can accumulate there, collapsing the lung and pressuring the mediastinum. If clamps are covered, there is the possibility of the clamped chest tube(s) being forgotten. If clamps are forgotten and left in place for too long, pressure can build up in the pleural space, causing a tension pneumothorax.
i. Keep petrolatum-infused gauze at the bedside.	To provide an airtight dressing to be used in case the chest tube is inadvertently pulled out of the chest cavity.
10. Examine the chest wound and dressing and change the dressing if needed. Protect the chest tube insertion site with a sterile dressing.	The dressing is removed and the site inspected for signs of infection unless protocol indicates that the physician will change the dressing. Redress the wound according to the procedure in Module 40, Providing Wound Care.
11. Complete the essential physical assessment.	
a. Assess the lungs.	The areas in which breath sounds are heard and the presence of adventitious sounds are important in determining how well chest tubes improve oxygenation.
b. Measure the vital signs (pulse, respiration, blood pressure, and temperature).	To assist in monitoring for potential infection and other complications related to chest tubes.
12. Assist the patient with moving and positioning in proper alignment. Encourage him or her to change positions frequently. When the patient is lying on the affected side, the tubing can be occluded by the patient's weight. To prevent this, place rolled towels beside the tubing.	Moving helps to prevent complications of immobility, such as hypoventilation, venous stasis, and postural hypotension.
13. Assist the patient with coughing and deep breathing at least once hourly.	To prevent **atelectasis** (lung collapse) and to assist in removing air or fluid from the pleural space.

(continued)

Action	Rationale
14. When appropriate, transport and/or ambulate the patient. Be sure to avoid clamping chest tubes to transport a patient to another department or to ambulate the patient. Instead, do the following:	
a. Keep the waterseal containers connected to the patient at all times, and detach the tubing from the suction device.	The waterseal prevents air from entering the pleural space. In general, suction is not needed for transport or ambulation. If it is, you will need to connect the pleural drainage system to a portable suction device.
b. Keep the container upright.	So that the waterseal is maintained.
c. Keep the container(s) below the level of the patient's chest.	Is so that gravity assists drainage and prevents back-flow of container contents into the pleural space.
d. Maintain an airtight system.	To prevent air from entering the system or the chest.
e. Keep the vent open (if present).	To ensure that pressure does not build up in the system.

EVALUATION

15. Evaluate using the individualized patient outcomes previously identified. **R:** Evaluation in relation to outcomes is essential for planning future care.
   a. Respiratory rate is within normal limits and lung sounds clear.
   b. Patient does not report pain or evidence anxiety.
   c. Integrity of system is maintained.
   d. Drainage type and amount are within expected range for type of procedure.
   e. Wound is healing without signs of infection.

DOCUMENTATION

16. Document information regarding the chest tubes including the following: time system checked, amount and description of drainage, suction level, that the system is intact, condition of the wound, and assessment of the patient's respiratory status, pain, and anxiety. **R:** Documentation is a legal record of the patient's care and therapy and communicates nursing activities to other nurses and caregivers.

POTENTIAL ADVERSE OUTCOMES AND RELATED INTERVENTIONS

1. Drainage is copious and bright red. Bleeding of more 100 mL/h is considered heavy bleeding.
Intervention: Measure vital signs, assess patient's physical status, and immediately contact the physician. A blood recovery device (sometimes referred to a "cell saver") may be attached to the chest drainage system to recover the blood, filter it, and prepare it for reinfusion to the patient. This is usually done for patients with a large amount of bleeding and limits the need for donor blood for blood replacement.

2. Drainage quickly fills the collection chamber.
Intervention: Obtain a new sterile drainage container. Fill the waterseal section with sterile water. Clamp the tube briefly, and connect to a new sterile system. Remove clamp, reinstate the suction, and dispose of old container appropriately.

3. Fluctuations and drainage stop.
Intervention: Mediastinal tubes will not fluctuate and will usually have minimal drainage. A gradual cessation of fluctuation or drainage in a pleural tube could indicate that the lung has re-expanded, and all fluid has been evacuated. With any type of tube, drainage cessation may indicate kinking of the tube, the patient lying on the tube, or a blood or **fibrin** clot within the tube. In such situations
   a. Make sure that the tubing is free of external obstructions.
   b. Keep in mind that if the patient has atelectasis or retained secretions, respirations may be shallow and may not create tidaling. Auscultate the chest to determine lung function. Have the patient deep breathe and cough. This may restore drainage.
   c. Remove any clots seen in the drainage because they have the potential to obstruct the tubing. Remove them into the drainage chamber by "milking" the tubing. Milking may be done in various ways, but it means compressing the tubing and then releasing it to create a pressure in

the tubing that will loosen the clot. Use the same motion in subsequent sections of the tubing, moving away from the patient's chest toward the drainage container. Because milking may create high negative pressure on the lung, the tubing should be milked only if there is evidence of clots that may obstruct drainage. If the tubing is in place to remove air only, there is no logical reason to milk the tube.

    d. If the lung does not re-expand and drainage is not restored, notify the physician.

4. The drainage bottle or plastic system has broken.
Intervention: Clamp the tubing close to the patient. Prepare a new sterile drainage container, and replace it as described previously.

5. The chest tube has pulled out.
Intervention: You must know whether air is entering the chest from inside the lung.

    a. If air is not entering from the lung, immediately place an occlusive dressing, such as a sterile petrolatum gauze pad (which should be available in the room), over the site to prevent room air from entering the pleural space. Cover the petrolatum gauze pad with a dry dressing and tape the dressing on all four sides to form an occlusive seal.

    b. If air is entering from the lung, make sure that this air can exit to prevent tension pneumothorax. Place the dressing over the wound, tape loosely on the top and two sides, and allow the fourth (bottom) side to be open. When the patient inhales, the dressing will be pulled against the wound, preventing room air from entering the chest. When the patient exhales, the dressing will be pushed away from the wound by the air exiting the chest.

    c. Assess the patient's respiratory status, and immediately notify the physician that the tube has pulled out.

6. Bubbling increases with inspiration and expiration.
Intervention: This is usually caused by a leak in the system. To identify a leak, do the following:

    a. Check the connections to be sure that they are firm. Retape connections if necessary.

    b. If the leak continues after connections are tight, there may be a crack in the drainage container or a pinhole leak in the tubing. To identify the location of the leak, place one of the clamps on the tubing close to the chest. If the excess bubbling continues, the leak is distal to the clamp. Gradually move the clamp toward the container. When the bubbling stops after placing the clamp, you know that the leak is between where the clamp is currently placed and the last placement of the clamp. A leak in the tubing may be sealed with occlusive tape. If the leak is in the drainage container, the container must be changed.

7. The patient's anxiety increases.
Intervention: Lack of oxygen creates a physiologic basis for anxiety. First, assess the patient's respiratory status. Next, check the drainage system for problems and correct any that you find. If the system is working properly, and respiratory status is stable, spend time with the patient. Explain how the drainage system works and why the sounds of the suction are important and beneficial.

8. Patient experiences moderate pain when moving.
Intervention: Medicate the patient based on the physician's order to provide pain relief adequate to facilitate easy movement. Remember to use nonpharmacologic means of pain relief as well to augment the effects of the medication (for instance, distraction and imagery). The patient must decide what level of pain relief is essential. Consult with the physician if ordered medications do not provide adequate pain relief.

PROCEDURE FOR ASSISTING WITH THE REMOVAL OF CHEST TUBES

To assist the physician with the removal of a chest tube, refer to Module 17, Assisting With Diagnostic and Therapeutic Procedures. The physician may order an analgesic premedication, or you can give the patient the ordered pain relief medication about 30 minutes before the chest tube is removed.

ASSESSMENT

1. Check the physician's order. **R:** An order is needed to remove the chest tube.
2. Note that a signed permission form is not needed for removal. **R:** The permission to insert chest tubes implies permission to remove them.
3. Assess the patient's status with emphasis on vital signs (pulse, respirations, and blood pressure). Also, assess the need for premedication. **R:** Vital signs provide a baseline measure, and premedication may help to maintain the patient's comfort.

ANALYSIS

4. Critically think through your data, carefully evaluating each aspect and its relation to other data. **R:** To determine the approach to the procedure that will best maintain patient comfort and safety.
5. Identify specific problems and modifications of the procedure needed for this individual. **R:** Planning for the individual must take into consideration the individual's problems.

PLANNING

6. Determine individualized patient outcomes in relation to the chest tube removal. **R:** Identification of outcomes guides planning and evaluation.
   a. Patient's vital signs are stable with respirations even and unlabored. **R:** This indicates that the patient is physiologically stable after the procedure.
   b. No indications of pneumothorax or **subcutaneous emphysema** are evident. **R:** Pneumothorax is indicated by sudden chest pain and shortness of breath. Subcutaneous emphysema is seen in puffy tissue around the tubing site that "crackles" when pressed.
   c. Patient states he or she is comfortable, allowing the patient to rest after the procedure.

7. Gather the necessary equipment, including the following. **R:** Obtaining all equipment in advance facilitates organization.
   a. Sterile gloves for the physician to wear to remove the chest tube
   b. Suture set (or sterile scissors and sterile forceps) to cut the sutures holding the chest tube in place
   c. Sterile petrolatum gauze to cover the chest tube removal site
   d. Skin closure material to close the chest tube removal site
   e. Dressing material to cover the chest tube removal site
   f. Wide tape, to hold the dressing in place

IMPLEMENTATION

Action	Rationale
8. Wash or disinfect your hands.	To prevent the transfer of microorganisms that may cause infection.
9. Identify the patient, using two identifiers.	To be sure you are performing the procedure on the correct patient.
10. Explain the procedure to the patient in general terms.	An explanation helps the patient to know what to expect, which facilitates relaxation and cooperation.
11. Close the door, pull the curtain around the bed, and set up the equipment.	To ensure privacy and readiness for the procedure.
12. Assist the patient into the proper position—either sitting at the edge of the bed or lying on the unaffected side.	These positions provide best access to the chest tube site.
13. Reassure, observe, and monitor the patient throughout the procedure.	Reassure the patient to decrease anxiety, continuously observe to determine tolerance to the procedure, and monitor to see if any complications develop.
14. Assist the physician as needed. Put on gloves before handling any equipment that might expose you to body secretions.	Assisting the physician facilitates the procedure. Wearing gloves prevents exposure to bloody secretions.
a. First, the physician removes any dressing materials and then cuts the sutures.	
b. The patient is asked to take a deep breath and bear down (Valsalva's maneuver).	To raise intrathoracic pressure and prevent air from entering the chest while the physician quickly pulls out the tube. Alternatively, the tube may be removed during expiration, to prevent air from being pulled

(continued)

Action	Rationale
	back into the pleural space during the removal of the tube.
c. After the tube is removed, the wound may be sutured or clipped closed and covered with the petrolatum gauze and dressing material, which is securely taped in place. Alternatively, the wound may simply be covered with petrolatum gauze and an occlusive dressing, which forms an airtight seal.	To prevent air from entering the chest.
d. A chest x-ray film usually is ordered when the procedure is complete.	To be sure the lung expanded and that no air entered the pleural space.
15. When the procedure is complete, reassess the patient.	
a. Recheck vital signs.	To determine if the patient is stable after the procedure.
b. Auscultate breath sounds and be alert for indications of pneumothorax (dyspnea, tachypnea, chest pain) and subcutaneous emphysema (air trapped in the subcutaneous tissue that crackles when palpated).	To identify complications that compromise the well-being of the patient and must be reported to the physician.
16. Properly care for equipment. Be sure to discard any sharps in sharps containers.	To dispose of equipment and maintain an orderly unit.
17. Wash or disinfect your hands.	To prevent the transfer of microorganisms that could cause infection.

EVALUATION

18. Evaluate using the individualized patient outcomes previously identified. **R:** Evaluation in relation to desired outcomes is essential for planning future care.
  a. Patient vital signs are stable with respirations even and unlabored.
  b. There is no indication of pneumothorax or subcutaneous emphysema.
  c. Patient states he or she is comfortable.

DOCUMENTATION

19. On the patient's record, document appropriate data, including physician's name, vital signs before and after the procedure, the patient's response, and any other significant observations. **R:** Documentation is a legal record of the patient's care and therapy and communicates nursing activities to other nurses and caregivers.

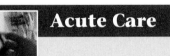

Acute Care

There are many options for pleural drainage systems in the acute care setting. Some new advances in pleural drainage systems include transport handles, fingertip suction adjustment, prepackaged water for creating the waterseal, and even waterless operating systems with a dry, one-way valve for patient protection. When new equipment is adopted, be sure to attend any education events to ensure that you have the competence needed for care of patients for whom this equipment is used.

Long-Term Care

Residents with a chest tube drainage system may be seen occasionally in the long-term care setting, particularly residents who may be receiving rehabilitation services through Medicare. Such residents may need less extensive care than is required in a hospital. However, a resident with a chest tube in a long-term care setting will need frequent monitoring by the nurse to prevent complications and ensure safety.

Home Care

There are now mobile pleural drainage systems available so that clients can return home sooner after hospitalization. Such clients will need reinforcement of chest tube care instruction from the home care nurse. These portable units allow the client freedom of movement because the units can be hung from the client's belt during ambulation. The Atrium Express includes such features as a positive pressure relief valve, a needleless access port, and an air leak window.

Ambulatory Care

Clients with chest tube drainage systems are seen more frequently in ambulatory care settings now that many healthcare procedures are performed and continued outside of hospitals. To provide proper and effective care, the ambulatory care nurse must understand how to care for clients with chest tubes and be aware of advances in pleural drainage systems.

LEARNING TOOLS

DEVELOP YOUR BACKGROUND KNOWLEDGE

1. Review the Learning Outcomes.

2. Read the material on the respiratory system in your assigned text, focusing on the anatomy and physiology of the respiratory system, especially the dynamics of breathing.

3. Look up Key Terms in the glossary.

4. Review the module as though you were preparing to teach the information to another person.

5. Mentally practice the specific procedure.

DEVELOP YOUR SKILLS

6. In the practice setting
   a. Examine chest tube insertion materials available, for example, trocars of various sizes and chest tubes of various sizes.
   b. Using your partner as a patient, simulate the explanation and positioning appropriate for chest tube insertion. Have your partner evaluate your performance.
   c. Examine any chest tube drainage containers or systems available.
   d. Explain to a partner how each of the above systems works.

DEMONSTRATE YOUR SKILLS

7. In the clinical setting
   a. Consult with your instructor for an opportunity to assist with insertion or removal of a chest tube.
   b. Consult with your instructor for an opportunity to care for a patient with chest drainage in place.

CRITICAL THINKING EXERCISES

1. Mr. M., who had surgery to the lower lobe of his left lung, returned from the postanesthesia recovery unit at 1500 hours. He has a chest tube in place on the left. The tube is attached to 20 cm of suction. You note that there is no drainage in the chest drainage system. Analyze what might be the cause of this. Determine what assessments you will make and what actions, if any, you will take.

2. Ms. R. had heart surgery yesterday. She has a mediastinal tube in place. You note there has only been 10 mL of drainage from the tube and that there is no evidence of tidaling in the waterseal section of the drainage system. Explain the significance of these observations and then determine what actions you should take.

SELF-QUIZ
SHORT-ANSWER QUESTIONS

1. List three reasons for insertion of chest tubes.

   a. _____

   b. _____

   c. _____

2. Define pneumothorax.

   _____

3. Where is a chest tube to remove air usually located and why?

   _____

   _____

4. List two reasons for locating the waterseal drainage system below the level of the patient's chest.

   a. _____

   b. _____

5. What is the function of the second bottle in the two-bottle system of waterseal drainage?

   _____

6. List three things to check when observing a chest drainage system.

   a. _____

   b. _____

   c. _____

7. What complication may happen if a clamp is left on a chest tube for too long?

   _____

8. Why is a chest x-ray film usually ordered after a chest tube is removed?

   _____

MULTIPLE CHOICE

_____ 9. What is the purpose of a mediastinal tube? (Choose all that apply.)
   a. To help the lung to re-expand
   b. To drain fluid from the mediastinal space
   c. To facilitate cardiac function
   d. To prevent infection

_____ 10. What problem will occur if the chest tubes are allowed to hang down off the side of the bed?
   a. Fluid may siphon back into the chest.
   b. Air will return to the chest.
   c. Air will be blocked from exiting the chest.
   d. Fluid will not drain from the chest.

_____ 11. What problem will occur if the chest drainage set is raised above the level of the chest?
   a. Fluid may siphon back into the chest.
   b. Air will return to the chest.
   c. Air will be blocked from exiting the chest.
   d. Fluid will not drain from the chest.

_____ 12. If the chest drainage container is accidentally crushed between the bed and a wheelchair, what should be the nurse's first action?
   a. Obtain a new chest tube set.
   b. Clamp off the chest tubes.
   c. Have the patient sit up.
   d. Have the patient lie flat and do Valsalva's maneuver.

Answers to the Self-Quiz questions appear in the back of the book.

MODULE 36

Emergency Resuscitation Procedures

SKILLS INCLUDED IN THIS MODULE

Performing CPR for Adults
  One-Rescuer CPR
  Using the Automated External Defibrillator (AED)
  Two-Rescuer CPR
Performing CPR for Infants and Small Children
Performing CPR in the Acute Care Facility
Clearing Foreign-Body Airway Obstruction in Adults
Clearing Foreign-Body Airway Obstruction in Infants and
  Small Children

PREREQUISITE MODULES

Module 1	An Approach to Nursing Skills
Module 2	Documentation
Module 4	Basic Infection Control
Module 6	Moving the Patient in Bed and Positioning
Module 11	Assessing Temperature, Pulse, and Respiration
Module 14	Nursing Physical Assessment

KEY TERMS

airway
automated
  external
  defibrillator
  (AED)
breathing
cardiac arrest
carotid pulse
circulation
compression-only
  CPR
defibrillation

foreign-body air-
  way obstruction
  (FBAO)
Heimlich maneuver
respiratory arrest
sternum
trachea
tracheostomy
ventricular
  fibrillation
xiphoid process

OVERALL OBJECTIVE

▸ To recognize the need for emergency resuscitation procedures and to perform them on adults, children, and infants in healthcare settings.

LEARNING OUTCOMES

The student will be able to
1. Assess the patient effectively to determine the need for cardiopulmonary resuscitation (CPR).
2. Assess the patient effectively to determine the need for the Heimlich maneuver.
3. Analyze assessment data to determine special problems or concerns that must be addressed to successfully rescue the patient.
4. Determine appropriate patient outcomes of the rescue procedure(s), and recognize the potential for adverse outcomes.
5. Perform CPR and/or the Heimlich maneuver correctly.
6. Use the automated external defibrillator (AED) correctly.
7. Evaluate the effectiveness of the procedure(s) for the specific patient.
8. Document the procedure and the patient's response in the record as appropriate.

Emergency resuscitation procedures encompass cardio-pulmonary resuscitation (CPR), which includes rescue **breathing** and cardiac compression, and the various maneuvers used to clear a foreign body obstruction from the **airway.** The nurse is expected to carry out emergency resuscitation procedures efficiently in a variety of healthcare settings and must be able to perform these lifesaving procedures—as a member of a team or alone—on adults, children, and infants. It is good practice to take a refresher course once a year to maintain expertise. Some healthcare agencies require this practice.

The following procedures are presented in a way that complements the formats used by the organizations that teach these procedures nationwide so that the rescuer can easily memorize the steps to call on in an emergency. As a nursing student reviewing the procedures, you may wish to identify for yourself which steps constitute assessment, analysis, planning, implementation, and evaluation.

DELEGATION

All personnel in healthcare facilities are taught emergency resuscitation procedures. Everyone must be able to do basic cardiopulmonary resuscitation and the Heimlich maneuver and be able to operate the automated external defibrillator (AED) if available. In most facilities, there are regular updates and competency checks to assure that staff are able to respond effectively.

INFECTION TRANSMISSION CONCERNS IN CARDIOPULMONARY RESUSCITATION

There is an extremely low likelihood of disease transmission during cardiopulmonary resuscitation practice and during actual performance of mouth-to-mouth resuscitation. However, in most healthcare settings, barrier devices are available for use during rescue breathing. Therefore, healthcare providers usually use barrier devices or bag-mask systems during resuscitation procedures (Fig. 36-1).

Gloves also will be available for your use during CPR in the workplace, providing protection in the event you are exposed to blood or body fluids during an emergency. It is prudent to carry gloves in your pocket at all times. In other settings, you may or may not have access to gloves.

CARDIOPULMONARY RESUSCITATION

CPR is a process of rescue breathing and chest compression that is provided to a person whose heart has stopped beating and who has stopped breathing. No matter where this person is, he or she needs immediate assistance to restore breathing and circulation. If the delay is longer than 4 minutes, the potential for permanent brain damage is great. Eventually, you may be involved not only in performing the skill but also in teaching it to professionals and laypeople as well.

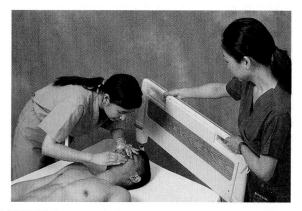

FIGURE 36-1 Position the barrier device (the mouth-to-mask device in this case) over the patient's mouth and nose, ensure an adequate seal, and initiate mouth-to-barrier device breathing.

Compression-only CPR (delivery of chest compressions without rescue breathing) is being studied. Current evidence indicates that the outcome of chest compressions without rescue breathing is significantly better than no resuscitation attempt at all (American Heart Association, 2000). Some countries are exploring the use of compression-only CPR for use by the lay public because of its ease of use. While it is not yet in general use in the United States, the appropriate use of this technique is outlined in Box 36-1.

PERFORMING CPR FOR ADULTS

One-Rescuer CPR

INITIATE THE PROCESS

1. Determine unresponsiveness (tap or gently shake the person and shout, "Are you all right?"). If you get no response, move to step 2.
2. Activate the emergency medical services (EMS) system in the healthcare facility or, if you are outside the healthcare facility, in the community. Because most adults with sudden nontraumatic **cardiac arrest** are found to be in **ventricular fibrillation,** a life-threatening cardiac dysrhythmia, survival is highly dependent on early **defibrillation** or early system access (American Heart Association, 2000).

AIRWAY

3. Position the person flat on the back on a firm, flat surface to facilitate moving on to cardiac compression. If you must roll the person over, try to move the entire body at once, as a single unit, to avoid worsening any injury to the neck, back, or long bones. Position yourself at the victim's side so that you can perform both rescue breathing and chest compressions if necessary. Open the airway, using one of the two methods below.
   a. Head-tilt/chin-lift maneuver: Tilt the patient's head back by placing the palm of one hand on the forehead and applying firm backward pressure. Place the fingers of the other hand under the bony part of the lower jaw near the chin and lift to bring the chin forward. This will clear the tongue out of the airway.
   b. Jaw-thrust maneuver: If a patient has been in an accident (a motor vehicle crash, a fall), and you suspect there is a neck injury, do not open the airway using the chin-lift method. Instead, grasp the angles of the victim's lower jaw, and lift with both hands, one on each side, displacing the mandible forward. Because this maneuver can usually be accomplished without extending the neck, it is the safest first approach to opening the airway of the child or adult with a possible neck injury (Fig. 36-2). Carefully support the head without tilting it backward or turning it from side to side. If mouth-to-mouth breathing is necessary, you can occlude the nostrils by placing your cheek tightly against them.

BREATHING

4. Assess breathing to determine inadequate or absent breathing. Place your ear close to the patient's mouth and do three things:
   a. *Look* for the chest to rise and fall.
   b. *Listen* for the sound of air leaving the lungs during exhalation.
   c. *Feel* for the flow of air against your cheek (Fig. 36-3).

      Note: Sometimes a person begins to breathe spontaneously after an airway has been estab-

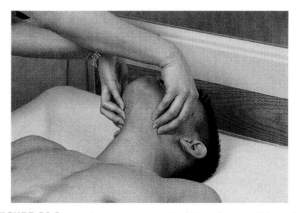

FIGURE 36-2 Jaw-thrust maneuver. Displacing the mandible is the safest way to open the airway for victims of all ages with suspected neck injury.

---

box 36-1 *Compression-Only CPR*

Indications for Compression-Only CPR

- When a rescuer is unwilling or unable to perform rescue breathing
- In situations where a 911 dispatcher is giving instructions by telephone to an untrained bystander (American Heart Association, 2000).

Compression-Only CPR Not Indicated

- In healthcare settings, because barrier devices and bag-mask ventilation equipment should be available and personnel are trained in CPR.

Technique

- Follow instructions for procedures in Adult CPR, but omit the rescue breathing.

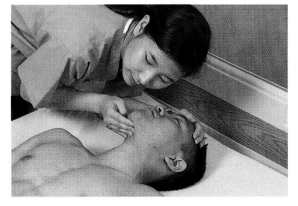

FIGURE 36-3 Checking for breathing. The airway is kept open by using the head-tilt/chin-lift maneuver.

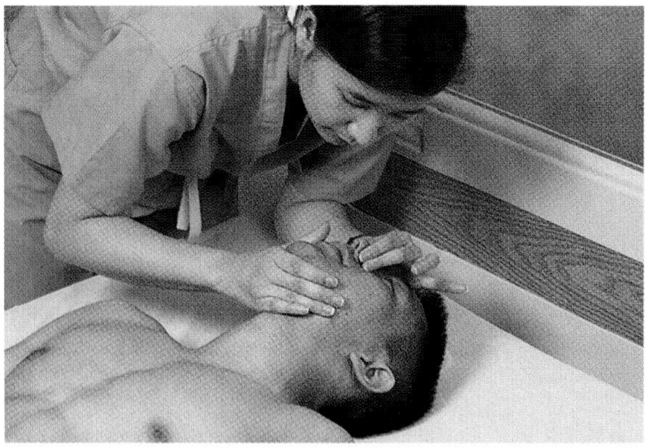

FIGURE 36-4 To occlude the nostrils, use the thumb and index finger of the hand on the forehead to gently pinch the nose closed.

lished. If breathing is absent or inadequate, you will need to provide rescue breathing.

5. Provide rescue breathing using mouth-to-mouth breathing (see below) or one of the alternative techniques shown in Table 36-1.

   a. Keeping the airway open by using the head-tilt/chin-lift maneuver, gently pinch the nose closed, using the thumb (Fig. 36-4). This will prevent air from escaping through the patient's nose.

   b. Take a deep breath, place your mouth over the patient's mouth, and make an airtight seal. Give two slow initial breaths of 2 seconds each. Be sure

the chest rises with each breath. Allow time for deflation of the patient's lungs between breaths. This technique should decrease the incidence of gastric inflation, regurgitation, and aspiration.

   c. After performing rescue breathing, if you observe the patient's chest rising and falling, showing that air has entered, proceed to step 6, Circulation (see below). If, however, you feel resistance when you try to breathe into the patient's mouth and the patient's chest wall does not rise and fall as you breathe, reposition the head and attempt to breathe again. If you still feel resistance, proceed with **foreign-body airway obstruction (FBAO)** maneuvers, discussed later.

CIRCULATION

6. Check for signs of **circulation.** While simultaneously assessing the patient for breathing, coughing, or movement, feel for the **carotid pulse** by locating the **trachea** and sliding your fingers off into the groove beside it. You should feel for the pulse on your side of the patient (Fig. 36-5) to avoid com-

table 36-1. Alternative Methods for Rescue Breathing	
Alternative	**Technique**
Mouth-to-barrier device	Although you may start rescue breathing using mouth-to-mouth breathing, barrier devices or bag-mask systems are used in healthcare settings. Two broad categories of barrier devices are currently available: mouth-to-mask devices and face shields. Mask devices often have a one-way valve to prevent exhaled air from entering the mouth of the rescuer. Most face shields have no such valve, and air often leaks around the shield. Position the barrier device over the patient's mouth and nose, ensure an adequate air seal, and initiate mouth-to-barrier device breathing using slow breaths as described.
Mouth to nose	If mouth-to-mouth breathing is not desirable or possible (for example, in cases of vomiting or injury to the mouth or jaw), mouth-to-nose breathing can be done by closing the mouth with one palm and breathing into the nose. The position of the head is the same as for mouth-to-mouth breathing.
Mouth to stoma	If the patient has a permanent **tracheostomy** or tracheal stoma, make an airtight seal around the stoma, breathe, and watch for the patient's chest to rise. You will need to remove your mouth from the stoma to permit passive exhalation.

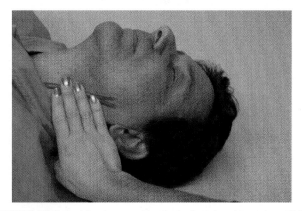

FIGURE 36-5 Feel for the carotid pulse by locating the trachea. Slide your hand towards yourself to avoid your hand from resting on the trachea, which could block ventilation.

pressing the other carotid artery with your thumb. Take no more than 5 seconds for this assessment.

7. If you locate a pulse, or other signs of circulation are present, perform rescue breathing (see below) at a rate of approximately 10 to 12 breaths per minute (or 1 breath every 5 seconds), rechecking the pulse after the first minute and every few minutes thereafter.

8. If you do not assess breathing, coughing, or movement and you cannot locate a pulse, attach an **automated external defibrillator (AED)** if one is available (see below), *or* immediately begin chest compressions.

9. Chest compressions:

   a. Kneel at the level of the patient's shoulders. You will then be in a position to perform both rescue breathing and chest compression without moving your knees. The patient should be on a hard surface to achieve best results. In a healthcare facility, place a cardiac board under the patient if he or she is in bed.

   b. Position your hands over the lower half of the **sternum,** using the method below or an alternative technique.

      (1) Locate the lower margin of the patient's rib cage on the side nearest you. Run the fingers of the hand nearest the patient's legs up along the rib cage to the indentation where the ribs meet the sternum (the xyphoid process).

      (2) Place the heel of the other hand on the lower half of the sternum, and then place the first hand on top of the second over the lower end of the sternum. Your hands should be parallel and directed away from you see (Fig. 36-6). This will keep the main force of compression on the sternum and decrease the chance of rib fracture. Your fingers may be either extended or interlaced, but they must be kept off the chest to avoid fracturing a rib (see Fig. 36-6).

   c. With your shoulders directly above the patient's chest, compress downward, keeping your arms straight. Move the sternum of an adult 1½ to 2 inches with each compression.

   d. Release the pressure after each compression to allow blood to flow into the heart. The time allowed for release should equal the time required for compression. Therefore, your motion should be a rhythmical 50% down and 50% up. Avoid quick, ineffective jabs to the chest that can increase the possibility of injury and may decrease the amount of blood circulated by each compression. Do not lift your hands from the chest or change their position in any way so that you do not lose correct hand position.

   e. Provide the proper ratio of compressions to breaths at the appropriate rate. The ratio and rate is 15 compressions to 2 breaths at a rate of 100 compressions per minute. You must maintain this rate to compensate for the compressions lost when you take time out to do the breathing. Move smoothly from one function to the other, keeping a steady rhythm.

Using the Automated External Defibrillator (AED)

An AED is a computerized defibrillator that can analyze the heart rhythm of a person in cardiac arrest, recognize a rhythm that will respond to electric shock, and tell the operator of the AED to push the "shock" button. These machines are widely available in the community in places such as airports, shopping malls, sports arenas, and churches, among others. They can be operated with very little training, and their use is easily integrated with CPR (Fig. 36-7). Although there are different types of AEDs, they operate in basically the same way:

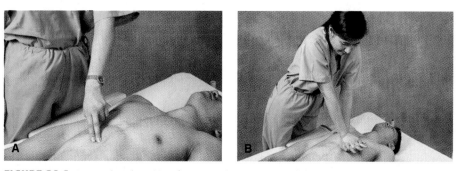

FIGURE 36-6 Correct hand position for external compression: (**A**) Locate the lower margin of the patient's rib cage on the side nearest you and run the fingers of the hand nearest the patient's legs up along the rib cage to the indentation where the ribs meet the sternum. Next, place the heel of the other hand on the lower half of the sternum. (**B**) Then place the first hand on top of the second over the lower end of the sternum. Your hands should be parallel and directed away from you. Your fingers should be interlaced above but not touching the chest to avoid fracturing a rib. This is the proper position for CPR of the adult.

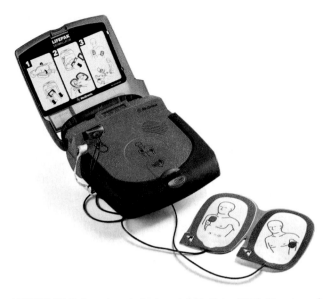

FIGURE 36-7 An automated external defibrillator (AED). (Courtesy of Medtronic, Inc.)

1. Turn on the POWER. This will start the voice prompts. To turn on the AED, press the power switch, or simply lift the cover (the AED comes on automatically when the AED is opened in some devices).
2. ATTACH the electrode pads to the chest of the patient. Stop compressions when you have removed any clothing from the person's chest and have the package of electrodes open and attached to the cables. Some AEDs come with the pads, cables, and AED unit already connected. Follow the diagram found on the machine to ensure correct placement. The electrodes have peel-off adhesive pads and should be attached directly to dry, bare skin.
3. State "STAND CLEAR OF THE PATIENT" to be sure no one is touching or attempting to move the patient during analysis. These actions will interfere with the analysis. Then PRESS the ANALYZE button (some AEDs start analyzing the rhythm automatically). Rhythm analysis takes 5 to 15 seconds. If ventricular fibrillation or ventricular tachycardia is present, the AED will indicate that a shock is needed.
4. CHARGE the AED, and press the SHOCK button if indicated. Many AED models begin charging automatically. A tone, voice message, or light will indicate that charging has begun. New machines move to the "shock" automatically if that is indicated, or the machine will advise you to "PUSH TO SHOCK." Again, be certain no one is touching the patient before you press the shock button.
5. If a "SHOCK" is not indicated, check the person's pulse and begin CPR.

   The benefits of early defibrillation have been established (American Heart Association, 2000). If

AEDs are available in the facility where you are employed, you need to know how to use them.

Two-Rescuer CPR

If a second rescuer arrives, he or she activates the EMS system (if this has not already been done by the first rescuer) and does one-rescuer CPR if the first rescuer has tired. If this is not needed, the second rescuer participates in the process by providing the rescue breathing and monitoring the victim while the initial rescuer continues with chest compressions. Thereafter, they may switch roles as indicated below.

1. *Assess the situation.* Determine responsiveness, breathing, and signs of circulation (steps 1 to 4c of one-rescuer CPR).
2. *Position yourselves on opposite sides of the patient.* Rescuer 1 is at the patient's side and provides chest compressions. Rescuer 2 is at the patient's head and maintains an open airway, monitors the carotid pulse, and provides rescue breathing (steps 5a to 5c).
3. *Provide compressions and rescue breathing.* Rescuer 1 should compress the sternum at a rate of 100 compressions per minute. Rescuer 2 maintains an open airway, monitors the carotid pulse for adequacy of chest compressions, and provides two breaths to the patient after every 15 compressions. A pause should be allowed for the ventilation (2 sec/breath). It is helpful if Rescuer 1 (the compressor) counts aloud to help both rescuers maintain the rate and ratio (steps 6 through 9e of one-rescuer CPR).
4. *Switch.* When Rescuer 1 (the person providing chest compressions) tires, the two rescuers should change positions with as little delay as possible.

MONITORING THE PATIENT

In two-rescuer CPR, Rescuer 2 assumes the responsibility for monitoring the patient's pulse and breathing. Rescuer 2 checks the carotid pulse during compressions to assess the effectiveness of Rescuer 1's external chest compressions. To determine whether the patient has resumed spontaneous breathing and circulation, chest compressions must be stopped for 10 seconds at about the end of the first minute of CPR and every few minutes thereafter.

TERMINATING CPR

Stop CPR when one of the following occurs:

- Breathing and spontaneous heartbeats are detected.
- An advanced life-support team arrives to take over the patient's care.
- A physician pronounces the patient dead and states that CPR can be discontinued.

- The rescuer(s) becomes physically exhausted and no replacement(s) is available. This is the most difficult reality for a rescuer to face, but there are limits to one's physical endurance. Fortunately, this seldom happens.

POTENTIAL ADVERSE OUTCOMES AND RELATED INTERVENTIONS

1. Gastric inflation related to rescue breathing (especially in children)

Intervention: Can be minimized by maintaining an open airway, limiting ventilation volumes to just the amount it takes to cause the chest to rise adequately, and making sure that the airway remains open during inspiration and exhalation

2. Regurgitation resulting from marked inflation of the stomach

Intervention: Turn the victim's body to the side, wipe out the mouth, return the body to the supine position, and continue CPR.

3. Rib fractures

Intervention: Can be minimized by correct hand position during chest compression

PERFORMING CPR FOR INFANTS AND SMALL CHILDREN

The procedure used with infants (younger than 1 year) and small children (younger than 8 years) is similar to that used with adults. However, there are some important differences.

INITIATE THE PROCEDURE

1. *Assess unresponsiveness with gentle stimulation.* Because the most common cause of arrest in the pediatric age group is primary **respiratory arrest** or an obstructed airway, assess the patient, and provide approximately 1 minute of rescue support—including opening the airway and delivering rescue breathing (see below)—*before* activating EMS (American Heart Association, 2000).

AIRWAY

2. *Open the airway.* Use chin-lift, jaw-tilt method described above.

BREATHING

3. *Look, listen, and feel for breathing* as described above.
4. *Provide rescue breathing* for an infant or a child.
   a. *Infant:* Cover both the mouth and the nose of the infant with your mouth to create a seal (Fig. 36-8). *Child:* If the patient is a larger child,

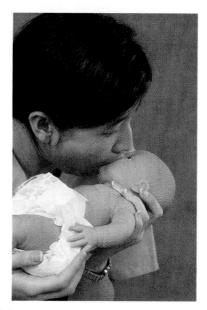

FIGURE 36-8 To breathe for an infant, cover both the mouth and the nose of the infant with your mouth.

occlude the nostrils with the fingers of the hand that is maintaining head tilt, and make a mouth-to-mouth seal.

   b. *Infant:* Provide breaths using only the amount of air needed to cause the chest to rise—usually just a mouthful of air is adequate. Because the volume of air in an infant's lungs is smaller than that in an adult's, watch carefully—as soon as you see the chest rise and fall, you are using the right volume of air. *Child:* A child has smaller lung volume than an adult, so do not use a full breath. Instead, watch carefully—as soon as you see the chest rise and fall, you are using the right volume of air.

   c. For an infant or child, breathe once every 3 seconds, or 20 times per minute. Give two slow breaths (1 to 1½ sec/breath), pausing between to breathe yourself.

CIRCULATION

5. Check for circulation.
   a. *Infant:* Locate the brachial artery and brachial pulse on the inside of the upper arm, between the elbow and shoulder. Placing your thumb on the outside of the arm, press gently with your index and middle fingers (Fig. 36-9). (The carotid artery is difficult to locate in an infant's short, chubby neck.)

   Note: Research suggests that lay rescuers cannot count pulses consistently, so you should not emphasize the pulse check when teaching CPR to laypersons. If a layperson finds an infant or child who is not breathing spontaneously, it is

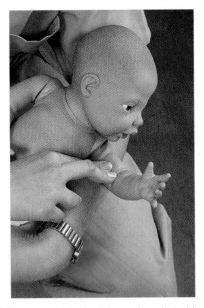

FIGURE 36-9 The brachial pulse is located on the inside of the upper arm of the infant.

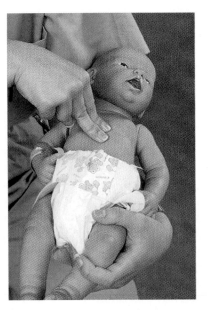

FIGURE 36-10 To identify finger position for chest compressions in an infant, locate an imaginary line between the nipples. Place the index finger of the hand farthest from the infant's head just under that line where it intersects with the sternum. The correct area for compression is one finger width below this intersection.

likely that the child has a slow heartbeat or is without heartbeat and needs cardiac compressions (American Heart Association, 2000).

b. *Child:* Locate and palpate the child's carotid artery. Locate the trachea (Adam's apple), and slide your fingers off into the groove beside it. Feel for the pulse on your side of the child to avoid compressing the other carotid artery with your thumb. Palpate for no more than 10 seconds.

6. Begin chest compressions *if signs of circulation are absent or the heart rate is less than 60 beats per minute with signs of poor perfusion.*

a. Infant

(1) Position the infant for performing compressions. The hard surface can be the palm of the hand that will not be used for performing the compressions. The weight of the infant's head and a slight lift of the shoulders then provide head tilt.

(2) Locate an imaginary line between the nipples over the sternum. Place the index finger of the hand farthest from the infant's head just under that line where it intersects with the sternum. The correct area for compression is one finger width below this intersection, where your middle and ring fingers are located. Be sure that you are not on or near the **xiphoid process.**

(3) Using two fingers, compress the sternum ½ to 1 inch at a rate of at least 100 times per minute (Fig. 36-10). A good rule of thumb is to compress the sternum of an infant or child approximately one-third to one-half the depth of the chest.

(4) Pause to deliver one breath after every fifth compression. Continue chest compressions and breaths at a ratio of 5:1 for one or two rescuers.

b. Child

(1) Position the child in a horizontal supine position on a hard surface as you would an adult.

(2) Position your hands correctly; the correct area for compressions is located in the same way as for an adult. Again, be sure that you are not on or near the xiphoid process.

(3) Use the heel of one hand to compress the chest 1 to 1½ inches at a rate of 100 times per minute (Fig. 36-11). A good rule of thumb is that the sternum of an infant or child is compressed approximately one-third to one-half the depth of the chest.

(4) Pause to deliver one breath after every fifth compression. Continue chest compressions and breaths at a ratio of 5:1 for one or two rescuers.

Note: If the child is large or older than 8 years, use the method previously described for adults.

PERFORMING CPR IN THE ACUTE CARE FACILITY

Acute healthcare facilities follow a specific procedure whenever emergency resuscitation procedures are nec-

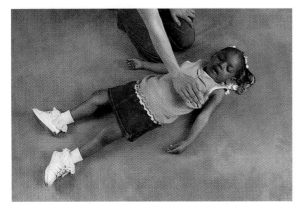

FIGURE 36-11 Correct hand position for chest compressions in a child. The correct area for compressions is located the same way it is for an adult, and the chest is compressed with the heel of one hand.

essary. In an acute care hospital, there will be a team that responds to all instances of cardiac or respiratory arrest. The designated code team consists of those with advanced cardiac life support expertise. These individuals may be notified by an overhead page but more commonly by pagers that are carried by the designated individuals. Most facilities designate a team of specially trained personnel (including a physician) to respond to all codes. This team arrives with special life-support equipment, including a defibrillator, emergency drugs, and breathing equipment (such as an Ambu bag), and takes over care completely. Information about Ambu bags and their use in ventilating patients can be found in Module 31, Administering Oxygen (Fig. 31-5).

1. *Establish that patient is unresponsive.* Shake the victim and shout, "Are you all right?" If the patient does not respond, proceed.
2. *Activate emergency medical services (EMS).* The person who discovers the patient's collapse activates the EMS system and calls for assistance. To simplify matters and to avoid alarming other patients, the EMS is activated using a designated code. In many facilities, this is done by dialing the code number on the bedside telephone. In critical care areas and emergency rooms, there may be a code button located on the wall that may be quickly pushed. The code designation differs from facility to facility, but "Code 99," "Code 199," and "Code Blue" are commonly used. You have a responsibility to ensure that your orientation includes the appropriate emergency codes in the facility.
3. *Verbally call for help.* Call for immediate help. This may mean calling out loud "Code 99 in Room XXX" or some other designated signal. This alerts other staff to your need for immediate help.
4. *Initiate CPR.* The discoverer or rescuer is the first responder and as such initiates CPR, following the above procedures for airway, breathing, and circulation.

5. *Work with the second responder.*
   a. The person who responds to the call for help gathers the emergency equipment (cardiac board, breathing bag, oxygen setup, emergency medications, and so forth) and takes it to the victim's location.
   b. The second responder then participates in emergency care and assists as necessary. This might include placing the cardiac board and participating in two-person CPR.
6. *Relinquish care to the code team.* Relinquish care to the code team members when they arrive. The first and second responders relinquish care to the team. They may stay to assist if that is part of the procedure for the facility, or they may return to their other duties.
7. *Assist with family support if needed.* If sufficient personnel are available, someone should provide support to any family members and any patients in the immediate area. Increasingly, it is becoming the role of a registered nurse or a chaplain to assist in addressing the psychosocial needs of families by allowing them to be present in the area where the CPR is taking place. Although not always practical, some believe the emotional benefits to the family outweigh the legal risks for the staff.
8. *Document the process.* Certainly, the initiation of CPR is of primary importance. But it is also a nursing responsibility to maintain a record of all resuscitation activities. Include the indication for and time of CPR initiation; the time and nature of all events that take place during resuscitation activities; assessment of the patient before, during, and after CPR; any medications given; the patient's response to all measures; and the time resuscitation activities are stopped. Most facilities have a flow sheet to simplify documentation of this detailed information (Fig. 36-12).

CLEARING FOREIGN-BODY AIRWAY OBSTRUCTION IN ADULTS

Foreign-body obstruction of the airway usually occurs during eating. Meat is a common cause of an obstruction in adults. Other foods and foreign bodies may be the cause in children and some adults. Choking on food may result from elevated blood alcohol level, poorly fitting dentures, or large, inadequately chewed food pieces.

RECOGNITION

1. A **foreign-body airway obstruction (FBAO)** can be partial or complete. If the victim's airway is only partially obstructed, some degree of air ex-

CARDIOPULMONARY ARREST RECORD

DATE	TIME OF ARREST	PATIENT DIAGNOSIS	PATIENT INTUBATED AT (TIME)
HOW WAS ARREST RECOGNIZED (ASYSTOLE, V TACH./, ETC)?			COMPLICATIONS

VENTILATION INITIATED AT (TIME)	MOUTH TO MOUTH/MASK ☐ YES ☐ NO	ANESTHESIA BAG AND MASK ☐ YES ☐ NO	
BY WHOM	EXTERNAL CARDIAC MASSAGE INITIATED AT (TIME)	PRECORDIAL THUMP ☐ YES ☐ NO	PATIENT INTUBATED PRIOR TO ARREST ☐ YES ☐ NO	ESTIMATED PERIOD OF APNEA

TIME	VITAL SIGNS	EPINEPH.	ATROPINE	LIDOCAINE	BICARB					IV DRIPS	RATE	PRE-SHOCK RHYTHM	WATT-SEC	RESULTING RHYTHM	COMMENTS (LAB RESULTS, LOC, PUPILS, RHYTHM, ETC.)

DEFIBRILLATION

COMMENTS:	PERSONNEL:
PRESUMED CAUSE / NATURE OF ARREST	
TERMINATION OF CPR (TIME / RATIONALE / RESULTS)	SIGNATURE - RECORDER
FAMILY NOTIFIED	SIGNATURE - PHYSICIAN IN CHARGE

FIGURE 36-12 Cardiopulmonary arrest record. The use of a flow sheet simplifies documentation of resuscitation activities.

change may be possible. If the air exchange is good, the victim may be able to cough forcefully. You should not interfere when inhalation and coughing are occurring. Encourage the victim to attempt to cough and breathe spontaneously.

2. If the victim has initial poor air exchange or good air exchange that has deteriorated to poor air exchange evidenced by ineffective cough, crowing noises when inhaling, and bluish color, manage as though it were complete airway obstruction.

3. Establish that the airway is obstructed. Ask the victim, "Are you choking?" The victim may know the universal distress signal for choking—clutching the neck with the hand(s) (Fig. 36-13). If the answer is an affirmative shake of the head, intervene immediately.

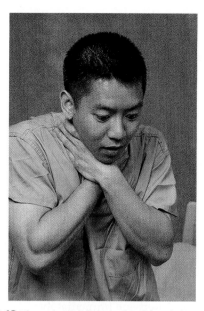

FIGURE 36-13 The universal distress signal for choking is the victim clutching the neck with his or her hand(s).

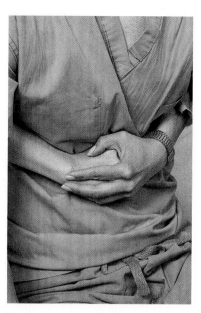

FIGURE 36-14 Correct hand position for manual thrusts. Make a fist with one hand and grasp the fist with your other hand. Use the thumb side of the fist for subdiaphragmatic abdominal thrusts.

MANAGEMENT

4. The **Heimlich maneuver** (subdiaphragmatic abdominal thrust maneuver) is recommended by the American Heart Association for relieving FBAO. Your hands should *not* be placed on the xiphoid process of the sternum or on the lower margins of the rib cage to prevent possible damage to internal organs. Your hands should be placed below this area but above the navel in the midline.

   a. Conscious victim
   (1) Stand behind the victim and wrap your arms around his or her waist. Then grasp one fist with your other hand, and place the thumb side of fist against the victim's abdomen in the midline slightly above the navel as described (Fig. 36-14).
   (2) Next, press into the victim's abdomen with a quick upward thrust (Fig. 36-15). Each thrust should be a separate and distinct movement.
   (3) Continue until the foreign body is expelled or the victim loses consciousness.

   b. Unconscious victim or conscious victim who becomes unconscious. (If a victim who was initially conscious loses consciousness, the muscles may become more relaxed, allowing for successful intervention.)
   (1) Activate the EMS system.
   (2) Position victim on the back (supine).
   (3) With the victim face up, use one hand to open the jaw by grasping the lower jaw and tongue between your thumb and fingers and lifting (tongue-jaw lift). This draws the tongue away from the back of the throat and away from any foreign body lodged there.

   (4) Insert the index finger of your other hand along the inside of the cheek, using a hooking action (finger sweep) to dislodge any foreign body, so it can be removed. Be careful not to push the foreign body further into the airway.
   (5) Open the airway and attempt to ventilate. If unsuccessful, reposition the head and try

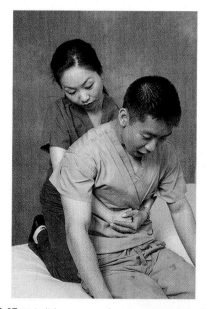

FIGURE 36-15 Heimlich maneuver for a conscious victim involves continual abdominal thrusts until the foreign body is expelled or the victim loses consciousness. For an unconscious victim, kneel astride his or her thighs and do up to five abdominal thrusts.

again. If still unsuccessful, kneel astride the victim's thighs and perform the Heimlich maneuver (Fig. 36-16).

(6) Place the heel of one hand against the victim's abdomen with the second hand directly on top of the first. Press into the abdomen with a quick upward thrust (see Fig. 36-16). Perform the Heimlich maneuver (up to five times).

(7) Chest thrusts are recommended only when the victim is in the late stages of pregnancy or when the Heimlich maneuver cannot be used effectively on the unconscious, very obese victim. In such cases, place the victim in the supine position and kneel at the victim's side. Using the same hand position as for external cardiac compression, deliver each thrust slowly and distinctly.

(8) Repeat the above sequence (tongue-jaw lift, finger sweep, and attempt to ventilate) until the obstruction is cleared.

CLEARING FOREIGN-BODY AIRWAY OBSTRUCTION IN INFANTS AND SMALL CHILDREN

Although the procedure for relieving FBAO in infants and small children is similar to that used for adults, there are some important differences to keep in mind. Airway obstruction in infants may be caused by an object, such as a small toy or a peanut, or by an infection that results in swelling of the airway. It is important to differentiate between the two. Seek treatment if the obstruction is caused by an infection. The procedure presented here is not effective in the case of infection and will only delay necessary treatment.

RECOGNITION

1. Establish that the airway is blocked.
   a. Infants
      (1) May be evidenced by weak or silent coughing, stridor (a high-pitched noisy sound), or wheezing.
      (2) The infant will demonstrate increasing respiratory difficulty.
      (3) The skin or lips may turn blue.
   b. Small child
      (1) If the child has good air exchange, encourage him or her to cough and breathe spontaneously.
      (2) If the child has poor air exchange, manage the situation as though it were complete airway obstruction.
      (3) Establish that the airway is obstructed. Ask the child, "Are you choking?" If answer is yes, intervene immediately.

MANAGEMENT

2. Clear the obstruction from the airway as directed below.
   a. Infants
      (1) Hold the infant prone over your forearm with the head lower than the trunk. The infant's legs will straddle your forearm. Support the head by firmly supporting the jaw (Fig. 36-17) and rest your forearm on your thigh to further support the infant. This is usually easier to do while seated but may be done while standing.
      (2) Deliver up to five back blows between the infant's shoulder blades, using the heel of the hand.

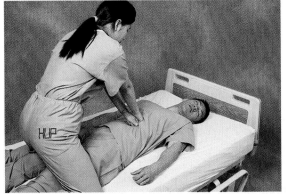

FIGURE 36-16 Proper position of rescuer for an adult. With your shoulders directly above the patient's chest, compress downward, keeping your arms straight.

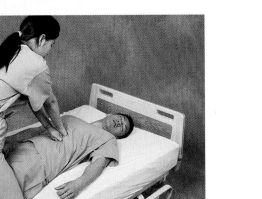

FIGURE 36-17 Relief of FBAO in the infant with back blows.

(3) Place your free hand on the infant's back so that the baby is "sandwiched" between your two hands (one supports the neck, jaw, and chest, while the other supports the back). Turn the infant as a unit and place him or her on your thigh, supine, with the head lower than the trunk.

(4) Deliver up to five thrusts in the same way as for external chest compressions, approximately one per second (Fig. 36-18).

(5) Open the airway, and if breathing is absent, attempt rescue breathing (see Performing CPR for Infants and Small Children, above).

(6) If the infant's chest does not rise, reposition the head and attempt rescue breathing again.

(7) Continue the sequence of up to five back blows and up to five chest thrusts and attempts to breathe until the object is removed or until the infant becomes unresponsive.

(8) Because a foreign body can easily be pushed further back in the airway and increase the obstruction, avoid blind finger sweeps in infants and children. If the victim is unconscious, open the mouth by lifting the lower jaw and tongue forward. If you can see the foreign body, remove it with your finger.

b. Conscious child, sitting or standing

(1) Stand behind the child, and wrap your arms around the torso.

(2) Deliver up to five subdiaphragmatic abdominal thrusts as you would for an adult, but more gently.

(3) Continue until the foreign body is expelled or the child loses consciousness.

c. Unconscious child, lying

(1) Position the child on his or her back.

(2) Open the child's airway using the tongue-jaw lift and look for the foreign body. If it is visible, remove it, but do not perform a blind finger sweep.

(3) Open the airway with the head-tilt/chin-lift and attempt rescue breathing. If the chest does not rise, reposition the head and try again.

(4) If the rescue breaths are still not effective, kneel beside the child or astride his or her hips and perform the Heimlich maneuver, delivering up to five subdiaphragmatic abdominal thrusts as you would for an adult, but more gently. Then repeat the sequence of Heimlich maneuver and attempts to breathe until the object is removed or rescue breathing is effective.

Acute Care

Patients who are hospitalized with serious illnesses usually have been asked whether or not they wish to have CPR carried out in the event of a cardiac or respiratory emergency. If the patient (or legally appointed substitute decision maker) has designated that no resuscitation or limited resuscitation is desired, the physician will write an order in the chart designating that the patient has "do not resuscitate" (DNR) status. Until this order is written, you are legally obligated to carry out resuscitation procedures if the patient suffers cardiac or respiratory arrest. You should be aware of the "code status" for each patient assigned to you as well as for those under your care when you are caring for another nurse's patients while he or she is at lunch or on a break. You should also be aware of the policy in your facility regarding family presence during CPR and other emergency procedures.

Long-Term Care

Many individuals who live in long-term care facilities have decided not to have CPR carried out when they stop breathing or when their heart stops. Just as in acute care, the appropriate decision maker determines whether resuscitation is desired, and the physician writes the order for "do not resuscitate" if that is desired. You should be aware of the code status of every resident for whom you are caring at any time. This will prevent residents from undergoing

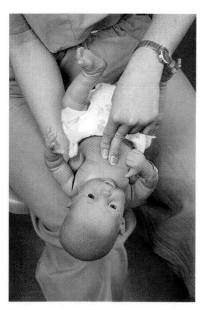

FIGURE 36-18 Relief of FBAO in the infant with chest thrusts.

CPR against their stated wishes or against the orders of the physician. In addition, the outcomes of CPR in very elderly individuals are exceedingly poor, sometimes resulting in increased longevity with decreased quality of life.

Home Care

Because the need for resuscitation or the removal of a foreign body commonly occurs outside of healthcare facilities, it is also important for people other than healthcare providers to be able to perform these skills. Ideally, someone in every household should be able to perform CPR; this is especially important in households where an individual(s) is particularly at risk for cardiac problems. If you are providing care in such a situation, you are responsible to identify the person or persons most able to learn and perform the necessary skills. Also, although everyone is potentially at risk for aspiration of a foreign body, the parents or care providers for infants and small children may be more likely to find it necessary to use the Heimlich maneuver. While providing care in the home or while doing discharge teaching, you have a unique opportunity to identify these needs and to suggest that appropriate individuals attend classes provided in your setting or in the community.

Some states have now enacted legislation that allows those receiving home care to establish "do not resuscitate" status. This may be done by completing specific documents and wearing a special identification bracelet. These documents provide legal protection to emergency response personnel in following the advance directives of individuals who do not wish to be resuscitated. In states or provinces where this is not a part of legislation, emergency response personnel may be obligated to carry out all resuscitation measures if they are called to the scene. Home care personnel need to be familiar with the relevant legal standards in their community to respond appropriately and to teach clients and families.

Ambulatory Care

Nurses who work in ambulatory care settings see clients of all ages in a variety of phases of illness. Emergency care policies, procedures, and equipment will vary. Most commonly, ambulatory care clinics call the community emergency response number of 911 and then initiate CPR until the emergency med-

ical technicians arrive and assume care. The person can then be transported to a hospital for acute care. If you work in a setting where clients with cardiac and respiratory disease are seen, you will be more likely to encounter emergency situations. In any event, you must be prepared to function according to the policies in your work place.

LEARNING TOOLS

DEVELOP YOUR BACKGROUND KNOWLEDGE

1. Review the Learning Outcomes.

2. Read the section on basic life support in your assigned text.

3. Look up the Key Terms in the glossary.

4. Review the module and mentally practice the techniques described. Study so that you would be able to teach CPR to another person.

DEVELOP YOUR SKILLS

1. In the practice setting, practice with a Resusci Annie or similar mannequin under your instructor's supervision.
   a. Establish an airway on the adult mannequin.
   b. Breathe 12 times per minute into the adult mannequin, allowing 2 seconds per breath, watching for the rise and fall of the chest wall, and allowing for "exhalation."
   c. Practice administering chest compressions on the adult mannequin at a rate of 100 compressions per minute, compressing the sternum 1½ to 2 inches each time.
   d. Establish an airway on an infant mannequin.
   e. Breathe 20 times per minute into the infant mannequin, allowing 1 to 1½ seconds per breath, using only the amount of air needed to cause the chest to rise.
   f. Practice administering chest compressions on the infant mannequin at a rate of 100 compressions per minute, using only the tips of your index and middle fingers to compress the sternum ½ to 1 inch each time.

DEMONSTRATE YOUR SKILLS

1. With a partner, practice CPR on adult, child, and infant mannequins, using the Performance Checklist on the CD-ROM in the front of this book as a guide. Take turns doing the breathing and administering the chest compressions. Have your instructor evaluate your performances.

2. With your partner as observer and evaluator, practice CPR alone on the adult, child, and infant mannequins, using the Performance Checklist as a guide. When you are satisfied with your performance, trade places, and have your partner demonstrate CPR on the adult, child, and infant mannequins with you observing and evaluating. When you are both satisfied with your performances, have your instructor evaluate them.

3. Working as a pair, simulate the recognition and management of foreign-body airway obstruction on each other or on an adult mannequin, using the Performance Checklist as a guide. Practice management of foreign-body airway obstruction on the infant mannequin as well. When you are satisfied with your performance, have your instructor evaluate you.

CRITICAL THINKING EXERCISES

1. You are the nurse assigned to care for the family during a code in the Emergency Department. Your facility's policy allows family members to be in the room when CPR is being administered. In this situation, the family of an accident victim has just arrived and you have been called. The patient has been severely disfigured as the result of the accident he has been in. Describe how you will handle the situation.

2. A resident in your long-term care facility has indicated to you that he doesn't want all that "folderol" if his heart stops; he just wants to be allowed to die in peace. You note that his record indicates that he has "full code" status (meaning use all possible resuscitation measures). If he has a cardiac arrest when you are present, what should you do? To ensure that his wishes are carried out, with whom would you consult? What needs to happen at this time?

3. You are beginning your orientation as a new registered nurse at a small community hospital. On the first day, you will be shadowing an RN to become acquainted with the layout of the unit and to develop your own list of information you would like to have covered in your orientation. What information on emergency procedures do you need immediately?

SELF-QUIZ
SHORT-ANSWER QUESTIONS

1. What is the first step you should take when you see an adult collapse?

2. Why is the first step in CPR different when the patient is an infant or child?

3. How do you position the victim's head if a neck injury is suspected?

4. How can you quickly locate the carotid pulse?

5. How is the brachial pulse located in an infant?

6. Where should the hands be placed for chest compressions on an adult?

7. What is the universal distress signal for choking?

8. Where are the hands positioned to correctly deliver the Heimlich maneuver?

9. Under what circumstances is the finger sweep maneuver used?

MULTIPLE CHOICE

_____ 10. Chest compressions should be delivered at the rate of 100/min in which of the following situations? (Choose all that apply.)
 a. One-rescuer CPR
 b. Two-rescuer CPR
 c. CPR for an infant
 d. CPR for a small child

_____ 11. The ratio of breaths to chest compressions is 15:2 in which of the following situations? (Choose all that apply.)
 a. One-rescuer CPR
 b. Two-rescuer CPR
 c. CPR for an infant
 d. CPR for a small child

Answers to the Self-Quiz questions appear in the back of the book.

REFERENCES AND SUGGESTED RESOURCES: UNIT 7

Ackerman, M. H., & Mick, D. J. (1998). Instillation of normal saline before suctioning in patients with pulmonary infections: A prospective randomized controlled trial. *American Journal of Critical Care, 7*(4), 261–266.

American Heart Association in collaboration with International Liaison Committee on Resuscitation. (2000). Guidelines 2000 for cardiopulmonary resuscitation and emergency cardiac care: International consensus on science. Dallas, TX: American Heart Association.

Ault, M. L., & Stock, C. (2004). Respiratory monitoring. *International Anesthesiology Clinics, 42*(1), 97–112.

Day, T., Farnell, S., Haynes, S. B., et al. (2002). Tracheal suctioning: An exploration of nurses' knowledge and competence in acute and high dependency ward areas. *Journal of Advanced Nursing, 39*(1), 35–45.

Deshpande, K. S., Tortolani, A. J., & Kvetan, V. (2003). Troubleshooting chest tube complications: How to prevent—or quickly correct—the major problems. *The Journal of Critical Illness, 18*(6), 275–280.

Goodfellow, L. T., & Jones, M. (2002). Bronchial hygiene therapy: From traditional hands-on techniques to modern technological approaches. *American Journal of Nursing 102*(1), 37–43.

Kinloch, D. (1999). Instillation of normal saline during endotracheal suctioning: Effects on mixed venous oxygen saturation. *American Journal of Critical Care, 8*(4), 231–242.

Kodali, B. S. (2005). Capnography: A comprehensive educational website. (Online.) Available at http://www.capnography.com/Homepage/HomepageM.htm. Retrieved April 14, 2005.

Pruitt, W., & Jacobs, M. (2003). Breathing lessons: Basics of oxygen therapy. *Nursing2003, 33*(10), 43–45.

Sole, M. L., Byers, J. F., Ludy, J. E., et al. (2003). A multisite survey of suctioning techniques and airway management practices. *American Journal of Critical Care, 12*(3), 220–230.

Sorenson, H. M. & Shelledy, D. C. (2003). AARC clinical practice guideline. Intermittent positive pressure breathing—2003 revision & update. *Respiratory Care, 48*(5), 540–546. (Online.) Available at http://www.guideline.gov/summary/summary.aspx?ss=15&doc_id=3753&nbr=2979. Retrieved April 14, 2005.

Tamburri, L. M. (2000). Care of the patient with a tracheostomy. *Orthopaedic Nursing, 19*(2), 49–60.

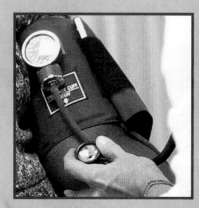

UNIT 8

Performing Special Therapeutic and Supportive Procedures

MODULES

Applying Bandages and Binders

SKILLS INCLUDED IN THIS MODULE

General Procedure for Applying Bandages and Binders
Specific Procedures for Applying Bandages or Binders
  Wrapping an Extremity
  Applying Elastic Compression (Antiembolic) Stockings
  Applying a Sequential Compression Device
  Applying a Stump Stocking or Wrapping a Stump
  Procedure for Applying Binders to Secure Dressings
  Applying an Arm Sling

PREREQUISITE MODULES

Module 1	An Approach to Nursing Skills
Module 2	Documentation
Module 3	Basic Body Mechanics
Module 4	Basic Infection Control
Module 5	Safety in the Healthcare Environment
Module 6	Moving the Patient in Bed and Positioning
Module 14	Nursing Physical Assessment

KEY TERMS

circular bandage
conformable
  gauze bandage
distal
elastic bandage
figure-eight
  bandage
net binders
proximal
recurrent-fold
  bandage

reverse-spiral
  bandage
roll bandages
sequential
  compression
  device
sling
spiral bandage
stockinette
T-binder

OVERALL OBJECTIVE

▸ To correctly apply commonly used bandages and binders.

LEARNING OUTCOMES

The student will be able to

1. Assess the patient effectively to determine the appropriate bandage or binder needed for the specific situation.
2. Analyze assessment data to determine special problems or concerns that must be addressed before applying a specific bandage or binder to a patient.
3. Determine appropriate patient outcomes regarding the application of a bandage or binder, and recognize the potential for adverse outcomes.
4. Apply a bandage or binder to the specific patient, using the appropriate equipment and adequate assistance.
5. Evaluate the effectiveness of the bandage or binder for the specific patient.
6. Document the application of the bandage or binder and the patient's response in the patient's plan of care and in the patient's record as appropriate.

Most bandages are made of a gauze material; some are made in a stretchable weave. Binders are often made of sturdy cotton cloth or elasticized fabric. There are a variety of reasons and, consequently, a variety of methods, for applying bandages or binders. Some protect an underlying wound or dressing; others provide pressure, warmth, support, or immobilization. It is important first to assess the needs of patients and then to select the device or material that best fulfills those needs. Physicians may order the specific type of bandage or binder to be used or may give only a general order. Box 37-1 outlines general guidelines for applying bandages and binders.

CIRCULATION, MOTION, AND SENSATION CHECKS

Approximately 30 minutes after you have applied a bandage or binder, check the patient for circulation, motion, and sensation (CMS). A bandage or binder that is too tight can interfere with circulation, causing swelling, numbness, tingling, or color changes in the area distal to the binder. Most bandages are applied on extremities from **distal** to **proximal** to facilitate venous return.

Tight bandages or binders that encircle an extremity can block venous return, leading to swelling. In addition, either the original bandage itself or the swelling may block arterial circulation to the distal extremity. This blocking of circulation may cause permanent nerve or other tissue damage. If this problem is discovered early, full recovery may occur. If it is allowed to continue, the damage may become permanent and interfere with function.

Circulation, motion, and sensation checks are designed to monitor for these problems. To check circulation, palpate pulses distal to the bandage to ensure that they are present. Capillary circulation is further assessed by pressing the tissue until it blanches (the blood has been pushed out and the skin pales) and then releasing the pressure. The pink color should return within 15 seconds. For patients with dark skin, circulation may be checked on the plantar surface of the foot, the palmar surface of the hands, and the nail beds where pigment is less prominent and will not mask the underlying capillary blood color in the tissue (see Box 21-1 in Module 21).

---

box 37-1 *Guidelines for Applying Bandages and Binders*

- Place all bandages over clean, dry surfaces *to prevent the harboring and growth of microorganisms.*
- Pad bony prominences *to prevent undue pressure that could lead to skin breakdown.*
- When dressings over open wounds are sterile, bandages or binders need not be *sterile if there are underlying sterile dressings to protect the wound.*
- Wrap in a manner that will be tight enough to hold yet loose enough to avoid constricting the body part in any way *to prevent circulation or nerve impairment.*
- Adequately cover all edges and corners with the bandage or binder *to keep the dressing clean.*
- Avoid bandaging or putting on a binder over wrinkled dressings, *which can produce pressure on the wound or skin.*
- Avoid applying a bandage or binder over a dressing that appears soiled, *which can provide a medium for the growth of infection-causing microbes.*
- Change bandages frequently *to maintain cleanliness.*

Assess motion by asking the patient to move the fingers and toes as much as possible. Decreased ability to move the fingers or toes may indicate the bandaging is too tight.

Assess sensation by asking the patient to report on sensations of numbness or tingling. It may also be assessed by asking the patient to identify a light "poke" with a fingernail. See Figure 37-1 for an example of a form used to document circulation, motion, and sensation checks.

NURSING DIAGNOSES

Nursing diagnoses that could apply to someone with a bandage or binder in place include

■ Acute Pain or Impaired Comfort: related to an unstable joint or conversely due to a bandage or binder that is too tight
■ Impaired Physical Mobility: related to injury or surgery on an extremity
■ Self-Care Deficits (feeding, bathing, dressing/grooming, toileting): related to inability to use an extremity
■ Deficient Knowledge: regarding applying own elastic bandages or elastic stockings
■ High Risk for Ineffective Peripheral Tissue Perfusion: related to elastic bandages or elastic dressings

DELEGATION

The application of many bandages and binders may be delegated to assistive personnel after the area to which the bandage or binder will be applied has been assessed by the nurse and after the assistive person has demonstrated to the nurse that he or she possesses the skill to apply the specific device. Assistive personnel must also be taught to observe and report any signs or symptoms that a bandage or binder is not accomplishing the purpose for which it was applied or that complications are occurring.

GENERAL PROCEDURE FOR APPLYING BANDAGES AND BINDERS

ASSESSMENT

1. Review the chart. **R:** A chart review identifies the patient's medical diagnosis, the part of the body to be supported, and the purpose of the particular bandage or binder for the patient.
2. If the patient has had a bandage or binder in place, assess it for its effectiveness. Note the length of time the bandage has been in place as well as the color, temperature, sensation, and skin condition of the extremity or area of the body. **R:** To identify complications or need for change in the procedure.

ANALYSIS

3. Critically think through your data, carefully evaluating each aspect and its relation to other data. **R:** This enables you to determine specific problems for this individual in relation to the application of the bandage or binder.
4. Identify specific problems and modifications of the procedure needed for this individual. **R:** Planning for the individual must take into consideration the individual's problems.

PLANNING

5. Determine individualized patient outcomes for the application of the specific bandage or binder, including the following. **R:** Identification of outcomes guides planning and evaluation.
   a. Bandage or binder is effective with regard to holding dressings in place or providing support.
   b. Circulation, motion, and sensation are intact distal to the bandage or binder.
   c. Patient reports no pain or discomfort related to the bandage or binder.
6. Plan the specific procedure to be used. **R:** Planning ahead allows you to proceed more safely and effectively.
7. Obtain the appropriate bandage or binder and, if needed, the fastening devices. **R:** Having all equipment readily available saves time and allows you to proceed efficiently.
8. Plan for intervals at which to recheck the bandage or binder. Assess circulation, motion, and sensation after 30 minutes and every 2 to 4 hours thereafter. After the first 8 hours, two checks per shift are usually sufficient. Binders around the trunk are less likely to cause circulatory problems but may become loose and wrinkle, causing discomfort. These bandages need less frequent checking. One check per shift is usually considered adequate. If the patient is conscious, the patient may be taught to check the bandage or binder and report discomfort, a decrease in circulation, or other symptoms of problems. **R:** Any bandage or binder that encircles an extremity must be checked more frequently because of the possibility that the device will compromise circulation.

		EXTREMITY								Circle Extremity Monitored LA (RA) LL RL					Initial

Fill in the parameters to be monitored. Refer to Standard & Individual Care Plans.
Parameter examples: Guaiac stools/emesis, urine fractionals, specific gravity, girth of limb/abd, bowel sounds, circulation of extremity, pedal pulses, frequent lab values.

Date	Time	COLOR 1.	CAPILLARY FILLING 2.	PULSE 3.	TEMPERATURE 4.	SENSATION 5.	MOTOR FUNCTION 6.	PAIN 7.	PAIN ON STRETCH 8.						Initial
3/12	20	B	<3	W	Wm	Nb	N	Mod	O						EA
3/12	22	B	<3	W	Wm	Nb	N	M	O						EA
3/12	24	B	<3	W	Wm	Nb	N	M	O						JW
3/13	04	N	<3	S	Wm	Nb/T	N	M	O						JW
3/13	06	N	<3	S	Wm	Nb/T	N	M	O					*feeling in all fingers*	JW

1. N Normal B Blue P Pale
2. < 3 Sec.   > 3 Sec.

3. S Strong   W Weak   A Absent
4. Wm Warm   H Hot   C Cool

5. N Normal T Tingle Nb Numb A Absent
6. N Normal W Weak A Absent

7. O None, M Mild, Mod Moderate, Sev Severe
8. O None, M Mild, Mod Moderate, Sev Severe

PARAMETER FLOW SHEET

Identify Initials with Signature:

		4.	8.
1.	*Ella Adams, RN*	5.	9.
2.	*Joy Williams, RN*	6.	10.
3.		7.	11.

ADDRESSOGRAPH:
McCarthy, Michael   M-76

Dr. Costello

HOSPITAL MEDICAL CENTER
SEATTLE, WASHINGTON

FIGURE 37-1 A form for the nurse to use in recording color, motion, and sensation after a bandage or binder has been applied.

IMPLEMENTATION

Action	Rationale
9. Wash or disinfect your hands.	To decrease the transfer of microorganisms that could cause infection.
10. Obtain any needed supportive devices or assistance.	To save time and maximize efficiency.
11. Identify the patient, using two identifiers.	Verifying the patient's identity helps ensure that you are performing the right skill for the right patient.
12. Pull the curtain around the bed and close the door.	To give the patient privacy.
13. Explain the purpose of the bandage or binder, how long it is to be in place, and how it should feel.	This permits the patient to participate knowledgeably in his or her own care by reporting discomfort or ineffective support.
14. Raise the bed to an appropriate working position based on your height.	To allow you to use correct body mechanics and protect yourself from back injury.
15. Position the patient so that the appropriate part of the body is exposed. Drape appropriately as necessary.	To facilitate the application of the bandage or binder and to protect the modesty of the patient.
16. Put gloves on and remove the soiled or used bandage or binder, if present. (A compression bandage over intact skin does not require gloves.)	To prevent the harboring and growth of microorganisms.
17. Apply the bandage or binder, using one of the specific techniques described below. Teach the patient or caregiver how to apply the device if indicated and appropriate.	The correct technique will accomplish the specific desired outcome. Teaching the patient increases the patient's ability to participate effectively in care.
18. Lower the bed.	To protect the patient by preventing a potential fall.
19. Wash or disinfect your hands.	To decrease the transfer of microorganisms that could cause infection.

EVALUATION

20. Evaluate using the individualized patient outcomes previously identified: Binder or bandage is effective with regard to holding dressings in place or providing support; circulation, motion, and sensation are intact in the extremity; and patient reports no pain or discomfort. **R:** Evaluation in relation to desired outcomes is essential for planning future care.

DOCUMENTATION

21. Document the procedure on the progress notes or flow sheet, including the following. **R:** Documentation is a legal record of the patient's care and therapy and communicates nursing activities to other nurses and caregivers.

   a. Time and type of bandage or binder applied; area to which bandage or binder was applied; and assessment of circulation, motion, and sensation as appropriate

   b. Length of time the device was off and the condition of the skin underneath, in cases of reapplication (see Fig. 37-1).

22. On the patient care plan, document a planned program of assessing circulation, motion, and sensation of the extremity and for teaching the patient needed self care. **R:** This measure promotes continuity of care.

◼ POTENTIAL ADVERSE OUTCOMES AND RELATED INTERVENTIONS

1. Patient develops edema distal to the bandage. *Intervention:* Remove bandage. Check circulation, motion, and sensation. Elevate extremity. Rewrap after edema is decreased. If edema continues, confer with physician.

2. Extremity is cool and cyanotic distal to the bandage. *Intervention:* Remove bandage. Check circulation, motion, and sensation. Notify physician of complications.

3. Patient states that he or she has begun having feelings of numbness or tingling in a wrapped extremity.

Intervention: Remove bandage. Have patient move extremity as much as possible to restore circulation. Replace bandage, making sure that there is room for your fingers underneath the bandage. Establish a monitoring plan for sensation in the extremity. Report the sensation change to the physician.

APPLYING ROLL BANDAGES

A variety of **roll bandages** are available. Often, the nurse chooses the type based on the particular situation. In some instances, the type of bandage is ordered by the physician.

TYPES OF ROLL BANDAGES

Roll gauze is available in ½-, 1-, 2-, and 3-inch widths. This material does not stretch but is soft, strong, and comfortable. It can be easily molded to a part of the body with proper bandaging technique. Roll gauze is used to hold dressings in place. It is available in both sterile and nonsterile forms.

Another type of **conformable gauze bandage** that comes in rolls is a soft, meshlike, flexible bandage that is stretchable, which facilitates shaping it to joints and curved body surfaces. This is often referred to as "Kling," which is a brand name. Several brands are available commercially in 2-, 3-, and 4-inch widths. Stretchable gauze can be used on extremities, the head, and the torso because of its conformability. It can be part of the primary dressing or used to hold other dressings in place and can be either sterile or nonsterile. When applying a stretchable gauze bandage, keep the patient's extremities in a functional position while they are wrapped to maintain correct alignment.

A third type of roll bandage is a heavier type of stretchable material commonly known as the **elastic bandage** and often referred to by the term "Ace" bandage. This, too, is a brand name, and there are many brands available. Elastic bandages are used to provide constant pressure over an area or to support an injured joint. On a lower extremity, these bandages also facilitate venous return.

METHODS OF APPLICATION

There are five general methods of applying roll bandages: circular, spiral, reverse-spiral, figure-8, and recurrent fold. The circular method is used to secure a dressing or to cover a confined area of an extremity. The spiral and reverse-spiral methods begin distally on an extremity and wind proximally, to provide comfort to a wider area. The figure-eight method is used over a joint to provide easy flexion. To bandage distal portions of extremities or a stump that has not been casted, the recurrent-fold technique best provides the correct pressure.

Before you begin to apply any type of roll bandage, make sure the bandage begins as a firm roll to facilitate smooth unrolling and wrapping. Always unroll it with the rolled-up portion on top (Fig. 37-2) to facilitate the process. Secure the bandage with a strip of cloth or paper tape over the loose end, fastened to the bandage, not the skin. If the material is porous, use a metal clip with sharp small teeth on the undersurface. Metal clips are commonly used with elastic bandages, but a safety pin or tape also may be used. Some elastic bandages have a self-adhering surface so that fastening devices are not needed.

CIRCULAR BANDAGE

Hold the end of the bandage with one hand while you unroll the bandage either toward you or laterally, hold-

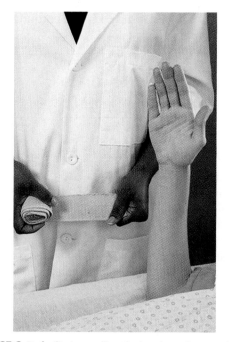

FIGURE 37-2 To facilitate unrolling the bandage, the nurse keeps the rolled portion on the top.

ing the loose end until it is secured by the first circle of the bandage (Fig. 37-3). Two or three turns may be needed to cover an area adequately. Hold the **circular bandage** in place with tape or a clip.

SPIRAL BANDAGE

Begin with the circular method. After securing with one or two complete overlaps, place the bandage to overlap one-half to two-thirds of the width, and in this manner, move up the extremity to provide even support (Fig. 37-4). Fasten the **spiral bandage** in place.

REVERSE-SPIRAL BANDAGE

Begin the **reverse-spiral bandage** as you would the spiral bandage. When the end is secured by the first turn, hold your thumb on the bandage as it approaches the side nearest you and fold over, reversing the direction downward (Fig. 37-5). Repeat this step with each turn, overlapping as before. When the desired area is covered, end with a circular wrap and secure the bandage with tape or a clip.

FIGURE-EIGHT BANDAGE

The **figure-eight bandage** is most often used on a joint. Make the first turns over the joint and secure the end by overlapping the bandage as you proceed. Make the next turn higher than, or superior to, the joint. Make the following turn lower than, or inferior to, the joint (Fig. 37-6). Continue working in this manner, one turn above and one below. The figure-eight pattern allows the joint to maintain its mobility without dislodging the bandage. Secure the bandage with tape or a clip.

RECURRENT-FOLD BANDAGE

The **recurrent-fold bandage** can be adapted for use on many parts of the body. It is used for the finger, hand, toe, or foot. This type of bandage is also useful as

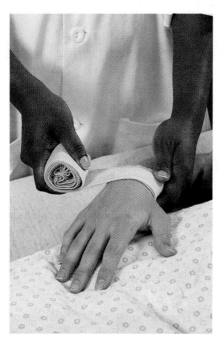

FIGURE 37-3 You may use a circular wrap for applying a bandage to a wrist.

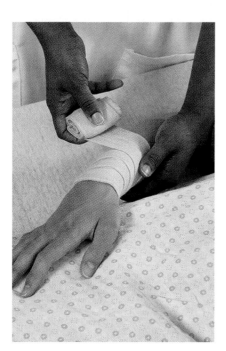

FIGURE 37-4 You may use a spiral wrap for applying a bandage to the wrist and forearm.

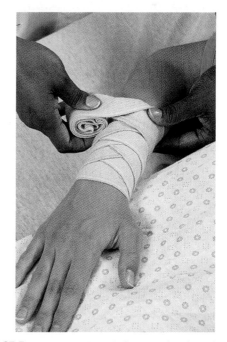

FIGURE 37-5 To use a reverse-spiral wrap to bandage the arm, hold the fold of the bandage in place with the thumb as you reverse the spiral and wrap with your other hand.

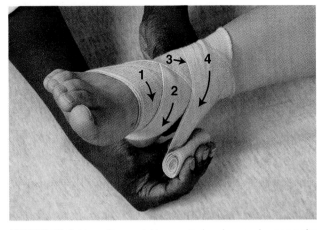

FIGURE 37-6 Use a figure-eight wrap to bandage and support the ankle.

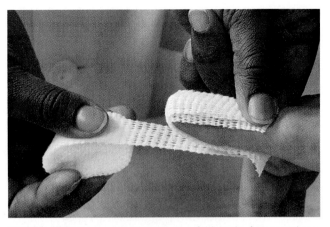

FIGURE 37-8 You can use the recurrent fold on the fingers and toes by following the same procedure as for the head.

a head dressing (Fig. 37-7) or as a wrap for the stump of an extremity.

To apply, hold the end of the bandage in place with one circular turn. Then, bring the roll down over the end of the body part (finger, hand, toe, foot, or stump) and back up behind. When used on the head, the circular turn is made, and then turns are made over and back across the top of the head. Subsequent turns are folded alternately to the right and left of the initial centerfold (Fig. 37-8). Keep your fingers in place at the top to secure the bandage until a circular turn or two can be made to complete it (Fig. 37-9). Clip or tape in place.

SPECIFIC PROCEDURES FOR APPLYING BANDAGES

For each procedure discussed, some steps of the General Procedure may be modified. Included completely are the modified steps as well as references to the steps of the General Procedure that remain the same.

Wrapping an Extremity

This procedure is based on applying the bandage over intact skin.

ASSESSMENT

1-2. Follow steps 1 and 2 of the General Procedure: Review the chart for diagnosis and orders, and assess bandage in place for effectiveness.

ANALYSIS

3-4. Follow steps 3 and 4 of the General Procedure: Think through your data, and identify specific problems and modifications.

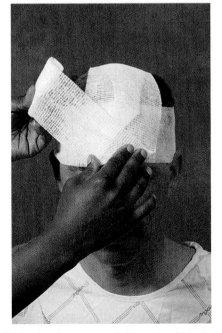

FIGURE 37-7 Using the recurrent fold on a head bandage. Hold the end of the bandage in place as you use your other hand to change directions and overlap. Continue overlapping to cover, making a final horizontal loop to secure the bandage.

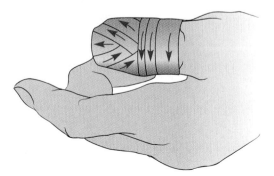

FIGURE 37-9 Recurrent bandages are secured with one or more circular/horizontal loops.

PLANNING

5. Determine individualized patient outcomes for the bandaging procedure, including the following. **R:** Identification of outcomes guides planning and evaluation.
   a. Bandage is effective with regard to holding dressings in place or providing support (depending upon the purpose).
   b. Circulation, motion, and sensation are intact distal to the bandage.
   c. Patient reports no pain or discomfort related to the bandage.
6-8. Follow steps 6 to 8 of the General Procedure: Plan the application of the ankle or wrist bandage; obtain the bandaging materials to be used; and devise a schedule for rechecks.

IMPLEMENTATION

Action	Rationale
9-16. Follow steps 9 to 16 of the General Procedure: Wash or disinfect your hands, obtain supportive devices or assistance, identify the patient (two identifiers), pull curtain and close door, explain the purpose of the bandage, raise the bed, position and drape the patient appropriately, and remove the soiled bandage, if present.	
17. Wrap the extremity.	
a. Keep the body part in a horizontal position for at least 15 minutes before bandaging.	To facilitate emptying of veins.
b. *For a lower extremity:* Secure the bandage around the instep of the foot with a single circular wrap, and form a figure-8 around the ankle itself. *For an upper extremity:* Secure the bandage around the wrist with a circular wrap.	To help make sure that the bandage will stay in place.
c. Wrap as far up the extremity as desired, using a spiral method. To continue the wrap above the knee or above the elbow, use a reverse-spiral method just below the knee or below the elbow to secure the bandage firmly. Always work from distal to proximal.	This, as well as the elastic quality of the bandage, promotes venous return.
d. Fasten in place.	To secure the bandage.
18-19. Follow steps 18 and 19 of the General Procedure: Lower the bed, and wash or disinfect your hands.	

EVALUATION

20. Follow step 20 of the General Procedure: Evaluate using the individualized patient outcomes previously identified: Bandage is effective with regard to holding dressings in place or providing support; circulation, motion, and sensation are distal to the bandage; and patient reports no pain or discomfort.

DOCUMENTATION

21-22. Follow steps 21 and 22 of the General Procedure: Document time; type of bandage applied; specific extremity involved; assessment of circulation, motion, and sensation; length of time bandage was off; and condition of skin, as well as plan for ongoing assessment.

ELASTIC OR COMPRESSION (ANTIEMBOLISM) STOCKINGS

Elastic compression stockings (also referred to as anti-embolic or antiembolism stockings) are used to provide firm support to the soft tissue of the leg, preventing venous blood from pooling and blood clots from developing in the deep veins. Elastic stockings are typically ordered preoperatively for patients to maintain venous return during the operation and to be kept in place during the postoperative phase as well. They are commonly used also when a patient's mobility is limited and sometimes to prevent or treat orthostatic hypotension. Elastic stockings usually are applied before the patient gets out of bed in the morning.

Among the many brands of elastic stockings are some that have openings to allow the toes to be examined and circulation to be checked, some that are knee-length, and some that are thigh-length. Thigh-length stockings usually have a nonconstrictive gusset set in at the inner aspect of the thigh.

Stockings are available in a variety of strengths of compression. The standard stockings used postoperatively commonly provide 8 to 15 mm of Hg compression to the legs. This provides support to veins and encourages venous return (Evan & Read, 2001). To provide adequate pressure at the right place without impairing blood flow, the correct size must be obtained. They are usually ordered in sizes of small, medium, large, or extra large. For individuals with venous insufficiency, higher compression stocking with 20 to 30 mm Hg may be specially ordered. Most provide greater pressure at the ankle and gradually decreasing pressure up the leg. A special measuring device is used to measure circumference at various points along the extremity as well as the length of the leg or arm in order to obtain the correct size.

Check the directions on the brand you are using to determine the size. Because they are so firm, elastic stockings are often difficult to apply using the usual techniques for putting on hose. Most manufacturers recommend an "inside-out" technique (Fig. 37-10).

Procedure for Applying Elastic Compression (Antiembolism) Stockings

ASSESSMENT

1-2. Follow steps 1 and 2 of the General Procedure: Review the chart for diagnosis and orders, and assess stockings in place (if present) for effectiveness.

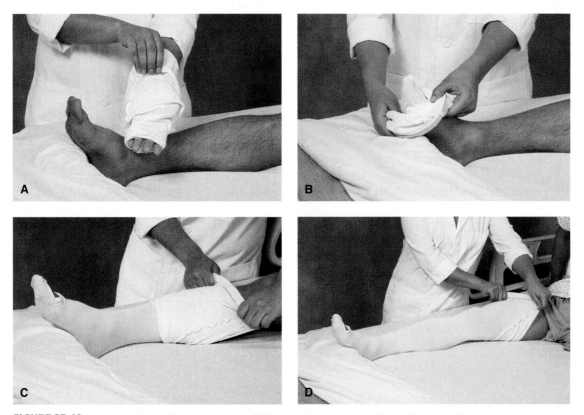

FIGURE 37-10 Putting elastic stockings on a patient. (**A**) Put hand inside the stocking and turn stocking wrong side out. (**B**) Stretch the stocking at the heel to facilitate putting it on. (**C**) Pull the stocking over the heel. (**D**) Pull the stocking up over the leg.

ANALYSIS

3-4. Follow steps 3 and 4 of the General Procedure: Think through your data, and identify specific problems and modifications.

PLANNING

5. Determine individualized patient outcomes in relation to applying elastic compression stockings.

    a. Stockings are smoothly in place.

    b. Circulation, motion, and sensation in the feet are within normal limits.

    c. Patient expresses comfort.

6-8. Follow steps 6 to 8 of the General Procedure: Plan the application of the elastic stockings, obtain the stockings, and devise a schedule for rechecks.

IMPLEMENTATION

Action	Rationale
9-16. Follow steps 9 to 16 of the General Procedure: Wash or disinfect your hands, obtain supportive devices or assistance, identify the patient (two identifiers), pull curtain and close door, explain the purpose of the stockings, raise the bed, position and drape the patient appropriately, and remove soiled stockings, if present.	
17. Apply the elastic stockings:	
a. Slide your hand into the foot of the stocking.	So that the stockings are applied smoothly and venous return is not restricted.
b. Turn the leg of the stocking down over your hand until the leg is inside out but the foot of the stocking is still right side out inside the leg.	
c. Remove your hand from the stocking and pull the foot of the stocking onto the patient's foot, carefully placing the heel of the stocking over the heel of the foot.	
d. Gradually pull the stocking up over the leg by turning it right side out onto the leg.	
e. Make sure that the stocking fits smoothly without wrinkles and that the foot is correctly positioned. Do not turn down the top edge; doing so may restrict venous return.	
f. Repeat steps a through e for the other stocking.	
g. At least every 8 hours, the stocking should be removed, the skin inspected, the legs elevated for 15 minutes, and the stockings reapplied.	To ensure that skin integrity has not been compromised and that capillary flow to leg tissue occurs.

(continued)

Action	Rationale
h. Cleanse the skin of the feet and legs at least every 24 hours.	To stimulate circulation to the skin and remove microorganisms that may grow under the stockings.
18-19. Follow steps 18 and 19 of the General Procedure: Lower the bed, and wash or disinfect your hands.	

EVALUATION

20. Follow step 20 of the General Procedure: Evaluate using the individualized patient outcomes previously identified: Stockings are smoothly in place; circulation, motion, and sensation in the feet are within normal limits; and patient expresses comfort.

DOCUMENTATION

21-22. Follow steps 21 and 22 of the General Procedure: Document time; type of stockings applied; assessment of circulation, motion, and sensation; length of time stockings were off and condition of skin, as well as plan for ongoing assessment.

▮ POTENTIAL ADVERSE OUTCOMES AND RELATED INTERVENTIONS

1. Impaired venous return. It is somewhat ironic that a treatment designed to improve venous return might impede it. However, if the stockings are too small for the patient's legs, the tight top of the stocking can have a serious constricting effect. This increases the potential for venous thrombosis (Shaughnessy, 2005). A properly fitted stocking can also constrict circulation if the top rolls down and creates a banding effect.
Intervention: Check measurements carefully to assure that the correct size is ordered. When stockings are applied, be sure that the tops are smoothly stretched to prevent banding. Teach the patient to check the stockings for proper placement and constriction. Institute a monitoring plan to assess compression stockings for constriction.

2. Ineffective therapeutic regimen management. Because compression stockings may be hot and uncomfortable, many patients who need to wear them as an ongoing preventive measure may stop wearing them.
Intervention: When a patient is initially prescribed compression stockings, the teaching plan should include a discussion of the lifestyle concerns about wearing them on an ongoing basis. When the patient comes to an ambulatory care setting, the nurse can assess whether the patient is managing the prescribed care and explore options that might increase the patient's willingness to wear the prescribed stockings regularly.

SEQUENTIAL COMPRESSION DEVICE

A **sequential compression device** is a mechanical device that provides intermittent compression over the lower leg or entire leg to promote venous return and prevent deep vein thrombosis and pulmonary embolism. Various forms of sequential compression devices exist, but the typical device usually consists of a vinyl "sleeve" that fits over the ankle and calf (some versions include the thigh) and fastens with hook-and-loop fasteners. A control unit, which may either hang on the bed frame or be placed on the floor under the bed, has a small pump that inflates and deflates channels in the sleeve to increase and decrease pressure (Fig. 37-11).

The compartments of the sleevelike device fill with air, gradually providing increasing pressure, and then deflate, removing the compression. Amounts of pressure exerted during the various phases of the cycle are adjustable and displayed on the control unit. It may be applied to one or both lower extremities. Such a device is contraindicated for patients with severe arterial disease of the lower extremities.

The device must be ordered in the appropriate size for the individual patient. Instructions for how to measure calf and thigh circumference and length are included with the device. In some cases, elastic stockings are applied beneath the sequential compression device for optimum clinical efficacy.

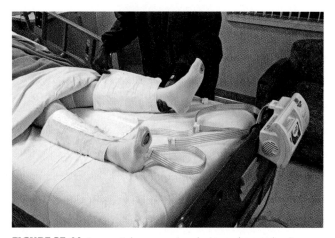

FIGURE 37-11 Sequential compression device and control unit.

Procedure for Applying a Sequential Compression Device

ASSESSMENT

1-2. Follow steps 1 and 2 of the General Procedure: Review the chart for diagnosis and orders, and assess stockings and/or sequential compression device, if present.

ANALYSIS

3-4. Follow steps 3 and 4 of the General Procedure: Think through your data, and identify specific problems and modifications.

PLANNING

5. Determine individualized patient outcomes for applying a sequential compression device. **R:** Identification of outcomes guides planning and evaluation.
   a. Device is accurately placed on legs and inflating and deflating in sequence.
   b. Circulation, motion, and sensation in the feet are within normal limits.
   c. Patient expresses comfort.

6-8. Follow steps 6 to 8 of the General Procedure: Plan the application of the sequential compression device, obtain the needed materials, and devise a schedule for rechecks.

IMPLEMENTATION

Action	Rationale
9-16. Follow steps 9 to 16 of the General Procedure: Wash or disinfect your hands, obtain supportive devices or assistance, identify the patient (two identifiers), pull the curtain and close the door, explain the purpose of the sequential compression device, position and drape the patient appropriately, raise the bed to an appropriate working position, and remove soiled bandages or stockings, if present.	
17. Apply the sequential compression device.	
a. Place the vinyl sleeve over the ankle and calf. If it is a tubular sleeve, slide it on over the foot, ankle, and calf. If it is a wrap style, align the leg on the open thigh-length sleeve according to the instructions included. Wrap the sleeve securely around the patient's leg and fasten the tabs, thigh section first.	Precise application of the device will promote optimum therapeutic effect.
b. Attach the connector on the sleeve to the correct end of the connector tubing. Check carefully to be certain there are no kinks in the tubing.	
c. Attach the other end of the connector tubing to the control unit.	
d. Turn the power on and adjust or monitor pressure according to your facility's protocol.	
e. Remove the device at least twice daily for 20 to 30 minutes each time.	This allows time for ambulation and bathing. *(continued)*

Action	Rationale
f. Replace immediately after ambulation or care.	For maximum therapeutic effect.
18-19. Follow steps 18 and 19 of the General Procedure: Lower the bed, and wash or disinfect your hands.	

EVALUATION

20. Follow step 20 of the General Procedure: Evaluate using the individualized patient outcomes previously identified: Device is accurately placed and functioning correctly; circulation, motion, and sensation in the feet are within normal limits; and patient expresses comfort.

DOCUMENTATION

21-22. Follow steps 21 and 22 of the General Procedure: Document time; type of device applied; specific leg(s) involved; assessment of circulation, motion, and sensation; length of time sequential compression device was off and condition of skin, as well as plan for ongoing assessment.

CARING FOR AN AMPUTATION STUMP

After amputation of a limb, the stump is commonly fixed in a cast. The cast compresses and molds the appendage and serves as the base for a device to which a temporary prosthesis can be attached. Once the cast is off, there is a concern that the stump will swell and the shape will distort. Therefore, the stump is covered with an elasticized stump stocking that helps to compress it and maintain the appropriate contours. In some instances, a stump stocking is not available and elastic bandages are used to wrap the stump to provide the needed compression and shape.

Applying a Stump Stocking or Wrapping a Stump

ASSESSMENT

1-2. Follow steps 1 and 2 of the General Procedure: Review the chart for diagnosis and orders, and assess wrapping or stocking in place, if present.

ANALYSIS

3-4. Follow steps 3 and 4 of the General Procedure: Think through your data, and identify specific problems and modifications.

PLANNING

5. Determine the individualized patient outcomes for wrapping a stump or applying a stump stocking. **R:** Identification of outcomes guides planning and evaluation.
   a. Stump stocking or elastic bandage is smoothly in place.
   b. Circulation, motion, and sensation in the stump are within normal limits.
   c. Patient expresses comfort.
6-8. Follow steps 6 to 8 of the General Procedure: Plan the wrapping of the stump or application of the stump stocking, obtain the needed materials, and devise a schedule for rechecks.

IMPLEMENTATION

Action	Rationale
9-16. Follow steps 9 to 16 of the General Procedure: Wash or disinfect your hands, obtain supportive devices or assistance, identify the patient (two identifiers), pull the curtain and close the door, explain what you plan to do, raise the bed, position and drape the patient appropriately, and remove soiled bandages or stocking, if present.	

(continued)

Action	Rationale
17. Apply the stump stocking or wrap the stump with an elastic bandage according to the method preferred by the surgeon.	
a. Turn the stump stocking inside out, placing the end of the tube against the end of the stump, and gradually invert the stocking over the stump (Fig. 37-12).	

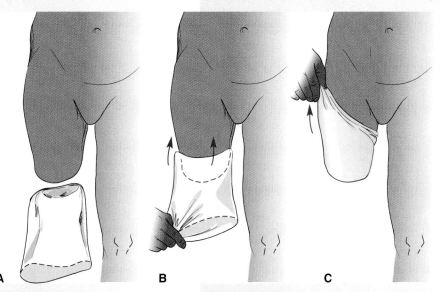

FIGURE 37-12 To apply the stump stocking, (**A**) turn the stocking inside out, (**B**) invert it over the end of the stump, and (**C**) gently pull it to its right side over the stump.

Action	Rationale
b. Be sure to put the shorter side of the stocking on the inner aspect of the thigh so that it stops at the groin. The longer side of the stocking fits on the outer, longer aspect of the thigh.	
c. Some stump stockings have buckles that fasten to a waist belt to help hold the stocking in place. Check the skin under the buckles carefully to make sure they are not causing irritation.	
d. To apply a recurrent and spiral elastic bandage: A recurrent bandage is placed on the stump first, and then a spiral is started at the distal end of the stump and moved up to the thigh (Fig. 37-13).	Decreasing pressure as you go up the stump, with slightly more pressure at the most distal portion of the stump, enhances venous return circulation and produces a smooth, even stump. *Note:* These wrapping techniques may be used on an upper extremity stump as well.

(continued)

Action	Rationale

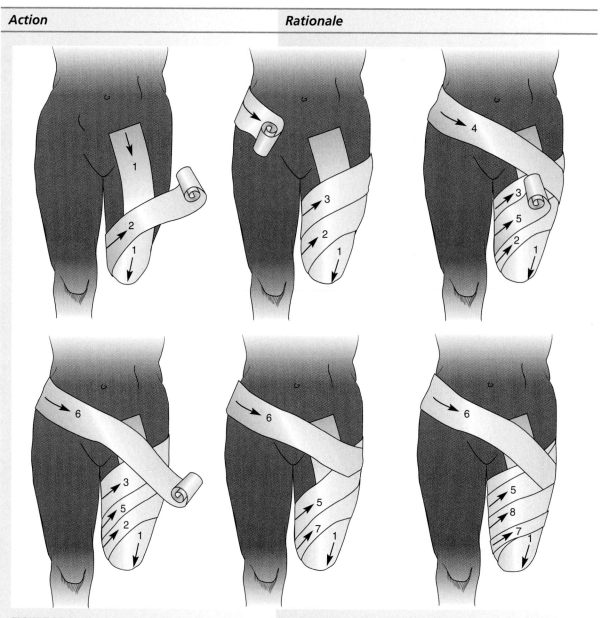

FIGURE 37-13 When bandaging a stump, use a recurrent bandage first, beginning at the end of the stump, and then wrap a spiral bandage up the thigh. (Courtesy University of Washington Department of Prosthetics-Orthotics, Seattle, Washington.)

e. Figure-eight bandage: Wrap the bandage in a figure-eight from the stump up and around the hip and waist and back down to the stump.

18-19. Follow steps 18 and 19 of the General Procedure: Lower the bed, and wash or disinfect your hands.

EVALUATION

20. Follow step 20 of the General Procedure: Evaluate using the individualized patient outcomes previously identified: Elastic bandage or stump stocking is smoothly in place; circulation, motion, and sensation in the stump are within normal limits; and patient expresses comfort.

DOCUMENTATION

21-22. Follow steps 21 and 22 of the General Procedure: Document time; specific wrapping or stump stocking applied; specific leg(s) involved; assessment of circulation, motion, and sensation; length of time wrapping was off and condition of skin; and the plan for ongoing assessment.

APPLYING BINDERS

Binders are generally used on the trunk of the body to hold dressings in place or to support tissues. They can be placed around the chest, the abdomen, or the pelvic area.

TYPES OF BINDERS

Binders are usually fashioned from a strong material such as heavy cotton or a heavy elasticized fabric that can hold dressings and provide support. They may be made of a wide strip of soft muslin, a strip of lightweight canvas material, an elastic fabric, or a stretch net fabric used to hold dressings in place. Some binders are lightweight and made from a tubular stretch mesh.

TUBULAR STRETCH NET BINDERS AND STOCKINETTE

Tubular stretch **net binders** hold a dressing in place without the need for tape; however, they do provide gentle support. Stretch net binders come in a variety of circumferences. They are usually used around the abdomen or chest but can be used on the extremities as well. Because the binders stretch and are available in different widths and lengths, you do not have to measure the body part. However, you do need to order a size you think is appropriate for the patient. Stretch net binders can be washed and dried easily, offer air circulation, and stretch to conform to the shape of the part being bound (Fig. 37-14).

Stockinette is a tubular-cotton, ribbed-knit material that comes in a several different diameters from 1 inch to 4 inches. This may be used to pull over dressings on a digit or an extremity and hold them in place. Stockinette has limited stretch but does conform to the shape of the extremity.

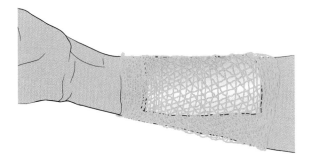

FIGURE 37-14 Stretch net binder. Gather and stretch net in your hands over the extremity.

T-BINDERS

T-binders are designed to hold perineal dressings or packs in place. Single T-binders are used for female patients; double T-binders are used for male patients so that the testicles are not unduly constricted (Fig. 37-15). Some T-binders are elastic with snap fasteners, some are muslin, and others are made of a disposable paper.

ELASTIC ABDOMINAL BINDERS

Most commercially made abdominal binders are a firm elastic fabric with hook-and-loop fasteners across the front that provide very firm support to the abdomen. They are ordered by the physician when extra abdominal support is needed after surgery. This is often used for the patient who is obese or at risk for wound dehiscence.

Procedure for Applying a Binder to Hold Dressings

ASSESSMENT

1-2. Follow steps 1 and 2 of the General Procedure: Review the chart for diagnosis and orders, and assess binder in place, if any.

ANALYSIS

3-4. Follow steps 3 and 4 of the General Procedure: Think through your data, and identify specific problems and modifications.

PLANNING

5. Determine the individualized patient outcomes for applying a binder to hold dressings in place. **R:** Identification of outcomes guides planning and evaluation.
   a. Dressings are held smoothly in place.
   b. Patient reports no pain or discomfort related to the binder.

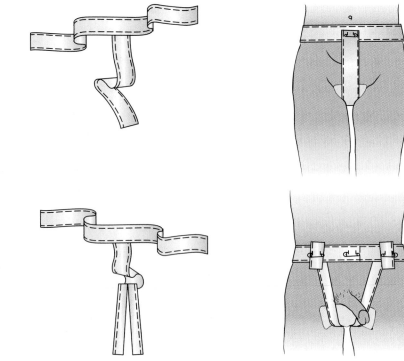

A

B

FIGURE 37-15 Disposable T-binders. To apply a T-binder, bring the waist tails around the patient's waist and the center tail (**A**) or tails (**B**) up between the patient's legs to hold the dressing in place. Secure the ends of the tail(s) with safety pins.

6. Follow step 6 of the General Procedure: Plan the application of the binder.

7. Obtain the type and size of binder for the location of the dressings. If you are unsure, call the Central Supply Department and ask for assistance. **R:** The correct size will facilitate holding the dressing in place.

8. Follow step 8 of the General Procedure: Devise a schedule for removal and reapplication of the binder.

IMPLEMENTATION

Action	Rationale
9-16. Follow steps 9 to 16 of the General Procedure: Wash or disinfect your hands, obtain supportive devices or assistance, identify the patient (two identifiers), pull the curtain and close the door, explain what you plan to do, raise the bed, position and drape the patient appropriately, and remove soiled binder and dressing, if present.	
17. Apply the binder.	
a. Tubular stretch net binder or stockinette:	
(1) Gather the net or the stockinette in your hands.	

(continued)

Action	Rationale
(2) *For the abdomen:* Stretch the net and slip it upward over the feet and legs to its position around the abdomen. Alternatively, slip it over the head and downward, surrounding the abdomen or chest. Use the technique that is most comfortable for the patient. When stretch net binders are used around the chest, they are usually pulled over the head (Fig. 37-16). *For an extremity:* Pull the mesh net or stockinette up from the end of the extremity to cover the dressings.	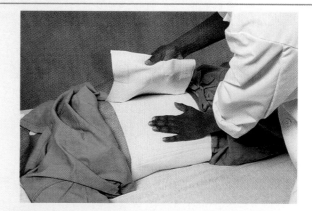 **FIGURE 37-16** Straight abdominal binder. With patient lying in the supine position, overlap the edges of the straight abdominal binder snugly over the abdomen. Secure with hook-and-loop fastener or safety pins.
b. Abdominal binder:	Smooth, even application promotes optimum support, safety, and comfort.
(1) Place the patient in the supine position. Ask the patient to lift the torso upward by using the legs, or roll the patient onto the binder. Apply the binder smoothly and evenly so that wrinkles do not cause pressure on the patient's skin.	
(2) Bring the ends of the binder upward around the patient's trunk.	
(3) Overlap the edges of the binder snugly over the abdomen.	
(4) Fasten using hook-and-loop fasteners or safety pins. Fasteners are more comfortable and safer for the patient than are the hard surfaces of pins (see Fig. 37-16).	
c. T-Binder:	This is for maximum comfort and binder security.
(1) Have the patient lift midsection, or turn patient side to side, and place the binder underneath the patient smoothly, with the waistband at waist level and the tails pointing down the midline of the back.	
(2) Bring the waist tails around the patient and overlap.	
(3) Bring the center tail (or tails) up between the patient's legs and over	*(continued)*

Action	Rationale
perineal dressings, taking care to touch only the outside of the dressings. Make sure the two tails of the double T-binder are on either side of the scrotum and penis.	
(4) Join the center tail(s) to the waistband and secure the ends with safety pins.	
18-19. Follow steps 18 and 19 of the General Procedure: Lower the bed, and wash or disinfect your hands.	

EVALUATION

20. Follow step 20 of the General Procedure: Evaluate using the individualized patient outcomes previously identified: Dressings are held smoothly in place; patient reports no pain or discomfort related to the binder.

DOCUMENTATION

21-22. Follow steps 21 and 22 of the General Procedure: Document time; application of the binder; specific area involved; assessment of circulation, motion, and sensation, as appropriate; length of time binder was off and condition of skin, as well as plan for ongoing assessment.

ARM SLING

A **sling** is used to rest the arm in a right-angle position. Slings may be commercially produced or made from fabric cut in a triangular shape.

Procedure for Applying an Arm Sling

ASSESSMENT

1-2. Follow steps 1 and 2 of the General Procedure: Review the chart for diagnosis and orders, and assess sling in place, if any.

ANALYSIS

3-4. Follow steps 3 and 4 of the General Procedure: Think through your data, and identify specific problems and modifications.

PLANNING

5. Determine the individualized patient outcomes for applying an arm sling. **R:** Identification of outcomes guides planning and evaluation.
   a. Arm is held securely, with the elbow at a right angle and the wrist supported.
   b. Circulation, motion, and sensation are intact.
   c. Patient reports no pain or discomfort related to the sling.
6. Follow step 6 of the General Procedure: Plan the application of the sling.
7. Obtain the sling. To make a sling from muslin, fold or cut (for less thickness) a 35-inch square of fabric diagonally. Or you may need to order the sling from the facility's Central Supply Department. **R:** Having the correct supplies available facilitates the procedure.
8. Follow step 8 of the General Procedure: Devise a schedule for removal and reapplication of the sling.

IMPLEMENTATION

Action	Rationale
9-16. Follow steps 9 to 16 of the General Procedure: Wash or disinfect your hands, obtain supportive devices or assistance, identify the patient (two identifiers), pull the curtains and close the door, explain	*(continued)*

Action	Rationale
what you plan to do, raise the bed, position the patient, and remove soiled sling and dressing, if present.	
17. Apply the arm sling, using one of the two following methods:	This is for maximum therapeutic effect, safety, and comfort for the patient.
a. *Method A: Triangular sling*	
(1) With the patient facing you, place the sling across the body and underneath the arms, as shown in Figure 37-17.	

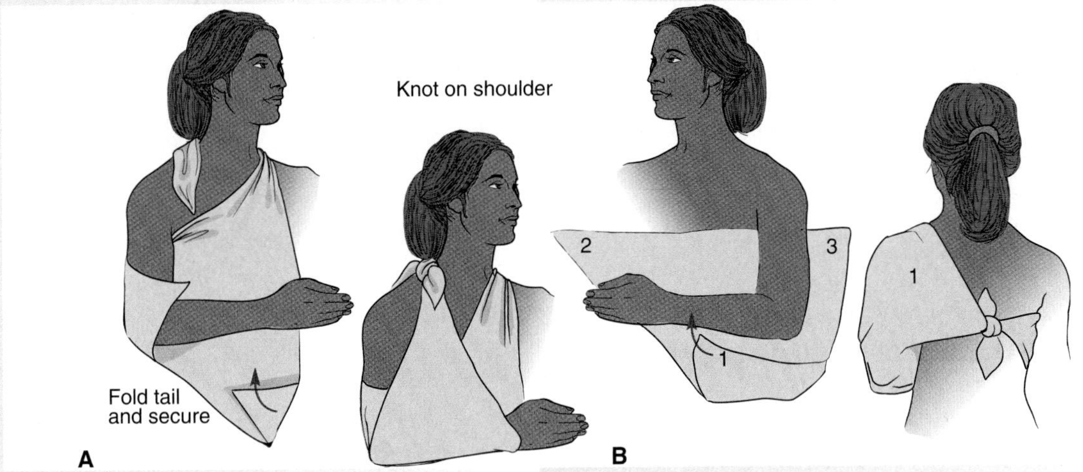

Knot on shoulder

Fold tail and secure

A

B

FIGURE 37-17 Arm slings. (**A**) Method A. Place one end of triangle over unaffected shoulder. Bring other end of triangle over affected shoulder. Tie or pin ends to one side of the neck. Fold corner flat at elbow and secure with safety pins. (**B**) Method B. Place triangle under the arms. Bring the corner that is under the unaffected arm up over the shoulder to the back and the corner under the affected arm around the body to the back. Tie the ends. Fold corner flat at the elbow and secure with safety pins.

Action	Rationale
(2) Bring the corner of the sling that is under the unaffected arm to the back.	
(3) Bring the lower corner up over the affected shoulder to the back and tie.	
(4) Fold the sling neatly at the elbow and pin.	
(5) Check the position—the hand should be supported in the sling.	
	For maximum therapeutic effect, safety, and comfort for the patient. *Note:* Method A is preferred because a sling applied using method B can pull or strain the neck muscles, even when it is tied at the neck. In method A, the entire shoulder bears the weight of the immobilized arm. *(continued)*

Action	Rationale
b. *Method B: Triangular sling*	
(1) With the patient facing you, place one end of the triangle over the unaffected shoulder.	
(2) Bring the long straight border under the hand on the affected side.	
(3) Loop upward, positioning the other end of the triangle over the affected shoulder.	
(4) Tie or pin the ends to one side of the neck, using a square knot, or pin smoothly, using a safety pin. Never secure a sling at the back of the neck, where pressure could be exerted.	
(5) Fold the corner flat and neatly at the elbow and pin.	
(6) Check the position—the hand should be supported in the sling (see Fig. 37-17).	
c. *Commercial sling* Some commercially made slings are made of a canvas-like material. They have a support pocket for the forearm and straps that go over the shoulder (Fig. 37-18).	

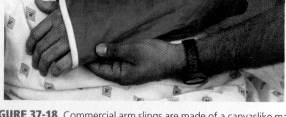

FIGURE 37-18 Commercial arm slings are made of a canvaslike material and have a pocket for the affected arm. They are supported by straps that go over the shoulder.

18-19. Follow steps 18 and 19 of the General Procedure: Lower the bed, and wash or disinfect your hands.

EVALUATION

20. Follow step 20 of the General Procedure: Evaluate using the individualized patient outcomes previously identified: Arm is held securely with the elbow at a right angle and the wrist supported; circulation, motion, and sensation are intact; patient reports no pain or discomfort related to the sling.

DOCUMENTATION

21-22. Follow steps 21 and 22 of the General Procedure: Document time; application of the sling; specific arm involved; assessment of circulation, motion, and sensation, if appropriate; length of time sling was off and condition of skin, as well as plan for ongoing assessment.

Acute Care

Bandages and binders are typically applied in the Emergency Department of acute care facilities, usually after a traumatic event. They are also applied and maintained postoperatively. In both cases, patients are usually sent home with a bandage or binder in place. Patients and caregivers need to be taught how to set up a schedule for checking the specific area for circulation, motion, and sensation and how to reapply the bandage or binder when needed. In many cases, the patient will be unable to perform these tasks independently.

Long-Term Care

The principles related to applying bandages and binders remain the same regardless of the setting in which they are used. However, the circulation of some older adults residing in long-term care facilities may be more compromised than that of younger people found in other settings. These residents may have decreased sensation as well and, therefore, they may be unaware of a bandage or binder that has become too snug. In addition, those who cannot communicate their distress are at added risk. Therefore, you may need to check circulation, movement, and sensation at more frequent intervals than in other settings.

Because of decreased mobility and poor venous return, many long-term care residents wear elastic stockings on a routine basis. These stockings need to be laundered frequently, which will lead to loss of elasticity and diminished effectiveness over time. This requires planning for sufficient pairs of stockings so that some are always available. The effectiveness of elastic stockings also needs to be evaluated frequently.

Home Care

Those who need to wear various types of bandages and binders at home need to know how to apply them safely and effectively and how often to check or change them. In some situations, the client will be able to do this without assistance. In other situations, a family member, friend, or neighbor may need to help.

Caution ambulatory clients who wear elastic stockings that these stockings may roll down, creating a constricting band and compromising circulation. Your teaching will be specific to a given situation, but do include teaching about how to change a sterile or clean dressing, how to assess circulation and skin condition, and principles of correct positioning. Encourage clients and their families to consult their care provider if questions or concerns arise.

Ambulatory Care

Bandages and binders frequently have their initial application in ambulatory care settings and even more frequently are reassessed and reapplied there. Reassessment includes the assessment of the client's or the caregiver's ability to manage the tasks involved in reapplication of the bandage or binder as well as their ability to make the observations necessary to ensure safe and effective use of the specific device.

LEARNING TOOLS

DEVELOP YOUR BACKGROUND KNOWLEDGE

1. Review the Learning Outcomes.

2. Look up the Key Terms in the glossary.

3. Review this module and mentally practice the techniques described. Study so that you would be able to teach these skills to another person.

DEVELOP YOUR SKILLS

1. In the practice setting
   a. Become familiar with the materials and available types of bandages and binders.
   b. With a partner, practice applying bandages, demonstrating each of the methods introduced, using the Performance Checklist on the CD-ROM in the front of this book. Explain the purpose for the bandage to the "patient" (partner) as it is applied.

c. Reroll the bandages and have your partner apply the bandages to you, using the described methods.

d. Together, evaluate one another's performance of steps b and c.

e. Again, with your partner, apply the straight abdominal binder, using the Performance Checklist. Again, explain the purpose for the binder to the "patient" (partner) as it is applied.

f. Have your partner apply this binder to you.

g. Apply an arm sling to your partner.

h. Have your partner apply an arm sling to you.

i. Together, evaluate one another's performance of steps e through h.

DEMONSTRATE YOUR SKILLS

1. In the clinical setting
   a. Consult with your instructor about opportunities to apply bandages and binders to appropriate patients.
   b. Consult with your instructor about an opportunity to observe or assist with the care of a patient using a sequential compression device.

2. Evaluate your performance with your instructor.

CRITICAL THINKING EXERCISES

1. A 14-year-old girl has sustained an injury that will require her to have her left arm in a sling for 2 weeks. Describe and demonstrate to the girl's mother an appropriate way to apply a sling. Write out instructions for the mother to take home.

2. Mr. D. sprained his ankle. It was wrapped in his physician's office, where you are employed. You are asked to teach his wife how to reapply the bandage. Write out the steps you will teach her, along with the rationale you will include. What observations will you teach her to make and how often will you suggest that she make them? Prepare a chart for Mrs. D. to document her observations.

SELF-QUIZ
SHORT-ANSWER QUESTIONS

1. List three reasons for applying bandages.
   a. _____
   b. _____
   c. _____

2. List five methods for applying bandages.
   a. _____
   b. _____

c. _____

d. _____

e. _____

3. What is one common use for the figure-eight method of bandaging?

_____

4. In what direction are bandages applied to extremities?

_____

5. You are applying a sequential compression device to the legs of a postoperative patient for whom you are providing care. What rationale will you provide for the use of this device?

_____

6. A sequential compression device should not be applied to someone with what problem?

_____

7. Abdominal binders are used primarily for what two purposes?
   a. _____
   b. _____

8. Name two advantages of stretch net binders for holding dressings in place.
   a. _____
   b. _____

9. Name one disadvantage of using safety pins as fasteners.

_____

MULTIPLE CHOICE

_____ 10. The recurrent-fold method would be used to bandage
   a. the arm.
   b. the elbow.
   c. a joint.
   d. a fingertip.

_____ 11. The arm sling is not tied behind the neck primarily because it
   a. obstructs the blood flow.
   b. does not hold firmly.
   c. places strain on neck muscles.
   d. compresses nerves.

Answers to the Self-Quiz questions appear in the back of the book.

MODULE 38

Applying Heat and Cold

SKILLS INCLUDED IN THIS MODULE

General Procedure for Applying Heat or Cold
Specific Procedures for Applying Heat
   Applying a Warm, Moist Compress
   Administering a Soak
   Administering a Sitz Bath
Specific Procedures for Applying Cold
   Applying an Ice Pack or Cold Pack

PREREQUISITE MODULES

Module 1	An Approach to Nursing Skills
Module 2	Documentation
Module 4	Basic Infection Control
Module 5	Safety in the Healthcare Environment
Module 11	Assessing Temperature, Pulse, and Respiration
Module 12	Measuring Blood Pressure
Module 14	Nursing Physical Assessment

The following module may be needed in some situations:

Module 24	Basic Sterile Technique: Sterile Field and Sterile Gloves

KEY TERMS

dilation	oxygenation
edema	suppuration
inflammation	vasoconstriction
metabolism	vasodilation

OVERALL OBJECTIVE

▸ To apply heat and cold appropriately, with emphasis on comfort and safety for patients.

LEARNING OUTCOMES

The student will be able to

1. Assess the patient effectively to determine the need for heat or cold treatment.
2. Analyze assessment data to determine special problems or concerns that must be addressed before applying heat or cold to a specific patient.
3. Determine appropriate patient outcomes of the specific heat or cold treatment and recognize the potential for adverse outcomes.
4. Apply heat and cold treatments correctly and safely.
5. Evaluate the effectiveness of the heat or cold treatment for a specific patient.
6. Document the treatment in the patient's record and the patient's plan of care as appropriate.

Applications of heat or cold are ordered for many different purposes and may be carried out in many different ways using a variety of equipment. It is essential that the nurse be aware of the indications and rationale for the application of heat and cold as well as safe and effective methods of application to carry out the procedures in ways that meet the needs of patients.

Policies regarding the application of heat and cold vary among healthcare settings. A doctor's order is usually required, although in some instances, there may be protocols that allow the nurse to apply heat or cold according to specific criteria. In any event, you must know the physiologic responses to and appropriate uses of heat and cold and then follow the policies and procedures in your agency.

NURSING DIAGNOSES

Nursing diagnoses that are important when applying heat or cold are

- Risk for Injury, because patients can incur tissue damage from an application that is either too hot or too cold or by one that is left in place for too long.
- Pain or Chronic Pain are nursing diagnoses for which applications of heat or cold may be ordered to relieve discomfort.
- Ineffective Thermoregulation, Hyperthermia, and Hypothermia are additional nursing diagnoses that may be related to the use of the thermal blanket.

DELEGATION

Heat and cold are applied by assistive personnel in healthcare facilities and by patients or family members in the home. The nurse must teach and supervise others in using these applications to assure both effectiveness and safety. This includes how to do the procedure correctly and what to report to the nurse. The nurse remains accountable for the assessment of the effectiveness of the specific treatment.

SAFETY GUIDELINES

To apply heat and cold safely, keep in mind the following approaches and principles.

ASSESS THOROUGHLY

Always assess the patient carefully both before you begin an application of heat or cold and throughout the process. Patients vary in their ability to tolerate heat and cold without experiencing discomfort, tissue damage, or systemic response. Factors that affect tolerance include age (very young and elderly persons are more susceptible to negative effects of heat and cold therapies), circulatory or neurologic deficiencies, level of consciousness, amount of body fat (areas with little body fat are more sensitive to heat and cold treatments), and the condition of the skin in the area being treated. The patient's diagnosis is also a factor to be considered, as is the particular type of heat or cold application. The length of time the body is exposed to heat or cold, as well as the size of the skin area being treated, affects the ability of the body to tolerate the treatment; that is, the briefer the exposure time to heat or cold and the smaller the area being treated, the better the tolerance.

The nurse should be particularly cautious when applying any heat or cold treatment to a patient with diminished sensory perception (the patient may be less aware of discomfort), diminished arterial or venous circulation (the patient is less able to recover from an injury caused by heat or cold), decreased alertness or awareness (the patient may move or tamper with the treatment), and to children or older adults, who are more sensitive to heat and cold. In all of these situations, lack of awareness of problems is more likely to lead to an injury.

EXPLAIN ACCOMMODATION TO HEAT OR COLD

A sensation of either warmth or coolness in a localized area of the body dissipates in a short time as the tissue accommodates to the temperature. Temperature receptors in the skin adjust rapidly to mild stimulation. Explain this phenomenon to the patient, so that the patient will not increase or decrease the temperature of the treatment to an unsafe level.

LIMIT DURATION OF HEAT AND COLD TREATMENTS

Neither heat nor cold treatments should last longer than 20 to 30 minutes (Stitik & Nadler, 1999, 1998). When heat is applied, maximum **vasodilation** occurs in 20 to 30 minutes. A rebound phenomenon can occur when a heat treatment is left in place too long, causing **vasoconstriction** and tissue congestion, thereby negating the therapeutic effects of the heat application. Explain the rebound effect to the patient to gain cooperation with the plan of care. When cold is applied, vasodilation begins after the temperature of the skin decreases to 59°F (15°C), again reversing the desired effect of the thermal application. Explain this phenomenon to the patient to ensure cooperation with the plan of care.

USE SPECIAL CARE WITH MOIST HEAT OR COLD

Moisture conducts heat better than air, so injuries are more likely. Because air is a poor conductor, it is used to insulate certain applications of heat and cold. For example, hot water bottles or ice packs are covered with a cloth before application. The air between the cloth and the bag provides insulation.

PHYSIOLOGIC RESPONSES TO HEAT AND COLD

When heat is applied to an area of the body, the blood vessels in that area undergo **dilation** (expansion), which increases blood circulation and **oxygenation** to the injured tissues, improving **metabolism.** When heat is applied systemically, as in the application of a hyperthermia blanket, the nurse should assess for increased respiratory rate and hypotension, which occur because of peripheral vasodilation (Box 38-1).

The application of cold constricts blood vessels in the affected area. This slows circulation, which retards the reabsorption of fluid into tissues. Because of this, **edema,** or swelling, may be prevented and **inflam-**

box 38-1 *Rationale for Applying Heat*

- To relieve pain from muscle spasms and painful joints
- To reduce swelling (and accompanying discomfort) by increasing circulation (fluid is more easily absorbed from the affected area)
- To increase circulation, which helps to eliminate any toxic waste products that have accumulated in the area of swelling or edema
- To promote **suppuration** (pus formation) in cases of infection
- To relax muscles
- To promote healing by increasing oxygen delivery to the tissues

mation reduced. If edema is already present in an area, the application of cold may slow the resolution of the edema because of the delayed reabsorption of fluid (Box 38-2).

DEVICES FOR APPLYING HEAT OR COLD

Water-flow pads (localized heat and cold-therapy systems), disposable instant packs, gel-filled packs, compresses, and thermal blankets may all be used to deliver either heat or cold treatments. Except for the localized heat and cold-therapy systems and the thermal blanket, the procedure is similar, regardless of the device used.

DISPOSABLE INSTANT HOT OR COLD PACK

Disposable instant hot or cold packs are used in the same way. They come in a variety of sizes and shapes, including a shape similar to an ice collar and those made especially for use in the perineal area. These packs deliver a specific amount of heat or cold for a specified length of time, as indicated by the manufacturer's instructions. Be certain to read these instructions carefully. To use a hot or cold pack, strike, shake, or knead the package. This creates a chemical reaction that releases the heat or cold. Disposable instant hot and cold packs are both convenient and safe when used properly. Some instant hot packs are reusable.

box 38-2 *Rationale for Applying Cold*

- To prevent swelling through vasoconstriction
- To relieve pain by slowing nerve transmission
- To decrease bleeding through vasoconstriction
- To stop the tissue injury in a burn

HOT OR COLD COMPRESSES

A compress is a wet dressing that is applied to an area to provide moisture. Although used more frequently to provide moist heat, a compress may be either hot or cold.

WATER-FLOW HEATING PAD WITH CONTROL UNIT/WATER-FLOW COLD-THERAPY SYSTEM

An order is usually needed for applying these heat or cold water-flow devices. Similarly designed, they consist of a distilled water reservoir control unit with two tubes that circulate temperature-regulated water to channels within a rubber or plastic pad. The single-patient-use pad has a soft, absorbent material on the inside next to the patient and waterproof material on the outside (Fig. 38-1 and Fig. 38-2). Newer units are equipped with audible and visual alarms to monitor both temperature and water level. These pads may be secured with a gauze wrap or tape. They should not be pinned because of the danger of puncturing the water channels. Because the unit is electrical, always check cords and controls to be sure they are in good repair.

THERMAL BLANKET: WARMING OR COOLING

The thermal blanket serves the dual purpose of either heating or cooling the body systemically. The blanket is similar to the water-flow heating pad except that it is larger—of blanket size. The thermal blanket is most commonly used for warming a patient after major surgery or trauma. Elderly patients and infants are among those most at risk for hypothermia.

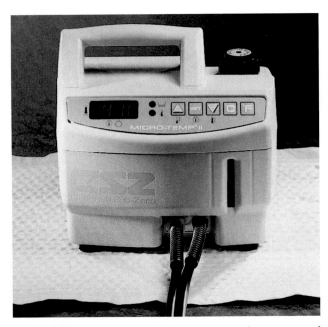

FIGURE 38-1 Water-flow–controlled heating unit. Photo courtesy of Cincinnati Sub-Zero.

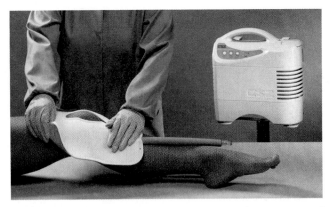

FIGURE 38-2 Water-flow cold therapy system. Photo courtesy of Cincinnati Sub-Zero.

When a thermal blanket is being used for cooling, it is commonly referred to as a hypothermia blanket. The hypothermia or cooling blanket is usually used for one of two primary purposes. Hypothermia may be induced as part of a surgical procedure to slow circulation and thus decrease the potential for bleeding or to decrease metabolic activity and thereby reduce oxygen requirements. The hypothermia blanket is also used to reduce persistent high fevers. In automatic operation, the patient's temperature is monitored with a sensor (a skin sensor or rectal probe with a sensor on the nursing unit and esophageal probe with a sensor in the operating room), and the blanket cools the patient to the desired body temperature and maintains that level.

ELECTRIC HEATING PAD

Electric heating pads are commonly used in the home because they are convenient for applying heat to small areas of the body and because they are relatively inexpensive. The wires that provide the heat must be covered by rubber or plastic insulation to ensure safety. Electric heating pads should never be used in the presence of moisture because of the danger of electric shock. Instruct the patient not to lie on top of the heating pad because heat may accumulate and cause a burn. In addition, it is essential that you follow the precautions already outlined for using electrical equipment.

WARM SOAKS AND SITZ BATHS

Soaks and sitz baths are commonly used to apply moist heat. A soak is used to apply moisture through immersion of a body part. A sitz bath is a way of providing heat to the perineal and rectal areas. Both are applied in healthcare settings as well as in the home.

ICE COLLAR/ICE PACK

An ice collar is a long, narrow bag made of rubber, plastic, or some other material that is moisture-proof. Some are made to be disposable; others are reusable. Some ice collars come with ties attached to make it easier to keep them in place. These devices are designed for use around the neck but can be used for other small areas of the body as well. An ice-filled glove may also be used as a substitute ice pack.

When a patient needs to continue cold packs at home on a short-term basis, a zippered plastic bag can be used. Simply place crushed ice or ice cubes and a small amount of water in a bag of the appropriate size, remove excess air, and zip shut. Cover with a light clean cloth and apply. A 16-oz bag of frozen peas or cut corn instead of ice also works well as an emergency cold pack and molds nicely to curved areas.

GENERAL PROCEDURE FOR APPLYING HEAT OR COLD

There is a general approach you can use to apply heat or cold. It can be modified as necessary according to the type of device being used.

ASSESSMENT

1. Check the order for the specific type of heat or cold treatment ordered. **R:** A physician's order is needed for heat and cold treatments.
2. Assess the patient:
   a. Assess the general condition of the patient, noting especially age, diagnosis, circulatory status, sensory perception in the area to be treated, level of awareness, and amount of body fat (areas with little body fat are more sensitive to external applications of heat and cold). **R:** To note any problems or concerns that may need to be resolved before beginning the procedure.
   b. Assess the vital signs. **R:** Vital signs provide baseline information for comparison.
   c. Assess the local site, noting especially the condition and color of the skin. **R:** This also provides

a baseline so that you will be able to identify changes.
   d. If the treatment has been given before, check the chart, or ask the patient for the patient's response to the preceding treatment. **R:** To help determine previous effectiveness of the treatment.
   e. Check the patient's room to see what equipment is already there and the space available for any temperature treatment device. **R:** To facilitate carrying out the procedure.

ANALYSIS

3. Critically think through your data, carefully evaluating each aspect and its relation to other data. **R:** To determine specific problems for this individual in relation to the specific heat or cold treatment ordered.
4. Identify specific problems and modifications of the procedure needed for this individual. **R:** Planning for the individual must take into consideration the individual's problems.

PLANNING

5. Determine individualized patient outcomes in relation to the specific application of heat or cold. Include the following as appropriate. **R:** Identification of outcomes guides planning and evaluation.
   a. Signs or symptoms of underlying problem are decreased.
   b. Patient states he or she is comfortable.
   c. No adverse outcomes result from the treatment.
6. Obtain the heating or cooling device you will use and any other supplies you will need. Some of the less complex heating and cooling devices are located on the nursing unit; others may be obtained from the Central Supply Department. **R:** Planning ahead allows you to proceed more efficiently and effectively.

IMPLEMENTATION

Action	Rationale
7. Wash or disinfect your hands.	To decrease the transfer of microorganisms that could cause infection.
8. Obtain assistance if needed.	To save time and promote efficiency.
9. Identify the patient, using two identifiers.	Verifying the patient's identity helps you be sure that you are performing the right procedure for the right patient.
10. Close the door to the room and pull the curtain around the bed.	To protect the patient's modesty.

(continued)

Action	Rationale
11. Explain to the patient what you plan to do, giving particular attention to the length of time the heat or cold application will be left in place and any condition about which the patient should notify you, such as any discomfort.	Explaining the procedure helps relieve anxiety or misperceptions that the patient may have about a procedure or activity and sets the stage for patient participation.
12. Raise the bed to an appropriate working position based on your height.	To allow you to use correct body mechanics and protect yourself from back injury.
13. Position the patient so that the heating or cooling device can be placed directly over the area to be treated. Expose only the area to be treated, uncovering as little of the rest of the patient's body as possible. If there is a dressing in place, remove it, using gloves if necessary.	To provide maximum therapeutic effect with minimum exposure of the patient's body. Use gloves to protect yourself from exposure to body fluids.
14. Place the specific heating or cooling device over the area to be treated, molding it to that area as closely as possible. Secure it in place appropriately.	So the device will remain directly over the area to be treated and so that it will have the maximum therapeutic effect.
15. Place the call signal where the patient can reach it easily to alert the nurse to any discomfort.	So that the patient can call for help if needed and to ensure minimum untoward effects.
16. Check the patient after the first 5 minutes and at least once during the remainder of the treatment.	To check for therapeutic or adverse effects and to be sure that the heating or cooling device is still placed properly.
17. Remove the heating or cooling device at the end of the ordered time or at a maximum of 20 to 30 minutes, if no length of time has been specified.	The desired effect of heat or cold therapy can be reversed if the heating or cooling device is left in place too long.
18. Examine the treated area.	Assess for pain, cyanosis, pallor, or irritation not present when treatment was initiated.
19. Replace any linen or clothing removed earlier. If a dressing was removed, replace it, using gloves if necessary. Leave the patient comfortable, warm, and dry.	To ensure that comfort and safety are maintained.
20. Lower the bed.	To promote safety.
21. Remove gloves if worn, and wash or disinfect your hands.	To decrease the transfer of microorganisms that could cause infection.

EVALUATION

22. Evaluate using the individualized patient outcomes previously identified, including the following. **R:** Evaluation in relation to desired outcomes is essential for planning future care.
    a. Signs or symptoms of underlying problem are decreased.
    b. Patient states he or she is comfortable.
    c. No adverse outcomes result from the treatment.

DOCUMENTATION

23. Document the treatment and the area treated as well as the length of time applied and the patient's response on the patient's record. **R:** Documentation

is a legal record of the patient's care and therapy and communicates nursing activities to other nurses and caregivers.

POTENTIAL ADVERSE OUTCOMES AND RELATED INTERVENTIONS

1. Patient complains of discomfort from heat treatment.
Intervention: Discontinue treatment. Assess skin at treatment site. Check with physician if necessary to reduce temperature or length of treatment.

2. Redness, tenderness, or blistering at treatment site at end of heat treatment.
Intervention: Report to physician. Assess skin for breakdown not present at beginning of treatment. Apply topical medication and dressing to area as ordered.

3. Patient complains of discomfort from cold treatment.
Intervention: Discontinue treatment. Assess skin at treatment site. Check with physician if necessary to increase temperature or reduce length of treatment.

4. Skin is mottled, dark red, or cyanotic at treatment site at end of the cold treatment.
Intervention: Report to physician. Assess skin for breakdown not present at beginning of treatment. Place treated area in dependent position if possible. Cover with a warm, light blanket.

SPECIFIC PROCEDURES FOR APPLYING HEAT

Applying a Warm, Moist Compress

A warm, moist compress provides moist heat to a specified area of the body.

ASSESSMENT

1-2. Follow steps 1 and 2 of the General Procedure: Check the order, and assess the patient (general condition, vital signs, local site, response to preceding treatment, and patient's room for equipment and space).

ANALYSIS

3-4. Follow steps 3 and 4 of the General Procedure: Think through your data, and identify specific problems and modifications.

PLANNING

5. Follow step 5 of the General Procedure: Determine individualized patient outcomes for the warm, moist compress.
   a. Signs or symptoms of underlying problem are decreased.
   b. Patient states he or she is comfortable.
   c. No adverse outcomes result from the treatment.
6. Obtain the material to be used for the compress.
   a. aquathermia pad or other heating device to maintain the heat of the compress, if necessary
   b. sterile procedure: Use sterile material (including sterile basin, sterile solution, and sterile gloves) and technique as necessary. Premoistened sterile compresses are available commercially. Follow package directions to heat the compress.
   c. clean procedure: A washcloth is commonly used when a small nonsterile compress is needed; a towel can be used for a larger area.
   d. plastic to cover the exterior of the warm pack; this may be in rolls of plastic wrap to cover clean packs. A moisture-resistant bed pad may also be used. Some sterile dressing materials have a moisture-proof exterior on one side.

IMPLEMENTATION

Action	Rationale
7-13. Follow steps 7 to 13 of the General Procedure: Wash or disinfect your hands and put on sterile gloves if necessary; obtain assistance if needed; identify the patient (two identifiers); close the door and pull the curtain around the bed; explain what you plan to do; raise the bed to an appropriate working position; position the patient, exposing only the area to be treated; and remove dressing if necessary.	

(continued)

Action	Rationale
14. Apply the warm, moist compress:	
a. Place a moisture-proof pad under the area to be treated.	To protect the bed from moisture.
b. Moisten the compress in hot water (105° to 115°F [40.5° to 46.1°C]) unless otherwise ordered and wring it out. The compress should remain moist but not dripping. In any event, the temperature of the compress should not be hotter than 115°F (46.1°C).	To keep surroundings dry. To prevent injury.
c. Apply the compress directly over the area to be treated.	To provide maximum therapeutic effect.
d. Cover the compress with plastic, and then cover with further insulation, such as a towel.	To protect the bed and to maintain the temperature of the compress.
e. Place a water-flow heating pad or other heating device on the outside, if necessary.	To maintain a constant temperature for the entire treatment.
f. Hold the compress, towel, and/or water-flow heating pad in place with ties or a gauze wrap.	The device needs to remain directly over the area to be treated so that it will have maximum therapeutic effect.
15-21. Follow steps 15 to 21 of the General Procedure: Place the call signal where the patient can reach it; check the patient after the first 5 minutes and at least once more; remove the compress; examine the treated area; replace any linen, clothing, or dressing removed earlier; lower the bed; remove gloves if worn; and wash or disinfect your hands.	

EVALUATION

22. Follow step 22 of the General Procedure: Evaluate using the individualized patient outcomes previously identified: Signs or symptoms of underlying problem are decreased, patient states he or she is comfortable, and no adverse outcomes result from the treatment.

DOCUMENTATION

23. Follow step 23 of the General Procedure: Document the treatment and the area treated as well as the length of time applied and the patient's response, including any adverse outcomes.

Administering a Soak

When a soak is administered, the specified body part is immersed in a solution. A soak is usually warm to provide moist heat.

ASSESSMENT

1-2. Follow steps 1 and 2 of the General Procedure: Check the order, and assess the patient (general condition, vital signs, local site, response to preceding treatment, and patient's room for equipment and space).

ANALYSIS

3-4. Follow steps 3 and 4 of the General Procedure: Think through your data, and identify specific problems and modifications.

PLANNING

5. Follow step 5 of the General Procedure: Determine individualized desired outcomes for the soak:

a. Signs or symptoms of underlying problem are decreased.

b. Patient states he or she is comfortable.

c. No adverse outcomes result from the treatment.

6. Obtain a basin. If a wound is involved, use sterile material (including sterile basin, sterile solution, and sterile gloves) and technique as necessary.

IMPLEMENTATION

Action	Rationale
7-13. Follow steps 7 to 13 of the General Procedure: Wash or disinfect your hands, and put on sterile gloves if necessary; obtain assistance if needed; identify the patient (two identifiers); close the door and pull the curtain around the bed; explain what you plan to do; raise the bed to an appropriate working position; position the patient, exposing only the area to be treated; and remove dressing if necessary.	
14. Administer the soak.	
a. Fill the basin half full with water, saline, or the medicated solution that has been ordered. The temperature of the water or solution is usually between 104°F (40°C) and 113.9°F (45.5°C), unless otherwise ordered. Remove the soaking body part from the basin if the solution cools to the extent that it becomes necessary to replace some of it with warmer solution. Before replacing the body part in the solution, measure the temperature of the solution to be sure it is not above 113.9°F (45.5°C).	To allow room for the body part to be soaked and for safety and maximum therapeutic effect.
b. Place a moisture-proof pad under the body part being treated if necessary. Place the basin on the pad.	To protect the bed or other surface where the basin will be placed.
c. Slowly place the body part to be treated into the basin. The duration of a soak is usually 15 to 20 minutes.	The body part needs to adjust to the temperature of the solution.
d. Make sure that the rest of the body is in good alignment and that there is no pressure on the part from the edge of the basin. You may need to pad the	To provide for comfort during the soak.

(continued)

Action	Rationale
edge of the basin with a towel to prevent pressure.	
15-21. Follow steps 15 to 21 of the General Procedure: Place the call signal where the patient can reach it; check the patient after the first 5 minutes and at least once more; remove the body part from the basin and gently pat it dry; examine the treated area; replace any linen, clothing, or dressing removed earlier; lower the bed; remove gloves if worn; and wash or disinfect your hands.	

EVALUATION

22. Follow step 22 of the General Procedure: Evaluate using the individualized patient outcomes previously identified: Signs or symptoms of underlying problem are decreased, patient states he or she is comfortable, and no adverse outcomes result from the treatment.

DOCUMENTATION

23. Follow step 23 of the General Procedure: Document the treatment and the area treated as well as the length of time applied and the patient's response. Include any adverse outcomes.

Administering a Sitz Bath

A sitz bath is a method of administering a soak to the perineal area. Disposable equipment that can be used on a toilet is used commonly (Fig. 38-3). Some facilities have special tubs or portable chairs designed for the purpose. These require meticulous cleaning and disinfection between use by different patients. Unless otherwise specified, the temperature of the water should be between 104°F (40°C) and 113.9°F (45.5°C), and the treatment should last 15 to 20 minutes.

ASSESSMENT

1-2. Follow steps 1 and 2 of the General Procedure: Check the order, and assess the patient (general condition, vital signs, local site, response to preceding treatment, and patient's room for equipment and space).

ANALYSIS

3-4. Follow steps 3 and 4 of the General Procedure: Think through your data, and identify specific problems and modifications.

PLANNING

5. Follow step 5 of the General Procedure: Determine individualized patient outcomes for the sitz bath:
   a. Signs or symptoms of underlying problem are decreased.
   b. Patient states he or she is comfortable.
   c. No adverse outcomes result from the treatment.

6. Gather the sitz bath equipment. In addition to the equipment for the bath itself, you will need a bath blanket and one or more towels. Place the bath blanket over the patient's shoulders to provide warmth and use the towel to dry the patient at the end of the treatment. Additional towels may be needed to pad the tub or chair to relieve pressure or to assist with body alignment.

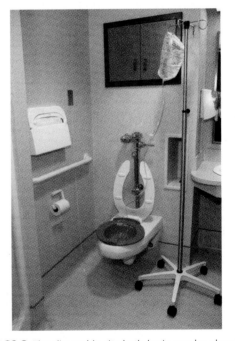

FIGURE 38-3 The disposable sitz bath basin can be placed on the toilet in a healthcare facility or in the home.

IMPLEMENTATION

Action	Rationale
7-9. Follow steps 7 to 9 of the General Procedure: Wash or disinfect your hands and put on gloves if necessary; obtain assistance if needed; identify the patient (two identifiers).	
10. Escort the patient to the bathroom where the sitz bath will be administered.	Most sitz baths are performed in the bathroom for access to water and the toilet for emptying the sitz bath.
11. Close the door to the room where the sitz bath is being administered.	To provide privacy.
12. Explain what you plan to do.	To facilitate the patient's cooperation.
13. Administer the sitz bath.	
a. Prepare the sitz bath. The water temperature should be between 104°F (40°C) and 113.9°F (45.5°C).	Accurate measurement of water temperature is necessary for safety and comfort.
(1) Disposable sitz bath: Place the disposable sitz bath on the toilet. Fill the attached bag with warm water of the desired temperature and hang it higher than the toilet. The water flows gradually into the basin, displacing the cooler water and maintaining a relatively constant temperature.	
(2) For a tub bath: Assist the patient to the tub room or bathroom. If the room is some distance away, assistive devices may be needed. Fill the tub or sitz bath chair with enough water to cover the area to be treated.	
(3) For a sitz bath chair: Move the chair to the bedside. Use a pitcher to fill it with warm water.	
b. Remove the patient's clothing as necessary and place the bath blanket over the patient's shoulders.	To provide for modesty and warmth.
c. Assist the patient into the tub or chair, providing padding as necessary.	To minimize pressure and to provide for good body alignment.
14. Place the call signal where the patient can reach it easily.	The patient can use the call signal to ask for help if needed.

(continued)

Action	Rationale
15. Return to the patient frequently during treatment. Monitor blood pressure and pulse after 5 minutes for hypotension, which could lead to dizziness or fainting. If the patient's condition warrants (first postoperative day, extremely fatigued or weak patient), stay in the room for the first 5 minutes or for the entire treatment.	To ensure safety.
16. Assist the patient out of tub or chair and dry the entire body.	For safety and comfort.
17. Help the patient to dress and return to room or bed.	To promote modesty, comfort, and safety.
18. Wash or disinfect your hands.	To decrease the transfer of microorganisms that could cause infection.

EVALUATION

19. Evaluate using the individualized patient outcomes previously identified: Signs or symptoms of underlying problem are decreased, patient states he or she is comfortable, and no adverse outcomes result from the treatment.

DOCUMENTATION

20. Document the treatment and the area treated, the length of treatment, and the patient's response including any adverse outcomes.

SPECIFIC PROCEDURES FOR APPLYING COLD

Applying an Ice Pack or Cold Pack

ASSESSMENT

1-2. Follow steps 1 and 2 of the General Procedure: Check the order, and assess the patient (general condition, vital signs, local site, response to preceding treatment, and the patient's room for equipment and space).

ANALYSIS

3-4. Follow steps 3 and 4 of the General Procedure: Think through your data, and identify specific problems and modifications.

PLANNING

5. Follow step 5 of the General Procedure: Determine individualized patient outcomes for the ice pack or cold pack.
   a. Signs or symptoms of underlying problem are decreased.
   b. Patient states he or she is comfortable.
   c. No adverse outcomes result from the treatment.
6. Obtain the materials to be used. Consider the size and shape of the area to be treated, the need for insulation, and the cold packs available in your facility. If you are using a commercially available pack, follow package directions carefully. Obtain a water-flow cold-therapy system to maintain the temperature of the pack, if necessary.

IMPLEMENTATION

Action	Rationale
7-13. Follow steps 7 to 13 of the General Procedure: Wash or disinfect your hands, and put on sterile gloves if necessary; obtain assistance if needed; identify the patient (two identifiers); close the door and pull the curtain around the bed;	*(continued)*

Action	Rationale
explain what you plan to do; raise the bed to an appropriate working position; position the patient, exposing only the area to be treated; and remove dressing if necessary.	
14. Apply the ice pack or cold pack.	
a. Place a moisture-proof pad under the area to be treated.	To protect the bed from moisture.
b. Apply the ice pack or cold pack directly over the area to be treated. If there is no dressing in place or other covering over the area, protect it with a wash-cloth, towel, or gauze wrap.	For comfort and safety and for maximum therapeutic effect.
c. Cover the compress with plastic, and then cover with further insulation, such as a towel, if necessary.	To protect the bed and to maintain the temperature of the pack.
d. Place a water-flow cold-therapy device on the outside, if necessary.	To maintain a constant temperature for the entire treatment.
e. Hold the compress, towel, and/or water-flow cold-therapy pad in place with ties or a gauze wrap.	To keep the device directly over the area to be treated, to promote maximum therapeutic effect, and to prevent puncturing the water-flow cold-therapy pad if used.
15-21. Follow steps 15 to 21 of the General Procedure: Place the call signal where the patient can reach it; check the patient after the first 5 minutes and at least once more; remove the cold pack after 15 to 20 minutes; examine the treated area; replace any linen, clothing, or dressing removed earlier; lower the bed; remove gloves if worn; and wash or disinfect your hands.	

EVALUATION

22. Follow step 22 of the General Procedure: Evaluate using the individualized patient outcomes previously identified: signs or symptoms of underlying problem are decreased, patient states he or she is comfortable, and no adverse outcomes result from the treatment.

DOCUMENTATION

23. Follow step 23 of the General Procedure: Document the treatment and the area treated as well as the length of time applied and the patient's response, including any adverse outcomes.

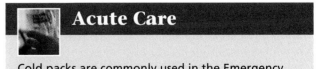

Acute Care

Cold packs are commonly used in the Emergency Department to decrease swelling and pain after acute orthopedic injuries. They are also used postoperatively following orthopedic surgeries.

Sitz baths, compresses, and soaks are also used for the patient with inflammation of an area as are water-flow heating and cooling pads and blankets for systemic warming and cooling.

Long-Term Care

In long-term care settings, it is not uncommon for heat or cold to be applied to relieve discomfort. Many older residents may have treated arthritic pain with heat even before they entered the facility and may wish to continue. Depending on the facility's policy, a physician's order may be needed.

The application of heat or cold poses increased risks for older persons because of changes in the skin, circulation, sensation, and perception. For example, prolonged exposure to heat or cold may damage the skin. Narrowed blood vessels and decreased cardiac output can intensify or localize heat to a given area because of the body's declining ability to dissipate the heat within the circulatory system. Of particular concern is the resident's decreased awareness of the degree of heat or cold being applied because of the decreased number of skin receptors. Therefore, apply heat or cold for only short periods, assess the resident frequently, and determine the safety of the procedure.

Home Care

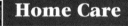

Many people have some type of device available at home for applying heat or cold. Some common devices include hot water bags (or bottles), electric heating pads, and various types of cold packs. All of the risks that exist in healthcare settings also are present in the home. A client of any age can sustain an injury if the procedure is misused. Also, clients may fail to seek medical consultation when the "home remedy" of heat or cold application has previously been successful.

Safety must be observed by the client, family members, or home care nurse. Electrical cords and outlets should be in good repair. Heat or ice should never be applied directly to the skin. Caution clients and caregivers to apply heat or cold treatments for no longer than 20 to 30 minutes and no more frequently than every 2 hours (Stitik & Nadler, 1999, 1998). Above all, conscientious and frequent assessments should be made.

Ambulatory Care

Applications of heat and cold are also commonly seen in ambulatory care settings. Clients may come in specifically for such a treatment, or it may be administered in response to an acute injury or illness. In any event, you may be responsible for teaching the client and/or family member how to safely administer the treatment at home. Of particular importance is information regarding assessments to make before and after the treatment is applied.

LEARNING TOOLS

DEVELOP YOUR BACKGROUND KNOWLEDGE

1. Review the Learning Outcomes.

2. Read the section on heat production, heat loss, and hypothermia in your assigned text.

3. Look up the Key Terms in the glossary.

4. Review this module and mentally practice the techniques described. Study so that you would be able to teach these skills to another person.

DEVELOP YOUR SKILLS

5. With a partner in the practice setting
   a. Prepare a warm, moist compress, and apply it to the inner aspect of your partner's forearm, protecting the bed and the "patient" from the moisture. Do this as a clean procedure (using medical asepsis).
   b. Reverse roles and repeat step a as a sterile procedure (using sterile technique).
   c. Evaluate one another's performance.
   d. Prepare an ice collar, pack, or glove, and apply and secure it to your partner's knee. Have your partner move around to see whether the pack stays in place.
   e. Reverse roles and repeat step d.
   f. Evaluate one another's performance.

DEMONSTRATE YOUR SKILLS

6. In the clinical setting
   a. Seek opportunities to observe the use of a water-flow heating/cold-therapy pad with control unit and a thermal blanket.
   b. Apply hot and cold treatments with supervision.
   c. Evaluate your performance with the instructor.

CRITICAL THINKING EXERCISES

1. Your patient, Mr. S., has a reddened intravenous site. The intravenous infusion has been discontinued, and the physician has ordered a hot pack to the area. Determine what assessment you will carry out. What physiologic benefits does the application of heat provide? Identify the hazards that exist in the application of heat and describe nursing actions that can prevent any untoward response. List the outcomes that you expect and that can be used for your evaluation.

2. J. B., a 16-year-old girl, sprained her ankle playing softball. The doctor has written orders for her to apply ice packs to the sprained ankle three or four times daily. What will you include in your instructions to her? What observations will you tell her to make before and after the ice pack applications?

SELF-QUIZ
SHORT-ANSWER QUESTIONS

1. List three principles to consider to safely apply heat and cold treatments.

   a. _____

   b. _____

   c. _____

2. What three items should be included in the documentation of a heat or cold treatment?

   a. _____

   b. _____

   c. _____

MULTIPLE CHOICE

_____ 3. The body's temperature receptors, which register sensations of warmth or coolness, are found in the
   a. skin.
   b. walls of internal organs.
   c. cortex of the brain.
   d. deep muscles.

_____ 4. Which of the following is the most important nursing diagnosis to use when applying heat or cold to the patient?
   a. Ineffective Thermoregulation
   b. Ineffective Individual Coping
   c. Risk for Injury
   d. Hyperthermia

_____ 5. Which of the following persons can best tolerate heat or cold with the fewest precautions?
   a. Elderly persons
   b. Infants
   c. Otherwise healthy adults
   d. Persons with circulatory problems

_____ 6. Heat causes blood vessels to
   a. constrict.
   b. dilate.
   c. become inflamed.
   d. become more elastic.

_____ 7. Heat reduces edema because
   a. it increases diaphoresis.
   b. output is increased.
   c. fluid is more easily absorbed.
   d. it increases the number of blood vessels to the part.

_____ 8. The application of cold can also decrease edema through which of the following actions?
   a. Increasing circulation
   b. Slowing circulation
   c. Narrowing capillaries
   d. Producing "shivering"

_____ 9. A sitz bath is generally administered for
   a. 5 to 10 minutes.
   b. 15 to 20 minutes.
   c. 30 to 40 minutes.
   d. 1 hour.

Answers to the Self-Quiz questions appear in the back of the book.

Administering Ear and Eye Irrigations

SKILLS INCLUDED IN THIS MODULE

General Procedure for Administering an Irrigation
Specific Irrigation Procedures
   Procedure for Ear Irrigation
   Procedure for Eye Irrigation

PREREQUISITE MODULES

Module 1	An Approach to Nursing Skills
Module 2	Documentation
Module 3	Basic Body Mechanics
Module 4	Basic Infection Control
Module 5	Safety in the Healthcare Environment

The following may be needed for some irrigations:

Module 6	Moving the Patient in Bed and Positioning
Module 24	Basic Sterile Technique: Sterile Field and Sterile Gloves
Module 45	Administering Medications by Alternative Routes

Note:
- Catheter/Bladder Irrigations are found in Module 27, Assisting the Patient Who Requires Urinary Catheterization.
- Nasogastric Tube Irrigation is found in Module 29, Inserting and Maintaining a Nasogastric Tube.

KEY TERMS

canthus	instill
cerumen	irrigant
concentration of	irrigate
solution	pinna
exudate	

OVERALL OBJECTIVES

▸ To know the purpose of a specific eye and ear irrigation.
▸ To plan the correct technique needed to accomplish that purpose.
▸ To carry out the irrigation safely and correctly.

LEARNING OUTCOMES

The student will be able to

1. Assess the patient effectively to determine the need for a specific irrigation.
2. Analyze assessment data to determine special problems or concerns that must be addressed to safely and successfully carry out a specific type of irrigation for the patient.
3. Determine appropriate patient outcomes of the specific irrigation procedure and recognize the potential adverse outcomes.
4. Determine the need for assistance to carry out the specific irrigation for the specific patient.
5. Position the patient correctly and effectively for the irrigation.
6. Carry out ear and eye irrigations, using appropriate equipment and the correct irrigating solution.
7. Evaluate the effectiveness of the irrigation for the specific patient.
8. Document the irrigation in the patient's record and on the patient's plan of care.

Generally, irrigations are done for two purposes. The first is to clean a passage or body area. The second is to **instill** medication. Small or large amounts of solution can be used to remove secretions, small clots, foreign material, and microorganisms. The solution used (the **irrigant**) may be one that simply flushes particles away or may contain special cleansing agents. A medication is given to exert a therapeutic effect such as antibacterial activity or as a soothing agent. Sometimes an irrigation serves both purposes at the same time (see Module 45, Administering Medications by Alternative Routes, regarding instilling medications).

Irrigations are usually specific to the needs of the patient and are usually ordered by the physician as part of medical therapy. Alternatively, nurses may initiate irrigations based on standing orders or protocols. There are many similarities in the way irrigations of ears and eyes are done, but the differences are critical. The nurse must be able to plan an appropriate procedure and to carry it out correctly.

NURSING DIAGNOSES

A number of nursing diagnoses may suggest the need for an irrigation. Examples are

- Disturbed Sensory Perception: Auditory as evidenced by decreased hearing related to accumulation of **cerumen** (earwax) in ear canals.
- Risk for Injury: Eye (specify), related to presence of small foreign body.

DELEGATION

Eye and ear irrigations are rarely delegated to assistive personnel. Eye irrigations require sterile technique and, therefore, are not delegated to assistive personnel. Assessment of the ear before an ear irrigation is done is critical and must be done by the physician or nurse caring for the patient. Irrigation procedures may be taught to patients or family members for use at home. In planning for this, the nurse must keep in mind the home environment and the differences in setting and equipment.

ASEPSIS

Sterile technique must be used for irrigations on any area of the body that is normally sterile. While the eyes are not normally sterile, sterile technique is also used for irrigations involving the eye because of the potential for serious injury from even a minor eye infection. Clean technique is used for irrigations of the ear.

SAFETY

The nurse wears clean gloves when performing most irrigations to provide protection from the patient's body secretions. Sterile gloves are worn when it is necessary to touch sterile equipment for irrigating the eye. A moisture-resistant gown or apron is needed if irrigant might come in contact with the nurse's uniform. Eye protection (goggles or face shield) is essential if there is potential for splashing irrigant into the eyes.

Most body tissue is sensitive to excessive pressure. Because fluid under pressure can cause actual tissue damage to a structure as sensitive as the eye, use gentle pressure only. If the patient feels discomfort, reduce the pressure. Remember that by decreasing the height of the container, you decrease the pressure.

Medications or chemicals may also irritate or cause tissue reaction. This is especially true if the wrong concentration is used for a particular tissue. Remember that the specific ingredients ordered at the correct strength or concentration must be accurate. Therefore, carefully check both the type and the **concentration of solution** used to make sure they are correct.

Many irrigations are done with solutions at room temperature. To increase the patient's comfort, you may need to warm solutions to body temperature. Do not use extreme temperatures, however. Very high temperatures can burn tissues. Low temperatures can produce a chilling or even a shock-like reaction as the body attempts to maintain homeostasis.

If medications are being instilled by irrigation, follow the directions in Module 45, Administering Medications by Alternative Routes.

GENERAL PROCEDURE FOR ADMINISTERING AN IRRIGATION

ASSESSMENT

1. Check the order to verify the following:
   a. Type of irrigation ordered to be sure you are carrying out the irrigation on the correct area. **R:** If you must **irrigate** an ear or eye, it is essential for you to know whether the irrigation is ordered for the right or for the left ear or eye or for both. If the order is unclear, you have a responsibility to clarify this before proceeding. Abbreviations for right eye (o.d.) and left eye (o.s.) or both eyes (o.u.) that were formerly used are no longer permitted in facilities because they were the source of confusion and errors. On occasion, these unclear abbreviations may be used. In these cases, always verify the correct eye with the prescriber by getting a specific designation of left eye or right eye or both eyes.
   b. Type, concentration, amount, and temperature of solution ordered. **R:** This information is needed to promote safety and maximum therapeutic effect.
2. Check the chart to determine whether the irrigation ordered has been done previously. Note any specifics about how the procedure was carried out and the patient's response to it. **R:** Checking the chart helps to facilitate continuity of care.

3. Assess what the patient knows about the procedure. **R:** Understanding what to expect will allow the patient to participate in his or her own care to the fullest extent.

ANALYSIS

4. Critically think through your data, carefully evaluating each aspect and its relation to other data. **R:** This enables you to determine specific problems for this individual in relation to the specific irrigation to be done.
5. Identify specific problems and modifications of the procedure needed for this individual. **R:** Planning for the individual must take into consideration the individual's problems.

PLANNING

6. Determine individualized patient outcomes for the specific irrigation procedure, including the following. **R:** Identification of outcomes guides planning and evaluation.
   a. Signs or symptoms of underlying problem are decreased.
   b. Patient expresses comfort.
7. Decide whether the irrigation is to be clean or sterile. **R:** Eye irrigations are always carried out using sterile technique, whereas ear irrigations may be done with clean technique.
8. Identify and gather the equipment needed for the specific irrigation, including the following.
   a. Solution. Check to ensure that the correct solution in the correct concentration and amount at the correct temperature is used. Use three checks for safety.
   b. Irrigating device. This may be specified in the physician's order. If not, use the equipment specified by your facility policy. **R:** The device determines your ability to direct the stream of fluid and the pressure that can be generated for instilling the fluid.
   c. Receptacle to contain used irrigating fluid
   d. Protective padding (towels or disposable waterproof pads). The padding will keep the patient and the environment dry.

   e. Clean or sterile gloves. **R:** Gloves protect you from contact with body secretions. It is also important to protect the patient from microorganisms that you may harbor in small cracks in your skin or on a minor abrasion. Sterile gloves are worn when sterile equipment must be touched.
   f. Gown or apron and eye protection if needed. Add these items to your supplies if there is potential for irrigant to splash or contact your uniform. **R:** This equipment protects you and your uniform from contamination, and planning ahead allows you to proceed more safely and effectively.

IMPLEMENTATION

Action	Rationale
9. Wash or disinfect your hands.	To decrease the transfer of microorganisms that could cause infection.
10. Obtain any needed supportive devices or assistance for the specific irrigation.	To save time and promote efficiency.
11. Identify the patient, using two identifiers.	Verifying the patient's identity helps ensure that you are performing the right skill for the right patient.
12. Close the door and pull the curtain around the bed as appropriate.	To provide privacy.
13. Explain the procedure you are about to perform.	Explaining the procedure helps relieve anxiety or misperceptions that the patient may have about a procedure or activity and sets the stage for patient participation.
14. Raise the bed to an appropriate working position based on your height.	To allow you to use correct body mechanics and protect yourself from back injury.
15. Position the patient as needed for the irrigation.	To facilitate the successful implementation of the irrigation.
16. Place protective padding where needed.	To protect the patient, his or her garments, and the environment.
17. Put on gloves and other protective garb needed.	To protect your uniform and your eyes from irrigant.
18. Carry out the irrigation according to the specific procedure outlined below.	
19. Make sure the patient is dry and comfortable.	To leave the patient feeling relaxed and able to rest.
20. Lower the bed.	To protect the patient.
21. Care for the used equipment, following the policy of your facility.	If the equipment is reusable, you may have to wash it thoroughly or return it to the Central Supply Department for processing. If it is disposable, discard according to your facility's policy.
22. Remove gloves if worn, and wash or disinfect your hands.	To decrease the transfer of microorganisms that could cause infection.

EVALUATION

23. Evaluate using the individualized patient outcomes previously identified.
   a. Signs or symptoms of underlying problem are decreased.
   b. Patient expresses comfort.

DOCUMENTATION

24. Document the following on a flow sheet, in the nursing care record, and/or on the nursing care plan. **R:** Documentation is a legal record of the patient's care and communicates nursing activities to other nurses and caregivers.

a. Type of irrigation
b. Type, concentration, amount, and temperature of solution used
c. Appearance of any secretions or drainage
d. Response of the patient, including comfort and any adverse outcomes

POTENTIAL ADVERSE OUTCOMES AND RELATED INTERVENTIONS

1. The patient experiences pain or discomfort from the irrigation.

Intervention: Stop the procedure and reassess the patient. Determine the cause of the pain if possible. Check to be sure that the correct irrigant is being used and that it is neither too warm nor too cold. If the pain is due to too much pressure, decrease the pressure (sometimes this is done by lowering the fluid container). Contact the physician if necessary.

SPECIFIC PROCEDURES FOR IRRIGATION

Procedure for Ear Irrigation

Before an ear can be irrigated, it must be examined with an otoscope to check the tympanic membrane. This may have been done by the physician, but if not, you should do it. If the tympanic membrane (eardrum) is not intact, do not irrigate the ear. The fluid could enter the middle ear and cause an infection. You should also inspect the **pinna** and the external ear canal for signs of infection, open areas, cerumen, or foreign objects.

An ear irrigation is most often used to remove cerumen or a foreign object in the ear. If an organic foreign body such as a bean or an insect is suspected, do not irrigate. The object may absorb the irrigating solution and swell, making it more difficult to remove.

An ear syringe is usually used to instill the fluid, although in some settings, you may find a commercial "ear wash" system. These devices are designed for cerumen removal and do not deliver pressures above a safe level. Because of the danger of injury to the eardrum or tissue of the ear canal from the hard dental tips, use of an oral water pressure device, commercially known as a Water Pik, is not recommended unless it has a special tip designed for earwax removal.

ASSESSMENT

1-3. Follow steps 1 to 3 of the General Procedure: Check the type of irrigation ordered and the type, concentration, amount, and temperature of the solution ordered; check whether the irrigation has been done previously; and assess what the patient knows about the procedure.

ANALYSIS

4-5. Follow steps 4 and 5 of the General Procedure: Think through your data, and identify specific problems and modifications.

PLANNING

6. Determine individualized patient outcomes of the ear irrigation, including the following. **R:** Identification of outcomes guides planning and evaluation.
   a. Cerumen or foreign object in the ear canal is removed.
   b. Patient states pain or discomfort is minimized.
7. Plan for clean technique. **R:** The ear is not a sterile environment and no open tissue is present.
8. Identify and gather the equipment needed for the ear irrigation, including the following.
   a. Solution ordered (commonly normal saline or water). For ear irrigations, the solution is warmed to body temperature. **R:** The solution does not need to be sterile but must be warmed because cold fluid striking the eardrum may cause dizziness and nausea.
   b. Irrigating device (usually a rubber bulb syringe) or a commercial ear wash device to deliver the solution or irrigant
   c. Basin or emesis basin to catch the used irrigating fluid. The shape of the emesis basin makes it ideal for this purpose (Fig. 39-1).
   d. Towels or other protective padding to protect the patient and the surroundings
   e. Clean gloves to protect you from contact with body secretions
   f. Gown or apron or eye protection if a Water Pik or other ear wash system is in use; these instruments provide higher pressure that is more likely to splash widely. **R:** Having all needed supplies available in advance will facilitate the procedure proceeding quickly and smoothly, with minimal disturbance to the patient.

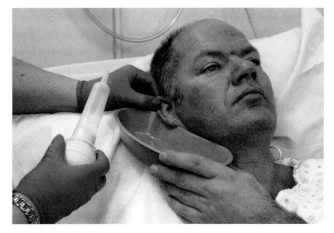

FIGURE 39-1 Equipment for ear irrigation: bulb syringe and emesis basin.

IMPLEMENTATION

Action	Rationale
9-14. Follow steps 9 to 14 of the General Procedure: Wash or disinfect your hands; obtain any needed supportive devices or assistance; identify the patient, using two identifiers; close the door and pull curtain around the bed; explain the procedure (especially the need to remain still during the irrigation); and raise the bed to an appropriate working position.	
15. Position the patient sitting or lying with the head tilted slightly forward and away from the side to be irrigated.	To make the ear accessible.
16. Place protective padding over the patient's shoulder.	To keep the patient dry because fluid from the ear is likely to drain onto the shoulder.
17. Put on clean gloves. (If a Water Pik or other ear wash system is used, eye protection and a gown are needed.)	This is for protection from exposure to body secretions.
18. Irrigate the ear as follows:	
a. Place the basin under the patient's ear. The patient may be able to hold the basin in place.	To collect the used irrigating solution.
b. Fill the syringe or other irrigating device with irrigating solution.	To be prepared to irrigate.
c. Straighten the ear canal, using the method appropriate for the patient's age. For an adult, pull the pinna upward and back. For a child, pull the pinna downward and back.	If a foreign body is lodged in the ear, straightening the canal may allow the object to fall out or to be removed easily. Straightening is accomplished by pulling the pinna in the direction of the canal, which in a child is more horizontal and in an adult is at a greater angle. Straightening also allows the irrigating solution to flow in more easily.
d. Direct the tip of the syringe toward the top of the patient's ear canal (Fig. 39-2), so that a circular current is set up with fluid flowing in along the top and out along the bottom.	With this action, cerumen or foreign material will be irrigated out.

Safety Alert *Be careful! Severe discomfort and dizziness can result from fluid directed onto the eardrum. Cold fluid increases the chance of adverse effects. Stop the procedure if the patient complains of severe pain.*

(continued)

Action	Rationale

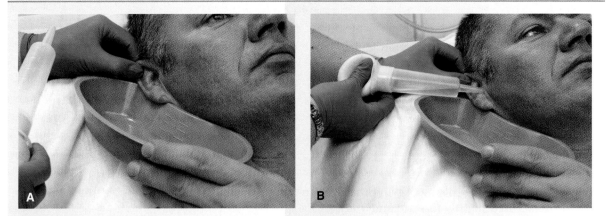

FIGURE 39-2 To irrigate the ear, the nurse (**A**) straightens the ear canal of an adult by gently pulling the pinna upward and back, and then (**B**) directing the flow from the bulb toward the upper part of the canal.

Action	Rationale
e. Irrigate until either the ear canal is clean or the ordered volume is used.	This is for maximum therapeutic effect.
19. Dry the ear with a clean sponge or towel and assist the patient to a comfortable position with the ear facing down on the affected side.	To drain excess fluid and to leave the patient comfortable.
20-22. Follow steps 20 to 22 of the General Procedure: Lower the bed, care for the used equipment, remove your gloves, and wash or disinfect your hands.	

EVALUATION

23. Follow step 23 of the General Procedure: Evaluate using the individualized patient outcomes previously identified.
    a. Cerumen or foreign object in the ear canal is removed.
    b. Patient states pain or discomfort is minimized.

DOCUMENTATION

24. Follow step 24 of the General Procedure: Document on a flow sheet, on the nursing care record, and/or on the nursing care plan.
    a. Ear that was irrigated (right or left)
    b. Type, concentration, amount, and temperature of solution used
    c. Appearance of any secretions or drainage
    d. Response of the patient

■ POTENTIAL ADVERSE OUTCOME AND RELATED INTERVENTIONS

1. An ear irrigation is ordered, and you see that the tympanic membrane is not intact.
Intervention: Do not carry out the procedure. Notify the physician.

Procedure for Eye Irrigation

Eye irrigation is a sterile procedure, because eyes are easily damaged by infection. Use a sterile syringe and sterile fluid. If both eyes are to be irrigated, use separate sets for each eye to prevent cross-contamination. An eye irrigation is most often used to remove a foreign body or injurious fluid that has splashed into the eye. It may also be used to remove secretions caused by infection.

ASSESSMENT

1-3. Follow steps 1 to 3 of the General Procedure: Check the type of irrigation ordered and the type, concentration, amount, and temperature of the solution ordered; check whether the irrigation has been done previously; and assess what the patient knows about the procedure.

ANALYSIS

4-5. Follow steps 4 and 5 of the General Procedure: Think through your data, and identify specific problems and modifications.

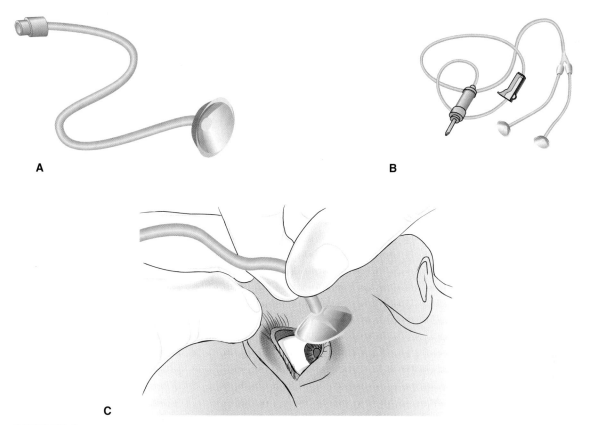

FIGURE 39-3 This eye irrigation system provides for continuous irrigation. (**A**) The eye shield. (**B**) Two eye shields attached to a Y-type intravenous tubing. (**C**) Placing the eye shield over the surface of the anesthetized eye for irrigation.

PLANNING

6. Determine individualized patient outcomes for the eye irrigation, including the following. **R:** Identification of outcomes guides planning and evaluation.
   a. Foreign body or contaminant is removed from the eye, or eye is clean and clear of **exudate.**
   b. Patient states pain or discomfort is minimized.
7. Plan for sterile technique. **R:** The eye is very susceptible to infection, and eye infections have the potential for serious consequences to vision.
8. Identify and gather the equipment needed for the eye irrigation. If both eyes are to be irrigated, separate equipment is used for each to prevent cross-contamination. **R:** Planning ahead promotes effective organization.

   a. Sterile solution ordered. Normal saline solution is most common, either in a pour bottle (for small volume) or in a 1,000-mL intravenous bag (for large volume).
   b. Irrigating device (sterile syringe or IV tubing). An IV stand will be needed for the latter.
   c. Emesis basin and a larger basin if a large volume is being used
   d. Sterile cotton balls or gauze squares
   e. Sterile gloves
   f. Absorbent padding to protect the bed and linens
   g. Eye shield (Fig. 39-3) and topical anesthetic eye drops if ordered for large-volume continuous flow method.

IMPLEMENTATION

Action	Rationale
9-14. Follow steps 9 to 14 of the General Procedure: Wash or disinfect your hands, obtain any needed supportive devices or assistance, identify the patient (two identifiers), close the door and pull the curtain around the bed, explain the procedure,	

(continued)

Action	Rationale
and raise the bed to an appropriate working position.	
15. Place the patient in the supine position. Turn the patient's head with the eye that is to be irrigated down. (The patient can be seated with the head tilted back and supported.)	This position allows the fluid to flow across the eye surface and not flow out toward the other eye.
16. Follow step 16 of the General Procedure: Place padding and an emesis basin beside and below the eye. It is wise to have a large bath basin available in which to empty the drainage basin halfway through the irrigation.	To prevent the solution from overflowing onto the patient.
17. Set up the irrigant and plan the method.	
a. *Small-volume syringe method:*	Used when a limited volume of fluid is ordered for removing secretion.
(1) Pour sterile saline solution into a sterile irrigation container.	
(2) Open sterile syringe.	
(3) Put on sterile gloves.	
b. *Large-volume continuous flow:*	Used when diluting chemical or particles in the eye.
(1) IV bag of appropriate fluid	
(2) IV tubing	
(3) eye shield if ordered	
18. Irrigate the eye(s) as follows:	
a. Hold the eye open with the thumb and forefinger of your nondominant hand. (Resting your hand on the patient's forehead may make this easier.)	
b. To use the *small-volume syringe method:*	
(1) Fill the syringe with 30 to 60 mL fluid.	The syringe method provides a way to administer precise volumes of irrigant.
(2) Gently release the fluid onto the lower conjunctival sac at the inner **canthus,** allowing the fluid to flow across the eye and then into the basin.	The fluid flows away from the other eye so that potentially contaminated fluid is not transferred from one eye to the other.

(continued)

Action	Rationale
(3) Repeat as needed. Continue the procedure until the eye is clean or until the fluid ordered has been used.	
c. To use the *large-volume continuous flow method:*	
(1) Adjust the IV stand to its lowest height.	To keep pressure low.
(2) Attach the IV tubing and hang the solution on the IV stand.	To prepare the solution for administration.
(3) Fill the tubing with fluid.	To eliminate the air, so it will flow evenly.
(4) Pull back the eyelids.	To expose the surface of the eye.
(5) Open the control valve or clamp on the IV tubing and allow the fluid to flow slowly across the eye from the inner to the outer canthus.	A continuous flow is important for thorough cleansing, but the pressure should never cause discomfort. Do not allow the hard irrigating tip of the IV line to touch the eye because doing so may cause injury.
d. To use the *large-volume eye shield method:* If an eye shield is ordered	
(1) Connect the eye shield to the IV tubing, keeping the eye shield sterile.	To protect the eye from potential infection.
(2) Open the eyelid and hold the lids back.	To provide access to the eye surface.
(3) Instill ordered topical anesthetic drops.	To prevent discomfort from the eye shield.
(4) Place the sterile eye shield over the eyeball, allowing the eyelids to close over the eye shield.	The eye shield device makes it unnecessary to hold the eye open and delivers fluid directly to the eye surface.
(5) Open the control valve on the IV tubing to allow the fluid to flow directly onto the eye through the eye shield.	A continuous flow is important for thorough cleansing, but the pressure should never cause discomfort.
19. Follow step 19 of the General Procedure: Remove equipment and dry the eyelid, wiping it from the inner canthus to the outer canthus, using a sterile cotton ball or 2- × 2-inch gauze pad. Use each cotton ball or gauze pad only once and discard.	This protects the opposite eye and moves any infected material away from either eye.
20-22. Follow steps 20 to 22 of the General Procedure: Lower the bed, care for the equipment, remove your gloves, and wash or disinfect your hands.	

EVALUATION

23. Follow step 23 of the General Procedure: Evaluate using individualized patient outcomes previously identified. **R:** Evaluation in relation to desired outcomes is essential for planning future care.
    a. Foreign body or contaminant was removed from the eye, or eye is clean and clear of exudate.
    b. Patient states pain or discomfort is minimized.

DOCUMENTATION

24. Follow step 24 of the General Procedure: Document on a flow sheet, on the nursing care record, and/or on the nursing care plan. **R:** Documentation is a legal record of the patient's care and communicates nursing interventions to other nurses and other disciplines.
    a. Type of irrigation done
    b. Type, concentration, amount, and temperature of solution used
    c. Appearance of the eye(s) irrigated
    d. Amount, color, consistency, and odor of any drainage or exudates
    e. Appearance of any secretions washed out with the irrigant
    f. Response of the patient

Acute Care

Eye irrigations are commonly done in the Emergency Department of most hospitals. People with eye injuries or who have come in contact with foreign bodies, harmful solutions, or other harmful substances often receive eye irrigations as a part of their therapy. In some cases, they will need to be taught how to continue eye irrigations at home. Ear irrigations may also be done in the Emergency Department, although often they do not require emergency treatment.

Long-Term Care

Performing irrigations is a common procedure in the long-term care facility. Older people may produce fewer tears with age (dry eye) so that small foreign bodies such as dust particles can enter the eye or other secretions can build up. Eye irrigations with normal saline solution can remove the cause of any irritation and are soothing.

The older adult also may produce an increased amount of cerumen (earwax), which can cause pain, hearing loss, or infection. Residents who wear canal-fitting hearing aids tend to build up more wax than those who do not wear such hearing aids because of the close contact of the aid with the auditory canal. This wax must be removed so that it does not interfere with the reception of sound. Knowledge and understanding of the irrigation procedure is essential for the nurse involved in long-term care.

Home Care

Irrigations have long been performed in the home by the home care nurse, the client, or a family member. For example, foreign bodies in the eye and simple ear infections may require the soothing effects of irrigation. The family may have an older member residing in the home who either has a hearing deficit or wears a hearing aid. Inspection for wax buildup should occur regularly and ear irrigation performed, if appropriate, to remove the wax.

Ambulatory Care

Clients who need eye and ear irrigations are seen frequently in ambulatory care settings. Most often, this is due to an urgent problem. Rather than visit an Emergency Department, the client with something in the eye or ear will usually visit an ambulatory care setting. The buildup of cerumen in the ear may have caused hearing loss. Attempts to remove the cerumen sometimes result in pushing it farther into the ear canal. An irrigation using a strong suction tip may be used in an office setting to remove impacted cerumen. Clients may need to be taught how to do irrigations at home.

LEARNING TOOLS

DEVELOP YOUR BACKGROUND KNOWLEDGE

1. Review the Learning Outcomes.
2. Read the section on the eyes and ears and sensory perception in your assigned text.
3. Look up the Key Terms in the glossary.

4. Review this module and mentally practice the techniques described. Study so that you would be able to teach these skills to another person.

5. Arrange for time to practice irrigations.

DEVELOP YOUR SKILLS

6. In the practice setting
   a. Review the equipment available for irrigations.
   b. Identify the various types of syringes used for irrigations and any prepackaged sets for ear and eye irrigations.
   c. Try using each piece of equipment to make sure you understand its function and can handle it. Review the instructions on the prepackaged irrigation sets.
   d. Review the recording of irrigations in sample situations given in the module. Use the Performance Checklist on the CD-ROM in the front of this book as a guide.

DEMONSTRATE YOUR SKILLS

7. In the clinical setting
   a. Consult with your instructor regarding the opportunity to observe irrigations done by others.
   b. Consult with your instructor regarding the opportunity to perform irrigations with supervision. Evaluate your performance with the instructor.

CRITICAL THINKING EXERCISES

Analyze the situations below to determine the assessment needed and what you should consider in your planning. Identify two different approaches to carrying out each procedure.

1. Mr. G. is a resident in a nursing home. He has bilateral hearing aids, but has experienced increasing difficulty hearing recently.

2. Mrs. R. brings her 12-year-old son to the Emergency Department. He has severe pain in his right eye from particles that blew into it when his chemistry set exploded. The physician orders an eye irrigation with 1,000 mL normal saline solution.

SELF-QUIZ
SHORT-ANSWER QUESTIONS

1. List two major purposes of irrigation.

   a. _____

   b. _____

2. Name one type of irrigation for which sterile technique must be used.

   _____

3. Name one type of irrigation for which clean technique is safe.

   _____

4. List three factors in an irrigation that can cause irritation or damage tissue.

   a. _____

   b. _____

   c. _____

5. Under what circumstances should an ear not be irrigated?

   _____

6. Why must each eye be irrigated separately?

   _____

7. When are protective eyewear and a gown or apron needed for performing an irrigation?

   _____

MULTIPLE CHOICE

_____ 8. You are checking an order for an eye irrigation. The order states "saline irrigation OD as needed for comfort." The safest nursing response to this order is to
   a. enter the correct eye or eyes in the plan of care based on your knowledge of the abbreviation.
   b. look up the abbreviation to assure that you are correct, and then enter the correct eye or eyes into the plan of care.
   c. ask the nursing supervisor to verify the correct eye with you, and enter the correct eye or eyes into the plan of care.
   d. contact the prescriber and ask for specific instructions using the terms right eye, left eye, or both eyes.

_____ 9. The nurse is instructing the patient's wife in irrigating the patient's ear to remove cerumen. The nurse should emphasize which of the following?
   a. Pull the pinna down and back to straighten the ear canal.
   b. Pull the pinna up and back to straighten the ear canal.
   c. Do not try to straighten the ear canal because this causes discomfort.
   d. Use the tip of the ear syringe to straighten the ear canal.

_____ **10.** Before beginning an ordered ear irrigation, the nurse examines the patient's ear with an otoscope and sees ragged tissue around the edges of where the tympanic membrane should be and no clear view of a tympanic membrane. The correct nursing response is to

a. plan to use very low pressure with the irrigation.

b. ask the patient if he has had an ear infection in that ear.

c. do not perform the irrigation; call the physician and explain the finding.

d. contact the supervisor to verify the condition of the ear before proceeding with the irrigation.

Answers to the Self-Quiz questions appear in the back of the book.

MODULE 40

Providing Wound Care

SKILLS INCLUDED IN THIS MODULE

General Procedure for Changing a Dressing
Specific Procedures Related to Wound Care
   Procedure for Shortening a Penrose Drain
   Procedure for Removing Skin Staples or Sutures
   Procedure for Emptying and Restarting a Wound
     Suction Device

PREREQUISITE MODULES

Module 1	An Approach to Nursing Skills
Module 2	Documentation
Module 3	Basic Body Mechanics
Module 4	Basic Infection Control
Module 5	Safety in the Healthcare Environment
Module 13	Monitoring Intake and Output
Module 14	Nursing Physical Assessment
Module 24	Basic Sterile Technique: Sterile Field and Sterile Gloves
Module 37	Applying Bandages and Binders

For colostomy pouching, see Module 28, Caring for the Patient With an Ostomy.
For tracheostomy dressings, see Module 34, Tracheostomy Care and Suctioning.
For central line dressings, see Module 49, Caring for Central Venous Catheters.

KEY TERMS

approximated	sanguineous
chronic wound	secondary
contamination	intention
debride	(second
epithelialization	intention)
exudate	serosanguineous
fistula	serous
healing ridge	shearing force
induration	slough
maceration	staging
Penrose drain	sterile
primary intention	tunneling
(first intention)	undermining
purulent	

OVERALL OBJECTIVE

▸ To provide care to patients with wounds, including complete wound assessment, changing dressings, and thorough documentation.

LEARNING OUTCOMES

The student will be able to

1. Assess the patient effectively with regard to the healing status of the wound and the effectiveness of the dressing materials in use.
2. Analyze assessment data to determine special problems or concerns regarding a wound that must be addressed when caring for the wound.
3. Determine appropriate patient outcomes for the patient with a wound and recognize the potential for adverse outcomes.
4. Plan appropriate strategies to ensure that the patient receives wound care that supports healing.
5. Implement wound care using appropriate clean or sterile technique.
6. Evaluate the effectiveness of the dressings applied and the progress of the wound healing.
7. Document wound care according to facility policies.

Wounds, such as surgical wounds, pressure ulcers, ulcers related to arterial or venous insufficiency, neuropathic ulcers, and burns, require care that will promote healing and prevent further injury or deterioration of the wound. Nurses choose the most appropriate dressing materials to promote healing and apply them in the most secure and comfortable way possible. Increasingly, nurses are being asked to consider the cost-effectiveness of the dressing materials chosen. In addition to caring for the wound itself, essential nursing responsibilities include assessing the whole patient in regard to the underlying causes of the wound and determining factors that will contribute to or interfere with healing. This module focuses on assessing the wound itself and managing the wound care.

NURSING DIAGNOSES

- Impaired Skin Integrity. This nursing diagnosis is specifically related to an open wound such as a pressure ulcer or an ulcer related to venous insufficiency that is in need of appropriate wound care.
- Acute Pain, related to the open wound. Individuals with open wounds may have pain related to the wound. This is often exacerbated by movement and by dressing changes.
- Fear, related to painful wound care. The nursing diagnosis of "Fear" related to painful wound

care procedures may be appropriate because of the cleaning techniques needed to help prepare the wound bed for healing.

- Imbalanced Nutrition: Less Than Body Requirements. This may be applicable to individuals with any type of wound. Adequate nutrition expedites the healing process.

DELEGATION

Wound care is not delegated to assistive personnel because of the need for informed assessment and planning and the use of special techniques in dressing the wound. Assistive personnel should be taught actions to prevent pressure ulcers and what skin changes to report to the nurse in order that developing pressure ulcers can be treated when they are just beginning.

OBSERVING AND DESCRIBING THE WOUND

Careful observation and accurate description of the wound are integral parts of changing a dressing. Observe the healing status of the wound. Healing status refers to the progress the wound is making toward healing.

HEALING STATUS OF SIMPLE SURGICAL WOUNDS

Simple surgical wounds have edges that are **approximated** (brought close together) and are sealed closed, although not healed, within 24 to 48 hours of surgery. When caring for a patient with a surgical wound, always examine the wound carefully. Are the edges approximated? Does the wound have a smooth contour? Are inflammation and edema (swelling) present? If so, to what degree? A wound with approximated edges, a smooth contour, minimal inflammation and swelling, and healing across all layers is said to be healing by **primary intention (first intention)**. Scarring is minimal with this type of healing (Fig. 40-1). Clean approximated surgical wounds are often left open to the air 24 to 48 hours after surgery. A simple clean dressing may be used to prevent abrasion over the still healing wound. After approximately 4 days, a **healing ridge** is visible along the incision. The body will "remodel" this into a flatter scar as healing progresses.

Any wound that is draining is still open. A wound with a drain in place is being kept open artificially to facilitate drainage. These wounds may heal by primary intention (first intention) as the drainage diminishes.

Historically, dressings over open wounds were always **sterile.** In current practice, however, many facilities have reviewed infection control data, healing rates, and costs and determined that clean technique is cost-effective and results in no increase in wound infections. Remember that using clean technique does not mean using less-careful technique. The dressing materials must be kept meticulously clean, and clean gloves are used on the hands. Instructions will be provided here for both clean and sterile technique. Patients in their home environment are almost always taught to use clean technique on an open wound.

HEALING STATUS OF OPEN, COMPLEX WOUNDS

Surgical wounds that have become infected, wounds created by pressure (pressure ulcers), wounds that result from vascular problems, and burns all are characterized by an open surface in which the edges cannot be closed together. If the edges were never closely approximated, the wound must heal from the base of the wound toward the outside and in from the edges. The gap gradually fills with granulation tissue. This pink, healing tissue that appears in the bed of the wound is fragile and easily damaged by antiseptic preparations or abrasion. This type of healing is called healing by **secondary intention (second intention).** Second intention healing takes longer and leaves a larger scar than healing by first intention.

Necrotic tissue in the wound may be eschar (hardened, blackened material) or soft, yellow matter that is referred to as **slough.** Slough of subcutaneous tissue is yellow with a fibrinous or threadlike appearance. Slough from muscle tissue tends to be thick and waxy, and this material does not wash off as thick drainage will. After describing surface characteristics, note the approximate percentage of the surface that each surface characteristic covers (Fig. 40-2).

All open wounds should also be inspected for **undermining**—a process characterized by extension of the open wound under the wound edges. **Tunneling** occurs when the wound creates an opening into deeper tissue. A **fistula** is like a tunnel that goes from the wound into another area, such as one that goes from a perineal wound into the vagina. Wounds that extend under other tissue provide a special challenge when applying dressings.

Note the length and width (in centimeters), depth (in centimeters), and the surface appearance. The dimensions of the wound can be measured with a disposable tape measure or a plastic grid designed for that purpose. Depth may be measured by using a sterile cotton swab stick, noting the depth on the stick and measuring the stick.

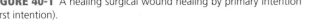

FIGURE 40-1 A healing surgical wound healing by primary intention (first intention).

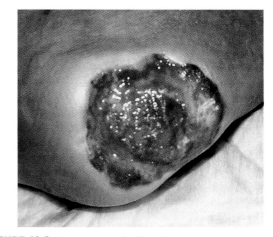

FIGURE 40-2 An open wound with eschar.

Large wounds that require intensive treatment are often photographed for the record. In such cases, a clear plastic measuring grid may be placed over the wound for measurement and marked with the patient's name, patient's medical record number, and the date, so these will appear in the picture. Then a Polaroid camera is used to take a photo that can be placed in the record. For electronic records, a digital camera may be used. There also are special "grid cameras" that overlay a grid on the picture. Photos facilitate accurate tracking of wound appearance and healing. Pictures are taken at intervals that vary based on the healing rate of the wound. See Figure 40-3 for an example of a form for recording ongoing assessment of an open wound.

Patient name _____ Date _____ Time _____

Ulcer 1
Site
Stage*_____
Size (cm)
   Length_____
   Width _____
   Depth _____   No   Yes

	No	Yes
Sinus tract	☐	☐
Tunneling	☐	☐
Undermining	☐	☐
Necrotic tissue		
Slough	☐	☐
Eschar	☐	☐
Exudate		
Serous	☐	☐
Serosanguineous	☐	☐
Purulent	☐	☐
Granulation	☐	☐
Epithelialization	☐	☐
Pain	☐	☐

Surrounding skin

	No	Yes
Erythema	☐	☐
Maceration	☐	☐
Induration	☐	☐

Description of ulcer(s)
_____
_____
_____

Ulcer 2
Site
Stage*_____
Size (cm)
   Length_____
   Width _____
   Depth _____   No   Yes

	No	Yes
Sinus tract	☐	☐
Tunneling	☐	☐
Undermining	☐	☐
Necrotic tissue		
Slough	☐	☐
Eschar	☐	☐
Exudate		
Serous	☐	☐
Serosanguineous	☐	☐
Purulent	☐	☐
Granulation	☐	☐
Epithelialization	☐	☐
Pain	☐	☐

Surrounding skin

	No	Yes
Erythema	☐	☐
Maceration	☐	☐
Induration	☐	☐

Description of ulcer(s)
_____
_____
_____

INDICATE ULCER SITES

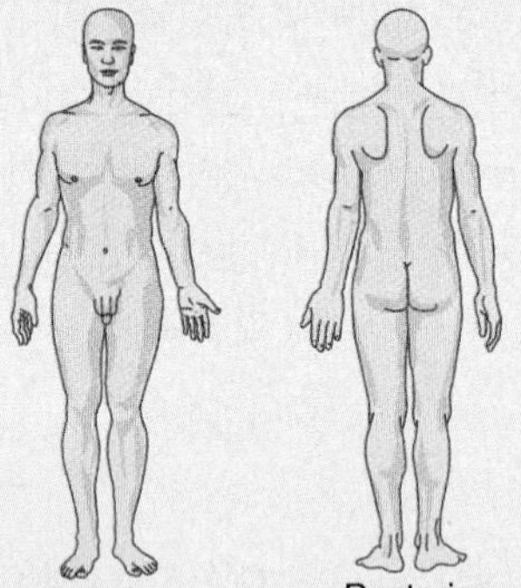

Anterior   Posterior
(Attach color photo of pressure ulcer)

*Classification of pressure ulcer

Stage I: Nonblanchable erythema of intact skin, the heralding lesion of skin ulceration. In individuals with darker skin, discoloration of the skin, warmth, edema, induration, or hardness may also be indicators.

Stage II: Partial thickness skin loss involving epidermis, dermis, or both.

Stage III: Full thickness skin loss involving damage to or necrosis of subcutaneous tissue that may extend down to but not through underlying fascia. The ulcer presents clinically as a deep crater with or without undermining adjacent tissue.

Stage IV: Full thickness skin loss with extensive destruction, tissue necrosis, or damage to muscle, bone, or supporting structures (e.g., tendon or joint capsule).

FIGURE 40-3 A visual wound assessment form. (Source: AHCPR. AHCPR Clinical Practice Guidelines #15. [1992]. Online at http://www.ncbi.nlm.nih.gov/books/bv.fcgi?rid=hstat2.section.6326. Retrieved Jan. 10, 2005.)

WOUND CLASSIFICATION

Open wounds may be classified by the tissue layers involved (Table 40-1).

PRESSURE ULCER STAGING

Pressure ulcers are wounds resulting from pressure on tissue over boney prominences. Pressure collapses blood vessels, resulting in the inability of the damaged cells to recover. Pressure ulcers are further advanced by **shearing force** and friction on tissue as well as poor underlying circulation. Inadequate oxygenation and poor nutrition are other factors that affect the tissue recovery.

An essential aspect of pressure ulcer assessment is called **staging.** Pressure ulcers are staged according to the standards of the National Pressure Ulcer Advisory Panel (NPUAP, 2000), which have become a widely adopted approach to evaluating pressure ulcers. (See Table 40-2 for an overview.) For complete information on staging pressure ulcers, consult the Agency for Health Care Policy and Research (AHCPR), Guideline for Treating Pressure Ulcers (AHCPR, 1994). (This agency has been renamed the Agency for Healthcare Research and Quality [AHRQ].) The 1994 guideline remains the standard for pressure ulcer assessment (but not for treatment). As pressure ulcers heal, the NPUAP advises that they not be "reverse" staged. The panel points out that the ulcer fills with granulation tissue that contracts to fill the space. The lost muscle, subcutaneous tissue, and skin layers are not restored. Therefore, the description should remain the stage originally present with the healing described in terms of lessening depth of the wound (NPUAP, 2005).

PERI-WOUND SKIN

Assessment of the peri-wound skin (skin around the wound) is important because the wound drainage, the tape used to secure dressings, failure of the healing process, and infection all can disrupt skin integrity. Thus, a wound that starts out as a small- or moderate-size wound can become a major wound if the surrounding skin begins to break down.

DRAINAGE

Drainage or **exudate** from the wound must be observed, described, and evaluated. Drainage may be primarily **serous** (composed of serum from the body), **serosanguineous** (composed of blood and serum), **sanguineous** (primarily blood), or **purulent** (containing pus). You must identify and document the color, amount, and odor of the drainage. Note the amount by stating the number of dressings saturated or stained by the drainage. If the color is yellow or tinged with green, it may reflect microorganisms growing in the drainage.

Describe how the wound drainage smells. The odor is assessed once the dressing is removed and the wound cleansed. Wound drainage accumulating in a dressing may have an odor as bacteria accumulate, but the wound itself may not have an odor. Be sure to differentiate this. Many wound products have characteristic odors that will affect the odor once the wound is uncovered. Odors are best described by comparing them with familiar smell such as urine, feces, ammonia, or a rotten onion, if that is possible.

All types of wound drainage support growth of microorganisms. Therefore, many measures are used to keep the wound surface clean and to move the drainage away from the wound bed itself. Drainage also can irritate and damage healthy skin around the wound, so heavily draining wounds may require special technique to protect healthy skin.

DRAINS

Drains are sometimes placed during surgery to enhance the flow of drainage from the wound, thus promoting wound healing. After surgery, a drain may also be used to help keep the surgical area dry. An example of such a drain is the **Penrose drain,** a soft latex tubing material. One end is placed in the bottom of the wound, and the other opens to the outside of the body, either through

table 40-1. Wound Classifications

Classification	Tissue Layers Involved	Healing Process
Superficial wound	Outer epidermis with potential cells for healing throughout the wound	Heals rapidly across whole wound.
Partial-thickness wound	Includes the entire epidermis, but hair follicles are in place and there are epidermal cells within the wound bed that will help healing to occur	Healing takes longer, but cells may granulate in the bottom of the wound as well as on the edges of the wound.
Full-thickness wound	All layers of the skin	Granulation tissue typically forms first at the edges and gradually moves across the surface.
Deep wound	Entire skin; extends into subcutaneous tissue and muscle	Heals very slowly from the edges. Unless very small, deep wound may require skin grafting to close.

table 40-2. **Stages of Pressure Ulcers**

Stage	Description
I	Nonblanchable erythema of intact skin, the heralding lesion of skin ulceration. In individuals with darker skin, discoloration of the skin, warmth, edema, **induration** (or hardness) may also be indicators.
II	Partial-thickness skin loss involving epidermis, dermis, or both. The ulcer is superficial and presents clinically as an abrasion, blister, or shallow crater.
III	Full-thickness skin loss involving damage to, or necrosis of, sub-cutaneous tissue that may extend down to, but not through, underlying fascia. The ulcer presents clinically as a deep crater with or without undermining of adjacent tissue.
IV	Full-thickness skin loss with extensive destruction, tissue necrosis, or damage to muscle, bone, or supporting structures (e.g., tendon, joint capsule). Undermining and sinus tracts also may be associated with stage IV pressure ulcers.

National Pressure Ulcer Advisory Panel (NPUAP). (2003). *Staging system from the 1989 Consensus Development Conference.* (Online.) Available at: http://www.npuap.org/positn6.html.

the wound itself or through a small surgical "stab" wound (a small puncture wound made by the surgeon) beside a larger wound. A sterile safety pin or other device is attached to the Penrose drain to prevent it from sliding down into the wound (Fig. 40-4). The drain may be withdrawn gradually and shortened to promote healing at the base of the wound. The procedure for shortening a Penrose drain is included in this module.

If a considerable amount of drainage is expected postoperatively, a closed wound suction device is placed at surgery. This portable system consists of a drainage tube with multiple openings that is placed within the wound and exits through the incision. The drainage tube is attached to a mechanical vacuum unit that gently suctions fluid from the wound. The Hemovac® is one example of this type of wound suction. It uses a spring

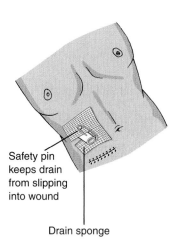

Safety pin keeps drain from slipping into wound

Drain sponge

FIGURE 40-4 A Penrose drain keeps the wound from sealing and provides an exit for drainage.

inside a cylinder to provide continuous suction to the tubing. Other brands have different methods of creating the suction. The Jackson-Pratt drain is a small plastic bottle that is opened, squeezed to remove the air inside, and then closed. The only opening goes to the drainage tubing, and as the plastic bottle seeks to recover its original shape, it creates suction in the tubing. These closed-wound suction devices, commonly used after breast, hip, or perineal surgery, help keep the wound dry. They move easily when the patient moves (Fig. 40-5).

WOUND PAIN

Some wounds are very painful while others are not (Reddy, Keast, & Fowler, et al., 2003). However, pain may accompany various dressing changes. While management of the patient's pain is not discussed in this module, the potential for pain must be considered, and any pain present must be addressed whenever a wound is being cared for.

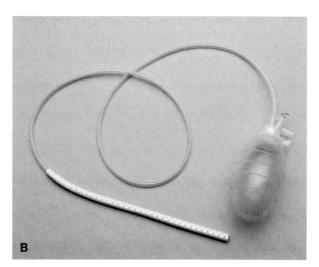

FIGURE 40-5 Wound suction devices remove excessive secretions: (**A**) Hemovac and (**B**) Jackson-Pratt.

DRESSING MATERIALS

Dressing materials vary from facility to facility. Dressing selection is based on wound assessment and the desired outcome for the wound. Some standard dressing materials may be selected by the nurse. Specialized dressing materials that are costly or contain medications require a medical order for use. Check the policies in your facility and see Table 40-3 for an overview of commonly used products. A comprehensive list of wound care products currently available in the United States is available online at http://www.medicaledu.com/prodindx.htm.

When a wound is not healing or is complex, a certified wound care nurse can provide expert consultation in planning for specialized wound care. If the wound care specialist does not have authority to write prescriptions for medical care, the specialist will confer with the physician when medical orders are needed.

CLEANING THE WOUND

If the wound has large amounts of drainage or exudate, it should be cleaned as part of the dressing change. The wound itself is usually cleaned with sterile saline solution to remove drainage and to loosen dressing materials. The solution may be applied with a sterile bulb syringe, with a piston syringe, or on gauze squares. Antiseptic agents applied directly to a wound surface interfere with healing by inhibiting granulation and **epithelialization.** When applied repeatedly to extensive open wounds, povidone-iodine (Betadine) compounds may be absorbed and cause iodine toxicity (AHCPR, 1994). Therefore, antiseptics should not be used on the open wound surface. Specific antimicrobial agents that do not inhibit epithelialization may be part of the medical orders.

In some facilities, the cleaning solution is available for individual use in small containers that are opened at the time of use. In other facilities, a large sterile container of the solution may be placed at the bedside. The solution can be poured into a sterile basin or directly onto sterile gauze dressings. If you open a large bottle of solution, be sure to label the bottle with the patient's name, the date and time, and your initials. This is especially important in rooms with more than one patient.

For cleaning around wounds, antiseptic-soaked swab sticks and small foil packages of antiseptic wipes are used. The most common antiseptic agents used for cleaning the skin around wounds are the iodophor compounds such as povidone (Betadine, ACU-dyne), which provide long-lasting antiseptic protection. Hydrogen peroxide and chlorhexidine (Hibiclens) may also be used. Chlorhexidine in an alcohol base (Chloraprep) is an excellent skin disinfectant but is also more costly.

Scrubbing with the disinfectant removes debris on skin and enables the disinfectant to come in contact with the folds of the skin. All should be allowed to dry to achieve maximum disinfection. These agents can cause skin reactions in some individuals, so when you are using them, assess the patient's skin carefully for signs of redness and edema.

SPECIAL DRESSING TECHNIQUES

Many different techniques are used to facilitate healing, particularly in situations where wounds are not healing well. These techniques are instituted as part of the medical orders for care and include the use of moisture, negative pressure, and compression.

WET-TO-MOIST OR WET-TO-DRY DRESSINGS

Wet-to-moist or wet-to-dry dressings may be used to **debride** (remove or clean away adherent material from) the wound surface. These dressings are based on the principle that moist gauze, which is placed in the wound, readily absorbs drainage and sloughed tissue. As it begins to dry, the dressing adheres to debris on the surface of the wound. When the dressing is removed, the surface debris is removed along with the dressing. This method is subject to many different interpretations. If allowed to dry completely (wet-to-dry technique), the dressing removes new granulation tissue as well as debris in the wound, which slows healing. If the dressing is removed while still moist (wet-to-moist technique), debridement is less effective but granulation tissue is preserved (Armstrong, 2004). Therefore, some individuals advocate the use of only wet-to-moist technique. Armstrong (2004) notes that it is common practice to use wet-to-moist technique even when the order reads "wet-to-dry." In fact, she found that many surgeons want wet-to-moist when they write an order for "wet-to-dry."

While wet-to-moist (or wet-to-dry) dressings have a long history, most wound care experts identify these as a poor method of wound debridement (Armstrong, 2004). They are minimally effective. Excess moisture may contribute to skin breakdown around the wound, and the development of new tissue is inhibited. The minimal expense of gauze and saline solution often contributes to the mistaken belief that they are the most cost-effective dressing. Because they are less effective and require more healing time and nursing care, they are actually quite costly. One research team has called this debridement method "nonselective, traumatic, painful, costly, and time consuming" (Sibbold, Williamson, Orsted, et al., 2000, p. 15). Many other more cost-effective methods of wound debridement are available (see list of wound care products in Table 40-3). Certainly,

table 40-3. Common Wound Care Products

Brand names appear in parentheses to help with identification.

Product	Description	Use
Adhesive barriers (Karaya, Stomadhesive)	The same products used to protect skin in patients who use ostomy pouches. Available as wafers, sheets, or paste.	Applied to skin around a draining wound to protect it from drainage as well as to provide a surface on which to tape dressings Also used when a profusely draining wound is pouched
Alginates (Kaltostat, Algiderm)	Alginates contain a seaweed product and water, saline solution, or a glycerin formed into sheets or ropes. As they absorb drainage, they become a gel. Available in single or multiple-use tubes or sheets	Maintain a moist wound environment. Used in minimal to moderately draining wounds Sheets may be chilled and placed over burns or used to hydrate the wound bed.
Enzymatic debriders (Collagenase, Elase)	Enzyme-based gel or ointment that is placed on the surface of the wound. The enzyme breaks down necrotic tissue. Action continues for 24 hours.	For open wounds with slough
Foams (plain or with an adhesive border) (3M Foam, Allevyn)	Absorbent foam that may be cut to fit the wound and covered with a secondary dressing	For draining wounds May be used under compression dressings.
Gauze	An open-weave absorbent cotton product Available in multiple shapes and sizes, including squares and rolls of material Available as sterile or nonsterile and in single or multi-use packages Examples are 4 × 4s, 2 × 2s, 3 × 3s, fluffs, roll gauze.	Used to clean wounds and to provide a protective covering for the wound bed Provides a delivery system for topical agents such as antibiotic cream or enzymatic preparations Fluffs are loose gauze used to fill open wounds. Roll gauze may be used to hold dressings in place or to fill a small wound.
Hydrocolloids (Duoderm, Restore)	Occlusive adhesive wafers that are easy to apply, moderately absorptive, and adherent to the intact skin surrounding the wound. For best results, there should be a 1- to 2-inch border over intact skin. Do not apply over cavity wounds. Available in various sizes and shapes.	Although hydrocolloids will absorb small amounts of drainage, they are best used with other materials if drainage is profuse. Also may be used around tubes or drains to hold them away from skin and prevent abrasion
Hydrogels (amorphous and sheets) (AquaSite, Tegagel, Hypergel, Vigilon)	Come in a variety of forms that are absorbent Do not block the movement of bacteria Fill spaces and maintain moist environment	Used for moderate drainage. Need to be covered with other dressing materials
Medication-impregnated dressing materials; antimicrobial (Acticoat, Actisorb)	A variety of dressing materials, such as alginates or polyurethane foam impregnated with antimicrobial agents, may be ordered for specific situations. These include materials with metallic silver and antibiotics.	Used for infected wounds
Moisture-vapor-permeable (MVP) transparent film (Bioclusive, Opsite, Tegaderm)	Look like thin sheets of plastic and are often called by their brand names One surface has an adhesive that adheres to dry, intact skin but not to a moist wound surface. The dressings are semipermeable and allow gases, such as moisture vapor and oxygen, to move through them. Larger molecules, such as those found in the drainage or in bacteria, do not pass through the material. Bacteria can move from the skin surrounding the dressing to the area under it through very small crevices in the skin that are not sealed off by the dressing. MVP dressings provide a moist surface that encourages epithelialization of the wound surface.	Used primarily over small wounds and sometimes for intravenous dressings May be placed over wounds with black eschar or necrotic debris because they help to liquefy the material, although this is a slow process. This is not desirable in immunocompromised people because the warm, moist environment may encourage infection to develop under the film.
Montgomery straps or ties	Large tapes with eyelet openings, which are laced or pinned closed. Device allows dressings to be changed without removing tape from the skin each time. Commercially available tapes may be cut to the desired width. Each tape includes one or more eyelets. Can be made from wide tape folded back, with holes cut for eyelets. Generally, twill tape, roll gauze, or rubber bands attached with safety pins are used to secure these straps or ties. Straps may remain on the skin until they come loose. Ties are changed when they become soiled.	Used to tie across large or bulky dressings that need frequent changing (see Fig. 40-9). This prevents the skin irritation caused by repeated tape removal.
Nonadherent dressings, impregnated (Vaseline gauze, Xerofoam); nonstick surface (Telfa)	Special sterile dressings that have a surface that will not stick to wound surfaces Impregnated nonadherent dressings have petrolatum, antimicrobials, or other agents on the woven material to prevent adherence.	Used directly on incisions or open wound surfaces to prevent injury to tissues when the dressing is removed

(continued)

table 40-3. Common Wound Care Products (Continued)

Product	Description	Use
Pouches	Other nonadherent dressings, such as Telfa, have a synthetic nonadherent material attached to one side of the gauze dressing. Telfa will lose its nonadherent properties when it is in contact with **sanguineous** (bloody) drainage. Available in different sizes and may be cut to a needed size Ostomy-type pouches or drainage bags whose adhesive barrier opening can be cut in the shape of the wound. They collect drainage and allow it be removed, thereby avoiding saturated dressings. This product uses an adhesive barrier to fix the pouch to the skin surface. Drainage bags may be connected to bedside drainage. The bags allow staff to measure drainage precisely and observe the wound. Pouch dressings control odor and moisture, making the patient more comfortable.	Used on a profusely draining wound or fistula
Starch co-polymer; available as paste, beads, or powders (Intra-site Gel) and embedded in dressings (Poly-Mem)	Absorbent and also promotes autolysis in the wound. Provides a moist healing environment	Used in wounds with minimal to moderate exudate Used with other products covering the wound
Tape; hypoallergenic tape (Hypafix, Metape, and Medipore)	Comes in a variety of materials (adhesive, plastic, paper, and other) and in widths from ¼ inch to 6 inches. Paper tape is generally considered hypoallergenic. Hypoallergenic tapes are less likely to create skin reaction and are especially useful for patients with fragile skin or tape sensitivities. Tape should not be stretched before placing on the skin because the pull of the stretched tape increases the risk of skin damage.	Used to fix dressings in place
Thick combination pads (ABDs, Combines)	Large, sterile or nonsterile, thick, absorbent pads (usually multiple layers of coarse gauze or other absorbent material covered by a smoother surface layer). Most have a moisture-resistant surface on one side to be used on the outside to prevent drainage from striking through.	Normally used over smaller dressing materials to absorb larger amounts of drainage and/or to pad a wound Insulates wound surface to preserve tissue temperature that promotes healing

Adapted from *World Wide Wounds.* (Online). Available at http://www.worldwidewounds.com/.

a wet-to-moist dressing should not be used on a wound that does not need debridement.

MOIST DRESSING

Some moist dressings are designed to provide a moist wound-healing environment and to prevent healing from occurring over the top of tunnels or pockets. Tunnels and pockets can become reservoirs for drainage, and abscesses may result. In these instances, saline-moistened gauze is loosely placed into the wound so that it is in contact with all wound surfaces. The intent is not to debride the wound, but to encourage granulation from the bottom up. The dressing is kept moist throughout treatment because wound healing occurs more rapidly in a moist environment. The dressing is covered with an absorbent combination pad (such as an ABD or Combine) to protect the wound, keep clothing and bedding dry, and maintain the warm temperature of the wound surface. Granulation occurs more effectively when the tissue can be kept at body temperature. Moist dressings must be remoistened frequently to prevent drying.

The greater cost of modern wound products that would keep the wound moist are often cited as reasons to use moist gauze on large wounds. Research shows that modern products that prevent evaporation of moisture from the wound surface and that insulate the tissue to maintain the optimum temperature for healing are cost-effective. Most of these dressing products need changing less often, and they do not increase infection rates. They are more comfortable for patients and encourage healing (Armstrong, 2004). Nurses who become knowledgeable about modern wound care products can advocate effectively for their use (see Table 40-3).

NEGATIVE PRESSURE WOUND THERAPY

Negative pressure wound therapy (NPWT) provides a means to manage large volumes of wound exudates, promote granulation, and decrease dressing frequency. This is also referred to as vacuum-assisted closure (VAC). The system consists of a porous foam material and a drain placed in the wound, covered with a transparent adhesive film, and attached to the wound vacuum device

(Thomas, 2001). The wound vacuum machine provides either intermittent or continuous suction to remove drainage, increase circulation to the wound bed, and promote healing. Follow the directions on the specific wound vacuum equipment to be used (Fig. 40-6).

COMPRESSION DRESSINGS

Compression dressings provide consistent pressure to an extremity, decreasing the fluid movement out of the vascular space into the interstitial spaces and promoting venous return. These dressings are most commonly used for ulcers on the legs caused by venous stasis. A variety of compression materials may be used for the dressing, which is wrapped by applying greater pressure at the ankle and decreasing pressure as it moves up the leg. Coverings over dressings, such as Unna's boot (which consists of a paste dressing of gelatin, zinc oxide, and glycerin that hardens in place), provide compression to the foot and lower leg for the ambulatory patient. Compression dressings are usually applied and left in place for up to 7 days. Some compression dressings have multiple complex layers and are applied by the wound care specialist or the medical care provider. Compression may also be achieved by the use of compression stockings over a dressing.

GENERAL PROCEDURE FOR CHANGING A DRESSING

This procedure is appropriate for surgical wounds and other simple wounds.

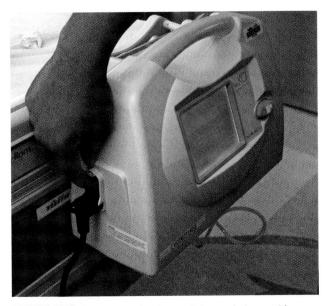

FIGURE 40-6 A vacuum-assisted wound closure device provides negative pressure at the wound surface.

ASSESSMENT

1. Check the orders for the dressing change. Sometimes the surgeon does the first dressing change after surgery and then writes an order: "Change dressing prn." Or you may be responsible for all dressing changes. If so, you must have a specific order for any dressing change performed. In any case, a dressing may be reinforced, meaning that you can apply additional dressings on top of dressings already in place to absorb drainage. Sterile dressings are used over a previous dressing to avoid introducing organisms. However, because they are placed on the contaminated exterior surface of the old dressing, they do not prevent the possibility of wound **contamination.**

   Note: Keep in mind that once drainage penetrates to the outside of a dressing, organisms may be carried to the wound through moisture.

2. Examine the current dressing. **R:** To determine the general size of the wound and the type and amount of dressing materials necessary. This information may be included in the nursing care plan.

3. Check the patient's unit for supplies and equipment already there. **R:** Once supplies are in the patient's room, they have been exposed to the microorganisms there and cannot be placed back in the supply storage area. This practice prevents the spread of microorganisms from one patient to another. Remember that dressing materials in packages that have been opened are no longer sterile because they have been exposed to the microbes in the air. If a dressing must be sterile, dressing materials from an open package must not be used.

ANALYSIS

4. Critically think through your assessment data, carefully evaluating each aspect and its relation to other data. **R:** To determine specific problems for this individual in relation to wound care.

5. Identify specific problems and modifications of the procedure that may be needed for the individual. For example, if you determine that the patient has an allergy to adhesive tape, you will need to plan for a hypoallergenic tape such as Hypafix, Metape, or Medipore. If the skin is irritated from frequent dressing changes, roll gauze, Montgomery straps, or a binder may be indicated. **R:** Planning for the individual must take into consideration the individual's problems.

PLANNING

6. Determine individualized patient outcomes in relation to changing dressing(s), considering the following. **R:** Identification of outcomes guides planning and evaluation.

a. Patient understands the purpose of the procedure and is able to cooperate.

b. The wound shows evidence of healing (forming granulation tissue, lessening size, and moving toward closure).

c. There is no evidence of wound infection (elevated temperature, elevated white blood count, redness, swelling, or drainage from the wound).

d. Dressing is securely in place.

e. Patient states he or she is comfortable after procedure.

7. Gather needed supplies. Some facilities use commercially prepared packages that include all the supplies commonly needed. Your facility may use a partially prepared dressing tray, in which case, you add the additional supplies needed. Most commonly, you must choose the individually packaged supplies needed. If a sterile dressing is required, choose sterile supplies for the items marked with an asterisk (*). Items you may need include

   a. scissors*

   b. thumb forceps (pickups)*

   c. 4- × 4-inch gauze squares, ABDs, and other dressing materials*. Take only the supplies necessary for the dressing to the room. If extra sterile supplies remain after the dressing is changed, place the sealed packages in a clean container where the next person will see them before bringing in more. If large packages of dressings are being used for a clean dressing, place them in a clean plastic bag or covered plastic container to keep them clean between dressing changes.

d. tape or other mechanism to secure the dressing in place

e. cleaning solution and cotton-tipped applicators or swabs with cleaning agent*

f. clean gloves—two pairs or one pair clean gloves and one pair sterile gloves for sterile dressing*

g. disposal bag for soiled dressing; some facilities have special disposal bags for soiled dressings. In others, the waste bag is used. If you follow the latter procedure, the bag should be discarded in the appropriate disposal container outside the patient's room and replaced immediately after the dressing is changed. Biohazard bags for disposal of heavily soiled dressings are recommended for infection control.

IMPLEMENTATION

Action	Rationale
8. Wash or disinfect your hands.	To decrease the transfer of microorganisms that could cause infection.
9. Identify the patient, using two identifiers.	To be sure you are performing the procedure for the correct patient.
10. Prepare the environment for changing the dressing.	
a. Close windows and door.	To eliminate drafts that might chill the patient or carry microorganisms into the open wound.
b. Pull the curtain around the bed.	To provide privacy.
c. Clear a working space. The overbed table serves this purpose well. Make sure the work surface is clean and dry.	To facilitate managing equipment and to prevent contamination of supplies.
d. Place a bag for soiled dressings within easy reach. The bag edges can be taped to the mattress edge for convenience.	To prevent contamination of the environment with wound drainage.
11. Explain what you intend to do. Allow the patient to ask questions to help ensure his or her cooperation. In the case of a very complex wound when pain is expected, arrange for pain medication before	Explaining the procedure helps relieve anxiety or misperceptions that the patient may have about the procedure and knowledge of what is to happen sets the stage for patient self-care after discharge.

(continued)

Action	Rationale
beginning the procedure. Ask the patient to keep his or her hands away from the dressing area and to avoid talking during the procedure.	To limit the number of microorganisms moving in the air.
Limit your own conversation to essential information while the open wound is exposed. In some situations, it may be necessary for both patient and nurse to wear masks during a dressing change.	To decrease microbes in the air.
12. Raise the bed and place the patient in a position that allows clear visibility of and access to the wound. Consider comfort for the patient during the procedure.	To facilitate assessment and prevent back strain while changing the dressing.
13. Expose the area of the wound and drape the patient. You can use a bath blanket or towel for this purpose.	For modesty and warmth.
14. Set up equipment and supplies (see Module 24, Basic Sterile Technique: Sterile Field and Sterile Gloves).	
a. Open all packages and leave the sterile equipment on the inner package surfaces.	To allow you to proceed efficiently. To maintain sterility.
b. Tear strips of tape in correct lengths and place them on the edge of an easily reached surface. Obtain a clean binder if the one in use is soiled. If you are applying or changing Montgomery straps, set them up at this time.	
c. Set up materials to clean the wound, if needed.	
d. Prepare dressings as needed. If a moist dressing is ordered, pour the solution into a sterile container. Another method is to open the container of sterile solution at this time and plan to hold the dressings in a gloved hand over the waste container as you pour the solution over the dressings using an ungloved hand on the bottle.	
15. Begin removing the dressing by loosening tape, starting from the outside and working toward the dressing; gently push the skin away from the tape. If body hair makes this activity uncomfortable for the	To allow you to handle the tape without gloves, which enables you to manage the skin-tape interface more effectively. To minimize pulling on the skin and wound.

(continued)

Action	Rationale
patient, you may want to clip the area with scissors before applying more tape. Some dressings are covered with an elastic or cloth binder, in which case you must unhook or unpin the binder before beginning to loosen tape.	Shaving has the potential for creating small nicks in the skin and increases the possibility for infections.
16. Put on clean gloves.	Wearing clean gloves to remove all dressings protects you from wound drainage.
17. Remove the dressings and immediately place them in the disposal bag. Take the outer dressings off by grasping them at the center (without applying any pressure) and removing them to the side. Notice how many of which type dressings are soiled. When all dressings have been removed, discard gloves into the bag with the dressings.	Placing soiled dressings in a bag limits the potential for spreading microorganisms. To indicate the amount of drainage when you document the dressing change in the patient's chart.
18. Wash or disinfect your hands.	To decrease the transfer of microorganisms that could cause infection.
19. Assess the wound bed for size, sinus tracts, undermining, tunneling, exudate, necrotic tissue, and the presence or absence of granulation tissue, epithelialization, and odor. Observe also for inflammation and edema, redness, and warmth around the wound. If the wound has drainage, debris, or odor, assess the wound again after cleaning it.	To enable you to accurately document the progress of wound healing.
20. Change the dressing, using the appropriate method below.	
a. *Sealed (closed) wound dressings:* If the wound appears sealed, place a simple dry dressing over the surface to protect it from abrasion.	The sealed wound does not have an avenue for microorganisms to enter the tissue nor does it leak moisture. The dry dressing will remain clean on its inside surface.
(1) Handle the dressing by the outside of the corners only.	To maintain sterility or cleanliness of the surface in contact with the wound.
(2) Place the dressing over the wound.	
(3) Tape dressing in place.	

(continued)

Action	Rationale
b. *Open wound dressings:*	
(1) Put on clean gloves or sterile gloves as determined by policy (see Module 24).	
(2) Clean the area around the wound with saline solution or antiseptic cleanser, using cotton balls or a prepared swab.	
(a) If the wound is small or is a surgical "stab" wound, clean in ever widening circles away from it, moving from the area it is most necessary to keep clean to the more contaminated (dirty) area (Fig. 40-7A). Scrub firmly.	To move microbes away from the open wound.

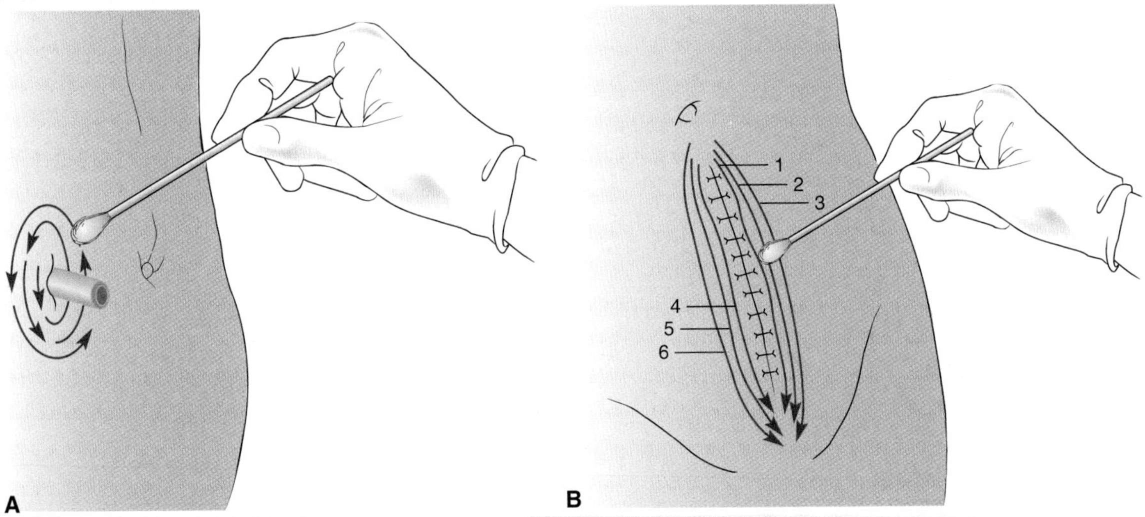

FIGURE 40-7 (**A**) To cleanse the small wound with or without a drain, move outward in concentric circles from the wound itself. (**B**) To cleanse a large wound, use lengthwise strokes and move outward from the wound. Use one sterile swab for the first three strokes and another sterile swab for the next strokes.

Action	Rationale
(b) For a longer wound, you may need to use consecutive long strokes, starting each stroke at the top of the wound and moving to the bottom. Each successive stroke is farther from the wound on that side. Use another swab to clean the other side of the wound, starting at the wound edges and gradually moving out (Fig. 40-7B). Use each swab only once.	To move microbes away from the wound.

(continued)

Action	Rationale
(c) If there are multiple wounds, such as a central incision with several drains, clean each wound separately, using fresh swabs. Clean the most complex site last.	To avoid moving microbes from one site to another.
(3) If debris and drainage are on the wound surface, gently clean the wound itself with sterile saline solution–moistened gauze squares or swabs. For large quantities of slough on the surface, a 35 mL syringe with a 19-gauge needle may be used to provide pressure irrigation to clean the wound bed.	Saline solution will remove most debris and will not harm granulation tissue. This size syringe and needle provides 8 psi pressure (Rodeheaver, 2001), which is within the 4 to 15 psi for irrigation recommended by the AHCPR (1994).
(4) Reassess the wound after cleaning.	Debris on the wound may interfere with accurate assessment of the wound surface. Once removed, accurate assessment is possible.
(5) If any topical agent is to be used on the wound, apply it at this time. Topical agents are usually applied with a clean 2- × 2-inch gauze square or a cotton-tipped swab.	Topical agents are ordered by the medical provider for specific actions in the wound such as preventing microbial growth or debridement.
(6) If the wound is deep and it is to be filled with dressing material, do that next. *Gauze filling:* Moisten the gauze and loosely fill the entire wound so that dressings contact all surfaces of the wound. While the term "wound packing" is often used, *avoid firmly packing* the site. For small wounds, ribbon gauze may be used for filling. For large wounds, "fluffs" of loose gauze are usually used. *Special absorptive filling materials* (see Table 40-3 for examples): Use according to package directions.	The loose filling prevents premature closure of areas, absorbs drainage and debris, and promotes healing from the bottom up. Firmly packing the wound puts pressure on the tissue, decreasing circulation to the granulation surface and interfering with healing.
(7) Place the outer dressing securely on the wound. *Gauze dressings:* Lighter-weight 4- × 4-inch gauze squares (4 × 4s) are used first and then covered with a larger ABD. Use materials in the order they were in when the old dressing was removed, if that	To keep all dressings in place and maintain the moist wound surface. It is also to promote healing and absorb drainage if large amounts of drainage are present.

(continued)

Action	Rationale
seemed effective. If not, change for greater effectiveness. *Specialized dressing products:* When using specialized dressing materials, follow the instructions for that dressing material, usually found on the package. These products may be cut or molded to the size of the wound.	
(8) If a drain is in place, the bulk of the absorbent dressing should cover the drain area, usually in a dependent position. Partially split a 4 × 4 with sterile scissors, or use a precut drain sponge, and place it snugly around the drain (Fig. 40-8A). A drain site may also be dressed with two 4-inch gauze squares. Open the squares and fold them in half lengthwise. By folding each at right angles, each can serve as two sides of the dressing (see Fig. 40-8B). Prenotched gauze squares are also available.	This arrangement absorbs drainage most effectively and prevents **maceration** of the skin around the drain site.

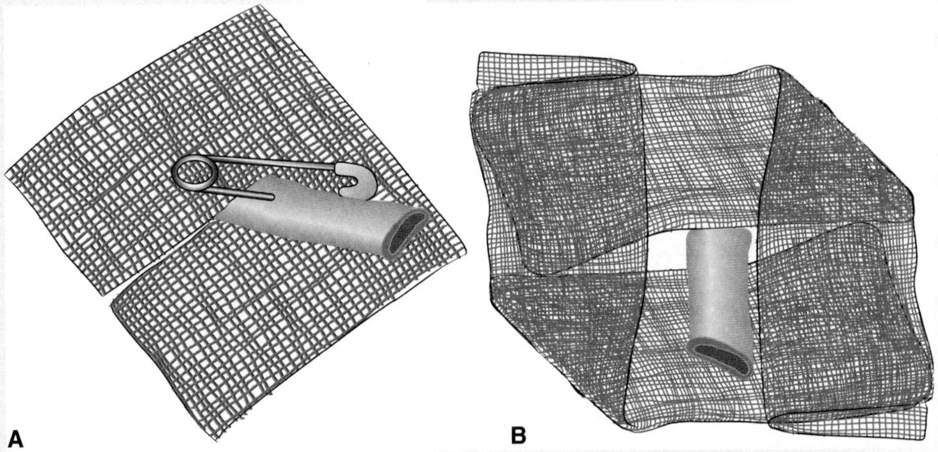

A **B**

FIGURE 40-8 Two kinds of dressing for a drain. (**A**) Pre-split (cut-to-fit) gauze sponge placed to surround a drain. (**B**) Two 4-inch gauze squares folded in half lengthwise, then folded again at right angles to closely surround a drain for best absorption.

Action	Rationale
21. Remove your gloves and place them in the bag of soiled dressing materials.	To prevent spreading body fluids or microorganisms.
22. Secure the dressing with tape or Montgomery straps (Fig. 40-9) or a binder as indicated. Use enough tape to hold the dressing in place, but not more than necessary. Avoid putting tension on the tape.	Excess tape increases the potential for damaging the skin. Tension on tape can create skin irritation and tape burns.

(continued)

Action	Rationale
	FIGURE 40-9 Montgomery straps tie and untie, thereby protecting the skin from repeated tape removal when checking or changing a dressing.
23. Assist the patient into a comfortable position and lower the bed.	For patient comfort and safety.
24. Put on clean gloves and care for the equipment. Remove the bag used for soiled dressings and other materials, and dispose of it in the appropriate place, commonly a special garbage receptacle in the soiled utility room. Rinse any glass or metal materials used to remove protein substances before sending them to the Central Processing Department. Dispose of gloves.	To prevent the spread of body fluids and microorganisms.
25. Wash or disinfect your hands.	To decrease the transfer of microorganisms that could cause infection.

EVALUATION

26. Evaluate using the individualized patient outcomes previously identified: Patient understands the purpose of the procedure and can cooperate; the wound shows evidence of healing; there is no evidence of infection in the wound; dressing is securely in place; patient stated he or she was comfortable after procedure. **R:** Evaluation in relation to desired outcomes is essential for planning future care.

DOCUMENTATION

27. Document the procedure on the patient's record, including the time the procedure was performed, observations of the wound, dressing and cleansing materials used, and the patient's knowledge and comfort. This information is sometimes entered on a flow sheet (Fig. 40-10). **R:** Documentation is a legal record of the patient's care and therapy and communicates nursing activities to other nurses and caregivers.

SPECIFIC PROCEDURES RELATED TO WOUND CARE

Shortening a Penrose Drain

The surgeon may order that a Penrose drain (described above) be shortened by a specific amount, usually to encourage the closure of the wound from the inside out. The drain is pulled out of the wound the specified distance, and its length inside of the wound is thus shortened. A sterile safety pin is commonly used to prevent the drain from slipping back inside the wound. Each

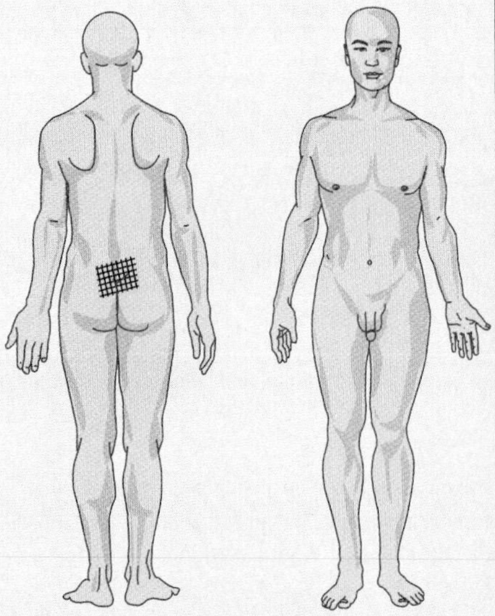

STAGE I	Skin is pink, red, or mottled; blanches on touch—lasting up to 15 min after pressure is released. Skin feels firm and warm.
STAGE II	Skin appears cracked, blistered, and broken. Surrounding area red.
STAGE III	Full thickness skin loss. May include subcutaneous tissue and produce serosanguineous drainage.
STAGE IV	Full thickness skin loss with deep tissue, muscle, or bone involved.
ESCHAR	If present, should be measured and documented.
POST-OP	Debridement, flap, rotation closure (sutures, staples, drains).

X Present on admission?   From ___Home___

THERAPEUTIC MEASURES/PHYSICIAN'S ORDERS FOR:

Present surface:

Alternating pressure	☐ PT _____	☐ Dietary assessment	
	☐ Range of motion exercise	☐ G Tube ☐ NG Tube	
X Elbow protectors	☐ Whirlpool therapy	☐ Protein supplement	
X Heel protectors	☐ Catheter	☐ Multi-vits/zinc/iron	
X Turn sched Q _2 hr_	☐ Hydration	☐ Current HGB/HCT	

Height 5'3"   Weight 50 kg   Ideal body wt _____

Other   *Clean and apply Duoderm as needed*

Illustrate position of affected area in red.
Utilize one sheet per affected area.

CULTURES DONE: Date _1-29-06_   Date _____   Date _____   Date _____

Date	#	Site	Stage	Length/width (cm)	Drainage/type	Treatment	MD notified
1-29-06	1	Coccyx	III	2 X 2.5	Yellow purulent	Cleaned with N.S. Duoderm applied	

Depth	Undermining/tunneling		Odor		Response	RN signature
2 mm	None		Musty	Red under drainage	States pain when cleansed	K. Lang

Comments

Date	#	Site	Stage	Length/width (cm)	Drainage/type	Treatment	MD notified

Depth	Undermining/tunneling		Odor	Color	Response	RN signature

Comments

FIGURE 40-10 Flow sheet for charting wound assessment and care information.

time the drain is shortened, the safety pin is moved. If a drain is stapled or sutured to the skin, remove the staple or suture before you shorten or remove the drain.

Shorten the drain during the dressing change, which is an open wound dressing change. The procedure for the dressing change is the same as above. Shorten the drain while the wound is exposed before redressing the wound.

ASSESSMENT

1-3. Follow steps 1 to 3 of the General Procedure for Changing a Dressing: Check the orders, examine the current dressing, and check the patient's unit for dressing supplies.

ANALYSIS

4-5. Follow steps 4 and 5 of the General Procedure: Critically think through your data, carefully evaluating each aspect and its relation to other data, and identify specific problems and modifications of the procedure needed for this individual.

PLANNING

6. Follow step 6 of the General Procedure: Determine individualized patient outcomes in relation to shortening a Penrose drain:
   a. Patient understands the purpose of the procedure and can cooperate.
   b. The wound shows evidence of healing.
   c. There is no evidence of infection in the wound.
   d. Penrose drain was shortened, and the end is securely fastened outside of the wound.
   e. Dressing is securely in place.
   f. Patient states he or she is comfortable after the procedure.
7. Gather supplies for changing the dressing and cleaning around the wound and also obtain a dressing set that includes a sterile pair of scissors.

IMPLEMENTATION

Action	Rationale
8-13. Follow steps 8 to 13 of the General Procedure: Wash or disinfect your hands, identify the patient (two identifiers), prepare the environment, explain what you intend to do, raise the bed, position the patient, expose the area of the wound, and drape the patient.	
14. Set up equipment and supplies.	
a. Set up supplies to clean around the wound and redress the wound.	
b. Open the package containing the sterile scissors.	The scissors used for cutting the drain must be sterile to avoid introducing microorganisms into the wound.
15-19. Follow steps 15 to 19 of the General Procedure: Loosen tape, put on clean gloves, remove and discard the dressing, wash or disinfect your hands, and observe the wound.	
20. Change the dressing as appropriate based on the General Procedure step 20b for open wound: Put on sterile gloves and clean around the wound and around the drain as appropriate. After cleansing, shorten the Penrose drain, and redress the wound.	
a. Grasp the Penrose drain with a pair of sterile forceps.	To maintain sterility of the drain.
b. Gently but firmly, pull the drain out the specified distance.	A gentle pull helps to guard against inadvertently pulling the drain too far.
c. If the sterile safety pin is to be replaced on the drain, handle it with sterile gloved hands. Remove and replace it at wound surface.	Doing so prevents the drain from sliding back into the wound, where a surgical incision would be needed to remove it.
d. Using sterile scissors, clip off the excess drain, making sure that 2 inches of drain remain visible outside the wound.	To ensure that there is enough outside to be able to grasp it when the drain is further shortened or removed.
e. Finish dressing the wound.	To provide an appropriate healing environment for the wound.
21-25. Follow steps 21 to 25 of the General Procedure: Remove gloves and place with soiled dressings, secure the dressing, assist the patient into a comfortable position and lower the bed, put on clean gloves, care for equipment, dispose of gloves, and wash or disinfect your hands.	

EVALUATION

26. Follow step 26 of the General Procedure: Evaluate using the individualized patient outcomes previously identified: Patient understands the purpose of the procedure and is able to cooperate; the wound shows evidence of healing; there is no evidence of infection in the wound; Penrose drain was shortened and securely fastened outside the wound; dressing is securely in place; patient states he or she is comfortable after procedure.

DOCUMENTATION

27. Document the procedure on the patient's record, including the time the procedure was performed; the amount the drain was shortened; observations of the wound, dressing, and cleaning materials used; and the patient's knowledge and comfort. This information is sometimes entered on a flow sheet.

Procedure for Removing Skin Staples or Sutures

Staples and sutures may be removed just prior to discharge. With short stays after surgery, they may be removed at a subsequent ambulatory care visit. Removal of sutures or staples may produce a pinching or pulling sensation but does not usually cause pain. If pain is present or anticipated based on the condition of the wound, give the patient the ordered pain relief medication about 30 minutes before the procedure is to be performed.

ASSESSMENT

1-3. Follow steps 1 to 3 of the General Procedure for Changing a Dressing: Check the orders, examine the current dressing, check the patient's unit for dressing supplies.

ANALYSIS

4-5. Follow steps 4 and 5 of the General Procedure: Critically think through your data, carefully evaluating each aspect and its relation to other data, and identify specific problems and modifications of the procedure needed for this individual

PLANNING

6. Follow step 6 of the General Procedure: Determine individualized patient outcomes in relation to removing skin staples or sutures:
   a. Patient understands the purpose of the procedure and can cooperate.
   b. The wound shows evidence of healing.
   c. Skin staples or sutures were removed without adverse outcomes.
   d. There is no evidence of infection in the wound.
   e. Dressing is securely in place.
   f. Patient states he or she is comfortable after procedure.

7. Gather supplies for changing the dressing and cleaning around the wound and also obtain a dressing set that includes a sterile pair of suture scissors or the package with a sterile staple remover.

IMPLEMENTATION

Action	Rationale
8-13. Follow steps 8 to 13 of the General Procedure: Wash or disinfect your hands, identify the patient (two identifiers), prepare the environment, explain what you intend to do, raise the bed, position the patient, expose the area of the wound, and drape the patient.	
14. Set up equipment and supplies.	
a. Set up supplies to clean around the wound and redress the wound.	
b. The suture removal kits and staple removers used in your facility may be either disposable or nondisposable. The latter type is sterilized and packaged in the Central Supply Department.	

(continued)

Action	Rationale
15-19. Follow steps 15 to 19 of the General Procedure: Loosen tape, put on clean gloves, remove and discard the dressing, wash or disinfect your hands, and observe the wound.	
20. Change the dressing as appropriate based on the General Procedure step 20b for open wound: Put on sterile gloves and clean around the wound and the drain as appropriate. After cleaning, remove the staples or sutures as follows:	
a. *Sutures:* If the patient's wound has been closed with sutures, gently lift each suture away from the skin with the pickup forceps. Then snip the suture close to the skin (Fig. 40-11). Pull it out by pulling in line with the suture that is still inside the tissue, so as not to traumatize tissue at the suture exit site. Remove every other suture first to determine whether the wound will remain closed. Then remove the remaining sutures.	Clipping close to the skin ensures that suture material that was outside the tissue is not pulled inside, which could contaminate the wound. 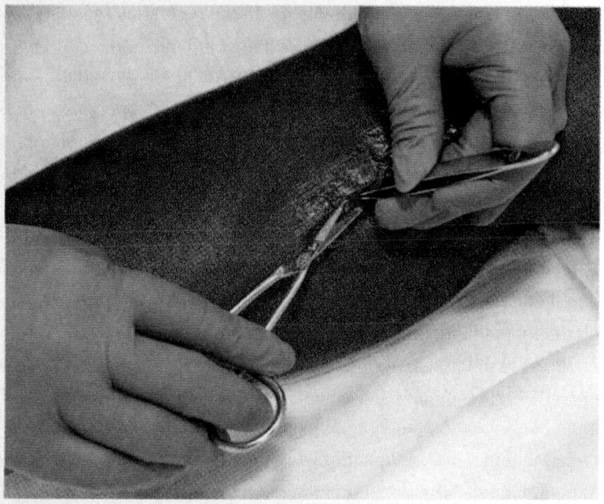 **FIGURE 40-11** Removing a suture by clipping close to the skin.
b. *Staples:* To remove skin staples or clips, slide the lower jaw of the staple remover under the staple, lift up on the staple, and squeeze the handles closed to exert pressure on the center of the staple. Remove every other staple first to determine whether the wound will remain closed. Then remove the remaining staples.	This motion raises the ends of the staple up and out of the tissue, allowing you to remove the staple easily.
c. Apply commercially available sterile tapes (Steri-Strips), if ordered or if included in the procedure at your facility.	Steri-Strips are usually used to provide extra support for holding the wound edges together after suture or staple removal.
d. Place a simple dry dressing over the wound if indicated.	To protect the wound.

(continued)

Action	Rationale
21-25. Follow steps 21 to 25 of the General Procedure: Remove gloves and place with soiled dressings, secure the dressing, assist the patient into a comfortable position, lower the bed, put on clean gloves, care for equipment, dispose of gloves, and wash or disinfect your hands.	

EVALUATION

26. Follow step 26 of the General Procedure: Evaluate using the individualized patient outcomes previously identified: Patient understands the purpose of the procedure and is able to cooperate; the wound shows evidence of healing; skin staples or sutures were removed without adverse outcomes; there is no evidence of infection in the wound; dressing is securely in place; patient states he or she is comfortable after procedure.

DOCUMENTATION

27. Follow step 27 of the General Procedure: Document the procedure on the patient's record, including the time the procedure was performed; the removal of the skin staples or sutures; the observations of the wound, dressing materials, and cleaning solution used; and the patient's knowledge and comfort. This information is sometimes entered on a flow sheet.

Procedure for Emptying and Restarting a Wound Suction Device

Many different brands of continuous wound suction devices are available. Three that are commonly used are the Hemovac, the Davol, and the Jackson-Pratt. These provide a much lower level of suction than do wall suctions or suction machines. They are lightweight and allow the patient to move freely.

ASSESSMENT

1. Identify the type of suction device and its location. **R:** This will enable you to plan the correct technique for emptying it.

2. Check the device. A check can determine whether the drainage chamber contains fluid and whether the suction container has re-expanded.

ANALYSIS

3. Critically think through your data, carefully evaluating each aspect and its relation to other data. **R:** This enables you to determine specific problems for this individual in relation to emptying and restarting a wound suction device.

4. Identify specific problems and modifications of the procedure needed for this individual. **R:** Planning for the individual must take into consideration the individual's problems.

PLANNING

5. Determine individualized patient outcomes in relation to emptying and restarting a wound suction device. **R:** Identification of outcomes guides planning and evaluation. Include
   a. Drainage is emptied, measured, and evaluated and shows no evidence of infection.
   b. Container is properly closed to prevent leaks.
   c. Suction is working in the device.

6. Obtain clean gloves, disinfectant wipe, clean towel or absorbent pad to protect the bed, and a container in which to measure the drainage. You will need to protect yourself and the bed from contact with the drainage and measure the drainage accurately. **R:** Planning ahead allows you to proceed more safely and effectively.

IMPLEMENTATION

Action	Rationale
7. Wash or disinfect your hands.	To decrease the transfer of microorganisms that could cause infection.

(continued)

Action	Rationale
8. Identify the patient, using two identifiers.	To be sure you are performing the procedure for the correct patient.
9. Pull the curtain around the bed and raise the bed to working height.	To provide privacy and protect you from back injury.
10. Explain what you intend to do and allow the patient to ask questions.	To help ensure understanding and cooperation.
11. Put on clean gloves.	To protect you from possible contact with drainage.
12. Expose the drainage container and place the absorbent pad under the opening.	To protect the bed from possible spilled drainage.
13. Clean the port with an alcohol or povidone-iodine wipe.	The drainage port provides a route for microorganisms to access the wound; therefore the port must be kept as clean as possible.
14. Open the drainage port, avoid contamination, and empty the contents into the container for measurement.	To keep the drainage contained.
15. Compress the suction chamber.	
a. For a Hemovac, press firmly down on the top of the chamber (see Fig. 40-5A).	To reestablish the vacuum and the suction.
b. For the bulb suction chamber, squeeze the bulb firmly to empty to bulb suction chamber (see Fig. 40-5 B). While pressing down or squeezing firmly, reseal the drainage port.	
16. Measure and empty the drainage and discard or clean the container.	Accurate measurement of drainage contributes to wound assessment.
17. Remove your gloves and wash or disinfect your hands.	To decrease the transfer of microorganisms that could cause infection.
18. Lower the bed and ensure that the patient is comfortable.	The low bed facilitates patient activity and prevents falls.

EVALUATION

19. Evaluate using the individualized patient outcomes previously identified: Drainage is emptied, measured, evaluated, and shows no evidence of infection; container is properly closed to prevent leaks; and suction is working in the device. **R:** Evaluation in relation to individualized outcomes is essential for planning future care.

DOCUMENTATION

20. Document the amount and describe the drainage on a flow sheet if one is available. If not, you can

add this information to the narrative progress notes. Also note the amount on the intake and output record, under "drainage." **R:** Documentation is a legal record of the patient's care and therapy and communicates nursing activities to other nurses and caregivers.

Acute Care

Most new postoperative patients will have a wound and a dressing. These wounds are expected to seal and heal rapidly. Dressings may be modest in size and changed only if grossly soiled. Other patients may be admitted for specialized treatment of wounds that have not healed. Expect that these wounds will need special dressing techniques.

Long-Term Care

In the long-term care setting, the most common types of wounds are ulcers created by circulatory problems or pressure. These wounds often take a long time to heal because of underlying physiologic deficits in circulation, nutrition, and oxygenation. The slow healing rate makes progress difficult to assess. The nursing care plan may specify the care techniques used, and documentation of wound status may be done on a weekly basis rather than daily. The nurse and the physician must work collaboratively on these difficult problems. To achieve the most successful outcomes, multiple products may be used on the long-term or **chronic wound.**

In addition to care of the wound itself, the nurse must be highly aware of the many factors involved in healing and strive to support the resident through nutrition, stress reduction, positioning, activity, oxygenation, and control of systemic factors, such as blood glucose concentration and blood pressure. Your nursing theory text provides more detailed information on the factors that affect wound healing.

Home Care

The client who returns home with a surgical wound may need little more than instructions to keep the area clean and dry until healing is complete. Occasionally, a client may return home with an extensive wound that requires complex manage-

ment. Before discharge, plan how this is to be done at home while there is still time to teach the client or a family member. Modification of technique may be necessary when hospital equipment and supplies are not available in the home.

For some long-term chronic wounds such as leg ulcers arising from poor circulation, clients will be instructed to use clean technique rather than sterile technique for home care. Sterile supplies are expensive and may not be unaffordable for a person on a limited income. Moreover, the body's own defenses may be adequate to prevent infection if the individual is at home without the threat of new and more virulent organisms that are frequently found in acute and long-term care facilities. Careful hand hygiene and use of meticulously clean supplies may be adequate protection in this setting.

The home care nurse can teach the client and any caregiver to assess the progress of the wound. Some of the same concerns regarding healing in the long-term care setting may also apply to the homebound person. Other physiologic problems interfere with healing, making attention to the whole person essential.

Ambulatory Care

Some clients with open wounds have wound dressing systems that remain in place for a week or longer. In some instances, these dressings are changed in a wound clinic where professional staff can assess the wound condition and ensure that dressing techniques are performed correctly. This is often the preferred method if the client needs specialized techniques such as compression dressings.

LEARNING TOOLS

DEVELOP YOUR BACKGROUND KNOWLEDGE

1. Review the Learning Outcomes.

2. Read the section on wounds and healing in your assigned text.

3. Look up the Key Terms in the glossary.

4. Review the anatomy of the skin.

5. Review this module and mentally practice the techniques described. Study so that you will be able to teach these skills to another person.

DEVELOP YOUR SKILLS

1. In the practice setting
   a. Inspect the dressing materials available. Note the differences in size, method of application, and purpose of each dressing material.
   b. Carefully read over the procedures and the Performance Checklists on the CD-ROM in the front of this book.

2. Working with two other students
   a. Simulate changing of a simple dressing and then a complex dressing using a mannequin. What adaptation would you make if a drain were present? If a drain were to be shortened? Give instructions and support to the mannequin as if it were an actual patient.
   b. Change roles so that each student has the opportunity to play the role of the nurse, the support person, and the evaluator.

3. Within your group of three or with the rest of the class, discuss the experience, focusing especially on what you learned from watching the other students.

4. Examine a suture removal kit. Practice using the forceps to pick up a small thread and clip it with the scissors.

5. Examine a staple removal kit. Note how the staple remover operates.

6. Examine a wound suction device. Practice opening, draining, and reestablishing the suction.

DEMONSTRATE YOUR SKILLS

1. In the clinical setting
   a. Examine the wound care products available in the clinical facility to which you are assigned.
   b. Consult with your instructor regarding the opportunity to observe changing a complex wound if possible.
   c. Consult with your instructor regarding the opportunity to care for a patient with a dressing you can change.

2. Validate your performance with the instructor.

CRITICAL THINKING EXERCISES

1. As you listen to the report, the nurse going off duty states that she has changed the patient's dressing every hour because of the volume of drainage. Based on this information, what are your concerns for the patient? Considering what you know about dressing materials, recommend some options for effectively dressing this wound. In addition to planning specific actions for wound care, what other nursing intervention will you undertake? Determine how you will evaluate the effectiveness of your interven-

tions. If your plan is successful, explain how you will communicate it to other nurses.

2. You are discharging a postoperative patient whose wound is still oozing a small amount of serosanguineous drainage. Based on this assessment data, what will you teach the patient about wound care at home?

SELF-QUIZ
SHORT-ANSWER QUESTIONS

1. List three reasons for applying dressings.

   a. _____

   b. _____

   c. _____

2. List three of the nurse's responsibilities with regard to dressing changes.

   a. _____

   b. _____

   c. _____

3. List four characteristics of drainage that must be noted when a dressing is changed.

   a. _____

   b. _____

   c. _____

   d. _____

4. List three characteristics of a wound that is healing by primary intention.

   a. _____

   b. _____

   c. _____

5. What is the term for a dressing that does not stick to the wound surface?

   _____

6. What type of tape is generally considered to be hypoallergenic?

   _____

7. Why are ostomy type supplies sometimes used for wound care?

   _____

8. What is the rationale underlying treatment of each wound site (drain wound, incision, etc.) separately when cleaning the wound area?

   _____

   _____

9. What is the purpose of a wet-to-dry or wet-to-moist dressing?

_____

MULTIPLE CHOICE

_____ **10.** In striving to prevent pressure ulcers, the nurse will address which factors in addition to pressure that contribute to their formation? (Choose all that apply.)
   a. Shearing force
   b. Poor nutrition
   c. Poor oxygenation
   d. Depression

_____ **11.** The wound is deep with undermining on the edges. The nurse is to choose a dressing material. What would best manage this wound?
   a. Transparent dressing (Opsite or Tegaderm)
   b. Dry gauze dressings
   c. Wet-to-moist dressings
   d. Moist gauze covered with dry dressings

_____ **12.** What is the purpose of a compression dressing on a wound?
   a. Increase venous return and lessen venous stasis
   b. Provide firm support to the dressing to hold it in place
   c. Prevent thrombophlebitis
   d. Decrease the need for multiple dressing changes

_____ **13.** When removing a Penrose Drain, why is a sterile safety pin used on the drain?
   a. To attach a drainage tubing to the Penrose Drain
   b. To secure Montgomery tapes to the dressing
   c. To prevent the drain from retracting into the tissue
   d. To prevent the drain from falling out of the wound

Answers to the Self-Quiz questions appear in the back of the book.

Providing Preoperative Care

SKILLS INCLUDED IN THIS MODULE

Procedure for the Preoperative Interview
Procedure for Preoperative Teaching
Procedure for Immediate Preoperative Care

PREREQUISITE MODULES

Module 1	An Approach to Nursing Skills
Module 2	Documentation
Module 4	Basic Infection Control
Module 11	Assessing Temperature, Pulse, and Respiration
Module 12	Measuring Blood Pressure
Module 14	Nursing Physical Assessment
Module 15	Collecting Specimens and Performing Common Laboratory Tests
Module 16	Admission, Transfer, and Discharge
Module 26	Administering Enemas
Module 32	Respiratory Care Procedures

KEY TERMS

ambulatory surgery	depilatory
anesthesiologist	hemostasis
antiembolism stockings	intraoperative
	NPO
antimicrobial	perioperative

OVERALL OBJECTIVES

▸ To integrate a preoperative nursing assessment with a preoperative checklist in patient's preparation for surgery.
▸ To facilitate patient's learning of perioperative routines, tests, and procedures.
▸ To effectively prepare a patient for surgery.

LEARNING OUTCOMES

The student will be able to

1. Assess the preoperative patient with special attention to allergies, past and current health status, and current signs and symptoms of illness.
2. Analyze assessment data, surgical procedure, and special patient concerns to determine needs that must be addressed to provide holistic perioperative care.
3. Determine appropriate patient outcomes related to perioperative care and recognize the potential for adverse outcomes.
4. Plan individualized care with emphasis on preventing adverse patient outcomes.
5. Implement a formal preoperative interview.
6. Implement individualized preoperative teaching.
7. Evaluate the effectiveness of preoperative care and teaching.
8. Document relevant data and patient outcomes.

Perioperative nursing practice includes activities performed by registered nurses during the preoperative, **intraoperative,** and postoperative phases of the patient's surgical experience. An important factor that contributes to a safe and successful perioperative experience and an uneventful convalescence is the conscientious and individualized preparation of the patient by the registered nurse. Remember that the patient is traumatized not only by the surgical procedure but also by exposure to anesthetic agents. In addition, surgery is emotionally stressful, causing varying degrees of fear and anxiety. Preoperative care, therefore, must include appropriate health teaching, physical preparation, and psychological support. Although portions of preoperative care may be undertaken by other members of the healthcare team, overall coordination and implementation remain the nurse's primary responsibilities. Perioperative care is truly interdisciplinary and collaborative (Table 41-1).

NURSING DIAGNOSES

- Deficient Knowledge: related to perioperative care. To participate in their own recovery, patients having surgery need to know what to expect and how they can participate. Anxiety is relieved by eliminating the unknown.
- Anxiety: related to potential pain or to previous experiences with surgery
- Fear: related to potential outcomes of the surgery and/or diagnosis

DELEGATION

Many aspects of general preoperative care may be delegated to assistive personnel. They often provide special

table 41-1. Perioperative Roles and Responsibilities

Role	Education	Responsibility
Circulating nurse	Must be registered nurse (RN); therefore, minimum of associate degree	Patient assessment, safety, and documentation
Scrub personnel	May be surgical technologist, LPN, or RN	Preparation, handling, and care of surgical instrumentation and surgical asepsis
Surgeon	Medical doctor (MD) or doctor of osteopathy with additional residency training in specialty	Medical diagnosis and surgical treatment, management of the surgical process
First assistant	May be RN, physician assistant (PA), or MD	Assists the surgeon in **hemostasis** (actions to stop bleeding), wound exposure, and suturing
Anesthesiologist	MD with additional residency training in anesthesia care	The anesthesiologist is a medical doctor whose specialty is administering local, regional, and general anesthetic agents. Many also have expertise in pain control procedures
Nurse anesthetist	RN with a master's degree in nurse anesthesia and certification in anesthesia administration	Monitoring, and administration of anesthetic agents

baths, measure vital signs, introduce the patient to the unit, and help the patient to put on a gown and get ready for the procedure. The majority of the tasks listed in the preoperative procedure cannot be delegated. Preoperative assessment, teaching, managing the legal aspects of care, and giving preoperative medications remain the responsibility of the nurse.

PLANNING PREOPERATIVE CARE

Preoperative care begins the moment a patient learns of an impending invasive procedure. Depending on the level of urgency of the procedure, some preoperative care will be done in surgeons' offices, preoperative testing units, day surgery units, or emergency settings. Surgeries scheduled in advance are called elective surgeries. In some instances, such as those in which complex preparations must begin the evening before surgery, patients may enter the hospital the day before the scheduled surgery.

To limit hospital costs by decreasing the length of stay, however, most patients enter the hospital on the morning of surgery. An "a.m. admission" often limits time for preoperative care. Nurses working in units with morning surgical admissions need excellent organizational and planning skills to complete all the preoperative care described in this module. Typically, more than one task is accomplished at the same time.

When patients have day surgery, also called **ambulatory surgery,** they commonly enter the hospital the day of surgery and are discharged later that same day or within 24 hours. This increases the importance of preoperative preparation regarding postoperative care. Much of the postoperative care may be performed independently by the patient and family. It is imperative to identify the patient's support systems and how the patient will be transported home from the surgical center because it is unsafe for patients to drive or use public transportation after receiving anesthetic or narcotic agents.

Preadmission outpatient visits are used in some settings to allow adequate time for preoperative procedures. This is especially true for patients scheduled for major surgery involving lengthy recovery periods and for children undergoing surgery. During these visits, the initial patient or family interview, laboratory work, and consent forms are completed. In addition, the nurse begins preoperative teaching. This may be done on a one-to-one basis, or special programs may be structured for groups of patients undergoing similar procedures. Family members may also be included. These programs are directly taught by nurses with special surgical and teaching skills.

Patients receive health teaching regarding what to expect preoperatively, intraoperatively, and postoperatively and how to participate in regaining independence. With the help of booklets and visual aids, they are taught deep-breathing exercises, leg and foot exercises, how to move in and out of bed, and measures for pain relief. They are also shown equipment that will be used in their postoperative care. Some programs include a tour of the surgical unit and introductions to the staff. Such programs are helpful in reducing anxiety and decreasing complications after surgery.

If the patient has not participated in a preadmission outpatient visit, the patient entering the preoperative unit has probably already been to the laboratory, where blood and urine samples have been collected for laboratory studies, such as a complete blood count (CBC) and urinalysis (UA). Other tests that may be necessary include an electrocardiogram, blood chemistry panel, chest x-ray, or other diagnostic imaging studies. In some settings, patients have no laboratory studies before surgery unless there is a recognized problem.

A consent form, which must be signed prior to any invasive procedure, may have been signed and witnessed in the surgeon's office. Often there will be multiple consents; for example, for surgery, anesthesia, or blood transfusions. These consents should be signed and dated. They usually list potential risks of the impending procedure. Sometimes, the preoperative nurse may need to obtain a signature for a consent; however, it is the surgeon's responsibility to provide the risks and complications of the procedure to the patient (Box 41-1). In addition, advance directives should be signed and secured on the chart prior to surgery. Preoperative care varies from facility to facility. At points throughout the module, you may have to check the policies of the facility in which you practice and adapt your care to those policies.

PROCEDURE FOR THE PREOPERATIVE INTERVIEW

The initial step in preoperative care is the preoperative interview. The nursing process phase of assessment is ongoing throughout this procedure because the nurse

---

box 41-1 *Possible Adverse Effects of Surgery*

Acute pain not relieved by pain management plan
Altered thermoregulation
Anxiety
Aspiration during perioperative period
Disturbed body image
Impaired tissue integrity (skin breakdown)
Injury during perioperative period
Latex allergy response
Postoperative infection

must integrate the patient's responses in the plan of care (AORN, 2004B). Usually, the preoperative interview fulfills many of the steps of the hospital physical assessment and the preoperative checklist. (See Module 14, Nursing Physical Assessment, and Module 16, Admission, Transfer, and Discharge.)

ASSESSMENT

1. Check the preoperative orders. Some surgeons use a stamp for their routine orders on a specific procedure and add any special orders for the individual patient. **R:** Checking orders helps to determine your responsibilities regarding preparing the patient for surgery.
2. Identify the type of surgery. **R:** Doing this helps you to plan for needs that the surgery will create.
3. Identify the required paperwork and any policies and procedures affecting preoperative care for the patient. Some facilities maintain a file listing the preferences of the surgeon and/or **anesthesiologist. R:** This helps to determine what you need to accomplish.
4. Check the patient's chart for the health history and physical examination (H&P), the signed consent form(s), patient's preferred speaking language, and results of any ordered laboratory tests, such as a CBC or a UA. **R:** Checking for these data will help you obtain data or records that are missing. The H&P and the completed consent form(s) must be on the record before surgery to protect the patient, the physician, and staff.

Safety Alert

Surgery cannot proceed (except in a life-threatening emergency) without a properly completed consent form. Know your facility's policy regarding informed consent.

ANALYSIS

5. Analyze the anatomic and physiologic implications of the procedure. For example, consider whether the patient will be able to stand, bend over, reach over the head, or use an extremity postoperatively. **R:** This analysis will help you integrate that information into your care plan.
6. Critically think through your data, carefully evaluating each aspect and its relation to other data. **R:** This enables you to determine specific problems for this individual in relation to preoperative care.
7. Identify specific problems and modifications of the procedure (such as the need for an interpreter) needed for this individual. **R:** Planning for the individual must take into consideration the individual's problems.

PLANNING

8. Identify the individualized patient outcomes for the preoperative interview, including the following. **R:** Identification of outcomes guides planning and evaluation.
   a. Required information is documented on the patient's record.
   b. Surgical site has been accurately marked.
   c. Patient states that all questions have been answered.
9. Arrange to complete the forms and procedures listed in step 4 if they are not on the record. **R:** Doing this will prevent a delay of surgery caused by lack of consent forms.
10. Inform laboratory personnel or the physician about missing data. **R:** These services need to know what data are missing so that they can be completed.
11. Plan sufficient uninterrupted time to carry out the preoperative interview. At times, the assistance of the family or an interpreter may be needed to obtain the necessary information. **R:** A rushed interview may fail to obtain essential data. Language barriers may result in failure to obtain accurate information.

IMPLEMENTATION

Action	Rationale
12. Using the appropriate form, interview the patient, making sure to include the following areas:	
a. Patient identity: Confirm the correct patient. Use two different patient identifiers. Ask the patient to state his or her full name *and* birth date; then compare that with the full name *and* birth date on the patient's record. Alternatively, compare the spelling of the name and	To ensure that the procedure will be performed for the correct patient and eliminate the chance that the wrong patient will undergo the wrong surgery (a major safety goal).

(continued)

Action	Rationale
the patient's number on the patient's record with the spelling of the name and the patient's number on the wristband (AORN, 2004A). *Note:* In the operating room before the procedure begins, there will be a halt in all activity while everyone focuses on ensuring patient identification, using two identifiers.	
b. Surgical procedure: Confirm the planned surgical procedure by asking the patient to state the planned procedure in his or her own words and compare that with the surgery listed on the patient's record.	To ensure that the correct patient undergoes the correct surgery and eliminate wrong-patient surgery (a major safety goal).
c. Record identification: Verify the patient's name and procedure on the consent form and on laboratory or radiology results.	To ensure that all documents included are on the right patient's record.
d. Surgical site confirmation: Confirm that the surgical site is marked. The operative site should be marked with a permanent marker. In some facilities, the patient is asked to independently mark the surgical site. The surgeon or the nurse may participate in this process with the patient. If the patient is not mentally competent to participate, then the surgeon usually marks the site. Follow the policy in your facility. *Note:* The correct surgical site will be rechecked immediately before the surgery when all in the operating room pause for this verification.	To prevent wrong-site surgery (a major safety goal).
e. General appearance: Describe the patient's general appearance and physical condition. Also record the patient's height and weight, which may be used to compute the amount of anesthetic agent administered. Note any sensory deficits. Include vital signs, **NPO** (nothing by mouth) status, skin condition, joint mobility or pain, and other relevant data.	To provide baseline data.
f. Allergies: Ask the patient about any allergies, including skin or contact, food, medication, and latex allergies.	The patient's allergies must be documented thoroughly to prevent contact with or use of products that create an allergic response or sensitivity. Latex sensitivity is especially critical because this will require that the entire operating room be made latex-free before the surgery. *(continued)*

Action	Rationale
g. Anxiety level: Determine the patient's anxiety level. Communication with the patient during the interview will usually indicate the patient's anxiety level. Look for restlessness, fidgeting, rapid respirations and pulse rate, and statements indicating anxiety.	To assist you in planning anxiety-reduction strategies.
h. Knowledge level: Identify the patient's knowledge level regarding current surgery. Ask the patient what he or she knows about the surgery. If the patient does not seem to recall information, give a general explanation. Direct any questions regarding specific points of the surgical procedure or expected results of surgery to the physician. Key your teaching to the patient's level of understanding.	Explicit details or unfamiliar terminology can raise the patient's anxiety level. Information necessary to informed consent, the specific surgical procedure, and the prognosis are all medical information and as such are given by the medical care provider.
i. Previous surgeries: Ask about previous surgeries and list all of them.	These may have physical and psychological consequences for the current surgery. Never assume that the patient who has had multiple surgeries needs less preparation. He or she may still be anxious and have inadequate knowledge. A previous negative experience may cause the patient to feel more anxious.
j. Chronic illnesses: Inquire about any chronic illness the patient may have.	Some illnesses, such as chronic lung disease, hypertension, kidney disorders, diabetes, heart or liver disease, may have implications for other aspects of care, including choice of anesthetic(s), medications ordered for pain and sleep, and respiratory care.
k. Smoking habits: Note whether the patient is a smoker or nonsmoker. Document pack years—multiplying the number of packs smoked per day by the number of years smoked.	The lung tissue of a smoker is more sensitive to anesthetic gases because of mild irritation. It is recommended that smoking cessation occur 1 month prior to a surgical procedure (Mangram, Horan, Pearson, et al., 1999). Many hospitals are nonsmoking environments; not being permitted to smoke may increase anxiety in some smokers.
l. Drug, alcohol, and caffeine intake: List all medications the patient is taking, including vitamin preparations, birth control pills, herbal agents, and non-prescription drugs. Some patients do not remember to mention long-term medications, such as diuretics or daily birth control pills or vitamin supplements. Emphasize the importance of a complete list.	Anesthetic agents and other medications ordered may interact with the medications or herbal agents the patient is already taking. Certain medications (for example, anticonvulsant drugs) will be continued throughout the operative period because interruption would cause adverse effects for the patient. A reliable alcohol history also is essential. Heavy use of alcohol has multiple effects on the body that can change the patient's response to anesthesia, surgery, and recovery. Additionally, knowing the patient's usual daily caffeine intake may be helpful, especially during the

(continued)

Action	Rationale
	immediate preoperative and postoperative phases. Some people experience severe headaches related to the sudden absence of caffeine.
m. Support-system data: List on the interview form the names and relations of close family members and friends and their telephone numbers.	The family and significant others are concerned about the patient, may be involved in the health teaching, and often care for the patient after discharge.
13. Encourage the patient and family to ask questions about the procedure, the policies of the facility, or aspects of care. If you do not know the answers to specific questions, consult the appropriate resource person.	The questions asked cue you to areas of deficient knowledge.
14. Provide emotional support: Convey a sense of confidence, use touch appropriately, and listen to the verbalization of concerns.	To relieve anxiety.

EVALUATION

15. Evaluate using the individualized patient outcomes previously identified. **R:** Evaluation in relation to desired outcomes is essential for planning future care.
   a. Required information is documented on the patient's record.
   b. Surgical site has been accurately marked.
   c. Patient states that all questions have been answered.

DOCUMENTATION

16. Attach the interview form to the patient's record where you and others can refer to it as you begin the written plan of care. **R:** This will assist the nursing care team in working effectively to ensure accuracy and continuity of care.

PROCEDURE FOR PREOPERATIVE TEACHING

Well-planned, individualized preoperative teaching prepares the patient for effective participation in the activities surrounding the surgery and results in fewer postoperative complications and a smoother postoperative course. After the surgery, the patient's ability to learn needed information will be impaired due to the effects of anesthesia, pain, and medications. Incorporate your knowledge of teaching and learning principles, implications of growth and development, the facility's routines, and the physician's orders to plan a teaching strategy to best meet the patient's needs and promote the best outcome. If the surgery is an emergency and time for teaching is short, you may be able to include only priority information.

ASSESSMENT

1. Carefully review the preoperative orders. **R:** Review of orders ensures that the information you share will be individualized, specific, and accurate.
2. Assess the patient's language level, educational background, growth and development stage, and anxiety level. If you interviewed the patient, you have some knowledge of these areas. If you have not yet met the patient, spend some time assessing these specific areas. **R:** This provides a baseline for planning.
3. If family members or significant friends are present, ask the patient if he or she would like to have them included in the preoperative teaching. **R:** During the postoperative period, these people can often reinforce what has been taught. Parents or guardians of small children should always be included because they will be the best source of information and they are legally responsible for the child.

ANALYSIS

4. Critically think through your data, carefully evaluating each aspect and its relation to other data. **R:** This enables you to determine specific challenges for this patient in terms of preoperative learning.

5. Identify specific problems and modifications of the procedure needed for this individual. **R:** Planning for the individual must take into account the individual's problems.

PLANNING

6. Determine individualized patient outcomes for the preoperative teaching, including the following. **R:** Identification of outcomes guides planning and evaluation.
   a. Patient can state in own words what will be done in the surgery and what specific postoperative care or procedures to expect following surgery.
   b. Patient can describe the expected postoperative care routines.
   c. Patient can state what he or she can do to assist with postoperative pain management.
   d. Patient can perform actions, such as deep breathing and coughing, moving about, and leg exercises, that he or she can do to prevent postoperative complications.
      Note: If you involve the family and significant others, their understanding of the preoperative teaching also will be important outcomes.
7. Allow sufficient uninterrupted time so that you will not be hurried in your instruction and the patient will feel more relaxed.

IMPLEMENTATION

Action	Rationale
8. Provide a quiet, nonstressful environment in which to teach. This includes providing comfortable chairs for those present, turning off the television set, and using an empty day room or conference room if the teaching could disturb a roommate.	Distractions may inhibit learning.
9. You may design your own teaching plan or use one provided in your clinical setting (Fig. 41-1), but be sure to include the following points as appropriate to the specific surgery planned.	
a. Preoperative routines: Outline the routines for the patient in clear, understandable terms. You may do this by body system, describing preoperative care of the gastrointestinal tract, skin, and so on, or by going through the preparation sequentially.	Understanding the procedures and processes will diminish anxiety and increase the patient's ability to participate.
b. Postoperative routines: Explain what will be done, with what frequency, and why.	
(1) Post-anesthesia care unit (PACU): Explain that the patient can expect to first be in the PACU, where constant surveillance is available until the patient is stable enough to be moved to a standard patient room.	Both patient and family may be alarmed by the delayed return to the room, assuming that it represents complications.
(2) Vital signs: Blood pressure, pulse, and respiration are checked every 15 minutes for at least the first hour after surgery and less frequently thereafter if they are stable.	Vital signs provide for early identification of problems, such as hypothermia or hyperthermia, hemorrhage, cardiac or respiratory complications.

(continued)

Action	Rationale

TEACHING MAY INCLUDE: Pathophysiology, Treatments, Nutrition, Medications, Side Effects, Procedures, Symptoms to report, Home Management, Preventative Health, etc.

TEACHING CONTENT PRE-OPERATIVE TEACHING	PATIENT RESPONSE			
	Indicates Understanding	Needs Reinforcement	Return Demonstration	Able to Perform Independently
1. Understands surgical procedure and expected outcome.	3/14 PB			
2. Immediate Post-op				
a. PACU	3/14 PB			
b. Frequent monitoring of vital signs	3/14 PB			
c. Return to floor/ICU	3/14 PB			
3. Diet				
a. Pre-op (i.e., clear liquids)	3/14 PB			
b. NPO after midnight	3/14 PB			
c. Progression after surgery	3/16 JE	3/14 PB		
4. Medications				
a. Sedation at H.S.	3/14 PB			
b. Pre-op medication day of surgery	3/14 PB			
c. Post-op medications (analgesics, antibiotics, other)	3/14 PB			
5. Pre-op Preparation				
a. Skin prep	3/14 PB			
b. Bowel Prep				
c. Other				
6. Equipment				
a. Intravenous	3/14 PB			
b. Foley catheter	3/14 PB			
c. Nasogastric tube				
d. Drains				
e. Dressings	3/14 PB			
f. Cast/splints				
g. Other				
7. Activity Post-Op				
a. Positioning				
b. Exercise	3/16 JE	3/14 PB	3/14 PB 3/16 JE	3/16 JE
c. Restrictions				
8. Pulmonary Care				
a. Turn, cough, deep breathe	3/14 PB		3/14 PB	3/14 PB

Identify Initials with Signature:	2. J. Ellison, R.N.	4.	6.
1. P. Boyd, R.N.	3.	5.	7.

ADDRESSOGRAPH:

HOSPITAL MEDICAL CENTER
SEATTLE, WASHINGTON

FIGURE 41-1 Patient education flow sheet.

(3) Dressing checks: These are made to observe the kind and amount of drainage.	Early recognition of bleeding is important to prevent shock.
(4) Progressive surgical diet: List the usual progression—from ice chips, to clear liquids, to full liquids, to a soft diet, and finally to a regular diet. The surgical patient can regain	Appropriate surgical diet may reduce nausea, vomiting, or complications related to paralytic ileus.

(continued)

Action	Rationale
normal eating patterns sooner if this progression is followed. For some less-extensive surgeries, the full progression will not be used.	
(5) Special procedures: Specific procedures (irrigation, respiratory therapy, casting, brace fitting, crutch walking, ostomy fitting) may be necessary for particular surgeries.	Early explanation of any special or unusual procedures that will be ordered may reduce patient anxiety and positively influence cooperation.
(6) Pain management: Instruct the patient to alert a nurse before pain becomes moderate or severe and explain the plan for pain management. Teach the patient about pain rating scales (for example, 0 is no pain and 10 is extreme pain), pain medications, patient-controlled analgesia (PCA), and other pain management strategies as appropriate.	Pain is considered a fifth vital sign and should be promptly assessed and interventions implemented. By encouraging the patient before the surgery to participate in planning for pain management, you help to relieve the patient's fear that pain will not be controlled.
(7) Postoperative appliances, tubes, and equipment: Inform the patient of any equipment or appliances that will be in place after surgery. These might include a catheter, an IV catheter for infusing medications and/or fluids, a nasogastric tube, or a wound suction apparatus.	Knowledge may decrease anxiety derived from the unknown or unexpected.
(8) Deep breathing and coughing: If the patient is going to have a general anesthetic, teach the patient how to breathe deeply and cough. (For instructions, consult Module 32, Respiratory Care Procedures.) In some hospitals, this teaching and that regarding the use of the incentive spirometer or other special equipment are done by a respiratory therapist.	Medications and immobility related to surgery will cause secretions to accumulate in the lungs. Deep-breathing and coughing assist the patient to expectorate these secretions and prevent postoperative atelectasis (collapsing of alveoli).
(9) Methods for moving: These methods include moving in bed and getting in and out of bed, as appropriate for the patient's postoperative condition and expected physician's orders. Consult appropriate modules to review the use of pillows for splinting, side rails for support, and body mechanics adaptations.	The purpose of teaching the patient to move with as little discomfort as possible is to encourage mobility. Turning in bed and getting in and out of bed prevent circulatory problems, stimulate the respiratory system, and decrease discomfort from gas.

(continued)

Action	Rationale
(10) Leg exercises: These exercises should be done 10 times each hour as soon as possible after surgery. If appropriate to the patient's surgery, active range-of-motion exercises can be substituted for these isometric exercises. Leg exercises are often augmented by the use of compression (antiembolism) stockings or sequential compression devices, which provide continuous support to the veins, decreasing venous stasis and promoting venous return. *Note:* When teaching leg exercises, first explain what you want the patient to do and why it is important. Then demonstrate for the patient. Finally, ask the patient to return the demonstration. Give positive feedback to the patient when the return demonstration is correct and encourage the patient if extra practice is needed. Three exercises are most commonly taught:	All these exercises facilitate venous return in the lower extremities and prevent venous stasis and clot formation.
(a) Calf or foot pumping. Instruct the patient to alternately dorsiflex and plantar flex the foot. Also inform the patient if a mechanical device will be applied perioperatively to facilitate this process.	
(b) Quadriceps setting. Instruct the patient to alternately contract the anterior thigh muscles and allow them to relax.	
(c) Gluteal setting. Instruct the patient to alternately contract the posterior thigh and gluteal muscles and allow them to relax.	

EVALUATION

10. Evaluate the effectiveness of your preoperative teaching using the individualized patient outcomes previously identified:
    a. Patient can state in own words what will be done in the surgery and what specific postoperative care or procedures to expect following surgery.
    b. Patient can describe the expected postoperative care routines.
    c. Patient can state what he or she can do to assist with postoperative pain management.
    d. Patient can perform actions, such as deep breathing and coughing, moving about, and leg exercises, that he or she can do to prevent postoperative complications.

Note: If family members were involved in the teaching, evaluate their understanding. **R:** Evaluation in relation to desired outcomes is essential for planning future care.

DOCUMENTATION

11. Most facilities have a preoperative form that provides space for noting preoperative teaching (see Fig. 41-1). If your facility does not have such a form, make an entry in the nurses' progress notes. **R:** Documentation is a legal record of the patient's care and therapy and communicates nursing activities to other nurses and caregivers.

PREOPERATIVE INTERVENTIONS

Depending on the surgical procedure planned, various interventions appropriate to that specific surgery may be ordered. For example, bowel preparation (usually consisting of enemas or laxatives) is routinely ordered for many abdominal procedures. Consult the appropriate modules for directions on the procedures needed. If a procedure does not have the outcomes expected, or the patient has an adverse response, be sure to notify the surgeon.

PREOPERATIVE SKIN PREPARATION

The effective preparation of the skin before a surgical procedure is an aspect of preventing infection in the postoperative patient. Because the skin—the first line of defense against invasion by microorganisms—will be opened, additional measures to prevent the entry of microbes are necessary. The main objective of preparing the skin is to remove dirt, oils, and microorganisms. A second objective is to prevent the growth of microorganisms that remain. A third objective is to leave the skin undamaged, with no irritation from the cleansing and hair removal procedure.

BATH

In most facilities, the preoperative patient is asked to shower or bathe, using an **antimicrobial** cleansing agent, on the evening before or the morning of surgery. If possible, the patient should shampoo at the time of the bath. Bathing removes gross contamination and soil and reduces colonization of typical wound pathogens that reside on the skin. The antimicrobial agent leaves a residue on the skin that decreases the overall bacterial count.

SCRUB OF THE SURGICAL SITE

Sometimes a surgeon orders that a surgical site be scrubbed for a predetermined length of time (for example, 5 minutes) prior to entering the surgical suite. This is most commonly done for elective orthopedic (bone) surgery because of the high risk of infection. The process results in a significantly lower bacterial count on the surgical site at the time of surgery. Because the procedure is so time-consuming and infection is not as frequent and serious in other kinds of surgeries, it is not performed routinely for most surgeries. A scrub procedure may also be ordered after an order for preoperative hair removal. The patient may be taught to do the preoperative scrub if the surgical site can be reached without strain and the patient can understand the procedure.

HAIR REMOVAL

Hair removal from a surgical site is a controversial topic because hair removal has been shown to increase surgical site infection rates. However, many surgeons prefer to have hair removed from the incisional area (Mangram, Horan, Pearson, et al., 1999). Shaving with a razor has the potential for injuring skin and thereby increasing the risk for infection. Recommended alternatives include clipping of hair or using a **depilatory** (Mangram, Horan, Pearson, et al., 1999). Consult the policies or procedures in your facility.

TIMING OF HAIR REMOVAL

The standard of care is to have hair removed immediately before the procedure (Mangram, Horan, Pearson, et al., 1999). If you have an opportunity to participate in the planning, you should understand the differences in infection rates that result from changes in timing of preoperative hair removal in relation to the time of surgery. Any time interval between the hair removal and the actual surgery allows hair to begin to regrow and microorganisms to multiply. Therefore, preoperative hair removal is carried out as close to the time of surgery as possible.

DEPILATORIES

Depilatories are chemicals that destroy the hair below the skin level, causing the hair to break off and leaving the skin cut-free and freer of hair than is possible with a razor. If a patient is not sensitive to depilatories, it is a safer method of hair removal than shaving. To use a chemical depilatory, read the instructions carefully and follow them exactly.

WET SHAVING

Although not recommended, wet shaves continue to be done. Dry shaves should not be done because they cause skin abrasions and increase the risk for infection

(Mangram, Horan, Pearson, et al., 1999). A wet shave is done using warm water and lather, causing fewer skin abrasions than dry shaves. Some facilities specify that clippers with a single-use head are to be used instead of a razor. Facility policy determines whether a wet shave or clippers are used, but the surgeon's order may take precedence over the usual policy.

PREOPERATIVE FASTING (NPO)

For many years, the custom in healthcare has been that the patient should be kept NPO (nothing by mouth) from midnight the day of surgery until the time of surgery. This time was adhered to even when the subsequent surgery was scheduled in the afternoon. The purpose of this practice was to prevent vomiting and subsequent aspiration. The problems associated with maintaining an NPO status for a prolonged period of time are primarily related to the relative dehydration that may occur. Moreover, patients who are accustomed to a significant caffeine intake may experience headache when they are NPO.

In 1999, the Task Force on Preoperative Fasting and the Use of Pharmacologic Agents to Reduce the Risk of Pulmonary Aspiration created guidelines for use in surgical settings (American Society of Anesthesiologists, 1999). These guidelines indicate that healthy adults may safely be given clear liquids up to 2 hours before a procedure that requires general anesthesia, regional anesthesia, or sedation/analgesia (often referred to as conscious sedation). The guidelines present evidence that the content of a meal is significant in determining how long the person should be NPO. A meal that contains fatty or fried foods or meat should be at least 8 hours before surgery. Milk or a light meal (without fatty foods) should be 6 hours before surgery. Based on these guidelines, some facilities are changing the directions given to preoperative patients. However, a nursing review of preoperative fasting in hospitals across the country demonstrated that many facilities had not updated their practice, and many nurses were unaware of changing guidelines (Crenshaw & Winslow, 2002). You will need to check the policy of your facility and the anesthesia orders regarding fasting to determine exactly how long the patient should be NPO.

PROCEDURE FOR IMMEDIATE PREOPERATIVE CARE

ASSESSMENT

1. Determine the precise time and type of surgery scheduled. **R:** Planning must take into consideration the schedule for surgery.
2. Check the chart for any changes or additions to orders. **R:** This review ensures that you are completing everything that is needed.
3. Check to be certain that the patient's informed consent has been given and the form signed. If it has not, notify the surgeon to obtain consent as soon as possible because this must be done before the patient receives any preoperative sedation. **R:** Keep in mind that the patient has the right to withdraw consent after it is given. Contact the surgeon if this occurs. Although the consent should have been checked on admission, repeat checks are done because accuracy is so critical.

ANALYSIS

4. Critically think through your data, carefully evaluating each aspect and its relation to other data. **R:** This enables you to determine specific problems for this individual in relation to preoperative care.
5. Identify specific problems and modifications of the procedure needed for this individual. **R:** Planning for the individual must take into consideration the individual's problems.

PLANNING

6. Determine individualized patient outcomes in relation to immediate preoperative care, including the following. **R:** Identification of outcomes guides planning and evaluation.
   a. All required procedures are completed prior to surgery (Fig. 41-2).
   b. The patient is ready for surgery at the scheduled time.
   c. All documentation (paper or computerized) is complete when the patient leaves the pre-surgical unit for surgery.
7. Plan ample time to complete the necessary tasks before the patient leaves the unit for surgery. **R:** Delays in completing preoperative care may result in delays for other patients as well.

IMPLEMENTATION

Action	Rationale
8. Measure and record the patient's vital signs. Blood pressure, pulse, and respirations may be increased because of anxiety,	To establish a baseline for future measurements and identify abnormal findings. An elevated temperature *(continued)*

Action	*Rationale*
but if the patient's temperature is even slightly elevated, report this to the surgeon at once. (Consult individual modules for specific procedures.)	may signal an infection, and the surgeon will need to decide whether or not to proceed with the surgery.
9. Document length of NPO (fasting) status.	Patients must fast, taking nothing by mouth, preoperatively to prevent a full stomach, which may trigger vomiting and subsequent aspiration with the induction of anesthesia.
10. Administer or assist the patient with oral care. Caution the patient not to swallow water, but only to rinse the mouth. You may have to perform oral care for some patients.	Oral care is necessary because the mouth tends to dry during the unconscious period with the administration of anesthetic gases.
11. Have the patient remove all items of clothing, including undergarments, and put on a clean gown. All prostheses, such as eyeglasses, contact lenses, hearing aids, and partial or complete dentures, should be removed and secured. Usually patients go to surgery without their dentures in place. If the patient has natural teeth or is a child, check for loose teeth that might be dislodged and aspirated during surgery. Note the presence of crowned or capped teeth or a permanent bridge.	Gowns are preferred in the operating suite for easy access to the patient's body, and valuables or prostheses can be lost. A tooth that comes out in surgery may obstruct the airway.
12. Remove and secure the patient's jewelry. Jewelry can be given to the family during surgery. Religious medals are often sent with the patient for comfort. If a patient does not want to have a wedding band removed, tape it in place to guard against loss. If the ring contains a stone, use a Band-Aid so that the stone is in contact with the gauze instead of with the sticky tape. Document the location and handling of all jewelry.	Any metal left on the body has a potential of serving as a path for electrical grounding. Valuable jewelry may slip off while the patient is unconscious.
13. Have the patient void, or insert a Foley catheter if ordered.	The bladder is emptied to avoid incontinence or injury during surgery. If the surgery is of short duration, voiding is usually sufficient. If a Foley catheter is ordered, consult Module 27. Some physicians prefer to have gastric intubation and catheterization performed after the patient has been anesthetized.
14. Remove colored nail polish and makeup.	This is so that the anesthesia provider can observe the nail beds and lips during surgery for circulatory assessment or use a pulse oximeter if indicated. Skin color and nail beds provide clues to hypoxia and can be readily observed during surgery.

(continued)

Action	Rationale
15. Remove hairpins and hairpieces.	These can cause pressure on the patient's scalp during the unconscious period.
16. Put **antiembolism stockings** or compression devices on the patient if ordered.	These stockings compress the peripheral leg tissue, increasing venous return during the immobile period, reducing blood stasis and risk for postoperative deep vein thrombosis.
17. Document the location or phone numbers of the patient's family or friends.	In case of an emergency or to provide progress reports, perioperative staff must be able to contact family and friends.
18. Check the chart for the preoperative medication orders. Review the preoperative checklist for completion prior to giving the medication.	Sometimes antianxiety, antibiotic, or antiemetic medications are ordered preoperatively. Most procedures should be done before the patient is sedated to allow for patient relaxation.
19. Prepare medications as ordered, administer them, and document.	Often more than one medication is given, and you must be certain all drugs are compatible, measured accurately, and documented (see Modules 44, 45 and 46). Postoperative infections are decreased by administering medications at precise times relative to the surgical procedure itself. Accuracy is critical to the safe administration of anesthesia.
20. Caution the patient to remain quiet in the bed after medication has been given. Put the side rails up for safety. Return the bed to the low position until the stretcher arrives. A lounge chair is used in some preoperative settings.	To prevent a fall and patient injury. A lounge chair promotes relaxation and lessens anxiety. It also facilitates transfer.
21. Place the call signal within the patient's reach.	This is so the patient has a method for contacting the nurse.
22. Follow the proper procedure for patient identification as the patient leaves the unit. In most facilities, the operating room transport person reads the patient's name and patient's number from the patient's wristband while another hospital employee checks that same information on the patient's record.	This is a safety precaution to verify identification and prevent "wrong patient" surgery.
23. Send the patient's record and any pertinent x-rays with the patient.	The surgeon may need to refer to the patient's record and x-ray films during surgery.

	YES	NO	N/A
1. Consent signed and witnessed	JE		
2. Time of last oral intake liquids _2400_			
solids _____			
3. Preop lab work	JE		
CBC _____			
Blood Ordered _____	—	JE	
Here _____			
Other			
_____			
_____			
_____			
Urinalysis	JE		
4. Preoperative bath or shower	JE		
5. Makeup and nail polish removed	JE		
6. Bobby pins, combs, hair pieces & wig removed	JE		
7. Rings, earrings, jewelry, watch (Disposition) c̄ husband	JE		
8. Prosthesis			
artificial eye— in - out			
contact lens— in - out			JE
pacemaker			
other			
9. Teeth			
natural _____	JE		
artificial upper _____			
lower _____			
bridges _____			
partial plate _____			
loose teeth			
10. Describe size and location of any skin lesion, burns, abrasions, etc. None JE			
11. Surgical Prep		JE	
12. Apparent preop mental condition of patient			
within normal limits _____ excited _____			
depressed _____ apprehensive _JE_			
irritable _____ other _____			

13. Location of family
   Rotunda _____
   Home _X-Will return at 1000_
   Office _____

14. Allergies   _None_

15. Pre-op vital signs
   TPR ___98⁴-88-24___
   B/P ___136/88___
   Wt. ___149#___

16. Voided
   Yes _0175_   No _____   NA _____

17. Retention Catheter
   Yes _____   No _JE_   NA _____

18. Pre-op Medication
   Ordered ___None___
   Given _____

Form completed by:

X   _Jean Estes R.N._
Signature

Date ___4/22/06___

Patient identification on unit
A. Person from surgery calling for patient
   1. Ask for patient by name & check identification band.
   2. Check patient's chart with nursing personnel on unit according to procedure.

Signature:

X   _Holly Martin LPN_
Nursing Unit

X   _John Peters_
Surgery Personnel

NURSING UNIT PREOPERATIVE CHECK LIST

FIGURE 41-2 Preoperative checklist.

EVALUATION

24. Evaluate using the individualized patient outcomes previously identified. **R:** Evaluation in relation to desired outcomes is essential for planning future care.
   a. All required procedures are completed prior to surgery.
   b. The patient is ready for surgery at the scheduled time.
   c. All documentation (paper or computerized) is complete when the patient leaves the pre-surgical unit for the operating room.

DOCUMENTATION

25. Document all pertinent data, including the following. The completed record must be ready to accompany the patient to surgery. **R:** Documentation is a legal record of the patient's care and therapy and communicates nursing activities to other nurses and caregivers.
   a. Preoperative checklist completed and signed (see Fig. 41-2). Check the form used in your facility to provide for continuity of care.

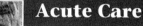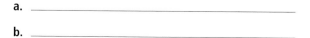

b. All nursing actions taken to prepare the patient for surgery and the patient's and/or family response

c. Any additional articles or devices sent with the patient to surgery

d. Time and mode of transportation to operating room

Acute Care

Most major surgeries occur in acute care hospitals where there are the facilities not only for the surgery itself but also for the postoperative care and treatment that may be needed. A large part of any hospital population is composed of surgical patients. Surgical patients have had steadily decreasing lengths of stay. Most of this results from a reduction in days spent in the hospital postoperatively, but part of it results from admitting patients the morning of surgery rather than the day or evening before as was historically done. These changes have greatly increased demands on the nurses in those settings.

Ambulatory Care

In the past 15 years, a steadily increasing percentage of surgeries are performed as ambulatory procedures. Some of these procedures are possible because of newer surgical techniques such as laparoscopy and the use of smaller incisions and less disruption of organs during the surgical procedure. Ambulatory procedures have created the need for very efficient use of time and excellent teaching of clients and families to enable them to manage their own postoperative care.

LEARNING TOOLS

DEVELOP YOUR BACKGROUND KNOWLEDGE

1. Review the Learning Outcomes.

2. Read the section on perioperative nursing in your assigned text.

3. Look up the Key Terms in the glossary.

4. Review this module and mentally practice the strategies described. Study so that you will be able to teach these strategies to another person.

DEVELOP YOUR SKILLS

1. In the practice setting, select a peer to implement a preoperative assessment and teaching on an abdominal surgery, a thyroid surgery, and a knee surgery. Compare the different types of information for each of these procedures.

2. Changing so that each has the opportunity to play the role of the patient, perform each of the following procedures. Those who are not participating at a given time can observe and evaluate the performances of the others.

Preoperative interview
Preoperative teaching
Immediate postoperative care

3. With the same group, change roles as you did before.

DEMONSTRATE YOUR SKILLS

1. In the clinical setting, consult with your instructor regarding the opportunity to work in a surgical admission department or to assist with preparing a patient for surgery. Evaluate your performance with the instructor.

CRITICAL THINKING EXERCISES

1. Consider how the growth and developmental needs of your patients will influence the teaching and learning strategies that you will implement for preoperative teaching. What might need to be changed for each developmental level?

2. What will you do if the patient informs you that he or she had breakfast on the morning of surgery, despite NPO status?

SELF-QUIZ
SHORT-ANSWER QUESTIONS

1. List two reasons why vital signs are taken during the immediate preoperative period.

a. _____

b. _____

2. Name three types of allergies that should be assessed for perioperative patients.

a. _____

b. _____

c. _____

3. List two reasons why you should know the family's location during surgery.

a. _____

b. _____

MULTIPLE CHOICE

_____ **4.** During the preoperative interview, you assess that the patient does not understand the expected outcomes of the scheduled surgery. The appropriate nursing action would be to
   a. explain the expected outcome of the surgery.
   b. notify the surgeon of the patient's lack of understanding.
   c. notify the anesthesiologist of the patient's lack of understanding.
   d. cancel the surgery.

_____ **5.** You note that the preoperative anesthesia orders include meperidine. During the preoperative interview, the patient tells you that she is allergic to meperidine. The correct nursing action would be to
   a. give it anyway because the doctor knows about the patient.
   b. hold the medication and put a note on the chart to that effect.
   c. notify the surgeon of the problem.
   d. notify the anesthesiologist of the problem.

_____ **6.** The patient expresses worry over the outcome of the upcoming surgery and states, "I guess I'm just scared that it will turn out to be cancer." The best nursing action in this situation is to
   a. sit down with the patient and encourage him or her to express his or her feelings.
   b. request a psychiatric consultation for the patient based on severe anxiety.
   c. ask the surgeon to visit the patient for reassurance.
   d. reassure the patient that it is unlikely to be cancer.

_____ **7.** The patient asks you why he or she cannot have anything to drink before surgery. Your best answer is
   a. because the surgeon ordered nothing by mouth.
   b. because it will cause nausea.
   c. to prevent the possibility of vomiting and aspiration while under anesthesia.
   d. to more closely monitor fluid balance through the use of intravenous fluids only.

Answers to the Self-Quiz questions appear in the back of the book.

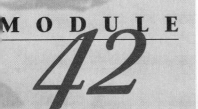

MODULE 42

Providing Postoperative Care

SKILLS INCLUDED IN THIS MODULE

Preparing the Postoperative Patient Care Unit
Immediate Care of the Postoperative Patient

PREREQUISITE MODULES

Module 1	An Approach to Nursing Skills
Module 2	Documentation
Module 4	Basic Infection Control
Module 9	Bedmaking and Therapeutic Beds
Module 11	Assessing Temperature, Pulse, and Respiration
Module 12	Measuring Blood Pressure
Module 14	Nursing Physical Assessment
Module 15	Collecting Specimens and Performing Common Laboratory Tests
Module 32	Respiratory Care Procedures
Module 41	Providing Preoperative Care

KEY TERMS

atelectasis
estimated blood loss (EBL)
paralytic ileus
postanesthesia care unit (PACU)

OVERALL OBJECTIVES

▸ To give comprehensive postoperative care designed to prevent complications.
▸ To identify promptly and report complications that may occur.
▸ To initiate appropriate interventions rapidly, thereby facilitating the surgical patient's return to health.

LEARNING OUTCOMES

The student will be able to

1. Assess the postoperative patient to identify any signs or symptoms of potential complications.
2. Analyze assessment data, surgical procedure, and special patient needs to identify particular problems or concerns that must be addressed to successfully provide holistic postoperative care.
3. Determine appropriate patient outcomes related to postoperative care, and recognize the potential for adverse outcomes.
4. Plan individualized care to prevent adverse patient outcomes.
5. Implement prevention strategies for potential postoperative problems.
6. Evaluate postoperative nursing care.
7. Document patient outcomes and objective data that will be used for discharge decisions.

Immediately after surgery, the patient is usually taken to the **postanesthesia care unit (PACU),** also known as the postanesthesia recovery room (PARR), where experienced nurses provide skilled care until the patient recovers from the anesthetic or can respond to stimuli. Usually, patients spend at least 1 hour in the PACU, but the time can be considerably longer. Patients who have had complex surgery or who develop complications may be taken to the intensive care unit for several days. This module discusses the care of patients who return to a regular nursing unit. For a more detailed understanding of the problems mentioned, consult a medical/surgical nursing text.

The nurse caring for any postoperative patient spends a large amount of nursing time teaching the patient and family or other caregivers how to manage at home. Topics might include activity, wound care, diet, hygiene, pain management, signs and symptoms of complications, and how to seek help if any problems arise. Standard instructions are often developed by the nursing staff to facilitate thorough and consistent teaching. When standard instructions are not available, the nurse is responsible for identifying the important teaching areas.

Written instructions are particularly important because this is a stressful time for those involved and complex instructions are easily forgotten or misunderstood. Many hospitals have standardized forms of home care instructions for common surgical procedures. These may be modified for the individual. If standard written instructions are not available, the nurse must write out the necessary information.

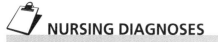

NURSING DIAGNOSES

- Fear: related to anesthesia, unknown surgical outcome, pain

- Anxiety: related to anesthesia, unknown surgical outcome, pain
- Acute Pain: related to inflammatory response resulting from surgical trauma
- Ineffective Airway Clearance: related to anesthetic gases, level of consciousness, immobility, pain
- Ineffective Breathing Pattern: related to sedation, pain, level of consciousness
- Ineffective Tissue Perfusion: related to hypovolemia, immobility, hypotension
- Impaired Skin Integrity: related to surgical incision, immobility, inadequate nutritional intake
- Impaired Physical Mobility: related to sedation, pain, or sequelae from surgical procedure
- Hypothermia: related to length of procedure, hypotension, stress response
- Hyperthermia: related to inflammatory response, pathology of malignant hyperthermia
- Imbalanced Nutrition: Less Than Body Requirements: related to pain, immobility, NPO status

DELEGATION

Preparation of the postoperative unit is frequently delegated. Immediate care of the postoperative patient should not be delegated to assistive personnel because the instability of the new postoperative patient requires the assessment and intervention skills of the professional nurse. After it has been determined that the patient is stable and assistive personnel have been apprised of symptoms that should be reported, measuring vital signs and other routine tasks may be delegated.

PROCEDURE FOR PREPARING THE POSTOPERATIVE PATIENT CARE UNIT

ASSESSMENT

1. Review the standard postoperative care needs related to the patient's surgery. **R:** To enable you to prepare the unit with all equipment needed.

ANALYSIS

2. Critically think through available data in relation to the patient who will be arriving in the unit. Carefully evaluate each aspect of the data and its relation to other data. **R:** To enable you to determine specific problems for the individual patient in relation to postoperative care.

3. Identify specific problems and modifications of the procedure needed for the individual patient. **R:** Planning for the individual must take into consideration the individual's problems.

PLANNING

4. Determine individualized patient outcomes in relation to the postoperative unit, including the following. **R:** Identification of outcomes guides planning and evaluation.

   a. Unit has all the equipment needed for a specific patient's care.

   b. Bed is prepared for easy transfer of the patient from the stretcher.

5. Identify and gather all the equipment and supplies needed for the patient's postoperative care. **R:** Obtaining and preparing needed equipment enables the nurse to care for the patient returning from surgery quickly and effectively.

   a. Tissues for cleaning drainage from nose and mouth

   b. Emesis basin in case of vomiting

   c. Thermometer, stethoscope, blood pressure cuff, and sphygmomanometer to measure vital signs

   d. Pulse oximeter for monitoring oxygenation

   e. IV stand to facilitate immediate transfer of IV fluids from stretcher to bedside

   f. Pencil and paper for making notes and/or flow sheet for documenting vital signs and care

   g. Special equipment appropriate to the type of surgery the patient has undergone; this might include traction equipment for a patient who has undergone an orthopedic procedure or a tracheostomy tray for a patient who has had thyroid surgery.

IMPLEMENTATION

Action	Rationale
6. Wash or disinfect your hands.	To prevent the spread of microorganisms.
7. Make the postoperative bed to receive the patient (see Module 9, Bedmaking).	The bed is arranged to make it easy to transfer the patient and to immediately cover the patient to prevent chilling (Fig. 42-1).

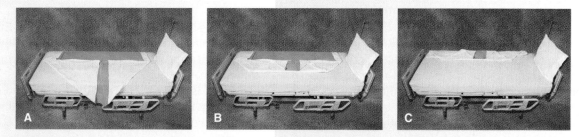

FIGURE 42-1 The bed for a postsurgical patient is prepared so that the patient can be transferred easily and then covered quickly to preserve body warmth. (**A**) Bed linens can be folded from the bottom and the top of the bed so that the linens come to a point at the middle of the mattress. (**B**) They are folded again toward the center of the bed and again (**C**) toward the far edge of the bed. When the patient arrives, the linens can be quickly unfolded to keep the patient warm.

a. Provide extra protection at the head, such as a pad or bath towel.	To make changing linens easier in case of vomiting.
b. Provide extra protection in the middle (plastic drawsheet, incontinence pad, or disposable moisture-proof pad).	To make changing linens easier in case of soiling by drainage or incontinence.

(continued)

Action	Rationale
c. Prepare turning sheet.	To provide assistance with positioning.
8. Place all the necessary equipment where it can easily be reached.	Placing this equipment appropriately prevents disorganization when the patient arrives.

EVALUATION

9. Evaluate using the individualized outcomes previously identified, including the following. **R:** Evaluation in relation to desired outcomes is essential for planning future care.
   a. Unit has all the equipment needed for a specific patient's care.
   b. Bed is prepared for easy transfer of the patient from the stretcher.

DOCUMENTATION

10. The preparation of the unit is not routinely documented.

PROCEDURE FOR THE IMMEDIATE CARE OF A POSTOPERATIVE PATIENT

You can use this general approach to care for any postoperative patient being received from the PACU. It can be modified as appropriate for the needs of a specific patient. This procedure begins with the data received from the PACU, the analysis of that information, planning to receive the patient, and initially receiving the patient. The procedure then immediately returns to assessment where the critical observations are listed. The analysis of the data obtained follows, and then there is planning for the ongoing care of the patient, the implementation of medical orders and nursing plans, the evaluation of the patient's status, and documentation. This demonstrates the flexibility of the nursing process in which ongoing assessment results in changes in planning and implementation.

ASSESSMENT

1. Receive the telephone call indicating that the patient will be transported to the unit. You should receive the key information below. **R:** Information allows you to be prepared to provide care as soon as the patient arrives. If conditions on the unit would interfere with providing appropriate care on the patient's arrival, the transfer time can sometimes be adjusted.
   a. Patient's identifying information for safety

   b. Exact surgery actually performed; this sometimes changes from what was originally planned.
   c. A general overview of the patient's status, including stability of vital signs, pain management in effect, level of awareness; this information will enable you to plan how long the patient will need one-on-one care.
   d. Identification of all equipment needed for care to allow you to obtain anything needed before the patient arrives
   e. Exact time the patient will be transported
2. Review the room. **R:** To assist in identifying any last-minute changes needed to receive the patient.

ANALYSIS

3. Critically think through available data in relation to the patient who will be arriving in the unit. Carefully evaluate each aspect of the data and its relation to other data. **R:** To enable you to determine specific problems for this individual in relation to postoperative care.
4. Identify specific problems and modifications needed for the individual patient. **R:** Planning for the individual must take into consideration the individual's problems.

PLANNING

5. Determine individualized patient outcomes in relation to postoperative care, including the following. **R:** Identification of outcomes guides planning and evaluation.
   a. Patient is transferred to the bed safely and comfortably without stress or changes in vital signs.
   b. Vital signs remain stable and within normal limits.
   c. Dressing is dry and intact.
   d. Intravenous fluids are as ordered and infusing at the prescribed rate.
   e. All equipment is ready for use and functioning correctly.
   f. Patient is oriented to person, place, and time.
   g. Patient states that pain is within the predetermined manageable range (for example, 3 on a 1-to-10 scale).
6. Obtain any necessary additional equipment not already in unit. **R:** To facilitate efficient and effective care.

IMPLEMENTATION

Action	Rationale
7. Wash or disinfect your hands.	To decrease the transfer of microorganisms that could cause infection. The postoperative patient is at a higher risk for infection.
8. Receive the patient from the PACU nurse or transporter.	
a. Identify the patient, using two identifiers.	To make sure that the patient's record and orders belong to the patient and that this is the patient you are expecting and that has been assigned to this room.
b. Move the patient carefully from the stretcher to the postoperative bed. Use a turning sheet or sliding board, if possible, and keep the patient covered.	Transfer devices make the move safer and more comfortable for the nurse and patient. Rough or precipitous handling can contribute to sudden changes in pulse and blood pressure, and the patient is easily chilled (see Module 18, Transfer).
9. Receive the report from the PACU nurse or transporter as to what has transpired since your telephone conversation.	This report along with the telephone report provides a baseline for your own assessment.
10. Make the following initial observations:	Careful initial observations and assessments help to identify early indicators of adverse outcomes.
a. Time of arrival on unit	
b. Responsiveness (what the patient responds to and how he or she responds, for example, to name call, touch, shaking, and arousal)	
c. Pulse oximetry value and vital signs: pulse, respirations, blood pressure, and temperature	
d. Skin color, temperature (warm or cool), and condition (dry or moist)	
e. Condition of dressing: intact, clean and dry, or drainage apparent	
f. Pooled blood or unusual drainage (Look and feel under patient to detect bleeding.)	
g. Presence of an intravenous infusion (see Module 47, Preparing and Maintaining Intravenous Infusions): type of solution, amount remaining, rate infusing	
h. Presence of urinary catheter: unclamped; connected to drainage bag; freely draining; color, clarity, and amount of urine	

(continued)

Action	*Rationale*
i. Presence of other drainage tubes: unclamped; attached appropriately to bottle or suction; tubes not kinked or under patient; characteristics and amount of drainage	
j. Safety and comfort: presence of pain, nausea, or vomiting; position appropriate for surgical procedure; side rails up; bed in low position; and call signal within reach	
11. Check the chart for the following information (some of which may have been included in the report from the PACU nurse). Some institutions use a PACU nursing record, which can be very helpful to the nurse who is taking over the care of the patient on the nursing unit (Fig. 42-2).	To plan effectively for care and identify any problems that may be occurring.
a. Surgical procedure and length of surgery	
b. Postoperative diagnosis	
c. Anesthetic agents used and type and duration of anesthesia	
d. **Estimated blood loss (EBL)**	
e. Blood or fluid replacement given during surgery and PACU stay	
f. Type and location of drains	
g. Vital signs when patient left PACU (for use as a baseline)	
h. Medications administered in the PACU: name of medication, time, type, amount, patient's response	
i. Output: urine, other drainage, emesis	
j. Physician's orders: frequency of measuring vital signs, diet, activity, IV fluid orders, medications (amount and frequency of pain and other medications), laboratory or respiratory therapy orders, orders specific to type of surgery or other problems of patient	
12. Identify any problems or potential problems that may be present. Integrate the pathophysiology of the surgical procedure with the patient presentation. Be alert to signs and symptoms that could indicate impending problems.	To detect any problems at the earliest time.

(continued)

Action	Rationale

POSTANESTHESIA RECORD

Schwartz, Mabel

Dr. Jenkins

ADMISSION 1410	DISCHARGE 1520	ANESTHESIA general

SURGERY cholecystectomy

NURSE I. Hubbard RN

OR TOTAL INTAKE	OR TOTAL OUTPUT	PERTINENT MEDICAL DATA	O₂ L/M 2 LPM

Fluid— 275 ml EBL— 350 ml

Blood— Ø Urine— 100 ml

No significant medical history

☒ AIRWAY dcd @ 1430   ☒ INTUBATED dcd @ 1420

VENTILATOR Ø

☐ ECG ☐ 12-LEAD ECG ☐ ART. LINE ☐ CVP ☐ SWAN GANZ ☐ X-RAY

NO	SOLUTION	VOL.	ADDITIVE	TIME	TOTAL ABSORBED	TUBES	LOCATION DESCRIPTION	INTAKE	OUTPUT
1	D5LR	1,000	—	1200	400 ml	FOLEY/CYSTO CATH.	—	—	75 ml
						CBI/IBI			
						HEMOVAC/JP			
						PLEUREVAC/EMERSON			
						NASO GASTRIC Ø			
						EMESIS Ø			
						DRESSINGS Ø			

ALDRETE SCORING

COLOR	AWAKE	VENTILATION	BP	MOVEMENT
2 PINK	2 AWAKE-AWARE	2 DEEP BREATHS & COUGHS	2 BP 20% ANESTH	2 MOVES 3 LIMBS
1 PALE-DUSKY-BLOTCHY	1 ROUSABLE-ORIENTED	1 SHALLOW BREATH AIRWAY	1 BP 20% - 50%	1 MOVES 2 LIMBS
0 CYANOTIC	0 NOT RESPONDING	0 APNEA/OBSTRUCTED	0 BP 50%	0 MOVES 0 LIMBS

ALLERGIES

COLOR:	2	2	2	2	2
AWAKE	0	0	1	1	2
VENTILATION	1	1	2	2	2
BP	1	2	2	2	2
MOVEMENT	0	1	1	2	2

MEDICATIONS

	AMT.	TIME
Demerol	50 mg	1425

VITAL SIGNS

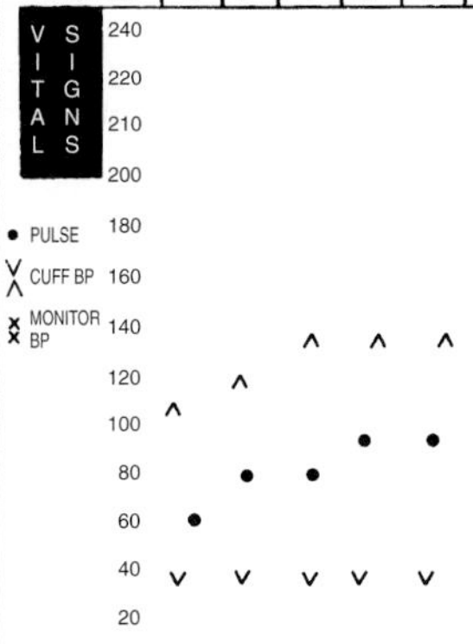

● PULSE
X∧ CUFF BP (V over ∧)
X MONITOR BP (X over X)

RESP.	14	16	16	18	18
TEMP.	97.6				
SAB					
CVP					
URINE					
PAIN	Ø	Ø	5	5	2

ABGS	PH	PCO²	PO²	% SAT	HCO³	B.E.	TESTS

FIGURE 42-2 Postanesthesia record.

(continued)

Action	Rationale
13. Determine any additional outcomes related to specific concerns or situation identified. For example, if this is a "day" surgery, identify the discharge criteria that must be met for the patient to leave. For common discharge criteria, see Box 42-1.	Outcome data evaluates the patient's progress.

box 42-1 *Common Discharge Criteria*

Vital signs stable
Swallow, cough, and gag reflexes present
Minimal nausea, vomiting, and dizziness
Adequate pain control
Absence of respiratory distress
Minimal swelling or bleeding at surgical site
Voiding without difficulties
Able to ambulate
Patient/significant other has received discharge instructions
Responsible adult to escort and care for patient at home

Action	Rationale
14. Determine the frequency for the systematic assessments—usually every 15 to 60 minutes after returning to the unit.	Frequent assessment provides for early recognition of adverse patient outcomes.
15. Plan actions to resolve or monitor problems identified.	Appropriate nursing interventions minimize adverse patient outcomes.
16. Carry out planned nursing actions related to specific physician's orders, assessment needed, or care related to surgery.	Ensuring the patient's safety and well-being during the postoperative period is a nursing responsibility.
17. Respond to problems encountered by initiating appropriate actions.	Early nursing response prevents problems from becoming severe.
18. Involve family members and significant others in the plan of care.	Family members or significant others of surgical patients may be important participants in the care of the patient if they understand the processes. They, too, often have anxiety and informational needs and are reassured by being included in teaching.

EVALUATION

19. Evaluate using the individualized patient outcomes previously identified.
  a. Patient is transferred to the bed safely and comfortably without stress or changes in vital signs.
  b. Vital signs remain stable and within normal limits.
  c. Dressing is dry and intact.
  d. Intravenous fluids are as ordered and infusing at the prescribed rate.
  e. All equipment is ready for use and functioning correctly.
  f. Patient is oriented to person, place, and time.
  g. Patient states pain is within the predetermined manageable range (for example 3 on a 1 to

10 scale). **R:** Evaluation in relation to desired outcomes is essential for planning future care.

DOCUMENTATION

20. Document patient responses and objective data appropriately on nursing flow sheet(s) or on the narrative record. **R:** Documentation is a legal record of the patient's care and therapy and communicates nursing activities to other nurses and caregivers.

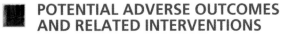

POTENTIAL ADVERSE OUTCOMES AND RELATED INTERVENTIONS

Table 42-1 provides an overview of the critical assessments in the postoperative period, the problems that may occur, and both prevention strategies and inter-

table 42-1. Ongoing Care of the Postoperative Patient

Functional Area	Nursing Diagnosis/ Collaborative Problems	Defining Characteristics	Selected Nursing Actions	
			Prevention	Treatment
1. Circulation Assess: Blood pressure, pulse, color of mucous membranes, peripheral circulation, temperature and color of lower legs, pain, and visible bleeding	a. Potential complication:* Hypovolemic shock related to blood loss	External or internal hemorrhaging; drop in blood pressure; rapid, weak pulse; cold, clammy skin	Avoid sudden movements; get patient up slowly; maintain IVs per physician's orders; keep warm.	Place flat with legs elevated; report changes in patient status to physician immediately; be prepared to administer medications, start oxygen, administer blood or IV fluids per physician's orders.
	b. Potential complication: Thrombophlebitis related to venous stasis	Localized pain, heat, and swelling, usually in lower extremities; positive Homans' sign	Encourage early ambulation or bed exercises, active or passive; encourage fluids; provide compression stockings or sequential compression device per physician's orders.	Provide bed rest; notify physician and prepare to apply hot, moist packs; administer drug therapy per physician's orders.
	c. Ineffective Tissue Perfusion: Peripheral venous stasis related to immobility	Legs immobile, dilated superficial veins, edema	Teach patient the importance of active exercise of legs while in bed and early ambulation; teach value of fluids in maintaining low blood viscosity.	Encourage early ambulation or bed exercises, active or passive; encourage fluids; provide elastic stockings per physician's orders.
	d. Fluid Volume Deficit related to inadequate fluid intake	Decreased urine output, dry mucous membranes, hypotension, fever, increased urine specific gravity, thirst	Maintain IV fluids at ordered rate; encourage adequate fluid intake as soon as oral intake permissible.	Readjust IV fluids based on policy and physician's orders; offer oral fluids of the patient's choice every hour.
	e. Fluid Volume Excess related to rapid infusion of IV fluids	Rapid, bounding, full pulse; moist sounds on auscultating lungs; puffy areas around eyes, sacrum, ankles	Maintain IV fluids at ordered rate.	Slow IV fluids according to policy or physician's orders; notify physician and be prepared to administer medications as ordered.
	f. Ineffective thermoregulation related to effects of anesthesia	Temperature fluctuates or remains low.	Monitor temperature; assess for signs and symptoms of shock; provide warm blankets.	Same as prevention.
2. Oxygenation/aeration Assess: Respiratory rate, depth, chest excursion, respiratory effort, breath sounds, pulse oximetry, and color of mucous membranes, nail beds, and conjunctiva	a. Potential complication: Pulmonary embolism	Rapid respirations, sudden chest pain, shortness of breath, anxiety, shock	Prevent thrombophlebitis (see above); do not massage lower extremities.	Notify physician. Administer drug therapy and oxygen per physician's orders; place patient in Fowler's position.
	b. Ineffective Breathing Pattern: Hypoventilation related to pain and immobility	Rapid, shallow breathing; diminished breath sounds	Preoperative teaching regarding the importance of deep breathing; pain management	Encourage turning, deep breathing, and coughing at least every 2 h. Encourage fluids and early ambulation.
	c. Ineffective Airway Clearance: Retained secretions related to painful coughing or decreased cough reflex secondary to narcotics	Presence of adventitious lung sounds; use of accessory muscles for respiration	Preoperative teaching regarding the importance of coughing up secretions; pain management; smoking cessation	Increase frequency of turning, deep breathing, and coughing; use suction if patient cannot cough out secretions. Notify physician for possible respiratory therapy.
	d. Potential complication: Atelectasis related to ineffective breathing pattern	Areas of absence of breath sounds, low-grade fever in first 24 h postoperatively; ineffective breathing pattern; ineffective airway clearance	All of the above treatments for ineffective airway clearance and ineffective breathing pattern	Notify physician for possible respiratory therapy; continue with treatment for ineffective airway clearance as above, increasing frequency.
	e. Potential complication: Hypostatic pneumonia	Rapid, noisy respirations; elevated temperature; increased pulse rate; restlessness; pain; cough	All of the above treatments for ineffective airway clearance and ineffective breathing pattern	Administer respiratory therapy and antibiotics per physician's orders.

(continued)

table 42-1. **Ongoing Care of the Postoperative Patient** (Continued)

Functional Area	Nursing Diagnosis/ Collaborative Problems	Defining Characteristics	Selected Nursing Actions	
			Prevention	**Treatment**
3. Comfort Assess: Patient subjective statements regarding comfort, pain rating scale, facial expressions, vital signs, willingness to engage in activities of daily living (ADLs); inspect for edema, tight dressings, or tight casts	a. Acute Pain related to incision/surgical procedure	Report of pain rating; grimacing; immobility (guarding wound); restlessness; blood pressure drop not accompanied by signs of blood loss	Administer pain medication before pain becomes severe; splint when moving; move slowly.	Administer medication per physician's orders; enhance pain medication with nursing measures (change of position, back rub, reassurance, information as to how long it will take pain medication to work).
	b. Nausea and vomiting related to anesthetic agents, pain medications	Complaint of nausea; emesis	Urge patient to breathe in and out through mouth; keep area well ventilated and free of odors.	Position patient on side to prevent aspiration; provide frequent oral care; give antiemetic medication before meals per physician's orders; NPO and nasogastric tube per physician's orders (for persistent vomiting).
	c. Impaired Comfort: Abdominal discomfort related to retained gas	Complaint of discomfort; drumlike distention of abdomen (palpate and percuss)	Encourage early ambulation.	Continue to encourage active movement and ambulation; encourage hot fluids (ice can increase problem); administer rectal tube, return-flow enema, or medication per physician's orders.
	d. Impaired Comfort: Hiccups (singultus) related to phrenic nerve stimulation secondary to dilation of the stomach or irritation of the diaphragm	Complaint of hiccups		Have patient rebreathe own carbon dioxide (inhaling and exhaling into paper bag held tightly over nose and mouth); administer medication per physician's orders.
4. Skin integrity/hygiene Assess: Wound appearance, temperature of skin around wound, and wound drainage	a. Risk for infection related to wound contamination or decreased resistance	Local signs of infection (redness, heat, swelling, pain, purulent drainage); generalized signs of infection (fever, increased pulse and respiratory rates)	Observe wound for signs of poor healing (wound edges not approximated, excess edema and inflammation). Keep dressing clean and dry; pay conscientious attention to caring for patient's hygiene needs; change linen at least daily; follow strict aseptic technique when changing dressing; administer antibiotics per physician's orders.	Administer antibiotics per physician's orders.
	b. Potential complication: Risk for dehiscence related to delayed healing	Separation of skin edges	Preop smoking cessation; adequate nutrition; apply abdominal binder per physician's orders.	Keep sterile dressings over wound; notify physician (surgical reclosure may be needed, or the wound may be left open to heal by second intention).
	c. Potential complication: Risk for evisceration related to delayed healing	Complaint of "giving" sensation in area of incision; sudden leakage of fluid from wound; wound open with abdominal contents protruding	Apply abdominal binder per physician's orders.	Cover open wound with sterile, warm saline packs; keep patient quiet; observe for signs of shock; notify physician; notify surgery (emergency surgical treatment usually required); stay with patient for psychological support.
	d. Impaired Skin Integrity related to surgical wound	Surgical wound not yet intact		Use sterile technique in care of wound; encourage optimum nutrition as permitted.

(continued)

table 42-1. Ongoing Care of the Postoperative Patient (Continued)

Functional Area	Nursing Diagnosis/ Collaborative Problems	Defining Characteristics	Selected Nursing Actions	
			Prevention	**Treatment**
5. Elimination Assess: Bowel tones, abdominal palpation, passing flatus?, stool appearance, urinary output, and color and clarity of urine	a. Constipation related to inadequate fluids and bulk, decreased activity, and effects of anesthesia and analgesics	Complaint of no bowel movement or small amounts of hard, dry stool; abdominal discomfort; abdominal distention	Encourage early ambulation; encourage fluids; administer stool softeners per physician's orders.	Administer enema per physician's orders (if no bowel movement in first 4 to 5 days); administer stool softeners per physician's orders.
	b. Potential complication: Paralytic ileus	Abdominal distention and discomfort, no flatus, absence of bowel tones, nausea	Encourage early activity and ambulation.	Notify physician; NPO and nasogastric tube per physician's orders (if paralytic ileus exists); administer medication to stimulate peristalsis per physician's orders.
	c. Potential complication: Urinary retention related to recumbent position, effects of anesthetic and narcotics	Urine output (measure); bladder distension (palpate); complaint of discomfort	Encourage early activity and ambulation.	Attempt measures to encourage voiding; insert urinary catheter per physician's orders (if no voiding 8–12 h after surgery).
	d. Potential complication: Risk for urinary tract infection related to catheterization or urinary stasis	Elevated temperature; cloudy or dark urine; burning on urination	Maintain adequate fluid intake; if catheter in place, give thorough catheter care.	Encourage fluid intake; administer medications per physician's orders.
6. Activity and rest Assess: Ability to move participate in ADLs	a. Impaired Physical Mobility related to general muscle weakness secondary to decreased mobility; pain and soreness secondary to surgical procedure	Weakness, dizziness, fatigue	Encourage early ambulation or active or passive range of motion if ambulation not possible; encourage adequate nutrition.	Same as preventive actions.
7. Psychosocial Assess: Ability to make decisions, willingness to assume responsibility for self-care, and ability to identify resources for support; expression of feelings, facial expressions, and body posture	a. Ineffective Coping related to diagnosis, physical status, hospitalization	Asocial behavior, malaise, listlessness, sleep disturbance	Encourage early ambulation; assist patient with personal needs; encourage patient's participation as appropriate; keep patient and patient's unit neat and free of odor; be available as listener; perform patient teaching.	Same as preventive actions; also arrange consultation per physician's orders.
	b. Anxiety related to pain and discomfort or possible outcome of surgery	Rapid pulse and respiration; elevated blood pressure; fidgety movement; states feels anxious or "nervous"	Provide preoperative teaching; stay with patient; encourage presence of significant others who are supportive; meet needs promptly.	Provide explanation and let patient know anxiety is normal response; encourage expression of feelings; help patient to name feelings; consider previous coping strategies; challenge unrealistic expectations of self; instruct in relaxation methods.
	c. Disturbed Self-Concept related to illness, surgery, change in body image, or effect of medications	Crying, withdrawal, sad appearance, indecision, apathy	Encourage participation in care; encourage use of support people; point out indications of progress; listen to concerns; teach about expected course of recovery.	Encourage activity as possible; point out progress in recovery; spend time with patient; encourage visits from significant others; inform that these feelings are common in postoperative period and resolve as recovery progresses.

*Potential complications must be identified and reported to the medical care provider for treatment.

ventions to correct problems. Some of the postoperative problems generate nursing diagnoses for which nurses will initiate care. Others are collaborative problems that require medical treatment as well as nursing interventions.

Home Care

To maintain safety, transportation home for a postoperative patient must be arranged taking into account his or her condition and the surgical procedure. The postoperative patient also may need a person(s) to assist in care because fatigue, pain, and disability usually limit the patient's ability to carry out ordinary self-care activities, such as shopping, meal preparation, and so forth. The nurse works with the family and patient to plan for this postoperative care. The nurse also must assess the learning needs of the patient and significant others to teach effective self-care practices. The family should be knowledgeable about wound care and signs and symptoms of infection. Other topics that should be addressed can be found in Module 41. Examples include leg exercises, early ambulation, importance of adequate nutrition and hydration, and smoking cessation, all of which promote wound healing and limit complications, such as **atelectasis** or **paralytic ileus.** A family member should know when and whom to notify for assistance or emergency care.

Ambulatory Care

The person having ambulatory surgery typically returns home within 24 hours of admission to the hospital. This is sometimes referred to as day surgery or same day surgery. Many hospitals now have a special unit for these patients. Here the patient is admitted and sent to surgery. The patient is received back from the PACU to the ambulatory surgery unit where he or she is monitored until stable and discharged home with planned transportation. At other facilities, the patient is monitored and discharged directly from the PACU. If complications occur or if the patient remains unstable, he or she is then admitted to the hospital for ongoing care.

The same guidelines for care apply as in inpatient surgery; however, the potential for problems is usually less. In particular, the patient is usually not immobile, so the problems of immobility that follow major surgeries are of less concern. A nurse from the facility usually makes a follow-up telephone call the day after the ambulatory surgery to see if any difficulties are being encountered and to answer questions.

LEARNING TOOLS

DEVELOP YOUR BACKGROUND KNOWLEDGE

1. Review the Learning Outcomes.

2. Read the section on postoperative nursing in your assigned text.

3. Look up the Key Terms in the glossary.

4. Review this module and mentally practice the techniques described. Study so that you would be able to teach these skills to another person.

DEVELOP YOUR SKILLS

1. In the practice setting, find and identify common equipment used for postoperative nursing care.

2. With two other students, go through a scenario in which one student is the patient, another the PACU nurse, and the third the receiving nurse on the general surgery unit. Go through the complete process of receiving the patient and initiating postoperative care.

3. Rotate roles so that each student has an opportunity to address the scenario.

DEMONSTRATE YOUR SKILLS

In the clinical setting

1. Consult with your instructor regarding the opportunity to care for a patient in PACU or a postoperative surgical unit.

2. Consult with your instructor regarding the opportunity to observe a nurse providing discharge teaching for a postoperative patient and significant others.

CRITICAL THINKING EXERCISES

1. You are caring for a 48-year-old woman who has a history of thrombophlebitis and has undergone a hysterectomy. Identify the potential complication that is of greatest concern for this woman. Determine what physician's orders you would expect relative to this potential complication.

2. You will be receiving a new patient who just underwent a thyroidectomy. What type of equipment will you have in the room? What are some nursing diagnoses that may apply to this patient? (Use whatever nursing texts are appropriate to complete this exercise.)

SELF-QUIZ

SHORT-ANSWER QUESTIONS

1. List four types of equipment that are usually included in the items gathered for a postoperative nursing unit.

    a. _____

    b. _____

    c. _____

    d. _____

2. List six general areas of concern that are included in the initial observation of the patient after his or her return from the postanesthesia care unit (PACU).

    a. _____

    b. _____

    c. _____

    d. _____

    e. _____

    f. _____

3. If a urinary bladder catheter is present when a patient returns from surgery, what three observations should you make?

    a. _____

    b. _____

    c. _____

4. List three actions that can help to prevent atelectasis.

    a. _____

    b. _____

    c. _____

5. List three nursing actions that should be taken if postoperative hemorrhage is identified.

    a. _____

    b. _____

    c. _____

MULTIPLE CHOICE

_____ 6. Mr. Smith is an 82-year-old single male admitted for gallbladder removal. He has a 60-pack-year smoking history and has continued to smoke. Which of the following nursing diagnoses or complications may apply to his situation?

    a. Potential for dehiscence

    b. Potential for atelectasis

    c. Imbalanced Nutrition: Less Than Body Requirements related to long-term nausea and abdominal pain after meals

    d. All of the above

_____ 7. Which assessment data informs you that your postoperative patient may not be ready for discharge?

    a. Respiratory rate of 12

    b. BP 112/82

    c. Pain rating of 3 on a scale of 1 to 10

    d. Slight serosanguineous drainage on the dressing

_____ 8. Which data may be indicative of a postoperative hemorrhage?

    a. Elevated BP

    b. Oral temperature of 97.4°

    c. Elevated hemoglobin

    d. Swelling and discoloration at the surgical site

_____ 9. Which of the following is a sign or symptom of a paralytic ileus?

    a. Active bowel sounds

    b. Abdominal distension

    c. Diarrhea

    d. Passing flatus

Answers to the Self-Quiz questions appear in the back of the book.

Providing Postmortem Care

SKILLS INCLUDED IN THIS MODULE

Procedure for Caring for the Body After Death

PREREQUISITE MODULES

Module 1	An Approach to Nursing Skills
Module 2	Documentation
Module 4	Basic Infection Control

Portions of the following modules may also prove useful:

Module 3	Basic Body Mechanics
Module 6	Moving the Patient in Bed and Positioning
Module 7	Providing Hygiene
Module 11	Assessing Temperature, Pulse, and Respiration
Module 12	Measuring Blood Pressure
Module 14	Nursing Physical Assessment
Module 18	Transfer

KEY TERMS

advance directive	morgue
algor mortis	mortician
autopsy	mortuary
deceased	next of kin
do not resuscitate (DNR)	organ/tissue donation
edema	postmortem examination
electroencepha-lography	repose
funeral director	rigor mortis
funeral home	shroud
livor mortis	sphincter
medical examiner	turgor

OVERALL OBJECTIVES

▸ To care for the patient's body after death in a skilled and respectful manner.
▸ To support the family in the pursuit of personal, religious, or cultural practices.

LEARNING OUTCOMES

The student will be able to

1. Assess the patient to verify that vital functions have ceased.
2. Analyze assessment data to determine special concerns that must be addressed in order to care for the patient and family after the patient's death.
3. Determine appropriate patient outcomes of postmortem care and recognize the potential for adverse outcomes.
4. Plan postmortem care based on patient and family wishes as well as facility policies and procedures.
5. Provide postmortem care with sensitivity and respect.
6. Evaluate the effectiveness of postmortem care for the specific patient based on patient desires and family responses.
7. Document all aspects of postmortem care according to facility policies.

In addition to the important task of giving comfort and emotional support to bereaved families and friends, the nurse also has the responsibility of caring for the patient's body after death. Postmortem care is a continuation of the quality of care a nurse gives patients before death. Essential to the task is an attitude of respect. In addition, survivors commonly view a body in the hospital or nursing home, and this makes postmortem care an even more important task.

To have patients clean and in **repose** after death not only comforts the bereaved, but is a nursing function that reflects personal involvement with the individual patient. Remember, patients are the nurse's responsibility from the time they enter the unit until the time they leave—whether in recovery or in death.

Care of the patient and family during the dying process is beyond the scope of this module. You are encouraged to consult other resources in your assigned texts and in nursing journals to help you develop skill in this area of patient care.

NURSING DIAGNOSES

- Disabled Family Coping, whether due to lack of physical, psychological, or cognitive resources.
- Decisional Conflict may be present for the family who must make decisions about the disposition of the body and perhaps of tissues and organs.
- Grieving is expected in the loved ones of the person who has died and should be supported.

DELEGATION

In some facilities, the physical aspects of postmortem care are carried out by nursing assistants. On many units, including the area of critical care, postmortem care often is given by nurses as part of the total care concept. The nurse must possess the skills and the sense of dignity necessary to care for a patient's body, to teach others to do it, or to supervise that care.

PRESENCE OF FAMILY AND FRIENDS AT TIME OF DEATH

The death of a patient in the healthcare facility has become much more personal in that the family and close friends are increasingly encouraged to be present and even to participate in giving care. The nurse should clearly determine how important it is to those who are significant to the patient that they be physically present at the time of death. If it is important, every effort should be made to have those persons present. Planning to accommodate the family or special friends in a sensitive manner can help offset later feelings of anger and guilt on the part of family and/or friends. It is also important for the patient to have a caring person present. The nurse can openly discuss the situation with the patient, family, or friends during the final stages of an illness. The wishes of those involved can be communicated by noting them on the care plan and by verbally relating them to the healthcare team. The same considerations are important when the dying patient is being cared for at home.

ORGAN OR TISSUE DONATION

Even though the willingness of people to donate their organs after death is increasing, there remains a large difference between the number of organs donated and the number of people waiting for organs. However, the number of persons whose life is prolonged or who gain renewed function of a body part or system through transplantation is increasing. Congress has recently passed legislation that requires hospital personnel to request organ and tissue from families of patients who are appropriate donors.

It is useful to remember that virtually anyone who dies can be considered a potential donor for some type of tissue. The donors of solid organs need to be supported on a ventilator after death is declared. Tissue donors do not need to be kept on a ventilator to maintain tissue viability. There is a continuous need for corneas, cadaver skin (used on burn areas until tissue regeneration occurs), bone, and connective tissue. Be aware of the patient's wishes before death regarding the donation of certain tissues and organs or of the wishes of the family after the patient's death. It is also useful to be aware of the views of various religious groups on organ and tissue donation. Anton and Johnson (2004) note that most major religions support organ and tissue donation. Even so, it may be helpful to have a member of the clergy participate in any decision-making process of the family. Many families find consolation in knowing that others will benefit from donated organs. In either case, signed permission is required.

To ensure the viability and usefulness of tissues, move promptly when you know that **organ or tissue donation** has been requested by the patient before death or by the family afterward. In most states, even when the patient has indicated a desire to donate organs, the family has to agree after the death for the organs actually to be removed. When death results from an accident and the patient's wishes are not known, family members can direct a donation of organs. The manner in which the family is approached may be a significant factor in the decision they reach.

Many acute care facilities have a transplant coordinator who manages the entire process, from discussions with the family to arrangements with the organ procurement agency. As soon as a nurse knows that a family is considering organ or tissue donation or when the healthcare team believes that the patient would be a suitable candidate for organ donation, the transplant coordinator should be contacted.

ADVANCE DIRECTIVES

Some patients, based on their own wishes or the decisions made by their families and physicians, are designated as "no code" or **do not resuscitate** (DNR), meaning that no heroic measures will be taken and resuscitation will not be attempted in the event of death. It is of utmost importance that you know the "code status" of each patient under your care. As a

nurse, you must understand that "no code" does not mean "no care." When a patient who has chosen not to be resuscitated is in the terminal stages of an illness, you should continue the high quality of care you would give to any patient until the moment of death.

As recent dilemmas in the definition of death for legal and organ retrieval purposes show, confusing situations can arise. To improve clarity in decision-making regarding end-of-life issues, the legislatures of an increasing number of states are enacting laws providing for advance directives. These are often titled a Natural Death Act. Unlike a living will, which is not legally binding, the Natural Death Act provides a legally binding mechanism whereby individuals may decline extraordinary measures to prolong life if more than one physician declares the person's condition to be terminal and irreversible. Another type of **advance directive,** the durable power-of-attorney for healthcare, may be used by individuals to designate a specific person to make decisions regarding end-of-life issues if they are not capable of decision-making. In 1991, the Patient Self-Determination Act became a federal law. This law requires healthcare agencies that participate in Medicare or Medicaid programs to inform patients, on admission to the agency, of their right to determine treatment by enacting an advance directive. Familiarize yourself with your responsibilities regarding this law in the setting in which you work.

DEFINING DEATH

A long-standing practical definition of death has been the point at which there is complete cessation of respiration, heartbeat, and blood pressure. Because peripheral pulses can subside long before the heart actually stops beating, check for apical heartbeat using a stethoscope. The heartbeat is usually the last vital sign to disappear.

When the patient's basic vital functions are being sustained by machines, identifying death is more complex. Death is then determined based on neurologic criteria. **Electroencephalography** most often is used to establish that the brain is no longer functioning. A complete discussion of this area is beyond the scope of this module. Always follow your facility's policies and procedures.

For patients without DNR orders and for whom you have determined that respiration and heartbeat have stopped, initiate resuscitation according to your facility's procedure (see Module 36, Emergency Resuscitation Procedures). Resuscitation measures continue until the patient recovers vital functions, or the physician pronounces the patient dead. Only after death has been pronounced and the option of organ donation is discussed with the family should machines supporting vital functions be turned off.

PRONOUNCEMENT OF DEATH

Once you have identified the cessation of vital functions, note the time, and call the physician. In most states, only a physician can legally pronounce a patient dead. Postmortem care begins after the physician has pronounced the patient dead.

Nurses can, however, legally determine and pronounce a patient dead in some states. In other states, there are certain specified situations (such as death in a long-term care facility or in a hospice setting when death has been expected for some time and is clearly imminent) in which the nurse may pronounce the patient dead and determine the time of death. The nurse then notifies the physician and completes appropriate records. In these cases, postmortem care is given, and the patient's body is removed from the unit. You should know the relevant law as well as the policy of the institution in which you work. The death certificate, which is the official record of death, is signed by a physician in all states.

REPORTING A DEATH TO THE MEDICAL EXAMINER

Some deaths must be reported to the **medical examiner** or equivalent legal authority to determine whether an investigation of the death will take place. An example of criteria for deaths that are to be reported to the medical examiner are shown in Box 43-1. If any of the circumstances listed exist, ensure that the appropriate person calls the office of your county's coroner or medical examiner. When in doubt, call and ask if a particular death should be reported. If the medical examiner considers an autopsy necessary, be sure that the patient's body is either held at the facility for examination or plans made to transfer the body to the medical examiner's office. The person responsible for reporting applicable deaths to the coroner or medical examiner varies from facility to facility. Read the policies where you practice to know your role and the specific procedure(s) to be followed.

CHANGES IN THE BODY AFTER DEATH

Several changes occur in the body immediately after death. These include rigor mortis, algor mortis, and livor mortis. If the body is not handled gently, skin indentation may also occur.

RIGOR MORTIS

Rigor mortis is the stiffening of a dead body accompanying the depletion of adenosine triphosphate in the muscle fibers. It occurs rapidly, sometimes within an hour if the patient has died suddenly while being active or exercising. In the chronically ill, bedridden patient, rigor mortis may not take place for some hours. The degree of rigor mortis differs greatly from one patient to another. It begins in the involuntary muscles but initially becomes noticeable in the muscles of the head and neck. It then travels downward to the trunk and finally to the lower extremities. Rigor mortis is most evident about 48 hours after death and subsides gradually after about 96 hours (a time lapse in which you are not involved).

ALGOR MORTIS

Algor mortis, or postmortem cooling, is the gradual decrease in body temperature that occurs as circulation slows and stops.

LIVOR MORTIS

Livor mortis is the skin discoloration that occurs after blood circulation stops because of the release of hemoglobin from the red blood cells that are breaking down. Gravity pulls the blood toward the dependent areas of the body after the heart stops pumping, so that discoloration is most apparent in those areas. Handle the body gently to prevent excessive discoloration, especially in areas that may be viewed later.

SKIN INDENTATION

Rough handling can also result in skin indentation. After death, the skin immediately loses its natural **turgor** and elasticity. Once this happens, the lightest pressure can indent the skin, a condition that is intensified if the patient had **edema.**

PROCEDURE FOR CARING FOR THE BODY AFTER DEATH

ASSESSMENT

1. Verify that vital functions have ceased. This includes complete absence of respiration, heartbeat, and blood pressure. Pronounce the patient dead if you are permitted to do so. If not, notify the physician. Record both the time of death and the time the patient is pronounced dead. **R:** Documenting this information confirms and records the death of the patient.

2. Notify the people and departments listed below. Be sure you have the necessary information at hand when you call. Policies and procedures vary from place to place. Follow the policies in your facility; check with your supervisor if you are unsure. **R:** In

box 43-1 *Criteria for Reportable Deaths**

1. **Persons who die suddenly when in apparent good health and without medical attendance within thirty-six (36) hours preceding death.** This category should be reserved for the following situations
   a. Sudden death of any individual with no known natural cause for the death
   b. Death during an acute or unexplained rapidly fatal illness, for which a reasonable natural cause has not been established
   c. Deaths of individuals who were not under the care of a physician
   d. Deaths of persons in nursing homes or other institutions where medical treatment is not provided by a licensed physician
2. **Circumstances indicate death caused entirely OR IN PART by unnatural or unlawful means.** This category includes, but is not limited to
   a. Drowning, suffocation, smothering, burns, electrocution, lightning, radiation, chemical or thermal injury, starvation, environmental exposure, or neglect
   b. Unexpected deaths during, associated with, or as a result of diagnostic or therapeutic procedures
   c. All deaths in the operating room whether due to surgical or anesthetic procedures
   d. Narcotics or other addictions, other drugs including alcohol or toxic agents, or toxic exposure
   e. Death thought to be associated with, or resulting from, the decedent's occupation. This includes chronic occupational disease such as asbestosis and black lung.
   f. Death of the mother caused by known or suspected abortion
   g. Deaths occurring from apparent natural causes during the course of a criminal act, e.g., victim collapses during a robbery
   h. Deaths that occur within 1 year following an accident even if the accident is not thought to have contributed to the cause of death

   i. Deaths following all injury producing accidents, if recovery was considered incomplete or if the accident is thought to have contributed to the cause of death (regardless of the interval between accident and death)
3. **Suspicious circumstances.** This category includes, but is not limited to, deaths under the following circumstances
   a. Deaths resulting from apparent homicide or suicide
   b. Hanging, gunshot wounds, stabs, cuts, strangulation, etc.
   c. Alleged rape, carnal knowledge, or sodomy
   d. Death during the course of, or precipitated by, a criminal act
   e. Deaths that occur while in a jail, prison, in custody of law enforcement, or other nonmedical public institutions
4. **Unknown or obscure causes.** This category includes
   a. Bodies that are found dead (see criteria #1 above)
   b. Deaths during or following an unexplained coma
5. **Deaths caused by any violence whatsoever, whether the primary cause or any contributory factors in the death.** This category includes but is not limited to
   a. Injury of any type including falls
   b. Any deaths due to, or contributed to, by any type of physical trauma
6. **Contagious disease.** This category includes only those deaths wherein the diagnosis is undetermined and a contagious disease, which may be a public health hazard, is a suspected cause of death.
7. **Bodies that are not claimed.** This category is limited to deaths where no next of kin or other legally responsible representatives can be identified for disposition of the body.
8. **Premature and stillborn infants.** This category includes only those stillborn or premature infants whose birth was precipitated by maternal injury, criminal or medical negligence, or abortion under unlawful circumstances.

*Source: Medical Examiner's Office, King County, State of Washington.

proceeding this way, you will be certain you are notifying all of the necessary people and departments.
a. The attending physician: In some settings, the attending physician is responsible for both pronouncing the patient dead and notifying the **next of kin** (nearest relative).
b. The nursing supervisor or other designated supervisory personnel: In some settings, the nursing supervisor is responsible for making some of the notification calls; for example, to the medical examiner when appropriate.
c. Next of kin or emergency contact person: This responsibility may not be yours to carry out, but it is your responsibility to be certain it has been done. In some facilities, the notification of the

next of kin is always the responsibility of the physician. It is prudent to ask whether the family will be coming in to view the body and collect the belongings as well as the name of the **mortuary** or **funeral home** to be notified. Next of kin have both a legal and ethical right to this information as soon as possible. **R:** You will need to ready the patient and the patient's unit for the family's visit.
d. Admitting or census department: This department is usually responsible for providing information on patients' conditions and should be notified as soon as possible.
e. The transplant coordinator or appropriate agency if any organ procurement is to take place.

f. The medical examiner, if appropriate: If you are uncertain whether the circumstances meet the criteria for reportable deaths, call the medical examiner's office for assistance.

g. The designated funeral home if the patient is not a medical examiner's case. **R:** Calling the funeral home may be the responsibility of the admitting or census department.

ANALYSIS

3. Critically think through your data, carefully evaluating each aspect and its relation to other data. **R:** This enables you to determine special considerations regarding this patient's postmortem care.

4. Identify specific concerns and modifications of the procedure needed for this individual. **R:** Planning for the individual must take into consideration the individual's problems.

PLANNING

5. Determine individualized patient outcomes in relation to postmortem care, including the following. **R:** Identification of outcomes guides planning and evaluation.

a. All necessary notifications carried out.

b. Body cared for and transported appropriately.

c. Family was able to carry out rituals, religious, or cultural practices, as well as viewing and spending time with patient as desired.

d. Family was offered the opportunity for organ and/or tissue donation if appropriate.

e. Possessions handled according to facility policy.

6. Plan for any special religious or cultural practices desired by the family that may need to take place before you begin the actual "after death" care. **R:** This promotes maximum participation and comfort of the family. Rituals cover a broad spectrum, from the Orthodox Jewish practice of washing the body to the Roman Catholic rite of anointing by a priest of the person before death occurs.

7. If the patient is not in a private room, and it is possible to do so, offer to transport any other patient(s) in the room to another location temporarily. Otherwise, pull the curtains around the unit and close the door. **R:** Doing this provides privacy for the family and friends of the **deceased** patient.

8. Place the "No Visitors—Check at Nurses' Station" sign on the door. **R:** This prevents visitors from walking in and disturbing the family or being unprepared for what they see.

IMPLEMENTATION

Action	Rationale
9. Wash or disinfect your hands.	To decrease the transfer of microorganisms.
10. Gather the equipment (a "**morgue** pack" may contain some of these items, including the **shroud,** identification tags, and sign for the door).	To proceed most efficiently and effectively.
a. clean gloves (at least two pairs)	
b. soap	
c. washcloth(s)	
d. towel(s)	
e. basin	
f. clean gown	
g. clean linen as needed for the bed if the patient is to be viewed	
h. clean dressings or ostomy bag if a wound or ostomy is present	
i. two disposable pads (ABDs, for example)	
j. a shroud or sheet	
k. identification tags	
l. masking tape	

(continued)

Action	Rationale
11. Obtain any needed assistance.	To save time and promote efficiency.
12. Identify the patient, using two identifiers.	To ensure proper identification of the body for transfer to the facility morgue, the autopsy room, and/or the funeral home.
13. Explain the procedure you are about to perform if family members are present.	Explaining the procedure helps relieve anxiety or misperceptions that the family may have about the care they will witness.
14. Raise the bed to an appropriate working position based on your height.	To allow you to use correct body mechanics and protect yourself from back injury.
15. Place the body in the supine position with the bed flat. Place the arms at the patient's side. Do not cross the hands.	Because the underlying hand will become discolored and indented.
16. Place a low pillow under the head.	To prevent blood from pooling in the face, which can cause discoloration.
17. Close the patient's eyes. Gently hold your index fingers on the eyelids for a few seconds.	This action will cause the eyes to remain closed.
18. Remove the patient's watch and jewelry. Ask the spouse or closest relative what to do with the patient's wedding band if one is worn. Make an itemized list of all the patient's possessions. Always chart the disposition of jewelry and obtain a signature from the family stating that the valuables of the deceased have been received.	Regardless of monetary worth, these items are often important as mementos for the family. Some prefer that the wedding band never be removed. If this is the situation, tape it carefully in place. Others may want to keep the ring; in which case, remove it and give it personally to the family. Taking care with the valuables of the deceased will prevent the loss of valuables and protect you legally.
19. Replace the patient's dentures.	This gives the person's face a more familiar and natural appearance if the patient is to be viewed by loved ones before being taken to the mortuary.
20. Do not attempt to replace the dentures if you encounter any resistance.	Marks or indentations can be left on the lips, jaw, or face if pressure is exerted. Place the dentures instead into a labeled container and send them with the body for the **mortician** to insert. Some facilities and funeral homes specify that dentures not be replaced.
21. Place a small towel under the patient's chin.	To support the mouth in a closed position.
22. Remove IV line(s), nasogastric tube, urinary catheter, and oxygen equipment. If the patient is to have an autopsy performed, or is to be examined by the medical examiner, and had special indwelling lines or catheters in place, cut the line or catheter approximately 1 inch from the body and tape the end to the skin.	This does not interfere with the viewing, and the insertion sites and functioning may prove important medically or legally in case of obscure causes of death. Some medical examiners insist that lines be neither cut nor removed, so check your facility's policy.

(continued)

Action	Rationale
23. Remove soiled dressings and ostomy bags, and replace them with clean ones.	To control odor and prepare the body for viewing.
24. Wash the soiled areas of the body. Pat the body dry. If the family rituals include bathing the body of the deceased person, relinquish care to the family at this time.	Brisk rubbing may cause undue discoloration of the tissues. Many cultures and religions include bathing the body in the mourning practices for families.
25. Place disposable pads (ABDs for example) in the perineal area.	To absorb any stool or urine released as the **sphincter** muscles relax.
26. Remove gloves, and wash or disinfect your hands.	To decrease the transfer of microorganisms.
27. Put a clean gown on the patient.	To prepare the body for viewing.
28. Check to be sure that the wrist identification remains in place. This usually is removed only if it is restricting the arm. (If the family has bathed the body and put the clean gown on the patient, the nurse makes sure that steps 27 and 28 are done after the bath is completed.)	The wrist identifcation serves as an excellent method of identifying the body. All pieces of identification should include the patient's name, hospital number, and physician's name. A hospital identification band will have other data, including the date of admission.
29. Attach a second piece of identification to the ankle or great toe. Follow the procedure in your facility.	It is prudent to have two pieces of identification attached to the body in case one becomes detached and lost. The ankle or great toe is an appropriate area because any marking on the skin in that location will not be noticeable when the body is viewed.
30. If the family and friends intend to view the body	
a. Replace the top linens (top sheet, spread, and pillowcase).	To give the bed a fresh and clean appearance.
b. Tidy the unit, caring for any equipment appropriately. If the family is to visit, provide chairs at the bedside.	To provide a comfortable setting for family and friends to sit with the body if they wish.
31. Dim the lights. Turn off all the ceiling lights and use the bedside lights, if possible.	This will soften the features of the deceased for viewing.
32. After the viewing, leave dentures in the patient's mouth, or place them in a denture container, according to facility and/or funeral home policy.	If the body is to be viewed at services later, the **funeral director** may request that dentures and eyeglasses be sent with the body. If the body is to be cremated, the funeral director will ask the family their wishes regarding these items.
33. Place the patient's personal effects in the container used by your facility. Include cards and letters received by the deceased.	To prevent loss of any patient's belongings.

(continued)

Action	Rationale
If possible, give these items to a family member and record the name of the recipient. If this is not possible, send these items to the department specified by your facility.	
34. Wrap the body in a shroud, or cover it with a clean sheet. Gently attach any masking tape needed to fasten the shroud or sheet closed.	To prevent indenting the body.
35. Attach an identification tag to the outside of the shroud. There may be a special tag to attach if the patient has been in isolation. Follow the policy in your facility.	For identification of the body and to alert those who will be handling the body to the need for special precautions.
36. Transport the body to the facility morgue, or leave it in the room until the funeral director arrives. In the latter case, open the windows, or turn down the heat.	To cool the room, thus retarding the discoloration of the tissue.
37. Close the doors of all other patient rooms before the cart bearing the body passes by if this is the policy in your facility.	To prevent distress on the part of other patients and their visitors.
38. Put away or dispose of equipment, supplies, linen, and garbage appropriately.	To prepare the room for the next occupant.
39. Wash or disinfect your hands.	To decrease the transfer of microorganisms.

EVALUATION

40. Evaluate using the individualized patient outcomes previously identified, including the following. **R:** Evaluation in relation to desired outcomes is essential.
    a. All necessary notifications carried out.
    b. Body cared for and transported appropriately.
    c. Family was able to carry out rituals, religious, or cultural practices, as well as viewing and spending time with patient as desired.
    d. Family was offered the opportunity for organ and/or tissue donation if appropriate.
    e. Possessions handled according to facility policy.

DOCUMENTATION

41. Document the postmortem activities, including the following. **R:** Documentation is a legal record of the patient's care and communicates nursing activities to other nurses and caregivers.

    a. Time vital signs ceased
    b. Persons notified and time of notification
    c. List and disposition of valuables and personal effects
    d. Time body transported from unit, destination (facility morgue, funeral home, medical examiner's office), and by whom transported
    e. Any other information required by your facility: in some places, there is a special form that indicates and includes spaces for all information required (Fig. 43-1).

POTENTIAL ADVERSE OUTCOMES AND RELATED INTERVENTIONS

None of the outcomes listed below should happen. Taking special care with the handling and identification of the body, the disposition of the patient's belongings, and the arrangements for transportation to the funeral home or medical examiner's office will help prevent them.

PATIENT EXPIRATION FORM

Date & Time of Death: _____

Attending Physician: _____

Pronounced By: _____ M.D. _____ R.N.

Signature of Persons filling out form:

Nursing: _____ Admitting: _____

I. NOTIFY IMMEDIATELY (to be completed by Nursing)

   A. Attending Physician _____ Time _____

   B. Patient Care Coordinator _____ Time _____

   C. Next of Kin_____ Phone Number _____
      and/or Emergency Notification Person
      Relationship to Deceased _____

      Who notified next of kin? Nurse _____ Physician _____

   D. Admitting Department _____ Time _____

II. PREPARATION OF THE BODY (to be completed by Nursing)
    Initial when Done _____

   A. Observe Religious Protocol _____

   B. Close eyes and replace dentures _____
      (If unable to do so, wrap, label and tape to body.)

   C. Clean and straighten the body _____

   D. Remove jewelry Yes_____ No_____
          (Rings taped at family's request) _____

   E. Remove tubes (*only if NOT* an M.E. case or autopsy) _____

   F. Remove gown; wrap in sheet/shroud _____

   G. Attach 4 tags   1) Morgue door log _____   2) Foot _____

               3) Sheet/Shroud _____   4) Chest (if applicable) _____

III. DISPOSITION OF THE BODY (to be completed by Nursing and Admitting)

   A. Medical Examiners Case Yes _____ No _____

      If yes, name of M.E. notified _____

      By whom at GHC? _____

      Case Number _____

      M.E. accepts body? Yes_____ No _____

      Is than an NJA case? Yes_____ NJA# _____ No_____

   B. Autopsy to be performed: Yes _____ No_____

      If yes, permit signed: Yes_____ No _____ By Whom_____

      Pathology Notified Yes_____ No _____ Time _____

      Autopsy completed Time _____ Date _____

> M.E. = Medical Examiner
> NJA = Non Jurisdictional Action

   C. Mortuary_____Phone_____

      Time and Date notified _____

      Morgue Release signed by _____

      Date and Time of Release _____

      Reception Clerk _____

IV. Circle which one VALUABLES/PERSONAL BELONGINGS (to be completed by Nursing and Admitting)

   A. List valuables: _____

      _____

      _____

      _____

      _____

   B. Released to: _____ Date & Time_____

   C. No family present, valuables secured by _____

      Location _____

V. ORGAN DONOR: Yes_____ No_____

   Which organ_____

   _____

   _____

VI. DOCUMENTATION

   A. Patient Expiration Notification form to the Admitting Office as soon as possible with two discharge cards (if applicable).

   B. Completed chart taken to Medical Records Department.

WHITE · INPATIENT'S CHART / CANARY · ADMITTING/PINK · NURSING
Patent Expiration Form

FIGURE 43-1 Patient expiration form.

1. The identification tab on the outside of the shroud is incorrect.

Intervention: Be sure that all tags attached to the body carry the same name as the wrist band. If an error is discovered after the body has left the unit or the facility, notify the funeral home or medical examiner's office immediately.

2. The patient's valuables are given to a person other than the legal next of kin.

Intervention: Before giving any of the patient's belongings to *anyone,* be certain you have correctly identified the person who is the legal next of kin. If this error is made, contact the person to whom the belongings were given and ask him or her to return the items immediately.

3. The body is injured during postmortem care.

Intervention: Notify your nursing supervisor and the physician.

4. The body is sent to the wrong funeral home.

Intervention: Notify the funeral home immediately and ask them to return the body.

DEATH OF AN INFANT

The death of an infant can be an especially sad and sensitive time. If you work in a labor and delivery area, you will need to be aware of your responsibility with regard to baptism in the event of infant death. Make sure the family knows they can see and hold the infant's body. If they wish to see the infant, wrap the child in a receiving blanket and carry the body of the baby as you would a living baby. Encourage the family to hold and examine the infant as desired. They may wish for you to unwrap the baby if they are not comfortable doing so. You may wish to provide a nursery crib if the family is not comfortable holding the baby. Offer the family the opportunity to be alone because they may feel inhibited with a nurse in the room.

AUTOPSY (POSTMORTEM EXAMINATION)

An **autopsy** is the examination of the body after death. Autopsies may be complete or partial. A complete autopsy consists of an examination of each of the body's organs, including the brain. A partial autopsy consists of an examination of only those organs of interest in determining the cause of death. Autopsies may serve several purposes: to ascertain the exact cause of death (in some cases, this may help the family recover insurance benefits or a legal settlement), to add to scientific knowledge, and to help in statistical data gathering. If an autopsy is done in the hospital at a physician's request, the family is usually not charged. On occasion, the family asks to have an autopsy performed, and a charge is then incurred. Check the specific policies in your facility.

It is the physician's responsibility to secure permission for an autopsy from the appropriate survivor. Standard forms are available; these should be made out in duplicate, with original signatures on each one.

In certain deaths, an autopsy is required by law; in which case, permission of the next of kin is not needed. County and state laws vary slightly in different areas. Know the law of the jurisdiction in which you practice. Cases requiring an autopsy are called coroner's or medical examiner's cases. The family is not charged for an autopsy that is required by law.

Acute Care

Deaths that occur in the Emergency Department of a hospital can be very difficult for all concerned because they often are unexpected—the result of accidents or violence. Specialized personnel may be available in some settings to assist with bereaved family and friends in these situations. When such personnel are not available, nurses who work in the setting may need to fulfill this role.

Deaths that occur after a long and difficult illness can be difficult for loved ones and staff persons alike. In some situations, staff members are encouraged to excuse themselves for short periods of time to attend to their own needs, if necessary. In these situations, a supervisor or staff person from another area will step in to assume the duties of the excused staff member.

Long-Term Care

Although some individuals are admitted to long-term care facilities for limited periods (for specific reasons such as rehabilitation), many more move to nursing homes with the clear expectation that they will live out the remainder of their lives there. In fact, it is the policy in many nursing homes to ask residents and their families on admission to indicate the mortuary they want notified when the resident dies. It is a legal requirement for the facility, if it receives Medicare or Medicaid funding, to offer each resident the opportunity to establish an advance directive on admission to the facility. Residents are also requested to indicate their wishes regarding donation of tissues and organs after death. It is especially important that the nurse know whether the resident wishes to be resuscitated, and, if so, exactly which components of resuscitation are to be included (cardiopulmonary resuscitation, drugs, mechanical ventilation, or a combination of these).

As a resident nears death, considerations regarding the presence and participation of family members are much the same as in an acute care facility. Nurses must be aware of the expressed needs of family and friends to be present at the moment of death so that they can honor those needs, if possible. Recall that in some states, registered nurses employed in long-term care facilities can legally pronounce a resident dead. The death certificate must be signed by a physician.

Staff members in long-term care facilities may have cared for some residents over a long period. For these staff members, the deaths of certain residents feel like deaths of a family member. In some facilities, brief memorial services are held on care units to help staff members work through their feelings of loss.

 Home Care

Increasingly, terminally ill individuals are choosing to die at home. In some cases, family and friends are able to provide much of the required care, with a home care nurse assisting as needed. In other situations, a hospice nurse supervises care, and in still others, caregivers other than family and friends provide most of the care. Depending on the situation, the nurse or the family must know the law regarding what is to be done and who is to be notified when death occurs in the home. As is true in healthcare agencies, an unexpected death in the home is handled differently than is an expected one, perhaps requiring notification of the coroner or medical examiner. It is always prudent to call when unsure.

LEARNING TOOLS

DEVELOP YOUR BACKGROUND KNOWLEDGE

1. Review the Learning Outcomes.

2. Read the section on care of the dying patient, death, and grief in your assigned text.

3. Look up the Key Terms in the glossary.

4. Review this module as though you were preparing to teach the concepts and skills to another person.

DEVELOP YOUR SKILLS

1. In the practice setting
   a. Demonstrate the proper positioning of a body by positioning a partner.
   b. Reverse roles and have your partner position you.
   c. Discuss the reasons for positioning with your partner.
   d. With your instructor as facilitator, join in a small group with three or four classmates. Explore together some of your feelings concerning the following:
      (1) touching and caring for a patient after death
      (2) interacting with the deceased patient's family members and friends
      (3) organ donation

DEMONSTRATE YOUR SKILLS

1. In the clinical setting
   a. Read your facility's policies and procedures regarding caring for the patient after death, the responsibility and process for reporting deaths to a medical examiner, and the organ donation procedure.
   b. Examine the various forms (for release of body, for autopsy) used in your facility.
   c. If an opportunity arises, arrange to observe a staff member discuss organ donation with the family of a dying patient. In postclinical conference, role-play discussing organ donation with a family.
   d. If death occurs, assist the instructor or a staff nurse for your first experience in giving care after death.
   e. When a subsequent opportunity arises, give care after death with the assistance and evaluation of your instructor.
   f. In postclinical conference, share with your classmates your experiences and feelings related to caring for a patient and his or her family after death.

CRITICAL THINKING EXERCISES

1. A patient for whom you are caring has just died. The family left the facility about 10 minutes ago and you know it will take them at least 45 minutes to get home. You do not know whether they will wish to see their loved one again. How will you proceed with caring for the body?

2. A woman you have cared for several times during a long illness has just died. She told you several times of her wish for others to benefit from any organs "that are any good." There is a signed donor card in her personal effects. How will you proceed? What

are the policies and procedures in the facility where you are assigned? Will you need permission from her family?

SELF-QUIZ
SHORT-ANSWER QUESTIONS

1. List three changes in the body after death.

   a. _____

   b. _____

   c. _____

2. Why should the arms be placed at the patient's side?

   _____

3. Name four types of treatment equipment that usually are removed from the body after death.

   a. _____

   b. _____

   c. _____

   d. _____

4. List two special considerations you should take when the patient is to be viewed in the hospital room by the family.

   a. _____

   b. _____

5. List two different considerations when the patient is an infant.

   a. _____

   b. _____

6. What is the benefit received by families who donate organs of their deceased loved one(s)?

   _____

7. Why is it important to report the availability of a donor promptly after death?

   _____

8. Name three instances when a death commonly must be reported to the coroner or medical examiner.

   a. _____

   b. _____

   c. _____

9. Define autopsy.

   _____

10. Name three reasons for performing autopsies.

    a. _____

    b. _____

    c. _____

MULTIPLE CHOICE

_____ 11. The last vital sign to disappear is usually the
   a. temperature.
   b. respiration.
   c. heartbeat.
   d. blood pressure.

_____ 12. In which situation would a medical examiner usually need to be notified? Choose all that apply.
   a. The patient died in the Emergency Department of a stroke.
   b. The patient died on the oncology unit of complications of chemotherapy.
   c. The patient died in the Emergency Department of a gunshot wound.
   d. The patient died at home without having had any medical care.

_____ 13. Why should the use of tape or ties for identification be avoided on the upper extremities?
   a. They would be mistaken for restraints.
   b. They can leave permanent marks that would be visible if the body is viewed in a funeral home.
   c. They could come loose and the identification be lost.
   d. They are too easily missed by the person checking for identity.

Answers to the Self-Quiz questions appear in the back of the book.

REFERENCES AND SUGGESTED RESOURCES: UNIT 8

Agency for Health Care Policy and Research. (1994). *Guideline for treating pressure ulcers. Clinical practice guideline No. 15.* Agency for Health Care Policy and Research, Public Health Service, U.S. Department of Health and Human Services. Publication No. 95-0652. (Online). Available at http://www.ncbi.nlm.nih.gov/books/bv.fcgi?rid=hstat2.chapter.5124. Retrieved October 19, 2005.

American Society of Anesthesiologists. (1999). *Practice guidelines for preoperative fasting and the use of pharmacologic agents to reduce the risk of pulmonary aspiration: Application to healthy patients undergoing elective procedures.* (Online). Available at http://www.asahq.org/publications AndServices/npoguide.html. Retrieved May 15, 2005.

Anton, M., & Johnson, K. (2004). The organ donation choice: Families need information and sensitivity. *NurseWeek, 5*(12), 30–32.

AORN, Inc. (2004a). *Correct site surgery tool kit: Building a safer tomorrow.* Denver, CO: Author.

AORN, Inc. (2004b). *Standards, recommended practices, and guidelines.* Denver, CO: Author.

Armstrong, M. H. (2004). Wet-to-dry gauze dressings: Fact and fiction. *MEDSCAPE.* (Online). Available at http://www.medscape.com/viewarticle/470257. Retrieved Jan. 10, 2005.

Bryant, R. A. (2000). *Acute and chronic wounds: Nursing management.* (2nd ed.). St. Louis: C. V. Mosby.

Crenshaw, J. T., & Winslow, E. H. (2002). Preoperative fasting: Old habits die hard: Research and published guidelines no longer support the routine use of "NPO after midnight," but the practice persists. *American Journal of Nursing, 102*(5), 36–44.

Evan, P., & Read, K. (2001). Graduated compression stockings for the prevention of post-operative venous thromboembolism. *Best Practice, 5*(2). (Online). Available at http://www.joannabriggs.edu.au/pdf/BPISstock.pdf. Retrieved October 19, 2005.

Joint Commission for the Accreditation of Healthcare Organizations (JCAHO). (2004). *Prohibited abbreviations.* (Online). Available at www.jcaho.org. Retrieved Aug. 15, 2004.

Mangram, A., Horan, T., Pearson, M., et al. (1999). Guideline for prevention of surgical site infection. *Infection Control and Hospital Epidemiology, 20*(4), 231–232. (Online). Available at http://www.cdc.gov/ncidod/hip/SSI/SSI_guideline.htm. Retrieved October 19, 2005.

National Pressure Ulcer Advisory Panel. (2000). *The NPUAP position statement.* (Online). Available at http://www.npuap.org/positn5.html. Retrieved May 25, 2005.

National Pressure Ulcer Advisory Panel (NPUAP). (2003). Staging system from the 1989 Consensus Development Conference. Adopted by the AHCPR Pressure Ulcer Guideline Panels. Published in both sets of AHCPR (now AHRQ) pressure ulcer clinical practice guidelines (1992, 1994). (Online). Available at http://www.npuap.org/positn6.html. Retrieved May 25, 2005.

Reddy, M., Keast, D., Fowler, E., et al. (2003). Pain in pressure ulcers. *Ostomy/Wound Management, 49*(4A), 30–35.

Rodeheaver, G. T. (2001). Wound cleansing, wound irrigation, and wound disinfection. In D. L. Krasnet, G. T. Rodeheaver, & R. G. Sibbald (Eds.), *Chronic wound care: A clinical source book for healthcare professionals.* (3rd ed., pp. 369–383). Wayne, PA: HMP Communication.

Shaughnessy, A. F. (2005). Compression stockings and post-thrombotic syndrome. *American Family Physician,* January. (Online). Available at http://www.findarticles.com/p/articles/mi_m3225/is_1_71/ai_n8704709. Retrieved October 19, 2005.

Sibbold, R. G., Orsted, H. L., Schultz, G. S., et al. (2003). Preparing the wound bed: Focus on infection and inflammation. *Ostomy/Wound Management, 49*(11), 24–51.

Sibbold R. G., Williamson, D., Orsted H. L., et al. (2000). Preparing the wound bed: Debridement, bacterial balance, and moisture balance. *Ostomy/Wound Management, 46*(11), 14–22, 24–28.

Stitik, T., & Nadler, S. (1998). When—and how—to use cold most effectively. *Consultant, 38*(12), 2881.

Stitik, T., & Nadler, S. (1999). When—and how—to apply the heat. *Consultant, 39*(1), 144.

Thomas, S. (2001). An introduction to the use of vacuum assisted closure. (Online). Available at http://www.worldwidewounds.com/2001/may/Thomas/Vacuum-Assisted-Closure.html. Retrieved May 25, 2005.

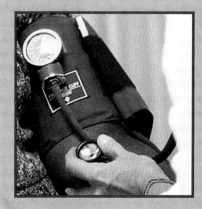

Administering Medications and Intravenous Therapy

MODULES

Administering Oral Medications

SKILLS INCLUDED IN THIS MODULE

Procedure for Administering Oral Medications

PREREQUISITE MODULES

Module 1	An Approach to Nursing Skills
Module 2	Documentation
Module 4	Basic Infection Control
Module 5	Safety in the Healthcare Environment
Module 14	Nursing Physical Assessment

The following modules may be useful in some specific situations:

Module 6	Moving the Patient in Bed and Positioning
Module 11	Assessing Temperature, Pulse, and Respiration
Module 12	Measuring Blood Pressure
Module 13	Monitoring Intake and Output
Module 30	Administering Tube Feedings

KEY TERMS

buccal	meniscus
capsule	pruritus
computerized order entry (COE)	route
	six rights
	stock supply
diversion	sublingual
dose	suspension
expectorate	syrup
generic name	tablet
medication administration	three checks
	trade (brand) names
medication administration record (MAR)	unit-dose

OVERALL OBJECTIVES

▸ To understand medication administration systems, how to administer medications to patients, how to record medication administration appropriately, and how to respond appropriately if a medication error occurs.

▸ To administer oral medications to patients and residents with accuracy and safety and to recognize and report adverse drug effects promptly and take corrective action.

LEARNING OUTCOMES

The student will be able to

1. Assess the patient in regard to the appropriateness of giving the oral medications prescribed.
2. Analyze data to determine whether any individual problems or concerns must be addressed before and/or during administration of oral medications.
3. Determine appropriate patient outcomes for the medications administered and recognize the potential for adverse outcomes.
4. Plan an appropriate strategy to ensure that the patient receives the prescribed medications.
5. Administer oral medications safely and accurately.
6. Evaluate the patient's response to medications administered.
7. Document medications administered and the patient's response according to facility policies.

One of the nurse's most routine and yet most critical responsibilities is the preparation and administration of medications. The responsibility extends beyond preparation and administration. The nurse must know how medicines act, the usual dosage, the desired effects, and potential side effects so that he or she can evaluate the effectiveness of the medication and recognize adverse effects promptly when they occur.

If you are giving medications, you must access and have available specific information about the drug, dosage, actions, desired effects, and side effects before you give the drug. When you are an experienced nurse, you may have memorized this information for drugs you commonly administer but will still need to look up new or unfamiliar drugs. As a student, you may be expected to have written notes on each medication you are to administer. You may be permitted to use commercially prepared medication cards or a drug book. However, once you have the information, you will need to individualize it to your specific patient by noting why this drug is being given to this patient (the desired effect) and what adverse effects to which the patient might be more susceptible.

Most medications given in healthcare facilities are administered by the oral **route.** A sizable number of oral medications may be ordered for a patient. Consequently, the nurse must be skilled in administering oral medications and incorporating sound knowledge, accuracy, and safety measures when administering each

drug. The nurse also must be skilled in recognizing side effects.

NURSING DIAGNOSES

■ Risk for Injury: The major nursing diagnosis to keep in mind when giving medications is Risk for Injury. Patients can be injured by medications given in the wrong dosage, at the wrong time, or by an incorrect route. They also can be injured by the omission of essential medications, the administration of an incorrect medication, and by incorrect documentation. Although this nursing diagnosis will not appear on the care plan, it applies to every situation in which a patient is being given medications.

■ Deficient Knowledge: Another nursing diagnosis frequently appropriate when administering medications is Deficient Knowledge. In this case, the deficit would be related to the patient being unaware of some aspect of the medication regimen; for example, the need to be aware of drug interactions between medications and antacids. This nursing diagnosis requires that the nurse provide health teaching so that the patient has basic information concerning the prescribed drug. With this knowledge, the patient can alert the staff to adverse reactions, such as **pruritus** (itching, hives, and the like), nausea, and others (see below).

- Risk for Aspiration: Another nursing diagnosis that is specific to oral medication administration is that of Risk for Aspiration. Swallowing deficits could lead to aspirating the medication into the bronchi, causing a life-threatening pneumonia.

- Disturbed Sensory Perception: Visual: It may be hazardous for a patient to self-administer oral medications for a variety of reasons. The patient may have adequate knowledge of a drug, but may be unable to see the medication well or read the label or instructions clearly. A nursing diagnosis of Disturbed Sensory Perception: Visual may be appropriate in this situation.

- Ineffective Therapeutic Regimen Management: If a hospitalized patient consistently refuses to take a medication that is necessary for treatment, or if a person at home fails to take or renew essential prescribed medications, a nursing diagnosis of Ineffective Therapeutic Regimen Management would be appropriate.

- Certain nursing diagnoses are associated with drug reactions. For example, a skin rash or eruption suggests a nursing diagnosis of Impaired Skin Integrity. Some medications interfere with sleep, causing Disturbed Sleep Pattern.

DELEGATION

Administration of oral medications is not delegated to assistive personnel in acute care settings. They may be asked to observe for and report specific effects (both desired and adverse) of medications the nurse has administered. Nursing assistants may also inform the nurse of situations in which a medication, such as an analgesic, may be needed. However, the nurse is responsible for assessing the need for prn (as needed) medication before administering it. The nurse is always responsible for evaluating the effect(s) of all medications administered.

Policies regarding delegation may vary in long-term care and federal institutions. Some states allow "medication aides" to give routine oral medications in long-term care settings. There may be legislation that permits the delegation of **medication administration** in community settings such as board and care homes. Medication administration may be delegated to personal care attendants in situations in which the disabled patient assumes responsibility for self-directed care but needs assistance in the physical tasks of opening containers, pouring water, and getting the medication to the mouth. In military installations, corpsmen have expanded roles that may include administering medications in certain situations. You will need to have specific information regarding the legal status of delegating medication administration in your state and setting.

READING MEDICATION ORDERS

Medications to be given in a healthcare facility must be ordered by a physician or other person with prescriptive authority such as a licensed dentist, nurse practitioner, or physician's assistant. A complete medication order should include the date, name of the drug, dosage, route of administration, frequency of administration, and signature of the prescribing person. In some facilities, the policy states that a medication is given by the oral route unless ordered differently. In those facilities, the route may not always be specified. If the order is incomplete, not clear, or does not conform to documented dosage ranges, the nurse should confer with the prescriber to clarify the order before giving the medication. The nurse also may find it helpful to consult the pharmacist. If the nurse believes that the order would be harmful or even dangerous as written, the nurse may refuse to give the medication but is obligated to follow appropriate facility protocols regarding conferring with a supervisor or other designated person.

Medications that are ordered to be given on a regular basis until the order is canceled are called routine orders. They may be given once a day, several times a day, every other day, at stated intervals, or on certain days of the week only (e.g., Tuesday, Thursday, and Saturday). Abbreviations are used to designate many of these times. Common abbreviations are listed in Table 44-1. Each facility has a list of approved abbreviations, and only the abbreviations that have been approved for use in that

table 44-1. Common Abbreviations Used in Medication Administration	
PO	by mouth
AC	before meals
PC	after meals
b.i.d.	twice a day
t.i.d.	three times a day
q.i.d.	four times a day
Stat	immediately
$\bar{c}$	with
$\bar{s}$	without
ss	one half
HS or hs	at bedtime
prn	as needed
QH or qh	every hour
Q2h or q2h	every 2 hours

facility may be used. The Joint Commission for the Accreditation of Healthcare Organizations (JCAHO) has published a list of abbreviations that should not be used because of their potential for error (JCAHO, 2004). These are listed in Module 2, Documentation. An individual facility may add abbreviations to this list.

Medications that are given when needed or requested only (a laxative for constipation, a narcotic for pain) are ordered on a prn basis. For example, "acetaminophen 500 mg by mouth q4h prn for pain." One-time-only medications are to be given on one occasion only at a specified time. Medications given prior to surgery or a diagnostic test are examples of one-time-only orders. For example, "triazolam 125 mcg at bedtime" might be ordered for a one-time **dose** of this sedative the evening before a surgery. These various types of orders are transcribed onto different parts of the **medication administration record (MAR)** or different screens in a computerized system.

A "stat" order means that the ordered medication is to be given immediately. The facility will have a policy as to how soon a stat order should be completed. For example, stat orders for a pain medication that is available on the unit might be given with 5 minutes. A stat order of a medication that must be dispensed by pharmacy might be given within an hour. A stat order is often used to initiate a new therapy or to address a specific patient problem. Sometimes, a stat order is combined with a subsequent routine order or prn order for continued management of the problem for which the stat medication was ordered. When stat orders are written, the nurse is responsible for ensuring that the medication is obtained and given promptly.

Although the prescriber orders the medication, the facility has standard times at which medications are administered. For example, medications ordered for four times a day may be given at 0900 (9 a.m.), 1300 (1 p.m.), 1700 (5 p.m.), and 2100 (9 p.m.) in some facilities, but at 0800 (8 a.m.), 1200 (12 noon), 1600 (4 p.m.), and 2000 (8 p.m.) in others. (*Note:* Most facilities use the 24-hour clock to avoid confusion between a.m. and p.m. times.) However, some medications ordered for four times a day must be given around the clock and, therefore, would be given at 0600 (6 a.m.), 1200 (12 noon), 1800 (6 p.m.), and 2400 (12 midnight). The nurse is responsible for identifying the appropriate times to give a medication based on its action in the body and the policy of the facility.

USING A MEDICATION ADMINISTRATION RECORD

Some healthcare facilities use a large notebook or a card index with a page or pages containing a listing of the medications for each patient. This is a permanent **rec-**ord and a guide as the medications are prepared and administered. The notebook or card index may be used for documenting the administration as well. In an increasing number of facilities, the entire MAR is computerized. The person writing the order completes a **computerized order entry (COE).** The nurse administering the medication checks the computer screen for medications to be given. All documentation may also be computerized. Some aspects may be computerized even if not all aspects are.

DRUG STORAGE AND DISPENSING SYSTEMS

Unit-dose medications are the most common method of storing drugs. The **unit-dose** system consists of the provision by pharmacy personnel of prepackaged and prelabeled individual doses of medications for patients. The individual doses are placed in that patient's medication drawer or cupboard. The unit-dose system is both accurate and convenient.

Drugs referred to as "scheduled" drugs (those with special control procedures mandated by federal law because of their potential for addiction or abuse) are usually kept in a single double-locked supply source for all patients on the unit (often referred to as a "**stock supply**"). They are then dispensed by nurses on the unit one dose at a time.

The traditional drug dispensing system consists of a medication cart with a drawer designated for each patient. The unit dosage medications for each patient are in the drawer. Tall bottles may be placed in a different place in the cart. The cart may also contain the double-locked drawer for the controlled drugs. The MAR is usually kept on top of the cart for ease of access and convenience of checking medications. The pharmacist may fill the drawers on a routine basis. In some facilities, there is a clinical pharmacist assigned to the unit who will dispense drugs into the patient drawers.

Many healthcare facilities now have computerized drug storage and dispensing systems such as the Omnicell or the Pyxis. These systems are stocked by the pharmacy with each patient's own drugs in his or her own drawer in the machine with certain drugs such as pain medications available from a stock supply in the machine. The nurse must access the system using a personal password and the patient's name or identification number. The machine then allows access only to that patient's medications or other medications ordered for the specific patient. The machine also keeps a record of who accessed the drawer and at what time. This process maintains tighter controls over supplies of all medications.

Most long-term care facilities have medications prepared by an off-site pharmacy. Many of these medications are received as "blister pack" cards. Each card has 1 month's supply of medication. Each **capsule** or **tablet** is in a clear blister on the front of the card, which is labeled with the resident's name and number, the name of the medication, and the dose of each tablet or capsule. These cards may be kept in a medication cart with a section for each resident.

LEGAL STANDARDS FOR THE ADMINISTRATION OF CONTROLLED DRUGS

Some drugs, such as those designated as narcotics or sedatives, are controlled by federal and state regulations and often referred to as "scheduled drugs" (because they appear on a document called a schedule) or controlled drugs (because of the various controls surrounding their use). These are drugs with a high potential for addiction and abuse. All doses are tracked from the manufacturer through to the individual patient to prevent the **diversion** of the drugs for an unintended or illegal use. Control processes to ensure that there is no unauthorized access to the drugs are mandated by federal legislation. Based on this legislation, both states and individual facilities establish policies regarding access and record keeping.

Controlled drugs are kept in a double-locked drawer or cupboard and must be signed out by the nurse administering the drug. The record indicates the patient for whom the dose was obtained, how many doses remain in the supply, the time the dose was removed, and the signature of the nurse. Removing a dose and making the appropriate documentation is often referred to as "signing out" the medication.

In most settings, narcotics are routinely counted at change of shift by two nurses, one from the departing shift and one from the oncoming shift. Anytime the supply is replenished, the drugs are usually recounted by a nurse on the unit and the pharmacist or pharmacy assistant who dispenses the drugs. If the amount of medication in the drawer does not agree with the record, the situation must be reported immediately. The nurses on the shift usually must remain until the count is reconciled. In some settings, narcotic control is computerized, and the drug is not released from the storage container until appropriate information is entered into the computer. When this is done, routine counting is not needed. Some units keep two separate supplies for frequently used drugs. One supply is the routinely used supply. The other is kept as the back-up supply. When the regular supply has been used, the back-up supply replaces it and a new back-up supply is ordered.

If you need to discard part or all of a controlled drug that is prepared and ready to give to a patient, you must have another nurse witness your action and co-sign the narcotic record.

Safety Alert

Never co-sign for a wasted drug that you did not observe being discarded. Follow the policy in your facility. All signatures for a wasted drug must be from individuals who are authorized to give the drug.

SAFETY IN MEDICATION ADMINISTRATION

Medication administration is a healthcare area in which errors commonly occur. These medication errors may be life-threatening. The Institute of Medicine (IOM) supported the research and publication of a major study of safety in the healthcare environment. This report makes recommendations for increasing safety (IOM, 2000). Medication safety was one of the major areas addressed in this report. The report noted that errors are costly in terms of life, health, and well-being of the patients. Additionally, errors are costly in terms of lost trust and are a major financial burden. This report suggested strategies for building a safer healthcare system. One was to set in place system-wide policies and procedures to promote safety. Another was to end a culture of blame when errors happen and instead focus on understanding the contributing factors and root causes of error and using this information to improve the system. Most healthcare agencies have established a system of policies and procedures to guard against error. All individuals must do their part to create a safer system.

AVOIDING SHORTCUTS AND "WORK-AROUNDS"

There is a tendency on the part of people to seek quicker and more efficient ways to complete their work. This is particularly true of nurses who typically face time pressure in their jobs. Some safety procedures may seem cumbersome and time-consuming. Unfortunately, while trying to be efficient may be useful in some areas, it may result in shortcuts or what have been termed "work-arounds." Shortcuts involve omitting some steps of the process; for example, not using two unique identifiers when identifying a patient. Work-arounds are processes that are quicker or more efficient but eliminate one or more of the safeguards instituted by the healthcare facility. This might be something as simple as taping a bar code wristband to the head of the bed so that it scans more easily than it would on a curved wrist. As soon as the wristband is removed from the patient, you have removed an essential safeguard.

Safety Alert

Guard against adopting any suggested "shortcut" or "work-around" that would eliminate an existing safeguard. If a consistent problem is present, such as difficulty making a bar code reader work on the wristband, then a system-wide correction is needed. Nurses can identify areas in which a system-wide improvement process is needed. Always follow facility procedures for safe medication administration.

AVOIDING DISTRACTIONS

Preparing medications requires that you make sure many small details are done accurately. Medication labels are often printed in small print, and there are containers that look alike. If someone stops you in the middle of the procedure, you may forget what has or has not been done. To be accurate, medication preparation requires your full attention. Do not hesitate to remind people not to distract you as you prepare medications and be careful not to distract others. Some clinical facilities are developing areas where nurses can work undisturbed to support the nurses' safe practice.

CALCULATING DRUG DOSAGES ACCURATELY

Before giving medications, you must have a satisfactory level of competence in mathematics of dosages and solutions. Many nursing programs test for a satisfactory level of proficiency in mathematics of dosages before permitting a student to give medications. Some clinical facilities routinely test those who will administer medications for mathematics proficiency. If you have concerns about this aspect of medication administration, plan to complete one of the many programmed instruction units available on mathematics of dosages and solutions. Consult your instructor for guidance.

However, calculating drug dosages remains a challenge for nurses throughout their careers. Skills that are used infrequently tend to be less well developed, and this leads to errors. Hospitals have many strategies in place to prevent these errors. In some facilities, when dosages must be calculated, they are done by a computerized program in the pharmacy with the information provided to the staff registered nurse. In other facilities, there is a policy that a nurse always has calculations double-checked by another nurse or by the pharmacy. If you are double-checking dosage calculations, each per-

son should set up and calculate the problem independently. The results are then compared. This provides a much more effective check on accuracy. Simply reviewing someone else's calculations may not reveal an error. Whatever the process, you will be accountable for accurate calculations to preserve patient safety.

MEASURING DRUGS PRECISELY

All drug doses must be accurate. Capsules are easy to count. Only scored tablets should be cut in half. Cutting unscored tablets is inaccurate; some doses may be too small, others too large, and in some cases, when the tablet is designed for extended release, large amounts of the drug may be released at one time.

Measuring liquid medications is a special procedure. To ensure accuracy, read the medicine glass or cup at eye level, with the thumbnail placed at the bottom of the **meniscus** at the correct level on the outside of the medicine container (Fig. 44-1). The liquid should be poured from the side of the opening that is opposite the label so that the liquid does not come in contact with the label and obscure it. Liquid amounts of less than 10 mL may be measured in a special oral syringe or medication-dispensing spoon.

THE SIX RIGHTS AND THREE CHECKS

Basic to the safe administration of medications are the **six rights** of medication administration. The right *drug*, the right *dose*, the right *route*, the right *time*, the right *patient*, and the right *documentation* are ensured by following careful procedures.

COMPLETING THE THREE CHECKS

The right *drug*, the right *dose*, the right *route*, and the right *time* are ensured by diligently completing the **three checks**: The name and dosage of the medication

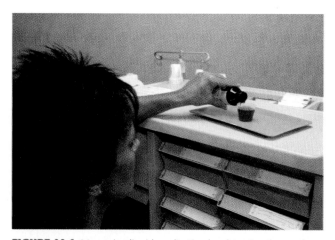

FIGURE 44-1 Measuring liquid medication by observing the meniscus at eye level. Note that the label is positioned so that medication will not drip on it.

as written on the drug label are checked with the MAR three times. This ensures the right drug and the right dose. In some facilities, the name of the drug is always the **generic name** that is assigned by the FDA. In other facilities, prescriptions may be written for **trade (brand) names** of drugs as well as for generic names. Most facilities have policies regarding the substitution of generic equivalents for many brand name drugs. These approved substitutions are usually listed in a manual, or the label from the pharmacy may specify that the generic equivalent may be used for the brand name.

The right dose should be listed clearly on the package. You need to be sure to read the measurement unit as carefully as the number. Be especially alert to decimal fractions.

The right route relates to whether the drug should be given orally, intramuscularly, or by some other route. When checking information, you should clearly differentiate the route because dosages differ based on route, and some drugs cannot be given by some routes.

The right time of administration is based on the ordered schedule and the facility policy regarding scheduling. In most facilities, the policy is that a drug may be given 30 minutes before or 30 minutes after the designated time and still be considered "on time." In some facilities, the policy is modified based on the frequency of drug administration ordered. For example, a daily medication might be designated on time if given within 60 minutes of the designated time, a drug given multiple times a day within 30 minutes, and a drug ordered every 2 hours or more frequently must be within 15 minutes to be considered on time.

The time at which the three checks are completed may differ somewhat depending on how the medications are stored and what the procedure is in the individual facility. Reading labels carefully three times may seem cumbersome, but medication names may be similar, dosages may differ from those ordered, and it is easy to "read" what you expect to be present if you only look one time. You will also check the correct time of administration on the MAR to ensure the right time. Commonly, the three times for checking are as follows:

1. When choosing the medication to take out of the drawer or cupboard, read the MAR and then locate the medication.
2. When the dose is in hand, hold the medication label and the MAR side by side to compare the label and the medication administration record (MAR).
3. When all drugs have been located and before leaving the medication cart or room for the patient's bedside, again compare the MAR and the label for each medication. In some facilities, this final check is done at the bedside (Fig. 44-2).

Keep all drugs in their individual dose package until you are at the patient's bedside. When discussing a med-

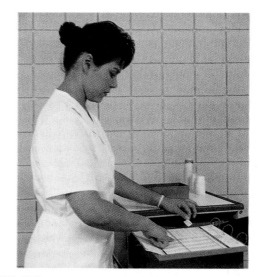

FIGURE 44-2 Compare the MAR with the medication label.

ication with a patient, you can then point out the labeled name of the drug as the patient observes its appearance. If the patient is not in the room or is unable to take the medication for some reason, you can return the medication, which is still in a labeled package, to the medication drawer for later administration because there is no chance of error in identification. This is one of the extra safeguards that the unit-dose method provides.

IDENTIFYING THE PATIENT

To ensure you have the right *patient*, carefully identify the patient, using two unique identifiers. This means that each identifier is both on the patient (or provided verbally by the patient) and also on the patient's chart, the MAR, or a special medication identification card. Acceptable identifiers, according to the JCAHO, include the patient's name, the patient's facility identification number, the patient's Social Security number, or the patient's date of birth. Some long-term care facilities use a photo of the resident as an identifier. Unique means that the identifiers are truly two different methods of identification. For example, if the patient says his name and you read the name on the wristband and compare that to the MAR, it is still one identifier—NAME. Getting it from two places such as the verbal statement and the wristband does not make it two unique identifiers. Using the name and patient identification number constitute two unique identifiers. When you are in the patient's room, you can compare the identification-card identifiers with the patient's wrist identification bracelet or ask the patient to state or spell his or her name while you check the identification card. When the patient is confused or unconscious, the use of the wristband is essential. Asking the patient to state his or her name or comparing numbers eliminates the possibility that the patient may respond casually to a "yes or no" question without truly hearing what you are asking. In an ambulatory care setting, the use of the client's name and birth date are common. The client is not wearing a wristband but is able to say or spell the name and tell you the birth date. The name and birth date will be a part of the client's record.

It is never acceptable to "remember" the patient's identification information and mentally compare this information with information found at the patient's bedside. No matter how long you have cared for a patient or how well you know the patient, these identification processes must never be omitted. When individuals are in a hurry or distracted, it is all too easy to enter the wrong room, approach the wrong bed, or approach the wrong patient sitting in a hallway.

COMPLETING DOCUMENTATION

The right *documentation* refers to documenting the medication administered in the correct format so that there is a legal record of the medication administration and other healthcare team members can respond appropriately. Failure to document or incorrect documentation is considered a medication error. It can lead to errors that may harm the patient such as the dose being repeated because there is no record that the appropriate dose was given.

Not only do nurses follow the six rights, these six rights are taught to family members and other caregivers and to medication assistants in places such as adult family homes and assisted living settings to ensure that the task is done correctly.

ADDITIONAL RIGHTS FOR SAFE AND EFFECTIVE MEDICATION ADMINISTRATION

In recent years, many suggestions have been made for expanding these six rights to seven, eight, or even nine rights. These additional aspects are all very important for the nurse who is administering medications and has professional responsibilities beyond the simple task of giving the medication. These additional rights include the right *patient assessment,* right *purpose,* right *knowledge of the drug's actions, interactions, and side effects,* and right *evaluation.* The registered nurse is responsible for these additional aspects of pharmacologic therapy even if someone else, such as a licensed practical nurse or even a medication assistant, is giving the medication.

Another safety factor is making sure that the patient has swallowed the medication. The patient should not be left alone until all medications have been swallowed. Although it is rare for a patient to deceive a nurse about taking medications, it does happen. A patient who has had a stroke may have a pill in the side of the cheek and not be aware that it was not swallowed. When you know this is the situation with the patient, you may need to ask to check the mouth to be sure that a pill is not lodged there. It is not appropriate to leave medica-

tions at the bedside for patients to take on their own unless so ordered by the prescriber or unless it is a policy for certain medications on a particular unit. Medications may be inadvertently misplaced, forgotten, or mistakenly picked up by another person if they are left at the bedside. Among the medications commonly self-administered are antacids, eye medications, and preparations that are inhaled. Medications that patients have been taking regularly at home, such as birth control pills, also may be the patient's responsibility.

The nurse who prepares a given medication should administer it. Stated another way, you should administer only drugs that you prepare. Only the person who prepared the drug can be sure that the all the checks were done. If a patient was unable to take a particular dose and it was returned to the medication drawer, another nurse would start by repeating the entire process.

REPORTING MEDICATION ERRORS

All medication errors must be reported both for the patient's well-being and in order for the system to improve. An error can result in serious adverse effects for the patient, depending upon the nature of the error and the action of the medication.

When an error occurs, the priority is assuring the well-being of the patient. The actions necessary for this vary, depending upon the nature of the medication. The nurse should use knowledge of the medication to determine what assessments to make immediately. The prescriber should be notified so that appropriate medications may be given to reverse the effect of an inappropriate drug or to re-establish an effective blood level. A special incident or quality assurance report is then completed. This report asks for the exact error and usually asks for information on contributing factors. The institution reviews these records to identify patterns and areas where processes should be improved. An important emphasis in the Institute of Medicine report was that reports of errors should not be used for disciplinary purposes but to determine the need for education and process change. If a punitive approach is used, medication errors may not be reported. This may result in more problems for the patient and the failure to correct processes that lead to errors. While from an ethical standpoint, nurses should always be truthful about medication errors, threats may intimidate individuals, making it hard to follow through on beliefs.

ASSISTING THE PERSON WITH SWALLOWING DIFFICULTIES

The nurse must consider the patient's ability to swallow when giving oral medications. Typically, it is sufficient to use a pill divider to split the solid pill into one or more pieces for easier swallowing.

Pills may be crushed using a mortar and pestle (Fig. 44-3) or a commercially produced pill crusher (Fig. 44-4). Pills should be crushed in their unit-dose packaging or in a closed paper medication cup to avoid contaminating them with the pestle. When using a pill crusher, place the pill in the circular area and pull the handle down. This action will crush the pill. Whole or split pills or capsules are sometimes given in a vehicle, such as a teaspoon of jelly. Unsweetened applesauce is a better vehicle for the patient with diabetes. When giving medications to children, never use an important food such as milk as a vehicle. If the medication tastes bad or is unpleasant in some other way, a child might refuse that food in the future.

Sometimes, it may be necessary to order a medication in liquid form; for example, a **syrup.** The pharmacy can provide an alternative to oral medication if it is available. Whether the nurse can independently order a different form of the medication is based on facility policy. It is also helpful to place the patient with swallowing difficulties in high-Fowler's or a sitting position and to provide sufficient fluid to assist swallowing. You might also use a small plastic glass designed to aid swallowing. It has a section of plastic slots inside to hold the medication in a midline position near the top of the glass. As the glass is tipped, the water facilitates easy swallowing.

OTHER METHODS OF ADMINISTERING MEDICATIONS BY MOUTH

In addition to medications that are swallowed, there are other techniques to ensure the absorption of medications.

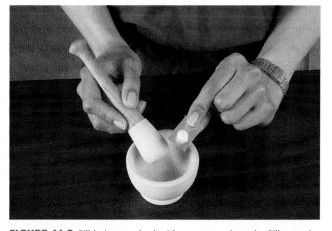

FIGURE 44-3 Pill being crushed with mortar and pestle. Pills may be crushed in their unit-dose packages or in a folded paper medicine cup.

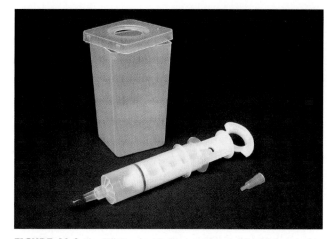

FIGURE 44-4 The Pill Crusher Syringe crushes solid tablets to a fine powder and then allows them to be administered to patients with feeding tubes. Courtesy of Welcon, Inc., Fort Worth, TX.

SUBLINGUAL AND BUCCAL MEDICATIONS

Some medications are ordered to be given by the **sublingual** route (placed under the tongue) or by the **buccal** route (placed between the cheek and gum). These medications are absorbed through the oral mucous membranes for rapid systemic effects. Instruct the patient not to swallow these medications, but instead to hold them in place until they dissolve completely. An alert and capable patient may place the sublingual or buccal tablet, or you may place it directly into the patient's mouth. If you place the medication, wear clean gloves to protect yourself from body secretions.

INSTANT DISSOLVING MEDICATIONS

There are some medications that are designed to dissolve rapidly in the mouth to facilitate swallowing. These medications are placed on the tongue, where they dissolve and then can be swallowed with little or no water. They may be helpful for those who are nauseated or simply cannot swallow pills.

ORAL MEDICATIONS ADMINISTERED AS RINSES

Some medications are used by the patient as a mouth rinse. After rinsing, the patient can either **expectorate** the rinse or swallow it as prescribed. If the medication is used as a rinse only, its effect is topical, with the purpose being to expose the oral mucous membrane to the drug for its local effect. After thoroughly rinsing the mouth, the patient expectorates into a basin or cup. Local anesthetic agents that are used for painful mouth lesions are examples of drugs that are used in this way. Other medications are used first as a rinse and then swallowed for additional systemic effect. These are commonly referred to on the order form or MAR as "S & S" (swish and swallow) medications. An antifungal medication used to combat a fungal infection of the mouth is an example of a drug used in this way.

Whether the medication is a rinse or one that is rinsed and swallowed, it should be administered last if there are other medications. This provides the greatest contact with the tissues and avoids removal of the agent by water taken with other drugs.

MEDICATIONS ADMINISTERED THROUGH A NASOGASTRIC TUBE

A patient with a nasogastric tube in place for the purpose of feeding is commonly given oral medications through the tube. The procedure is the same as for giving other oral medications, except that the medications must all be in a liquid or **suspension** form so that they can pass through the tube. Tablets are crushed and dissolved as much as possible in water. Capsules are emptied into water. Because the granules in capsules commonly do not dissolve thoroughly, it is important to follow them with water to flush the suspended medication completely out of the tube; otherwise, the medication can occlude the tube and the patient will not receive the intended dose.

Remember that a product that is designed to be sustained or released a portion at a time (timed release) cannot be crushed or emptied from the capsule. Another medication form must be ordered. Gel medications, such as some stool softeners, can be liquefied quickly by placing them in a plastic or paper cup and microwaving for a few minutes on a low setting. After cooling, they can be introduced into the nasogastric tube. Some medications can be obtained from the pharmacy as liquids or suspensions. The nurse can measure these medications in a syringe and then administer them directly from the syringe. All medications must be thoroughly flushed through the tube with at least 30 mL of clear water. If this is not done, the medication may remain in the tubing and the patient does not receive the dose. The medication may also clog the tube, making its replacement necessary.

When giving the medications, follow the procedure in Module 30, Administering Tube Feedings, for checking the placement of the tube and putting the medication in the tube. Do not put medications in the tube feeding solution because it is impossible to know whether the entire dose is administered at the appropriate time. If a continuous feeding is being administered, stop the feeding, give the medications, flush the tubing, and resume the feeding.

GENERAL PROCEDURE FOR ADMINISTERING ORAL MEDICATIONS

This procedure will be used as the General Procedure for learning the administration of medications by other routes as well.

ASSESSMENT

1. Review the medication record used in your facility to identify whether any medications are to be given to an individual patient during your shift. **R:** To determine whether you need to look medications up and to plan for the appropriate time to give medications. Generally, medications should be given within 30 minutes of the time ordered. Exceptions to this include preoperative medications and medications given every 2 hours or more frequently. These medications must be given within 15 minutes.

2. Examine the MAR for accuracy and completeness as prescribed by your facility. Check the patient's name and room number, name of the medication(s), dosage, route of administration, and time(s) the medication is to be given. Determine whether the ordered medications have already been given or are to be held. Often that information is noted at the place in the record where you would indicate having given the drug. **R:** Many factors can cause changes in prescribed medications that might not be reflected in the MAR. In some facilities, the MAR is compared with the medication orders each day. In other facilities, the procedure for verifying the MAR may include a double-check system at the time the order is noted, in which case it may not be necessary to check against the orders again. In this procedure, as in all others, follow the policy at your facility.

3. Review information about the medication(s) to be administered, including indication, usual dosage range, the expected effects, any contraindications, the potential side effects, and special instructions regarding administration. Be sure to check whether any specific assessment, such as measuring pulse or blood pressure, is required before administering the medication. **R:** It is the nurse's responsibility to always have reviewed the information regarding each medication and to plan for nursing assessment and evaluation relative to the medication's effect. The nurse also plans teaching based on this information.

4. Assess the patient's ability to take the medications as ordered. **R:** In order to plan for problems such as inability to swallow, decreased level of consciousness, or disorientation, or whether another factor (such as nausea and vomiting) might interfere with giving an oral medication.

5. Assess the patient's need for any prn medications. **R:** To administer prn medications in a time-efficient manner and ensure that the patient's immediate problems are addressed.

ANALYSIS

6. Critically think through your data, carefully evaluating each aspect and its relation to other data.

R: To determine specific problems for this individual in relation to medication administration.

7. Identify specific problems and modifications of the procedure needed for this individual. **R:** Planning for the individual must take into consideration the individual's problems.

PLANNING

8. Determine the individualized patient outcomes in relation to the medication(s) administered, including the following. **R:** Identification of outcomes guides planning and evaluation.
   a. The right *patient* receives the right *medication* in the right *dose* by the right *route* at the right *time*.
   b. The patient experiences the desired effect(s) from the medication(s) administered.
   c. The patient experiences no undesired effect(s) from the medication(s) administered.

9. Plan for any special procedures that may be needed before medication administration, such as measuring the blood pressure or assessing the apical pulse, or for special equipment and supplies needed for administration. **R:** Planning ahead allows you to proceed more safely and effectively. Assessment of vital signs can be done when you enter the room to administer the medication but might also be done as a part of routine care at an earlier time.

IMPLEMENTATION

Action	Rationale
10. Wash or disinfect your hands.	To decrease the transfer of microorganisms that could cause infection.
11. Obtain the official medication administration record, or access that record on the computer.	To provide you with an accurate listing of all medications to be administered to the patient.
12. Read from the record the name of the medication to be given. In some facilities, the MAR is on the computer screen.	The medication administration record provides the legal document showing which medications are ordered for the patient.
13. Access the medication supply and check the labels on the medications. Compare the medications to the MAR and choose the correct one before picking it up. Be sure to read the *name* of the medication and the *dosage* available.	This is the first of the three checks.
14. Pick up the medication and check the label again, comparing it with the MAR. If the medication is in a container, do this check before you remove the medication from the container. Again compare both the name of the medication and the dosage. Some facilities use a bar code reader to check the MAR and the unit-dose package in a computerized documentation system. If the bar code shows that this is the correct drug in the correct dose to be given at this time, then the computer shows this. Even when bar code systems are in place, do not omit reading the medication label yourself. The bar code system is a safety check but does not eliminate the need for an individual nurse to critically think about the process.	This is the second of the three checks.

(continued)

Action	Rationale
15. Remove the correct amount of medication for the individual dose to be given at this time. In some instances, the dose will be more than one unit-dose package.	You will be taking only the individual dose to the bedside. Unit-dose medications are opened at the bedside in order to further safeguard the correct medication and dose. The bottle containing liquid medication must be kept clean in order for the label to be legible. The third check must be done when the medication container with information on the dose is still where it can be seen.
a. For a unit-dose medication, place packages containing the correct number of tablets or capsules in the medication cup or on the tray. Do not open the packages at this time. For unit-dose medications, you may do the third check at this time, or wait and do the third check for all unit doses at the same time.	
b. For medication prepared in "blister packs" with multiple doses on the cardboard	
(1) Pop the capsule or tablet through the thin covering on the back of the "blister" containing the capsule.	
(2) Place the capsule or tablet in a medicine cup.	
(3) Complete the third check before replacing the "blister pack" card in the drawer.	
c. For a liquid	
(1) Place the bottle cap upside down on the countertop.	To prevent contamination.
(2) With the medicine cup at eye level, pour the liquid to the desired level in the cup, using the bottom of the concave meniscus as your guide (see Fig. 44-1).	
(3) Pour with the label facing up.	To prevent medication from running onto and distorting the label.
(4) Wipe the neck of the bottle with a clean paper towel before replacing the cap.	To prevent the cap from adhering and being difficult to remove.
(5) Complete the third check before putting the medication bottle away.	
16. Prepare any additional medications to be given at this time repeating steps 12 to 15 for each medication ordered.	All medications will be taken to the bedside together.

(continued)

Action	Rationale
17. With all medications out, check each unit-dose medication label with the MAR once again, comparing both the name of the medication and the dose.	This is the third of the three checks.
18. Obtain the patient's identification to be taken to patient's bedside as prescribed by your facility's policy. This may be the MAR itself, or it may be a separate identification label. Check this label carefully to be sure that it shares at least two identifiers with the MAR that can also be expected to be available at the patient's bedside. Some facilities use a bar code scanner at the bedside to scan the unit-dose package and the patient's wristband. The scanner is connected to the computerized documentation system. If the unit-dose, the patient, and the time do not match, a warning is displayed on the computer screen. If all match, then a notification to proceed is provided.	This provides a means to check two unique identifiers with the patient at the bedside.
19. Identify the patient, using two identifiers. By identifying the patient before you begin the rest of the procedure, you avoid causing distress by mistakenly offering medication that is intended for someone else. Although you prevent an error if you check the identification after offering the medication, the patient may feel that a mistake was almost made and may thus feel anxious. You can walk into the room and simply say, "Hello. May I check your wristband?" Another approach is to look at your identification record and say, "Hello. Would you please spell your last name for me?" or "Hello. Would you please state your full name for me?" When that matches the record, check the second identifier.	Verifying the patient's identity helps ensure that you are giving the right medication to the right patient.
20. Explain how the medication is to be taken and provide any other appropriate teaching regarding the medication.	Explaining the procedure helps relieve anxiety or misperceptions that the patient may have about a medication, and knowledge of the medication sets the stage for patient self-care after discharge.
21. Administer the medication.	
a. Give the patient a glass of fresh, cold water. If the medication has an unpleasant flavor, you can give it with juice instead of water, as long as this is not contrary to the patient's diet order	To facilitate the patient being able to swallow the medication. Fluids are important for dilution of many medications as they dissolve. Cold water tends to lessen any bad taste of a medication. *(continued)*

Action	Rationale
or the drug manufacturer's directions. If the patient has a favorite juice, indicate it on the record, so other nurses who administer the medication will know and will not have to ask the patient again.	
b. Watch the patient take the medication. If you are not certain it has been swallowed, or if there seems to be a problem with swallowing, have the patient open his or her mouth and look inside to see if the medication is still there.	To ensure that the patient receives the prescribed medication.
c. Sometimes a patient will ask you to leave a medication to be taken later. Do not do this.	This is not appropriate because you would not be able to document that the patient actually took the medication. When you refuse the request, you might say, "No, I am responsible for it, so I don't want to leave it. If you can't take it now, I will come back with it later." If the medication is needed immediately, explain why it should be taken promptly.
d. If a tablet or a capsule falls to the floor, discard it and obtain a replacement.	Anything that touches the floor is considered contaminated.
22. Leave the patient in a comfortable position.	This contributes to the patient's ability to rest and to feelings of well-being.
23. Discard any medication containers and packaging.	To maintain a neat environment for the patient.
24. Wash or disinfect your hands.	To decrease the transfer of microorganisms that could cause infection.

EVALUATION

25. Evaluate using the individualized patient outcomes previously identified, including the following. **R:** Evaluation in relation to desired outcomes is essential for planning future care.
  a. The patient receives the right *medication* in the right *dose* by the right *route* at the right *time*.
  b. The patient experiences the desired effect(s) from the medication(s) administered.
  c. The patient experiences no undesired effect(s) from the medication(s) administered.

DOCUMENTATION

26. Documentation should show that right *patient* received the right *medication* in the right *dosage* by the right *route,* at the right *time,* and it was documented in the right *way* with an appropriate signature. This may be directly on the MAR, in a computerized documentation system, or on a separate medication administration form. In facilities that use bar coding to identify medications and patients, the administration may be automatically documented when the patient's wristband and the unit dose are scanned at the bedside. Be especially careful with documentation of drugs that are given on unusual schedules such as every other day, twice a week, or monthly. If a drug was given at other than designated time because a patient was away from the unit or having a diagnostic test, there will be a specific way to record this information. **R:** To provide the legal record of care administered and communicate with the healthcare team.

27. Document your evaluation of the patient's response to the medication as appropriate for the drug and according to facility policy. **R:** Evaluating the patient's response to pharmacologic therapy is a nursing responsibility. Facility policy may indicate that only responses to prn drugs, adverse responses, and responses to new drugs are routinely documented.

POTENTIAL ADVERSE OUTCOMES AND RELATED INTERVENTIONS

1. The patient experiences an adverse response to a medication.
Intervention: Notify the prescriber and do not give further doses of the drug until you have had an opportunity to confer with him or her. Document your assessment of the adverse response and that further doses of the medication were held.

2. The patient is nauseated and/or vomiting.
Intervention: Hold the medication. Document that the medication was held and the reason in the manner required by your facility. If an antinausea medication has been ordered, give that medication and wait until it is effective; then administer the medication, noting the time it was actually administered. If this is not successful, notify the prescriber, and consult regarding a different route of administration. Document the process, including the exact times the actions were taken.

3. The patient refuses the medication.
Intervention: Explain the rationale for the medication and how it will benefit the patient. If the patient continues to refuse the medication, document that the medication was not given, the patient's refusal as well as your teaching, and notify the prescriber.

Acute Care

Because of the high acuity of patients in hospitals and the rapid rate at which they are admitted and discharged, the potential for medication errors is very high. A study done by the Institutes of Medicine (IOM, 2000) identified medication errors as a serious problem in the healthcare system. Preventing these errors requires that prescribers, nurses, and pharmacists work collaboratively. Each provides a check on the accuracy of the others. Communication between them is essential to accuracy. Nurses need to be assertive if orders are not clear or if there is a conflict between medications, allergies of the patient, or potential adverse responses are occurring. The environment should be one that fosters respect for all participants in the process and sets the stage for accuracy.

Long-Term Care

Because of the number and frequency of medications to be given, the number of residents, and the kinds of physical, cognitive, and psychosocial alterations that may affect the residents (e.g., swallowing difficulties or inability to understand the medication actions or medication procedure), the nurse in long-term care must be especially adaptable when giving medications. The nurse typically administers oral medications to many residents, making identification of each individual resident and accuracy of administration a more challenging responsibility. Identifying residents who may move about the facility and who may be cognitively impaired provides an additional challenge. Nurses in long-term care typically must find ways to assist residents with swallowing difficulties or those whose coordination makes handling medications difficult.

For various reasons, older adults are more susceptible to the adverse effects of medications. For instance, kidney and liver function in the older adult may be decreased, so dosages that are therapeutic for younger people can be toxic. The circulatory system may be compromised, decreasing medication distribution to the cells and metabolism. Chronic illness may also affect drug metabolism.

Home Care

It is sometimes appropriate to monitor the oral medication regimen for clients living at home. As a home care nurse, you should review the medication list with the client, focusing on several aspects such as instructions, drug names and expiration dates, medication times, and OTC (over-the-counter) medications. You would also be assessing whether the client was taking the medications as prescribed, and seek solutions to managing any medication problems.

Some medications have instructions printed in very small type, making it difficult for people to read. Suggest using a simple magnifying glass as a visual aid. Medications may have confusing brand names, so a client may unknowingly take two medications at the same time that have the same purpose. Clearly identify all medications and explain the purpose of each to the client. Instruct the client to check the expiration dates of medications because the action of outdated drugs is less effective.

Without "reminders," medication times may be completely missed, causing inconsistent dosages.

Inexpensive plastic containers with designated times and sections for storing medications are available. Some pharmacies provide these without charge. Also, half of an egg carton can be marked and used for this purpose.

 Ambulatory Care

Assess both any prescribed and any OTC (over-the-counter) medication(s) the client is taking to be sure there is no conflict with other prescribed medications. Instruct clients never to "lend" medications or give them to another person for whom they were not prescribed. Also instruct clients to make sure that all medications are stored out of the reach of children. With the assistance of health teaching, clients and any family members assisting can continue administration of oral medications safely and effectively.

LEARNING TOOLS

DEVELOP YOUR BACKGROUND KNOWLEDGE

1. Review the Learning Outcomes.

2. Read the section on administering medications in your assigned text.

3. Look up the Key Terms in the glossary.

4. Review this module and mentally practice the techniques described. Study so that you would be able to teach these skills to another person.

DEVELOP YOUR SKILLS

1. In the practice setting, select another student to work with.

2. Changing so that each has the opportunity to play the role of the patient, administer pseudo-medications to one another using the Performance Checklist on the CD-ROM in the front of this book. If groups of three are used, the one who is not participating at a given time can observe and evaluate the performances of the others.

3. With the same group, change roles as you did before until all have had the opportunity to play the role of the patient and the nurse administering medications.

DEMONSTRATE YOUR SKILLS

In the clinical setting

1. Review the medication administration record and procedures used in your facility.

2. Go through the procedure step by step, referring to the Performance Checklist as necessary. Use the appropriate procedures for your facility.

3. Consult with your instructor regarding the opportunity to administer oral medications in the clinical setting.

4. Evaluate your performance with the instructor.

CRITICAL THINKING EXERCISES

Use your medication reference book to assist with these exercises.

1. Your patient has these oral medication orders:

   digoxin (Lanoxin) 0.125 daily
   furosemide (Lasix) 20 mg bid
   folic acid 1 mg daily
   levothyroxine sodium (L-thyroxine) 0.05 daily
   amoxicillin 250 mg q8h
   nystatin 10 mL (S&S) tid.
   docusate sodium (Doss) 250 mg daily
   triazolam (Halcion) 0.125 mg HS prn

   Formulate a general medication plan for this patient, using columns indicating the times you would be giving these medications. Note the meaning of the abbreviations on the sample MAR (above) and in the first column, write down the time, and identify why these are the appropriate times to administer each of these medications. In the second column, specify any side effects that may determine what time is most appropriate. In the third column, recommend any special health teaching that needs to be done.

2. Your patient has complained of "chest pain." The prescriber has ordered one nitroglycerin tablet to be administered sublingually. The patient has never had this medication before. Describe how this medication would be administered. Determine what explanation you would give the patient. Describe the drug's action and the expected patient response from the drug. Explain how you would document its administration.

SELF-QUIZ
SHORT-ANSWER QUESTIONS

1. List the six rights.

   a. _____

   b. _____

   c. _____

d. _____

e. _____

f. _____

2. When does the nurse check the name and dosage of the medication against that ordered?

_____

3. Name two methods of identifying the patient before giving medications.

a. _____

b. _____

MULTIPLE CHOICE

_____ 4. Which of the following nursing diagnoses is most important to the safety concerns of administering an oral medication?
   a. Impaired Communication
   b. Risk for Activity Intolerance
   c. Impaired Skin Integrity
   d. Risk for Aspiration

_____ 5. When pouring a liquid medication, you should measure from
   a. the top edge of the meniscus.
   b. the bottom of the meniscus.
   c. neither of these.
   d. It makes no difference.

_____ 6. Which of the following nursing actions is most helpful for the patient with swallowing difficulties?
   a. Placing the patient in a sitting position
   b. Mixing the medication with food
   c. Turning the patient toward you
   d. Dissolving the medication in a glass of water

_____ 7. When giving medication through a nasogastric tube, water is instilled afterward to
   a. provide the patient with additional fluid.
   b. dissolve the medication.
   c. flush the tube.
   d. check the patency of the tube.

_____ 8. When giving an oral medication contingent on pulse or blood pressure measurement,
   a. measure the pulse or blood pressure within 1 hour of giving the medication.
   b. have two people do the measurements.
   c. keep this medication separate from any others.
   d. carry out all measurements with the patient in the sitting position.

_____ 9. If a medication is in unit-dose form,
   a. open it immediately.
   b. only open at the bedside.
   c. remove the label and place it on a tray.
   d. have the patient open the package.

_____ 10. Which of the following is the most appropriate vehicle in which to administer oral medication to a diabetic patient with a swallowing problem?
   a. Milk
   b. Unsweetened applesauce
   c. Ice cream
   d. A small amount of jelly

_____ 11. It is important not to leave medication at the bedside because
   a. you will be unable to document that the patient actually took the medication.
   b. it may fall on the floor.
   c. the patient may forget to take it.
   d. it takes time to return and check with the patient later.

_____ 12. Buccal medications are those
   a. placed between the cheek and the gum.
   b. placed under the tongue.
   c. injected into the buttocks.
   d. swallowed without water.

_____ 13. Oral rinses have which of the following actions?
   a. Systemic effect when swallowed
   b. Decrease microorganisms and tooth decay
   c. Increase the ability to taste
   d. Local effect through exposure to the mucous membrane

_____ 14. Which of the following is an example of an S & S (swish and swallow) oral medication?
   a. Anesthetic agents
   b. Mouthwashes
   c. Antifungals
   d. Antibiotics

_____ 15. Oral medications for the elderly may produce toxicity because of
   a. poor eyesight.
   b. decreased kidney function.
   c. increased incidence of allergy.
   d. increased blood pressure.

Answers to the Self-Quiz questions appear in the back of the book.

MODULE 45

Administering Medications by Alternative Routes

SKILLS INCLUDED IN THIS MODULE

Procedure for Instilling Ophthalmic Medications
Procedure for Instilling Otic Medications
Procedure for Instilling Nasal Medications
Procedure for Administering Medications Using a Metered-Dose Inhaler
Procedure for Applying Topical Medications
Procedure for Administering Transdermal Medications
Procedure for Administering Vaginal Medications
Procedure for Administering Rectal Medications

PREREQUISITE MODULES

Module 1	An Approach to Nursing Skills
Module 2	Documentation
Module 4	Basic Infection Control
Module 5	Safety in the Healthcare Environment
Module 6	Moving the Patient in Bed and Positioning
Module 14	Nursing Physical Assessment
Module 24	Basic Sterile Technique: Sterile Field and Sterile Gloves
Module 39	Administering Ear and Eye Irrigations
Module 44	Administering Oral Medications

Review of the anatomy and physiology of the eye, ear, nose, skin, vagina, rectum, and respiratory system.

KEY TERMS

aspiration pneumonia	ophthalmic
canthus	otic
conjunctival sac	Parkinson's position
dorsal recumbent position	pinna
ethmoid sinus	Proetz position
eustachian tubes	Sims' position
eye drops	sphenoid sinus
frontal sinuses	suppository
instillation	suppurating
intraocular medication disk	systemic
	topical
	transdermal
liniment	tympanic membrane
maxillary sinuses	vaginal
ointment	

OVERALL OBJECTIVE

▶ To prepare and administer medications safely, using ophthalmic, otic, nasal, inhalation, topical, vaginal, and rectal routes.

LEARNING OUTCOMES

The student will be able to

1. Assess the patient with regard to the specific medication and route ordered.
2. Analyze assessment data to determine special problems or concerns that must be addressed to successfully administer the medication ordered by the route ordered.
3. Determine appropriate patient outcomes for the medication(s) administered and recognize the potential for adverse outcomes.
4. Plan appropriate strategies to assure that the patient receives the medication ordered by the route ordered.
5. Administer medications safely and accurately using the ophthalmic, otic, nasal, inhalation, topical, vaginal, and rectal routes.
6. Evaluate the patient's response to the medication(s) administered.
7. Document the medications administered and the patient's response according to facility policies.

Drugs can be administered by various routes, depending on the patient's condition, the drug, and the desired effect. The nurse must be able to prepare and administer drugs correctly using various routes, keeping in mind the basic concepts of safe administration and those related to the special routes. The nurse's knowledge of the anatomy and physiology related to the organ being treated and of the actions, usual dosage, desired effects, and potential side effects of the drug being administered are imperative for safe practice.

NURSING DIAGNOSES

- Risk for Injury: The major nursing diagnosis to keep in mind when giving medications is Risk for Injury. Patients can be injured by medications given in the wrong dosage, at the wrong time, or by an incorrect route. Patients also can be injured by the omission of essential medications or the administration of an incorrect medication. Although this nursing diagnosis will not appear on the care plan, it applies to every situation in which a patient is being given medications.
- Deficient Knowledge: Another nursing diagnosis frequently appropriate when administering medications is Deficient Knowledge. Knowledge may be deficient related to some aspect of the medication regimen; for example, the exact

manner in which to self-administer the drug, the desired effects to evaluate, and the potential side effects to report.

DELEGATION

Administration of medications by any route is not delegated to assistive personnel in acute care settings. They may be asked to observe for and report specific effects (both desired and adverse) of medications the nurse has administered. Nursing assistants may also inform the nurse of situations in which a medication, such as a medication for a rash or for a breathing problem, may be needed. However, the nurse is responsible for assessing the need for prn medication before administering it. The nurse is always responsible for evaluating the effect(s) of all medications administered.

In home care settings, assisted living settings, and long-term care settings in some states, nursing assistants are taught to administer certain topical, vaginal, and rectal medications. They may assist the competent patient in managing a metered-dose inhaler. The nurse needs to be aware of the legal requirements of the setting in which he or she practices in order to make an appropriate decision about delegation. If one of these types of medications is delegated, the nurse must specifically teach the assistant about each medication and its proper administration and evaluate the individual's ability to administer it correctly. A nurse who delegates in these settings remains accountable for assessment and the evaluation of a medication's effects.

PROCEDURES FOR ADMINISTERING MEDICATIONS BY ALTERNATIVE ROUTES

For each specific medication route discussed, some steps of the General Procedure for Administering Oral Medications in Module 44 may be used and others may be modified. References to the steps of the General Procedure that remain the same are included. Modified steps are completely described.

PROCEDURE FOR INSTILLING OPHTHALMIC MEDICATIONS

Ophthalmic medications are those used in the eye. They are used to soothe irritated tissue, dilate or constrict the pupil, treat eye disease, or provide anesthesia. Medications used in the eye are always sterile. In addition to the six rights discussed in Module 44, you must be certain you are medicating the correct ("right") eye. The correct eye should be designated by "right eye" or "left eye" or "both eyes." If the order does not use this clear terminology, the prescriber should be contacted and the designation clarified and written in these terms. (*Note:* The abbreviations for right eye [OD] and left eye [OS] and both eyes [OU] that were formerly used are no longer permitted in some facilities because they were the source of confusion and errors. These abbreviations have now been eliminated by the majority of healthcare facilities.) To instill ophthalmic medications, follow the General Procedure for Administering Oral Medications, Module 44, as modified below.

ASSESSMENT

1. Follow step 1 of the General Procedure: Review the medication administration record (MAR) for medications to be administered.

2. Examine the MAR for accuracy and completeness as prescribed by your facility. When verifying the medication order for an eye medication, identify whether the medication is to be given in the right eye, the left eye, or both eyes. **R:** On occasion, unclear abbreviations may be found on the medication order because they were formerly acceptable.

3-5. Follow steps 3 to 5 of the General Procedure: Review medication information, assess the patient's abilities, and assess the need for medications given prn.

ANALYSIS

6-7. Follow steps 6 and 7 of the General Procedure: Critically think through your data, carefully evaluating each aspect and its relation to other data, and identify specific problems and modifications of the procedure needed for this individual.

PLANNING

8. Determine the individualized patient outcomes in relation to the ophthalmic medication(s) administered, including the following. **R:** Identification of outcomes guides planning and evaluation.

   a. The right *patient* receives the right *medication* in the right *dose* by the right *route* (and into the correct eye) at the right *time*.

   b. The patient experiences the desired effect(s) from the medication(s) administered.

   c. The patient experiences no undesired effect(s) from the medication(s) administered.

9. Plan for any special procedures, equipment, or supplies that may be needed before medication administration, including the following. **R:** Planning ahead allows you to proceed more safely and effectively.

   a. Clean gloves to protect yourself from contact with body secretions

   b. Cleansing supplies (gauze squares or a clean washcloth) to clean the exterior surface of the eyelid before administering the eye medication if the eye is **suppurating** (weeping matter)

   c. A tissue, gauze square, or cotton ball to wipe away any medication that gets on the exterior of the eye

IMPLEMENTATION

Action	Rationale
10. Wash or disinfect your hands.	To decrease the transfer of microorganisms that could cause infection.
11-14. Follow steps 11 to 14 of the General Procedure: Access the official MAR; read the name of the medication to be given;	Observing all safety measures helps to ensure the right *medication*. *(continued)*

Action	Rationale
access the ophthalmic medication, and check the label on the medication; compare the medication to that on the MAR and choose the correct one before picking it up; pick up the medication and check the label again.	
15. Remove the correct amount of medication for the individual dose to be given at this time.	
a. *Multiple-dose containers:* Remove the entire container.	Eye medications often are dispensed from dropper-top bottles or from tubes of **ointment.** The entire bottle of eye drops or tube of ointment is removed from the drawer. This will be taken to the bedside to administer the medication. The actual dose of liquid medication must be measured directly into the eye as drops from the dropper bottle. The dose of an ophthalmic ointment is simply the length of ointment extruded that fits in the **conjunctival sac** (see directions in the procedure below).
b. *Single-dose packages:* Remove from the drawer the correct number of individual packages to equal the dose ordered for both eyes and take the unopened packages to the bedside.	All medications provided in single-dose packages are taken to the bedside in their original individual packages. Some eye drops and ointments are dispensed in individual dose packages that are taken to the bedside and discarded after administering the medication. Intraocular medication disks used to deliver eye medications are individually packaged with one disk in each package.
16-20. Follow steps 16 to 20 of the General Procedure: Prepare any additional medications to be given at this time, check each medication label with the MAR once again, obtain the patient identification to be taken to patient's bedside as prescribed by your facility's policy, identify the patient (two identifiers), and explain how the medication will be administered.	
21. Administer the eye medication.	
a. Wash or disinfect your hands, and put on clean gloves just before administering the eye medication.	To decrease the transfer of microorganisms that could cause infection and protect yourself from eye secretions.
b. Clean the eyelids and lashes if necessary.	Secretions that could harbor microorganisms may have accumulated and dried. Moving from inner canthus to outer canthus prevents contamination of the opposite eye as well as the lacrimal duct.

(continued)

Action	Rationale
(1) Use a clean washcloth, gauze squares, or cotton balls moistened in tap water. If secretions are dried and crusted, you may need to leave the moist washcloth or cotton ball in place for a few minutes to soften them.	If gloves contact exudate, they are contaminated. Only clean gloves should handle the eye medication containers.
(2) When cleaning, move from inner **canthus** to outer canthus, using each cotton ball for only one wipe.	
(3) Removed contaminated gloves. Cleanse the hands and put on clean gloves.	
c. Have the patient tip the head slightly backward. This can be done with the patient lying in bed or sitting in a chair.	This provides access to the eye.
d. Have the patient look up.	The cornea will be partially protected by the upper eyelid, and the patient is less likely to blink while looking up.
e. Remove the cap from the dropper bottle or tube, hold the container in your dominant hand, and rest your hand on the patient's forehead. For an intraocular disk, open the package, press your gloved finger gently against the convex surface of the disk, and pick it up. The disk should adhere to your finger. If the disk will not adhere to your glove, you may need to moisten your glove with sterile saline solution.	This prepares the medication for administration, and stabilizing your hand prevents you from inadvertently striking the patient in the eye.
f. Hold a tissue, cotton ball, or gauze square in your other hand and use that to pull down on the lower lid of the eye to be medicated.	This will expose the lower conjunctival sac, and the tissue, cotton ball, or gauze square will catch any excess medication that may escape from the eye.
Choose the correct technique from g through i described below.	
g. Instill **eye drops:** Hold the container tip down, close to but not touching the eye, and squeeze the bottle to drop the ordered number of drops into the middle of the exposed conjunctival sac. Do not touch the dropper tip to the eye (Fig. 45-1).	Touching the eye with the dropper tip will contaminate the tip and allow microorganisms to grow and contaminate the medication. It also is uncomfortable for the patient.

(continued)

Action	Rationale

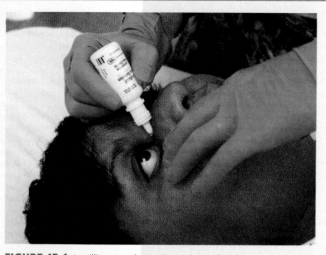

FIGURE 45-1 Instilling eye drops. Drop the ordered number of drops into the middle of the lower conjunctival sac.

h. Instill eye ointment:

(1) Squeeze out a ribbon of medication along the entire lower conjunctival sac, moving from inner canthus to outer canthus (Fig. 45-2).	To distribute the medication evenly across the eye.

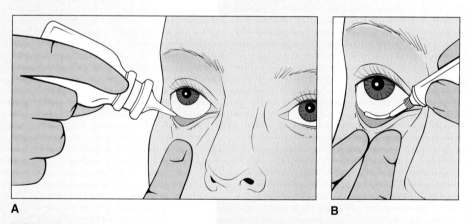

A   B

FIGURE 45-2 (**A**) Drops placed in lower conjunctival sac. (**B**) Ribbon of medication squeezed out along the entire lower conjunctival sac.

(2) Discontinue the ribbon of ointment by twisting or turning the tube.	Twisting the tube will prevent the entire line of ointment from lifting back out of the eye as you remove the tube.
i. Insert and remove **intraocular medication disk:**	If a disk is being replaced, remove the old disk before inserting the new disk.
(1) To remove the disk, gently pull the lower eyelid downward. Pinch the disk between the thumb and forefinger of your opposite hand and lift it out of the eye.	To expose the disk and facilitate its safe removal.

(continued)

Action	Rationale
(2) Gently place the disk in the conjunctival sac and pull the lower eyelid out and up over the disk.	To secure the disk in place and ensure that the medication will be delivered.
j. Ask the patient to close the eye gently. If eye drops were instilled, have the patient move the eyeball around while it is closed. If ointment was used, have the patient keep the eye closed a full minute following the **instillation.** Use a tissue or gauze square to wipe away any excess medication. If a disk was inserted, you should not be able to see it. If you can, pull the lower eyelid up and over the disk a second time.	If the eye is squeezed tightly shut, the drops or ointment may be pushed out. Moving the eyeball around will help disperse the drops. Keeping the eye closed for a full minute will allow the ointment to melt and disperse over the eye.
k. When administering eye medications that may have **systemic** effects, apply gentle pressure to the nasolacrimal duct using a clean tissue or clean washcloth (Fig. 45-3).	To prevent the medication from being absorbed into the general circulation.

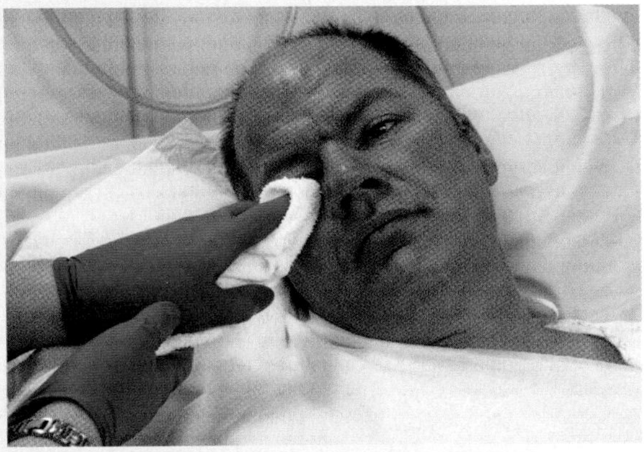

FIGURE 45-3 When administering eye medication that has systemic effects, apply gentle pressure to the nasolacrimal duct using a clean tissue.

Action	Rationale
22. Follow step 22 of the General Procedure: Leave the patient in a comfortable position.	
23. Wipe any excess medication from the dropper bottle or tube with a clean tissue, replace the cap, and discard tissues and single-dose containers appropriately.	Medication left on the outside may make the cap difficult to remove and soil the medication drawer. Used supplies that are not discarded appropriately may be a place for microbes to grow and also contribute to an unpleasant environment for the patient.
24. Follow step 24 of the General Procedure: Remove your gloves, and wash or disinfect your hands.	

EVALUATION

25. Follow step 25 of the General Procedure: Evaluate using the individualized patient outcomes previously identified:
    a. The right *patient* received the right *medication* in the right *dose* by the right *route* (and into the correct eye) at the right *time*.
    b. The patient experienced the desired effect(s) from the medication(s) administered.
    c. The patient experienced no undesired effect(s) from the medication(s) administered.

DOCUMENTATION

26-27. Follow steps 26 and 27 of the General Procedure: Complete right *documentation*. Document the medication, the dose, the route (as well as the eye medicated), the time, and your signature according to the facility policy. Also document your evaluation of the patient's response to the medication as appropriate for the drug and according to facility policy.

POTENTIAL ADVERSE OUTCOMES AND RELATED INTERVENTIONS

1. Patient complains of pain. Eye appears irritated and bloodshot.
Intervention: Eye may have been touched with dropper tip. Document and continue to observe. If it continues, patient may be experiencing a reaction to the medication. Do not administer further doses until after conferring with the prescriber.
2. Patient experiences systemic effects of eye medication administered.
Intervention: Notify prescriber. Stay with patient. Do not administer further doses of medication.

PROCEDURE FOR INSTILLING OTIC MEDICATIONS

Otic medications are used in the ear. They can be introduced into the ear to soften wax, relieve pain, or treat disease. The instillation of medication to the ear is a clean procedure, *except* when the **tympanic membrane** is not intact, in which case sterile technique is used. To instill otic medications, follow the General Procedure for Administering Oral Medications, Module 44, as modified below.

ASSESSMENT

1. Follow step 1 of the General Procedure: Review the MAR for medications to be administered.
2. Examine the MAR for accuracy and completeness as prescribed by your facility. When verifying the medication order, identify whether the medication is to be given in the right ear, the left ear, or both ears.
3-5. Follow steps 3 to 5 of the General Procedure: Review medication information, assess the patient's abilities, and assess the need for prn medications.

ANALYSIS

6-7. Follow steps 6 and 7 of the General Procedure: Critically think through your data, carefully evaluating each aspect and its relation to other data, and identify specific problems and modifications of the procedure needed for this individual.

PLANNING

8. Follow step 8 of the General Procedure: Determine the individualized patient outcomes in relation to the otic medication(s) to be administered. Include
    a. The right *patient* receives the right *medication* in the right *dose* by the right *route* (and into the correct ear) at the right *time*.
    b. The patient experiences the desired effect(s) from the medication(s) administered.
    c. The patient experiences no undesired effect(s) from the medication(s) administered.
9. Follow step 9 of the General Procedure: Plan for any special procedures that may be needed before medication administration or supplies needed, including a tissue, cotton ball, gauze square, and clean gloves to wipe away any medication that drains out of the ear. Gloves protect your hands from possible drainage and from contact with the medication.

IMPLEMENTATION

Action	Rationale
10. Wash or disinfect your hands.	To decrease the transfer of microorganisms that could cause infection.

(continued)

Action	Rationale
11-14. Follow steps 11 to 14 of the General Procedure: Access the official MAR; read the name of the medication to be given; access the otic medication and check the label on the medication; compare the medication to the MAR and choose the correct one before picking it up; pick up the medication and check the label again.	
15. Remove the correct amount of medication for the individual dose to be given at this time. Ear medications often are dispensed in dropper-top bottles. Remove the entire bottle of ear drops from the drawer and take it to the bedside to administer the medication. You will measure the actual dose directly into the ear as drops from the dropper bottle.	
16-20. Follow steps 16 to 20 of the General Procedure: Prepare any additional medications to be given at this time, check each medication label with the MAR once again, obtain the patient identification to be taken to patient's bedside as prescribed by your facility's policy, identify the patient (two identifiers), and explain how the medication will be administered.	
21. Administer the ear medication:	
a. Warm the medication to body temperature by holding the container in your hand for a short time or by placing the container in warm water.	Cold medication touching the eardrum may cause the patient to feel dizzy and may be painful.
b. Have the patient lie on the side, with the ear to be medicated facing up.	This allows the medication to reach all parts of the canal. The direction of pull should be relative to the direction of the ear canal, and that direction changes during growth to adulthood.
c. Put on gloves if there is drainage from the ear and straighten the ear canal. In an adult, gently pull the **pinna** upward and backward (Fig. 45-4). In an infant or small child (under 3 years old), gently pull the pinna downward and backward.	To protect yourself from potentially contaminated secretions.
d. Instill the correct number of drops, directing them toward the side of the ear canal. Do not touch the dropper tip to the ear.	From the side of the ear canal, they will run down onto the eardrum. Touching the ear tissue will contaminate the dropper and allow microorganisms to grow and contaminate the medication. *(continued)*

Action	Rationale
	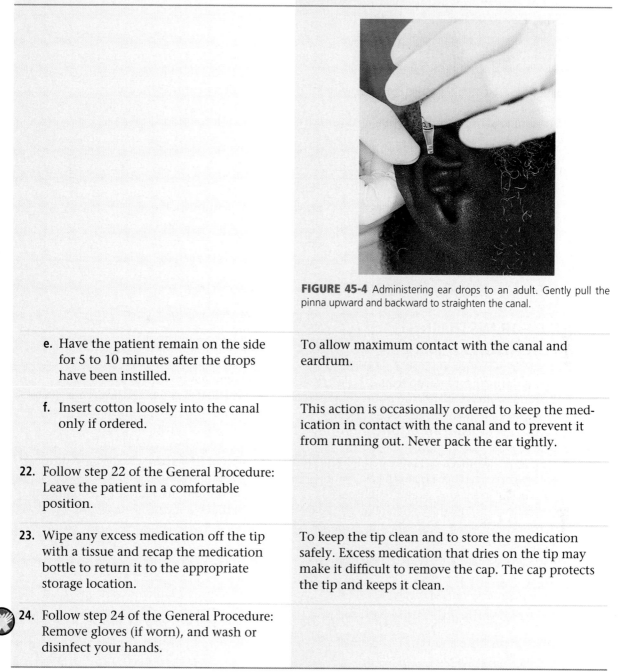 **FIGURE 45-4** Administering ear drops to an adult. Gently pull the pinna upward and backward to straighten the canal.
e. Have the patient remain on the side for 5 to 10 minutes after the drops have been instilled.	To allow maximum contact with the canal and eardrum.
f. Insert cotton loosely into the canal only if ordered.	This action is occasionally ordered to keep the medication in contact with the canal and to prevent it from running out. Never pack the ear tightly.
22. Follow step 22 of the General Procedure: Leave the patient in a comfortable position.	
23. Wipe any excess medication off the tip with a tissue and recap the medication bottle to return it to the appropriate storage location.	To keep the tip clean and to store the medication safely. Excess medication that dries on the tip may make it difficult to remove the cap. The cap protects the tip and keeps it clean.
24. Follow step 24 of the General Procedure: Remove gloves (if worn), and wash or disinfect your hands.	

EVALUATION

25. Follow step 25 of the General Procedure: Evaluate using the individualized outcomes previously identified:

   a. The right *patient* received the right *medication* in the right *dose* by the right *route* (and into the correct ear) at the right *time*.

   b. The patient experienced the desired effect(s) from the medication(s) administered.

   c. The patient experienced no undesired effect(s) from the medication(s) administered.

DOCUMENTATION

26-27. Follow steps 26 and 27 of the General Procedure: Complete right *documentation.* Document the medication, the dosage, the route (as well as the ear medicated), the time, and your signature according to the facility policy. Also document your evaluation of the patient's response to the medication as appropriate for the drug and according to facility policy.

POTENTIAL ADVERSE OUTCOMES AND RELATED INTERVENTIONS

1. Ear canal is occluded or partially occluded with cerumen (earwax).
Intervention: Do not attempt to instill ear medication. If there is no standing order, consult with prescriber regarding the need for ear irrigation to remove cerumen.
2. Ear canal is inflamed and tender to touch.
Intervention: Medication may not be effective. Document continuing symptoms, and notify prescriber.
3. Patient reports itching and ear appears irritated.
Intervention: The patient may be experiencing a reaction to the medication. Confer with prescriber before administering further doses.

PROCEDURE FOR INSTILLING NASAL MEDICATIONS

Nasal medication is normally ordered to relieve nasal or sinus congestion and is often given in the form of nose drops. Nose drops and nasal sprays are water soluble because of the danger of **aspiration pneumonia** with oil-based solutions. The administration of nasal medication is not a sterile procedure, but careful clean technique should be practiced because of the close and direct connection between the nose and the sinuses. To instill nasal medications, follow the General Procedure

for Administering Oral Medications, Module 44, as modified below.

ASSESSMENT

1-5. Follow steps 1 to 5 of the General Procedure: Review the medication record to determine whether medications are to be administered, examine the MAR for accuracy and completeness, review medication information, assess the patient's abilities, and assess the need for prn medications.

ANALYSIS

6-7. Follow steps 6 and 7 of the General Procedure: Critically think through your data, carefully evaluating each aspect and its relation to other data, and identify specific problems and modifications of the procedure needed for this individual.

PLANNING

8. Follow step 8 of the General Procedure: Determine the individualized patient outcomes in relation to the nasal medications to be administered. Include
  a. The right *patient* receives the right *medication* in the right *dose* by the right *route* at the right *time.*
  b. The patient experiences the desired effect(s) from the medication(s) administered.
  c. The patient experiences no undesired effect(s) from the medication(s) administered.
9. Follow step 9 of the General Procedure: Plan for any special procedures that may be needed before medication administration and supplies (such as tissues) that will be needed.

IMPLEMENTATION

Action	Rationale
10. Wash or disinfect your hands.	To decrease the transfer of microorganisms that could cause infection.
11-14. Follow steps 11 to 14 of the General Procedure: Access the official MAR; read the name of the medication to be given; access the nasal medication and check the label on the medication; compare the medication to the MAR, and choose the correct one before picking it up; pick up the medication and check the label again.	
15. Obtain the medication. Usually, the medication will be in a dropper bottle or in the form of a nasal spray, which will be taken to the bedside.	

(continued)

Action	Rationale
16-20. Follow steps 16 to 20 of the General Procedure: Prepare any additional medications to be given at this time, check each medication label with the MAR once again, obtain the patient identification to be taken to patient's bedside as prescribed by your facility's policy, identify the patient (two identifiers), and explain how the medication will be administered.	
21. Administer the nasal medication.	
a. Have the patient blow gently into a tissue and clear the nasal passages.	This allows the medication to contact the mucous membrane and also opens the **eustachian tubes.**
b. Position the patient according to the area you want to medicate and the type of administration device. Help support the head with one hand.	Each position allows access to the nostrils and facilitates the medication reaching the desired location. Supporting the head prevents strain on the neck muscles.
(1) To instill drops into the **ethmoid** and **sphenoid sinuses:** Place the patient in the **Proetz position,** flat on the back with the head hanging straight back over the edge of the bed (Fig. 45-5A).	

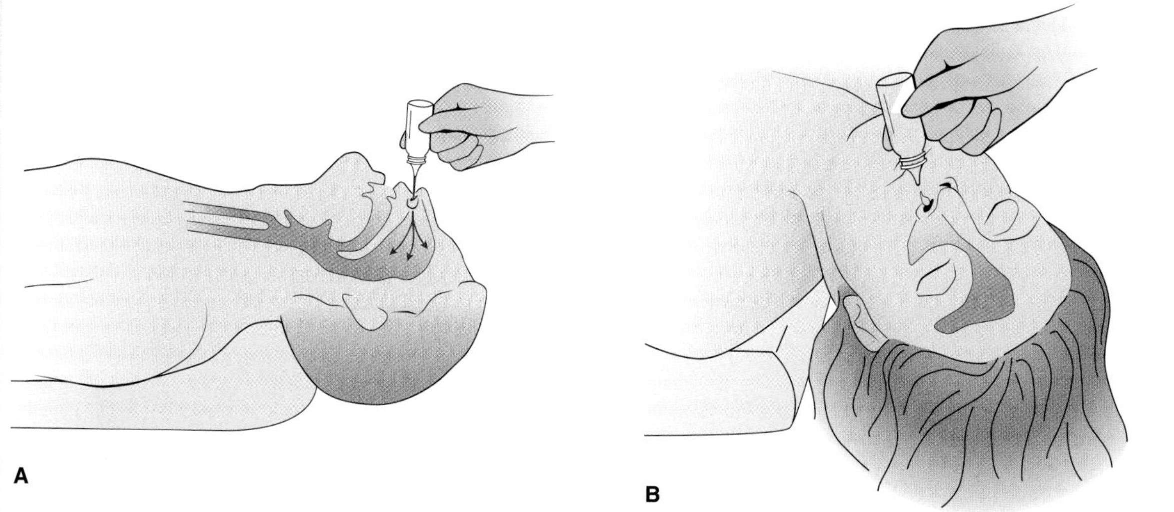

FIGURE 45-5 (**A**) Proetz position for instilling nose drops. The patient is flat on the back with the head hanging straight back over the edge of the bed. (**B**) Parkinson's position for instilling nose drops. The head is slightly over the edge of the bed and turned toward the affected side.

(continued)

Action	Rationale
(2) To instill drops into the **frontal and maxillary sinuses:** Place the patient in **Parkinson's position,** flat on the back with the head slightly over the edge of the bed and turned toward the affected side (Fig. 45-5B).	
(3) Nasal spray: Position the patient in a chair, with the head tilted back.	
c. Instillation by dropper bottle:	
(1) Invert the dropper bottle, and with the tip of the dropper about ⅜ of an inch inside the nostril, instill the ordered number of drops into each side. Be careful not to touch the side of the nostril.	Touching the side of the nostrils could cause the patient to sneeze and will contaminate the dropper bottle.
(2) Have the patient remain as positioned for 5 minutes after instilling the medication. Caution the patient not to "sniff" the medication.	To allow gravity to assist the medication to reach desired areas.
d. Instillation by nasal spray:	
(1) Have the patient hold one nostril closed as you spray the medication into the other nostril.	To facilitate maximum distribution of medication.
(2) Instruct the patient to inhale as the spray is being administered.	
(3) Repeat on the other nostril.	To promote maximum distribution of medication. *Note:* Patients often administer their own nasal sprays.
(4) Keep the patient's head back for 1 to 2 minutes.	
22. Follow step 22 of the General Procedure: Leave the patient in a comfortable position.	
23. Recap the medication bottle and return it to the appropriate storage location.	To keep the tip clean and to store the medication safely.
24. Follow step 24 of the General Procedure: Wash or disinfect your hands.	

EVALUATION

25. Follow step 25 of the General Procedure: Evaluate using the individualized patient outcomes previously identified:
   a. The right *patient* received the right *medication* in the right *dose* by the right *route* at the right *time*.
   b. The patient experienced the desired effect(s) from the medication(s) administered.
   c. The patient experienced no undesired effect(s) from the medication(s) administered.

DOCUMENTATION

26-27. Follow steps 26 and 27 of the General Procedure: Complete right *documentation*. Document the medication, the dosage, the route, the time, and your signature according to the facility policy. Also document your evaluation of the patient's response to the medication as appropriate for the drug and according to facility policy.

POTENTIAL ADVERSE OUTCOMES AND RELATED INTERVENTIONS

1. Patient is not experiencing expected outcome of medication and is not able to breathe easily through nose.
Intervention: Stop medication. Notify prescriber. Patient may be experiencing rebound effect due to frequent use of the medication.

2. Nasal passages appear inflamed and irritated. Patient is complaining of pain and discharge.
Intervention: Medication may not be effective. Notify prescriber with description of patient's response to medication.

PROCEDURE FOR ADMINISTERING MEDICATION USING A METERED-DOSE INHALER

Inhaled medications are ordered for their local effect in the lungs. They may be administered with an atomizer or nebulizer attached to oxygen or air under pressure or by a metered-dose inhaler (MDI). For the nebulizer, the medication is placed in the device, the device is attached to the oxygen or compressed air, and the patient simply breathes in the mist through the device until all of the medication is gone. Usually these medications are administered by respiratory therapy personnel.

The MDI is a metal canister with the drug and a propellant inside that fits into a plastic inhaler. MDIs are small and portable and do not require compressed air or oxygen for delivery. When the canister is pressed down into the inhaler, the MDI delivers a precise dose of medication. A specific number of puffs is ordered. Each puff is a precise medication dose.

Use of an MDI requires considerable coordination of effort; it is not uncommon for much of the medication to be deposited in the mouth and upper airway rather than in the lower airway where it is needed. Because incorrect use of the MDI can result in a wrong dose of medication or in the medication not getting into the lower respiratory tract, you must carefully assess the patient's ability to follow the directions. Even young children can be taught to manage and use their own MDI.

A "spacer" is recommended for use with the MDI. The spacer attaches to the MDI and serves as a reservoir for the drug as it is dispensed from the MDI. The patient breathes in the medication from the spacer. Use of a spacer results in a more consistent dosage and less medication deposited in the tissues of the mouth and is much easier for most individuals to use. Some MDIs come with a built-in spacer. For others, the spacer is separate and the MDI is attached to the spacer each time it is used.

The MDI and spacer must be kept clean and free of dust or particles that could be inhaled into the lungs. At home, the patient should clean out the mouthpiece once a week, using a cotton-tipped applicator moistened with tap water. The MDI should always be stored with the mouthpiece cover in place.

Some MDIs are manufactured with a counter that shows the numbers of doses remaining in the device. This facilitates ordering a new MDI before one is empty. For the majority of MDIs without a built-in counter, the manufacturers recommend keeping notations of doses used. In the healthcare agency, it is relatively easy to count the number of doses that have been used since the MDI was started because that is part of the patient's record. In the home, most patients do not do this. Instead they can calculate the number of doses per day, and divide that into the number of doses the label states that the inhaler contains. They can then calculate the number of days the inhaler can be used. This allows them to order a prescription refill before the MDI is empty. The refill date may be marked directly on the canister with a permanent marker. There are suggestions for measuring the amount of remaining medication by putting the canister in water to determine how high in the water it floats. The higher it floats, the less medication remains. The manufacturers state that this is not a reliable indicator.

To administer medications using a metered-dose inhaler, follow the General Procedure for Administering Oral Medications, Module 44, as modified below.

ASSESSMENT

1-5. Follow steps 1 to 5 of the General Procedure: Review the MAR to identify whether any inhaled medications are to be given, examine the MAR for accuracy and completeness, review medication information, assess the patient's abilities, and assess the need for prn medications.

ANALYSIS

6-7. Follow steps 6 and 7 of the General Procedure: Critically think through your data, carefully evaluating each aspect and its relation to other data, and identify specific problems and modifications of the procedure needed for this individual, paying particular attention to the patient's ability to follow directions.

PLANNING

8. Follow step 8 of the General Procedure: Determine the individualized patient outcomes in relation to the inhaled medications to be administered. Include
  a. The right *patient* receives the right *medication* in the right *dose* by the right *route* at the right *time.*
  b. The patient experiences the desired effect(s) from the medication(s) administered.
  c. The patient experiences no undesired effect(s) from the medication(s) administered.

9. Follow step 9 of the General Procedure: Plan for any special procedures that may be needed before medication administration, and gather the supplies needed, including tissues. If a spacer is being used, be sure you obtain the spacer. The spacer may be stored in the medication drawer or in a clean plastic bag in the patient's room.

IMPLEMENTATION

Action	Rationale
10. Wash or disinfect your hands.	To decrease the transfer of microorganisms that could cause infection.
11-14. Follow steps 11 to 14 of the General Procedure: Access the official MAR; read the name of the medication to be given; access the medication and check the label on the medication, compare the medication to the MAR, and choose the correct one before picking it up; pick up the medication and check the label again.	
15. Remove the labeled MDI from the drawer and take it to the bedside to administer the medication. The actual dose will be inhaled directly into the lungs from the MDI. If a spacer is in the drawer, take it as well.	
16-20. Follow steps 16 to 20 of the General Procedure: Prepare any additional medications to be given at this time, check each medication label with the MAR once again, obtain the patient identification to be taken to patient's bedside as prescribed by your facility's policy, identify the patient (two identifiers), and explain how the medication will be administered. You may need to demonstrate the use of the MDI if the device is new to the patient.	
21. Administer the medication, using the MDI as follows. If more than one MDI is ordered, one is usually a bronchodilator. Administer the bronchodilator first.	A bronchodilator will open airways, which will facilitate the flow of other medications throughout the airways. The MDI must be used correctly in order to achieve the maximum therapeutic effect.

(continued)

Action	Rationale
a. Holding the MDI so that you have one finger over the top of the canister, vigorously shake the MDI three or four times.	Shaking mixes the medication inside the canister with the propellant.
b. Take the cap off the inhaler. If this is a new MDI, follow the directions for first time use and release puffs into the air.	The cap protects the mouthpiece of the MDI, but must be removed for use. For first time use, usually at least one puff is released into the air to clear the chambers. Some manufacturers recommend two to four puffs be released, shaking between, in order to prime the device.
c. Instruct the patient to hold the inhaler in one of the following three ways, which are listed in order of preference.	For maximizing medication reaching the lower airways.
(1) If the MDI has a spacer, insert the MDI into the spacer (Fig. 45-6). Instruct the patient to hold the MDI with spacer attached so that the mouthpiece of the spacer is inside the teeth and the lips are closed around the mouthpiece. A spacer may have a mask instead of a mouthpiece.	The spacer serves as a reservoir. The spacer has air intake openings near the MDI. Keeping the lips closed allows air to be drawn into the spacer through its air vents, and the air moves the medication ahead of it into the lungs.

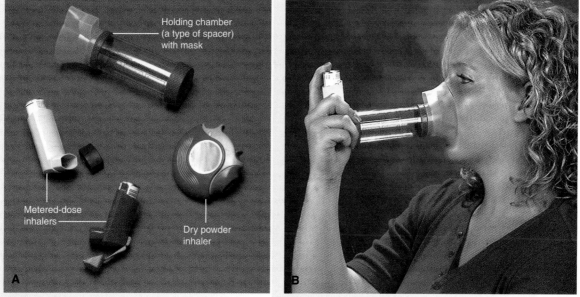

FIGURE 45-6 (**A**) Various kinds of inhalers. (**B**) A metered-dose inhaler with holding chamber (a kind of spacer). The patient holds the device to the face, pushes down, and inhales the medication dispensed in the holding chamber. If the inhaler does not have a spacer, the patient holds the mask inhaler against the face, pushes down, and breathes in.

(2) With the MDI mouthpiece 1 to 2 inches in front of the opened mouth.	If a spacer is not used, the recommended method is method (2) because it increases the likelihood of the medication being delivered to the lower airways, rather than being deposited in the mouth and upper airways. Air entering around the mouthpiece tends to continue moving the medication further into the lungs.
(3) With the MDI mouthpiece inside of the teeth and the lips closed loosely around it.	

(continued)

Action	Rationale
d. Have the patient take a deep breath and breathe out normally.	To ready the airway to receive the medication.
e. With the MDI positioned, have the patient push down once on the canister and breathe in slowly. Instruct the patient to start inhaling as the puff is dispensed and to continue to breathe around the device, which acts to push the mist deeper into the lungs. For the confused or less-dexterous patient, you may need to hold the MDI in place and push down on the canister when you say "Inhale."	To allow the air to help move the medication into the affected airways.
f. Instruct the patient to hold his or her breath for a few seconds and then breathe out very slowly.	Holding the breath will give the medication time to flow deeper into the airways, and breathing out slowly keeps the small airways open.
g. Instruct the patient to wait 1 to 2 minutes before taking the next puff.	To allow the medication to be absorbed into the tissue.
h. Repeat the process for additional ordered puffs.	The ordered number of puffs provides the correct dose of the medication. Additional puffs may result in an overdose and side effects of the medication.
i. Have the patient rinse the mouth to remove medication deposited on the mouth surface, if indicated by the medication instructions.	Some medications may cause adverse effects if left on the mouth tissue.
22. Follow step 22 of the General Procedure: Leave the patient in a comfortable position.	
23. Replace the cap on the MDI and return it to the appropriate storage location.	To keep the mouthpiece clean and to store the medication safely.
24. Follow step 24 of the General Procedure: Wash or disinfect your hands.	

EVALUATION

25. Follow step 25 of the General Procedure: Evaluate using the individualized patient outcomes previously identified:
  a. The right *patient* received the right *inhaled medication* in the right *dose* by the right *route* at the right *time.*
  b. The patient experienced the desired effect(s) from the medication(s) administered.

  c. The patient experienced no undesired effect(s) from the medication(s) administered.

DOCUMENTATION

26-27. Follow steps 26 and 27 of the General Procedure: Complete right *documentation.* Document the medication, the dosage, the route, the time, and your signature according to the facility policy. Also document your evaluation of the patient's response to the medication as appropriate for the drug and according to facility policy.

 ## POTENTIAL ADVERSE OUTCOMES AND RELATED INTERVENTIONS

1. Patient symptoms are not relieved by medication. *Intervention:* Assess patient's use of MDI. Report to prescriber for possible change of medication.

2. Patient experiences severe bouts of coughing after MDI use. *Intervention:* Patient may not be using the MDI correctly, resulting in medication being deposited in mouth and upper airways. Reassess patient's use of device. Contact prescriber for possible change in delivery method.

PROCEDURE FOR APPLYING TOPICAL MEDICATIONS

Medications applied to the skin for local effect are commonly in the form of lotions, ointments, or **liniments** and occasionally powders. Lotions protect, soften, soothe, and provide relief from itching. Ointments have an oil base, and body heat causes them to melt after application. Medications that fight infection or soothe inflamed tissues are usually available in ointment form. Liniments, which are applied by rubbing, provide relief for tight aching muscles. Powders are applied for their soothing, drying action. To apply medications to the skin or mucous membranes, follow the General Procedure for Administering Oral Medications, Module 44, as modified below.

ASSESSMENT

1-5. Follow steps 1 to 5 of the General Procedure: Review the MAR to identify whether any topical medications are to be administered, examine the MAR for accuracy and completeness, review medication information, assess the patient's abilities, and assess the need for prn medications.

ANALYSIS

6-7. Follow steps 6 and 7 of the General Procedure: Critically think through your data, carefully evaluating each aspect and its relation to other data, and identify specific problems and modifications of the procedure needed for this individual.

PLANNING

8. Follow step 8 of the General Procedure: Determine the individualized patient outcomes in relation to the topical medications to be administered. Include
  a. The right *patient* receives the right *medication* in the right *dose* by the right topical *route* at the right *time*.
  b. The patient experiences the desired effect(s) from the medication(s) administered.
  c. The patient experiences no undesired effect(s) from the medication(s) administered.

9. Plan for any special procedures that may be needed before medication administration and for supplies needed for the specific medication, such as clean or sterile gloves, applicators, or gauze squares. **R:** You may need clean gloves to apply any **topical** medication that can be absorbed through the skin to protect yourself from the medication itself or to protect yourself from any medication that could stain your skin. Clean gloves will also be needed to protect you from body secretions if medication is applied to mucous membranes. You will need sterile gloves if the skin is open. For small areas, cotton-tipped applicators may be needed to apply medication. Although cotton balls and gauze squares may be used, they tend to absorb large amounts of medication, and this may increase cost. Tongue blades should be avoided if possible because they can be harsh to skin.

IMPLEMENTATION

Action	Rationale
10. Wash or disinfect your hands.	To decrease the transfer of microorganisms that could cause infection.
11-14. Follow steps 11 to 14 of the General Procedure: Access the official MAR; read the name of the medication to be given; access the medication and check the label on the medication; compare the medication to the MAR, and choose the correct one before picking it up; pick up the medication and check the label again.	

(continued)

Action	Rationale
15. Obtain the medication. Most skin medications are in tubes that are taken to the bedside for use. If the medication is in a jar, use a tongue blade to remove enough for the individual application and place it in a medication cup. If the medication must remain sterile for application, place it in a sterile medication cup or on a sterile gauze square. Discard any excess when the medication has been administered; it cannot be returned to the jar.	
16-20. Follow steps 16 to 20 of the General Procedure: Prepare any additional medications to be given at this time, check each medication label with the MAR once again, obtain the patient identification to be taken to patient's bedside as prescribed by your facility's policy, identify the patient (two identifiers), and explain how the medication will be administered.	
21. Apply the topical medication as follows.	Topical medications must be applied appropriately to achieve maximum therapeutic effect.
a. Close the door, pull the curtain around the bed, raise the bed if necessary, and drape to expose only the area to be treated.	To avoid exposure and embarrassment for the patient and to protect your back from injury.
b. Provide adequate lighting.	For maximum visualization of the area.
c. Position the patient so that the area to be treated is accessible. In some cases, you may need assistance, for example, with the support of an arm or leg.	So area to be treated is accessible.
d. Be sure the area to be treated is clean so that the medication contacts the skin. Skin medications are typically applied immediately after a bath or shower.	For maximum absorption of medication.
e. Apply the medication to the area to be treated with a gloved hand.	Using gloves wastes less medication and is less irritating than using gauze.
(1) Apply the ointments, creams, or lotions in thin, even layers unless otherwise ordered. Take care that you do not increase discomfort through pressure or rubbing areas that are inflamed or painful. In some situations, teach patients how to apply the medication to	The medication in contact with the skin is the effective treatment. Some lotions are absorbed into the skin. Thick layers merely waste medication.

(continued)

Action	Rationale
their own skin, especially when the area to be treated is in easy view and reach.	
(2) To apply powder, instruct the patient to turn his or her head away. Sprinkle powder on your gloved hand. Spread the powder lightly and evenly, taking care not to let it accumulate between skin folds. Avoid shaking the powder directly over the patient.	To prevent the patient from inhaling the powder and to distribute the powder over the whole area.
f. Use a light dressing to cover the area only if ordered by the prescriber.	A dressing may hold the medication on the skin but it also increases skin temperature, which increases itching. Some medications should not be covered.
22-24. Follow steps 22 to 24 of the General Procedure: Lower the bed, and leave the patient in a comfortable position, care for the equipment, remove your gloves, and wash or disinfect your hands.	

EVALUATION

25. Follow step 25 of the General Procedure: Evaluate using the individualized patient outcomes previously identified:
   a. The right *patient* received the right *topical medication* applied to the right *area,* in the right *dose* by the right *route* at the right *time.*
   b. The patient experienced the desired effect(s) from the medication(s) administered.
   c. The patient experienced no undesired effect(s) from the medication(s) administered.

DOCUMENTATION

26-27. Follow steps 26 and 27 of the General Procedure: Complete right *documentation.* Document the medication, the dosage, the route, the time, the area treated, the appearance of the area before treatment, and your signature according to the facility policy. Also document your evaluation of the patient's response to the medication as appropriate for the drug and according to facility policy.

■ POTENTIAL ADVERSE OUTCOMES AND RELATED INTERVENTIONS

1. Area being treated is not improving as expected. *Intervention:* Describe condition of affected area as well as any patient comments in documentation. Contact prescriber if condition appears to be worsening.

PROCEDURE FOR ADMINISTERING TRANSDERMAL MEDICATIONS

Some medications are available in a form that is readily absorbed from the skin to provide systemic effects. These are called **transdermal** medications. Examples of these are nitroglycerin, which is given for cardiac problems; scopolamine, which is given for vertigo and nausea; and fentanyl, which is an opioid pain medication. The dosage of these medications must be as precise as the dosage of any other medication given for systemic effect.

The correct dose may be impregnated in a small patch-type bandage. The backing is removed from the tape surface, and the patch is then applied to clean skin. The medication is absorbed gradually. The patch is removed when the next dose is applied to the skin, and a new site is used for application to avoid skin irritation from the tape or the medication. Follow specific directions regarding such matters as showers and shampoos.

When the medication is an ointment, the order may call for a certain number of inches of ointment. A special pad of measuring strips in which each sheet is marked in inches comes with the tube of ointment so that the nurse (or the patient) can carefully measure a line of ointment the diameter of the mouth of the tube and the ordered length onto the measuring strip. The paper is then placed on the skin, ointment side down, and secured around the edges with tape. To apply transdermal medications, follow the General Procedure for Administering Oral Medications, Module 44, as modified below.

ASSESSMENT

1-5. Follow steps 1 to 5 of the General Procedure: Review the MAR to identify whether any transdermal medications are to be administered, examine the MAR for accuracy and completeness, review medication information, assess the patient's abilities, and assess the need for prn medications.

ANALYSIS

6-7. Follow steps 6 and 7 of the General Procedure: Critically think through your data, carefully evaluating each aspect and its relation to other data, and identify specific problems and modifications of the procedure needed for this individual.

PLANNING

8. Follow step 8 of the General Procedure: Determine the individualized patient outcomes in relation to the transdermal medications to be administered. Include

   a. The right *patient* receives the right *medication* in the right *dose* by the right *route* at the right *time.*

   b. The patient experiences the desired effect(s) from the medication(s) administered.

   c. The patient experiences no undesired effect(s) from the medication(s) administered.

9. Plan for any special procedures that may be needed before medication administration and gather the supplies needed for the specific medication. You will need clean gloves. You also may need a washcloth, a basin with warm water, mild soap, and a towel if you need to remove an ointment previously applied. **R:** The nurse may absorb medication if it is in contact with skin. Medication from the last dose administered should be removed to prevent potential overdose. Planning ahead allows you to proceed more safely and effectively.

IMPLEMENTATION

Action	Rationale
10. Wash or disinfect your hands.	To decrease the transfer of microorganisms that could cause infection.
11-14. Follow steps 11 to 14 of the General Procedure: Access the official MAR; read the name of the medication to be given; access the medication and check the label on the medication; compare the medication to the MAR, and choose the correct one before picking it up; pick up the medication and check the label again.	
15. Obtain the medication. Medication patches are packaged individually. Take a medication patch to the bedside in the package. For medications such as nitroglycerin packaged as an ointment in a tube, you also will need a medication-measuring strip. Measuring strips are usually on a tear-off pad with the tube of ointment. If you are administering nitroglycerin ointment, take the tube of ointment along with one measuring strip to the bedside.	
16-20. Follow steps 16 to 20 of the General Procedure: Prepare any additional medications to be given at this time, check each medication label with the MAR once again, obtain the patient identification to be taken to patient's bedside as prescribed by your facility's policy, identify the patient (two identifiers), and explain how the medication will be administered.	

(continued)

Action	Rationale
21. Administer the transdermal medication.	
a. Write the date, time, and your initials and/or other information as indicated by the policy at your facility on the patch or measuring strip for the ointment before applying the new transdermal medication to the patient's skin.	To prevent medication errors.
b. Put on clean gloves.	To protect yourself from systemic effects of the medication.
c. Remove previous transdermal patch or nitroglycerin strip, fold it in half medication side in, place it in the trash container, and wash the site where it was placed. If you do not see the previous application, do a complete skin assessment seeking the former patch.	Cleaning prevents skin irritation from the medication itself or from the adhesive material on the patch. Patients have received overdoses of medications from having previous patches inadvertently left in place when they were in a less-visible site.
d. Choose a site for the new transdermal patch or nitroglycerin strip. The site should be clean and dry, hairless, and without calluses or cuts. The chest, clavicular area, abdomen, and thigh are frequently used.	For maximum therapeutic effect and for minimum skin irritation. The best absorption occurs from areas on the trunk.
e. Apply the transdermal medication.	
(1) *For a transdermal patch:* Remove the protective covering and apply the patch to the site chosen (Fig. 45-7). Apply firm pressure to the patch, especially around the edges.	To ensure contact with the skin and to prevent having the patch come loose or fall off.

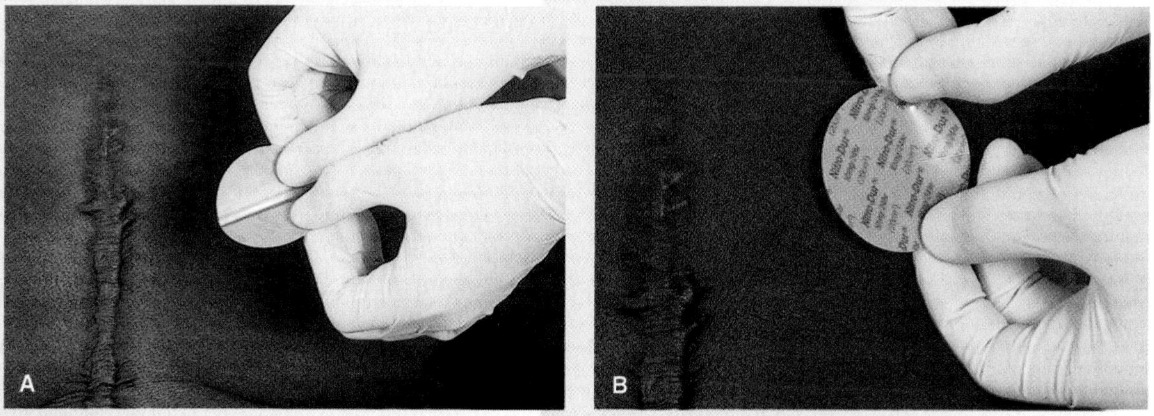

FIGURE 45-7 When applying a transdermal patch, (**A**) bend the patch to open the seal, then (**B**) remove the protective backing and apply to clean skin.

(continued)

Action	Rationale
(2) *For nitroglycerin ointment:*	
(a) Apply even pressure to the tube of ointment and squeeze the ordered dosage onto the measuring strip. Be sure to carefully follow any package instructions. Do not allow medication to come into contact with your skin.	To ensure an accurate dose of medication. If medication comes in contact with your skin, you could experience systemic effects of nitroglycerin.
(b) Turn the measuring strip over and place it directly on the new site. Do not massage or rub in ointment.	Massaging or rubbing the area will increase absorption and could interfere with sustained action.
(c) Tape measuring strip in place with tape on all four edges. Apply an occlusive dressing if ordered.	To prevent strip from becoming dislodged. An occlusive dressing will prevent medication from oozing out from under the measuring strip.
22-24. Follow steps 22 to 24 of the General Procedure: Leave the patient in a comfortable position, care for the equipment, remove your gloves, and wash or disinfect your hands.	

EVALUATION

25. Follow step 25 of the General Procedure: Evaluate using the individualized patient outcomes previously identified:

a. The right *patient* received the right *transdermal medication* applied to the right *area,* in the right *dose* by the right *route* at the right *time.*

b. The patient experienced the desired effect(s) from the medication(s) administered.

c. The patient experienced no undesired effect(s) from the medication(s) administered.

DOCUMENTATION

26-27. Follow steps 26 and 27 of the General Procedure: Complete right *documentation.* Document the medication, the dosage, the route, the time, the condition of the skin where the patch was removed, the location of the new patch, and your signature according to the facility policy. Also document your evaluation of the patient's response to the medication as appropriate for the drug and according to facility policy.

■ POTENTIAL ADVERSE OUTCOMES AND RELATED INTERVENTIONS

1. Skin irritation from prolonged contact with the medication and tape.

Intervention: Change sites for each dose. Clean skin after site is used. Confer with prescriber about the use of ointment or cream on irritated skin area.

2. Medication overdose from inadvertent placement of more than one transdermal patch at the same time.

Intervention: When symptoms of an overdose appear, remove the patch and notify the prescriber. Institute actions to prevent the problem, including the following: Document the site of any transdermal medication. Do not place a new patch or medication until you have removed the previous one. For a newly admitted patient, ask the patient about previous transdermal medications and their location in order to remove them before applying new ones. If the patient is not cognitively aware or reliable, inspect the skin carefully to be sure a previous transdermal medication is not in place.

PROCEDURE FOR ADMINISTERING VAGINAL MEDICATIONS

Creams, gels, and suppositories are used to administer **vaginal** medications. Vaginal medications may be needed to treat infection, relieve discomfort, or alter pH to maintain normal flora. Use clean technique when inserting vaginal medications. Be especially alert to the patient's feelings of embarrassment. To insert vaginal medications, follow the General Procedure for Administering Oral Medications, Module 44, as modified below.

ASSESSMENT

1-5. Follow steps 1 to 5 of the General Procedure: Review the medication record to identify whether any vaginal medications are to be administered, examine the MAR for accuracy and completeness, review medication information, assess the patient's abilities, and assess the need for prn medications.

ANALYSIS

6-7. Follow steps 6 and 7 of the General Procedure: Critically think through your data, carefully evaluating each aspect and its relation to other data, and identify specific problems and modifications of the procedure needed for this individual.

PLANNING

8. Follow step 8 of the General Procedure: Determine the individualized patient outcomes in relation to the vaginal medications to be administered. Include
   a. The right *patient* receives the right *medication* in the right *dose* by the right *route* at the right *time*.
   b. The patient experiences the desired effect(s) from the medication(s) administered.
   c. The patient experiences no undesired effect(s) from the medication(s) administered.

9. Plan for any special procedures that may be needed before medication administration, and gather the supplies needed, including clean gloves, applicator, and lubricant if needed. If the medication you are administering is in **suppository** form, you may also need lubricant. If the medication is a cream, you should be sure you know how the applicator for the medication works. If this is the first dose, the applicator will be in the package. Read the directions on the package carefully. If previous doses have been administered, the applicator should have been washed and left in the patient's room. **R:** Planning ahead allows you to proceed more safely and effectively.

IMPLEMENTATION

Action	Rationale
10. Wash or disinfect your hands.	To decrease the transfer of microorganisms that could cause infection.
11-14. Follow steps 11 to 14 of the General Procedure: Access the official MAR; read the name of the medication to be given; access the medication and check the label on the medication; compare the medication to the MAR, and choose the correct one before picking it up; pick up the medication and check the label again.	
15. Obtain the medication and prepare the dose using the applicator as indicated in the package directions.	Although similar, applicators may have differences in construction and method of use.
16-20. Follow steps 16 to 20 of the General Procedure: Prepare any additional medications to be given at this time, check each medication label with the MAR once again, obtain the patient identification to be taken to patient's bedside as prescribed by your facility's policy, identify the	

(continued)

Action	Rationale
patient (two identifiers), and explain how the medication will be administered.	
21. Insert the vaginal medication.	
a. Close the door, pull curtain around the bed, and raise the bed.	To prevent exposure and embarrassment and to protect yourself from back injury.
b. Provide adequate lighting.	For maximum visualization of the area.
c. Place the patient in the **dorsal recumbent position,** with knees flexed and spread as for catheterization (see Module 27). **Sims' position** also can be used.	So medication can be administered easily.
d. Drape the patient with perineum exposed.	To allow for maximum visualization for the nurse and minimal exposure and embarrassment for the patient.
e. Put on clean gloves.	To protect yourself from contact with body secretions and microorganisms.
f. Instill the medication.	
(1) *Vaginal creams:* Introduce creams with a narrow, tubular applicator that has a plunger attached.	The applicator ensures the correct dose of the medication and places it high in the vagina where it will melt and contact all the tissue.
(2) *Suppositories:* Introduce suppositories with the special suppository inserter that comes with the medication or with a gloved and lubricated finger.	The inserter places the suppository high in the vagina where it is more likely to melt and contact all the tissue.
g. Have the patient lie quietly for 20 minutes after inserting the medication.	To allow the medication to reach all surfaces. In many instances, a patient can be taught to administer vaginal medications to herself.
22. Follow step 22 of the General Procedure: Lower the bed, and leave the patient in a comfortable position.	
23. Care for the equipment. If an applicator was used, wash it thoroughly with soap and water each time it is used, and store it dry. It is always stored at the bedside or elsewhere in the patient's room.	An applicator is used for the entire time the package of medication is being used. It is not returned to the medication storage area because of the potential for cross-contamination.
24. Follow step 24 of the General Procedure: Remove your gloves, and wash or disinfect your hands.	

EVALUATION

25. Follow step 25 of the General Procedure: Evaluate using the individualized patient outcomes previously identified:

a. The right *patient* received the right *medication,* administered by the right *method,* in the right *dose* by the right *route* at the right *time.*

b. The patient experienced the desired effect(s) from the medication(s) administered.

c. The patient experienced no undesired effect(s) from the medication(s) administered.

DOCUMENTATION

26-27. Follow steps 26 and 27 of the General Procedure: Complete right *documentation.* Document the medication, the dosage, the route, the time, and your signature according to the facility policy. Also document your evaluation of the patient's response to the medication as appropriate for the drug and according to facility policy.

◼ POTENTIAL ADVERSE OUTCOMES AND RELATED INTERVENTIONS

1. Vaginal area appears inflamed and irritated. There is discharge present.

Intervention: Administer medication. Report inflammation and discharge.

2. Patient experiences pain during insertion of medication.

Intervention: Add additional lubrication to suppository or applicator. Have patient breathe in and out through the mouth for relaxation.

PROCEDURE FOR ADMINISTERING RECTAL MEDICATIONS

Rectal medications are usually given for their local effect, but some (e.g., aspirin suppositories) are given for systemic effect. Suppositories are most common, although creams and retention enemas also can be used. Clean technique is appropriate for all. To administer rectal medications, follow the General Procedure for Administering Medications, Module 44, as modified below.

ASSESSMENT

1-5. Follow steps 1 to 5 of the General Procedure: Review the MAR to identify whether any rectal medications are to be administered, examine the MAR for accuracy and completeness, review medication information, assess the patient's abilities, and assess the need for prn medications.

ANALYSIS

6-7. Follow steps 6 and 7 of the General Procedure: Critically think through your data, carefully evaluating each aspect and its relation to other data, and identify specific problems and modifications of the procedure needed for this individual.

PLANNING

8. Follow step 8 of the General Procedure: Determine the individualized patient outcomes in relation to the rectal medication to be administered. Include

a. The right *patient* receives the right *medication* in the right *dose* by the right *route* at the right *time.*

b. The patient experiences the desired effect(s) from the medication(s) administered.

c. The patient experiences no undesired effect(s) from the medication(s) administered.

9. Plan for any special procedures that may be needed before medication administration or supplies needed including clean gloves and a lubricant. **R:** The gloves will protect you from contact with body excretions and microorganisms, and the lubricant makes the process more comfortable for the patient. Planning ahead allows you to proceed more safely and effectively.

IMPLEMENTATION

Action	Rationale
10. Wash or disinfect your hands.	To decrease the transfer of microorganisms that could cause infection.
11-14. Follow steps 11 to 14 of the General Procedure: Access the official MAR; read the name of the medication to be given; access the medication and check the label on the medication; compare the medication to the MAR, and choose the correct	

(continued)

Action	Rationale
one before picking it up; pick up the medication and check the label again.	
15. Obtain the medication and prepare the medication for administration. If a cream is to be administered, the applicator will be cleaned and kept in the patient's room, not returned to the medication storage area.	To prevent the potential for cross-contamination.
16-20. Follow steps 16 to 20 of the General Procedure: Prepare any additional medications to be given at this time, check each medication label with the MAR once again, obtain the patient identification to be taken to patient's bedside as prescribed by your facility's policy, identify the patient (two identifiers), and explain how the medication will be administered.	
21. *Administer the rectal medication:*	
a. Close the door, pull the curtain around the bed, and raise the bed.	To prevent exposure and embarrassment for the patient and to protect your back from injury.
b. Provide adequate lighting.	For maximum visualization of the area.
c. Place the patient in the side-lying position. If this position is difficult for the patient, have him or her assume the dorsal recumbent position with the knees flexed.	To provide access to the rectum for the nurse and comfort for the patient.
d. Drape the patient with the rectum exposed.	To allow for maximum visualization for the nurse and minimal exposure and embarrassment for the patient.
e. Put on clean gloves.	To protect yourself from body excretions.
f. Insert the medication.	
(1) *Suppository:*	
(a) Open the package and lubricate the suppository if it is not prelubricated.	Lubrication eases insertion and provides comfort for the patient.
(b) Ask the patient to breathe in and out through the mouth while you are inserting the suppository.	To help relax the sphincter muscles.
(c) Using a gloved, lubricated finger, insert the suppository beyond the internal sphincter.	At this location, it is unlikely to be expelled, and there will be maximum absorption and therapeutic effect. *(continued)*

Action	Rationale
(2) *Rectal cream:*	
(a) Introduce the cream with the special tip attached directly to the tube of cream.	The tip is designed to enter the rectum without injuring the mucosa and penetrate beyond the sphincter to apply medication to internal tissue.
(b) Remove the tip and clean it after each use.	To decrease transfer of microorganisms and prepare for the next use.
(3) *Retention enema containing medication:* Administer the enema after the patient has a bowel movement. Instruct the patient to avoid defecating.	For maximum effect of the medication. (See Module 26 for the necessary equipment and procedure.) To prevent loss of medication.
g. Clean the anal area with tissue.	To remove the lubricant.
22. Follow step 22 of the General Procedure: Lower the bed, and leave the patient in a comfortable position.	
23. Care for the equipment. If an applicator was used, wash it thoroughly with soap and water each time after use, and store it dry in the patient's room.	The same applicator is used for the entire time the package of medication is being used. Storing it clean and dry decreases microbial growth.
24. Follow step 24 of the General Procedure: Remove your gloves, and wash or disinfect your hands.	

EVALUATION

25. Follow step 25 of the General Procedure: Evaluate using the individualized patient outcomes previously identified:
   a. The right *patient* received the right *medication,* administered by the right *method,* in the right *dose* by the right *route* at the right *time.*
   b. The patient experienced the desired effect(s) from the medication(s) administered.
   c. The patient experienced no undesired effect(s) from the medication(s) administered.

DOCUMENTATION

26-27. Follow steps 26 and 27 of the General Procedure: Complete right *documentation.* Document the medication, the dosage, the route, the time, and your signature according to the facility policy. Also document your evaluation of the patient's response to the medication as appropriate for the drug and according to facility policy.

■ POTENTIAL ADVERSE OUTCOMES AND RELATED INTERVENTIONS

1. Patient experiences extreme pain when administration of rectal medication is attempted.
Intervention: Apply more lubricant and try again. Contact prescriber if rectal route seems contraindicated.
2. Patient reports that symptoms for which medication is ordered are not relieved.
Intervention: Discuss with patient. Notify prescriber for possible change of medication.

Acute Care

Patients in acute care facilities may need to receive medications by one or more of the several alternative routes described here. You must be prepared to administer eye, nasal, or transdermal medications to a patient hospitalized, for example, for orthopedic surgery, because the medication(s) is/are a part of the patient's medication regimen on a daily basis.

Alternatively, the medication may be needed on a short-term basis only. You also need to be prepared to teach patients and/or their caregivers how to administer any new medication(s) prescribed if they need to take the medication(s) at home.

Long-Term Care

Nurses in long-term care facilities administer ophthalmic, otic, nasal, and transdermal medications frequently to manage chronic or acute problems among their elderly residents. In addition, skin problems are frequent in this population. Knowing how to administer medications by alternative routes skillfully will assist you in timely completion of these tasks.

Home Care

Many people who care for themselves at home take medications by various alternative routes on a routine basis. You may need to monitor this activity to ensure accuracy or to teach others in the setting to do so. You also may be engaged in evaluating the effectiveness of the drugs or the dosage. In all cases, familiarity with drugs given by alternative routes and the procedure(s) used to administer them is essential.

Ambulatory Care

Those who work in office, clinic, and outpatient surgery settings also need to know how to administer and monitor medications being given by alternative routes. Whether they are being given on a one-time basis, for a short period of time, or routinely, the nurses must be able to explain what they are doing, carry out the processes skillfully, and teach others (clients and caregivers) as well.

LEARNING TOOLS

DEVELOP YOUR BACKGROUND KNOWLEDGE

1. Review the Learning Outcomes.

2. Read the section on administering medications in your assigned text.

3. Look up the Key Terms in the glossary.

4. Review this module and mentally practice the techniques described. Study so that you would be able to teach these skills to another person.

DEVELOP YOUR SKILLS

1. In the practice setting: With another student playing the role of the patient, do the following:
   a. Simulate the instillation of eye drops. If artificial tears are available, your instructor may want you to use these or a sterile normal saline solution.
   b. Simulate the instillation of ear drops in an adult's ear. Do not use any actual drops.
   c. Simulate the instillation of nose drops and nasal sprays. Do not use any actual drops or sprays. Position your partner appropriately for the administration of a nasal spray and in the three positions described for nose drops.
   d. Using a mannequin, practice the explanation and positioning for administration of a vaginal cream. Teach your "patient" self-administration.
   e. Using a mannequin, practice the explanation and positioning for insertion of a rectal suppository.
   f. Practice the explanation for having patients take inhaled medications. Simulate the use of a metered-dose inhaler (MDI) if one is available.
   g. Change roles with your partner and repeat steps 1a through f.
   h. Evaluate each other's performance. Use the Performance Checklists on the CD-ROM in the front of this book as a guide.

DEMONSTRATE YOUR SKILLS

In the clinical setting
1. Seek opportunities to administer medications given by alternative routes.

CRITICAL THINKING EXERCISES

1. Mrs. Wilson, an elderly woman, came to the clinic because of a rash on her back. The prescriber prescribed a medicated cream to be used on the rash. Before leaving the clinic, Mrs. Wilson stops to ask if you will teach her husband how to apply the cream. He is in the waiting room and has not heard the prescriber's instructions. Determine what information you should gather before giving instructions and identify some of the factors that you will need to consider. Then formulate two alternative approaches that you might take.

2. Joel Hanson is an elderly resident of the assisted living facility where you are employed. He visited his prescriber today and came back with a newly prescribed inhalant bronchodilator. He brings it to you and says, "I'm not sure I understand how this works! It hardly seems that pushing down once on

that thing gives you much medicine. Should I hold it down like you do for that mouth spray stuff?" Consider what you should include in your teaching. Identify the information and skills Mr. Hanson needs. Identify the potential administration errors his remarks reveal, then develop a plan for safe administration.

SELF-QUIZ
SHORT-ANSWER QUESTIONS

1. Why are nose drops and nasal sprays water soluble?

   _____

2. The Proetz position is used to reach which sinuses?

   _____

3. List three reasons for the administration of lotions.

   a. _____

   b. _____

   c. _____

4. Name two positions that can be used to insert vaginal medication.

   a. _____

   b. _____

5. How far should a rectal suppository be inserted?

   _____

6. Why is it helpful to have the patient breathe in and out through the mouth when you are inserting a rectal suppository?

   _____

7. How can the patient make sure that an inhaled medication reaches the lungs?

   _____

MULTIPLE CHOICE

_____ 8. Administration of which of the following requires the use of sterile medication? (Choose all correct responses.)
   a. Ophthalmic medications
   b. Nasal medications
   c. Vaginal medications
   d. Rectal medications

_____ 9. Eye drops are instilled into which part of the eye?
   a. Cornea
   b. Inner canthus
   c. Conjunctival sac
   d. Outer canthus

_____ 10. When administering ear drops to an infant, how do you straighten the ear canal?
   a. By pulling the pinna upward and backward
   b. By pulling the pinna downward and backward
   c. By pulling the pinna upward and forward
   d. By pulling the pinna downward and forward

Answers to the Self-Quiz questions appear in the back of the book.

Administering Medications by Injection

SKILLS INCLUDED IN THIS MODULE

Procedure for Withdrawing Medication From a Vial
Procedure for Withdrawing Medication From an Ampule
Procedure for Mixing Powdered Medication for Injection
Procedure for Mixing Medications in a Syringe
General Procedure for Administering Medications
by Injection
  Procedure for Administering Medications by
    Subcutaneous Injection
  Procedure for Administering Medications by
    Intramuscular Injection
  Procedure for Using the Z-Track Technique for an
    Intramuscular Injection
  Procedure for Administering Medications by
    Intradermal Injection

PREREQUISITE MODULES

Module 1	An Approach to Nursing Skills
Module 2	Documentation
Module 4	Basic Infection Control
Module 5	Safety in the Healthcare Environment
Module 6	Moving the Patient in Bed and Positioning
Module 14	Nursing Physical Assessment
Module 24	Basic Sterile Technique: Sterile Field and Sterile Gloves
Module 44	Administering Oral Medications

The following modules may be useful in some specific situations:

Module 11	Assessing Temperature, Pulse, and Respiration
Module 12	Measuring Blood Pressure
Module 13	Monitoring Intake and Output

KEY TERMS

ampule	parenteral
aspirate	particulate matter
barrel	plunger
bevel	prefilled cartridge
diluent	reconstituted
gauge	shaft
heparinoid	subcutaneous
hub	syringe
infuser	taut
intradermal	vial
intramuscular	viscosity
Luer-Lok	wheal
lumen	Z-track
needle	

OVERALL OBJECTIVE

▸ To prepare and administer medications safely, using subcutaneous, intramuscular, and intradermal routes.

LEARNING OUTCOMES

The student will be able to

1. Assess the patient with regard to the medication and injection route ordered.
2. Analyze assessment data to determine special problems or concerns that must be addressed to successfully administer the medication ordered by the injection route ordered.
3. Determine appropriate patient outcomes for the medication(s) administered and recognize the potential for adverse outcomes.
4. Plan appropriate strategies to ensure that the patient receives the medication ordered by the injection route ordered.
5. Administer medications safely and accurately using the subcutaneous, intramuscular, and intradermal routes.
6. Evaluate the patient's response to the medication(s) administered.
7. Document the parenteral medication administered, including the injection site, route, and the patient's response according to facility policies.

Medications that are given by injections or infusions directly into body tissues are termed **parenteral** medications. All injections are considered parenteral administration of medications. The safe preparation and administration of **subcutaneous, intramuscular,** and **intradermal** medications is an important nursing responsibility that requires dexterity; sterile technique; knowledge of the actions, usual dosage, desired effects, and potential side effects of the drug being given; and knowledge of correct identification of site for giving the injection. Not only are drugs given by these routes absorbed more quickly than those given by mouth, but they also are irretrievable once injected. Therefore, the nurse must have a firm mathematics foundation and conscientiously practice using the three checks and the six rights.

NURSING DIAGNOSES

■ Risk for Injury is a priority nursing diagnosis when giving injections. Patients can be injured by injections given incorrectly or given at the wrong time, by an incorrect route, or injected into an incorrect site. Although this nursing diagnosis will not appear on the nursing care plan, it applies to every situation in which an injection is being administered.

■ Deficient Knowledge is another nursing diagnosis that is commonly appropriate when administering injections. The knowledge deficit may be related to some aspect of the medication regimen; for example, the need to learn how to safely administer injections to oneself or to a family member.

■ Noncompliance With the Therapeutic Regimen is a nursing diagnosis that can be appropriate if the patient consistently refuses, for any reason (for example, fear of pain or a reaction), an injectable medication that is essential to treatment and that cannot be administered using another route.

DELEGATION

Administration of parenteral medications is not delegated to assistive personnel in acute care settings. However, they may be asked to observe for and report specific effects (both desired and adverse) of medications the nurse has administered as well as for pain at the injection site. Nursing assistants may also inform the nurse of situations in which a medication, such as an analgesic, may be needed. However, the nurse is responsible for assessing the need for prn medication before administering it. The nurse is always responsible for evaluating the effect(s) of all medications administered.

ADVANTAGES AND DISADVANTAGES OF ADMINISTERING MEDICATIONS BY INJECTION

Medications administered by injection have several advantages over the oral method of administration. First, if the patient has adequate circulatory status, you can depend on rapid, almost complete absorption of the medication given by injection, although it is usually faster from the subcutaneous site than from the intramuscular site. Second, medication can be given by injection even when there is a gastrointestinal disturbance. Third, the patient does not have to be conscious or rational to receive an injection.

The greatest disadvantage of administration by injection is that it penetrates the body's first line of defense, the skin. Thus, it is imperative that sterile technique be used for the patient's safety. Another disadvantage relates to the need for adequate circulation to the tissue.

When circulation is impaired, absorption is impaired, and the medication may not be available when it is needed. In fact, poor circulation to a muscle could result in the medication staying in the muscle and being absorbed only when circulation improves. If several injections were given while circulation was impaired, inadequate medication may have been delivered during that time and the absorption of several doses later might then result in an overdose. Injections are also painful and cause distress to the patient. Some medications given by injection are irritating to tissue so that the discomfort goes beyond that caused by the needle stick and includes ongoing pain at the site.

EQUIPMENT

To give any injection, the nurse needs to choose an appropriate syringe and needle to give the medication as ordered.

SYRINGES

Syringes are available in various sizes, shapes, and materials. Several commercially made syringes are designed for use with specific **prefilled cartridges.**

GLASS SYRINGES

Once the mainstay of every healthcare facility's syringe supply, glass syringes (Fig. 46-1) are rarely used now that plastic disposable syringes are available. Some glass syringes are still used in some settings, however, because

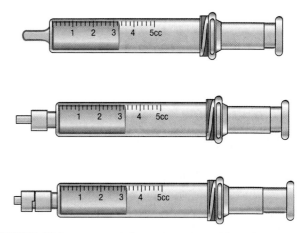

FIGURE 46-1 A variety of glass syringes is available, although they have been replaced in large part by disposable plastic syringes.

they can be sterilized and included in surgical, obstetric, and treatment setups. Glass syringes are available in 2-mL, 5-mL, 10-mL, 20-mL, and 50-mL sizes. They can be secured with special control handles, which are sometimes used to administer local and regional anesthetics. Some syringes have a specialized tip on the syringe that attaches the needle to the syringe by a threaded seal. This makes the connection more secure than the friction connection of a standard syringe. It may be referred to as **Luer-Lok**, twist-on, or screw-on.

DISPOSABLE PLASTIC SYRINGES

Disposable plastic syringes are widely used and are available in various sizes, with or without needles attached. They are usually prepackaged, either in a paper wrapper or in a rigid plastic container and are available in 0.5-mL, 1-mL, 3-mL, 5-mL, 10-mL, 20-mL, and 50-mL sizes.

One-milliliter syringes are often referred to as "tuberculin" syringes because one major use is for tuberculin testing. One-milliliter syringes are usually chosen for administering very small amounts of medication because they are marked in 0.01-mL increments. The accuracy of the syringe allows you to measure small quantities precisely, making these syringes ideal for infant and pediatric use (Fig. 46-2).

Insulin syringes are marked in units specifically to measure doses of insulin (Fig. 46-3). U-100 insulin means that there are 100 units of insulin in 1 mL. The syringe holds 1 mL and is marked directly in units. A small syringe, which holds 0.5 mL or 50 units, is also available for giving doses of less than 50 units. When given a choice, the 0.5 mL syringe should be used for injecting less than 50 units to increase accuracy.

Most plastic syringes have a plain straight **hub** to which needles fit by friction when pushed straight on. The needle cover is removed by pulling it straight off. Needles are removed by twisting. There are also plastic

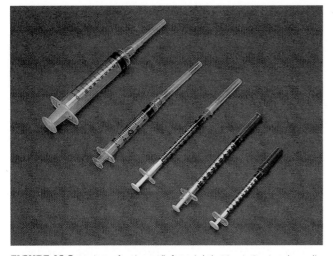

FIGURE 46-2 Variety of syringes (left to right): 10 mL, 3 mL, tuberculin (1 mL), insulin, and low-dose insulin.

syringes that have a threaded hub. The needle attaches to the syringe by turning it on, in the same way that a lid turns onto a jar.

Syringes with needles already attached are convenient and time-saving if the needles are the correct size and length. Those packaged with needles attached have the needle most commonly used with that size or type of syringe.

PREFILLED SYRINGES AND CARTRIDGES

Prefilled syringes come with a single dose of medication already in the syringe and usually come with appropriate needles attached and with directions for use.

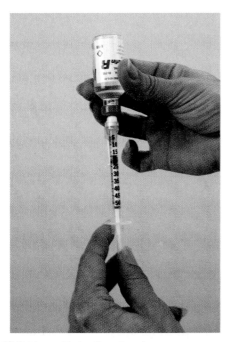

FIGURE 46-3 Disposable insulin syringe in use.

Especially helpful are syringes prefilled with drugs for emergency use. Prefilled syringes are disposable.

Prefilled cartridges contain medication and have appropriate needles attached. The disposable cartridge and needle are designed to fit into a nondisposable metal or plastic cartridge holder or injector device. The cartridge must be screwed into the device to secure it in place and the **plunger** of the holder must be screwed into the stopper of the cartridge so that you can **aspirate** (to determine whether the needle is in a blood vessel) when you administer the injection (Fig. 46-4). Drawing up the medication is eliminated, which does make the preparation easier and faster. However if the drug in the cartridge must be mixed with another drug, the preparation can be more difficult.

NEEDLES

Needles for use with syringes come in standardized lengths (0.5 to 5 inches) and gauges (13 to 27). **Gauge**

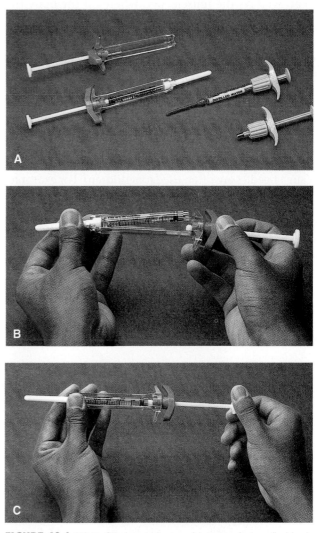

FIGURE 46-4 (**A**) Prefilled cartridges and injector devices (holders). (**B**) Cartridge inserted into injector device (holder). (**C**) Cartridge screwed into place.

refers to the diameter of the needle **lumen.** The length and gauge of disposable needles are indicated on the outside of the packaging. Sometimes color coding is used to indicate needle size. Because this practice is not standardized from one company to another, you must be cautious when moving from one healthcare facility to another. Both disposable and reusable versions of syringes are available, although most are disposable. Needles currently used are disposable to prevent the transmission of infection. Needles usually have a plastic hub and metal **shaft.** Figure 46-5 shows the parts of a needle.

The length of the needle usually varies from ⅜ to 5 inches and is chosen based on the purpose for which it will be used. Needles intended to reach from the surface into the dermis or into subcutaneous tissue are usually ⅜ to ½ inch long. Needles that are intended to reach from the surface to muscle tissue may be 1 to 3 inches long. The choice is made based on how large the person is, the thickness of the subcutaneous tissue that overlays the muscle, and where on the body the muscle is located. The most common length for intramuscular use is 1½ inches.

The most common needle gauges are 18 to 25. The lumen size is indicated on the hub. The greater the needle's gauge, the smaller the lumen. On insertion, a needle with a small lumen is less painful to the patient. The choice of a needle gauge is based on the relative **viscosity** or thickness of the medication, the length of the needle (very long needles may be unstable if they are a very small gauge), and size of the patient (smaller gauge needles are often used for children). For example, most clear fluid solutions can be given intramuscularly with a 22- or 23-G needle. Subcutaneous injections of these kinds of fluids can be given with a 25- or 26-G needle. More viscous opaque medications given intramuscularly may require a 20- or 21-G needle. Larger

needles are used primarily for drawing blood and administering blood transfusions.

Safety needles are structured to prevent accidental needle sticks. The federal Occupational Health and Safety Act requires that healthcare agencies monitor needle-stick injuries and have in place a needle-stick prevention program that includes engineering safety. This means that safety is not simply a matter of changing the behavior of the employees because errors will always happen in a busy healthcare setting. Engineered controls prevent needle-stick injuries by having covered needles or needleless connector systems when those are appropriate. See Box 46-1 for a summary of the National Institute for Occupational Safety and Health (NIOSH) recommendations (NIOSH, 1999).

The manufacturer of each brand of syringe has developed its own approach to needle safety. Some separate needles have a cover that can be flipped over the needle by the thumb of the hand holding the syringe. Other safety needles are packaged as a unit with a syringe. Some have a needle that retracts into the syringe **barrel** after the medication is injected. NIOSH has suggested the desirable characteristics of safe devices (Box 46-2). Figure 46-6 shows several safety syringes and needles.

---

box 46-1 *Recommendations for Healthcare Workers to Prevent Needle-Stick Injuries*

To protect themselves and their coworkers, healthcare workers should be aware of the hazards posed by needle-stick injuries and should use safety devices and improved work practices as follows:

1. Avoid the use of needles where safe and effective alternatives are available.
2. Help your employer select and evaluate devices with safety features.
3. Use devices with safety features provided by your employer.
4. Avoid recapping needles.
5. Plan safe handling and disposal before beginning any procedure using needles.
6. Dispose of used needle devices promptly in appropriate sharps disposal containers.
7. Report all needle-stick and other sharps-related injuries promptly to ensure that you receive appropriate follow-up care.
8. Tell your employer about hazards from needles that you observe in your work environment.
9. Participate in bloodborne pathogen training and follow recommended infection prevention practices, including hepatitis B.

National Institute for Occupational Safety and Health (NIOSH). (1999). *NIOSH Alert: Preventing needlestick injuries in healthcare settings.* DHHS (NIOSH) Publication No. 2000-108. (Online). Available at www.cdc.gov/niosh/2000-108.html. Retrieved Sept. 10, 2004.

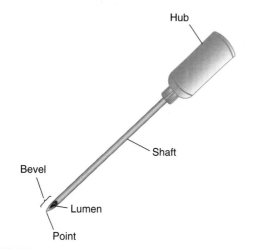

FIGURE 46-5 The parts of a needle. Most needles in current use are disposable.

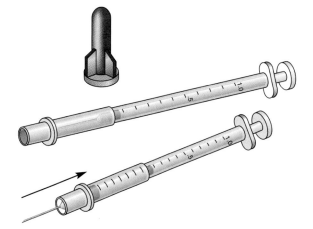

FIGURE 46-6 Safety syringes and needles (with shields) protect health-care workers from needle-stick injuries.

MEDICATION CONTAINERS

Two types of containers for injectable medications are the **vial** (either multiple dose or single dose) and the **ampule** (Fig. 46-7). A vial is a small, glass, round container with an airtight rubber stopper sealed to the glass by a metal rim. An ampule is an all-glass container that has a narrow neck. The top of the ampule must be broken off to remove the medication.

WITHDRAWING SOLUTIONS FROM CONTAINERS

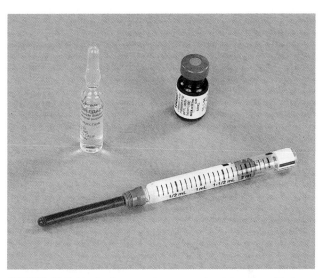

FIGURE 46-7 Medication containers: ampule, vial, and prefilled cartridge. (Photo by Rick Brady.)

The procedure for drawing the medication into the syringe is the same for all types of injections. It is presented here as a separate skill that you will integrate into the overall procedure.

When the exact measurement of a medication is crucial—for example, a dose of insulin or heparin—it is common practice to have two qualified individuals check the dose together. The medication record and the filled syringe, still attached to the medication container if possible, are presented to the person who is doing the checking. Review the policy of the healthcare facility where you practice.

PROCEDURE FOR WITHDRAWING MEDICATION FROM A VIAL

IMPLEMENTATION

Action	Rationale
1. Wash or disinfect your hands.	To prevent the spread of infection.
2. Using an alcohol or other type of antiseptic wipe, clean the rubber top of the	This provides both mechanical cleansing and maximum antiseptic action of the alcohol. The covered

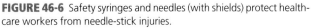

(continued)

Action	Rationale
vial with a firm circular motion, and allow the alcohol to dry. If you are using a vial that has not been previously opened, you may simply remove the plastic cap and insert the needle.	rubber top of a new vial is still sterile and does not need to be cleaned with an alcohol wipe.
3. Discard the wipe.	To maintain a clear work environment.
4. Prepare the syringe and safety withdrawal device or needle; select the correct type of syringe. Be careful to keep the safety withdrawal device or needle, the syringe tip, the inside of the barrel, and the side of the plunger sterile. If using a safety withdrawal device, remove the needle in its cap from the syringe and set it aside for later use.	The syringe must be suited to the type of medication, the type of injection, and the size of the patient. A safety withdrawal device is used to prevent needle-stick injuries to nursing staff. It will need to be removed and replaced with a needle to administer the injection. Careful handling prevents contamination of the equipment (Fig. 46-8). 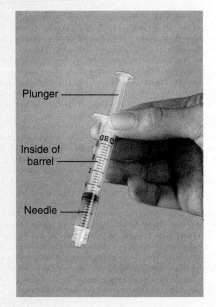 **FIGURE 46-8** Parts of a syringe to be kept sterile. If your fingers touch the sides of the plunger, they can then contaminate the inside of the barrel.
5. Draw as much air into the syringe as the volume of solution you have calculated you will need. *Note:* Calculating the dosage is part of the entire process of administering an injection. For practice purposes, plan to use 1 mL of fluid.	The air will replace the volume of fluid to be drawn out of the vial.
6. With the vial resting on the work surface, remove the "needle" guard and insert the safety device/needle through the rubber top of the vial.	Resting the vial on the work surface as you do this increases safety from a needle stick because the "target" remains still.

(continued)

Action	Rationale
7. Inject the air into the vial by pushing the plunger of the syringe into the barrel.	To prevent a vacuum when you withdraw the medication and allows the medication to flow easily into the syringe.
8. Pick up the vial in your nondominant hand and hold the vial upside down at eye level. Many persons find it easier to hold the vial between the index and middle fingers (Fig. 46-9). The medication also may be withdrawn from a vial while it rests on the work surface. Practice these techniques until you feel comfortable with one.	Holding the vial upside down places the fluid at the neck of the vial near the stopper where the tip of the safety device/needle may be kept under the surface of the fluid. When leaving the vial on the work surface, be sure to keep the tip under the fluid surface. You may need to tip the vial to withdraw all of the fluid in the vial.

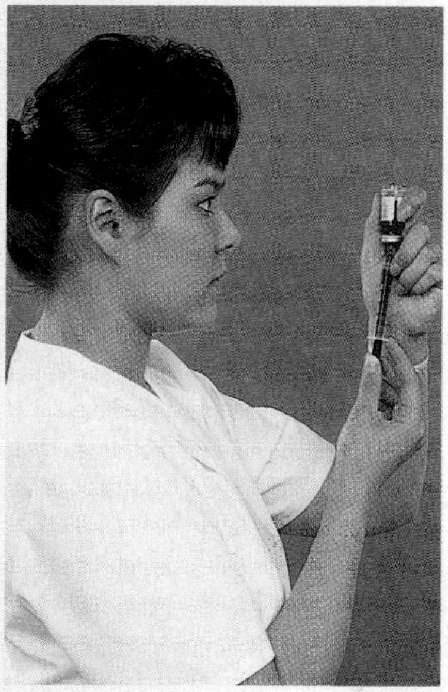

FIGURE 46-9 Holding the vial upside down at eye level helps you to ensure that the needle is under the surface of the fluid in the vial.

Action	Rationale
9. Pull the plunger down to withdraw the necessary amount of medication. Make sure the tip is beneath the fluid level in the inverted vial and that you do not touch the sides of the plunger as you withdraw medication.	The sides of the plunger will touch the inside of the barrel as you manipulate to expel air and get the exact dosage. If you have touched them, they can then contaminate the inside of the barrel.
10. Examine the medication for air bubbles and remove any that are present by keeping the syringe vertical and flicking your index finger (or a pen) against the side of the syringe over the air bubble to make the bubble rise to the base of the needle. If the bubble does not rise when the syringe is tapped, you may have to push the medication back into the vial and draw the medication again.	The vibration will usually cause the bubble to break loose and rise to the top. You can then push up on the plunger and expel the air into the vial without expelling the fluid.

(continued)

Action	Rationale
11. Once all air is removed from the syringe, make sure that you have the exact volume of medication needed. Needles and syringes are marked so that the volume in the needle and hub is considered dead space. This means that this space is full of medication when you begin to give the injection, and it is still full when the injection is completed. Therefore, the exact dose measured in the syringe is given. Modern syringes have a very small dead space so that medication is not wasted. The practice of drawing an air bubble into the syringe to clear the medication from the needle actually creates a dose error by expelling the medication that is in the dead space.	The dose must be exact.
12. Remove the needle from the vial and replace the needle guard using a one-handed technique. Keep your hand that is not holding the syringe completely away from the needle guard. One method is to simply place the needle guard in a convenient place on the work surface or medicine cart and "scoop" it on. Some facilities use syringes that come housed in a case that becomes a vertical holder for the needle guard after the syringe is removed. Be sure to touch the needle to the inside of the needle guard only. A needle that touches the outside of the needle guard is contaminated and must be replaced. If a safety withdrawal device was used, you will need to remove it and replace it with a needle for the injection.	To protect yourself from needle-sticks, never place the needle guard over the needle with your hand. A needle must be covered to be transported to the patient beside. Although a used needle should not be recapped and should be disposed of directly into a sharps container, a clean, sterile needle does not pose the threat of bloodborne infection, so it can be recapped. However, even a sterile needle stick in the finger can open the way for an infection from the environment in a healthcare worker's hand.
13. If there is medication left in the vial, mark it with the patient's name, the date it was opened, and your initials. Then store it appropriately.	To ensure that the medication is available for future doses for the patient for whom it was ordered and to be sure that it is not used after the expiration date. Parenteral medications are expensive, and when intended to be used for multiple doses, proper storage is essential to maintaining medication potency and effectiveness.

PROCEDURE FOR WITHDRAWING MEDICATION FROM AN AMPULE

IMPLEMENTATION

Action	Rationale
1. Wash or disinfect your hands.	To prevent the spread of infection.
2. If the medication is in the upper part of the ampule, move it down into the lower part by flicking the tip of the ampule with	Flicking the ampule creates a vibration in the fluid, thereby moving it down. The shake uses centrifugal force to move the fluid.

(continued)

Action	Rationale
your index finger. Another method is to grasp the ampule by the tip, and shake it firmly downward (Fig. 46-10).	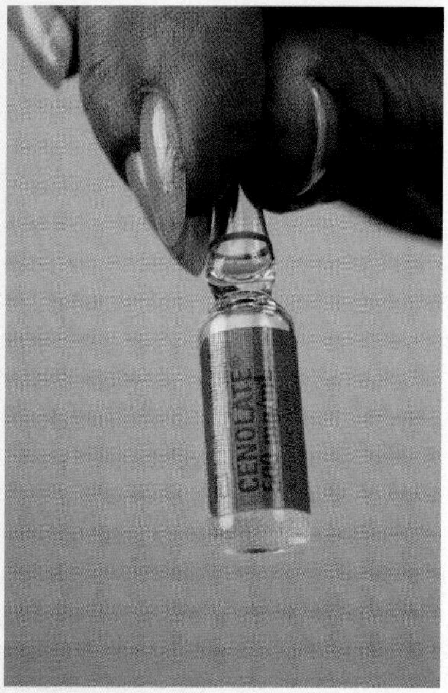 **FIGURE 46-10** Shaking fluid to the bottom of an ampule. Grasp the ampule by the top and shake it firmly downward. (Photo by Rick Brady.)
3. Using an alcohol or other type of antiseptic wipe, clean the narrowest part of the ampule with a firm circular (twisting) motion.	For infection control.
4. Prepare the syringe and safety withdrawal device or needle, using the procedure appropriate to the type of syringe used in your facility. Always use sterile technique. Many facilities provide special filter needles to withdraw medications from ampules. If using a filter needle, remove the standard needle from the syringe and set it aside to put back on the syringe after the medication is drawn up. Then put the filter needle on the syringe.	The filter needle prevents the aspiration of **particulate matter** into the syringe. The filter needle must not be used for injection and must be replaced with an appropriate needle after the medication has been drawn up.
5. Wrap an alcohol wipe or gauze square around the neck of the ampule. Break off the top of the ampule away from yourself. To do this, hold the base of the ampule in one hand, grasp the top firmly with the other hand, and exert pressure (Fig. 46-11).	The swab protects your hands from the glass edges as the ampule breaks. On occasion an ampule crushes. Holding the ampule away from you prevents glass particles from scattering toward you.
6. Discard the top in the sharps container.	The sharp edge is a hazard to others if left in the environment.
7. Remove the needle guard and place it aside.	If the needle is to be used for the injection, you will need to replace it to transport the needle and syringe to the bedside.

(continued)

Action	Rationale
	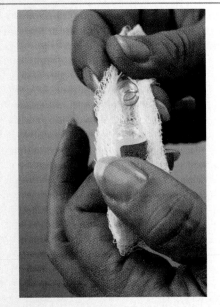 **FIGURE 46-11** Breaking the neck of an ampule. Cover the neck of the ampule with a swab or gauze square to protect yourself from cuts. Hold the ampule away from yourself with one hand, and break the top off with the other. (Photo by Rick Brady.)
8. Invert the ampule, holding it between two fingers, or hold it firmly in your non-dominant hand, resting on the work surface. Insert the safety device/needle into the open end of the ampule, being careful to touch the ampule with the safety device/needle on the inside only (Fig. 46-12). *Do not* inject air into an ampule.	As a beginner, you are less likely to stick your own hand or contaminate the needle if the ampule is held firmly in one place and not moving. Touching the outside of the ampule would contaminate the needle. Injecting air into an ampule causes the fluid to bubble up out of the ampule if it is resting on a work surface and to flow out of the ampule if it is upside down.
9. Pull the plunger of the syringe back gently to draw medication into the syringe. Be careful to keep the tip of the needle or safety withdrawal device in the solution.	If the ampule is held upside down in the hand, the surface tension will hold the fluid in the ampule and it can be withdrawn. Air will move around the needle into the ampule, enabling the fluid to be drawn up smoothly. Keeping the needle under the fluid level prevents drawing air into the syringe.
10. Withdraw the needle from the ampule when you have drawn up slightly more than the amount of solution needed. Most ampules are slightly overfilled to allow sufficient medication.	To enable exact measurement.

(continued)

Action	Rationale

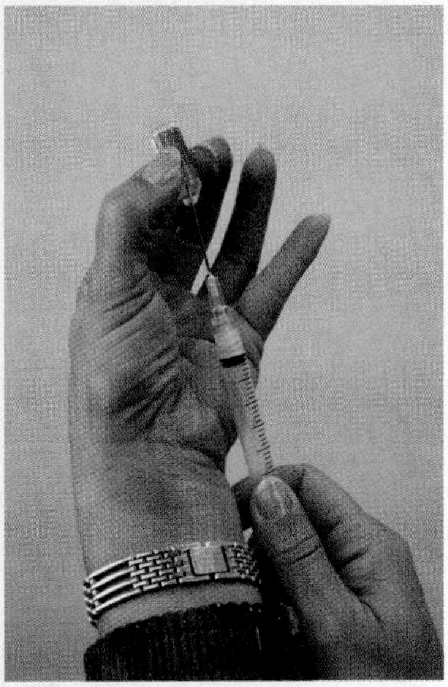

FIGURE 46-12 Withdrawing fluid from an inverted ampule. Keeping the needle in the solution, pull back the plunger and withdraw the amount needed. (Photo by Rick Brady.)

Action	Rationale
11. With the needle pointing vertically, pull back slightly to aspirate the fluid from the needle into the syringe, and push the plunger gently into the barrel until 1 drop of medication appears at the point of the needle. This drop can be removed with a gentle shake of the syringe and needle over a sink or container.	Doing this prevents the medication from being on the outside of the needle and irritating the tissues as the needle is inserted. Removing the drop from the tip over a sink or container prevents medication from being expelled into the environment.
12. Make sure you have the exact volume needed. If extra fluid must be ejected, the syringe can now be pointed downward over a sink or receptacle, so excess medication does not flow back over the needle.	The dose must be exact.
13. If you used a safety device or filter needle when drawing up the medication, remove it and replace with an appropriate needle.	The filter needle should not be used for injection because the particulate matter would be pushed out of the filter into the tissue. The safety device will not pierce the skin.
14. Replace the needle guard using a one-handed scoop technique. Be careful to touch the needle to the inside of the needle guard only.	The scoop technique protects you from a needle stick. Touching the outside of the guard contaminates the needle, which must then be replaced.

PROCEDURE FOR MIXING POWDERED MEDICATION FOR INJECTION

Some injectable medications come as a powder in a vial. The powder must be **reconstituted** as a fluid. The appropriate **diluent,** in the correct volume, must be injected into the vial, the contents mixed, and the medication then withdrawn.

IMPLEMENTATION

Action	Rationale

1. Read the label to determine the
 	
   a. appropriate diluent
 	
   b. quantity of diluent to be used
 	
   c. resulting strength of the prepared medication
	Each medication has specific requirements that must be followed for precise dosage. The powdered medication adds to the volume of the diluent, so the label must be consulted to know the concentration of the resulting dissolved solution.

2. Obtain the needed equipment: alcohol wipe, diluent, and appropriate syringe.	Having necessary equipment at hand helps you proceed more efficiently.
3. Clean the top of both the vial of diluent and the vial of powder with an alcohol wipe and allow to dry.	To decrease the potential for contaminating the needle and solution.
4. Inject air into the diluent vial and withdraw the appropriate volume of diluent, using the directions given for withdrawing medication from a vial. Remove the needle or safety withdrawal device from the diluent vial.	Injecting air into the vial prevents a vacuum when you withdraw medication and promotes accurate measurement.
5. Insert the safety device/needle through the rubber stopper of the medication vial and instill the diluent toward the inside glass of the vial.	Some medications foam on direct contact with the diluent and then do not mix well.
6. Withdraw the safety device or needle and recap it, using a one-handed technique.	To protect yourself from needle-stick injury.
7. Mix the medication by gently rotating the vial between the palms of your hands.	The medication must be well mixed for accurate dosage. Shaking creates bubbles, which are difficult to remove from the syringe.
8. Draw up the appropriate dose of medication from the vial, using the directions given above.	To ensure the correct dose.
9. If sufficient medication remains in the vial to warrant saving it and if the medication is stable, label the vial with the patient's name, date, the strength of the prepared solution, and your initials. Store it appropriately.	To ensure that the medication is available for future doses for the patient for whom it was ordered and to be sure that it is not used after the expiration date. Parenteral medications are expensive, and when intended to be used for multiple doses, proper storage is essential to maintaining medication potency and effectiveness.

PROCEDURE FOR MIXING MEDICATIONS IN A SYRINGE

More than one injectable medication may be prescribed to be given at the same time. It is possible to combine medications to give one injection if the medications are compatible and the total volume is not too large. The important point is not to contaminate the medication in one vial with the medication from the other.

IMPLEMENTATION

Action	Rationale
1. Determine whether the two medications are compatible when mixed. Obtain this information from a drug reference book or the pharmacy.	Incompatible medications may precipitate in the syringe or form ineffective compounds.
2. Determine the total volume of fluid that you will give if the drugs are mixed and given together. If the volume is larger than 2.5 mL for an adult, you will need to plan for separate injections.	The total volume will be needed to measure the drugs accurately. In the adult, a large muscle, such as the ventrogluteal, may be able to effectively absorb 2.5 mL of medication. Any larger amount causes pain and will not be readily absorbed. Check a pediatric reference in regard to any injection for a child.
3. Determine which medication you will draw up first. If one medication is in a multiple-dose vial and the other is in an ampule, draw from the vial first. If both are from ampules or one-dose vials or both are from multiple-dose vials, the order in which you draw up the medication is not important except in the case of insulin, for which the clear is drawn up before the cloudy.	The multiple-dose vial must be kept uncontaminated because it will be used again.
4. Obtain equipment: alcohol wipes, appropriate syringe, and appropriate needle.	Organizing your supplies helps you to proceed more efficiently.
5. Prepare vials or ampules as described previously.	Cleaning assists with infection control. Opening the ampule correctly protects you from injury and maintains infection control.
6. *If using two vials:*	
a. Draw an amount of air equal to the combined volume needed.	Each vial must be injected with an appropriate amount of air to facilitate withdrawing the medication.
b. Inject the correct amount of air into each vial, first injecting air into the last medication you plan to draw up.	If the exact amount is injected into the vial, the exact amount will be easy to withdraw without having excess come out.
c. After injecting the air into the medication to be drawn up first, withdraw the exact volume of that medication needed, as described above. Be sure all air is out of the syringe.	To ensure an exact dose of the first medication.

(continued)

Action	Rationale
d. Withdraw the needle from the first vial, and insert the needle into the second vial, keeping the needle from touching anything as the transfer is made.	To maintain infection control.
e. Make sure that the needle is under the surface of the fluid before beginning to aspirate. Turning the vial upside down may make it easier to withdraw the fluid but is not necessary.	Because you will be unable to push bubbles out of the syringe without contaminating the second medication with the first medication, thereby making it impossible to ensure an exact dose of each medication.
f. Draw medication into the syringe until you have the precise volume needed for the combined medications.	The medications will mix in the syringe immediately, and you cannot expel any excess without making the dose incorrect.
g. Withdraw the needle from the vial, and recap the needle using a one-handed scoop technique.	To enable you to carry the needle and syringe to the bedside and protect yourself from a needle stick.
7. *If using a vial and ampule:*	
a. Draw the amount of air to equal the medication to be removed from the vial.	The air will allow medication to be removed from the vial. No air is injected into an ampule.
b. After injecting the air into the vial, withdraw the exact volume of that medication needed, as described above. Be sure all air is out of the syringe. Then remove the syringe from the vial.	To ensure the exact dose of the first medication.
c. Insert the needle into the ampule, and draw out medication as described above to the level of the total volume of the two drugs.	This provides the exact drug amount of the second drug.
8. Recap the needle, using a one-handed scoop technique.	To prevent needle-stick injury, to provide safety while transporting the syringe, and to prevent contamination of the needle.

GENERAL PROCEDURE FOR ADMINISTERING MEDICATIONS BY INJECTION

The General Procedure for Administering Medications by Injection is based on Module 44's Procedure for Administering Oral Medications. It will be used as the basis for separate procedures for giving subcutaneous, intramuscular, and intradermal injections. The modi-fied steps for giving injections as well as references to the steps of the General Procedure for Administering Oral Medications that apply are included.

ASSESSMENT

1. Follow step 1 of the General Procedure for Administering Oral Medications: Review the medication record used in your facility to identify whether any medications are to be given to an individual patient during your shift.

2. Examine the MAR for accuracy and completeness as prescribed by your facility. When verifying the medication order, identify the route to be used for the injection. **R:** To ensure that the medication is given by the correct injection route. See Table 46-1 for more information on injection routes.

3-5. Follow steps 3 to 5 of the General Procedure for Oral Medications: Review medication information; assess the patient's abilities, especially the ability to change position; and assess the need for prn medications.

ANALYSIS

6-7. Follow steps 6 and 7 of the General Procedure: Critically think through your data, carefully evaluating each aspect and its relation to other data, and identify specific problems and modifications of the injection procedure needed for this individual.

PLANNING

8. Determine the individualized patient outcomes in relation to the injection(s) to be administered, including the following. **R:** Identification of outcomes guides planning and evaluation.
   a. The right *patient* receives the right *medication* in the right *dose* by the right *injection route* at the right *time*.
   b. The patient experiences the desired effect(s) from the medication(s) administered.
   c. The patient experiences no undesired effect(s) from the medication(s) administered.

table 46-1. Comparing Different Injection Routes

Route	Needle Size	Syringe Size/Type	Injection Angle
Subcutaneous	⅜ to ½ inch long, 25 gauge or higher	1 mL, insulin, 2 mL	90 degrees, 45 degrees for very thin person
Intramuscular	1 inch for arm or thigh, 1½ inches or longer for gluteal sites	2–3 mL	90 degrees
Intradermal	⅜ to ½ inch long, 25 gauge or higher	1 mL	10–15 degrees

   d. The patient experiences minimal discomfort from the injection.
9. Follow step 9 of the General Procedure: Plan for any special procedures that may be needed before administering the injection, such as measuring blood pressure or assessing the apical pulse, or for special equipment and supplies needed for administration. Necessary supplies include the appropriate needle and syringe, alcohol wipes to use in preparing the medication and in giving the injection, and clean gloves. The needle must be the correct length for the type of injection, and the size of the patient and the syringe must be the correct size to measure medication accurately.

IMPLEMENTATION

Action	Rationale
10. Wash or disinfect your hands.	To decrease the transfer of microorganisms that could cause infection.
11-14. Follow steps 11 to 14 of the General Procedure: Access the official MAR; read the name of the medication to be given; access the ordered parenteral medication, and check the label on the medication; compare the medication to the MAR, and choose the correct one before picking it up; pick up the medication, and check the label again.	
15. Prepare the parenteral medication.	
a. Calculate the volume of medication needed.	Most medication orders are written in terms of milligrams of the drug. You will need to read the label to determine how many milligrams are found in each milliliter to calculate how many milliliters you are to give.

(continued)

Action	Rationale
b. Draw up the correct dose using one of the specific techniques above.	To ensure an accurately measured, sterile product.
16-20. Follow steps 16 to 20 of the General Procedure: Prepare any additional medications to be given at this time, check each medication label with the MAR once again, obtain the patient identification to be taken to the patient's bedside as prescribed by your facility's policy, identify the patient (using two identifiers), explain how the medication will be administered, and identify which site was used for the previous injection, if there was one, to rotate to a different site and avoid excessive use of one area. *Note:* When giving an injection to a child, you may wish to conceal the syringe with your hand to avoid frightening the child as you enter the room. In all cases, verbally prepare any child who is old enough to understand before giving the injection. Then give the injection immediately.	
21. Give the injection.	
a. Close the door, pull the curtain around the bed, and raise the bed. Make sure there is adequate lighting, and position the patient for access to the injection site.	To provide privacy and enable you to see the injection site. The bed is raised to allow you to use correct body mechanics.
b. Put on clean gloves.	To protect yourself from contact with blood.
c. Select the appropriate injection site.	The site used is based on the type of injection and any plan for rotating sites.
d. Clean the site with an alcohol wipe, using a circular motion and moving from the middle of the site outward, and allow the skin to air-dry.	The circular motion provides mechanical cleansing of the site, moving microbes away from the puncture site. Drying allows for maximum effect of the alcohol in disinfecting the skin.
e. Place the wipe between the third and fourth fingers of your nondominant hand. If you find this awkward, place the wipe on the outer portion of the swab wrapper to maintain cleanliness.	This positions the wipe so that it is conveniently available when needed after the injection.
f. Remove the needle guard, being careful to pull it straight off and away from the needle. Again, the needle should touch only the inside of the guard.	To keep the needle sterile and prevent sticking yourself.

(continued)

Action	Rationale
g. Using your nondominant hand, stretch the skin, so it is **taut** over the injection site.	An injection is less painful if the skin is taut when pierced. Also, tautness allows the needle to enter the skin more easily.
h. Hold the syringe like a dart (the barrel between the thumb and index finger of your dominant hand).	To allow you to use a smooth dart-like motion to enter the skin.
i. Insert the needle through the skin with a quick dart-like thrust at the correct angle. Transfer your nondominant hand to the plunger of the syringe.	Quickly piercing the skin is less painful to the patient. The length of needle combined with the angle and size of the patient determines where the end of the needle is located—either subcutaneously or intramuscularly or intradermally. Moving your hands steadies the syringe and prepares you to inject the medication.
j. Pull back gently on the plunger of the syringe (aspiration) if appropriate to the type of injection. If no blood is aspirated into the syringe, continue with step k.	There are moderate-size blood vessels in muscle tissue. Injection of a medication into a blood vessel can injure the vessel (the medication may not be appropriate for intravenous administration) and can produce a more immediate and considerably stronger effect than desired, possibly leading to serious complications. While intramuscular injection sites are chosen because there are seldom blood vessels in the injection areas, it is a possibility. If blood appears in the syringe, the needle is in a blood vessel. Withdraw the needle, obtain new sterile equipment, and repeat the entire procedure. Blood vessels in the subcutaneous tissue and skin are so small that they do not pose a risk of injecting medication into a vessel.
k. Inject the medication by pushing the plunger into the barrel with slow, even pressure.	Slow infusion allows the medication to move into intracellular spaces, making room for additional fluid and reducing pain from pressure on the tissue.
l. Using your nondominant hand, steady the tissue immediately adjacent to the puncture site, and quickly remove the needle.	To prevent the skin from painfully dragging on the needle as it is removed.
m. Gently massage the injection site with the alcohol wipe unless this is contraindicated for the specific medication, and discard the wipe.	To facilitate absorption of the medication.
22. Lower the bed, and leave the patient in a comfortable position.	For patient safety and comfort.
23. Discard the syringe and needle in the closest sharps container without replacing the needle guard.	To prevent the needle from being a hazard to yourself or to other healthcare workers.
24. Follow step 24 of the General Procedure: Remove your gloves, and wash or disinfect your hands.	

EVALUATION

25. Evaluate using the individualized patient outcomes previously identified:
    a. The right *patient* received the right *medication* in the right *dose* by the right *injection route* at the right *time*.
    b. The patient experienced the desired effect(s) from the medication(s) administered.
    c. The patient experienced no undesired effect(s) from the medication(s) administered.
    d. The patient experienced minimal discomfort from the injection.

DOCUMENTATION

26. Complete the right *documentation*. In addition to documenting the standard items (name of medication, dose, route, time, and signature), record the site of the injection. **R:** All documentation helps to ensure safety by avoiding erroneously repeating doses. This practice allows nurses to plan site rotation.
27. Also document effectiveness of medication given and presence of any side effects. **R:** To provide a legal record of care and communicates with other healthcare team members.

ADMINISTERING MEDICATIONS BY SUBCUTANEOUS INJECTION

Subcutaneous injections are administered into the subcutaneous tissue that is under the skin and over the muscle layer (Fig. 46-13). Subcutaneous is often abbreviated SC or SQ or Sub-Q. There has been concern about the use of these abbreviations being misunderstood, and for a time, the abbreviation SC was on the JCAHO's list of prohibited abbreviations. Extra caution is appropriate to be sure that you clearly understand the medication order and the route being prescribed.

ADVANTAGES AND DISADVANTAGES

Subcutaneous injections of medication have several advantages over the oral method of administration. First, if the patient has adequate circulatory status, you can depend on rapid, almost complete absorption of the medication. Second, gastric disturbances do not affect medication given subcutaneously. Third, the patient does not have to be conscious or rational to receive the medication.

The greatest disadvantage of subcutaneous administration is that it penetrates the body's first line of defense, the skin. Thus, it is imperative that sterile technique be used for the patient's safety.

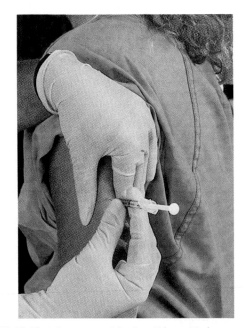

FIGURE 46-13 Subcutaneous injection. Either a 90-degree angle or a 45-degree angle may be used for subcutaneous injection if adequate subcutaneous tissue is present.

SELECTING THE EQUIPMENT

In most instances a 25-G, ⅜- to ½-inch needle is used for subcutaneous injections. An extremely thin or especially obese patient may need individual variations in choice of needle or injection technique. For insulin injections, a 27-G needle is used to decrease discomfort.

The maximum amount of solution that can be comfortably given subcutaneously is from 0.5 mL to 2.0 mL. In many facilities, the smallest regular syringe available is 3.0 mL. Insulin syringes, 1-mL syringes, and 0.5-mL syringes can be used for smaller amounts.

SELECTING THE SITE AND ANGLE

Subcutaneous tissue lies directly below the skin. In many cases, there is sufficient subcutaneous tissue to use a 90-degree angle. In very thin patients, you may need to use a 45- to 60-degree angle. The angle of insertion depends on the individual patient's size and on the needle length. In all cases, the end of the needle must lie in the subcutaneous tissue (see Fig. 46-13).

The site you select will vary with individual patients and circumstances. Generally, areas are selected so that the medication is injected below the dermal layer of the skin. Avoid any areas that are tender or have signs of scarring, swelling, or inflammation. Several sites can be used, such as the upper arms, anterior aspects of the thighs, upper back, and the abdominal wall (Fig. 46-14). It is important to rotate sites for patients who receive subcutaneous injections frequently to decrease any local site irritation.

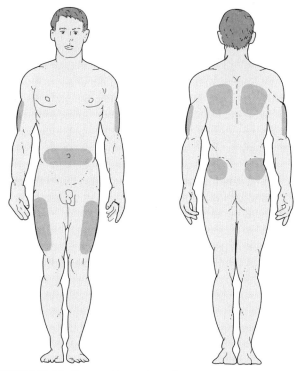

FIGURE 46-14 Sites used in rotating subcutaneous injections.

SPECIAL CONCERNS FOR SUBCUTANEOUS INJECTIONS

Some medications that are frequently given by subcutaneous injection require special attention to technique.

ADMINISTERING HEPARIN AND HEPARINOIDS

Heparin and **heparinoids** are drugs that are commonly given by subcutaneous injection. The preferred site is the abdomen for patient comfort, but other sites may also be used. Research on efficacy (drug effectiveness) and bruising indicated that there were no significant differences when the drug was injected in the abdomen, thigh, or arm (Fahs & Kinney, 1991). Zeraatkari and colleagues (2005) identified that while bruising did not differ significantly when the abdomen, thigh, or arm was used for heparin injections, patients reported less pain when the abdominal site was used (Zeraatkari, Karimi, Shahrzad, et al., 2005). In a study by Chan (2001), slowing the injection resulted in less bruising and less discomfort as reported by the patients receiving heparin injections. When giving this drug, do not aspirate or massage the site afterward. These actions might increase the capillary damage and contribute to bruising. In addition, apply firm pressure to the injection site until all blood has stopped oozing to help prevent bruising. For patients who bleed or bruise easily,

ice sometimes is applied to the site for 15 to 30 minutes before the injection. Doing this causes vasoconstriction and hastens clotting.

ADMINISTERING INSULIN

Insulin is also administered by subcutaneous injection. Because insulin may be a lifetime need, sites must be rotated with great care to avoid damage to subcutaneous tissue. A pattern is established and followed by the patient and others giving insulin injections (see Fig. 46-14).

When mixing different types of insulin, the clear insulin is always drawn up first, and any cloudy insulin is drawn up second. Clear insulins are fast acting and designed for immediate needs. Cloudy insulins contain substances that delay absorption of the insulin, creating a therapeutic pattern of availability. The goal is to avoid contaminating the fast-acting insulin so that its availability is not changed.

Patients are taught to give their own insulin injections. They should have opportunities for practice under supervision before being expected to take on this responsibility independently. To make self-administration of insulin easier, insulin is now available in multiple-dose "pens." The correct dose can be dialed into the pen, and then the insulin is injected. The needle may be changed to allow the pen to be used for multiple doses. An insulin pen is especially useful for the person whose diabetes management plan includes frequent testing for blood glucose followed by fast-acting insulin given based on the test result.

Insulin is also administered through an insulin pump. The insulin pump is filled with fast-acting insulin. A tubing connects the pump with a subcutaneous needle that is inserted over the abdomen and taped in place. The insulin pump can be programmed to provide a consistent dosage of insulin throughout the day (basal rate) with the ability to give bolus doses when a blood test shows a glucose level higher than desired or at predetermined times such as meal-times. The pump is refilled daily. The needle is commonly changed every 2 days. There are newer pumps in which there is a plastic cannula inside the needle. After insertion, the needle can be withdrawn, leaving only the plastic catheter in place. These may remain in place for a longer period of time, depending upon the individual's response.

Insulin may also be administered through a subcutaneous **infuser.** An infuser has a needle or catheter that is inserted into the subcutaneous tissue like the insulin pump. However, instead of a pump, there is a device taped to the skin that is a portal for injecting insulin. The infuser may remain in place for up to 72 hours (depending upon the individual's response). The infuser decreases the number of injections per day when trying to maintain close control of the blood glucose level through frequent blood testing and insulin injection.

Procedure for Administering Medications by Subcutaneous Injection

Use the General Procedure for Administering Medications by Injection as the basis for the Procedure for Administering Medications by Subcutaneous Injection, with the modifications noted below.

ASSESSMENT

1-5. Follow steps 1 to 5 of the General Procedure for Administering Medications by Injection: Review the medication administration record (MAR) to identify whether any medications are to be given to an individual patient during your shift; examine the MAR for accuracy and completeness and injection route as prescribed by your facility; review medication information; assess the patient's abilities, especially the ability to change position; and assess the need for prn medications.

ANALYSIS

6-7. Follow steps 6 and 7 of the General Procedure: Critically think through your data, carefully evaluating each aspect and its relation to other data, and identify specific problems and modifications of the subcutaneous injection procedure needed for this individual.

PLANNING

8. Follow step 8 of the General Procedure: Determine the individualized patient outcomes in relation to the injection(s) to be administered: Include

   a. The right *patient* receives the right *medication* in the right *dose* by the right *injection route* at the right *time*.

   b. The patient experiences the desired effect(s) from the medication(s) administered.

   c. The patient experiences no undesired effect(s) from the medication(s) administered.

   d. The patient experiences minimal discomfort from the injection.

9. Follow step 9 of the General Procedure: Plan for any special procedures that may be needed before administering the injection, such as monitoring blood glucose or prothrombin time, or for special equipment and supplies needed for administration. Necessary supplies include the appropriate needle and syringe, alcohol wipes to use in preparing the medication and in giving the injection, and clean gloves.

   a. The needle for a subcutaneous or intradermal injection is short (⅜ to ½ inch) and of a small (25 to 27) gauge. **R:** This length of needle will usually enter the subcutaneous tissue or skin and not the muscle. A small gauge causes less tissue discomfort.

   b. When planning to administer insulin, choose an insulin syringe, 1-mL syringe, or 3-mL syringe. **R:** An insulin syringe must be used to accurately measure insulin. A small syringe is more accurate for measuring the amount of other medications to be given subcutaneously.

IMPLEMENTATION

Action	Rationale
10-14. Follow steps 10 to 14 of the General Procedure: Wash or disinfect your hands, access the official medication administration record; read the name of the medication to be given; access the ordered parenteral medication, and check the label on the medication; compare the medication to the MAR, and choose the correct one before picking it up; pick up the medication, and check the label again.	
15-20. Follow steps 15 to 20 of the General Procedure: Prepare the parenteral medication as follows: Calculate the volume of medication, and draw up the correct dosage; prepare any additional medications to be given at this time; check each	*(continued)*

Action	Rationale
medication label with the MAR once again; obtain the patient identification to be taken to the patient's bedside as prescribed by your facility's policy; identify the patient (using two identifiers); explain how the medication will be administered; and identify which site was used for the previous injection, if there was one.	
21. Give the injection.	
a-b. Follow steps 21a and 21b of the General Procedure: Close the door, pull the curtain around the bed, and raise the bed. Make sure there is adequate lighting, position the patient for access to the injection site, and put on clean gloves.	
c. Select a correct injection site. For subcutaneous injections, the site is commonly the upper outer arm, across the abdomen, or the thigh, although they may also be given across the upper buttock or on areas under the scapulae (see Fig. 46-14).	The site used is based on the type of injection and the plan for rotating sites. Sites chosen for subcutaneous injections are easily accessible and usually have sufficient subcutaneous tissue.
d-g. Follow steps 21d to 21g of the General Procedure: Clean the skin with an alcohol wipe, using a circular motion and moving from the middle of the site outward, and allow the skin to air-dry; place the swab between the third and fourth fingers of your nondominant hand; remove the needle guard (being careful to pull it straight off and away from the needle); and, using your nondominant hand, make the skin taut over the injection site.	
h. Hold the syringe like a dart (the barrel between the thumb and index finger of your dominant hand). For the subcutaneous route, a 90-degree angle is usually used. For the very thin person, a 45-degree angle may be needed to ensure that the end of the needle does not pierce the muscle.	The subcutaneous tissue at the sites used is thicker than ½ inch in the average person.
i-m. Follow steps 21i to 21m of the General Procedure: Insert the needle through the skin with a quick dart-like thrust at the correct angle; transfer	

(continued)

Action	Rationale
your nondominant hand to the plunger of the syringe; do NOT aspirate; inject the medication by pushing the plunger into the barrel with slow, even pressure; using your nondominant hand, steady the tissue immediately adjacent to the puncture site, and quickly remove the needle; gently massage the injection site with the alcohol swab unless this is contraindicated for the specific medication; and discard the swab.	
22-24. Follow steps 22 to 24 of the General Procedure: Lower the bed and leave the patient in a comfortable position; discard the syringe and needle in the closest sharps container without replacing the needle guard; remove your gloves and wash or disinfect your hands.	

EVALUATION

25. Follow step 25 of the General Procedure: Evaluate using the individualized patient outcomes previously identified: The right *patient* received the right *medication* in the right *dose* by the right *injection route* at the right *time;* the patient experienced the desired effect(s) from the medication(s) administered; the patient experienced no undesired effect(s) from the medication(s) administered; the patient experienced minimal discomfort from the injection.

DOCUMENTATION

26-27. Follow steps 26 and 27 of the General Procedure: Complete the right *documentation.* Document the name of medication, dose, route, time, signature, and the site of the injection. Also document the effectiveness of the medication given and the presence of any side effects.

■ POTENTIAL ADVERSE OUTCOMES AND RELATED INTERVENTIONS

1. Lipodystrophy. Changes in the subcutaneous tissue in which there are hardened areas and some areas of tissue atrophy.
Intervention: When the first sign of tissue changes are observed, the rotation cycle of insulin administration should be examined and altered to provide greater rest to the tissue between injections.

2. Allergic response manifested by flushing, rapid heart rate, and breathing difficulties is an emergency.
Intervention: There should be a protocol for administering epinephrine to provide immediate relief of symptoms. The prescriber should then be notified. Antihistamines and/or steroids may be prescribed for continuing treatment.

ADMINISTERING MEDICATIONS BY INTRAMUSCULAR INJECTION

Intramuscular injections pose a variety of challenges to the person administering the injection. There are both advantages and disadvantages and particular concerns regarding site selection.

ADVANTAGES AND DISADVANTAGES OF INTRAMUSCULAR INJECTIONS

In addition to the general advantages of medications administered by injection, irritating drugs may be given intramuscularly because very few nerve endings are in deep muscle tissue. In addition, the tissue is larger and can absorb a larger volume.

The major disadvantages include the possibility of nerve damage, pain that may linger after the injection, and the potential for abscesses. Nerve damage may occur if the healthcare provider is not careful about site selection and also if the patient has an aberrantly located nerve. Pain may linger because of the localized effect of the medication on the muscle tissue. Because the medication amount is usually larger, if circulation is inadequate, the material may form a sterile abscess. If contamination occurs, an infection at that site may become an infected abscess. In addition, more complex patient teaching is necessary for the individual and/or family member who needs to administer an intramuscular medication after discharge.

SELECTING THE EQUIPMENT FOR INTRAMUSCULAR INJECTION

A 19- to 22-G needle is used for intramuscular injections. The choice will depend on the viscosity of the medication. The needle length depends on the patient's size, but it is usually 1 to 1½ inches long. A 22-G, 1½-inch needle is most commonly used.

Syringe size varies, but generally a 3-mL syringe is used. In most facilities, no more than 3 mL of medication is injected into any one intramuscular site at a time.

SELECTING THE INTRAMUSCULAR INJECTION SITE

Because large blood vessels and nerves run through muscles, selecting an intramuscular site requires careful attention to anatomic landmarks.

VENTROGLUTEAL SITE

The ventrogluteal site has several advantages over the other intramuscular sites (see below). No large nerves or blood vessels are in the area, it is generally less fatty, and the patient on bed rest neither needs to turn to receive the injection nor lie directly on the injection site afterward. The patient can be placed in one of several positions to receive the injection; while side-lying is preferred, either prone or supine can be used. In addition, because the gluteus medius muscle used for the dorsogluteal site is not completely developed in small children, the ventrogluteal site is essential until a child is walking.

The landmarks of the ventrogluteal site are the greater trochanter, the crest of the ilium, and the anterior superior iliac spine. To identify the site, first locate these landmarks on the patient. Then place the heel of your palm on the greater trochanter. Point one finger toward the anterior superior iliac spine and an adjacent finger toward the crest of the ilium, forming a triangle with the iliac bone. (The size of your hand and the patient's bone structure may require small adjustments in hand position to form this triangle.) Use your nondominant hand to locate the site so that your dominant hand is free to manipulate the syringe. The injection site is near the middle of this triangle, approximately 1 inch below the iliac bone (Fig. 46-15A). When the site is located, pro-

ceed with the injection, pointing the needle slightly toward the iliac bone as you insert it.

DORSOGLUTEAL SITE

The dorsogluteal site was once widely used but is no longer because of the greater potential for injury to nerves or blood vessels. However, it may sometimes be the only site available. Great care must be taken to accurately identify the site. The injection is given in the gluteus medius muscle with the patient in the side-lying or prone position. The area should be adequately exposed (that is, all clothing must be moved away) to aid site identification. The landmarks for the dorsogluteal site are the greater trochanter and the posterior iliac spine. Draw an imaginary line between the greater trochanter of the femur and the posterior superior iliac spine (see Fig. 46-15B). An injection given laterally and superiorly to this line is away from the sciatic nerve because the line runs lateral to the nerve.

VASTUS LATERALIS SITE

The lateral thigh is relatively free of major nerves and blood vessels and is accessible in the dorsal recumbent or sitting position. This site is recommended particularly for infants and small children, whose gluteal muscle is still undeveloped.

In adults, the superior boundary is a hand's breadth below the greater trochanter. The inferior boundary is a hand's breadth above the knee. On the front of the leg, the midanterior thigh serves as a boundary. On the side of the leg, the midlateral thigh is the boundary. The result is a narrow band (approximately 3 inches wide) that is suitable for intramuscular injection (see Fig. 46-15C).

Insert the needle to a depth of only 1 inch, and hold it parallel to the surface of the bed. This site is particularly well suited for large or obese patients. Small or slender persons experience some degree of discomfort when this site is used.

DELTOID SITE

The deltoid muscle of the arm can also be used as a site for intramuscular injection if the muscle is well developed. Although it is easily accessible, its use is limited because this smaller muscle is not capable of absorbing large amounts of medication. Another, possibly more critical, limitation on the use of this site is danger of injury to the radial nerve.

The deltoid site is rectangularly shaped. The upper boundary is two to three fingerbreadths down from the acromion process on the outer aspect of the arm. The lower boundary is roughly opposite the axilla. Lines parallel to the arm, one-third and two-thirds of the way around the outer lateral aspect of the arm, form the side boundaries (see Fig. 46-15D).

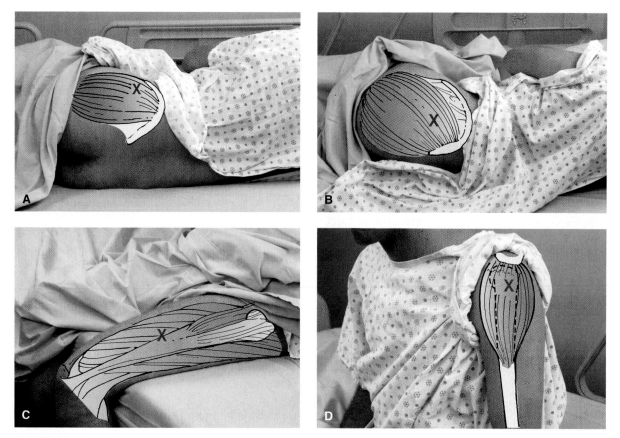

FIGURE 46-15 Sites for intramuscular injections: (**A**) ventrogluteal; (**B**) dorsogluteal; (**C**) vastus lateralis, which is recommended particularly for infants and small children whose gluteal muscle is underdeveloped; and (**D**) deltoid (the amount of medication injected at this site should be no more than 2 mL). (Photos by Rick Brady.)

Although the size of the muscle varies with the size of the person, the amount of medication injected at this site should be limited to a maximum of 1 mL, preferably of nonirritating medication.

Procedure for Administering Medications by Intramuscular Injection

Use the General Procedure for Administering Medication by Injection as the basis for the Procedure for Administering Medications by Intramuscular Injection, with the modifications noted below.

ASSESSMENT

1-5. Follow steps 1 to 5 of the General Procedure for Administering Medications by Injection: Review the medication administration record (MAR) to identify whether any medications are to be given to an individual patient during your shift; examine the MAR for accuracy and completeness and injection route as prescribed by your facility; review medication information; assess the patient's abili-

ties, especially the ability to change position; and assess the need for prn medications.

ANALYSIS

6-7. Follow steps 6 and 7 of the General Procedure: Critically think through your data, carefully evaluating each aspect and its relation to other data, and identify specific problems and modifications of the procedure needed for this individual.

PLANNING

8. Follow step 8 of the General Procedure: Determine the individualized patient outcomes in relation to the injection(s) to be administered: Include
   a. The right *patient* receives the right *medication* in the right *dose* by the right *injection route* at the right *time*.
   b. The patient experiences the desired effect(s) from the medication(s) administered.
   c. The patient experiences no undesired effect(s) from the medication(s) administered.
   d. The patient experiences minimal discomfort from the injection.

9. Follow step 9 of the General Procedure: Plan for any special procedures that may be needed before medication administration, and obtain the supplies needed, including the appropriate needle and syringe, alcohol wipes to use in preparing the medication and in giving the injection, and clean gloves.
a. The needle for an intramuscular injection is long (1 inch for the very thin person, 1½ inches for the average person, and up to 3 inches for the very heavy person). A 22-G needle is commonly

used. **R:** The end of the needle must reach through the subcutaneous tissue into the main muscle mass. The amount of subcutaneous fat affects the length of needle needed. A long needle must be a somewhat larger gauge in order to not bend.
b. A 3-mL syringe with a 22-G, 1½-inch needle is commonly used. **R:** The dosage of most intramuscular medications can be accurately measured in a syringe of that size.

IMPLEMENTATION

Action	Rationale
10-14. Follow steps 10 to 14 of the General Procedure: Wash or disinfect your hands; access the official medication administration record; read the name of the medication to be given; access the ordered parenteral medication, and check the label on the medication; compare the medication to the MAR, and choose the correct one before picking it up; pick up the medication, and check the label again.	
15-20. Follow steps 15 to 20 of the General Procedure: Prepare the parenteral medication, including calculating the volume of medication and drawing up the correct dosage; prepare any additional medications to be given at this time; check each medication label with the MAR once again; obtain the patient identification to be taken to patient's bedside as prescribed by your facility's policy; identify the patient (using two identifiers); explain how the medication will be administered; and identify which site was used for the previous injection, if there was one, to rotate to a different site and avoid excessive use of one area.	
21. Administer the injection.	
a-b. Follow steps 21a and 21b of the General Procedure: Close the door, pull the curtain around the bed, and raise the bed. Make sure there is adequate lighting, position the patient for access to the injection site, and put on clean gloves.	

(continued)

Action	Rationale
c. Choose a correct intramuscular site for the amount of medication to be administered.	For intramuscular injections, use the deltoid or vastus lateralis for volumes of 1 mL or less of nonirritating medication, the ventrogluteal (or the dorsogluteal if the ventrogluteal is not accessible) for amounts more than 1 mL or for irritating medications. These sites have sufficient muscle mass for the amounts indicated.
d-g. Follow steps 21d to 21g of the General Procedure: Clean the skin with an alcohol wipe, using a circular motion and moving from the middle of the site outward, and allow the skin to air-dry; place the swab between the third and fourth fingers of your nondominant hand; remove the needle guard, being careful to pull it straight off and away from the needle; and using your nondominant hand, make the skin taut over the injection site.	
h. Hold the syringe like a dart (the barrel between the thumb and index finger of your dominant hand). The needle should be at a 90-degree angle in order for it to enter muscle.	The muscle tissue often lies more than 1 inch below the skin, and the needle must penetrate to the main muscle mass.
i. Follow step 21i of the General Procedure: Insert the needle through the skin with a quick dart-like thrust at the correct angle. Transfer your nondominant hand to the barrel of the syringe, and transfer your dominant hand to the plunger.	
j. Pull back gently on the plunger (aspiration) for the intramuscular injection.	To be sure the needle is not in a blood vessel.
k. If *no* blood appears in the syringe, inject the medication by pushing the plunger into the barrel with slow, even pressure.	No blood indicates that the needle is not in a blood vessel. Slow infusion allows the medication to move into intracellular spaces, making room for additional fluid and reducing pain from pressure on the tissue.
l-m. Follow steps 21l to 21m of the General Procedure: Using your nondominant hand, steady the tissue immediately adjacent to the puncture site, quickly remove the needle, and then gently massage the injection site with the alcohol wipe (unless this is contraindicated for the specific medication), then discard the alcohol wipe.	

(continued)

Action	Rationale
22-24. Follow steps 22 to 24 of the General Procedure: Lower the bed, and leave the patient in a comfortable position; discard the syringe and needle in the closest sharps container without replacing the needle guard; and remove your gloves, and wash or disinfect your hands.	

EVALUATION

25. Follow step 25 of the General Procedure: Evaluate using the individualized patient outcomes previously identified: The right *patient* received the right *medication* in the right *dose* by the right *injection route* at the right *time;* the patient experienced the desired effect(s) from the medication(s) administered; the patient experienced no undesired effect(s) from the medication(s) administered; the patient experienced minimal discomfort from the injection.

DOCUMENTATION

26-27. Follow steps 26 and 27 of the General Procedure: Complete the right *documentation.* Document the name of the medication, dose, route, time, signature, and the site of the injection. Also document the effectiveness of the medication(s) given and presence of any side effects.

USING THE Z-TRACK TECHNIQUE FOR INTRAMUSCULAR INJECTION

The **Z-track** technique of intramuscular injection is used when a drug such as injectable iron preparations stains the tissues, or when a drug is extremely irritating such as several central nervous system drugs. Correct use of the Z-track technique prevents a drug from leaking back up through the needle track and staining the skin or causing irritation to the subcutaneous tissue. The technique also may be used for any intramuscular injection to decrease discomfort and bruising. The equipment used for this procedure is generally the same as for routine intramuscular injections, except that a 1½-inch needle is desirable.

Procedure for Using the Z-Track Technique

To give a Z-track injection, modify step 21 (above) as follows:

- Locate the ventrogluteal site (or dorsogluteal if the ventrogluteal is not accessible) for a Z-track injection using the techniques described in Figures 46-15 and 46-16. These sites have a large muscle with significant overlying subcutaneous tissue.
- Place the outer surface of your nondominant hand firmly at the site to be used for the injection, and pull the skin and subcutaneous tissue firmly

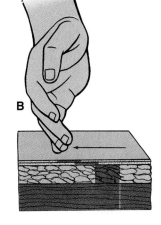

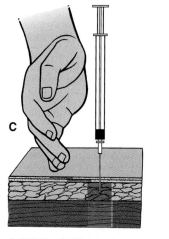

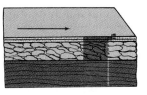

FIGURE 46-16 Z-track technique. (**A**) Normal skin and tissues. (**B**) When skin is pulled taut to one side, (**C**) needle can be inserted at a 90-degree angle. (**D**) After aspiration and injection, the needle is withdrawn and displaced tissue can return to normal position. The Z-track method of injection prevents medication from escaping from the muscle tissue.

to the side (Fig. 46-16). Doing this displaces the subcutaneous tissue overlying the muscle.

- Follow steps 21d to 21l of the General Procedure: Clean the site with an alcohol wipe, and allow the skin to air-dry; place the swab between the third and fourth fingers of your nondominant hand; remove the needle guard by pulling it straight off and away from the needle; and using your nondominant hand, keep the skin taut over the injection site. Holding the syringe like a dart (the barrel between the thumb and index finger of your dominant hand), insert the needle through the skin at a 90-degree angle with a quick dart-like thrust. Pull back gently on the plunger (aspiration) for the intramuscular injection. If no blood appears in the syringe, inject the medication by pushing the plunger into the barrel with slow, even pressure. Using your nondominant hand, steady the tissue immediately adjacent to the puncture site, and quickly remove the needle.
- Release the tissue that has been held to the side. **R:** Doing this tends to close the needle pathway through the tissue and prevent leakage of medication into the subcutaneous tissue.
- All other steps remain the same.

POTENTIAL ADVERSE OUTCOMES AND RELATED INTERVENTIONS

1. Nerve damage from needle contact with the nerve or the effect of irritating medication. The patient may complain of pain that radiates down the leg. *Intervention:* Notify the physician immediately. Unfortunately, there is no remedy that will reverse the problem if the nerve has been damaged. The nerve may recover through the body's healing processes.
2. Abscess in the muscle. This may be an infection but also may be a sterile abscess that is a reaction to the medication. The patient will experience localized pain, and a lump may be felt in the tissue. *Intervention:* Notify the physician immediately. Warm compresses are often ordered to increase circulation and help with absorption of the medication.

USING THE INTRADERMAL ROUTE

The intradermal route is commonly used for diagnostic purposes, usually for diagnosing allergies and sensitivities and for administering the tuberculin test. It has the longest absorption time of all the parenteral routes.

SELECTING THE EQUIPMENT AND SITE

Because a very small amount of drug is used, a 1-mL, or tuberculin, syringe is used, with a short (¼- to ⅜-inch), fine-gauge (25-G to 27-G) needle.

Intradermal literally means "between the skin layers," and the injection is administered just under the epidermis. The inner surface of the forearm is the most common site, although the subscapular region of the back can be used as well.

Procedure for Administering Medications by Intradermal Injection

Use the General Procedure for Giving Injections as the basis for the Procedure for Administering Medications by Intradermal Injection, with the modifications noted below. Because intradermal injections are commonly given in outpatient settings, you may have to adapt this procedure accordingly. For example, the patient may be sitting in a chair in an office rather than resting in a bed.

ASSESSMENT

1-4. Follow steps 1 to 4 of the General Procedure for Giving Injections: Review the MAR to identify whether any medications are to be given to an individual patient during your shift; examine the MAR for accuracy and completeness and injection route as prescribed by your facility; review medication information; and assess the patient's abilities.
5. Intradermal medications are rarely given when other medications are being given and thus assessing the need for prn medications is not necessary.

ANALYSIS

6-7. Follow steps 6 and 7 of the General Procedure: Critically think through your data, carefully evaluating each aspect and its relation to other data, and identify specific problems and modifications of the procedure needed for this individual.

PLANNING

8. Follow step 8 of the General Procedure: Determine the individualized patient outcomes in relation to the injection(s) to be administered: Include
   a. The right *patient* receives the right *medication* in the right *dose* by the right *injection route* at the right *time*.
   b. The patient experiences the desired effect(s) from the medication(s) administered.

c. The patient experiences no undesired effect(s) from the medication(s) administered.
d. The patient experiences minimal discomfort from the injection.

9. Obtain the supplies needed, including the appropriate needle and syringe, alcohol wipes to use in preparing the medication and in giving the injection, and clean gloves.

a. A short (⅜- to ½-inch), fine-gauge (25- to 28-G) needle is needed. **R:** This length of needle will usually enter the dermis and not the subcutaneous tissue when used at the correct angle. A small gauge causes less tissue discomfort.
b. A 1-mL syringe is used to accurately measure the small volume used for intradermal injections.

IMPLEMENTATION

Action	Rationale
10-14. Follow steps 10 to 14 of the General Procedure: Wash or disinfect your hands; access the official medication administration record; read the name of the medication to be given; access the ordered parenteral medication, and check the label on the medication; compare the medication to the MAR, and choose the correct one before picking it up; pick up the medication, and check the label again.	
15-20. Follow steps 15 to 20 of the General Procedure: Prepare the parenteral medication, including calculating the volume of medication and drawing the correct dosage; prepare any additional medications to be given at this time; check each medication label with the MAR once again; obtain the patient identification to be taken to patient's bedside as prescribed by your facility's policy; identify the patient (two identifiers); explain how the medication will be administered; and identify which site was used for the previous injection, if there was one, to rotate to a different site and avoid excessive use of one area.	
21. Administer the injection.	
a-b. Follow steps 21a and 21b of the General Procedure: Close the door, and raise the bed, or position yourself at the same level as the patient if he or she is sitting in a chair. Make sure there is adequate lighting, position the patient for access to the injection site, and put on clean gloves.	
c. Select the appropriate injection site (often the inner surface of a forearm).	The inner aspect of the forearm is easily visible to examine the skin reaction.

(continued)

Action	Rationale
d-g. Follow steps 21d to 21g of the General Procedure: Clean the skin with an alcohol wipe, using a circular motion and moving from the middle of the site outward, and allow the skin to air-dry; place the wipe between the third and fourth fingers of your nondominant hand; remove the needle guard, being careful to pull it straight off and away from the needle; and using your nondominant hand, make the skin taut over the injection site.	
h. Hold the syringe barrel between the thumb and index finger of your dominant hand. The needle should be **bevel** up at a shallow (10- to 15-degree) angle (Fig. 46-17).	To allow you to enter the skin but not go through it.

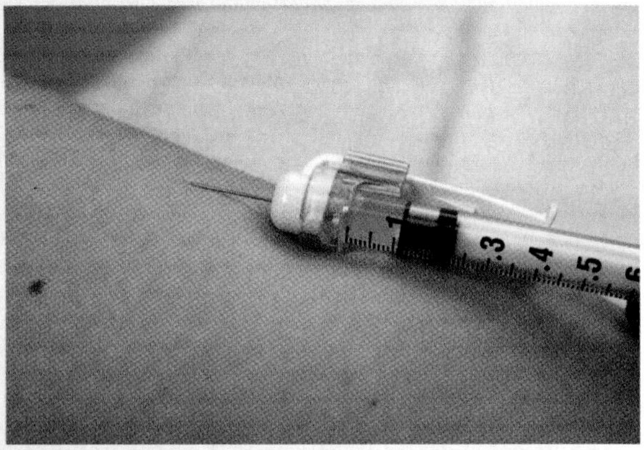

FIGURE 46-17 Intradermal injection technique. The syringe is held at a 10- to 15-degree angle, almost level with the skin, with the bevel of the needle facing up.

Action	Rationale
i. Insert the needle through the skin just until the bevel is no longer visible. Transfer your nondominant hand to the barrel of the syringe, and transfer your dominant hand to the plunger.	To ensure that the medication will be in the correct area. Moving your hands steadies the syringe.
j. Inject the medication by pushing the plunger into the barrel with slow, even pressure. For an intradermal medication, a small **wheal** of fluid should become apparent within the skin.	The skin has no extra space, and so the fluid will create a wheal.
k. Using your nondominant hand, steady the tissue immediately adjacent to the puncture site, and quickly remove the needle.	To prevent the skin from dragging on the needle as it is removed, which causes pain. (*Note:* The site is not massaged because absorption is not desired.)

(continued)

Action	Rationale
22-24. Follow steps 22 to 24 of the General Procedure: Lower the bed (if it was raised), leave the patient in a comfortable position, discard the syringe and needle in the closest sharps container without replacing the needle guard, and wash or disinfect your hands.	

EVALUATION

25. Follow step 25 of the General Procedure: Evaluate using the individualized patient outcomes previously identified: The right *patient* received the right *medication* in the right *dose* by the right *injection route* at the right *time;* the patient experienced the desired effect(s) from the medication(s) administered; the patient experienced no undesired effect(s) from the medication(s) administered; the patient experienced minimal discomfort from the injection.

DOCUMENTATION

26-27. Follow steps 26 and 27 of the General Procedure: Complete right *documentation.* Document the name of medication, dose, route, time, signature, and site of the injection. The site of the injection must be documented very specifically in order to facilitate evaluation of any reaction at the site.

> *Note:* Results of skin tests are usually read 24 to 48 hours after the test is done. A positive response is indicated by redness and induration (swelling). The area of induration is measured in millimeters for reporting the result. A negative test is indicated by no or very limited reaction, such as an area of redness without induration or induration less than a specified size. Consult the manufacturer's instructions to determine how and when to read the results.

POTENTIAL ADVERSE OUTCOMES AND RELATED INTERVENTIONS

1. Extreme reaction to the substance injected. A person who is very sensitive may develop a large, painful, itching area of reaction.
Intervention: Notify physician. An anti-inflammatory medication may be prescribed to decrease the severity of the symptoms.

Acute Care

In acute care settings, there are many patients who require subcutaneous insulin and subcutaneous heparin and heparinoids during their stay. For patients with diabetes, the nurse should consult with the patient regarding the maintenance of any site rotation plan. Many diabetics ask that injections while they are hospitalized be done in sites they themselves cannot reach. This provides an opportunity for the sites they commonly use to have longer recovery periods. Because heparin and its analogues affect clotting times, it is important to prevent bruising by careful attention to the size of the needle and pressure after the injection.

Because hospital stays are often short, and many patients have an intravenous line in place during much of their stay, there are few intramuscular injections given in most acute care settings. The majority are for pain medications. The nurse should be aware that in patients with diminished circulation, intramuscular drugs may be poorly absorbed. This results in a lack of effective action. If the circulation is subsequently restored, and there are multiple unabsorbed or poorly absorbed doses in the muscle tissue, an overdose of the medication may be absorbed.

Long-Term Care

Many residents in long-term care settings have diabetes and require insulin injections on a regular basis. Others receive periodic intramuscular injections of vitamin preparations. The nurse must take into account several considerations when administering injections to elderly persons.

- First, these persons may be receiving multiple medications, some orally, which may interact with the drug being injected.

- Second, elderly persons typically have less muscle mass than younger persons, so the technique used may have to be altered to suit the particular individual.
- Third, an older person's metabolism may not be as vigorous as a younger person's, so the nurse must closely monitor drug effects.
- Fourth, a confused person may be resistant to having an injection, and the nurse may need considerable skill and sometimes the assistance of another person.

Home Care

It is essential that those caring for clients in the home setting, whether professionals or lay persons, carry out the administration of injections with the same high quality of performance as that offered in any healthcare facility. An additional responsibility is the safe disposal of syringes and needles. An alternative to purchasing the type of container used in a professional setting is to use a disposable container commonly found in the home. A plastic, disposable soft drink bottle resists puncture, can be capped tightly, and does not burst under pressure. Syringes and needles can be placed there as they would be placed in the sharps container in the hospital. The container must be stored where children cannot reach it and must be capped before disposal.

Nonlicensed persons who are caring for clients at home sometimes are permitted by law to administer subcutaneous injections. It may be your responsibility to teach this skill to these persons. Areas for emphasis include sterile technique, accurate dose measurement, and effective injection procedure. You will also need to teach what specific side effects to observe for and when to contact the nurse.

Ambulatory Care

In the ambulatory care setting, the most common injections are immunizations. Most of these are given intramuscularly in the deltoid for adults and in the vastus lateralis for children. Antibiotics may also be given intramuscularly if the client has not responded to oral medications. In the ambulatory care setting, newly diagnosed diabetics may be taught to self-administer insulin. This is an important skill and must be evaluated carefully. Allergy testing and testing for possible tuberculosis exposure are the common intradermal injections given in ambulatory care settings.

LEARNING TOOLS

DEVELOP YOUR BACKGROUND KNOWLEDGE

1. Review the Learning Outcomes.
2. Read the section on injections in your assigned text.
3. Look up the Key Terms in the glossary.
4. Review this module and mentally practice the techniques described. Study so that you would be able to teach these skills to another person.

DEVELOP YOUR SKILLS

1. In your home study setting and the practice setting
   a. Observe and become familiar with the assortment of needles and syringes available in your program and in your facility.
   b. To increase your manual dexterity before actually giving an injection, practice the sequence of movements involved: finding and cleansing the site, taking the needle cover off the needle, inserting the needle, aspirating, injecting the medication, and withdrawing the needle without giving an injection. You may practice these movements using a syringe and needle or simply using a pen with a cap and an alcohol wipe over a table. Doing this will help you to feel comfortable handling the equipment and also to remember the sequence when you are actually giving the injection.
   c. In your home setting, you may have a family member or friend who would permit you to identify injection sites using anatomic landmarks. Each person is slightly different, and the more different persons you practice this skill on, the more comfortable you will become with your own technique.

2. In the practice setting, practice using the equipment.
   a. Using a 3-mL syringe and a 1½-inch needle, draw up 1 mL solution from a multiple-dose practice vial.
   b. Using the same equipment, draw up all the solution from a practice ampule containing 1 or 2 mL solution.
   c. Change a needle as you would if the first one had been contaminated.
   d. Draw up the equivalent of 65 units of U-100 insulin in an insulin syringe that would hold 100 units total. Then draw up 5 units of U-100 insulin in an insulin syringe that would hold just 50 units total.

3. In the practice setting, practice subcutaneous injections using the Performance Checklists on the CD-ROM in the front of this book as a guide. Practice

until you can do each procedure smoothly without referring to the written guide.

   a. Give 1.0 mL solution to a simulation pad as though you were giving it subcutaneously.

   b. Give a subcutaneous injection using a mannequin where you must choose a site. Continue practicing until you feel confident of your technique.

   c. When you feel prepared, ask your instructor to evaluate your performance.

   d. *Under supervision,* give a subcutaneous injection of 0.5 mL sterile saline solution to another student (if this is accepted policy).

4. In the practice setting, practice intramuscular injections using the Performance Checklists on the CD-ROM in the front of this book as a guide. Practice until you can do each procedure smoothly without referring to the written guide.

   a. Give 1.0-mL solution to a simulation pad as though you were giving it intramuscularly.

   b. Give two intramuscular injections to a mannequin where you must choose a site. Give one in the ventrogluteal site and one in the dorsogluteal site.

   c. Give two intramuscular injections using the Z-track technique to a mannequin where you must choose a site. Give one in the ventrogluteal site and one in the dorsogluteal site. Continue practice until you feel confident of your technique.

   d. When you feel prepared, ask your instructor to evaluate your performance.

   e. *Under supervision,* give an intramuscular injection of 0.5 mL sterile saline solution to another student (if this is accepted policy).

5. In the practice setting, practice intradermal injections using the Performance Checklist as a guide. Practice until you can do the procedure smoothly without referring to the written guide.

   a. Give 1 mL solution to a simulation pad as though you were giving it intradermally.

   b. Give an intradermal injection using a mannequin where you must choose a site. Continue practice until you feel confident of your technique.

   c. When you feel prepared, ask your instructor to evaluate your performance.

   d. *Under supervision,* give an intradermal injection of 0.5 mL sterile saline solution to another student (if this is accepted policy).

DEMONSTRATE YOUR SKILLS

In the clinical setting

1. Consult with your instructor regarding the opportunity to give injections to patients.

2. Evaluate your performance with the instructor.

CRITICAL THINKING EXERCISES

1. You are to give an intramuscular injection of pain medication to a patient who has had her gallbladder removed. As you enter her room, you observe that she is lying on her back moaning. Describe your interaction with this patient, and identify the site and technique that would be most appropriate.

2. You are to teach a 60-year-old patient how to give a subcutaneous self-injection. Using the steps of the nursing process, create a teaching plan. Consider your interaction with the patient (or family), explanations of the equipment, technique to be used, and evaluation and documentation.

SELF-QUIZ
SHORT-ANSWER QUESTIONS

1. Name four types of available syringes.

   a. _____

   b. _____

   c. _____

   d. _____

2. What does U-100 insulin mean?

   _____

3. Needles are sized according to what two attributes?

   a. _____

   b. _____

4. Name two types of containers that are commonly used for injectable solutions.

   a. _____

   b. _____

5. Air is injected before removing the solution when which type of parenteral medication container is used?

   _____

6. List three advantages of subcutaneous medication administration over oral medication administration.

   a. _____

   b. _____

   c. _____

7. What needle size is most commonly used for subcutaneous injections?

   _____

8. Name three anatomic areas that are acceptable for subcutaneous injections.

   a. _____

   b. _____

   c. _____

9. Absorption is most rapid in which of the three routes: intradermal, subcutaneous, or intramuscular?

   _____

10. What needle length is most commonly used for intramuscular injections?

   _____

11. Name three anatomic landmarks that are used to identify the ventrogluteal site.

   a. _____

   b. _____

   c. _____

12. Name three advantages of the ventrogluteal site over the dorsogluteal.

   a. _____

   b. _____

   c. _____

13. What are two disadvantages of using the deltoid site for intramuscular injection?

   a. _____

   b. _____

14. When doing an intramuscular injection, why do you aspirate immediately after the insertion of the needle?

   _____

MULTIPLE CHOICE

_____ 15. In a very thin person, which of the following angles would be most appropriate for subcutaneous injection?
   a. 45-degree angle
   b. 60-degree angle
   c. 90-degree angle
   d. The angle is not critical.

_____ 16. After which of the following injection techniques is massage not indicated? (Choose all that apply.)
   a. Intradermal
   b. Subcutaneous
   c. Intramuscular
   d. Z-track technique

Answers to the Self-Quiz questions appear in the back of the book.

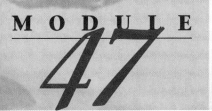

MODULE 47

Preparing and Maintaining Intravenous Infusions

KEY TERMS

air embolus	microdrip
cannula	needleless system
embolus	nonvolumetric
extravasation	osmolarity
infiltration	phlebitis
infusion	thrombophlebitis
intravenous	volumetric
macrodrip	

OVERALL OBJECTIVE

▶ To prepare and maintain intravenous infusions accurately, with comfort and safety for patients.

LEARNING OUTCOMES

The student will be able to

1. Assess the patient to prepare and maintain appropriate intravenous (IV) therapy.
2. Analyze assessment data to determine special needs or concerns that must be addressed to provide safe IV infusion therapy for the individual patient.
3. Describe the criteria necessary to support safe provision of IV infusion therapy.
4. Determine appropriate patient outcomes of the IV infusion therapy and recognize the potential for adverse outcomes.
5. Administer or discontinue (as ordered) the IV infusion therapy, utilizing appropriate supplies and equipment in a safe, effective manner.
6. Evaluate the effectiveness and safety of the IV infusion therapy.
7. Document the infusion therapy and nursing care provided in the patient's plan of care and in the patient's record.

Intravenous **infusion** therapy is an important responsibility of the nurse. The proper initiation and maintenance of therapy is vital to the care of the patient, as is the proper discontinuance. Many patients require **intravenous** (IV) therapy, some for long-term therapy and some for very brief intervals. Accuracy, safety, and comfort should guide all nursing actions related to IV infusion therapy.

Intravenous infusions are used when patients need fluids, electrolytes, medications, or nutritional supplements that cannot be taken orally or need to be given continuously. Because the infusion provides direct access to the bloodstream, it involves many hazards: It provides an optimum entry for infectious organisms; it can allow foreign material, including air, to be introduced and to act as emboli; it can cause bleeding; and both the equipment and the solution can irritate the tissue. The nurse is responsible for protecting the patient from these hazards.

In addition, ensuring that the infusion flows at the correct rate is a critical nursing responsibility. Too rapid a flow can create a fluid volume overload of the circulatory system, potentially resulting in death if not corrected. A flow that is too slow may deprive the patient of needed fluid, electrolytes, or medication. The nurse must monitor and maintain the correct infusion rate. The nurse also is responsible to make sure that the correct fluid is administered, using appropriate equipment. Knowledge of fluid and electrolyte balance is essential for the nurse who is responsible for managing intravenous therapy. That information will be found in your assigned theory text.

NURSING DIAGNOSES

■ Risk for Injury: The primary nursing diagnosis to consider when administering IV therapy is

Risk for Injury. Administration of IV fluids involves utilizing the proper type of IV fluid, providing it over the correct length of time, and ensuring that there are no signs of skin or venous irritation.

■ Risk for Infection is another important nursing diagnosis. Because the first line of defense for the immune system has been disrupted by the introduction of an IV access device, infection can occur. Also, the fluids, medication, and other equipment utilized can be a potential source of infection from contamination. Remember that proper hand hygiene is the first step in protecting the patient.

■ Risk for Imbalanced Fluid Volume, usually fluid volume excess, is a third concern of infusion therapy. An IV that infuses too rapidly or a total amount that is too great for the patient's heart and kidneys to manage may result in a fluid volume excess. Proper IV fluid administration requires careful monitoring of administration rate. In addition to the IV itself, the nurse also should be aware of the patient's total intake and output in relation to fluid needs. IV infusion pumps/controllers are often the standard for continuous infusions and for some types of intermittent infusions to ensure the correct volume will be delivered at the desired rate.

■ Impaired Comfort for the patient should always be considered when providing IV infusion therapy. A well-functioning IV should not be painful. However, the decreased mobility caused by an IV device in an arm may create muscle or joint discomfort. The additional fluids may create the need for more frequent toileting, which can cause discomfort. Discomfort at the site may be related to complications.

- Acute Pain can have many causes. Some of the more common causes of acute pain are cold fluids being infused rapidly and causing vasospasm; medications that are irritating due to pH, **osmolarity,** or rapid infusion; and the positioning required for adequate infusion such as prolonged joint extension.
- Other nursing diagnoses may apply as well, for example, Anxiety, Risk for Latex Allergy Response, and Impaired Tissue Integrity in certain populations.

DELEGATION

The preparation and maintenance of IV infusions are not delegated to assistive personnel because ability to use sterile technique and skill in calculating infusion rates are both necessary. However, assistive personnel may care for patients receiving IV therapy and must know how to provide basic care without disturbing the IV. The nurse should also inform the nursing assistant of signs and symptoms of problems that need to be reported immediately.

EQUIPMENT

INTRAVENOUS FLUID SOLUTIONS

Intravenous solutions are available in 50-mL, 100-mL, 150-mL, 250-mL, 500-mL, and 1,000-mL volumes. The most common volume is 1,000 mL. IV solutions, regardless of volume, are comparable in cost, so it is not a great saving to the patient to supply fluid from a small-volume bag as an interim if a larger bag is ordered but has not arrived on the unit.

GLASS BOTTLES

Some IV fluids come in glass bottles. Glass bottles are used primarily for the infusion of medications that are unstable in plastic bags. For the fluid to flow out of the bottle, there must be some kind of mechanism to allow air to enter the bottle. This can be a vent incorporated into the drip chamber of the tubing set (Fig. 47-1). The air vent usually has a filter that prevents contaminants from the air entering the bottle.

PLASTIC BAGS

Most IV fluids are now supplied in plastic bags (see Fig. 47-1). Because the plastic bag collapses as fluid is removed, no air vent is needed. This prevents nonsterile air from coming in contact with the IV fluid.

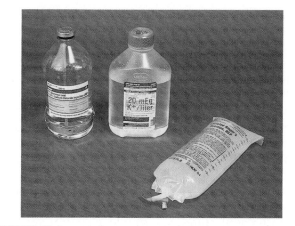

FIGURE 47-1 IV solution containers include glass and plastic bottles and flexible plastic bags as well. There must be an air vent in the solution bottle.

Safety Alert

Plastic bags have a characteristic that is of special concern to nurses. They can absorb some types of ink and transport the ink to the fluid. For this reason, it is appropriate to do all marking on tapes or labels that can be adhered to the bag and not to use any type of ink marker on the plastic. It is also advisable not to use felt-tip pens, both because the ink may penetrate the surface of the plastic bag and because it may become illegible if it comes into contact with moisture. To minimize the potential for infection and possible complications, the nurse should closely inspect all bags before administration. Check for leaks, cracks, damaged caps, particulate material, and expiration date.

Another concern focuses on medications or additives in IV solutions that adhere to the inner surface of a plastic bag. The result is that the patient does not receive an accurate amount of the additive. For this reason, IV solutions with these additives are prepared in glass bottles.

ADMINISTRATION SETS

The conventional administration set consists of plastic tubing with multiple parts attached. At the top is a plastic spike that is inserted into the IV bag or bottle. The spike must be kept sterile.

Below the spike is a drip chamber, which allows the rate of fluid administration to be monitored by counting the drops falling into the chamber. The drip chamber must be kept half full of fluid to avoid trapping air into the fluid and infusing air. If an infusion pump or controller is in use, the drip rate within the drip chamber may be monitored by a sensor.

Administration sets are constructed so the orifice in the drip chamber delivers a predictable number of drops for each milliliter of fluid. The drop factor (drops per mL) for an individual set is usually found on the packaging supplied with the product.

The most common type of set is the macrodrip set that delivers 10 to 20 drops/mL (Fig. 47-2). Remember that this figure is correct for regular, water-type fluids (crystalloids). When viscous fluids such as those containing amino acids and fats (colloids) are given, the number of drops per milliliter can vary. Because of this, most facilities use an infusion control device to deliver these solutions.

Most manufacturers also supply microdrip sets (Fig. 47-2). These sets deliver 60 drops/mL and can be identified by the fine metal orifice in the drip chamber. The package specifies the number of drops per mL for the specific set being used.

Most IV sets are nonvented and designed to be used with an IV bag that will collapse as fluid exits. When a glass bottle is used, air must enter the bottle for the fluid to exit. An intravenous tubing with an integral air vent above the drip chamber is used. If vented tubing is attached to an IV bag, the fluid will still flow, although the plastic bag may not collapse evenly because of the air entering the bag. Review the procedure for the equipment used in your facility.

There is a roller clamp on the tubing that is used to control the flow rate. A screw clamp or a slide clamp is also found on tubing, but its primary purpose is to turn the flow on or off. It does not provide an accurate way to control a flow rate manually.

The distal part of the tubing connects into the hub of the needle in the vein. This part is referred to as a syringe tip or male adapter tip. Often a screw-on system, or locking collar, is incorporated into administration set connections to prevent disconnection. Most sets have one or more entry ports that can be accessed for medication

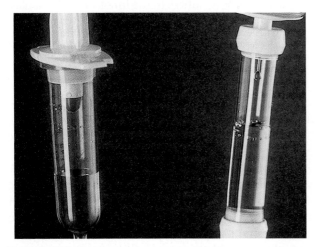

FIGURE 47-2 Regular (macrodrip) IV administration set and microdrip administration set.

administration into the IV tubing. Most entry ports are designed for needleless entry devices. Some are designed for a needle entry, in which case a special shielded needle is used.

Special tubing with an additional cartridge-like chamber is used with volume-controlled infusion devices. The cartridge serves as a volume meter (volumeter), so that the device delivers a programmed volume within a specified period (see the following section on pumps and controllers).

Blood administration sets are specially designed to deliver blood safely. They include a large built-in filter in the drip chamber, which removes any clots or precipitates in the blood. See Module 52 for information on administering blood and blood components.

SECONDARY SETS

A secondary set is designed to connect a second IV container into the primary (main) IV. A secondary set is often used to administer an intravenous medication and therefore often connected to an infusion pump or controller to ensure proper rate infusion. Most infusion pumps are programmed to deliver the secondary fluid at the prescribed rate as set by the nurse, and then the primary fluid will resume infusing when the secondary fluid is completed.

When a pump or controller is not used, the secondary set can be attached using one of three methods. Using a *tandem setup,* the secondary set with its attached bag is connected to the primary set at an entry port on the bag. The bag on the secondary set is hung higher than the one on the primary set. The bag on the secondary set (farthest from the patient) empties first, because the bag and the fluid volume are located higher. If the secondary fluid is in a glass bottle, air will enter through the air filter to displace the fluid. In a tandem setup, there is mixing of fluid from the secondary set with the fluid in the primary bag.

The second method is the *piggyback setup.* The secondary set is used to attach the second bag to the tubing port on the primary set rather than to the bag itself. Using the piggyback setup, either bag can be made to run by shutting off the tubing to one bag above the junction and keeping the tubing to the other bag open (Fig. 47-3). The piggyback setup is most commonly used to deliver small volumes of fluid containing medications. In this situation, both lines are left open and the piggyback bag is hung higher than the original bag. The higher bag finishes first. When that bag is empty, the lower bag will start infusing.

Two bags can also be hung at the same time by using a *Y-type* administration set (Fig. 47-4). When both arms of the Y are open, the bag with the fluid at a higher level empties first and then the other bag empties. The Y set can also be used to alternate solutions.

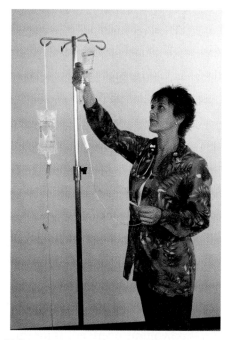

FIGURE 47-3 Secondary piggyback set. When the piggyback bag is empty, in some types of tubing, a special valve at the piggyback entry port allows the lower bag to start running again.

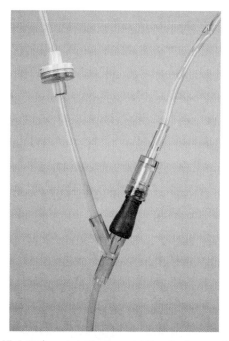

FIGURE 47-4 Y-type administration set. When both arms of the Y are open, the bag at the higher level empties first.

Safety Alert

In glass bottle infusions, if the tubing does not contain a special stop valve for the bottle that empties first, the infusion must be closely monitored. The branch to the bottle emptying first must be turned off while fluid remains in the tube. If air, which enters through the air vent port, is allowed to enter one arm of the Y, it will be pulled into the fluid stream coming from the second bottle and could cause a significant air embolus.

SAFETY NEEDLES AND NEEDLELESS DEVICES

The National Institute for Occupational Safety and Health (NIOSH) recommends that needle use be eliminated wherever possible (NIOSH, 1999). Determine if your facility uses a **needleless system** or if needles may be used to puncture the administration ports on the IV tubing. If needles are allowed for medication injection into the IV tubing, only the special soft rubber or latex ports can be utilized; use of needles anywhere else along the tubing will cause a leak.

When needles are used, the preferred needle is one that has a needle guard surrounding it that will decrease the potential for needle-stick injury. The needle is surrounded with rigid clear plastic that slides over the injection port, guides the needle into the injection port, and secures the needle in place (Fig. 47-5A).

A variety of needleless systems are commercially available. Some use a plastic **cannula** that punctures a specially designed IV lock device and others use a unit with a mechanical valve recessed in a plastic covering. Any male connector can then be used to access this latter system (Fig. 47-5B). These devices may be referred to as adaptors, connectors, access devices, pins, or other names depending on the manufacturer's terminology. Most facilities utilize a screw-on type method to prevent disconnection.

EXTENSION TUBING

Extension tubing is a length of IV tubing with a male adapter on one end and a female adapter on the other, so it can be attached to the main set to create longer tubing. Some extension tubing has a clamp. Extension tubing is commonly added to allow a patient greater mobility. Some kinds of extension tubing also provide filters, stopcocks, and additional access ports.

STOPCOCKS

Stopcocks are typically used to provide multiple entries into the infusion system or to provide an emergency access to the system. They can be part of the extension tubing or applied separately. Use is most common in critical care or procedural areas. The sterility of additional ports is a concern. If additional ports of access are open female receptors, they must be kept capped when not in use and care should be taken to prevent contamination by placing a sterile cap over each port after each use.

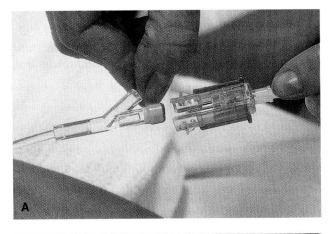

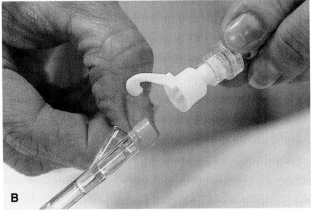

FIGURE 47-5 (**A**) Safety needle is surrounded with rigid clear plastic, which slides over the injection port, guides the needle into the injection port, and secures the needle in place. (**B**) Needleless system in which a blunt plastic cannula enters a prepared injection site. Device has a locking clamp that holds the apparatus in place.

FILTERS

Filters are devices that prevent the passage of undesired particulate matter such as foreign objects, bacteria, fungi, and air. Filters are available in different sizes and have different purposes. Intravenous fluids are usually filtered through a 0.2-micron filter. These filters are considered bacteria-retentive and air-eliminating of particles that are 0.2 microns or larger.

Filters may be used as part of in-line filters in tubing, used separately as add-on filters, or used as filter needles or straws. Filters as in-line tubing are an integral part of the tubing and are positioned near the end that connects the tubing and the needle. An in-line filter, which can be seen in Figure 47-4, looks like white filter paper in a plastic tube, but some manufacturers color code the plastic tube to indicate the size of the particulate material to be filtered. When the IV infusion is being initiated or during tubing changes, the in-line filters should be saturated with IV fluid and any air bubbles should be eliminated from the filter to prevent infusion problems.

Total parenteral nutrition (TPN) should be administered by a set that has a 1.2-micron filter unless specified

otherwise by the pharmacy. Filter needles are recommended for use when preparing IV medications that are drawn from glass ampules or when the medication is to be administered intravenously and cannot be administered through an in-line filter. Filter needles or straws prevent particles from 1 to 5 microns from passing through the filter (Alexander & Corrigan, 2004).

CONTROLLED-VOLUME SETS

Controlled-volume administration sets (Fig. 47-6) consist of an IV tubing with a 100- to 250-mL chamber, which is located just below the spike into the IV bag or bottle. The drip chamber is below this chamber. These sets usually deliver a **microdrip,** or 60 drips/mL. Some controlled-volume administration sets deliver a **macrodrip,** or regular drip, at 15 drips/mL. Check the package to make sure you know the correct drop factor. Controlled-volume sets are used when medication must be added to a limited fluid volume or when there is high risk for fluid volume overload, as for the pediatric patient. Some common brands are Peditrol, Soluset, and Volutrol.

IV POLES

IV poles or stands can be attached to a bed, placed on casters on the floor (Fig. 47-7), or suspended from the ceiling with chains or hooks. When the gravity method of infusion is used, the height of the fluid container affects the flow rate. The higher the fluid container, the greater the pressure and the faster the rate.

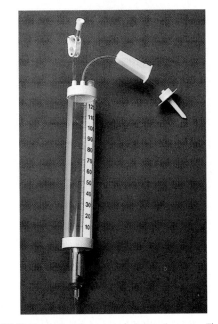

FIGURE 47-6 Controlled-volume administration sets. These sets are often used when medication must be added to a limited fluid volume or for administering fluids to children.

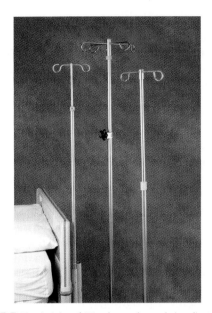

FIGURE 47-7 The height of IV poles and stands is adjustable so that the flow rate of an infusion can be regulated.

EXTENSION HANGERS

Various metal wires or plastic hooks may be used to hang one bottle on an IV pole lower than the other. The higher bottle then flows in first.

ARMBOARDS

An armboard is a rigid plastic or cardboard device used to immobilize a joint to ensure that an IV site is not disrupted. Commercially produced armboards may be for single patient use and disposable or designed for multiple patient use. The latter are commonly used in procedural areas. Disposable armboards are usually made of heavy cardboard material that is foam-padded (Fig. 47-8).

Armboards are used only when necessary because they interfere with the motion of the joint. Veins away from

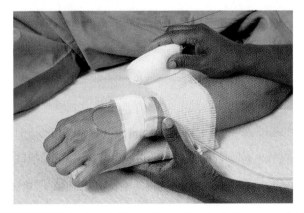

FIGURE 47-8 Armboard. It is best to use the shortest board available to keep from disrupting the IV site while maintaining maximum mobility of nearby joints.

areas of frequent movement are selected for use whenever possible. Hand and forearm veins are preferable to wrist or elbow veins. Occasionally, when IVs must be started over areas of frequent movement or the patient is restless or confused, an armboard is used. Armboards come in various lengths; use the shortest board to accomplish the task so that maximum mobility can be maintained. If the need for an armboard arises and none is available, the nurse may improvise with cardboard padded with cloth or a soft disposable paper drape.

INFUSION CONTROL DEVICES

Healthcare facilities are increasing their use of infusion control devices. These devices provide safer IV therapy for patients and save valuable staff time. Many manufacturers are making infusion control devices; you need to become familiar with the type(s) used by your facility and carefully follow the specific instructions for their use. For purposes of this module, these devices are discussed in general terms.

In some facilities, flow control devices are used for the majority of IVs. In other facilities, flow control devices are used for specific high-risk situations. A control device adds a margin of safety when the IV fluid contains a medication and a precise rate of administration is necessary to maintain a therapeutic blood level. A control device also contains warning systems that may be important when the fluid contains an additive that might have adverse effects if given too rapidly (such as a high concentration of glucose or amino acids or when the patient cannot tolerate any excess fluid volume). Warning signals typically sound if the fluid flow stops, if the resistance to flow is increased, or the fluid flow increases beyond the set rate.

Two types of electronic infusion devices are available to regulate the flow rate of an IV infusion—controllers and pumps. Regardless of which is used, it is essential for the nurse to know that the roller clamp is left open while the tubing is in the machine and the machine is regulating the flow. When the tubing is released from the machine, there is no control and the fluid will begin flowing freely into the vein, unless it is manually regulated by using a clamp. This free flow may result in a sudden excess of any additive in the fluid and excess fluid in a short time. Critical errors in IV administration have occurred when tubing was removed from a controller or pump and the patient received a dangerous dose through the free-flowing tubing. Newer IV controllers provide "free-flow protection"; they include a mechanical or electronic safety mechanism that prevents free flow. Even when devices are used that have free-flow protection, the rate must still be adjusted and regulated by roller clamp when disconnected from the controller. You need to become familiar with the devices in use where you practice.

Both controllers and pumps can be either **volumetric** or **nonvolumetric.** Volumetric devices deliver a specific desired *volume* over a specified period. An example is the administration of parenteral nutrition. Devices that are nonvolumetric are designed to deliver a constant *rate* over a specified period. One example is the administration of medications to patients with heart irregularities or seriously low blood pressure where the rate of administration is critical, not the volume of fluid.

INFUSION CONTROLLERS

The least complex type of IV fluid control uses a controller that regulates the flow rate in drops per minute. This type of device has a drop counter and a mechanism for applying pressure to the tubing. It is set for the desired number of drops per minute. A controller can be volumetric or nonvolumetric. The deciding factor is whether a sensor counts drops only or measures volume. Some can convert the drops into volume but depending on the fluid infusing, this can vary.

In the controller, gravity is responsible for the pressure in the tubing. Changing the height of the fluid container changes the pressure and thus the flow. If the IV fluid infiltrates the tissue, the flow will eventually slow and stop because the pressure of gravity is less than the tissue pressure that will build up as the fluid infiltrates. This feature makes the controller the preferred device when the fluid contains a medication that could cause tissue damage if infiltration occurs. Depending on the patient's condition (e.g., fluid status, skin turgor, and IV site location), a significant amount of fluid/medication could still be infiltrated. Therefore, the IV site should be checked frequently and regularly.

The controller can deliver a constant rate of flow but will not necessarily deliver a precise volume of flow, because variations in IV tubing and fluid viscosity affect the size of the drop. This feature makes the controller appropriate for situations in which rate of flow is important for titrating medication dosage but the exact volume of fluid delivered is not critical.

ELECTRONIC INFUSION PUMPS

Three basic types of electronic infusion pumps include the syringe, peristaltic, and cassette. Most modern pumps can be either volumetric or nonvolumetric. The computer system in the pump allows the "mode" to be set. Most of the time, you will find electronic infusion pumps set in the volumetric pump mode. Volumetric pump mode *must* be set for central lines in which there is pressure in the vein to be overcome.

Of the electronic infusion pumps, syringe pumps are designed to deliver measured doses of medications and are discussed in Module 48, Administering Intravenous Medications. Peristaltic pumps deliver IV solutions by a squeezing action on the tubing. Cassette pumps col-

lect a small, specified amount of solution in a reservoir and then deliver that volume.

Pump rates are set for milliliters per hour and the fluid is then delivered at that rate. Because of their high degree of accuracy in terms of volume administered, these devices are best suited to situations in which the volume administered is critical, as in infants or TPN therapy.

Pumps do not depend on gravity to maintain a flow rate. Pressure is provided by a mechanism within the system. This positive pressure allows fluid to be administered into an arterial line, where pressure is needed to overcome the arterial blood pressure, or into a venous system. The same pressure is a disadvantage when infiltration occurs. The machine can continue to pump fluid into the tissue, causing extensive infiltration if the patient is not assessed, or monitored, frequently.

All pumps have multiple alarm systems that indicate when the infusion device is occluded, when air is in the system, when the desired infusion volume has been reached, and when the battery system needs to be charged. Alarms may alert you to other problems too, depending on the type of device(s) in use in your facility. Always test the alarm system to verify that the alarms are set to be audible because some devices can be set to silence the alarm. Multiple electronic infusion devices may be in use when the patient is an acutely ill individual receiving a variety of fluids and medications.

Some infusion control devices include a combination pump and controller (the user chooses the function desired) within one system. There are also pumps that deliver infusions through two separate channels with separate controls for each line (Fig 47-9).

Most pumps for ambulatory patients are designed to be very lightweight, less than 1 pound, and are programmed by microprocessors. These devices are commonly used in home care and pain management. Patients sometimes return to the hospital with their home medications infusing or with a need for assistance with infusion problems. Be sure to check the manufac-

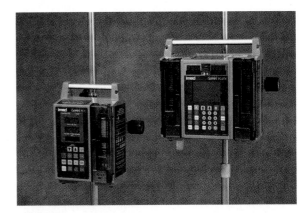

FIGURE 47-9 Volumetric electronic infusion controller/pumps. A single controller/pump may be used for primary infusions with a setting for secondary infusions or a dual-chamber controller/pump can be utilized for multiple infusions.

turer's directions for specific information on operating any individual pump.

There are also mechanical infusion devices that are called pumps that are not electronically dependent. Of the mechanical infusion devices, there are elastomer balloon types, spring-coil piston syringe types, and spring-coil container types (Alexander & Corrigan, 2004). These mechanical devices are more often used by patients in home infusion care to administer single-dose medications.

PROCEDURE FOR MONITORING AND MAINTAINING AN INFUSION

Monitoring involves looking for signs and symptoms of adverse outcomes and complications, such as **phlebitis** (or **thrombophlebitis**), **infiltration** (or **extravasation**), and obstruction of flow. These are discussed in detail below. Thus, most of the actions implemented are for the purpose of assessment. Maintaining the infusion includes taking actions to ensure patency, adjusting the rate, changing the site dressing, and changing the IV bag or bottle and tubing. These actions are needed to ensure appropriate outcomes of IV therapy and to avoid complications.

ASSESSMENT

1. Review the form used to monitor IV infusions in your facility, noting the following. **R:** This will identify whether an individual patient has IV fluids infusing.
   a. Number (dose or bag) of the IV infusing
   b. Ordered contents of the fluid container
   c. Time the IV container was hung
   d. Time the IV infusion is to be completed

2. Examine the IV therapy record for accuracy and completeness as prescribed by your facility. Note also if another IV infusion is to follow the one currently infusing. **R:** This determines when a new bag must be prepared.

3. Review information about the particular IV fluid infusing. **R:** This helps you to anticipate any complications that may result from the fluid.

ANALYSIS

4. Critically think through your data, carefully evaluating each aspect and its relation to other data. **R:** You need to determine specific problems for the patient in relation to IV therapy.

5. Identify specific problems and modifications of the procedure needed for the patient. **R:** Planning for the individual must take into consideration the individual's problems.

PLANNING

6. Determine individualized patient outcomes in relation to intravenous therapy. **R:** Identification of outcomes guides planning and evaluation. Include
   a. The right *patient* receives the right *intravenous fluid(s)* in the right *volume* at the right *rate* administered at the right *time.*
   b. The patient experiences the desired effect(s) from the IV fluid(s) administered.
   c. The patient experiences no adverse effect(s) from the IV fluid(s) administered.
   d. The patient experiences no discomfort at the IV site.

7. Plan your approach to monitoring the IV infusion and secure any equipment you will need, based on your assessment of the IV record. **R:** Planning ahead allows you to proceed more safely and effectively.

IMPLEMENTATION

Action	Rationale
8. Wash or disinfect your hands.	To decrease the transfer of microorganisms that could cause infection.
9. Identify the patient, using two identifiers. Each identifier is both on the patient (or provided verbally by the patient) and also on the patient's record, the medication administration record (MAR), or a special medication identification card. Acceptable identifiers include the patient's name, the patient's facility identification number, the patient's social security number, or birth date.	Verifying the patient's identity helps ensure that the right patient is receiving the right IV fluids.

(continued)

Action	Rationale
10. Explain that you are monitoring the IV infusion.	Explaining the procedure helps relieve anxiety or misperceptions that the patient may have about a procedure or activity and sets the stage for patient participation. This is a good opportunity for patient education.

11. Review the entire system. Check the following:
   a. IV bag or bottle
     (1) Note the date and time.
     (2) Verify that the number of the bag or bottle is correct.
     (3) Verify that the correct solution is infusing.
     (4) Note the fluid level in the bag or bottle. Verify that, at the current rate, the fluid will be infused at the designated time.
   b. Inspect the drip chamber.
     (1) Check that the drip chamber is filled to an appropriate level. There is usually a mark on the drip chamber indicating the level to which it should be filled.
     (2) Check that the fluid is dripping.
     (3) Check that the rate is correct.
   c. Check the tubing over its entire length for kinks or obstructions.
	These checks enable you to identify whether the current IV infusion is functioning according to the orders for therapy and to identify problems with the system.

12. Assess the IV site for signs and/or symptoms of phlebitis or infiltration:
   a. skin color and temperature
   b. swelling
   c. patient indicates or reports pain at the site
	The site should be smooth without marked pallor, redness, coolness, or edema. See Tables 47-1 and 47-2 for more information about complications.

13. If an armboard is being used, remove it periodically to provide range of motion to the arm or leg. Then replace the armboard.	This helps prevent stiffness in the joint and allows you to assess for discomfort, skin irritation, and circulatory impairment.
14. Critically think through the data gathered when examining the IV and identify specific problems for this individual.	This enables you to determine specific problems for this individual in relation to his or her IV infusion therapy.
15. If problems are detected, refer to the chart on troubleshooting IV problems (Table 47-3) and plan an appropriate course of action.	Planning ahead allows you to proceed more safely and effectively.
16. Carry out the action planned.	
17. Wash or disinfect your hands.	To decrease the transfer of microorganisms that could cause infection.

table 47-1. Evaluation and Treatment of IV Phlebitis

Assessment Grading Criteria	Interventions
1+ Pain at site*	1. Assess severity of phlebitis.
2+ Pain at site or along vein	2. Discontinue IV catheter.*
Mild erythema localized at site	3. Apply warm pack to site assessed 3+ or greater.
3+ Pain at site or along vein	4. Determine if drug/fluid is causative factor of phlebitis. Arrange for drug dilution or rate change, if
Erythematous at site and streaking along vein	appropriate.
4+ Pain and severe erythematous streak along vein	5. 3+ and 4+: Initiate QA Problem Record
Palpable cord or induration of vein area	6. 4+: Report problem to physician; obtain order for K-Pad treatment. Notify unit RN if he or she is to
	be involved in treatment plan.

*1+ Phlebitis—Intervention steps 3 and 4 may be initiated first to determine if mild pain relieved without removing IV catheter: reassess site in 1–2 h.
QA, quality assurance.
Courtesy of Swedish Hospital Medical Center.

table 47-2. Evaluation and Treatment of IV Infiltration

Assessment Criteria	Interventions
1+ Small area of swelling at or above IV site	1. Determine if infiltrated fluid/medication is a vesicant; refer to treatment of extravasation.
2+ Area of swelling around IV site >1″ and <2″	2. Assess severity of infiltrate: discontinue IV catheter.
3+ Area of swelling >2″; involves one surface or extremity	3. Grade 3+ and 4+: Elevate extremity on two pillows.
Skin cool over swollen area	4. Grade 4+: Notify unit RN and initiate QA Problem Record.
4+ Gross infiltrate involving circumference of extremity	
Skin very tight and cold to touch	

QA, quality assurance.
Courtesy of Swedish Hospital Medical Center.

EVALUATION

18. Evaluate using the individualized patient outcomes previously identified. **R:** Evaluation in relation to desired outcomes is essential for planning future care.
   a. The right *patient* received the right *intravenous fluid(s)* in the right *volume* at the right *rate* administered at the right *time*.
   b. The patient experienced the desired effect(s) from the IV fluid(s) administered.
   c. The patient experienced no adverse effect(s) from the IV fluid(s) administered.
   d. The patient experienced no discomfort at the IV site.

DOCUMENTATION

19. Complete right *documentation*. On the flow sheet, note that the correct IV infusion is running, (number and contents of bag or bottle), the rate at which it is running, and the appearance of the site. See Figure 47-10 for an example of a flow sheet. If a new IV bag or bottle was hung during your shift, indicate the time it was hung and the time it should be completed. **R:** Careful documentation ensures accuracy of IV administration by all nursing staff.

20. If any problems were identified and corrected, note them on the nurses' notes on the flow sheet, as prescribed by your facility. **R:** Documentation is a legal record of the patient's care and therapy and communicates nursing activities to other nurses and caregivers.

POTENTIAL ADVERSE OUTCOMES AND RELATED INTERVENTIONS

1. The patient experiences phlebitis. Phlebitis (inflammation of the vein) can be present with or without a clot in the vein. When there is a clot, the condition is technically thrombophlebitis. In practice, the two terms are used interchangeably. Phlebitis is characterized by redness, warmth, pain, and swelling at the IV site. It results from direct irritation of the vessel and seems to occur more rapidly when electrolytes (especially potassium) are in the solution and when antibiotics are being administered through the IV set.
Intervention: Assess the site utilizing the information in Table 47-1. When phlebitis occurs, the course of action is determined by the degree of the problem. See Table 47-1 regarding evaluation and treatment of IV phlebitis. The IV infusion may need to be stopped and then restarted at a new site. Use warm compresses on the site if this is part of your facility's protocol.

table 47-3. Troubleshooting IV Problems

Problem	Action	Rationale
1. IV off schedule	a. Calculate rate to finish IV over remaining time. If new rate is over 3 mL/min for adult or drastically changed (more than 20% increase), consider patient's condition, and consult with prescriber before increasing rate. b. Reset flow.	a. Fluid is absorbed and used over time. Too-rapid infusion will simply result in high urine output. If a patient's cardiovascular system is inadequate, fluid overload may occur. b. If fluid is behind schedule, infusing at original rate will result in inadequate fluid intake for 24-h period. c. Calculating new rate provides adequate fluids in an evenly distributed pattern. d. Exact rate may be critical to patient and should be determined by prescriber.
2. Incorrect solution	a. Slow rate to minimum. b. Initiate change to correct solution. c. Assess patient. d. Follow incident procedure for facility. e. Notify prescriber.	You may want to minimize amount of incorrect solution given without losing access to the vein. In some instances, the type of solution is critical, and laboratory tests may be necessary to determine action.
3. Tubing kinked	Straighten tubing and check flow rate again.	Kinked tubing slows flow rate. When kink is removed, rate may increase significantly.
4. Flow stopped	Take the following steps to reestablish flow: a. Look for obstruction of tubing and correct if present. b. Open regulator completely, move to new position, and regulate again if flow begins. c. Reposition arm. d. Place container lower than IV site to see if blood flows back, indicating cannula and tubing are patent. e. Gently raise cannula hub. If this starts flow, support hub with cotton ball or 2- × 2-inch gauze square. f. Note height of IV bag and adjust if it is not at least 3 feet above IV site. g. Obtain sterile syringe with needleless tip as used at your facility. Clean injection port closest to IV site with alcohol. Pinch off tubing above syringe and aspirate. Then open flow.	a. Pressure of arm, side rails, and other equipment can obstruct IV tubing. b. Changes in position or "fatigue" of plastic may alter flow rate. c. Flexing or twisting the forearm can obstruct vein proximally to IV site, stopping flow. d. Pressure in vein causes blood backflow when pressure in tubing is reduced. e. Cannula tip may be against wall of vein or a valve, obstructing flow. f. The force of gravity may not be adequate to overcome the pressure of the blood in the vein. g. Aspiration can remove clogged fluid. (Clot or clog moves into syringe and is removed, so it is not hazardous to patient.)
5. Bubbles in tubing	a. For a few small bubbles high in tubing: (1) Turn off flow. (2) Stretch tubing taut downward. (3) Flick tubing with fingernail. Bubbles will flow up to drip chamber. (4) Start flow, and regulate. b. For large amounts of air high in tubing: (1) Turn off flow. (2) Clean injection port with alcohol and insert syringe with needleless tip as used at your facility. (3) Open flow slowly. When air reaches the syringe, aspirate gently to remove the air. (4) Start flow and regulate. c. For air low in tubing, below last port: (1) Turn off flow. (2) Obtain sterile syringe with needleless tip as used at your facility. (3) Clean injection port with alcohol and insert syringe tip into port closest to the IV site. (4) Pinch tubing distal to port and close it off. (5) Aspirate air into syringe. Blood will return into tubing. (6) Start flow rapidly to flush out blood. (7) Regulate flow.	a. Air is lighter than fluid and therefore rises. b. Because air is lighter than fluid, it rises out of tubing when it reaches opening. c. Aspiration creates suction, pulling contents of tubing—including air—into syringe.
6. Drip chamber full of fluid, so drip is not visible	For flexible drip chamber: a. Pinch off tubing. b. Invert IV bag. c. Squeeze fluid back into IV bag. d. Hang up IV bag. e. Release tubing.	With drip chamber full, it is not possible to monitor fluid rate. When no fluid is squeezed into IV bag, air at top of bottle can enter drip chamber.

(continued)

table 47-3. Troubleshooting IV Problems (Continued)

Problem	Action	Rationale
7. Solution falls below drip chamber and fluid container is empty	a. If tubing is scheduled to be changed: (1) Slow drip rate. (2) Follow directions for changing IV bag and tubing. b. If tubing does not need to be changed: (1) Obtain next IV bag and syringe with needleless tip as used at your facility. (2) Connect tubing in use to new bag. (3) Fill drip chamber. (4) Clean injection port with alcohol and aspirate column of air through port on tubing. (5) Regulate flow rate.	a. Prevent IV from clotting off. b. Aspiration creates suction, pulling contents of tubing—including air—into syringe.

2. The patient experiences infiltration. Infiltration means that fluid moves into the tissue. It is also referred to as extravasation, which means the leaking of IV fluid out of the vein. Pallor, swelling, coolness, pain at the site, and usually a diminished IV flow rate are all indications of infiltration. Infiltration is caused most often by a cannula that dislodged and penetrated a vein wall. The term "cannula" refers to metal needles and various plastic IV access devices, although metal needles are not recommended for infusion purposes. Infiltration can occur around a cannula that has been in place for an extended period, has had fluids infusing at a high rate, or contained irritating fluids (such as those with high osmolarity, high or low pH, or high viscosity).

Intervention: Stop the infusion. Apply warm compresses and elevate the IV site if possible. The infusion will

IV FLOW RECORD

IV START DC	START : SITE	Ⓛ Hand		
	TIME / # ATTEMPTS	1100 / 1	/	/
	GAUGE / LENGTH	18 / 1 1/2"	/	/
	TYPE	Angiocath		
	D/C : TIME / SITE EVAL.	/	/	/
	CATHETER INTACT			
	CONVERTED TO HEP LOCK : TIME			
A B G	SITE / ALLENS TEST	/	/	/
	ECCHYMOSIS/HEMATOMA	/	/	/
	INITIALS	JL		

IV		2300 - 0700	0700 - 1500	1500 - 2300
	SITE EVALUATION TIME/CONDITION			1600 OK
	HOURLY BOTTLE CHECK	00-01-02-03 04-05-06-07	08-09-10-11 12-13-14-15	16-17-18-19 20-21-22-23
	DRESSING Δ / TUBING Δ	/	Ø / Ø	Ø / Ø
	INFUSION DEVICE:		Ø	Ø
	SITE EVALUATION TIME/CONDITION			
	HOURLY BOTTLE CHECK	00-01-02-03 04-05-06-07	08-09-10-11 12-13-14-15	16-17-18-19 20-21-22-23
	DRESSING Δ / TUBING Δ	/	/	/
	INFUSION DEVICE:			
	INITIALS		JL	EK

DATE	IV#	AMOUNT AND SOLUTION	ADDITIVES	INITL'S	TIME IV HUNG	TIME IV COMPLT	FLOW RATE CC/HR	INFU-SION DEVICE	SHIFT CHANGE STATUS TIME	IV#	#CC LEFT TO CNT
6/23/06	1	1000 ml LR		JL	1100	2100	100	Ø			
	2	1000 ml D5NS		EK	2100		100	Ø	22	2	900

FIGURE 47-10 IV flow record portion of 24-hour flow sheet. Space for nurse's signature is on another part of form.

need to be restarted in a new site. This may be done by a unit staff nurse or by an IV nurse depending upon hospital protocol.

3. The patient experiences infiltration (or extravasation) of a fluid containing a vesicant medication. Vesicant medications are highly irritating and damaging to the tissue.

Intervention: Stop the infusion. Aspirate any remaining fluid from the IV catheter. Leave the catheter in place until the prescriber has been contacted. Notify the prescriber and anticipate possible injection of medication to counteract the medication that is still in the IV catheter. Medication(s) also may be ordered for injection subcutaneously or intradermally around the IV site to further alleviate tissue damage. If no medication is ordered to be injected at the site, discontinue the IV catheter and arrange for the infusion to be restarted in another appropriate location. Depending on the medication, warm or cool compresses may be indicated. Verify treatment with a pharmacist or facility protocol.

4. The patient experiences an embolism. An embolism is a moving particle within the blood stream. The most common embolism is a clot. Air bubbles and small particles such as the end of an IV catheter that breaks off may also become emboli. Emboli in the venous system move toward the heart and are most likely to move through the heart and lodge in pulmonary blood vessels.

Intervention: Assess the type and cause of embolism. If the cause is air, place the patient in reverse Trendelenburg position and turn the patient to the left side. A large air embolism may lodge in the right side of the heart or the pulmonary vasculature, interfering with blood circulation to the lungs. Notify the prescriber. Provide oxygen to increase oxygenation of areas not affected by the embolism and comfort measures as needed. Anticipate further testing procedures such as chest x-ray or echocardiogram. If a foreign body embolism occurs, apply a tourniquet proximal to the IV site, if possible, to compress the affected vein and prevent movement of the **embolus** toward the heart. Be careful not to compromise arterial circulation to the entire extremity. Notify the prescriber. Anticipate the need for further testing and procedures to retrieve the embolic material.

5. The patient experiences leakage at the IV site. Leakage of the fluid around the site onto the skin and dressings may occur.

Intervention: Determine the cause of leakage. Check for loose connections at the needle hub with the IV tubing. Leaking also can be caused by infiltration or thrombophlebitis. If leakage continues, arrange for the infusion to be restarted at another location. Continue to observe the IV site for additional problems, such as bleeding, swelling, or tissue weeping.

6. The patient has signs of an allergic reaction. Local allergic reactions include rash and pruritus around the site. A systemic allergic response may include a rash anywhere on the body, shortness of breath, wheezing, and a cough.

Intervention: Assess severity, type, and cause of reaction. If allergic reaction is due to infusion or medication, stop the infusion or medication immediately. Change IV tubing and keep vein open with normal saline solution. Notify the prescriber. Anticipate medication administration to counteract the reaction. If allergic reaction is due to materials being used in IV infusion therapy, such as latex, immediately discontinue any offending supplies and replace with latex-free articles. Notify the prescriber and treat the reaction according to symptoms.

CALCULATING THE INTRAVENOUS INFUSION RATE

The IV drip rate must be regulated in drops per minute to provide the ordered quantity of fluid over the ordered period. Many manufacturers provide tables with this information, but the nurse should know how to compute the rate when tables are not available. Below are three methods of calculation. Try each of them and determine which works best for you. To calculate the rate using any of the methods, you need three pieces of information.

- Volume of fluid to be infused
- Length of time this volume of fluid is to run
- "Drop factor" (number of drops per milliliter) for the administration set, which is commonly found on the package. (Most administration sets provide 10 gtt/mL, 15 gtt/mL, or 20 gtt/mL. Microdrip sets and some controlled-volume sets provide 60 gtt/mL.)

METHOD 1

1. Divide the total volume by the number of hours to obtain the *milliliters per hour.*

$$\frac{\text{Total volume in mL}}{\text{Time in hours}} = \text{mL/hour}$$

Example: $\dfrac{1,000 \text{ mL}}{10 \text{ hours}} = 100 \text{ mL/hour}$

Note: This is the volume that would be set on most pumps. If you are regulating an infusion that is being controlled with an infusion pump or controller, consult the instructions for the specific device. Most pumps or controllers have to be programmed to the correct rate and total amount in the "reset mode," then turned to "operate" to start the flow.

If manually setting a drip rate, continue on.

2. Divide the milliliters per hour by 60 to obtain the *milliliters per minute.*

$$\frac{mL/hr}{60\ min} = mL/min$$

Example: $\dfrac{100\ mL/hr}{60\ min\ in\ 1\ hour} = 1.67\ mL/minute$

(round to 1.7)

3. Multiply the milliliters per minute by the drop factor to obtain the *drops per minute.*

$$mL/min \times drop\ factor = drops/min$$

Example: 1.7 mL/min × 15 drops/mL

= 25.5 drops/min (round to 26)

Note: The drop rate of microdrip sets that deliver 60 drops/mL is always equal to the number of milliliters per hour. Try a few examples using the method above to check this.

METHOD 2

A calculator is often used with this method because it involves large numbers.

Use the following formula:

Volume in mL × drop factor = Total drops
Hours to run × 60 minutes = Total time in minutes
Divide total drops by total time in minutes to find
 drops per minute.

METHOD 3 (DIMENSIONAL ANALYSIS)

To use the dimensional analysis method, you need the same information. The advantage of this method is that it helps you keep track more clearly of all units as well as numbers.

1. First, identify the amount of solution to be infused, the time over which it is to run, and the "drop factor" or number of drops that equal 1 mL of solution (found on the administration set package).

   For this example, the amount of solution is 1,000 mL over 8 hours, and the drop factor is 10 drops/mL. You need to set the rate in drops per minute.

2. Second, set up the problem by placing each of the values in a proportion. This proportion is set up with matching units above and below the line. For the example below, the 1,000 mL per 8 hours is the first part of the equation. Then choose a ratio that includes hours. The only ratio that would include hours is the relation between hours and minutes. There are 60 minutes in each hour. Put the hours above the line and the minutes below the line: 1 hour per 60 min. Then take the next set of num-

bers. You have drops per mL still to account for. The only mL is above the line so put that ratio with the mL below the line opposite the other mL you have in the equation, 10 drops per mL. Your final equation would be:

$$\frac{1,000\ mL}{8\ hour} \quad \frac{1\ hr}{60\ min} \quad \frac{10\ drops}{1\ mL}$$

3. Next, cancel out numbers and units from the upper and lower levels of the equation. Start with the numbers. The 1's above and below the line cancel one another out. The numbers 10 above the line and 60 below the line also cancel, as follows:

$$\frac{1,000\ mL}{8\ hour} \quad \frac{\cancel{1}\ hour}{\underset{6}{\cancel{60}}\ min} \quad \frac{\overset{1}{\cancel{10}}\ drops}{\cancel{1}\ mL}$$

4. Then cancel other numbers if possible. For example, the 1,000 and 8 cancel as follows:

$$\frac{\overset{125}{\cancel{1,000}}\ mL}{\underset{1}{\cancel{8}}\ hour} \quad \frac{\cancel{1}\ hour}{\underset{6}{\cancel{60}}\ min} \quad \frac{\overset{1}{\cancel{10}}\ drops}{\cancel{1}\ mL}$$

5. The goal is to end with the smallest number possible below the line. You can further cancel the numbers by dividing 6 into the 6 below the line and dividing 6 into the large number (125) left above the line. In any dimensional analysis, you can continue canceling numbers as long as possible. The goal is to end with the number one below the line if possible. The *numbers* further cancel as follows:

$$\frac{\overset{20.8}{\cancel{125}}}{\underset{1}{\cancel{8}}\ hour}\ \frac{\overset{1,000}{\cancel{1,000}}\ mL}{\underset{1}{\cancel{8}}} \quad \frac{\cancel{1}\ hour}{\underset{\underset{1}{6}}{\cancel{60}}\ min} \quad \frac{\overset{1}{\cancel{10}}\ drops}{\cancel{1}\ mL}$$

The *units* cancel as follows:

$$\frac{\overset{20.8}{\cancel{125}}}{\underset{1}{\cancel{8}\ hour}}\ \frac{\cancel{1,000}\ \cancel{mL}}{} \quad \frac{\cancel{1}\ \cancel{hour}}{\underset{\underset{1}{6}}{\cancel{60}}\ min} \quad \frac{\cancel{1}\ drops}{\cancel{1}\ \cancel{mL}}$$

6. Multiply each level across. You are left with 20.8 drops on top and 1 minute below.

$$\frac{20.8\ drops}{1\ min}$$

The answer is 20.8 drops per minute.
Note: Round up to 21 drops per minute because you cannot count tenths of a drop.

PROCEDURES FOR CHANGING THE IV BAG OR BOTTLE, TUBING, AND DRESSING

ASSESSMENT

1. Review the prescriber's orders. Pay particular attention to the type of fluid and solution concentration and to the infusion rate. Many abbreviations are used; three of the most common are for concentration of dextrose or saline solutions:

   5% dextrose in water = D_5W or 5% D/W
   5% dextrose in normal saline solution = D_5N/S or 5% D/NS
   Half-strength normal saline solution = ½ N/S

   If the prescriber's orders are unclear, verify with the prescriber. **R:** Thorough understanding of the orders helps to ensure safety and accuracy.
2. Verify when the tubing, dressing, and container were last changed. **R:** This will enable you to plan for changes at appropriate times. According to Infusion Nursing Standards of Practice, (Hankins, Lonsway, Hedrick, et al, 2001), continuous peripheral and central primary sets and secondary administration sets should be changed every 72 hours. However, if phlebitis rate is higher than 5%, or there is any increase in rate of catheter-related bacteremia, a return to 48 hour administration set changes should be implemented. The Infusion Nurses Society (INS) further recommends that IV dressings be changed with the administration set change whenever possible. Fluid containers should be changed every 24 hours. Follow the policy in your facility.

ANALYSIS

3. Critically think through your data, carefully evaluating each aspect and its relation to other data. **R:** You will need to determine specific problems for this individual in relation to IV therapy.
4. Identify specific problems and modifications of the procedure that are indicated for this individual. **R:** Planning for the individual must take into consideration the individual's problems and strengths.

PLANNING

5. Determine the individualized patient outcomes in relation to changing the IV bag or bottle. **R:** Identification of outcomes guides planning and evaluation.

a. The right *patient* is receiving the right *solution,* infusing at the right *rate.*
b. The tubing and IV bag or bottle are changed with no contamination.
c. The IV site is observed, and the dressing is replaced and dated.

6. If any specific problems or modifications are indicated, prepare your supplies and equipment accordingly. **R:** Planning ahead allows you to proceed more safely and effectively. Select the equipment:

   a. Fluid: Obtain the ordered fluid, using the three checks used in all medication administration situations (check the name and strength of the medication when obtaining the fluid, when the fluid is in hand, and just before administering the fluid). **R:** Recall that the right *drug,* the right *dose* (for IVs, strength and volume), the right *route,* and the right *time* are ensured by diligently completing the three checks. The name and dosage (strength and volume) of the fluid as written on the label are checked with the prescriber's orders or the IV fluid administration record three times. This ensures the right fluid and the right volume. In this situation, you will know that the route of administration is IV. These three times may differ somewhat depending on how the IV fluids are stored and what the procedure is in the individual facility. Reading labels carefully three times may seem cumbersome, but labels may be similar, and it is easy to "read" what you expect to be present if you look only one time. You will also check the correct time of administration on the IV fluid administration record to ensure the right time.
   b. Infusion set: Consider the volume of fluid to be administered and the rate. **R:** If a very slow rate is needed, a microdrip set will provide more accurate regulation. If medications are to be given, a set with multiple injection ports may be needed. For an infant or child, the use of a controlled-volume set is usually routine. When certain types of fluids are being administered or when certain routes are being utilized (central venous lines), protocols may require the use of a controlled-volume pump that requires specific tubing.
   c. Extension tubing if needed. **R:** Extension tubing gives the patient more mobility or allows for more access ports.
   d. Tape, if needed. **R:** To tape the IV line in place.
   e. Clean gloves. **R:** To protect yourself from exposure to blood.
   f. If you will be changing the dressing, gather the items you will need to redress the site according to your facility's procedure.

IMPLEMENTATION

Action	Rationale
7. Wash or disinfect your hands.	To decrease the transfer of microorganisms that could cause infection.
8. Identify the patient, using two identifiers.	Verifying the patient's identity helps ensure that you are performing the right procedure for the right patient.
9. Explain the procedure you are about to perform.	Explaining the procedure helps relieve anxiety or misperceptions that the patient may have about a procedure or activity and sets the stage for patient participation.
10. Raise the bed to an appropriate working position based on your height.	This allows you to use correct body mechanics and protect yourself from back injury.
11. Set up the IV bag and tubing.	
a. Examine the IV bag or bottle against a light to check for cracks or perforations, cloudiness, particulate matter, or other evidence of contamination. Check a plastic bag for leakage by squeezing lightly.	Careful inspection of the IV bag or bottle is critical for safe IV fluid administration. If abnormalities are present, the solution is potentially contaminated and should not be used. If in doubt, do not use the fluid. Select another container and save the potentially contaminated bag or bottle to be returned to the pharmacy or the central processing department. Squeezing will force fluid out if even a pinpoint hole is in the bag. Dampness on the outside of plastic bags is usually condensation from the sterilization procedure and is expected.
b. Open the package containing the tubing. Be sure to maintain the sterility of the connectors. If the connectors are covered with plastic caps, leave the plastic caps in place until you are ready to connect the tubing. Check the drop factor of the tubing.	To prevent contamination and to ensure using the correct drop factor when calculating the rate.
c. Open the entry area of the IV bag or bottle according to the manufacturer's directions. You should see evidence that the bag or bottle was sealed, which ensures sterility. Be careful not to contaminate the entry port. If medication was added to the bag or bottle by the pharmacy department, there should be a foil or plastic covering over the port that indicates medication has been added. Medication ports are usually separate from the entry port.	To provide correct access to the IV bag or bottle without contamination.
d. Follow the manufacturer's directions about cleaning the entry port with an alcohol wipe. Most IV bags are sealed, so the entry area is sterile and does not need to be cleaned if not contaminated.	To prevent fluid contamination if area entered by spike is not sterile.

(continued)

Action	Rationale
e. Close the regulator on the tubing.	So you do not inadvertently fill the tubing with air and spill fluid on the floor.
f. Insert the spike of the tubing into the IV bag or bottle through the correct entry port.	The spike of the tubing is designed to enter the entry port but not the port for adding medication.
g. Invert the IV bag or bottle with the tubing hanging down. It is convenient to hang the bag on a hook or IV pole at this time.	This action allows you to use gravity to fill the tubing.
h. For a flexible plastic drip chamber, squeeze the chamber to fill it half full with fluid. A rigid drip chamber usually fills when the fluid container is inverted.	A drip chamber half-full allows the drip rate to be monitored. If the chamber is full, it is impossible to monitor the drip rate.
i. Hold the end of the tubing over a basin or a waste container. Open the regulator gradually to allow the tubing to fill and to eliminate air in the tubing. Remove the cap if necessary to allow fluid to flow. Be sure all large bubbles are eliminated. Carefully replace the cap to prevent contamination when the tubing is full.	If the end of the tubing is tightly capped and does not have a cap that allows air to exit, the air in the tubing will not allow the fluid to flow. The cap must be carefully removed to allow the air to exit as the fluid fills the tubing. Some caps allow air to exit, but as soon as the fluid touches them, they seal. Large air bubbles can create an air embolus. Very tiny bubbles that together do not constitute a large bubble cannot cause an embolus that is dangerous, so there is no need for alarm if a small bubble is inadvertently administered. However, it is not wise practice to knowingly administer any air. Patients are often frightened if any air bubbles are administered and may need reassurance.
12. Hang the new bag or bottle on the IV pole beside the current container. Place a towel under the arm.	The towel will protect the linen from any spills.
13. Put gloves on.	To protect yourself from exposure to blood.
14. Change the IV bag or bottle and tubing.	
a. Gently remove the tape and dressing on the IV site to expose the hub of the cannula.	To avoid dislodging the cannula and facilitate observation.
b. Examine the IV site for signs of swelling or inflammation.	To check for phlebitis or infiltration.
c. When the hub is exposed, shut off the IV flow.	To prevent spilling.

(continued)

Action	Rationale
d. Hold the hub of the cannula firmly and remove the tubing with a slight twisting and/or pulling motion to disconnect.	To prevent dislodging the cannula.
e. Continue holding the hub of the cannula with one hand while you remove the cap of the new tubing and insert it firmly into the hub with the other; be careful not to push the hub further into the vein. Very slight pressure directly over the vein just medial to the tip of the catheter will help minimize blood spill. A sterile gauze pad placed at the front of the hub will catch any inadvertent blood spill.	The catheter hub must be stabilized to properly connect the tubing and to prevent patient discomfort. Light pressure over the vein will prevent blood flow. The gauze helps contain any blood spill.
f. Immediately start the new IV infusion at the appropriate rate.	The IV should be halted only briefly to prevent blood clotting or spilling.
g. Label the tubing according to facility policy.	The label should be current and reflect the information that is required by policy. Date changed, date to change next, time, and nurse's initials are commonly recorded. Some labels are color coded to reflect the day of the week changed, but the nurse should not rely on the color-coding system alone. Proper documentation is essential for good communication.
15. Change the dressing on the IV site according to your facility's procedure. If your facility has no specific guidelines, use the following:	
a. Clean the site. If the skin is obviously soiled, wash the area with soap and water. Alcohol should then be used to cleanse as an antiseptic and to remove debris, skin oils, or other contaminants. Next, utilize povidone-iodine solution as a bactericidal agent. Allow the solution to dry.	The antiseptic prepares the skin for the bactericidal agent. This three-step approach to skin prep will help prevent a skin-contaminant infection. Drying increases the bactericidal effect.
b. Apply an occlusive, or airtight, seal over the IV site with a transparent dressing. If the patient does not want to see the IV site, clean gauze may be applied over the transparent dressing, but it must be easy to remove so that the nurse can assess the site. Apply the transparent dressing up to but not over the cannula hub so that tubing changes can occur without dressing changes if necessary.	The transparent dressing is meant to keep the IV site free from contamination and to stabilize the IV site. The fewer times it is removed or changed, unless it is loose, soiled, or nonocclusive, will help to prevent contamination around the IV site.

(continued)

Action	Rationale
c. Stabilize the IV catheter hub with tape and secure the IV tubing with tape to minimize movement of the catheter and tubing. Remove and discard gloves.	Movement of the catheter hub and/or tubing could cause displacement of the IV, bleeding at the IV site, and discomfort to the patient.
d. Write the date, time of dressing change, and your initials directly on the tape to facilitate future assessment. The date and time of starting the IV may also be recorded on the tape each time the dressing is changed. In some facilities, a special adhesive label is used for this purpose.	Dressing changes should occur with each new IV start and as needed if the site is soiled or the dressing is nonocclusive. Anyone caring for the patient should be able to see by looking at the dressing label when the IV was started and when dressing changes have occurred.
16. Verify that the IV fluid is infusing at the correct rate.	IVs can be positional and cause alteration in IV infusion rate.
17. Dispose of any used supplies appropriately and wash or disinfect your hands.	Blood contaminated supplies should be disposed of according to facility policy. Red bags are often used for disposal of IV supplies. Any catheter or needle should be disposed of in a sharps container.

EVALUATION

18. Evaluate using the individualized patient outcomes previously identified. **R:** Evaluation in relation to desired outcomes is essential for planning future care.
   a. The right *patient* is receiving the right *solution,* infusing at the right *rate.*
   b. The tubing and IV bag or bottle were changed with no contamination.
   c. The IV site was observed and dressing is replaced and dated.

DOCUMENTATION

19. Complete right *documentation:* Document observations of the IV site and position as appropriate. Document according to your agency policy on the nursing care plan, the medication administration record, the IV flow sheet, and/or the patient's record. The exact time of the IV start and stop, dressing changes, and observations made should be documented in the patient's record. Document the volume of IV fluid taken in the area for intake on the I & O record area. Note the patient's response or any problems or complications related to therapy. **R:** Documentation is a legal record of the patient's care

and therapy and communicates nursing activities to other nurses and caregivers.

PROCEDURE FOR CHANGING THE IV BAG OR BOTTLE ONLY

ASSESSMENT

1. Review the prescriber's orders to determine the type of fluid.
2. Verify when the tubing and dressing were last changed. This helps you determine that there is no need for a tubing or dressing change at this time.

ANALYSIS

3. Critically think through your data, carefully evaluating each aspect and its relation to other data. **R:** This enables you to determine specific problems for this individual in relation to IV therapy.
4. Identify specific problems and modifications of the procedure that are indicated for this individual. **R:** Planning for the individual must take into consideration the individual's problems and strengths.

PLANNING

5. Determine individualized patient outcomes in relation to changing the IV bag or bottle, including the following. **R:** Identification of outcomes guides planning and evaluation.

a. The right *patient* receives the right *IV fluid* at the right *time*.

b. The correct *IV fluid* is infusing at the right *rate*.

c. The IV dressing is intact, and the site is clear.

6. Obtain the correct bag or bottle of fluid, using the three checks. The three checks ensure that it is the correct fluid ordered.

IMPLEMENTATION

Action	Rationale
7. Wash or disinfect your hands.	To decrease the transfer of microorganisms that could cause infection.
8. Identify the patient, using two identifiers.	It is essential to verify the patient's identification before administering any medications or IV fluids.
9. Explain what you are going to do, if appropriate. There may be no need to waken the patient if he or she is asleep because you can change the container without disturbing the patient (if you can safely identify him or her).	Explaining what you do will help to alleviate the patient's anxiety or fear. It is an excellent time for patient teaching also.
10. Remove the cover from the entry port and place the IV bag or bottle on the bedside stand or table.	So it will be within easy reach for connection.
11. Turn off the IV flow using the slide or screw clamp, or if the IV is on a pump, turn the pump to the correct mode.	To avoid the drip chamber emptying while in the process of changing the bag.
12. Invert the old IV bag or bottle.	To prevent any remaining fluid from spilling on the floor.
13. Remove the tubing spike from the old IV bag. Be careful not to contaminate the tubing spike by touching it.	Contamination of the tubing will contaminate the fluid.
14. Insert the tubing spike into the new IV bag or bottle.	To gain access to the fluid in the new IV bag or bottle.
15. Invert the new bag and hang it on the IV pole.	For convenience and safety.
16. Turn on the flow and regulate the rate.	With every IV bag or bottle change, the IV rate should be verified and checked so that the IV is infusing at the ordered rate.
17. Dispose of the old IV bag or bottle appropriately.	To prevent clutter at the bedside.
18. Wash or disinfect your hands.	To decrease the transfer of microorganisms that could cause infection.

EVALUATION

19. Evaluate using the individualized patient outcomes previously identified. **R:** Evaluation in relation to desired outcomes is essential for planning future care.
  a. The right *patient* received the right *IV fluid* at the right *time.*
  b. The right IV fluid is infusing at the right *rate.*
  c. The IV dressing is intact, and the site is clear.

DOCUMENTATION

20. Complete right *documentation.* **R:** Documentation is a legal record of the patient's care and therapy and communicates nursing activities to other nurses and caregivers. Document
  a. time of IV fluid change and exact contents of new IV bag or bottle
  b. volume of fluid infused from old IV bag or bottle
  c. assessment of IV site and dressing as facility policy requires

PROCEDURE FOR CHANGING A GOWN OVER AN IV LINE

Changing the gown of a patient with an IV infusion running can present a challenge. In some facilities, gowns with shoulder seams that open and close with snap fasteners are available for patients with IVs. If such gowns are not available, use the following procedure:

Removing a Soiled Gown

1. Remove the gown from the free arm and chest. Gather the sleeve on the IV arm until it forms a compact circle of fabric. Hold this circle firmly (Fig. 47-11).
2. Move the sleeve down over the arm, being particularly careful as you pass over the IV site. The sleeve should now be around the tubing, not around the arm.
3. Move the gown up the tubing toward the IV bag or bottle.
4. Remove the IV bag or bottle from the IV pole.
5. Slip the gown over the IV bag or bottle.
6. Rehang the IV bag or bottle.

Putting on a Clean Gown

Proceed in the opposite direction.
1. Gather the appropriate sleeve of the gown into a firm circle and remove the IV bag or bottle from the IV stand.
2. Carefully move the gown over the tubing and onto the arm.
3. Remove the IV bag or bottle from the IV stand.
4. Slip the gown over the IV bag (see Fig. 47-11).
5. Rehang the IV bag.

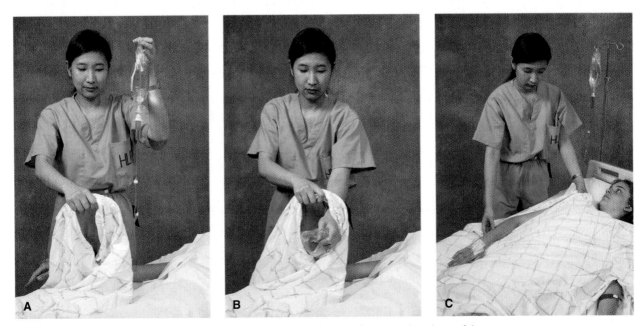

FIGURE 47-11 To change a patient's gown with an IV line in place, (**A**) gather the appropriate sleeve of the gown into a firm circle and remove the IV bag or bottle from the IV pole or stand. (**B**) Slip the gown over the IV bag and tubing and rehang the IV bag. (**C**) Take the fresh gown and reverse the process.

6. Carefully move the gown over the tubing and onto the arm.
7. Adjust the gown on the IV arm.
8. Place the patient's other arm in the gown and fasten the gown.

PROCEDURE FOR DISCONTINUING AN IV INFUSION

ASSESSMENT

1. Check the orders carefully. **R:** It is painful as well as expensive for patients to have an IV restarted after it has been discontinued by mistake.

ANALYSIS

2. Critically think through your data, carefully evaluating each aspect and its relation to other data.

R: This enables you to determine specific problems for this individual in relation to IV therapy.

3. Identify specific problems and modifications of the procedure that are indicated for this individual. **R:** Planning for the individual must take into consideration the individual's problems and strengths.

PLANNING

4. Determine individualized patient outcomes in relation to discontinuing the IV, including the following. **R:** Identification of outcomes guides planning and evaluation.
   a. The intravenous infusion is discontinued.
   b. Any bleeding is controlled.
   c. The catheter or cannula removed is intact.
5. Select the necessary equipment. **R:** Planning ahead allows you to proceed more efficiently and effectively.
   a. Sterile 2- × 2-inch gauze square
   b. An adhesive bandage or tape
   c. Clean gloves

IMPLEMENTATION

Action	Rationale
6. Wash or disinfect your hands.	To decrease the transfer of microorganisms that could cause infection.
7. Identify the patient, using two identifiers.	Proper patient identification is necessary to ensure you are treating the correct patient.
8. Explain to the patient what you plan to do.	To alleviate anxiety and fear and to provide an opportunity for patient teaching.
9. Shut off the IV flow.	To prevent IV fluid from dripping out of the IV catheter.
10. Carefully remove the tape and dressing.	Skin that is fragile requires special care to prevent tearing. Hair is likely to be pulled, and moistening the area with a wet cloth or alcohol swab will help to remove the dressing. Some facilities provide adhesive remover swabs for dressing removal.
11. Put on clean gloves.	To protect against blood exposure.
12. Hold the sterile 2- × 2-inch gauze square above the entry site. Be ready to apply pressure as soon as the needle is out.	Pressure after catheter removal will help prevent bleeding, but pressure during catheter removal can damage the blood vessel.
13. Pull IV cannula out and immediately put pressure on the site.	To control bleeding.

(continued)

Action	Rationale
14. Keep pressure on the site until bleeding is controlled.	People may bleed easily depending on medications they take or on their medical condition. Observe closely for any signs of continued bleeding or hematoma formation.
15. Put an adhesive bandage or tape over the site.	A light dressing will help to prevent and contain bleeding.
16. Remove all the equipment from the bedside. Be sure to note the volume of fluid remaining in the IV bag.	Remove equipment to prevent clutter at the bedside. Note fluid remaining to record intake accurately.
17. Wash or disinfect your hands.	To decrease the transfer of microorganisms that could cause infection.

EVALUATION

18. Evaluate using the individualized patient outcomes previously identified. **R:** Evaluation in relation to desired outcomes is essential for planning future care.
    a. Intravenous infusion was discontinued.
    b. Bleeding was controlled.
    c. The catheter or cannula removed was intact.

DOCUMENTATION

19. Complete right *documentation.* **R:** Documentation is a legal record of the patient's care and therapy and communicates nursing activities to other nurses and caregivers.
    a. On the flow sheet or nurses' notes, document that the IV infusion was discontinued with catheter intact, your assessment of the site, and the time.
    b. On the intake and output sheet, document the intake from the IV infusion that occurred on your shift. To do this accurately, check whether any fluid was administered on the previous shift and subtract that amount from the total amount of fluid administered from the discontinued bag.

skill in accessing the venous system is required. For care of critically ill patients over long periods of time, long-term IV access is often achieved with a central venous line, peripherally inserted central catheter (PICC), or even implanted ports (IPs). These are discussed in more detail in Module 49.

Long-Term Care

Because an increased number of people are being admitted to long-term care facilities for rehabilitation or transitional care before returning home, IV infusions and electronic infusion control devices are being seen with greater frequency in these settings. Although the procedures themselves vary little from those used in acute care settings, fragile residents need especially careful monitoring. Increased susceptibility to peripheral infections, fragility of veins, and risk for fluid volume overload demand more frequent and meticulous inspection of IV sites and schedules.

Acute Care

In acute care settings, IV therapy is usually required as part of the nursing care. Often, patients are admitted to acute care settings primarily to receive medications, tests, or treatments that necessitate the administration of IV fluids. In emergency situations, nursing

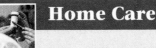

Home Care

Home infusion therapy has become quite common and is related to early discharge from hospitals as well as the need for IV therapy or medications in the treatment of many chronic conditions. In addition, the recognition that hospitalization can be a stressful and disruptive event for clients, especially children, has led hospitals, home health agencies, and private enterprises to set up programs for home infusion therapy.

If you are employed in an acute or chronic care facility and are aware that the individual for whom you are caring will be going home on IV fluids, you will need to coordinate your teaching with that of the agency responsible for overseeing this aspect of care. Generally, the focus of the teaching program is to prepare clients, family members, or other caregivers to administer the required IV therapy safely and independently, using the equipment required.

Teaching requires a careful assessment of caregiver ability, equipment required, and the home setting. Physical, learning or mental disabilities, fear, language barriers, and distance from supervising agencies can play a part in problems that can be encountered in home infusion therapy.

Ambulatory Care

In many respects, ambulatory infusion care is like home infusion care. Home care often involves clients who are considered home-bound, but ambulatory clients are often active and may even work outside the home if their condition allows. They may be given care at an infusion center or may self-administer their therapy at home. These clients need support to allow maximum mobility and convenience for the duration of their infusion therapy. Because their therapy may be for very long periods of time, periodic evaluations at home or at the infusion center are necessary because of increased risk of complications over time (Weinstein, 1997).

LEARNING TOOLS

DEVELOP YOUR BACKGROUND KNOWLEDGE

1. Review the Learning Outcomes.

2. Read the section on preparing and maintaining IV infusions in your assigned text.

3. Look up the Key Terms in the glossary.

4. Review this module and mentally practice the techniques described. Study so that you would be able to teach these skills to another person.

5. Think about how to change a patient's gown if two fluids are infusing through a controller or pump.

6. Practice the documentation for infusion therapy skills as required by your facility.

DEVELOP YOUR SKILLS

In the practice setting

1. Examine the IV equipment available. Identify as many of the following as possible:
   a. microdrip (pediatric) sets and macrodrip sets; differentiate between the two
   b. secondary administration sets (piggybacks)
   c. safety needles and needleless devices
   d. extension tubing
   e. filters
   f. controlled-volume sets (Peditrol, Soluset, Volutrol)
   g. IV poles
   h. IV bags and bottles
   i. any infusion control devices available
   j. armboards

2. Read the directions on the package regarding how to set up the equipment you will be using.

3. Working in pairs, do each of the following. Be sure each student has the opportunity to perform each skill.
   a. Set up an IV line as if it were to be started. Pay particular attention to maintaining sterility.
   b. Attach the end of the IV line to another fluid container, so the fluid will run from the first container to the second. This will simulate an ongoing IV line.
   c. Regulate the drip rate by manual control and by using an infusion control device:
      (1) to 32 drops/minute
      (2) to whatever rate would be needed to deliver the fluid remaining in the IV bag in 4 hours. You will need to figure the drip rate. Consult the tubing package to identify the drops per milliliter delivered by the tubing.
   d. Change the IV bag or bottle only.
   e. Change the IV bag or bottle and IV tubing and redress.
   f. Set up an IV using a pump or controller. Set the rate for 125 mL per hour, using the device according to the manufacturer's directions. Change the rate to 42 mL per hour. Occlude the tubing by bending it close to where it enters the arm. See how the alarm responds and use the various controls to correct the occlusion problem. Empty the drip chamber. See how the alarm responds to this problem and use the various controls to correct the air in the system problem.

g. Using a mannequin, remove and replace a gown with the IV in place.

h. Remove the IV from the mannequin's arm as if you were discontinuing the IV.

4. Practice documentation for the following situations. Compare your work with that of your partner.

a. You have hung an IV, 1,000 mL D₅W, to be given over 8 hours from 4:00 p.m. to 12:00 midnight.

b. You are maintaining an IV, and it is the end of your shift. On the previous shift, 1,000 mL D₅W was started. When your shift began, 100 mL had been given; 50 mL remain now. (Simulate any observation data that would be needed.)

c. You are carrying out an order to discontinue an IV. The entire amount, 500 mL normal saline solution, has been given.

DEMONSTRATE YOUR SKILLS

In the clinical setting

1. Consult with your instructor regarding the opportunity to regulate an IV using gravity, a controller, and a pump; set up an infusion to be administered; change a glass bottle and tubing; change an IV bag and tubing; change an IV dressing; and discontinue an IV under supervision. Document each skill. Have your instructor evaluate your performance.

CRITICAL THINKING EXERCISES

1. It is the beginning of your shift and you are doing a routine assessment of all IVs for which you are responsible. When you inspect Mr. Bear's IV site, you find it to be cool and edematous. You find that the infusion is infusing slower than the prescribed rate. Explain what you think is the problem and how to take corrective action if indicated.

2. Infusion therapy is ordered for your female patient who is febrile and dehydrated. She states that she has never had an IV infusion before and she doesn't understand why she needs it. What teaching will you do with this patient?

SELF-QUIZ
SHORT-ANSWER QUESTIONS

1. What type of administration set is best to use for administering fluids to a young child?

2. What type of set is used to administer a "piggy-back" IV medication?

3. What is one advantage, in terms of sterility, of the plastic bag over the glass bottle?

4. What is the proper action if the fluid in the IV bag or bottle has particulate material?

5. If two IV bags are to be hung on a Y set, what are the two ways to make sure that the appropriate one empties first?

a. _____

b. _____

6. Calculate the drop rate for each of the following problems:

a. 1,000 mL to be given over 8 hours; the drop factor is 15 gtt/mL.

b. 650 mL to be given over 4½ hours; the drop factor is 10 gtt/mL.

c. 200 mL to be given over 2 hours; the drop factor is 20 gtt/mL.

d. 100 mL to be given over 3 hours using a micro-drip set, which delivers 60 gtt/mL.

7. How often should the entire IV setup be changed?

8. Why is it important to regulate the drip rate exactly?

9. What are two measures that will stop bleeding after an IV is discontinued?

a. _____

b. _____

10. Give five possible causes of IV flow obstruction.

a. _____

b. _____

c. _____

d. _____

e. _____

11. What are four common symptoms of phlebitis at the IV site?

    a. _____

    b. _____

    c. _____

    d. _____

12. What are five common symptoms of infiltration of the IV?

    a. _____

    b. _____

    c. _____

    d. _____

    e. _____

13. List six major elements that are part of a routine assessment of an IV.

    a. _____

    b. _____

    c. _____

    d. _____

    e. _____

    f. _____

MULTIPLE CHOICE

_____ 14. Factors that may contribute to thrombophlebitis include which of the following? (Choose all that apply.)
    a. Viscosity of solution
    b. pH of solution
    c. Size of catheter

_____ 15. Common sources of bacterial contamination causing IV associated infections may include which of the following sources? (Choose all that apply.)
    a. Skin
    b. Hair
    c. Blowing respirations

_____ 16. To prevent fluid volume overload, the nurse should consider which of the following actions? (Choose all that apply.)
    a. Administer the fluid at the prescribed rate.
    b. Have the patient sit upright at all times.
    c. Check the IV volume infused at frequent, regular intervals.
    d. Utilize the roller clamp to regulate the flow at the drops per minute required to deliver the prescribed rate.

_____ 17. Preparation for the IV infusion includes which of the following steps? (Choose all that apply.)
    a. Verifying prescriber orders
    b. Verifying patient identification
    c. Patient teaching

_____ 18. Stopcocks are utilized for which of the following purposes? (Choose all that apply.)
    a. To allow multiple injection sites
    b. To control flow of fluids or medications
    c. To prevent bacterial contamination

_____ 19. Screw-on devices assist in IV therapy because they provide which of the following? (Choose all that apply.)
    a. A secure connection between tubings
    b. A filter to eliminate air
    c. A back valve to prevent backflow of fluids and medication

Answers to the Self-Quiz questions appear in the back of the book.

MODULE 48

Administering Intravenous Medications

SKILLS INCLUDED IN THIS MODULE

General Procedure for Administering Intravenous Medications
Specific Procedures for Administering Intravenous Medications
  Administering Medication by IV Push Into an Infusing IV
  Administering Medication Into an Intermittent Infusion Adapter (IV Lock)
  Using a Small-Volume Parenteral Drug Delivery System
  Using a Syringe Infusion Pump
  Using a Patient-Controlled Analgesia Pump
  Using a Controlled-Volume Administration Set
  Adding Medication to a New IV Bag or Bottle
  Adding to an Infusing IV Bag or Bottle

PREREQUISITE MODULES

Module 1	An Approach to Nursing Skills
Module 2	Documentation
Module 4	Basic Infection Control
Module 5	Safety in the Healthcare Environment
Module 11	Assessing Temperature, Pulse, and Respiration
Module 12	Measuring Blood Pressure
Module 13	Monitoring Intake and Output
Module 14	Nursing Physical Assessment
Module 24	Basic Sterile Technique: Sterile Field and Sterile Gloves
Module 44	Administering Oral Medications
Module 46	Administering Medications by Injection
Module 47	Preparing and Maintaining Intravenous Infusions

KEY TERMS

additive	IV lock
bolus	laminar airflow
compatible	hood
diluent	phlebitis
flashback	piggyback
heparin lock	psi
intermittent	thrombophlebitis
infusion adapter	venipuncture

OVERALL OBJECTIVE

▸ To prepare and administer intravenous (IV) medications, using an IV access device that is in place and one of the following methods: a controlled-volume administration set, a small-volume container, a syringe infusion pump, a patient-controlled analgesia (PCA) infuser, or an intermittent infusion adapter (IV lock or heparin lock).

LEARNING OUTCOMES

The student will be able to

1. Assess the patient regarding the need for administration of intravenous (IV) medications.
2. Analyze the assessment data to determine special needs or concerns that must be addressed to administer IV medications safely.
3. Determine appropriate patient outcomes of the IV medication administered and recognize the potential for adverse outcomes.
4. Administer IV medication(s) accurately, using appropriate supplies and equipment, while maintaining comfort and safety for the patient.
5. Evaluate the effectiveness and safety of the IV medication administered.
6. Document the IV medication administered and the care provided in the patient's record as appropriate.

The use of intravenous (IV) medications is common in patient care. There are numerous reasons for IV medications to be given. Among them are to give rapid onset of action, to avoid discomfort of frequent intramuscular or subcutaneous medication, or to maintain a blood level of medication, or the medication prescribed is only formulated for IV use. Often, critically ill patients need IV access for emergency drug use in the event of rapid physiologic changes. Sterile technique must be faultless to prevent infection, and all aspects of the procedure must be performed correctly. Of course, careful attention to the three checks and six rights (see Module 44) is always necessary for safety.

NURSING DIAGNOSES

- Risk for Injury: The major nursing diagnosis to keep in mind when administering IV medications is Risk for Injury. Patients can be injured by IV medications given in the wrong dose, at the wrong time, or at an incorrect rate of speed. They also can be injured by the omission of essential medications, the administration of an incorrect medication, or inaccurate documentation. Patients also are at risk for injuries related to tissue irritation from the equipment or the medication being administered. Although this nursing diagnosis will not appear on the nursing care plan, it applies to every situation in which a patient is receiving an IV medication.
- Deficient Knowledge: Another nursing diagnosis to consider for administration of IV medication is Deficient Knowledge. Patients need to know about the medications they are receiving. Basic information includes the purpose of the medication, the expected effect(s) of the medication, side effects that are common to the medication, what adverse effects to report to their caregiver, and what general care considerations need to taken. More in-depth education can be provided as the patient is ready for it.

An example of giving the basic information could be as follows: "Mrs. Green, this is the IV medication to help bring your blood pressure down. You may feel slightly warm or drowsy and tired as it takes effect in the next few minutes. Please tell me if you develop a headache, changes in vision, or any other problems. I will be checking your blood pressure every 5 minutes for the next 15 minutes or until your blood pressure returns to the desired level."

DELEGATION

Administration of IV medications is not delegated to assistive personnel in any care facility. They may be asked to observe for and report specific effects (both desired and adverse) of medications the nurse has administered. Nursing assistants may also inform the nurse of situations in which a medication, such as an analgesic, may be needed. However, the nurse is responsible for assessing the need for a prn medication before administering it. The nurse is always responsible for evaluating the effect(s) of all medications administered.

Patients are discharged with IV medications to be given at home. The patient, a family member, a partner, or a close friend may be taught to give an IV medication. In these situations, the nurse is responsible for teaching the specific technique for the specific patient for the use of a specific drug. Usually, a home health nurse is accessed to provide oversight, assessment, and evaluation.

HAZARDS OF ADMINISTERING INTRAVENOUS MEDICATIONS

The nurse must be aware of the potential hazards of IV medications. The medication that rapidly has a positive effect may also exhibit a negative effect rapidly. An IV medication is circulated rapidly throughout the body (average circulation time ranges between 18 and 24 seconds), and adverse systemic reactions may be life threatening. The major danger is from reactions that interfere with respiratory, circulatory, or neurologic functions. Whenever a medication is given intravenously, observe for a change in respirations or pulse rate, chills or flushing, rash, nausea, or headache. These can be early signs of severe reaction. If any of these occur, discontinue the medication, carefully assess the patient, and notify the prescriber. In addition to these general symptoms, be aware of the possible adverse reactions specific to the medication being given and of possible adverse effects of drugs that affect only certain people.

PHLEBITIS AND THROMBOPHLEBITIS

Many IV medications irritate the vein and can cause skin redness and swelling over the vein, a condition known as **phlebitis.** This may involve the formation of a clot, which is then termed **thrombophlebitis.**

The rate of instillation also can affect the degree of irritation to the vein, which can cause the patient discomfort. Administering the medication slowly allows the drug to become diluted by the flow of blood in the vein, which makes it less irritating and less painful.

DRUG INCOMPATIBILITIES

Drug incompatibilities can alter or negate the effects of drug(s) or, more seriously, cause the patient to experience adverse reactions. Factors that can affect compatibility are concentration of the drug, length of time in contact, ionic or electrolyte strength, and pH level.

Drug incompatibilities can be physical or chemical. A physical incompatibility is visible and may be evidenced by precipitation, color change, cloudiness, or the formation of gas bubbles. Chemical incompatibilities can cause the drugs to become inactive or toxic. For example, antibiotics often become unstable when the pH of a solution is very high or very low. Important ways to prevent incompatibilities include always checking a reference for this information before administering an IV medication and becoming knowledgeable about the drug classes that are likely to cause this problem.

The appropriate speed of instillation can be related to the effect of the medication, either a desired or adverse effect. For example, if the patient has suddenly become seriously ill, the prescriber may order a drug to be given as rapidly as possible to achieve the desired effect. In other situations, a slow administration allows for gradual adaptation of the body to the effect and limits such problems as a drop in blood pressure related to the medication.

The literature accompanying the medication (package insert information) is an excellent source of information about incompatibilities and about the appropriate **diluent** (diluting fluid), amount of diluent, and how slowly or rapidly to give the medication. If the literature is not available or does not answer your questions, consult a drug reference book for nurses, or contact a pharmacist for assistance.

CARDIOVASCULAR OR NEUROLOGICAL RESPONSE

Many medications when given intravenously may precipitate a sudden drop in blood pressure, cardiac irregularities, and a shock-like response. This is more likely to occur if the medication is given too rapidly. Other medications can cause dizziness, light-headedness, and even a decreased level of consciousness when given too rapidly. The rate of administration is critical to safe administration of IV medications. Always inject according to manufacturer's guidelines, but if none are given, a general rule may be that no syringe-held bolus should be given faster than 1 mL per minute.

ADMINISTRATION EQUIPMENT

There are many kinds of equipment used to administer IV medications. The equipment chosen depends on one or more of the following factors: the medication itself, the volume needed, and the speed with which it is to be administered.

EQUIPMENT FOR BOLUS OR PUSH IV MEDICATIONS

IV medications are sometimes ordered to be given as a **bolus,** or push, which means that a measured amount of medication, diluted or undiluted, is manually instilled directly into the vein by **venipuncture** or through some type of IV device that is in place. When this is the case, the basic equipment is the same as for an intramuscular injection.

SYRINGE SELECTION

To begin, select the size of syringe appropriate for the quantity of medication. A small syringe exerts greater pressure measured as **psi** (pounds per square inch) and a larger syringe exerts less pressure (lower psi). A very small syringe may create enough pressure to damage the vein if the plunger is depressed rapidly. Therefore, the rate of administration should be adjusted based on the syringe size.

SAFER ACCESS DEVICES

Most facilities require the use of needleless devices for medication administration. In 1999, it was reported that up to 40 percutaneous injuries (needle sticks) occurred per 100 occupied beds for teaching hospitals and 34 per 100 for nonteaching facilities (Shelton & Rosenthal, 2004). As a result of many healthcare workers suffering needle sticks and some contracting bloodborne infections from these needle sticks, in November 2000, the U.S. Congress passed the Needlestick Safety and Prevention Act. This act requires all health facilities receiving Medicare or Medicaid funds to monitor and track all needle-stick injuries; involve healthcare workers in the selection and evaluation of new, safer alternatives to needles; and develop needle-stick prevention plans. As a result of the demand created by this legislation, many products have become available. Nurses should participate in selecting effective equipment and become familiar with the devices available at their facilities.

Several types of devices that protect the staff from accidental needle sticks are available for use when drawing up medications and for injecting medications into IV access devices. Needleless devices use a short male adapter that fits into a hub on the IV lock or on the IV line. The needle-lock-type device has a needle with a rigid clear plastic cover that slides over the injection port, guides the needle into the injection port, and secures the needle in place while protecting fingers from potential contact with the needle.

A needleless device is preferred for drawing up and administering any medication, but the principles of administration are the same whether a needle or needleless device is used. A small-gauge device may deliver medication but restricts flow and may not be appropriate for a viscous medication. A large-gauge device will deliver the medication and facilitate the injection of a more viscous medication.

Not all needleless systems are **compatible;** this can be problematic when patients are admitted from home to a facility that uses different products or when patients are transferred between facilities that do not use compatible products. If the nurse plans to continue using the existing IV site, the current products can be removed from the cannula hub and replaced with products that are compatible with those in use at the receiving facility.

INTERMITTENT INFUSION ADAPTORS

An **intermittent infusion adapter,** also called an **IV lock** (saline lock or **heparin lock**) is designed to provide ready access to a vein without having an IV infusing continuously. A cannula is placed in the vein. Attached to the cannula hub is a cap that can be accessed by use of a male adapter (usually with a screw-type connection), or it may have a very short tubing with an entry port at the end. Normal saline or dilute heparinized saline solution is injected through the port to fill the IV cannula and associated tubing and port. This solution prevents blood from entering the cannula and coagulating and blocking the needle. Whenever the lock is used, it must be refilled with fresh normal saline or heparinized saline solution. If heparinized saline solution is used, most

facilities use 10 IU (International Units) of heparin in 1 mL of solution and instill up to 3 mL of solution.

Positive-pressure flush technique is very effective in maintaining patency of IV tubing when saline solution alone is used. However, research in pediatric IV therapy indicates increased patency and less tenderness when IV tubing is flushed with heparinized saline solution; studies focused on neonatal IV therapy showed no patency differences between use of saline solution alone or heparinized saline solution as long as the IV line was flushed every 4 hours (Hankins, Lonsway, Hedrick, et al, 2001). Each facility has a policy regarding flushing IV locks.

CLEANSING AGENTS AND TAPE

An alcohol wipe is needed to clean any surface being punctured to access the venous system. Tape has often been used to reinforce the attachment of an access device in the cannula hub. Because the sticky residue left by tape may attract microorganisms, needleless devices with a screw-type connector or needle-lock devices at points of attachment are preferred.

EQUIPMENT FOR ADDITIVE IV MEDICATIONS

The IV bag or bottle has a special entry port for adding medications. In some facilities, medications are added to IV fluids only in the pharmacy where an area of minimal contamination from microorganisms is maintained through the use of a **laminar airflow hood.** If an IV **additive** is added on the nursing unit, the nurse is responsible to add the medication to the container in an area that is as free from potential contamination as possible.

When adding medications to IV fluids, the nurse takes precautions to ensure that the medication and the fluid are thoroughly mixed. If a medication is lighter or heavier than the solution, it tends either to float or to fall to the bottom of the container, which means that the patient receives a concentrated dose of the added medication rather than the desired mixture. To prevent this, thoroughly agitate the IV bag or bottle before administering. If the added medication has a lipid or oil base, shake the container every 15 to 30 minutes during the infusion. Commercially prepared solutions with a lipid or oil base are prepared as emulsions and do not require the frequent agitation of the infusion.

A small-volume container holds 50 to 100 mL of solution containing the prescribed drug. It is used to administer a small volume of medication that must be diluted. The medication is added to the container in the pharmacy or on the nursing unit, and the container is then hung from an IV pole as a secondary administration set.

A controlled-volume administration set (Peditrol, Soluset, Volutrol) is attached to a regular, large IV bag or bottle. This set allows a measured volume of fluid to be withdrawn from the large container. The medication can then be added to the controlled-volume reservoir and given at the appropriate rate.

GENERAL PROCEDURE FOR ADMINISTERING INTRAVENOUS MEDICATION

Use the General Procedure for Administering Oral Medications, Module 44, as the basis for the General Procedure for Administering Intravenous Medications, with the modifications noted below.

ASSESSMENT

1. Verify the prescriber's orders for the medication. **R:** Verification confirms the need for administering an IV medication.
2. Examine the medication administration record (MAR). Check the patient's name and room number, the name of the medication, the dosage, and the time(s) the medication is to be given. Check for any medication allergies. Note especially whether the ordered medication has already been given or is to be held. **R:** Doing this ensures accuracy and completeness as prescribed by your facility.
3. Assemble information on the drug, including its *effects*, whether or not it needs to be *diluted*, and if so, with *what diluent*; *amount of diluent*; *rate of administration*; and *compatibility* with other IV fluids or medications being given. Also check the expected actions and potential adverse reactions. **R:** This ensures that the medication can be given safely with the current IV fluid being given or with heparinized saline solution (if it is in the IV lock) and that you are prepared to act promptly should an adverse response occur.
4. Assess the patient to see what type of IV access is present—that is, whether an existing IV infusion is running, whether an IV lock is in place, or whether a venipuncture must be performed to administer the medication. **R:** To enable you to select the correct equipment.

5. Follow step 5 of the General Procedure for Administering Oral Medications: Assess the patient for the need for prn medications. **R:** This enables you to give all medications in an organized manner.

ANALYSIS

6. Critically think through your data, carefully evaluating each aspect and its relation to other data. **R:** This enables you to determine concerns in relation to administration of this particular IV medication.
7. Identify specific problems and modifications of the IV medication procedure needed for this individual. **R:** Planning for the individual must take into consideration the individual's problems.

PLANNING

8. Determine the individualized patient outcomes in relation to the medication(s) to be administered, including the following. **R:** Identification of outcomes guides planning and evaluation.
   a. The right *patient* receives the right *medication* in the right *dose* by the right *route* at the right *time*.
   b. The medication is given over the correct length of time.
   c. The patient experiences the desired effect(s) from the medication(s) administered.
   d. The patient experiences no adverse effect(s) from the medication(s) administered.
9. Determine the equipment you will need for the specific technique to be used. If the patient has been receiving IV medications, there may be some equipment in the room. Always plan to use a sterile device for accessing the venous system. **R:** Often, the prescriber's orders specify the method of IV administration. Alternatively, the pharmacist may make that decision based on the medication (Box 48-1). If access to the vein is not present, the medication must be given by a nurse skilled in venipuncture. When multiple IV push medications are needed, the nurse may request an order for an IV lock from the prescriber. **R:** Planning ahead allows you to proceed more safely and effectively.

IMPLEMENTATION

Action	Rationale
10-14. Follow steps 10 to 14 of the General Procedure: Wash or disinfect your hands; access the official medication administration record; read the name of the medication to be given; access the ordered parenteral medication and check the label on the medication; compare the medication to the MAR and choose the correct one before picking it up; pick up the medication and check the label again.	

(continued)

box 48-1 *Types of IV Drug Delivery Systems*

- **IV additive.** An order for "add to IV" indicates that medication should be placed in the large-volume bag or bottle to be administered for the time designated for the fluid. Medications given this way must be stable in solution for the length of time the infusion is to run and must be mixed thoroughly to ensure even distribution throughout the fluid.
- **Small-volume parenteral.** Many medications are administered intermittently. These are diluted and mixed in small volumes of solution and are usually prepared in the pharmacy and sent to the units clearly labeled for individual patients. The IV bag or bottle may be hung piggyback style, using a secondary administration set attached to an injection port of the primary IV set, or the container may be attached to a primary tubing to be given into an IV lock. When rate is critical, the small-volume set may be connected to a volumetric IV pump.
- **Ready-to-mix IV drug systems.** These systems use minibags filled with a diluent solution, along with vials containing com-

monly used drugs in powder form. The nurse attaches the vial containing the ordered medication to a port with a breakaway seal on the minibag. Next, the nurse squeezes solution into the vial and squeezes and releases the bag to transfer the solution and dissolve and mix the medication.

This system allows reconstitution as needed on the clinical unit. The system has no exposed spikes or needles.

- **Syringe infusion pump.** This is a small battery-run device that can be hung on an IV stand, placed on a bedside table, or carried by an ambulatory patient.

The medication-filled syringe, prepared either in the pharmacy or by a nurse on the unit, is attached to small-diameter tubing and placed in the pump. The tubing is attached to the IV access. An alarm on the device alerts the nurse when all the medication has infused. Follow the policy in your facility regarding frequency for tubing change.

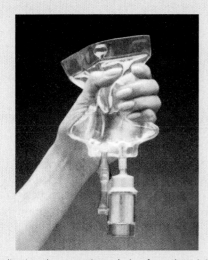

Mixing medications by squeezing solution from the minibag to half fill the vial. Courtesy of Baxter Healthcare.

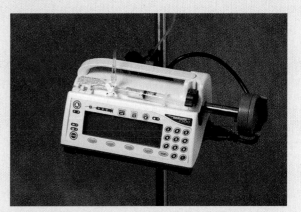

Syringe infusion pump.

Action	Rationale
15. Prepare the medication and other needed solutions using sterile technique. Follow the facility policy to properly label a medication drawn up; this usually includes the name of the medication, dose, date, time, and nurse's initials. See specific procedures for other solutions that are needed in specific situations.	All solutions must be kept sterile to prevent infection.
16-20. Follow steps 16 to 20 of the General Procedure: Prepare any additional medications to be given at this time, check each medication label with the MAR once again, obtain the patient identification to	*(continued)*

Action	Rationale
be taken to patient's bedside as prescribed by your facility's policy, identify the patient (two identifiers), and explain how the medication will be administered.	
21. Administer the medication in the appropriate manner.	
a. Establish that the IV access is patent. If IV fluids are being administered, confirm that they are infusing as ordered. Examine the site for evidence of infiltration or phlebitis. If there is a doubt about the patency of the IV access device, aspirate for blood return if the patient has an IV lock; if the patient has an ongoing IV, lower the bag to see if blood returns into the tubing (referred to as **flashback**).	To ensure that you are not injecting medication into the tissue surrounding the vein.
b. Cleanse the access site to the system or to an IV container by scrubbing with an alcohol wipe. Then allow it to air-dry.	Scrubbing mechanically removes contaminants, and as the alcohol dries, it disinfects the site.
c. Follow the specific procedure for administering the medication with emphasis on using the correct rate of administration.	Rate of administration of IV medications is critical to avoid adverse responses.
d. Observe the patient carefully for adverse effects while you are administering the medication.	Observing for patient's response will help to detect any problems or complications early.
22. Follow step 22 of the General Procedure: Leave the patient in a comfortable position and safe environment.	
23. Discard syringes and alcohol wipes into the sharps container and place any used bags in the appropriate biohazard container.	To prevent others from inadvertently contacting blood or body secretions.
24. Follow step 24 of the General Procedure: Wash or disinfect your hands.	

EVALUATION

25. Follow step 25 of the General Procedure. Evaluate using the individualized patient outcomes previously identified:
    a. The right *patient* received the right *medication* in the right *dose* by the right *route* at the right *time*.
    b. The medication was given over the correct length of time.
    c. The patient experienced the desired effect(s) from the medication(s) administered.
    d. The patient experienced no adverse effect(s) from the medication(s) administered.

DOCUMENTATION

26-27. Follow steps 26 and 27 of the General Procedure: Complete the right *documentation*. Document the medication, the dose, the route, the time, and your signature according to the facility policy, and document your evaluation of the patient's response to the medication as appropriate for the drug and according to facility policy.

POTENTIAL ADVERSE OUTCOMES AND RELATED INTERVENTIONS

1. The patient experiences an adverse response to a medication such as blood pressure dropping, pulse changing greatly, flushing, sweating, or change in level of awareness.

Intervention: Stop administration of the medication. Keep the vein open by aspirating the catheter to remove any remaining medication. Flush the IV catheter with sterile normal saline solution and restart IV fluids, or lock the IV. Notify the prescriber and document the effect of the medication. Hold any further doses of the drug until you confer with the prescriber.

2. The patient experiences pain or discomfort at the IV site or along the vein path with the IV medication administration.

Intervention: Try to determine the cause of the pain or discomfort. Is the IV site patent and working well? If it is not, the IV needs to be restarted. Is the medication likely to be irritating to the vein because of its composition? If this is the case, the medication may need to be diluted more or given more slowly. In some cases, dilating the veins with a warm compress will help the discomfort. Is the medication cold? If the medication is given rapidly and is cold, painful venospasm can occur. In this situation, administer the medication more slowly, and dilate the veins with a warm compress. In most cases, administering the medication more slowly and dilating the vein path will help if the IV site is patent and working.

3. Infiltration of medication occurs.

Intervention: Stop administering the medication. A new IV site will be needed to complete the medication. Apply warm, moist compresses according to facility policy. Document the appearance of the site, action(s) taken, and patient's response.

4. Extravasation of a vesicant medication occurs. A vesicant is a "blistering agent" and causes tissue damage when in the interstitial spaces.

Intervention: Stop the administration of the medication. Aspirate any remaining medication from the cannula and leave the cannula in place with a sterile male adapter in the hub until the prescriber is notified and gives further orders. Medication to counteract the effects of the extravasation may need to be instilled through the cannula. Depending on the medication that was extravasated, warm or cool compresses may be required. Verify with the prescriber and/or pharmacist which type of compress to use.

5. The patient refuses the medication.

Intervention: Explain the rationale for the medication and how it will benefit the patient. If the patient continues to refuse the medication, document that the medication was not given, the patient's refusal as well as your teaching, and notify the prescriber.

SPECIFIC PROCEDURES FOR ADMINISTERING INTRAVENOUS MEDICATIONS

Administering Medication by IV Push Into an Infusing IV

To administer medication by IV push into an infusing IV, follow the steps of the General Procedure for Administering IV Medications as modified below.

ASSESSMENT

1-2. Follow steps 1 and 2 of the General Procedure for Administering IV Medications: Verify the prescriber's orders and examine the MAR for accuracy and completeness.

3. Review information about the medication(s) to be given. Especially note the recommended speed of injection and the dilution and diluent, if appropriate, and whether the medication is compatible with IV fluid being administered. **R:** This ensures that the medication is administered at the appropriate strength and rate and is not mixed with an incompatible fluid.

4-5. Follow steps 4 and 5 of the General Procedure: Verify the type of IV access present and if there is a need for prn medication.

ANALYSIS

6-7. Follow steps 6 and 7 of the General Procedure: Critically think through your data, carefully evaluating each aspect and its relation to other data, and identify specific problems and modifications of the procedure needed for this individual.

PLANNING

8. Follow step 8 of the General Procedure: Determine the individualized patient outcomes in relation to the particular IV medication that has been prescribed for the patient. Include

   a. The right *patient* receives the right *medication* in the right *dose* by the right *route* at the right *time*.

   b. The medication is given over the correct length of time.

   c. The patient experiences the desired effect(s) from the medication(s) administered.

   d. The patient experiences no adverse effect(s) from the medication(s) administered.

9. Determine and select the appropriate equipment:
   a. syringe, large enough to accommodate the medication and correct amount of diluent, if any is needed
   b. needleless access device to draw up the medication

   c. needleless access device to access the IV system
   d. alcohol wipes
   e. syringe with 5 mL normal saline solution if the existing IV fluid is not compatible with the medication

IMPLEMENTATION

Action	Rationale
10-14. Follow steps 10 to 14 of the General Procedure: Wash or disinfect your hands; access the official medication administration record; read the name of the medication to be given; access the ordered parenteral medication and check the label on the medication; compare the medication to the MAR and choose the correct one before picking it up; pick up the medication and check the label again.	
15. Prepare the medication and flush solutions using sterile technique. Follow the facility policy to properly label the medication drawn up, usually including name of medication, dose, date, time, and nurse's initials. See specific procedures for other solutions that are needed for specific situations.	Flush solution is needed if the medication is not compatible with the existing IV. All solutions must be kept sterile to prevent infection.
16-20. Follow steps 16 to 20 of the General Procedure: Prepare any additional medications to be given at this time, check each medication label with the MAR once again, obtain the patient identification to be taken to patient's bedside as prescribed by your facility's policy, identify the patient (two identifiers), and explain how the medication will be administered.	
21. Administer the medication by IV push into the existing IV infusion.	
a. Verify patency of the IV line and identify the injection port closest to the patient.	To best control the rate of medication administration.
b. Clean the port with an alcohol wipe.	For infection control.
c. If saline flush solution is needed, insert the needleless device attached to the 5-mL syringe of saline firmly into the IV access port.	The access port will seal itself and prevent leakage of fluids and medication.
d. Pinch off the primary IV tubing between the injection port and the primary IV bag.	To prevent retrograde infusion (away from the patient) and dilution.

(continued)

Action	Rationale
e. Inject 2.5 mL of the saline solution.	To remove the incompatible IV fluid from the port, line, and cannula.
f. Remove the saline syringe and insert the medication syringe into the port, maintaining sterility of the access devices.	All equipment accessing the venous system must be sterile to prevent infection.
g. Inject the medication at the correct rate, taking into account the amount of tubing between the injection port and the IV insertion site.	The closer the injection port to the patient, the more accurately you can control the infusion of the medication. The further the injection port is from the patient, the greater chance there is for the medication to remain in the tubing and infuse at a different rate than intended.
h. Remove the medication syringe and reinsert the saline syringe if the fluid is incompatible with the medication, again maintaining sterility of the access device on the saline syringe.	To enable you to flush the line before the incompatible fluid can come into contact with the medication.
i. Inject the saline flush solution, or release the IV line to flow at the same speed at which you injected the medication.	There is still medication in the line and in the port; therefore, you are still administering medication to the patient.
j. Observe the patient for immediate effects or side effects.	You need to determine if the medication is having intended effects, to be able to intervene on any side effects, and to detect any complications at the IV site. There should be no swelling or coolness, and the patient should report no pain.
k. Release the tubing when the injection is completed and restore the IV fluid rate.	To ensure that the primary fluid is flowing at the desired rate.
l. Withdraw the needleless device from the injection port.	The medication was given. If the syringe is allowed to stay in the access port, the primary fluid could fill the syringe and push the plunger out, causing a spill of IV fluid and possible occlusion or bleeding from the IV site.
22-24. Follow steps 22 to 24 for General Procedure: Leave the patient in a comfortable position, dispose of used syringes in the sharps container, and wash or disinfect your hands.	

EVALUATION

25. Follow step 25 of the General Procedure: Evaluate using the desired patient outcomes previously identified:
   a. The right *patient* received the right *medication* in the right *dose* by the right *route* at the right *time.*
   b. The medication was given over the correct length of time.
   c. The patient experienced the desired effect(s) from the medication(s) administered.
   d. The patient experienced no adverse effect(s) from the medication(s) administered.

DOCUMENTATION

26-27. Follow steps 26 and 27 of the General Procedure: Complete right *documentation*. Document the medication, dose, route, time, and your signature according to the facility policy. Also document your evaluation of the patient's response to the medication as appropriate for the drug and according to the facility policy.

Administering Medication Into an Intermittent Infusion Adapter (IV Lock)

An intermittent infusion adaptor (IV lock) is a small male IV catheter plug designed to seal the IV access while allowing a syringe or IV tubing to be inserted whenever needed to administer medications or fluids. When not in use, the device is filled with saline or heparinized saline solution (depending upon facility policy) to prevent blood backup into the catheter and to maintain patency. To administer medication into an IV lock, follow the steps of the General Procedure for Administering IV Medications as modified below.

ASSESSMENT

1-2. Follow steps 1 and 2 of the General Procedure for Administering IV Medications: Verify the prescriber's orders and examine the MAR for accuracy and completeness.

3. Review information about the medication(s) to be given. Especially note the recommended speed of injection, the dilution and diluent if appropriate, and whether the medication is compatible with heparin if there is heparinized saline in the lock. **R:** This ensures that the medication is administered at the correct strength and rate and is not mixed with an incompatible fluid.

4-5. Follow steps 4 and 5 of the General Procedure: Verify the type of IV access present and if there is a need for prn medication.

ANALYSIS

6-7. Follow steps 6 and 7 of the General Procedure: Critically think through your data, carefully evaluating each aspect and its relation to other data, and identify specific problems and modifications of the procedure needed for this individual.

PLANNING

8. Follow step 8 of the General Procedure: Identify the individualized patient outcomes in relation to the particular IV medication that has been prescribed for the patient.
   a. The right *patient* receives the right *medication* in the right *dose* by the right *route* at the right *time*.
   b. The medication is given over the correct length of time.
   c. The patient experiences the desired effect(s) from the medication(s) administered.
   d. The patient experiences no adverse effect(s) from the medication(s) administered.

9. Determine and select the appropriate equipment.
   a. Syringe large enough for medication and diluent if needed
   b. Needleless access device
   c. Separate syringe for normal saline or heparinized saline solution to fill the lock after completion
   d. Separate syringe with normal saline flush solution if the lock is heparinized and the medication is not compatible with heparin. If more than one medication is to be given, prepare or obtain enough normal saline solution to flush between each medication and before the heparinized saline solution is injected.
   e. Enough alcohol wipes for the number of medications and flushes to be administered.

IMPLEMENTATION

Action	Rationale
10-14. Follow steps 10 to 14 of the General Procedure: Wash or disinfect your hands; access the official medication administration record; read the name of the medication to be given; access the ordered parenteral medication and check the label on the medication; compare the medication to the MAR and choose the correct one before picking it up; pick up the medication and check the label again.	

(continued)

Action	Rationale
15. Prepare the medication and heparinized saline and flush solutions, using sterile technique. Follow the facility policy to properly label the medication drawn up; this usually includes name of medication, dose, date, time, and nurse's initials.	Heparinized saline solution prevents clotting in the cannula. Normal saline may also prevent clotting in the cannula. Flush solution is needed if the solution is not compatible with the medication being administered. All solutions must be sterile to prevent infection.
16-20. Follow steps 16 to 20 of the General Procedure: Prepare any additional medications to be given at this time, check each medication label with the MAR once again, obtain the patient identification to be taken to patient's bedside as prescribed by your facility's policy, identify the patient (two identifiers), and explain how the medication will be administered.	
21. Prepare and administer the medication using an intermittent infusion adaptor.	
a. Locate the IV lock and assess the site for signs of phlebitis.	If phlebitis is present, it may not be wise to give the medication at this site.
b. Clean the IV lock port with an alcohol wipe.	For infection control.
c. Insert the syringe with the saline solution into the IV lock and flush the IV lock with approximately half of the saline solution, gently aspirate for blood return, and finish the flush while assessing for any swelling, discomfort, or coolness at the site.	To determine patency of the IV lock and clear the heparinized saline solution (if present) from the port. Sometimes blood will not return until a small amount of fluid has been injected.
d. Remove the saline syringe and again clean the access port of the IV lock with an alcohol wipe.	For infection control.
e. Administer the medication at the correct rate.	To reduce the chance of an untoward response of the patient or irritation of the vein.
f. Remove the medication syringe and clean the access port of the IV lock with an alcohol wipe again.	For infection control.
g. Insert the syringe with the saline solution, gently flush and check for signs of infiltration.	To finish injecting the medication and prevent blood from clotting the IV lock.
h. If heparinized saline solution is to be used, clean the access port with an alcohol wipe and follow the second saline flush with the heparinized saline solution.	Some facilities use heparinized saline solution to help prevent blood from causing occlusion in the IV catheter.

(continued)

Action	Rationale
22-24. Follow steps 22 to 24 of the General Procedure: Leave the patient in a comfortable position, discard used syringes in the sharps container, and wash or disinfect your hands.	

EVALUATION

25. Follow step 25 of the General Procedure: Evaluate using the individualized patient outcomes previously identified:
   a. The right *patient* received the right *medication* in the right *dose* by the right *route* at the right *time*.
   b. The medication was given over the correct length of time.
   c. The patient experienced the desired effect(s) from the medication(s) administered.
   d. The patient experienced no adverse effect(s) from the medication(s) administered.

DOCUMENTATION

26-27. Follow steps 26 and 27 of the General Procedure: Complete the right *documentation*. Document the medication, the dosage, the route, the time, and your signature according to the facility policy. Also document your evaluation of the patient's response to the medication as appropriate for the drug and according to the facility policy.

Using a Small-Volume Parenteral Drug Delivery System

A small-volume parenteral drug delivery system contains 50 to 100 mL of fluid as a vehicle for delivering an IV medication. It may be referred to as a partial-fill, a minibottle, or a piggyback. A **piggyback** is a technique of attaching a second container to an ongoing IV line. A small-volume parenteral system may be attached to an ongoing IV line or placed in an IV lock. To administer medication using a piggyback, follow the steps of the General Procedure for Administering IV Medications as modified below.

ASSESSMENT

1-5. Follow steps 1 to 5 of the General Procedure for Administering IV Medications: Verify the prescriber's order; examine the MAR for accuracy and completeness; assemble information on the drug to be given and whether or not it is compatible with other medications being given or with heparinized saline solution; determine what type of IV access is present; and assess the patient for the need for prn medication.

ANALYSIS

6-7. Follow steps 6 and 7 of the General Procedure: Critically think through your data, carefully evaluating each aspect and its relation to other data, and identify specific problems and modifications of the procedure needed for this individual.

PLANNING

8. Follow step 8 of the General Procedure: Determine the individualized patient outcomes in relation to the particular IV medication that has been prescribed for the patient. Include
   a. The right *patient* receives the right *medication* in the right *dose* by the right *route* at the right *time*.
   b. The medication is given over the correct length of time.
   c. The patient experiences the desired effect(s) from the medication(s) administered.
   d. The patient experiences no adverse effect(s) from the medication(s) administered.
9. Determine and select the equipment needed.
   a. For an IV lock (saline lock or heparin lock), you will need regular long IV tubing, a needle, needle-lock device or needleless access device, and an alcohol wipe. Tape may be needed.
   b. For attaching to an existing infusion, you will need a secondary administration set. Most manufacturers include an extension hanger in the secondary set package. You also will need an alcohol wipe and tape.
   c. For attaching a new container to an existing secondary or conventional line, you will need a new needleless access device, an alcohol wipe, and tape. Be sure to change the access device to the IV line each time because contamination could occur and would not be known when the next infusion is hung.

IMPLEMENTATION

Action	Rationale
10-14. Follow steps 10 to 14 of the General Procedure: Wash or disinfect your hands; access the official medication administration record; read the name of the medication to be given; access the ordered parenteral medication and check the label on the medication; compare the medication to the MAR and choose the correct one before picking it up; pick up the medication and check the label again.	
15. Prepare flush solutions if the medication is not compatible with any IV fluid infusing or with heparinized saline solution, if in use.	Flush solution prevents the medication from mixing with an incompatible solution. All solutions must be sterile to prevent infection.
16-20. Follow steps 16 to 20 of the General Procedure: Prepare any additional medications to be given at this time, check each medication label with the MAR once again, obtain the patient identification to be taken to patient's bedside as prescribed by your facility's policy, identify the patient (two identifiers), and explain how the medication will be administered.	
21. Administer the small-volume parenteral medication.	
a. If the container did not come from the pharmacy as a premixed and labeled medication, follow the directions on the medication for preparing it and instilling it into the bag through a port. Then agitate the bag to mix the medication. Label the container with the medication, dose, time, and your initials. This must be done in a clean medication preparation area before going to the patient room.	Accurate labeling is essential to safe medication administration. Follow your agency policy for labeling the bag. In most agencies, a small-volume parenteral will be prepared by the pharmacy.
b. *If you are using a new tubing set, do the following.*	
(1) Open the tubing set and close the regulator on the tubing.	To prevent spilling the fluid and medication as you set it up.
(2) If the container is a bottle, clean the top with alcohol; if the container is a soft plastic bag, remove the access port covering (it usually pulls off).	For infection control and preparation.

(continued)

Action	Rationale
(3) Insert the spike on the administration set into the IV bag or bottle.	To provide a means of administering the fluid and medication.
(4) Place the access device or connector on the end of the administration set.	To provide a means to attach the secondary administration set to the primary administration set.
(5) Hang the small-volume parenteral and fill the chamber half full of fluid.	This allows you to see the fluid and medication drip and to regulate the flow rate.
(6) Remove the cover of the access device and open the regulator to expel air from the secondary administration set. When the air is expelled, close the regulator.	The air must be expelled to prevent an air embolus from occurring.
(7) Clean the entry port on the primary administration set with alcohol where you will access the secondary administration set.	For infection control.
(8) Insert the access device from the secondary administration set into the port on the primary administration set.	To attach the two administration sets together.
(9) Place the primary or main IV bag or bottle on an extension hanger.	The primary IV bag or bottle must be lower than the secondary one for the piggyback to flow.
(10) Open the regulator on the piggyback and use the regulator on the primary line to set the drip rate.	The rate must be set correctly, so the patient receives the medication over the proper length of time. If the rate is too fast, it could be dangerous and painful. If the rate is too slow, it could be ineffective and disruptive to the schedule of the primary fluid infusion. By using the primary line to set the rate, when the secondary set is empty and the bag has collapsed, fluid will flow from the primary line. Thus, IV fluid administration does not stop.
(11) Secure the connection where the secondary administration set enters the primary administration set. There is usually a screw-type connector or safety needle.	To prevent inadvertent disconnection and spilling of fluid and medication.
c. *If you are using an infusing secondary line, do the following.*	
(1) Identify the correct used small-volume parenteral bag and tubing. If multiple medications are being given by secondary set and the	Mixing incompatible medications or fluids will cause precipitation and the IV will not infuse. The IV site may need to be restarted.

(continued)

Action	Rationale
drugs are incompatible, a different tubing is used for each. The tubings are changed every 48 to 72 hours or according to your facility policy.	
(2) If the medication is in a bottle, clean the top with alcohol; if it is in a soft plastic bag, remove the access port covering (it usually pulls off).	For infection control and to prepare the bag or bottle for access.
(3) Turn the regulator off.	To prevent the fluids and medication from spilling.
(4) Remove the old small-volume parenteral from the IV pole and detach it from the tubing.	To prepare to hang the new small-volume parenteral.
(5) Insert the spike of the used tubing into the proper access port of the new small-volume parenteral.	To connect the previous tubing to the new piggyback set.
(6) If the needleless access device is still attached to the primary set, you do not need to take the needle out of the access port. If the access device was not attached but was hanging loose and the sets were not attached to each other, change the needleless access device.	For infection control.
(7) If there is air in the tubing, open the regulator and lower the piggy-back bag or bottle below the level of the primary fluid; the fluid will backfill into the secondary line. Fill the tubing and the drip chamber half full. Some tubings have valves that do not allow backfilling. If this is the case, squeeze the drip chamber to fill it half full, and disconnect the tubing from the primary line long enough to allow the air to exit. Avoid dripping if at all possible, but hold it over a waste container in case dripping occurs.	To prevent instilling air into the IV line. Backfilling prevents the potential for medication escaping into the environment. Allowing medication to flow into the ambient air increases the potential for contact of healthcare personnel with the medication. This can sensitize them to the medication. Antibiotics in the environment can increase the presence of resistant organisms.
(8) Hang the piggyback bag or bottle on the IV pole and the primary IV one on the lower extension tubing.	To provide for a higher pressure in the piggyback to cause it to flow first.

(continued)

Action	Rationale
(9) Set the correct drip rate for the medication by using the regulator on the main IV.	The rate must be set correctly, so the patient receives the medication over the proper length of time. If the rate is too fast, it could be dangerous and painful. If the rate is too slow, it could be ineffective and disruptive to the schedule of the primary fluid infusion. When the medication has finished running, the main IV will begin to drip at the same rate as the small bag or bottle. You may need to return to the room to regulate the IV to its previous rate.
d. *If you are administering it into an IV lock, do the following.*	
(1) Prepare the medication and tubing using primary tubing. You may be using new tubing or using existing tubing as described in steps a and b.	
(2) Locate the IV lock device and check for phlebitis.	
(3) Clean the access port with an alcohol wipe.	
(4) Insert the syringe with the saline flush into the port.	
(5) Gently flush the port to remove heparinized saline solution and verify patency.	
(6) Remove the flush syringe and clean the port.	
(7) Insert the access device into the medication tubing.	
22-24. Follow steps 22 to 24 of the General Procedure: Leave the patient in a comfortable and safe environment, discard single-use or disposable supplies correctly, and wash or disinfect your hands.	

EVALUATION

25. Follow step 25 of the General Procedure: Evaluate using these criteria:
    a. The right *patient* received the right *medication* in the right *dose* by the right *route* at the right *time*.
    b. The medication was given over the correct length of time.
    c. The patient experienced the desired effect(s) from the medication(s) administered.
    d. The patient experienced no adverse effect(s) from the medication(s) administered.

DOCUMENTATION

26-27. Follow steps 26 and 27 of the General Procedure: Complete the right *documentation*. Document the medication, dosage, route, time, and your signature according to the facility policy. Complete the intake and output record: If you administered 50 to 100 mL of fluid, add this amount to the intake record. Also document your evaluation of the patient's response to the medication as appropriate for the drug and according to the facility policy.

Using a Syringe Infusion Pump

The infusion pump is used for small volumes of medication, usually 50 mL or less. In many facilities, syringes containing the medication in a predetermined level of solution are prepared in the pharmacy. When the pump is activated, the medication is delivered at the correct rate (see Box 48-1). To administer medication using a syringe infusion pump, follow the steps of the General Procedure for Administering IV Medications as modified below.

ASSESSMENT

1-2. Follow steps 1 and 2 of the General Procedure for Administering IV Medications: Validate the prescriber's orders and examine the MAR for accuracy and completeness.

3. Review information about the medication(s) to be administered. **R:** If more than one medication is being administered using the syringe infusion pump, determine whether or not the same tubing can be used for both medications, that is, whether or not they are compatible.

4-5. Follow steps 4 and 5 of the General Procedure: Verify the type of IV access present and the need for prn medication.

ANALYSIS

6-7. Follow steps 6 and 7 of the General Procedure: Critically think through your data, carefully evaluating each aspect and its relation to other data, and identify specific problems and modifications of the procedure needed for this individual.

PLANNING

8. Follow step 8 of the General Procedure: Determine the individualized patient outcomes in relation to the particular IV medication that has been prescribed for the patient. Include
  a. The right *patient* receives the right *medication* in the right *dose* by the right *route* at the right *time.*
  b. The medication is given over the correct length of time.
  c. The patient experiences the desired effect(s) from the medication(s) administered.
  d. The patient experiences no adverse effect(s) from the medication(s) administered.

9. Follow step 9 of the General Procedure: Select the supplies and equipment needed.
  a. Infusion pump, if not already at the bedside: If this is a new order, you will need to order the pump (usually from the central processing department of the facility).
  b. Special administration tubing designed for the specific infusion pump
  c. Sterile needleless access device, syringe, alcohol wipe, and tape
  d. Syringe from the pharmacy containing the medication: Check to make sure you have the right *medication* for the right *patient* in the right *dose* at the right *time,* or draw up the medication in the predetermined amount of solution. (See Module 46 for detailed instructions.) When the medication is prepared in the pharmacy, it may come with a small air bubble in the syringe to prevent loss of medication during transport and storage.

IMPLEMENTATION

Action	Rationale
10-14. Follow steps 10 to 14 of the General Procedure: Wash or disinfect your hands; access the official medication administration record; read the name of the medication to be given; access the ordered parenteral medication and check the label on the medication; compare the medication to the MAR and choose the correct one before picking it up; pick up the medication and check the label again.	

(continued)

Action	Rationale
15. Prepare the medication and flush solutions if needed using sterile technique. Follow the facility policy to properly label the medication drawn up; this usually includes the name of medication, dose, date, time, and nurse's initials.	Heparinized saline and flush solution is needed if the medication is not compatible with the existing IV, if one is infusing. All solutions must be kept sterile to prevent infection.
16-20. Follow steps 16 to 20 of the General Procedure: Prepare any additional medications to be given at this time, check each medication label with the MAR once again, obtain the patient identification to be taken to patient's bedside as prescribed by your facility's policy, identify the patient (two identifiers), and explain how the medication will be administered.	
21. Administer the medication using the syringe infusion pump.	
a. *If you are setting up the infusion pump, do the following.*	
(1) Attach the end of the tubing that has a female adapter with a screw-on end to the syringe.	To ensure that the medication syringe is securely connected to the tubing.
(2) Purge the air from the tubing by manually flushing the syringe to expel the air in the tubing and connecting device. Sometimes this can be done without removing the cap on the end if the cap is permeable to air. If a cap needs to be removed to purge the air, do so, and then carefully replace the cap.	To prevent infusing air through an IV, which can cause an air embolus, and to maintain sterility of the connectors.
(3) Attach a label to the tubing indicating the date, time, and your initials.	Follow your facility policy regarding tubing labels.
(4) Place the syringe into the pump according to the directions on the specific brand of syringe pump being used. Secure the flange of the plunger so that it will be pushed by the mechanism.	To ensure that the syringe engages the mechanism that regulates the infusion rate.
(5) Hang the pump on the IV pole, the bedside rail, or place on the bedside table where it is secure and will not fall.	To prevent damage to the pump, syringe dislocation, or pulling on the IV site.

(continued)

Action	Rationale
(6) Use an alcohol wipe to clean the access port on the primary IV line to which the syringe pump tubing will be connected, and attach the tubing to the catheter hub.	For infection control.
(7) Attach the tubing to the catheter hub, IV lock, or port and secure the access device to the primary tubing or directly to the patient's catheter hub/tubing.	To prevent inadvertent disconnection of the syringe pump tubing.
(8) Turn the switch of the pump on and set the alarms. Watch for the indicator light to flash, showing that the pump is working properly and that the medication is infusing.	To properly begin the infusion. Alarms contribute to increased patient safety as well as convenience for the nurse.
(9) When the medication has infused, the pumping action will stop; solution will remain in the tubing. Remove the access device and cover it with a sterile cap or another sterile access device. Turn the syringe pump switch off.	To disconnect the patient from the syringe pump.
(10) Flush the IV lock with saline or restart the IV.	
b. *If you are using an existing infusion pump, do the following.*	
(1) Check the tubing for the date and verify if the medication in the tubing is compatible with the medication to be given next.	To administer with a current tubing and prevent precipitation of medication that could cause occlusion of the IV.
(2) Remove the used syringe and discard it.	To prepare for the next syringe and keep the room tidy.
(3) Attach the tubing to the new syringe.	To connect the medication syringe to the tubing.
(4) Replace the access device with a new sterile access device.	For infection control.
(5) Place the syringe in the pump with the syringe flange and clamps in proper position.	To properly administer the medication.
(6) Clean the access port on the primary tubing or IV lock with alcohol and connect the syringe pump tubing to the catheter hub, IV lock, or IV port.	For infection control.

(continued)

Action	Rationale
(7) Follow steps 21a(7) through 21a(10) above: Hang the pump on the IV pole or the bedside rail, or place on the bedside table where it is secure and will not fall; cleanse the access port with alcohol and attach the tubing; turn the switch of the pump on and set for use of the alarms; secure the access device to the primary tubing or directly to the patient's catheter hub/tubing; and when the medication has been infused, remove the access device and cover it with a sterile cap or another sterile access device. Turn the syringe pump switch off.	
22-24. Follow steps 22 to 24 of the General Procedure: Leave the patient in a comfortable and safe environment, discard used syringe into the sharps container and single-use or disposable supplies correctly, and wash or disinfect your hands.	

EVALUATION

25. Follow step 25 of the General Procedure: Evaluate using the individualized patient outcomes previously identified:
   a. The right *patient* received the right *medication* in the right *dose* by the right *route* at the right *time*.
   b. The medication was given over the correct length of time.
   c. The patient experienced the desired effect(s) from the medication(s) administered.
   d. The patient experienced no adverse effect(s) from the medication(s) administered.

DOCUMENTATION

26-27. Follow steps 26 and 27 of the General Procedure: Complete the right *documentation.* Document the medication, dosage, route, time, and your signature according to the facility policy. This may be directly on the MAR, in a computerized documentation system, or on a separate medication administration form. Also document your evaluation of the patient's response to the medication as appropriate for the drug and according to the facility policy.

USING A PATIENT-CONTROLLED ANALGESIA PUMP

Patient-controlled analgesia (PCA) is a system for administering IV pain medications. The patient can activate the system when the need for medication arises. PCA is available in two major types—mechanical or electronic. Mechanical PCA devices are utilized mainly in home care and are not discussed here. Electronic PCA pumps are used most often in the acute care settings and often in the home as well.

The electronic version of PCA delivers pain medication through a computer-controlled infusion pump. The unit can be programmed to deliver a continuous infusion (basal rate), an adjustable patient-controlled dose (bolus), or both. A lockout interval also may be specified. During that time, the machine will not deliver another dose. In addition, a 4-hour dosage limit may be set. The nurse programs the PCA pump according to the prescriber's orders.

The continuous infusion is ordered to provide the patient with a baseline amount of medication continuously that will maintain a steady blood level of medication. The patient-controlled dose is the number of milliliters of fluid that is to be given for each individual dose. The prescriber orders the number of milligrams of drug in each milliliter, or the pharmacy may provide a standardized solution. Morphine sulfate with 1 mg/mL and meperidine with 10 mg/mL are common solutions. The individual injection dose is then calculated to match the prescriber's prescription. The lockout interval is ordered to prevent the patient from receiving too much medication. It can be adjusted to specify a period from several minutes to several hours. The 4-hour limit is set to limit the total volume to be infused over any consecutive 4-hour period.

The PCA pump holds a syringe or bag of medication inside a locked case. This syringe or bag is attached to a port on the patient's IV line by a small-diameter tubing that is less flexible than a regular administration set. It has an antireflux valve to prevent fluid from moving retrograde (up the tubing) and mixing with the medication. The medication in the syringe is administered when the patient pushes a control button attached to the machine (Fig. 48-1).

The PCA pump computer contains a clock and a rechargeable battery so that the device can be unplugged for transport or ambulation. The computer records each attempt by the patient to receive medication and each dose of medication given. By programming a code on the machine, it is possible to get a complete history of the use of the pain medication, including the total number of milliliters used from the current syringe, the number of attempts, and the number of injections given during each hour, and to verify the settings for the dose and intervals programmed into the machine.

Patients using PCA pumps are receiving IV narcotics; therefore, careful assessment of respiratory status, sedation level, and analgesic effect is essential. Figure 48-2 gives an example of a flow sheet used to record the monitoring of a patient on a PCA.

For the PCA to be effective, the patient must be alert and oriented. Careful teaching is needed for the patient to use the PCA effectively. It is important to emphasize that the administration is safe because the machine is programmed to give only the prescribed dose and can-

not give the patient too much medication or too many injections. It is also important to encourage the patient to use the medication to maintain comfort and not to wait a specified time to seek more medication. Even small children can learn to use a PCA properly and effectively.

In evaluating the effectiveness of PCA, the nurse should consider whether the patient is frequently attempting to get injections unsuccessfully. This may indicate that the patient is not feeling adequate pain relief. Excessive sedation or respiratory depression may indicate that the individual dose is too large for the patient or that the interval between injections is too brief.

To set up a PCA pump, refer to the specific directions for the brand used in your facility. Also, refer to your facility's policies and procedures for guidelines on managing the narcotics used in the machine and monitoring the patient. Some facilities require that two nurses check the set-up of a PCA to decrease the potential for error.

Using a Controlled-Volume Administration Set

Controlled-volume administration sets are most commonly used in pediatric settings and in situations in which the patient can tolerate only small amounts of fluid. These also are used instead of small-volume parenterals to dilute medication and deliver it intravenously over short periods of time, usually 30 to 60 minutes. To administer medication using a controlled-volume administration set, follow the steps of the General Procedure for Administering IV Medications as modified below.

ASSESSMENT

1-3. Follow steps 1 to 3 of the General Procedure for Administering IV Medications: Verify the prescriber's orders and examine the MAR for accuracy and completeness; assemble information on the medication(s).

4. Determine whether the medication is compatible with the intravenous fluid being administered. **R:** A controlled volume set will mix the IV fluid and the medication together. Compatibility is critical to safety.

5. Assess the need for any prn medication ordered.

ANALYSIS

6-7. Follow steps 6 and 7 of the General Procedure: Critically think through your data, carefully evaluating each aspect and its relation to other data, and identify specific problems and modifications of the procedure needed for this individual.

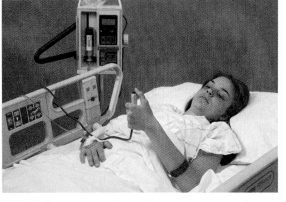

FIGURE 48-1 PCA pump. The medication is administered when the patient pushes a control button attached to the machine.

Start new record daily at 2400.

DATE   *6-12-06*

PCA

MEDICATION *morphine sulfate*			CONCENTRATION (mg / ml) *1 mg/ ml.*							
TIME	*0015*	*0200*								
BOLUS DOSE (ml)	*1 ml.*	∅	∅	∅	∅	∅	∅	∅	∅	∅
PCA DOSE (ml)	*.5 ml.*	→	→	→	→	→	→	→	→	→
INTERVAL (min.)	*10 min.*	→	→	→	→	→	→	→	→	→

EPIDURAL

TIME										
PF MORPHINE										
FENTANYL										

CONTINUOUS INFUSION

MEDICATION			CONCENTRATION (mg / ml)							

INITIALS										

CONTINUOUS INFUSION / EPIDURAL / PCA (Please Circle)				
SHIFT	**2200 0600**	**0600 1400**	**1400 2200**	**24 HR TOTAL**
TOTAL ATTEMPTS	*40*	*36*	*30*	
TOTAL INJECTIONS	*40*	*36*	*30*	
TOTAL ml USED	*20*	*18*	*15*	
TIME SYRINGE CHANGE	∅	∅	*2100*	
ml DISCARDED	∅	∅	*4 ml*	
INITIALS	*ML*	*DB*	*MK*	

INITIAL	SIGNATURE
ML	*M.Lewis RN*
DB	*D. Baker RN*
MK	*M.Keithly RN*

PATIENT CARD IMPRINT

Memorial Hospital

PAIN MANAGEMENT FLOW SHEET

FIGURE 48-2 Flow sheet for administering PCA IV medication.

PLANNING

8. Follow step 8 of the General Procedure: Determine the individualized patient outcomes in relation to the medication(s) to be administered. Include

   a. The right *patient* receives the right *medication* in the right *dose* by the right *route* at the right *time*.

   b. The medication is given over the correct length of time.

   c. The patient experiences the desired effect(s) from the medication(s) administered.

   d. The patient experiences no adverse effect(s) from the medication(s) administered.

9. Follow step 9 of the General Procedure: Determine and select the appropriate equipment.

   a. A controlled-volume administration set to attach to the existing IV bag or bottle (if this is a new order)

   b. Syringe and needleless device to draw up the medication and an alcohol wipe to prepare the injection port

IMPLEMENTATION

Action	Rationale
10-14. Follow steps 10 to 14 of the General Procedure: Wash or disinfect your hands; access the official medication administration record; read the name of the medication to be given; access the ordered parenteral medication and check the label on the medication; compare the medication to the MAR and choose the correct one before picking it up; pick up the medication and check the label again.	
15. Prepare the IV medication using sterile technique. Follow the facility policy to properly label the medication drawn up; this usually includes the name of the medication, dose, date, time, and nurse's initials.	All solutions must be kept sterile to prevent infection.
16-20. Follow steps 16 to 20 of the General Procedure: Prepare any additional medications to be given at this time, check each medication label with the MAR once again, obtain the patient identification to be taken to patient's bedside as prescribed by your facility's policy, identify the patient (two identifiers), and explain how the medication will be administered.	
21. If the controlled-volume set is not already in place, change the existing IV tubing for the controlled-volume set with tubing (see Module 47). Then administer the medication using the controlled-volume administration set.	
a. Open the inlet to the controlled-volume chamber. Fill with 50 to 100 mL of IV solution, depending on the dilution suggested by the drug manufacturer	To provide the correct dilution.

(continued)

Action	Rationale
(100 mL is commonly used for an adult unless the patient has a fluid restriction).	
b. Tightly close the inlet to the chamber.	To prevent overfilling.
c. Check the chamber. If it is hard plastic, make sure the air vent is open.	The chamber can develop negative pressure, which would prevent fluid from dripping out.
d. Turn on the drip from the chamber; if it drips properly, turn the drip off.	To verify that the system does not have an airlock and will work properly.
e. Clean the entry port of the fluid chamber with an alcohol wipe.	For infection control.
f. Insert the syringe with needleless device or needle (depending on the port) through the entry port, and inject the medication. Agitate the fluid gently.	To mix the medication with the fluid in the chamber.
g. Calculate the drip rate and regulate the flow. Remember that the controlled-volume set usually has a microdrip orifice. In all sets that deliver 60 drops/mL, the drip rate is the same as the number of milliliters per hour. Monitor the drip and volume closely.	The fluid will infuse according to the drip rate that is set. Monitor closely so that the controlled-volume chamber and tubing do not completely empty (which may result in occlusion).
h. Label the chamber with the name and amount of medication, date, time, and your initials according to facility policy.	To facilitate verification of the contents of the IV bag or bottle.
22-24. Follow steps 22 to 24 of the General Procedure: Leave the patient in a comfortable and safe environment, discard used syringe into the sharps container and other disposable supplies correctly, and wash or disinfect your hands.	

EVALUATION

25. Follow step 25 of the General Procedure: Evaluate using the individualized patient outcomes previously identified:
   a. The right *patient* received the right *medication* in the right *dose* by the right *route* at the right *time*.
   b. The medication was given over the correct length of time.
   c. The patient experienced the desired effect(s) from the medication(s) administered.
   d. The patient experienced no adverse effect(s) from the medication(s) administered.

DOCUMENTATION

26-27. Follow steps 26 and 27 of the General Procedure: Complete right *documentation*. Document the medication, dose, route, time, and your signature according to the facility policy. Also document your evaluation of the patient's response to the medication as appropriate for the drug and according to the facility policy.

Adding Medication to a New IV Bag or Bottle

Medications, vitamins, and electrolytes may be added to the main IV bag or bottle to be administered over many hours. Medications given this way provide for a stable blood level. Vitamins and electrolytes given in this manner are available to the body as they are needed. To add medications, vitamins, or electrolytes to a new IV bag or bottle, follow the steps of the General Procedure for Administering IV Medications as modified below.

ASSESSMENT

1-2. Follow steps 1 and 2 of the General Procedure for Administering IV Medications: Verify the prescriber's orders and examine the MAR for accuracy and completeness.

3. Review information about the medication, vitamin, or electrolyte to be added. **R:** To validate that the additive is compatible with the fluid in the main IV container.

4-5. Follow steps 4 and 5 of the General Procedure: Determine what type of IV access device is in place, and identify any need for prn medication.

ANALYSIS

6-7. Follow steps 6 and 7 of the General Procedure: Critically think through your data, carefully evaluating each aspect and its relation to other data, and identify specific problems and modifications of the procedure needed for this individual.

PLANNING

8. Follow step 8 of the General Procedure: Determine the individualized patient outcomes in relation to the particular IV medication that has been prescribed for the patient. Include
  a. The right *patient* receives the right *medication* in the right *dose* by the right *route* at the right *time*.
  b. The medication is given over the correct length of time.
  c. The patient experiences the desired effect(s) from the medication(s) administered.
  d. The patient experiences no adverse effect(s) from the medication(s) administered.

9. Determine and select the equipment needed.
  a. Large-volume IV bag or bottle containing the ordered IV fluid: Check carefully because all medications are not compatible with all IV fluids. Your facility may stock 1,000-mL bags of certain IV fluids with potassium chloride 20 mEq or 40 mEq already added for convenience and safety.
  b. Alcohol wipe to prepare the medication injection port
  c. Needleless device (or needle) and a syringe of the appropriate size to draw up the medication or additive
  d. Medication to be added
  e. Appropriate diluent for medication if it comes in a powder form
  f. Label for IV bag or bottle

IMPLEMENTATION

Action	Rationale
10-14. Follow steps 10 to 14 of the General Procedure: Wash or disinfect your hands; access the official medication administration record; read the name of the medication to be given; access the ordered parenteral medication and check the label on the medication; compare the medication to the MAR and choose the correct one before picking it up; pick up the medication and check the label again.	
15. Prepare the additive medication and IV fluid in a clean environment.	Areas adjacent to the corridor or where many individuals congregate are more likely to have air currents that move microorganisms that could contaminate the IV solution.

(continued)

Action	Rationale
a. Complete a label for the IV container that identifies the medication you are about to add and attach it to the IV fluid container.	Labeling allows the contents of the solution to be verified by other caregivers.
b. Prepare the parenteral medication based on instructions in Module 45, using the appropriate type and volume of diluent according to manufacturer's directions.	To ensure accurate medication administration.
c. Open the top of the new IV bag or bottle, identify the injection port, and instill the medication into the injection port. The port may be designated by the word "Add" or by a triangle on the rubber top. On a plastic bag, the injection port usually appears as a conventional soft rubber injection port, which is self-sealing. Then apply the label to the container.	The medication must be injected through a sealable port, or leakage and contamination will occur. All IV fluids must be labeled for contents to permit verification of the medication.
d. Tilt the fluid container back and forth to mix the additive thoroughly.	If the additive is not mixed, it may concentrate in the bottom of the container (if of a high specific gravity) or in the top of the fluid (if of a low specific gravity). Either causes some of the fluid to have a higher concentration of the medication, which may precipitate an adverse response.
16-20. Follow steps 16 to 20 of the General Procedure: Prepare any additional medications to be given at this time, check each medication label with the MAR once again, obtain the patient identification to be taken to patient's bedside as prescribed by your facility's policy, identify the patient (two identifiers), and explain how the medication will be administered.	
21. Hang the solution containing the additive medication.	
a. Follow the steps in Module 47 with regard to hanging a new fluid container: Turn off the IV flow, remove the spike from the old IV bag or bottle, spike the entry port of the new bag or bottle with tubing, invert the bag or bottle and hang it on the IV pole, squeeze to fill the drip chamber, and expel the air from the tubing.	To ready the fluid and medication for infusion.

(continued)

Action	Rationale
b. Regulate the flow.	The IV flow rate must be regulated to the correct infusion rate for the patient's safety.
(1) If you are using an infusion control device, thread the tubing through the device, according to manufacturer's instructions and set the controls to the desired milliliters per hour.	
(2) If you are not using an infusion control device, slowly open the roller clamp and regulate the manual roll clamp to set the desired rate.	
22-24. Follow steps 22 to 24 of the General Procedure: Leave the patient in a comfortable and safe environment, discard used syringe into the sharps container and single-use or disposable supplies correctly, and wash or disinfect your hands.	

EVALUATION

25. Follow step 25 of the General Procedure: Evaluate using the individualized patient outcomes previously identified:
   a. The right *patient* received the right *medication* in the right *dose* by the right *route* at the right *time*.
   b. The medication was given over the correct length of time.
   c. The patient experienced the desired effect(s) from the medication(s) administered.
   d. The patient experienced no adverse effect(s) from the medication(s) administered.

DOCUMENTATION

26-27. Follow steps 26 and 27 of the General Procedure: Complete right *documentation*. Document the medication, dosage, route, time, and your signature according to the facility policy. Document your evaluation of the patient's response to the medication as appropriate for the drug and according to facility policy.

Adding to an Infusing IV Bag or Bottle

Occasionally, it will be necessary to add a medication, vitamin, or electrolyte to an infusing IV bag or bottle. Be sure to verify precisely the amount of fluid left in the IV to ensure accurate calculation of administration rate. To add medications, vitamins, or electrolytes to an infusing IV bag or bottle, follow the steps of the General Procedure for Administering IV Medications as modified below.

ASSESSMENT

1-2. Follow steps 1 and 2 of the General Procedure for Administering IV Medications: Verify the prescriber's orders and examine the MAR for accuracy and completeness.

3. Review information about the medication, vitamin, or electrolyte to be added. **R:** This review verifies that the additive is compatible with the fluid in the infusing IV bag or bottle.

4-5. Follow steps 4 and 5 of the General Procedure: Determine what type of IV access device is in place, and identify any need for prn medication.

ANALYSIS

6-7. Follow steps 6 and 7 of the General Procedure: Critically think through your data, carefully evaluating each aspect and its relation to other data, and identify specific problems and modifications of the procedure needed for this individual.

PLANNING

8. Follow step 8 of the General Procedure: Determine the individualized patient outcomes in relation to

the particular IV medication or additive that has been prescribed for the patient. Include

a. The right *patient* receives the right *medication or additive* in the right *dose* by the right *route* at the right *time*.

b. The medication or additive is given over the correct length of time.

c. The patient experiences the desired effect(s) from the medications(s) or additive(s) administered.

d. The patient experiences no adverse effect(s) from the medication(s) or additive(s) administered.

9. Follow step 9 of the General Procedure: Determine what equipment is needed and select it.

a. Alcohol wipe to prepare the medication/additive injection port

b. Needleless device (or needle) and a syringe of the appropriate size to draw up the medication or additive

c. Medication or additive to be added

d. Appropriate diluent for medication or additive if it comes in a powder form

e. Label for IV bottle or bag

IMPLEMENTATION

Action	Rationale
10-14. Follow steps 10 to 14 of the General Procedure: Wash or disinfect your hands; access the official medication administration record; read the name of the medication or additive to be given; access the ordered parenteral medication or additive and check the label on the medication or additive; compare the medication or additive to the MAR and choose the correct one before picking it up; pick up the medication or additive and check the label again.	
15. Prepare the medication or additive and IV fluid in a clean environment.	
a. Complete a label for the IV bottle or bag that identifies the medication or additive you are about to add, and attach it to the IV fluid container.	Labeling allows the contents of the solution to be verified by other caregivers.
b. Prepare the parenteral medication or additive based on instructions in Module 45, using the appropriate type and volume of diluent according to manufacturer's directions.	To ensure the accuracy of the medication or additive dose.
16-20. Follow steps 16 to 20 of the General Procedure: Prepare any additional medications to be given at this time, check each medication or additive label with the MAR once again, obtain the patient identification to be taken to patient's bedside as prescribed by your facility's policy, identify the patient (two identifiers), and explain how the medication or additive will be administered.	

(continued)

Action	Rationale
21. Inject the medication, vitamin, or electrolyte to the infusing IV.	
a. Turn off the IV flow.	To contain the solution without risk of medication or additive being administered before dilution.
b. Invert the IV bag or bottle.	To pool the fluid and give easier access to the injection port.
c. Clean the medication port with an alcohol wipe.	Alcohol is an antiseptic and helps prevent infection.
d. Inject the medication or additive into the appropriate medication port on the IV bag or bottle.	The self-sealing port will prevent leaks.
e. Tilt the container back and forth.	To mix the medication or additive thoroughly.
f. Attach the prepared label to the container.	To facilitate verification of the contents of the IV bag or bottle.
g. Rehang the IV container approximately 3 feet overhead.	To facilitate flow.
h. Regulate the flow rate as ordered.	To administer the fluid at the prescribed rate.
22-24. Follow steps 22 to 24 of the General Procedure: Leave the patient in a comfortable and safe environment, discard used syringe into the sharps container and single-use or disposable supplies correctly, and wash or disinfect your hands.	

EVALUATION

25. Follow step 25 of the General Procedure: Evaluate using the individualized patient outcomes previously identified:

a. The right *patient* received the right *medication or additive* in the right *dose* by the right *route* at the right *time*.

b. The medication or additive was given over the correct length of time.

c. The patient experienced the desired effect(s) from the medication(s) or additive(s) administered.

d. The patient experienced no adverse effect(s) from the medication(s) or additive(s) administered.

DOCUMENTATION

26-27. Follow steps 26 and 27 of the General Procedure: Complete right *documentation*. Document the medication or additive, dosage, route, time,

and your signature according to the facility policy. Also document your evaluation of the patient's response to the medication or additive as appropriate for the drug and according to the facility policy.

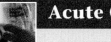

Acute Care

Most patients who are admitted to hospitals will receive an IV during their hospital stay. Many of those patients will receive IV medications; some will receive multiple medications with varying dosages and varying schedules. The medications may require different diluents and different times over which they are to be infused. Given that patients may have same or similar names, and medications may have same or similar names, the potential for medication error is great. The Joint Commission on Accreditation of Healthcare Organizations (JCAHO, 2004) has recognized that medication errors are a widespread problem in hospitals. Handwriting that is difficult to read and inappropriate use of abbreviations also lead to errors in medication administration. The nurse must be diligent in following all facility policies to help ensure safe IV medication administration.

hospitalization or home care. The nurse will need to be alert to the individual needs of the client and monitor closely while the client is in the facility. The facility policy will indicate how long the client should stay after receiving the medication. Discharge instructions for the client must include emergency information in the event of delayed adverse effects.

Long-Term Care

Intravenous (IV) medication administration is common in many long-term care agencies. Residents are often treated for chronic and end-of-life problems with IV medications. This population often presents special problems, such as disturbed sensory perception, impaired memory, and confusion, which can add to the challenge. Decreased cardiac output and decreased peripheral circulation also can be factors in how IV medications will act. The nurse must be alert to safety issues such as the resident's tendency to bleed, adverse medication effects that the resident does not report, and drug and diet interactions.

Home Care

Initial IV medications provided for clients being cared for at home should always be given by a nurse. After a program of client and caregiver education, the client may self-administer, depending on the specific medication. Many factors should be considered before home IV medication administration can be allowed. The client and caregiver must be able to understand and follow instructions regarding the necessary care. The environment should be clean with an appropriate place for storage of supplies or equipment that is needed. In some cases, a reliable method of refrigeration is needed for medication storage. Some healthcare agencies will send nurses to the home for every IV medication administration, but this often depends on the client's insurance coverage and benefits.

Ambulatory Care

Infusion centers provide nursing care for IV medication administration. Some primary care centers will give IV medications for clients who do not need

LEARNING TOOLS

DEVELOP YOUR BACKGROUND KNOWLEDGE

1. Review the Learning Outcomes.

2. Read the section on administering IV medications in your assigned text.

3. Look up the Key Terms in the glossary.

4. Review this module and mentally practice the techniques to be performed.

5. Review the policy for IV medication administration in the facility to which you are assigned.

DEVELOP YOUR SKILLS

In the practice setting

1. Draw up medication as you would for an intramuscular injection, using the needleless device available in your practice setting.

2. Working in pairs, perform each of the following procedures:
   a. Administer a medication through an IV lock.
   b. Administer a medication by syringe pump.
   c. Administer a medication using a minibag as a piggyback.
   d. Have one student play the role of a patient with an infiltration of IV medication. Provide care for him or her and then switch roles. Any students who are not participating at a given time can observe and evaluate the performances of the others.

DEMONSTRATE YOUR SKILLS

In the clinical setting

1. Consult with your instructor regarding the opportunity to administer IV medication with supervision:
   a. Add medication to a new IV bag.
   b. Administer medication using a controlled-volume administration set.
   c. Administer an IV push into an infusing IV.
   d. Administer a medication by IV lock.
   e. Administer a medication by syringe pump.

2. Consult with your instructor regarding the opportunity to observe or participate in the care of a patient-controlled analgesia infuser.

CRITICAL THINKING EXERCISES

1. You are preparing to administer a routine medication at the prescribed time to a patient. The patient states that her IV site is painful and that the last medication given has made her whole arm sore. What actions will you take?

2. The patient has been ordered to have a medication for nausea. You see that the medication is ordered to be given as an IV push and is supplied in a 1-mL vial. However, your research on the drug reveals that the medication is very irritating to the vein and painful during injection. What actions should you take and why?

SELF-QUIZ

SHORT-ANSWER QUESTIONS

1. If there is no designated speed of injection for an IV push medication, how fast should it be injected and why?

   _____

   _____

2. When adding medications to a small- or large-volume IV bag or bottle, why should you agitate the solution to mix it thoroughly?

   _____

   _____

3. What are two effects of drug incompatibilities?

   a. _____

   b. _____

4. What are two resources for determining the actions and possible incompatibilities of drugs?

   a. _____

   b. _____

5. What is the purpose of an IV lock?

   _____

6. Why must the premeasured syringe of medication be accurately placed in the infusion pump?

   _____

7. Why is normal saline or heparinized saline solution left in the IV lock?

   _____

8. How many milliliters of fluid are usually used to dilute the medication in a controlled-volume administration set?

   _____

MULTIPLE CHOICE

_____ 9. The nurse has mixed a small-volume bag of IV fluid with the premeasured antibiotic as supplied by the manufacturer. The nurse's next action immediately after admixture of the two components is which of the following?
   a. Identify the patient.
   b. Place a tubing label on the tubing.
   c. Check the bag for particulate matter.
   d. Rotate the medication bag gently.

_____ 10. The nurse has just administered an IV medication for pain and nausea to the postoperative patient. Which of the following medication effects should the nurse report to the prescriber? (Choose all that apply.)
   a. Feeling warm
   b. Sudden, severe shortness of breath
   c. Itching all over
   d. Feeling drowsy

Answers to the Self-Quiz questions appear in the back of the book.

MODULE 49

Caring for Patients With Central Venous Catheters

KEY TERMS

air embolism
Broviac catheter
catheter
central venous
   catheter (CVC)
cephalic vein
Groshong catheter
Hickman catheter
Infus-a-port
midline catheter
peripherally
   inserted central
   catheter (PICC)

Port-a-cath
right atrium
sclerosed
septicemia
subclavian vein
subcutaneous
   catheter port
superior vena cava

OVERALL OBJECTIVE

▸ To care for a patient with any of the various types of central venous infusion catheters by assisting with insertion, changing dressings, providing intravenous (IV) therapy, and drawing blood.

LEARNING OUTCOMES

The student will be able to

1. Assess the patient to determine the type of central venous catheter (CVC) in use and any related complications.
2. Analyze assessment data to determine if any specific problems related to the CVC are present.
3. Determine appropriate patient outcomes of therapy that uses a CVC and recognize the potential for adverse outcomes.
4. Plan for the care of the specific CVC and for administering various therapies via the catheter.
5. Access the specific CVC appropriately for the type of catheter in order to administer medications, draw blood, and maintain patency.
6. Care for the exit site of a CVC effectively.
7. Evaluate the status of the CVC and entry site and identify whether desired patient outcomes for therapies using the CVC were achieved.
8. Document the care of the catheter and exit site and all therapies using the CVC.

In modern healthcare settings, many patients receive intravenous (IV) medications, such as chemotherapy and nutritional solutions. Many of these products irritate small veins but are tolerated without local irritation in larger vessels that have a high-volume blood flow, allowing for rapid dilution of the product. A **central venous catheter (CVC)** is often in place in these patients before therapy begins. For other patients, small vessels that have been used repeatedly for standard IV products have become irritated or **sclerosed** (scarred) or in other ways unusable. For patients in all these situations, the CVC offers an effective route for the administration of needed therapy. Because of the direct access to the central circulation, the special dynamics of blood flow in the large central veins, and the difficulty in replacing CVCs, specialized care techniques are required.

NURSING DIAGNOSES

■ Risk for Infection is a major nursing diagnosis assigned to patients with central lines. First, the solution is flowing directly into the central circulation. Any bacteria introduced with the fluid circulate freely, and generalized **septicemia** may result. Second, the **catheter** enters through the skin and provides a direct path that microbes may follow from the surface, along the

outside of the catheter, and into the central circulation, also creating the potential for septicemia. Many of the steps in the procedures for care are designed to guard the patient against this high infection risk, and much of the assessment is designed to identify infection at the earliest point.

■ Disturbed Body Image may be related to the feelings about having a CVC in place for long-term use. It may be visible under clothing; limits the clothing that can be worn because of its appearance; and prevents activities such as swimming. The individual may struggle between the desire to maintain a "normal" appearance and the need to let others know about the CVC and the health condition that necessitates its use.

■ Ineffective Therapeutic Regimen Management is a concern for those patients who must manage the care of a CVC over time. The care seems demanding and requires knowledge and its omission may have serious consequences. Teaching strategies are aimed at preventing this problem from occurring.

Various collaborative problems may occur with CVCs. These are discussed in "Potential Adverse Outcomes and Related Interventions" below.

DELEGATION

Care of CVCs is not delegated to assistive personnel in healthcare settings. However, in the home setting, the patient, family, or significant others may be providing this care. In those instances, the nurse teaches the appropriate caregiver how to provide this care. Written directions are important references for family caregivers. The nurse plans for follow-up to make sure that care is being completed correctly and to answer questions.

TYPES OF CENTRAL VENOUS CATHETERS

Several types of central venous infusion catheters are in use. The various standard CVCs, the surgically inserted CVC, the subcutaneous central venous port, and the **peripherally inserted central catheter (PICC),** which has a peripheral exit site, are discussed briefly. Other types of central IV lines may be used in your facility. By analyzing the type of line in use, you should be able to adapt these procedures to your situation as necessary.

STANDARD CENTRAL VENOUS CATHETERS

The standard CVC is inserted by a physician or specially trained nurse using a sterile procedure in which an introducer is used to thread a catheter directly into a central vein. The catheter, which may be short or long, is sutured or otherwise secured to the skin at the exit site. The most common insertion site is the right or left **subclavian vein,** but the right **cephalic vein** or the right or left internal jugular vein also may be used (Fig. 49-1). These central catheters are suitable for shorter-term use. In long-term use, their entry sites are more likely to become infected than other types discussed below.

The long CVC is inserted in a minor bedside surgical procedure by a physician, usually a surgeon. The catheter introducer is inserted into the subclavian area, a large central vein is accessed, and the catheter threaded from the entrance site until the tip rests in the **superior vena cava** outside the **right atrium.** The location of the catheter is verified by x-ray image before it is used. These catheters have a single lumen. This type of line may be used to administer medications and transfusions and to measure central venous pressure. The standard CVC is not usually used for drawing blood because its small lumen is more easily occluded than the lumens of larger catheters.

The long catheter insertion is a complex procedure and has the potential for complications such as piercing the vein and creating bleeding (hemothorax) or piercing the lung in the insertion process, creating a pneumothorax.

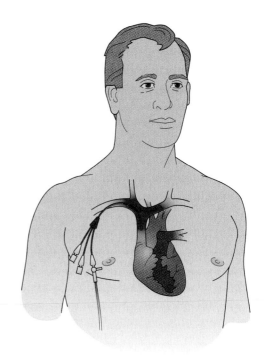

FIGURE 49-1 Subclavian central venous catheter in place. The tip of the catheter is positioned in the right atrium.

Short CVCs are designed for insertion through the internal jugular vein. These include the Arrow and Hon brands among others. These are inserted in the same way as a standard IV cannula with an inside-the-needle catheter. Internal jugular catheters are often inserted in surgery by an anesthesiologist, although in some facilities, nurses are certified to insert internal jugular catheters by completing special classes.

Internal jugular catheters may have single, double, or triple lumens. The multiple-lumen catheter has separate color-coded ports, each going to a different lumen. Each lumen exits separately from the other lumens. It is therefore possible to designate each lumen for a separate purpose. For example, the triple-lumen catheter can have one lumen designated for nutritional solutions, another for drawing blood, and the third for intermittent medication. Any one, any two, or all three may be capped and filled with heparinized saline or other saline solutions for intermittent use.

PERIPHERALLY INSERTED CENTRAL CATHETERS

The peripherally inserted central catheter is referred to as a PICC or sometimes as a central catheter with a peripheral exit site. This is a long central IV catheter that is inserted into a vein in the arm through an intracatheter needle. The catheter is then threaded from a spool through the needle into the subclavian vein until its tip rests outside the superior vena cava (Fig. 49-2). An x-ray

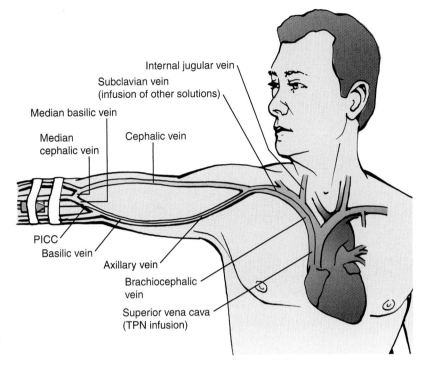

FIGURE 49-2 The peripherally inserted central venous catheter (popularly called a PICC).

image is used to verify its position. In some facilities, PICC catheters are inserted by registered nurses certified to do so. PICC lines may be left in place for a prolonged period of time. The catheter volume is 0.4 mL.

The PICC facilitates administration of fluids and medications that can be infused only into the large central veins without the use of the more complex procedure necessary to insert a conventional CVC or the surgical procedure to implant a catheter. This type of line also may be used to measure central venous pressure and to draw blood.

In most facilities, care is identical to that given for the standard CVC. In some facilities, the care is the same as that given for other peripheral IV lines unless nutrient solutions are being administered. Be sure to check the policy in your facility.

Clear lines of communication must be established so that members of the healthcare team are aware that this is not a peripheral IV line. In addition to recording this information in the patient's permanent record and on the nursing plan of care, it is wise to note the type of line being used by writing directly on the dressing or on a piece of tape placed over the dressing. Then, even if someone does not thoroughly read the patient's record, the information will be immediately apparent when the line is used or given care.

ASSISTING WITH THE INSERTION OF A CENTRAL VENOUS CATHETER

Most CVC insertion procedures occur at the bedside. Maximal barrier precautions, including the use of sterile gloves, masks, and sterile drapes around the area are rec-

ommended for the insertion procedure (O'Grady, et al., 2002). The nurse usually obtains the equipment and sets up the environment for this procedure. Use the general procedure in Module 17.

SURGICALLY INSERTED CENTRAL VENOUS CATHETERS

Central venous catheters, such as the tunneled catheters and subcutaneous ports that are used for patients being treated for cancer or other major illnesses, are resistant to displacement and infection for a prolonged time. These types of catheters are inserted in the operating room as a minor surgical procedure.

SUBCUTANEOUS CATHETER PORTS

The implanted or **subcutaneous catheter port** (examples include **Port-a-cath,** Mediport, PasPort, **Infus-a-port,** or Hickman Port) is surgically implanted. The catheter end is in a large central vein and is connected to a reservoir that has a rubber diaphragm for a top and is implanted under the skin (most often in the subclavicular area of the chest). To access it, the nurse uses a noncoring 45° angle needle (sometimes referred to as a Huber needle) inserted through the skin and then through the rubber diaphragm into the port. The needle must be secured to the skin with tape. The subcutaneous port can be filled with heparinized saline solution and used intermittently or connected to IV fluids and/or IV medications.

These devices appear to be more susceptible than other central lines to clotting closed when used for drawing blood. This is probably due to the size and shape of the reservoir under the diaphragm and the potential for some blood to remain in the reservoir. Therefore, the nurse must take extra care to be sure that the entire port is adequately flushed after every blood drawing. Because the port has no exit site, the potential for infection is decreased if the site is not being used. However, a needle puncture is needed each time the port is accessed. When the port has an access needle attached for ongoing delivery of fluids and medications, there is a concern about infectious agents migrating into the catheter from the skin. A port that has been accessed is cared for as if it were a standard central IV line, except that a larger volume of heparinized saline solution (5 mL) is needed when flushing the port (Fig. 49-3).

TUNNELED CENTRAL CATHETERS

The tunneled catheter is surgically inserted into the chest and into a central vein. It is tunneled under the chest tissue after it exits from the vein so that the exit site at the skin is a distance from the exit from the vein. In the subcutaneous tunnel, the catheter is surrounded by a Dacron cuff, which allows tissue to grow into the material, forming a seal against microbes. It takes approximately 3 weeks for the catheter to thoroughly heal into place. This time varies depending on the patient's health and healing ability.

The **Hickman catheter** (Fig. 49-4) was the first of several brands of tunneled central catheters. Frequently,

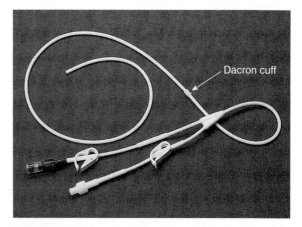

FIGURE 49-4 Double-lumen Hickman catheter with ports and clamps in place.

the term "Hickman" is used as a generic term to refer to standard tunneled catheters. The internal diameter of the Hickman catheter is 1.6 mm, which is large enough to allow withdrawal of blood and infusion of fluid into the vein. This type of catheter may be kept open with a continuous infusion or may be capped and filled with heparinized saline solution to be used as an intermittent access to the vein. The Hickman catheter may have one, two, or three lumens. Each lumen is heparinized independently of the others. Another brand of tunneled catheter, the **Broviac catheter,** is a single-lumen catheter and has an internal diameter of 1 mm, so it cannot be used for drawing blood. It is used only for infusing fluids.

The double-lumen Hickman catheter is actually a fusion of two standard Hickman catheters or of a Broviac (smaller lumen) catheter and a single large-lumen catheter (see Fig. 49-4). The double-lumen catheter is used principally to allow adequate nutrients to be infused without interruption, while allowing medications to be given and blood to be drawn intermittently. A continuous infusion of a nutritional solution is administered through the smaller lumen, while the larger lumen is used for drawing blood samples (with the smaller lumen temporarily clamped) and for infusing medications (may be administered simultaneously with the infusion of the nutrient solution). When both lumens are the large size (Hickman diameter), either lumen may be used for all purposes, although for convenience, the lumens may be dedicated to certain specific purposes.

Care is the same for all tunneled catheters. The insertion site is dressed using sterile technique until the site heals. The exit site is dressed using sterile technique until the catheter cuff heals into place because this is a fresh surgical wound and the patients are often immunocompromised. After healing, clean technique is usually used (see the procedures below).

When the line is used intermittently, it must be filled with heparinized saline solution to prevent coagula-

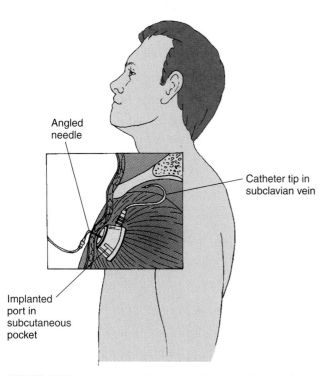

FIGURE 49-3 Implanted central venous catheter port. The IV catheter is threaded into the right atrium. The catheter exits the vein and attaches to the metal reservoir, which has a resealable rubber diaphragm on the top. The port can be accessed with a Huber-style 90-degree angle needle.

tion at the catheter tip, which would occlude the line. Because these lines are intended for long-term use, the patient and the family must be taught to carry out the care at home. A clamp must be kept on the catheter whenever fluid is not being infused to guard against inadvertent separation of the cap and line and the resulting risk of **air embolism.** Plastic clamps are part of most CVCs.

SPLIT-TIP TUNNELED CATHETERS

The split-tip tunneled catheter (often referred to by the brand name **Groshong catheter**) is a surgically implanted CVC made of silicone. It is inserted through a tunnel in a manner similar to a standard tunneled catheter (Hickman). It has a specially designed tip that allows the pressure of fluid being instilled to open the tip and administer fluid. The tip also can be opened by the negative pressure created by a syringe and, therefore, can be used for drawing blood. However, the tip will not open from the blood pressure in the central vein, so no blood can get into the catheter and form a clot. In addition, the patient is protected from air embolism because the tip does not allow the negative pressure in the chest to be transmitted to the catheter lumen. This catheter is filled with normal saline solution when not in use. Because no heparin is administered to keep it open, it is safer for the patient who should not receive heparin. However, some facilities do use heparin solution in Groshong catheters. Follow the procedure in your facility.

MIDLINE CATHETERS

To be accurate, a **midline catheter** is not truly a CVC because the tip does not lie in the great central veins. However, in many institutions, the care of the midline catheter is the same as the care of the CVC and, therefore, it is discussed in this module. The midline catheter is most frequently inserted into a large vein in the arm either immediately above or immediately below the antecubital fossa. The catheter is threaded into the vein and its tip lies in the proximal area of the extremity where the vessels are becoming larger with greater blood flow. A midline catheter is usually between 4 and 8 inches long. While not designed for long-term use in situations such as chemotherapy, it is possible to continue to use a midline catheter for 2 to 4 weeks. It is used for solutions that do not require the large blood flow of the central veins.

PREVENTING AIR EMBOLISM

If there is an open end to the CVC, it is possible for negative pressure at the catheter's tip caused by intrathoracic pressure changes to draw air into the catheter and create an air embolism. As a precaution against accidental opening of the central IV line to a potential air embolism, an integral clamp is usually in place on the catheter itself. The catheter can be clamped before any action is taken that would require the catheter to be opened.

The surgically inserted catheter may not have an integral clamp; instead, an extension tubing with an integral clamp is used. The extension tubing is considered a permanent part of the line. The intravenous fluid line must be secured to the IV catheter through a twisting screw-type device on the end of the tubing to prevent accidental separation of the tubing and the catheter. The nurse must choose the appropriate tubing that has the screw-type tip.

CHANGING THE CENTRAL VENOUS CATHETER DRESSING

Most facility protocols specify use of sterile technique for changing dressings over nontunneled CVCs. Sterile technique may also be used for dressings over an implanted port that has an access needle in place and over a newly inserted tunneled catheter before healing occurs around the catheter. Clean, "no touch" technique, in which clean gloves are worn and sterile swabs used for cleaning may also be used for these catheters (Pellowe, Pratt, Harper, et al., 2003). Be sure to check the facility protocol in regard to technique. Protocols are usually based on a study of infection rates in the facility itself. All these types of central catheters have access for bacteria from the dressing and skin, along the needle and catheter directly into the central circulation. The dressing change permits careful assessment of the insertion site, thorough cleansing of the area, removal of any debris that might foster microbial growth, application of antiseptic or antimicrobial agents to decrease future growth of microbes when appropriate, and application of new sterile dressing materials.

For the healed, tunneled catheter, clean no-touch technique is used. The same process for cleansing around the catheter and for applying a new dressing is used, but clean gloves instead of sterile gloves are worn while cleansing the site with swabs and applying the new dressing. These gloves protect the nurse from contact with secretions and prevent transferring microorganisms from the outside of the old dressing to the wound area itself. The cleansing swabs and dressing materials are still in sealed sterile packages. The clean gloves also protect your hands from contact with the antibacterial materials. The swab handles protect the wound, and dressings are handled from the edges that will not touch the insertion site.

The frequency with which these dressings are changed is not standardized. In some facilities, where standard gauze and tape dressings are used, the dressings are changed daily or every other day. In other facilities, such dressings are changed three times weekly on a prescribed schedule. In some facilities, where transparent, moisture-vapor-permeable (MVP) dressings such as OpSite and Tegaderm are used, dressings are left in place until they begin to loosen or for 1 week, whichever comes first. This method saves nursing time, is effective for assessing the site, and protects the site. The use of a MVP dressing is recommended (Pellowe, Pratt, Harper, et al., 2003). In addition to regularly scheduled changes, the dressing is changed if it pulls loose or becomes wet, because these situations increase the potential for contamination of the entry site.

No specific recommendation on the type of dressing or frequency of change has been made by the Centers for Disease Control and Prevention at this writing. It would be appropriate to watch the literature closely for research results and specific recommendations. Meanwhile, continue to follow the procedure designated in your facility.

PROCEDURE FOR CHANGING THE CENTRAL VENOUS CATHETER DRESSING

ASSESSMENT

1. Check the date and time of the last dressing change and the specific type of central line in use. **R:** This review determines when the catheter dressing should be changed.
2. Review the facility procedure. **R:** Procedure dictates which dressing materials are appropriate to use for the type of CVC in place.

ANALYSIS

3. Critically think through your data, carefully evaluating each aspect and its relation to other data. **R:** This enables you to determine specific problems for this individual in relation to the CVC.
4. Identify specific problems and modifications of the procedure needed for this individual. **R:** Planning for the individual must take into consideration the individual's problems.

PLANNING

5. Determine individualized patient outcomes in relation to the CVC dressing. **R:** Identification of desired outcomes guides planning and evaluation.
   a. Dressing remains intact and clean between dressing changes.
   b. Entrance site is clear and free of infection or skin breakdown.
   c. The IV line is intact with flow not obstructed, rate correctly set, and all connections secure.
   d. Patient does not experience discomfort.
6. Obtain the necessary supplies, including
   a. one pair of clean gloves and one pair of sterile gloves if sterile technique is being used. Two pairs of clean gloves if clean technique is being used. **R:** Gloves protect your hands from body secretions and protect the site.
   b. trash bag. **R:** This container is for the soiled dressing, which will thereby prevent potential contamination of supplies by the soiled dressing during the dressing change.
   c. a prepared CVC dressing tray or the cleansing agents obtained separately; agents vary from facility to facility. Use what is prescribed by facility policy. **R:** Cleansing agents remove microorganisms and drainage from the site. The common agents are
      (1) A 2% alcohol chlorhexidine-based disinfectant is recommended as the preferred disinfectant (Chaiyakunapruk, Veenstra, Lipsky, et al., 2002).
      (2) Povidone-iodine solution, povidone-iodine swab sticks, tincture of iodine, and alcohol 70% sticks are considered acceptable substitutes for chlorhexidine (O'Grady, 2002). Gauze squares are needed if the solution does not come on swab sticks. *Note:* In the past, acetone was used. This was shown to increase skin reactions and contribute to site infections and is not recommended.
      (3) Skin protectant. This usually comes as a pad saturated with the protectant in a foil wrapper. **R:** Skin protectant provides a barrier over the skin where the tape will be placed and decreases skin irritation and reactions to tape.
      (4) Dressing material: 2- × 2-inch gauze squares and nonallergenic tape such as paper tape are used if there is drainage from the wound, *or* if there is no wound drainage, transparent dressing material may be used (Pellowe, Pratt, Harper, et. al., 2003). Use the material designated by your facility. **R:** These materials protect the site from microorganisms and from contacting bedding and clothing that might pull the catheter out. The gauze absorbs drainage to lessen skin irritation. The transparent dressing usually lasts longer, resists moisture more effectively, and allows for assessment of the site without removing the dressing.

      Note: Povidone-iodine ointment or other antiseptic ointment may be used at the catheter exit site in some facilities; however, the current recommendation is to avoid using ointments. The ointment, when used, is designed to provide both a mechanical and chemical barrier to microorganisms. Reactions to the ointment and trapping of moisture against the skin increase the incidence of fungal infections. In addition, the ointment can make it difficult to assess the site through the transparent dressing (O'Grady, 2002).

IMPLEMENTATION

Action	Rationale
7. Wash or disinfect your hands.	To decrease the transfer of microorganisms that could cause infection.
8. Identify the patient, using two identifiers.	Verifying the patient's identity helps ensure that you are performing the right skill for the right patient.
9. Close the door and pull the curtain around the bed.	To provide privacy.
10. Explain the procedure you are about to perform.	Explaining the procedure helps relieve anxiety or misperceptions that the patient may have about a procedure or activity and sets the stage for patient participation.
11. Raise the bed to an appropriate working position based on your height.	To allow you to use correct body mechanics and protect yourself from back injury.
12. Open the catheter dressing set or open the various dressing materials.	So that they are accessible without contaminating your sterile gloves.
13. Put on clean gloves and position the waste container conveniently.	To protect yourself from possible contact with body substances.
14. Expose the dressing site, pull tape loose carefully, and remove the old dressing cautiously. Discard the dressing in the waste container.	It is possible to damage skin by pulling tape off rapidly rather than slowly and carefully. Some central lines are sutured in place, but others are not, so great care must be taken not to dislodge a catheter while removing the dressing.
15. Remove and discard your gloves in the waste container.	To keep any soiled material away from the clean site.
16. Wash or disinfect your hands, and put on the second pair of clean gloves or sterile gloves.	To remove any bacteria that have built up while the hands were in the previous gloves and to protect the site from microorganisms that could be on your hands.
17. Clean around the catheter, using the disinfectant cleansing swabs. Clean in a spiral manner, beginning at the catheter itself and moving out approximately 2 inches in all directions. Also clean the section of the catheter that will be under the dressing. Use a scrubbing action.	The disinfectant cleanser removes microorganisms and crusts or secretions around the catheter. The scrubbing action on the skin mechanically moves microorganisms.

(continued)

Action	Rationale
18. Repeat cleansing with a new disinfectant swab. If using alcohol or an iodine compound, allow the area to dry for 2 minutes before proceeding.	This further removes microorganisms. Allowing the area to dry thoroughly provides maximum disinfection (Pellowe, Pratt, Harper, et al., 2003). *Note:* If the facility policy requires an ointment or if one is being used because of a documented infection, apply it at this time.
19. Apply the skin protectant to the area where the tape will be applied and allow it to dry.	The dried protectant forms a barrier that protects the skin as dressings are repeatedly changed.
20. Place dressing materials over the exit site and secure them in place. a. Gauze squares are usually placed with one square under the tubing and one square over the tubing. The dressing is secured on all sides with tape (Fig. 49-5). b. Transparent dressings are molded around the tubing where it leaves the dressing (Fig. 49-6).	To provide a sealed dressing that protects against contamination.

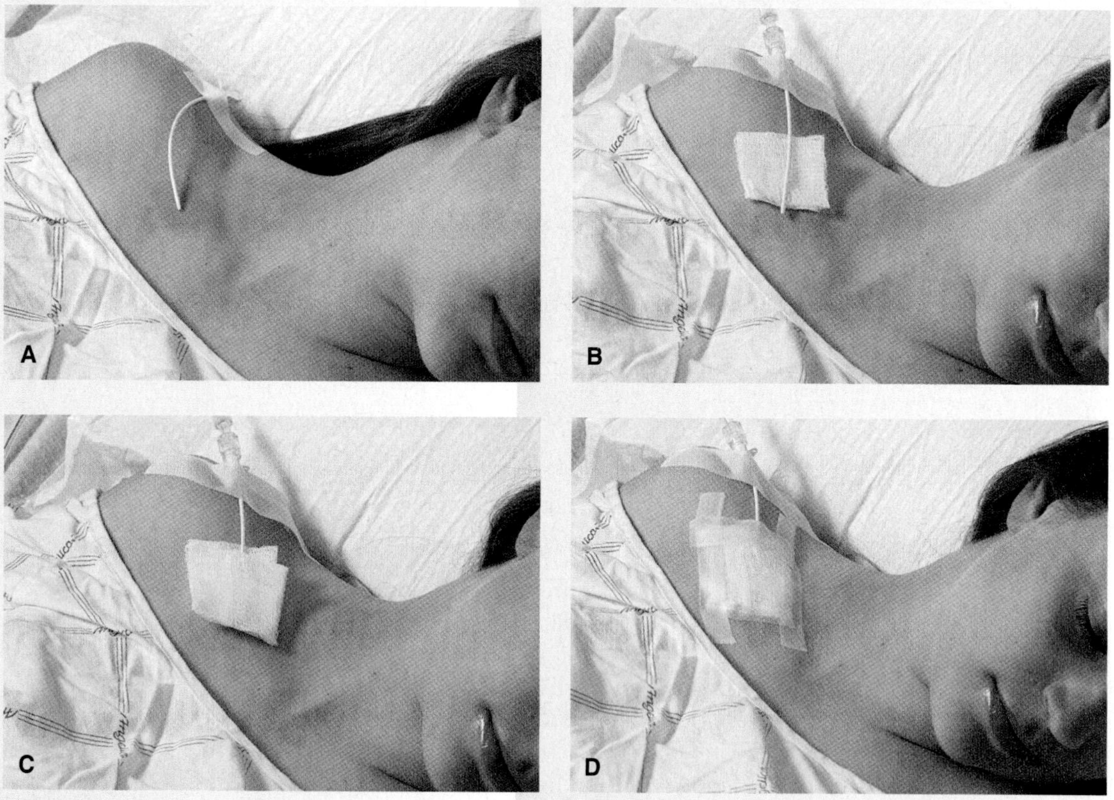

FIGURE 49-5 Using gauze squares as a dressing for a subclavian central venous line. (**A**) Catheter and insertion site. (**B**) The first gauze square is placed under the catheter. (**C**) The second gauze square is placed over the catheter exit site. (**D**) The edges are taped down to form a seal on all sides. Note how the tape is placed around the catheter.

(continued)

Action	Rationale
	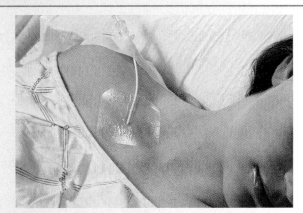 **FIGURE 49-6** Dressing the subclavian central venous line with a transparent, moisture-permeable dressing, such as OpSite.
c. Commercial dressings are available that protect the site and make it visible (Fig. 49-7).	**FIGURE 49-7** Commercial dressing for a central venous catheter. The line is connected to the IV tubing with a screw connection. Note the plastic clamp on the line.
21. Tape the catheter to the skin.	To protect the catheter from inadvertently being pulled.
 **22.** Remove and discard gloves and package wrappings.	To prevent contact between soiled gloves and other materials.
23. Wash or disinfect your hands.	To decrease the transfer of microorganisms that could cause infection.
24. Return the patient's bed to a low position and make the patient comfortable.	For patient safety and comfort.

EVALUATION

25. Evaluate using the individualized patient outcomes previously identified: dressing intact and clean; entrance site clear and free of infection or skin breakdown; IV line is intact with flow not obstructed, rate correctly set, and all connections secure; and patient does not experience discomfort. **R:** Evaluation in relation to desired outcomes is essential for planning future care.

DOCUMENTATION

26. Document the dressing change. **R:** Documentation is a legal record of the patient's care and therapy and communicates nursing activities to other nurses and caregivers. Document the following:
    a. dressing change
    b. appearance of exit site
    c. patient comfort

■ POTENTIAL ADVERSE OUTCOMES AND RELATED INTERVENTIONS

1. Infection of the catheter entry site.
Intervention: Report to the physician. A topical antibiotic may be ordered to treat the infection.

2. Bacteremia (systemic infection) originating in central catheter. The patient exhibits high fever, often has chills, and is flushed. The patient may appear very ill. The CDC only recognizes catheter-related bloodstream infections with bacteremia and labels those infections without bacteremia as colonization; therefore, bacteremia is diagnosed from blood cultures (CDC, 2002).
Intervention: Prevention is the first line of defense against bacteremia. Change the cap on the central line at regular intervals to prevent multiple puncture sites from allowing the entrance of microorganisms. Because no references identify exactly how many punctures of an IV cap are safe, check with the product manufacturer for individual recommendations. The larger the needle or needleless access device, the larger the openings. The more often the cap is punctured, the more likely microorganisms will enter (Pellowe, Pratt, Harper, et al., 2003).

Safety Alert ▲

The Occupational Safety and Health Administration (OSHA) requires hospitals to eliminate needles whenever possible; however, if needles must be used, 20- to 25-G needles 1 inch or less in length are the least likely to damage the cap or catheter and the most likely to reseal.

If bacteremia is suspected, notify the physician immediately. Blood cultures are drawn from a site other than the suspected catheter. The catheter is usually discontinued, with the tip sent in an appropriate container to the laboratory for culture and sensitivity testing. The patient will be started on appropriate antibiotic therapy based on the results of testing.

3. Occlusion of the central catheter. Occlusion may occur from medications that precipitate in the catheter, from blood clotting at the end, or from fibrin sheaths that form across the end of the catheter.
Intervention: Prevention is the most important approach to this adverse outcome. Use adequate amounts and types of flushing materials to prevent precipitation of materials in the tubing and to wash the blood out of the tubing. However, the fibrin sheath may not be entirely preventable. Often the fibrin sheath allows material to be instilled into the tube but prevents aspiration of blood from the catheter. When the catheter appears to be blocked, notify the physician. Some medications may be tried to dissolve clots or fibrin. When ordered, they are used in the manner prescribed by institutional protocol (Bunce, 2003).

4. Air embolism occurs when a large volume of air enters the central circulation and forms a bubble, which functions as an embolism. The patient experiences severe shortness of breath. When the embolus is large enough to lodge in the heart near a cardiac valve, a "cog-wheel" sound that is related to valve attempts to close is heard on auscultation of the heart.
Intervention: Immediately turn the patient onto the left side. This may trap the air embolus in the ventricle, preventing its movement into the lungs, where it will interfere with oxygenation of the blood. Notify the physician immediately. The air embolus may gradually be absorbed if it is not too large, but emergency treatment may be required.

CHANGING THE IV BAG OR BOTTLE AND THE TUBING

When changing an IV bag or bottle connected to a central line, use the same technique as for changing a bag or bottle on a conventional IV line (see Module 47). Remember that the tubing must be clamped during the changing of the bag or bottle and the tubing to prevent the potential for air embolus.

ESTABLISHING AN INTERMITTENT INFUSION LOCK ON A CENTRAL VENOUS CATHETER

When any CVC is being used for intermittent infusion and blood withdrawal, the catheter itself or the access tubing for an implanted port must be capped with a screw-type needleless injection cap. As in the regular IV lock, the catheter must be filled with heparinized saline solution to prevent clots from forming at the tip of the catheter and occluding it. A solution of 10 to 100/units heparin per milliliter of normal saline solution is the most common mixture. The heparin solution is injected at least twice a day to maintain patency of the catheter. Some facilities are experimenting with using a stronger heparin solution (100 to 500 units/mL) and allowing longer intervals between additions of new solution. Consult the policy in your facility.

PROCEDURE FOR ESTABLISHING AN INTERMITTENT INFUSION LOCK ON A CENTRAL VENOUS CATHETER

ASSESSMENT

1. Check the order for discontinuing IV fluids and establishing a heparin lock on a central line. **R:** This helps you be sure that the patient no longer needs continuous fluid administration.
2. Check the facility procedure for the type, amount, and strength of solution to be used to keep the lock open. **R:** Facilities vary in their policies in regard to the solution to be used.
3. Check the type of central IV line in place and the number of milliliters of fluid necessary to fill it. **R:** The flush solution must fill the catheter, plus there must be enough extra to flush through the tip.

ANALYSIS

4. Critically think through your data, carefully evaluating each aspect and its relation to other data. **R:** This enables you to determine specific problems for this individual in relation to establishing the intermittent infusion lock.

5. Identify specific problems and modifications of the procedure needed for this individual. **R:** Planning for the individual must take into consideration the individual's problems.

PLANNING

6. Determine individualized patient outcomes in relation to this procedure. **R:** Identification of desired outcomes guides planning and evaluation. Include
   a. Catheter clamp is secure on the catheter.
   b. Adapter is securely fastened to the catheter hub.
   c. The correct amount and type of solution are in the catheter and lock.
7. Gather the necessary equipment.
   a. Sterile needleless access screw-type cap. **R:** Needleless devices protect staff from the potential for needle-stick injuries and infection transmission. A screw-on cap is secure.
   b. 10-mL syringe with solution to keep lock open and a special tip for accessing the needleless device. If syringes do not come prefilled, use a needle to fill the syringe, and then change the needle for a needleless tip. **R:** The 10-mL syringe has an internal diameter that provides the pressure needed for turbulence in the catheter that thoroughly flushes through the tubing. There are newer flushing syringes that hold smaller volumes of fluid but have the same diameter as the 10-mL syringe. The Hickman catheter has an internal volume of 2 mL. An extra 0.5 mL (2.5 mL total) is usually added to make sure the tip of the catheter is free of clots. Surgically implanted ports hold 5 mL of solution. Some facilities use a larger volume to irrigate the catheter or port to ensure that all blood is flushed out. Follow the procedure in your facility.
   c. Alcohol wipes to disinfect the connection site

   d. Clean gloves to protect yourself from possible exposure to blood

IMPLEMENTATION

Action	Rationale
8. Wash or disinfect your hands.	To decrease the transfer of microorganisms that could cause infection.
9. Identify the patient, using two identifiers.	To be sure you are performing the procedure for the correct patient.
10. Close the door and pull the curtain.	To provide privacy.
11. Explain the procedure to the patient.	Explaining the procedure helps relieve anxiety or misperceptions that the patient may have about a procedure or activity and sets the stage for patient participation.

(continued)

Action	Rationale
12. Turn off the IV infusion and clamp the catheter.	To prevent fluid from flowing onto the area when it is disconnected and protect the patient from possible air embolus.
13. Put on gloves.	To protect yourself from coming in contact with any blood returning through the catheter.
14. Scrub the junction of the catheter and the tubing with an alcohol wipe for 1 minute and allow the solution to dry before proceeding.	To decrease the number of microbes in the immediate area when the tubing is opened. The period of time to allow drying creates the most effective antimicrobial activity.
15. Open the package containing the sterile cap. Hold the cap carefully by the outside rim of the rubber injection cap.	To preserve sterility, do not touch the end that will be placed in the central IV line.
16. Loosen the IV tubing connector by twisting it, remove the IV tubing, and insert the injection cap screwing it on firmly. Be careful to maintain sterility of the ends of the catheter and the cap.	Excessive force will make the cap difficult to remove. If the injection cap falls out, or the ends are touched, the system is open to contamination.
17. Insert the needleless connector of the filled syringe into the cap. Follow the instructions for the specific needleless connector being used.	For most needleless systems, the tip is pushed firmly into the opening.
18. Release the clamp and inject the prescribed solution into the catheter, clamping as you finish injecting.	Be sure that the clamp is open so that excess force is not exerted against the walls of the catheter. Clamping at the end of instillation keeps a positive pressure in the tubing.
19. Remove the syringe from the cap and discard it into the sharps container.	All used syringes are considered biohazardous material and discarded.
20. Remove gloves, and wash or disinfect your hands.	To decrease the transfer of microorganisms that could cause infection.

EVALUATION

21. Evaluate using the individualized patient outcomes previously identified. **R:** Evaluation in relation to desired outcomes is essential for planning future care.
    a. Catheter clamp secure on the catheter.
    b. Adapter securely fastened to the catheter hub.
    c. The correct amount and type of solution are in the catheter.

DOCUMENTATION

22. Discontinuing the continuous infusion and placing the lock on the central line are typically noted on the IV flow sheet. If this is not the case in your facility, make a brief note on the progress record. **R:** Documentation is a legal record of the patient's care and therapy and communicates nursing activities to other nurses and caregivers.

DRAWING BLOOD THROUGH A CENTRAL VENOUS CATHETER

Most CVCs may be used for drawing blood because the diameter is large enough for blood flow and they can be flushed clear of blood. Some small-diameter catheters are more easily occluded if used for drawing blood. Check the policy in your facility for which central catheters may be used for drawing blood.

PROCEDURE FOR DRAWING BLOOD THROUGH A CENTRAL VENOUS CATHETER

ASSESSMENT

1. Check the order for blood tests to be done. **R:** Checking the order ensures that you are completing the procedure for the correct tests and have the information needed to enable you to select correct supplies.

2. Check the facility protocols to determine which types of blood collection tubes should be used for the test(s) ordered. **R:** Blood collection tubes are characterized by different colors of rubber stoppers. Each color identifies a particular preservative in the tube (or that a tube has no preservative). Each blood test has particular requirements for the type of tube and for handling as it is transported to the lab.

3. Check the type of CVC that is in place. **R:** The type of CVC determines whether there is fluid running that must be restarted after blood drawing or whether it is locked, and the central line must be relocked after the blood is drawn.

ANALYSIS

4. Critically think through your data, carefully evaluating each aspect and its relation to other data. **R:** This enables you to determine specific problems for this individual in relation to drawing blood from a CVC.

5. Identify specific problems and modifications of the procedure needed for this individual. **R:** Planning for the individual must take into consideration the individual's problems.

PLANNING

6. Determine individualized patient outcomes for this procedure, including the following. **R:** Identification of desired outcomes guides planning and evaluation.
   a. Sufficient blood is drawn and placed in an appropriate, labeled test tube for each test ordered.
   b. Catheter is patent.
   c. Tubing or adaptor port is securely fastened to the catheter hub.
   d. The correct amount and type of solution are in the catheter if the catheter is being used intermittently.

   e. The correct fluid is flowing at the correct rate for a catheter in current use.

7. Gather the necessary equipment.
   a. One empty 5-mL syringe without a needle or an extra 5-mL test tube without anticoagulant for the blood collection device. **R:** To remove and discard the fluid that is currently in the line.
   b. A blood collection device that holds blood sample tubes and an appropriate connector or one syringe large enough to aspirate the amount of blood required for the laboratory test(s) ordered. **R:** Blood collection devices that hold the blood sample tubes so that no transfer of blood is needed are the recommended method. This decreases the chance of contact with blood during the process. Because the sealed vacuum tubes must be punctured to fill them, a syringe must be fitted with a needle to fill the tube, putting the staff member at higher risk. The vacuum in the tubes withdraws the blood.
   c. Test tubes of the appropriate type and number needed for the tests to be done; be sure to attach test tube labels. **R:** Using the correct tube supports accurate test results. Labeling of the test tube ensures that the data is recorded for the correct patient.
   d. Two 10-mL syringes with saline solution to flush blood from the line; if syringes do not come prefilled, fill the syringe, and then change the needle for a needleless tip. **R:** The 10-mL syringe has an internal diameter that provides the pressure needed for turbulence in the catheter that thoroughly flushes through the tubing. There are newer flushing syringes that hold smaller volumes of fluid but have the same diameter as the 10-mL syringe to provide the flow turbulence but do not require as much saline solution. Some facilities use a larger volume to irrigate the catheter or port. Follow the procedure in your facility.
   e. One syringe with the amount of heparinized or normal saline solution (depending upon the type of line and facility policy if a locked line is in place. **R:** This equipment helps in making sure the entire line, including the tip of the catheter, will remain free of clots.
   f. A sterile needle or needleless connector in its cover to hold the cap or to place on the end of an IV tubing to protect it from contamination
   g. Povidone-iodine or alcohol wipe to cleanse the connection and the access port; the povidone may leave a sticky residue. In some facilities, after the povidone has dried, the surface is wiped with alcohol to remove residue.

h. Clean gloves to protect your hands from possible exposure to blood

i. Eye protection to protect your eyes from the possibility of blood splashing from an accident with the syringe or the blood tube; face shields and goggles are the best eye protection because they completely shield the eyes from all directions. Regular eyeglasses may be considered adequate eye protection in some instances, but they do not protect from the side. Check the policy in your facility as to whether or not eyeglasses may be used for eye protection.

j. Alcohol wipes to clean the outside of the tubing/catheter connection

k. Plastic bag to protect transport and laboratory people when blood tubes are sent to the laboratory

IMPLEMENTATION

Action	Rationale
8. Wash or disinfect your hands.	To decrease the transfer of microorganisms that could cause infection.
9. Identify the patient, using two identifiers.	To be sure you are performing the procedure for the correct patient.
10. Close the door and pull the curtain.	To provide privacy.
11. Explain the procedure to the patient.	Explaining the procedure helps relieve anxiety or misperceptions that the patient may have about a procedure or activity and sets the stage for patient participation.
12. Turn off the IV infusion.	To prevent fluid from draining onto the surroundings when disconnected.
13. Put on gloves.	To protect yourself from the possibility of contact with blood.
14. Clamp the catheter in the off position.	To prevent air from entering as the tubing is disconnected and fluid from spilling onto surroundings.
15. Scrub the junction of the catheter and the tubing (or the junction of the catheter and the cap) with the povidone-iodine or alcohol wipe. Allow the solution to dry before proceeding.	To decrease the number of microbes in the immediate area when the tubing is opened.
16. Remove the IV tubing connector or the cap by twisting it and cover the end of the cap or tubing with a sterile needle or needleless connector.	To keep it sterile while you are working. Experienced nurses may hold this between two fingers but this is not recommended for the beginner because contamination is too likely.
17. Connect the empty 5-mL syringe or the collection device to the catheter.	To allow you to aspirate the contents of the catheter.
18. Release the clamp on the catheter.	To allow fluid to be aspirated.

(continued)

Action	Rationale
19. Aspirate 5 mL fluid from the catheter, or engage an extra test tube into the collection device to aspirate blood for discard. For some patients (such as children or those with a very low red blood count) removing blood is not appropriate. In these instances, use the "pull—push" method to clear the line. Aspirate into the syringe, and then push the fluid and blood back into the patient. Do this three times and you will have rinsed all the fluid out of the tubing, and it will be filled with undiluted blood. *Note:* If the syringe will not aspirate with ease, have the patient turn. Turning will move the tip of the catheter in the vein, and if it was against the wall of the vein or a valve, will allow it to move away. Gently aspirate again. If you still cannot aspirate, stop the procedure, and notify the physician.	The heparinized saline solution or IV fluid must be completely removed from the catheter, and the catheter filled with undiluted blood for test accuracy.
20. Clamp the tubing and put aside the syringe with blood or the blood tube to be discarded into the sharps container. If an extra test tube is used, discard it immediately so that it is not confused with an actual sample at a later time.	The sharps container is considered a biohazard container.
21. One at a time, place the blood collection tubes into the collection device and allow them to fill. If a syringe is to be used, attach the large syringe and aspirate the amount of blood needed.	The vacuum in the tubes draws the correct amount of blood into the tube for the amount of preservative in the tube. Each tube can be set aside.
22. Reclamp the catheter, and then disconnect the syringe or collection device.	To prevent air from entering as the syringe or collection device is disconnected.
23. Flush the line. The recommended amount of flush solution after withdrawing blood is 20 mL normal saline solution in two 10-mL syringes. a. Connect the first saline solution–filled syringe into the catheter. b. Release the clamp and inject the saline solution into the catheter, clamping as you finish injecting. c. Remove the syringe from the catheter and repeat with the second saline solution-filled syringe.	Making sure that the clamp is open while injecting flush solution prevents excess force from being exerted against the walls of the catheter. Clamping at the end of injection keeps a positive pressure in the tubing. Thorough flushing prevents clotting in the line.

(continued)

Action	Rationale
d. Be sure to clamp the catheter before removing the syringe.	
e. If a syringe was used to withdraw blood, fill the test tubes at this time. Agitate each one gently to mix in the preservative.	The drawn blood must be placed in the appropriate container before the blood begins clotting.
24. Restart the IV flow at the correct rate, or fill the lock according to facility policy.	
a. *For IV fluid:* Uncover the tip of the IV tubing and attach it to the catheter, being careful to maintain sterility of the ends of the catheter. Unclamp the catheter and then set the IV pump for the correct rate.	Restarting the IV fluid prevents clotting in the catheter.
b. *For lock:* Insert the needleless connector into the catheter. Screw the connection device in securely by hand. Release the clamp and inject prescribed heparinized solution into the catheter, clamping as you finish injecting. Remove the syringe from the cap and discard into the sharps container.	The heparinized saline solution prevents clotting in the catheter.
25. If blood has been collected in a syringe, fill the tubes. Place labeled blood test tubes in the plastic bag and attach the requisition.	For safe transport to the laboratory and clear identification of the correct patient.
26. Remove gloves, and wash or disinfect your hands.	To decrease the transfer of microorganisms that could cause infection.

EVALUATION

27. Evaluate using the individualized patient outcomes previously identified. **R:** Evaluation in relation to desired outcomes is essential for planning future care.
    a. Sufficient blood was drawn and placed in appropriate, labeled tube for each test ordered.
    b. Catheter is patent.
    c. Tubing or adaptor port is securely fastened to the catheter hub.
    d. The correct amount and type of solution are in the catheter if the catheter is being used intermittently.
    e. The correct fluid is flowing at the correct rate for a catheter in current use.

DOCUMENTATION

28. A note may be made of the blood drawn and sent to the lab. This may be on the narrative record, or there may be a place on the laboratory documen-tation to note blood drawn. **R:** Documentation is a legal record of the patient's care and therapy and communicates nursing activities to other nurses and caregivers.

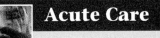

Acute Care

In the acute care environment, you are more likely to be working with the newly inserted CVC. Assessment is particularly critical at this point because initial complications may become apparent early. These patients often have multiple IV medications as well as total parenteral nutrition (TPN). When heparin is used in CVCs, the nurse must take the responsibility for calculating how much heparin is being given in a 24-hour period in order to consult with the physician regarding whether the patient is receiving enough heparin to alter bleeding and clotting times.

Long-Term Care

Central venous catheters are rarely used for residents in long-term care environments except for terminally ill individuals who have had catheters placed earlier for therapy. The CVC may continue to be used for pain management in the terminally ill person.

Home Care

Most clients with long-term needs for a CVC for chemotherapy or TPN go home with these catheters in place. When possible, the client is taught how to provide self-care. When that is not possible, a caregiver may be taught how to care for the catheter. The home care nurse usually visits initially to help the client and caregiver determine the best way to manage the various procedures in the home. Thereafter, the home care nurse makes periodic visits for assessment if the client is not returning to a clinic on a regular basis.

Ambulatory Care

Ambulatory clinics treating people with serious chronic illnesses such as cancer administer medications through existing CVCs. The nurse in the clinic provides the assessment, answers client or caregiver questions, and helps to make sure that the catheter remains patent and effective for the purpose for which it was inserted. In some instances, new CVCs are inserted in day procedures where the client will be discharged immediately. In such cases, the teaching plan is often carried out in advance to be sure that the client can manage self-care at home.

LEARNING TOOLS

DEVELOP YOUR BACKGROUND KNOWLEDGE

1. Review the Learning Outcomes.

2. Read the section on central venous catheters in your assigned text.

3. Look up the Key Terms in the glossary.

4. Review the module as though you were preparing to teach the contents to another person. Mentally practice the skills.

DEVELOP YOUR SKILLS

In the practice setting
1. Examine the various central venous catheters (CVCs) used in the facility in which you practice.

2. Review the following procedures in your facility:
   a. CVC dressing change
   b. CVC care
   c. tunneled catheter care (Hickman or Broviac)
   d. subcutaneous catheter port (Port-a-cath, Infus-a-port) care

3. Choose a partner. Change so that each has the opportunity to play the role of the patient and practice each of the following procedures. A chest mannequin with various central venous catheters may also be used. Those who are not participating at a given time can observe and evaluate the performances of the others.
   a. CVC dressing change
   b. establishing an intermittent lock on a CVC
   c. drawing blood through a CVC
   d. When you have mastered these procedures, select another student and critique each other's performance. Use the Performance Checklist on the CD-ROM in the front of this book as a guide.
   e. Arrange for your instructor to evaluate your performances.

DEMONSTRATE YOUR SKILLS

In the clinical setting, do the following:
1. Identify patients with CVCs in place.

2. Consult with your instructor regarding the opportunity to observe and/or assist with the care of these patients.

3. Ask your instructor for an opportunity to carry out the specific care needed by the patient.

CRITICAL THINKING EXERCISES

1. Jeff Madison has had Crohn's disease for many years. Because his recent exacerbation was particularly severe, a CVC for total parenteral nutrition (TPN) is to be inserted. The procedure is scheduled for tomorrow morning. As you plan for Jeff's care, determine what concerns he might have about this procedure and how the procedure is carried out. Specify what teaching will be needed and what concerns he might have. Describe what you will need to do to assist with such a procedure in your setting. Identify your immediate concerns for the patient after the procedure and decide how you will address these concerns in your planning.

2. Margaret Sand, age 83, was admitted with severe pneumonia. Because her veins were so poor, the physician decided that a PICC line should be

inserted to provide IV access for fluids and antibiotics. The certified IV nurse has just inserted the PICC line. Specify what concerns you will have and what monitoring you should do. When can the PICC line be used to start the ordered fluids and antibiotics? What care guidelines should you establish? Explain whether Mrs. Sand's age has any influence on your care planning.

SELF-QUIZ
SHORT-ANSWER QUESTIONS

1. What are two common reasons for the use of CVCs?

   a. _____

   b. _____

2. Name two major adverse outcomes of CVCs.

   a. _____

   b. _____

3. List three purposes for changing the dressing on a CVC.

   a. _____

   b. _____

   c. _____

4. What is the purpose of applying an antiseptic or antimicrobial ointment to the catheter insertion site?

   _____

5. Why should a right atrial catheter with a peripheral exit site be labeled as a CVC directly on the dressing?

   _____

6. What is the difference between the Hickman catheter and the Broviac catheter?

   _____

7. Why is the cap removed from the CVC for drawing of blood?

   _____

8. Why is a tunneled CVC always clamped when not in use?

   _____

9. What type of needle is used to access an implanted subcutaneous central venous port such as a Port-a-cath, and why?

   _____

MULTIPLE CHOICE

_____ 10. Which products are appropriate to use for cleaning a CVC site? (Choose all that apply.)
   a. Acetone
   b. Iodophor iodine
   c. Tincture of iodine
   d. Chlorhexidine

_____ 11. When you cannot aspirate from a central line, your first action should be to
   a. reclamp the catheter, and notify the physician.
   b. use the declotting protocol in the facility.
   c. get a larger syringe to put more suction on it.
   d. ask the patient to turn, and try again.

_____ 12. Which kind of CV catheter is most often associated with an insertion site infection?
   a. Implantable port
   b. Hickman catheter
   c. Standard CVC
   d. PICC

Answers to the Self-Quiz questions appear in the back of the book.

SKILLS INCLUDED IN THIS MODULE

Procedure for Initiating Intravenous Access
Procedure for Converting an Intravenous Infusion to an
Intravenous Lock

PREREQUISITE MODULES

Module 1	An Approach to Nursing Skills
Module 2	Documentation
Module 4	Basic Infection Control
Module 5	Safety in the Healthcare Environment
Module 13	Monitoring Intake and Output
Module 14	Nursing Physical Assessment
Module 24	Basic Sterile Technique: Sterile Field and Sterile Gloves
Module 44	Administering Oral Medications
Module 46	Administering Medications by Injection
Module 47	Preparing and Maintaining Intravenous Infusions

*Review of the anatomy and physiology of
the vascular system.*

KEY TERMS

antecubital space	patent
armboard	Penrose drain
bevel	percutaneous
bifurcation	peripherally
butterfly	inserted central
infiltration	catheter (PICC)
IV cannula	phlebitis
laminar airflow	tourniquet
hood	venipuncture

OVERALL OBJECTIVE

▶ To initiate intravenous (IV) therapy safely and comfortably for patients, using the equipment correctly and maintaining safety for the nurse.

LEARNING OUTCOMES

The student will be able to

1. Assess the patient to determine an appropriate site to insert an intravenous (IV) access device.
2. Analyze assessment data to determine special problems or concerns that must be addressed to successfully start the IV infusion.
3. Determine appropriate patient outcomes related to starting the IV infusion and recognize the potential for adverse outcomes.
4. Determine and select appropriate equipment and supplies for starting the IV infusion for a specific patient.
5. Initiate IV therapy in a safe, effective, and comfortable manner.
6. Convert an IV infusion to an IV lock.
7. Evaluate the effectiveness of the IV access in relation to its purpose as well as the patient's response to it.
8. Document the procedure in the patient's record.

Depending on the policies of the facility, unit nurses may or may not insert intravenous (IV) access devices (commonly referred to as "starting an IV"). If the nurse will be hanging IV fluids after the IV access is established, the nurse must follow the six rights and three checks in relation to the fluid (see Module 47). If specially trained IV nurses are responsible for starting IV infusions, the unit nurse must still be sufficiently familiar with the equipment and the procedure to be of assistance.

NURSING DIAGNOSES

Patients who require IV therapy may have a variety of nursing diagnoses. Among them are the following:

■ Risk for Deficient Fluid Volume or the actual problem of Deficient Fluid Volume related to fasting (NPO) status, nausea, and/or vomiting.
■ Risk for Infection related to breach of normal body defenses.

The various potential complications of IV therapy, such as **phlebitis** and **infiltration,** also are a concern and are discussed later in the module.

DELEGATION

Initiation of IV therapy is not delegated to assistive personnel. They may care for individuals receiving IV infusions and should be aware that signs of complications, such as pain and swelling, should be reported immediately.

PSYCHOLOGICAL IMPLICATIONS

The knowledge that they are about to have an IV inserted is threatening to some patients. Some may feel the procedure implies serious illness. Others are frightened by the threat of pain, discomfort, and immobility. Still others fear contracting infections, such as acquired immunodeficiency syndrome (AIDS). Previous experience can help make the patient less apprehensive, assuming the experience was positive. For others, the memories of problems related to IV infusions make the impending experience more frightening.

Explain the procedure just a few minutes before the IV is to be started. This prepares the patient without providing a long time for worry. In addition, keep the equipment out of the room until you actually begin.

The use of an intradermal or topical anesthetic agent makes it easier for the patient to cooperate and removes most of the pain and discomfort associated with the insertion. However, the anesthetic sometimes makes it more difficult to identify the vein in challenging situations. In some facilities, the policy is to use 0.1 to 0.2 mL of a local anesthetic intradermally to numb the skin and the vein before starting an IV. An alternative is EMLA cream (lidocaine and prilocaine) applied to the planned IV site. This, however, must be applied 60 minutes before beginning and covered with an occlusive dressing. Check the manufacturer's literature for specific directions. Before using an intradermal anesthetic or applying EMLA cream, you must check the patient's history for allergies. Individual healthcare facilities may have specific policies governing the use of a local anesthetic before **venipuncture.**

INDICATIONS FOR INTRAVENOUS ACCESS

Intravenous access enables IV fluids to be given for many different reasons, such as meeting the daily requirements for fluid in the patient who is NPO (fasting) or who is nauseated and vomiting, replacing lost fluid in the postoperative patient, and providing large amounts of fluid rapidly for a patient who is severely dehydrated. Intravenous access also facilitates the administration of many medications, such as pain medications and antibiotics. In emergency situations, IV administration of medications is essential for rapid achievement of therapeutic effects.

Intravenous fluids are ordered by the physician specifically to meet the needs of the individual patient. Refer to Module 47, Preparing and Maintaining Intravenous Infusions, for a discussion of the variety of solutions available and the procedure for administering them.

An IV access device or IV lock is inserted and maintained when there is need for IV access without need for IV fluids. Examples of such situations are the need for IV antibiotic therapy and the need for access for prn (as needed) drug therapy. Advantages of an IV lock include greater patient mobility and reduction in cost of care. Module 48, Administering Intravenous Medications, includes a discussion of IV locks.

PREVENTING INFECTIONS ASSOCIATED WITH INTRAVENOUS DEVICES

One aspect of preventing healthcare-acquired infections is the prevention of infections among healthcare workers. The current recommendation is that gloves be worn during any invasive procedure to protect the healthcare worker (Pellowe et al., 2003). Gloves protect the caregiver from the possibility of contamination by the patient's blood through skin breaks.

Gloves do not protect from inadvertent needle sticks. Needle sticks present more of a risk for bloodborne infections than do blood spills because the skin is penetrated. The larger the device, the more blood it can carry, and the greater the potential of transmitting infection. Because of this risk, there is a general move to the use of safety IV access devices that protect the caregiver from accidental needle sticks. These are referred to as "engineering controls" by the Occupational Safety and Health Administration (OSHA) and include non-needle sharps or a needle with a built-in safety feature or mechanism that effectively reduces the risk of an exposure incident (OSHA, 2001).

The Agency for Health Research and Quality of the Centers for Disease Control and Prevention (CDC) has created the National Guideline Clearing House for the dissemination of evidence-based guidelines in healthcare. Among those documents are two addressing the prevention of healthcare-associated patient infections related to IV devices (O'Grady, et al., 2002; & Singapore Ministry of Health, 2002). These comprehensive documents review research and other evidence worldwide and make recommendations based on the strength of the evidence. Some of the central recommendations for preventing infection of IV sites include effective disinfection of the site before cannula insertion, not palpating the site after it has been cleansed, and caring for the site appropriately. The most common source of infection associated with IV devices is the IV cannula wound. The terminology **IV cannula** refers to all types of **percutaneous** devices used for vascular access, including small steel needles (as found on **butterfly** and scalp vein devices) and plastic catheters. The IV access device is a direct conduit between the world external to the patient and the bloodstream.

INTRAVENOUS EQUIPMENT

No single type of IV equipment is ideal; each has advantages and disadvantages. Most facilities select a single manufacturer of IV solutions and equipment as their supplier. You will become familiar with this equipment with time. Types of IV bags and bottles and administration sets are discussed in Module 47.

A peripheral IV is inserted into a vein in an extremity or in the case of an infant, in the scalp. A central IV is inserted into a major central vein such as the internal jugular or subclavian. A **peripherally inserted central catheter (PICC)** is inserted in a peripheral vein but threaded into the vein until the tip reaches a central vein. See Module 49 for more detailed information about central venous catheters. This module focuses on inserting peripheral IVs.

When choosing equipment, consider the purpose of the IV access; the type of IV solution or medication ordered for the patient; the patient's diagnosis and history of IV therapy; the length of time the equipment will be in place; and the patient's age, mobility, and vein condition and structure. Then compare these factors to the characteristics of the equipment and make your choice. For each situation, select the catheter with the shortest length and the smallest diameter that allows for appropriate administration of the fluid or other therapy prescribed. Soft plastic cannulas cause less irritation to the vein than metal cannulas. Steel cannulas are recommended only when the IV therapy is planned to last no more than a few hours. Their movement in the vessel is more likely to lead to phlebitis than a catheter made of another material (Singapore Ministry of Health, 2002).

The winged-tip infusion set comes with plastic "wings" that are attached to the cannula hub for easier manipulation during insertion. Like a handle, the wings can be held at an angle to the vein for inserting the cannula, and after the vein has been entered, the wings lie flat against the skin and provide a means for securing the needle and tubing (Fig. 50-1).

A winged-tip device consisting of an over-the-needle (plastic) catheter (ONC) with attached tubing (e.g., Angio-set/Intima IV catheter) is the preferred access device (Fig. 50-2) for most standard applications. From ¾ to 1 inch long, these devices are available in gauges from 16 to 24. The smaller sizes are particularly useful for infants' scalp veins and for patients with small, fragile, or rolling veins. The nurse inserts the needle and catheter. When blood returns, the needle is removed, leaving only the flexible catheter in place. Steel winged-tip or butterfly devices (often referred to as scalp vein needles) are also available.

Over-the-needle IV access devices also are available with protective needle shields that prevent needle-stick injuries. These shields are activated after the IV cannula is in place and the nurse is ready to remove the needle.

SELECTING A VEIN

Selection of a vein depends on a number of factors, including the reason for the IV, the length of time it is expected to be needed, the condition of the patient's veins, and the patient's comfort and safety. If you have a choice, it is preferable not to use the dominant hand or arm and it is better to change sides with subsequent IVs. Your choices are commonly limited by the diagnosis, the condition of the patient's veins, or the presence of additional equipment. IV lines are not started on an arm with a dialysis access or on the side of a mastectomy because of concern regarding circulation on that side.

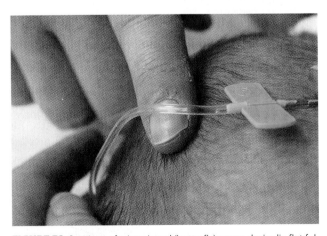

FIGURE 50-1 Wings of wing-tipped (butterfly) access device lie flat following insertion of the cannula.

Leg veins in adults are a poor choice because they are associated with higher rates of infections (O'Grady, et al., 2002).

Although it is usually easy to start an IV in the branches of either the cephalic or the basilic vein located near the **antecubital space** (inner aspect of the elbow), these veins are usually not a good choice. In addition to limiting the patient's mobility in that arm, laboratory technicians often rely on these veins for blood samples. Also, these veins are the preferred site for PICC access. They should be used as a last resort and in emergency situations only. Leg veins are avoided because of the danger of thrombus formation and subsequent pulmonary emboli.

The scalp veins are used in infants because there is less movement there and hence less chance of dislocation. Scalp vein IV devices, however, are esthetically unpleasant, and parents may object to their use. Another excellent site in infants or nonambulatory small children is the portion of the saphenous vein that crosses or is anterior to the medial malleolus. When initiating IV therapy for infants and children, avoid a child's thumb-sucking hand, the dominant hand of an older child, or the feet of children who are ambulatory.

For the adult patient, start IVs in a hand if possible. If hand veins are not accessible, the lower branches of the basilic and the cephalic veins of the forearm (Fig. 50-3) can be used. Then, if you are unsuccessful, or if the IV comes out later, you can choose a vein proximal to or higher than the first one. A site where there is **bifurcation** may be easier to enter if you can enter from below. Compare the length of the device you plan to use with the available vein.

Select the vein by looking, palpating, and attempting to distend any veins in the area. A clearly visible vein that can be palpated and that has a straight section for entry is most desirable. If one is not visible, look for the faint outline of a blue vein under the skin to determine where to begin. If not even an outline is visible, you must begin to distend the veins to make them visible or palpable.

To distend the veins, place a **tourniquet** (a length of **Penrose drain** will suffice if no commercial tourniquet is available) a few inches above the area where you want to start the IV and ask the patient to "pump" (opening and closing the fist). Generally, these maneuvers distend the vein, making it easier to locate and enter. If you still cannot locate a vein, place the arm in a dependent position for 5 to 10 minutes or apply warm wet packs to the area (Fig. 50-4). Veins that are not visible but are palpable can be used.

Some veins can be entered without using a tourniquet, which is advisable when a patient's veins are particularly fragile or rolling. The extra distention produced by a tourniquet can cause a vein to rupture or roll even more. In these cases, some nurses prefer to use a blood pressure cuff instead of a tourniquet. Inflate the cuff to

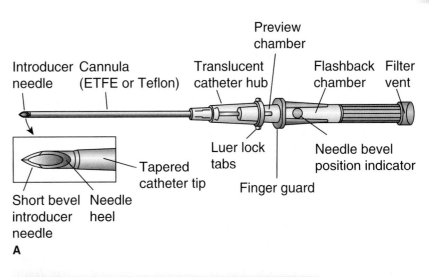

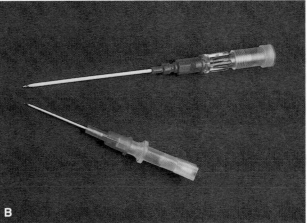

FIGURE 50-2 Various styles of over-the-needle IV access devices. (**A**) Diagram of the ONC device (**B**) and appearance of the ONC device.

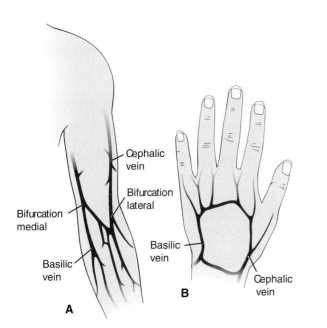

FIGURE 50-3 Suitable veins for starting an IV in an adult arm. (**A**) Forearm. (**B**) Hand.

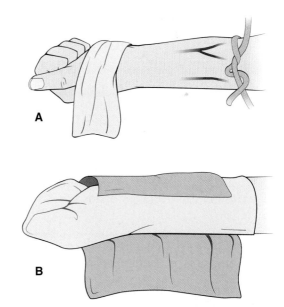

FIGURE 50-4 Ways to distend a vein. (**A**) Tourniquet. (**B**) Moist heat.

just below the diastolic pressure to dilate the vein, but not cause excessive distention.

If you have tried two times and have been unable to enter a vein, it is best to get assistance. The procedure is uncomfortable for the patient, and it is unwise to use up all the available veins. If no member of the nursing staff can start the IV, it may be necessary to ask the anesthesia department for assistance (depending on the policies in your facility), or the physician may elect to insert a central venous catheter.

PROCEDURE FOR INITIATING INTRAVENOUS ACCESS

ASSESSMENT

1. Validate the physician's orders for placement of an IV or facility policy regarding changing the site. If IV fluids are to be infused, the orders will include the type and amount of solution and the length of time over which it should run. The physician also may order additional medications to be added to the solution. Depending on the policies of the facility in which you work, you may add them yourself, or they may be added in the pharmacy under a **laminar airflow hood** (see Module 48, Administering Intravenous Medications). **R:** Validation is a way to verify the accuracy of the infusion to be started. Based on the CDC recommendations, peripheral IV lines are commonly changed every 72 to 96 hours and additives are instilled into the solution in the pharmacy to decrease infections (O'Grady, et al., 2002).

2. Check the patient's record for notes regarding previous IV infusions, any limitations to site selection, and/or complications noted. **R:** The patient's record helps determine if any adjustments need to be made with regard to equipment, site selection, and the like.

ANALYSIS

3. Critically think through your data, carefully evaluating each aspect and its relation to other data.

R: This will enable you to determine specific problems for this individual in relation to IV therapy.

4. Identify specific problems and modifications of the procedure needed for this individual. **R:** Planning for the individual must take into consideration the individual's problems.

PLANNING

5. Determine individualized patient outcomes in relation to initiating IV access, including the following. **R:** Identification of desired outcomes guides planning and evaluation.
   a. IV access device is **patent.**
   b. IV access device is secured in place with appropriate dressing.
   c. Hand or arm is positioned for comfort without obstructing potential IV fluid flow.
   d. IV fluids are infusing as prescribed, or an IV lock is in place.

6. Determine and select equipment to set up and start the IV infusion. Much of this equipment may be in an "IV start" package or may be kept together in a box or on a cart. This is a convenient practice because you may not know which device you will use until you examine the patient. Be sure that this box or cart is kept well stocked. **R:** Planning ahead allows you to proceed more safely and effectively. You will need the following:
   a. tourniquet
   b. chlorhexidine swab
   c. IV access device of choice
   d. tape (tear four 6-inch strips and place them conveniently at hand)
   e. dressing materials used in your facility; transparent occlusive dressings are commonly used.
   f. **armboard**
   g. clean gloves
   h. sterile IV solution if ordered, along with tubing and an IV pole (pole may be in the room) *or* IV lock and syringe with saline solution (or heparinized saline solution depending upon facility policy) for instillation into the lock.

IMPLEMENTATION

Action	Rationale
7. Wash or disinfect your hands.	To decrease the transfer of microorganisms that could cause infection.
8. Set up the IV fluid or the IV lock in the medication preparation area.	To avoid increasing any anxiety the patient might have about having an IV infusion.

(continued)

Action	Rationale
a. Set up the IV fluid and tubing as described in Module 47.	
b. For an IV lock, draw up the solution to fill the lock.	
9. Identify the patient, using two identifiers.	Verifying the patient's identity helps ensure that you are performing the right procedure for the right patient.
10. Explain the procedure to the patient. Just a few minutes before you plan to start the IV, tell the patient that IV therapy has been ordered and why. (See the section on Psychological Implications, and refer to Module 47.)	Explaining the procedure helps relieve anxiety or misperceptions that the patient may have and sets the stage for patient participation.
11. Adjust the lighting. Be sure you have adequate lighting, which is extremely important and often overlooked. If the room lights are inadequate, locate a portable lamp for temporary use.	To better visualize potential IV sites.
12. Prepare the patient physically.	
a. Close the door to the room and pull the curtain around the bed.	To provide for privacy.
b. Prepare the patient for IV therapy. Look at the gown or pajamas the patient is wearing and help the patient change to more convenient clothing if necessary. You may have to remove the patient's watch or change the position of the identification band if either is in the way.	A pajama top with narrow sleeves or a long nightgown may be difficult if not impossible to remove once the IV line is in place. A patient gown with a shoulder snap opening is often the easiest and best garment for the patient to wear. The identification band and watch are frequently where they will interfere with inserting or dressing the IV.
c. Position the patient as comfortably and conveniently as possible and place a towel under the arm.	To provide comfort for the patient, to facilitate initiation of the IV infusion, and to protect the bed.
13. Raise the bed to an appropriate working position based on your height.	To allow you to use correct body mechanics and protect yourself from back injury.
14. Wash or disinfect your hands, and put on clean gloves.	To decrease the transfer of microorganisms that could cause infection and to protect you from blood spills.
15. Set up the equipment. **a.** Hang the IV fluids on the pole if they are to be used.	To ensure that you are ready to proceed once the IV access is in place.
b. Arrange the other equipment on the bedside stand so that it can be easily accessed.	

(continued)

Action	Rationale
c. If using an IV lock, prepare it for ease of use. An extension tubing is usually attached and the lock and extension tubing filled with saline solution or heparinized saline, depending upon facility policy. The syringe with needleless connector is left attached so that the remainder of the flush solution can be used to flush the cannula after connection.	
16. Position yourself for good visibility of the arm and ability to manipulate your dominant hand in starting the IV. Some nurses sit in a chair at the bedside; others put the bed in high position and stand; still others sit on the bed.	Starting an IV is a fine motor skill that requires manual dexterity and clear vision. This is facilitated by a comfortable, non-strained position. Policies in your facility may limit the range of choices.
17. Locate a vein in which to start the IV. Examine both hands and forearms and select a suitable site using the criteria of straight, visible, or palpable, as distal as possible, and in patient's nondominant hand or arm. (See "Selecting a Vein," above.) Keep in mind that there may not be an ideal site.	To allow the patient greater self-care and to preserve higher veins for other uses.
18. Place a tourniquet 5 to 6 inches above the area where you want to start the IV.	To cause the vein to distend. Do not use a tourniquet if the veins are extremely fragile or rolling because the extra distention may cause the veins to burst or roll more. Do not use a latex tourniquet if the patient has a latex allergy.
19. Initiate other methods to promote venous distention if the tourniquet alone is not successful.	
a. Ask the patient to open and close the fist.	To promote an increase in the amount of blood in the extremity.
b. Tap the vein lightly.	The vein may respond by dilating, which also helps increase its visibility.
c. Place the arm in a dependent position (lower than the heart).	Gravity promotes venous filling and distention.
d. Apply warm, moist packs to the area.	Increases blood supply.
20. Release the tourniquet.	To allow blood flow to return to the extremity and promote patient comfort.

(continued)

Action	Rationale
21. Clean the area thoroughly with a 2% chlorhexidine-based preparation (preferred). Tincture of iodine, an iodophor, or 70% alcohol are acceptable substitutes. Using a back-and-forth motion, apply friction for 30 seconds (O'Grady, et al., 2002). If the area is especially hairy, clip the hair. Clean the area after the hair has been removed.	Hair is removed to facilitate cleaning and to prevent the tape from pulling. Because of the risk of nicking the skin and thus increasing the potential for infection, most facilities do not permit shaving IV sites. The antiseptic agent used for cleaning is usually indicated by unit or facility policy. Chlorhexidine gluconate (Chloraprep) is preferred because of its effectiveness in reducing skin microorganisms, but 70% isopropyl alcohol can be used (Centers for Disease Control, 1987; Singapore Ministry of Health, 2004). The Intravenous Nurses Society (INS) recommends disposable single-use no-touch applicators (Intravenous Nurses Society, 2000). *Do not touch the area after it has been cleaned.*
22. If it is the policy in your facility to anesthetize the area, do so now. Be sure to check first to determine if the patient is allergic to local anesthetics.	To decrease the patient's sensation of pain.
23. Reapply the tourniquet.	To distend the vein, re-identify the vein selected, and facilitate entry.
24. If using a device with a catheter, inspect the device and catheter for defects.	To prevent injury to the patient from a part of the catheter becoming detached or from a sharp or uneven tip.
25. Insert the needle. Using the thumb of your nondominant hand, gently retract the skin away from the site. Hold the needle at a 15- to 30-degree angle with the **bevel** up.	Retracting the skin makes it taut and facilitates piercing the skin. A low angle of approach decreases the potential for pushing a needle through the vein and piercing the far side.

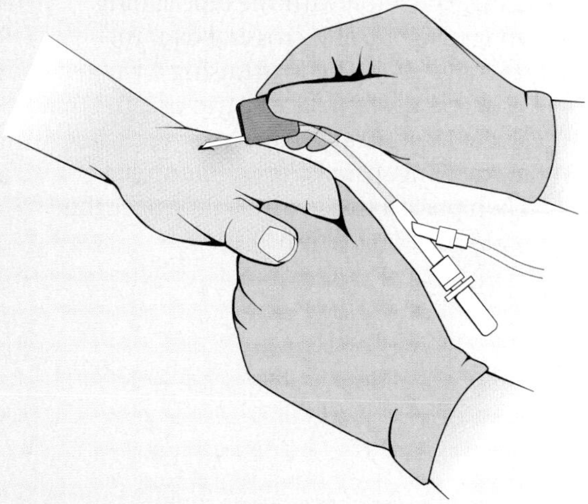

   a. *Direct method:* Pierce the skin immediately over the selected vein and direct the needle toward the vein. Advance the needle until it enters the vein.

   b. *Indirect method:* Pierce the skin immediately beside the selected vein (Fig. 50-5). When the needle is through the skin, decrease the angle until it is almost parallel with the skin, and enter the vein.

   c. When blood comes back into the cannula hub or tubing (depending on the device you are using), insert the needle to almost its full length. Advance the cannula according to package instructions and facility policy for the device you are using.

FIGURE 50-5 With skin retracted and needle bevel up, pinch wings on IV access device together and hold at a 15- to 30-degree angle to pierce the skin, followed by a decreased angle for entering the vein.

(continued)

Action	Rationale
26. Holding the needle or catheter steady with your dominant hand, gently release the tourniquet with your other hand.	Reestablishes venous flow and prevents excessive backflow of blood through the catheter.
27. If using an ONC access device, apply gentle pressure 1½ to 2 inches above the catheter insertion site. Remove the stylet of the ONC device. Secure the safety device over the stylet according to package instructions.	To remove the metal needle from the vein, leaving the plastic catheter in place and to protect yourself against possible needle-stick injury.
28. Quickly connect the tubing: Remove the protective cap from the IV tubing (maintaining sterile technique), connect it securely to the cannula, and open the regulator to initiate a moderate flow. If inserting an IV lock, insert the lock into the hub, and flush the cannula slowly with saline or heparinized saline solution, following the policy at your facility.	To prevent the patient's blood from clotting and occluding the cannula.
29. Remove your gloves.	To facilitate handling tape.
30. Tape the cannula securely and dress the site. This should be done according to unit or facility procedure. If you have no procedure, use one of the three following methods, which usually include taping the hub of the needle down and covering with a dressing.	
a. *Chevron tape:* Tape the hub into place, using a chevron with the tape sliding under the hub and crossing over the top (Fig. 50-6). If you are using a winged IV access device, place a strip of tape under the hub and down over each side of the wing, parallel to the cannula. Then place a third strip of tape over the wing itself (Fig. 50-7A & B).	To secure the cannula so that it does not move out of the vein and protect the site from contamination. 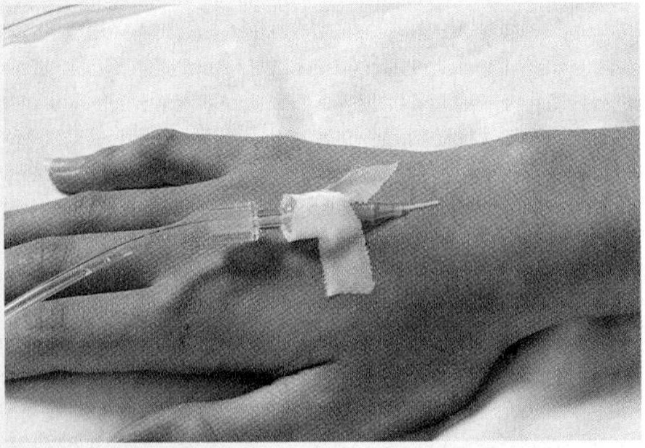

FIGURE 50-6 Chevron tape in place.

(continued)

Action	Rationale

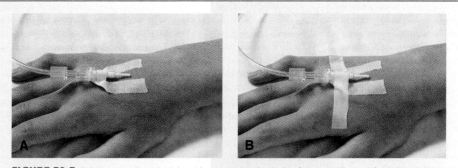

FIGURE 50-7 (**A**) Tape is placed sticky side up under the hub of the needle and folded to adhere along each side of the hub. (**B**) A second strip of tape is placed across the hub and first piece of tape.

b. Put the dressing over the site.

(1) *Transparent occlusive dressing* (Fig. 50-8): Transparent, moisture-vapor–permeable adhesive dressings (OpSite, Tegaderm) are the recommended dressing material. Follow specific package directions. Seal the dressing around the cannula hub and secure all the edges.	The transparent occlusive dressing resists moisture from the outside, allows for assessment of the site without manipulation, and can be left in place until the site must be changed unless it comes loose. The dressing covers the IV site and seals snugly around the hub of the cannula, leaving the hub out for ease of tubing change.

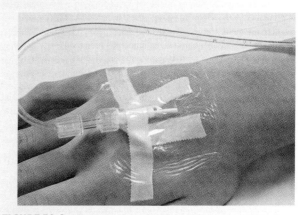

FIGURE 50-8 Transparent dressings are used to cover IV sites in many healthcare facilities.

(2) *Gauze dressing:* Place a sterile 3- × 3-inch or 2- × 2-inch gauze square open over the IV site and tape it securely in place. A 2-inch square may be folded and placed under the hub to support it if needed (Fig. 50-9). There is no evidence of a difference in infection rates based on the dressing used; however, a gauze dressing is preferable if the site is oozing or if the patient is diaphoretic (O'Grady, et al., 2002).	To protect the site.

(continued)

Action	Rationale

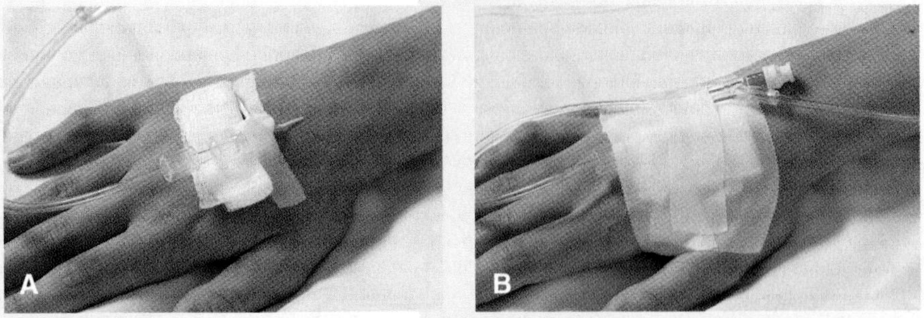

FIGURE 50-9 (**A**) Gauze square under hub to support position. (**B**) 2- × 2-inch gauze square dressing placed over the site and taped in place.

Action	Rationale
c. Make a loop of tubing near the point of entry and tape the loop in place, using paper tape.	This helps prevent the weight of the tubing from dislodging the cannula. Paper tape is less traumatic to skin than other types.
d. Tape the armboard in place if necessary.	To prevent an IV device inserted near a joint from becoming dislodged due to excess movement.
31. Write the date, time, type of device, catheter gauge, and your initials on the tape or label.	To facilitate appropriate care by other nurses.
32. If a bag or bottle of IV solution was hung, adjust the flow rate. (See Module 47.)	To make sure that the solution is being administered at the prescribed rate.
33. Put on gloves and care for the equipment appropriately. Any catheter or needle should be disposed of in a sharps container.	Blood-contaminated supplies are considered biohazard waste. Catheters and needles have the potential for injury to other hospital personnel. Red bags are often used for disposal of IV supplies.
34. Remove and dispose of your gloves, and wash or disinfect your hands.	To decrease the transfer of microorganisms that could cause infection.
35. Lower the bed.	For patient safety.

EVALUATION

36. Evaluate using the individualized patient outcomes previously identified. **R:** Evaluation in relation to desired outcomes is essential for planning future care.
   a. IV access is patent.
   b. IV access is secured in place with appropriate dressing.
   c. Hand or arm is positioned for comfort without obstructing potential IV fluid flow.
   d. IV fluids are infusing as prescribed, or an IV lock is in place.

DOCUMENTATION

37. Document the IV insertion. Usually a special form is used for this purpose (see Module 47). Include the date, time the IV was started, type of IV solution, any additives, where the IV was started, and by whom. Intake and output is usually monitored for a patient with an infusing IV. **R:** Documentation is a legal record of the patient's care and therapy and communicates nursing activities to other nurses and caregivers.

POTENTIAL ADVERSE OUTCOMES AND RELATED INTERVENTIONS

1. Blood begins to flow out of the vein into the tissue when the needle is inserted, causing a hematoma. *Intervention:* The attempt to initiate the IV infusion was unsuccessful. Release the tourniquet, remove the needle, and apply pressure over the insertion site with a gauze square. Choose another site, in the opposite arm if possible.

2. Two attempts to initiate IV therapy are unsuccessful. *Intervention:* Notify another skilled nurse to attempt to start the IV. If that nurse determines that success is not likely, notify the physician. In some facilities, personnel from the Anesthesia Department are available to assist. If they are unsuccessful too, it may be necessary to consider a central venous catheter.

3. The IV infusion fluid infiltrates. *Intervention:* Stop the IV infusion and discontinue therapy. Elevate the affected arm. Restart the IV infusion on the opposite arm if possible. See Table 47-2 in Module 47.

4. The patient develops phlebitis. *Note:* Phlebitis is a long-term complication and will not be immediately evident. *Intervention:* Stop the IV infusion and discontinue therapy. Place a warm, moist pack over the affected area. If another IV infusion is indicated, start it in the opposite arm, if possible. See Table 47-1 in Module 47.

PROCEDURE FOR CONVERTING AN INTRAVENOUS INFUSION TO AN INTRAVENOUS LOCK

When the need for IV fluids is absent but the need for IV access remains, you may be asked to convert an IV infusion to an intermittent IV access device (commonly called an IV lock).

ASSESSMENT

1. Validate the orders for the IV infusion to be converted to an IV lock. **R:** Validation ensures that there is no current need for IV fluids.

2. Assess the IV site for signs and symptoms of phlebitis, infiltration, and obstruction of flow. **R:** If there is any evidence of phlebitis, infiltration, or obstruction of flow, discontinue the IV, and establish a new site for the IV lock.

ANALYSIS

3. Critically think through your data, carefully evaluating each aspect and its relation to other data. **R:** To determine specific problems for this individual in relation to converting the infusing IV to an IV lock.

4. Identify specific problems and modifications of the procedure needed for this individual. **R:** Planning for the individual must take into consideration the individual's problems.

PLANNING

5. Determine individualized patient outcomes in relation to converting the infusing IV to an IV lock. **R:** Identification of desired outcomes guides planning and evaluation.
   a. The IV lock is securely in place and the catheter is patent.
   b. There is no swelling, pallor, or inflammation at the IV site.
   c. The patient is comfortable.

6. Identify and select the equipment needed. **R:** Planning ahead allows you to proceed more safely and effectively.
   a. IV lock adapter. **R:** The adapter has a male tip to fit into the cannula hub.
   b. 1 mL heparinized saline or normal saline solution in a syringe with the appropriate adaptor to fit into the IV lock available. **R:** One milliliter is adequate to completely fill the lock and a peripheral IV cannula. The solution is determined by facility policy. Saline solution eliminates the potential for adverse responses to heparin. Needleless adapters are preferred to protect staff from needle-stick injuries.
   c. Dressing and taping materials to secure the lock in place
   d. Clean gloves to protect yourself from potential contact with blood

IMPLEMENTATION

Action	Rationale
7. Wash or disinfect your hands.	To decrease the transfer of microorganisms that could cause infection.
8. Identify the patient, using two identifiers.	Verifying the patient's identity helps ensure that you are performing the right procedure for the right patient.
9. Fill the IV lock adapter with heparinized or normal saline solution, using sterile technique.	To keep the lock patent when no IV fluids are infusing.
10. Expose the IV catheter hub and remove or loosen any tape holding IV tubing in place.	To prepare the IV site for conversion to an IV lock.

(continued)

Action	Rationale
11. Put on clean gloves.	To protect yourself from blood spills.
12. Turn off the existing IV and disconnect it at the hub of the catheter.	To prevent spilling of fluid and to prepare the hub for the IV lock adaptor.
13. Attach the IV lock adapter and instill the remainder of the heparinized or normal saline solution.	To install the IV lock and to keep the IV catheter patent.
14. Dress and tape the IV lock according to facility policy, or refer to step 30 under Procedure for Starting an Intravenous Infusion.	To secure the IV lock into the hub of the IV catheter and to protect it from being dislodged.
15. Observe and document the amount of fluid remaining in the IV bag or bottle.	To maintain accurate intake records.
16. Dispose of the IV tubing and container, following your facility policies.	To avoid clutter in the patient's room.
17. Dispose of your gloves, and wash your hands.	To decrease the transfer of microorganisms that could cause infection.

EVALUATION

18. Evaluate using the individualized patient outcomes previously identified, including the following. **R:** Evaluation in relation to desired outcomes is essential for planning future care.
    a. The IV lock is securely in place and the catheter is patent.
    b. There is no swelling, pallor, or inflammation at the IV site.
    c. The patient is comfortable.

DOCUMENTATION

19. Document the conversion of the IV infusion to an IV lock on the IV record or as appropriate in your facility. Record the IV fluid intake in the appropriate place(s). **R:** Documentation is a legal record of the patient's care and therapy and communicates nursing activities to other nurses and caregivers.

Acute Care

Many acute care facilities have IV teams because of the data demonstrating a reduction in IV complications when a designated team does all IV starts. Members of these teams start most IV infusions in the facility and are available to assist the nursing staff when IV therapy presents unusual challenges. Nevertheless, registered nurses are responsible for converting IV infusions to IV locks and for facilitating positive patient outcomes for those who have IV fluids infusing.

Long-Term Care

Because an increasing number of individuals with higher acuity levels are receiving care in long-term care facilities, there is an increasing need for IV access devices to be placed and used for fluid and medication therapy. Again, individual facilities will have chosen specific equipment and will have policies in place regarding individuals who are responsible for initiating and caring for IV infusions. The procedures remain the same.

Home Care

IV fluid and medication therapy are being administered to increasing numbers of individuals receiving care at home. Although clients or their caregivers are commonly successful at maintaining the prescribed therapy, skilled home care nurses are needed to assist with trouble-shooting IVs and restarting IVs that are no longer functional. Again, individual agencies choose specific equipment and have policies in place regarding who initiates and cares for those receiving IV therapy. The procedures remain the same.

Ambulatory Care

Individuals coming into ambulatory care centers for IV medications may have had their IV started while hospitalized. Some individuals have long-term IV therapy initiated in an ambulatory setting. Those settings employ nurses able to insert both peripheral devices and peripherally inserted central IV lines.

LEARNING TOOLS

DEVELOP YOUR BACKGROUND KNOWLEDGE

1. Review the Learning Outcomes.

2. Read the section on administering fluids intravenously in your assigned text.

3. Look up the Key Terms in the glossary.

4. Review the module as though you were preparing to teach the concepts and skills to another person. Mentally practice the skills included.

DEVELOP YOUR SKILLS

1. In the practice setting, do the following:
   a. Examine the various IV access devices available in your setting. All are available in various sizes. Identify each of the following:
      (1) a winged-tip or butterfly needle
      (2) an IV catheter over a needle
      (3) any other available devices
   b. Read the package instructions accompanying each of the previous devices. Handle the equipment, and attempt to follow the instructions.
   c. Using a mannequin or IV "arm," start an IV with a 21-G butterfly needle or a 22-G over-the-needle IV device. Do the complete procedure, including the explanation to the "patient," the taping, and the dressing. Review Module 47, Preparing and Maintaining Intravenous Infusions, and, if time permits, set up the IV as well. Use the Perfor-

mance Checklist on the CD-ROM in the front of this book as a guide. When you feel you have had sufficient practice, ask your instructor to evaluate your performance.
   d. If sterile equipment is available, and school policy permits, practice starting an IV with another student as the patient. Carry out the entire procedure and have the student evaluate your performance.
   e. Practice documenting, using the form used in the facility to which you are assigned, and a narrative note, SOAP, or FOCUS note.

DEMONSTRATE YOUR SKILLS

1. In the clinical setting, do the following:
   a. Ask your instructor to arrange for you to observe an IV infusion being started.
   b. Ask your instructor to arrange for you to start an IV under supervision in your facility, if the facility's policies permit. For your first experience, a patient with "good" veins (for example, a young male) is preferable.
   c. If your facility employs an IV nurse, ask your instructor if arrangements can be made for you to observe. If time permits, ask if you can practice locating a suitable vein, and have the nurse evaluate your choice. If policy permits, ask if you can start an IV on a patient with good veins.

CRITICAL THINKING EXERCISES

1. You are to start an IV infusion for a 64-year-old woman who has just been hospitalized for pneumonia. She also had a left radical mastectomy 2 weeks ago and is dehydrated. Identify the sites commonly used for peripheral IVs and explain which of these you will consider. Justify your choices. Tell which sites you will not consider and the reasons why.

2. Margaret Seder will be having a minor surgical procedure this morning. You have been assigned to set up IV access for IV medication administration. Given this purpose, identify what equipment you will use and what site(s) you will consider first. How will you determine if this IV line is patent when a medication is ordered?

SELF-QUIZ
SHORT-ANSWER QUESTIONS

1. List three reasons why patient may fear IV infusions.

   a. _____

   b. _____

   c. _____

2. List two reasons why a patient might be receiving IV fluids.

   a. _____

   b. _____

3. Where is an IV usually started in an infant?

   _____

   Why?

   _____

4. List four methods that can be used to distend a vein.

   a. _____

   b. _____

   c. _____

   d. _____

5. What antiseptic agent is recommended for cleaning the intended IV site?

   _____

6. Describe how the IV site should be cleaned.

   _____

7. List five items of documentation that should be included on the tape that secures the IV dressing in place.

   a. _____

   b. _____

   c. _____

   d. _____

   e. _____

8. Name two reasons for an infusing IV to be converted to an IV lock.

   a. _____

   b. _____

MULTIPLE CHOICE

_____ 9. Where is an IV usually started in an adult patient?
   a. Antecubital space
   b. Scalp vein
   c. Hand or forearm
   d. Lower leg

_____ 10. Which of the following should be avoided when selecting a site for an IV? (Choose all that apply.)
   a. A site distal to an IV just removed
   b. On the same side as a mastectomy surgery
   c. On the same side as a dialysis access site
   d. Antecubital fossa

Answers to the Self-Quiz questions appear in the back of the book.

MODULE 51

Administering Parenteral Nutrition

SKILLS INCLUDED IN THIS MODULE

General Procedure for Administering Parenteral Nutrition
Specific Procedure for Administering Fat Emulsions
(Lipids)

KEY TERMS

amino acids	infusion pump
cyclic TPN	lipids
cycling	lumen
dextrose	parenteral
fat emulsions	partial parenteral
finger stick	nutrition
hyperalimentation	piggyback
hyperglycemia	positive nitrogen
hypertonic	balance
hypoglycemia	test dose

OVERALL OBJECTIVES

▸ To safely administer parenteral nutrition through an existing intravenous line or a central venous catheter (CVC).
▸ To meet nutritional, fluid, and electrolyte needs of the patient.

LEARNING OUTCOMES

The student will be able to

1. Assess the patient to determine the need for parenteral nutrition.
2. Analyze data to determine specific needs, problems, or concerns related to administering parenteral nutrition.
3. Determine appropriate patient outcomes for administering total parenteral nutrition and recognize the potential for adverse outcomes.
4. Choose the appropriate equipment and procedure for administering parenteral nutrition.
5. Demonstrate the proper procedure and techniques for administering all types of parenteral nutrition.
6. Evaluate the effectiveness of administration of parenteral nutrition.
7. Document the procedure in the patient's plan of care and specific observations of any adverse findings in the patient's record as appropriate.

Parenteral nutrition involves the provision of carbohydrates, proteins, lipids, vitamins, electrolytes, and minerals intravenously. A greater number of individuals are receiving parenteral nutrition in the hospital, in the long-term care setting, and in the home because of the improvements in central venous lines, the availability of intravenous (IV) nutritional solutions, and the increasing number of people with long-term illnesses that interfere with normal nutrition. The complexity of the procedure and the potential for complications demand a high level of nursing skill.

NURSING DIAGNOSES

Patients who are candidates to receive parenteral nutrition to treat malnutrition or to prevent nutritional deficits may have a variety of nursing diagnoses. Examples are

- Imbalanced Nutrition: Less Than Body Requirements: related to inadequate intake to meet caloric needs
- Risk for Infection: related to central venous catheter (CVC) insertion
- Impaired Skin Integrity: related to CVC insertion
- Risk for Excess or Deficient Fluid Volume: related to altered infusion rates

DELEGATION

The administration of parenteral nutrition is not delegated to assistive personnel in healthcare settings. They can, however, care for patients receiving parenteral nutrition and can be taught to observe for adverse reactions to the procedure and to report them immedi-

ately. If the patient is receiving parenteral nutrition at home, the nurse teaches the appropriate caregiver how to provide this care. Written directions are important references for family caregivers. The nurse plans for follow-up to ensure that care is being completed correctly and to answer questions.

TOTAL PARENTERAL NUTRITION

Total parenteral nutrition (TPN) involves supplying all nutrients needed by the body intravenously. Several terms are used for this therapy including **hyperalimentation** (sometimes referred to as "hyperal" or HA). Patients receiving TPN are usually those who cannot eat for a long time because of major trauma or a critical illness; disease of the intestinal tract; anorexia nervosa; or long-term illness, such as cancer, acquired immunodeficiency syndrome (AIDS), burns, or sepsis. Other patients who receive TPN are those who cannot eat normally and, therefore, cannot take in sufficient nutrients.

Although standard IV solutions provide water, calories, and some electrolytes, they do not provide the calories or the nitrogen to meet the body's daily requirements. Therefore, policies usually require that after 3 to 5 days without oral food intake, an alternate method must be provided to meet nutritional needs to avoid protein depletion and malnutrition.

The nutrients supplied by TPN include **dextrose,** protein, electrolytes, **amino acids,** vitamins, minerals, and trace elements. These substances are mixed with sterile water into a **hypertonic** solution. The maximum dextrose concentration for total parenteral nutrition solutions is 50%, although the usual is 20% to 25%. Because of the high osmolarities of the dextrose and amino acid solutions, these fluids must be delivered through a central high-flow vein, where they are diluted in a large volume of blood to prevent chemical phlebitis, blood clot formation, and hemolysis. (For details about the position of central venous lines and their care, see Module 49, Caring for Patients With Central Venous Catheters.) Many patients also receive **fat emulsions (lipids)** in a separate solution that piggybacks into the TPN line. For guidelines on this procedure, see Module 48, Administering Intravenous Medications.

PARTIAL PARENTERAL NUTRITION (PPN)

Somewhat diluted solutions of the same nutrients discussed under TPN can be provided through peripheral veins for short times as **partial parenteral nutrition.** Some patients who are unable to eat adequate amounts for an extended time and who are nutritionally depleted may receive partial parenteral nutrition as a temporary adjunct to their oral nutritional intake. These patients can ingest some foods and fluids but not enough to meet needs for healing and recovery. In partial parenteral nutrition, the solution is infused through a peripheral IV line. This route is not recommended for any length of time because the solution irritates the veins and can lead to phlebitis. The limiting factor for PPN is the high osmolarity of the solution. A high osmolarity irritates peripheral veins and can result in phlebitis. The dextrose concentration should not exceed 10%. Dextrose solutions exceeding 10% must be delivered through a CVC. Peripheral parenteral nutrition is used more frequently to prevent nutritional deficits rather than correct them. The peripheral veins can also accommodate lipids.

COMPLICATIONS OF PARENTERAL NUTRITION

There are potential complications with either total or partial parenteral nutrition. The most common complications are inflammation and sepsis of the catheter insertion site. Strict aseptic techniques are used during catheter manipulations, dressing changes, tubing changes, and bottle/bag changes (see Module 49). The administration of these solutions, particularly those containing lipids, does not increase the risk of developing sepsis of the central catheter (O'Grady, et al., 2002). However, the nurse should carefully assess the catheter site each time parenteral nutrition is administered and document any signs of inflammation or infection. Any drainage, if present, should be cultured to assist in deciding whether the catheter needs to be removed.

TPN bypasses the normal regulatory processes involved in digestion and metabolism. Therefore, complications related to the blood level of TPN components are a concern. TPN infusion rates should always be monitored and regulated by an electronic infusion device in order to avoid too-rapid administration of electrolytes and other TPN components.

One common complication is **hyperglycemia.** The solutions contain large amounts of dextrose, which is not rapidly metabolized and which may elevate the volume of glucose in the blood. If hyperglycemia is allowed to continue, the patient may become dehydrated and confused and the level of consciousness may decrease. Patients receiving parenteral nutrition are assessed on a continuing basis for hyperglycemia through glucose monitoring with blood from a **finger stick** and a glucometer (see Module 15, Collecting Specimens and Performing Common Laboratory Tests, for use of a glucose monitor). When therapy is initiated, the infusion rate is usually graduated upward over 24 to 48 hours. If hyperglycemia is a problem, a small amount of insulin may be prescribed and added to the solution or given subcutaneously. On the other hand, **hypoglycemia** may occur when TPN is discontinued if the rate is not properly tapered downward (see "Discontinuing TPN" below).

During the early phases of parenteral nutrition, fluid and electrolyte imbalances also can occur. The nurse is responsible for scheduling the periodic laboratory tests (usually daily) ordered by the physician to detect any potential fluid or electrolyte problems. Changes are then made in the solution to correct any imbalance.

Because patients receiving TPN lack adequate amounts of vitamins K and B_{12}, bleeding and anemia can occur. These complications are prevented by adding the vitamins to the parenteral solution weekly.

SOLUTIONS USED FOR PARENTERAL NUTRITION

The solutions prepared for parenteral nutrition follow a standard for the facility with individualized adaptations for the specific needs of the patient. Figure 51-1 is a sample form listing the content of routine total parenteral nutrition solutions. The physician, who may consult with the pharmacist, nutritionist, or nurse specialist, orders the formula, and the prescription is reviewed daily with special consideration given to electrolyte, fluid, and **positive nitrogen balance.** A thorough nutritional assessment is required to determine the TPN therapy. Some nurses specialize in caring for patients receiving parenteral nutrition and teach the procedure to the patient and the family when appropriate.

INITIATION OF TPN — ADULT

☐ 1. STANDARD CENTRAL VENOUS FULL-STRENGTH TPN SOLUTION
D50W 500ml (850 Calories) + Amino Acids 10% 500ml (50 Grams Protein)
Final Concentration = Dextrose 25% & Amino Acids 5%

NaCl	30 mEq	Reg. Insulin ___0___ u.
KCl	25 mEq	Multivitamins (MVI) 1 pack (10ml) daily
KPhos	15 mEq	Multitrace Elements (MTE) 1 ml daily
CaGluc	8 mEq	Vitamin C 500mg daily
MgSO4	8 mEq	(except BMT = 16 mEq)	Vitamin K 10mg weekly (Sundays)

2. RATE: TO INFUSE AT _____ ml/hr TO PROVIDE A TOTAL OF _____ liters(s)/day.

☑ 3. NON-STANDARD CENTRAL OR PERIPHERAL FORMULA (Note: Non-standard TPN material and labor costs ae higher than for the standardized solution above.)

SPECIFY: A) solution type, strength and amount   B) additives and amounts

D10W _____ ml   Amino Acid 8.5% _____ ml   NaCl ___7___ mEq   Reg Insulin ___Ø___
D20W _____ ml   Amino Acid 10% _500_ ml   NaAcet _____ mEq   Multivitamins (MVI) ___1___
D40W _____ ml   Hepatamine 8% _____ ml   KCl ___40___ mEq   Multitrace Elements (MTE) ___1___
D50W _500_ ml   KPhos ___20___ mEq   Vitamin C ___500___
D70W _____ ml   CaGluc ___8___ mEq   Vitamin K _____
                                                  MgSO4 ___16___ mEq   Other _____

C) FINAL Concentration Dextrose ___25___ % & Amino Acids ___5___ %

4. RATE: TO INFUSE AT ___40___ ml/hr TO PROVIDE ___1___ liter(s)/day.

☑ 5. INTRAVENOUS FAT EMULSION

___✓___ 10% (1.1 calories/ml) ___50___ ml/hr over ___10___ hours (minimum 4 - 6 hours)
_____ 20% (2.0 calories/ml) _____ ml/hr over _____ hours (minimum 8 - 10 hours)

6. Non-BMT and Non-ICU Patients: Begin fat infusion after TPN (Hyperal) Screen is drawn and before 0600.

7. Infuse initial dose slowly. 10%: begin at 60ml/hr x 30 min.; 20%: begin at 30ml/hr x 30 min.
(Note: some patients may react adversely to subsequent exposures.)

The following orders are standard for all non-bone marrow transplant patients. Delete only if crossed out by physician.

PRE-TPN ORDERS

8. Central venous catheter placement verification: (circle one)
　　(a.) CXR asap for placement needed
　　 b. Catheter tip location: _____ ; may begin TPN infusion.

9. Baseline Lab: ZINC, COPPER, TRIGLYCERIDES, TPN (Hyperal) SCREEN I (CBC w/diff, Protime, Ca, P04, Mg, GOT, Bilirubin, Lytes, BUN, Glucose, Albumin, Prealbumin)

TPN INITIATION AND MAINTENANCE ORDERS

(10.) Initiate TPN Nursing Protocol.

(11.) Nutritional Assessment – notify Unit Dietitian.

12. TPN LAB:
Lab Draw Time: ICU Patients – draw TPN labs in AM;   Non-ICU Patients – draw TPN labs in the evenings before 1900

✓ Daily x 1st 3 Days: lytes & glucose (already included in Monday & Thursday labs)

✓ Mondays: TRIGLYCERIDES, if IV fat administered.
　　　TPN (Hyperal) SCREEN I (includes CBC w/diff, Protime, Ca, PO4, Mg, GOT, Bilirubin, Lytes, BUN, Glucose, Albumin, Prealbumin)

✓ Thursdays: TPN (Hyperal) SCREEN II (includes CBC, Lytes, Glucose, Ca, PO4, Mg)

✓ Chemstick: Q 8 hrs x 1st 48 hours.   Thereafter, urine fxs Q 8 hrs on fresh specimen – Chemstick for trace or greater.
Chemstick Results: Chemstick > 240 notify MD if no sliding scale ordered
　　　　　　　　　　 Chemstick > 400 notify MD & obtain stat glucose
　　　　　　　　　　 Chemstick for S/S hypoglycemia: < 60 notify MD & obtain stat glucose

(13.) Daily Weight; Strict I & O

Date ___7/15/06___ MD Signature ___A. Bryant, M.D._____

HOSPITAL MEDICAL CENTER

FIGURE 51-1 TPN order form that is filled out by the physician.

The solutions are prepared under sterile conditions in the facility's pharmacy. The usual concentration is 25% dextrose solution and 4.25% amino acids. The caloric count is 1 Kcal/mL solution. Standard electrolytes are added to each bag and include sodium, potassium, calcium, magnesium, chloride, phosphate, and acetate. The standard multivitamin additive is MVI-12, which is added every day. The solution has a clear, pale yellow appearance after the addition of multivitamins. Vitamin K 10 mg is added weekly. Trace elements, such as zinc, copper, manganese, and chromium, are also added to the solution (Fig. 51-2).

Fat emulsions (lipids) appear as a white milky solution and are provided in glass bottles because lipids react

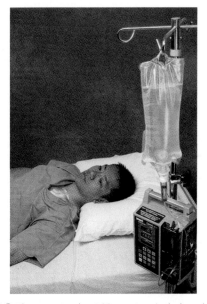

FIGURE 51-2 The parenteral nutrition set-up includes a bag of nutrients usually hung from an IV pole or stand, a pump for regulating delivery of nutrients, and the IV line that transports the nutrients to the patient's CVC.

with plastics and their components. They are used as a caloric source and to prevent essential fatty acid deficiency. Lipids are available as a 10% product, which is 1.1 Kcal/mL, and a 20% product, which is 2.0 Kcal/mL (ASPEN, 2001). Only the more dilute 10% emulsion is given by the peripheral route. Lipid solutions are administered simultaneously with other nutritional solutions via a Y-connector, into a port in the CVC, or (if the more dilute solution) through a peripheral line. They must be connected below the filter because the lipids will clog the filter. The typical administration of lipids is 500 mL of 10% dilution over 4 to 6 hours one to three times weekly. The lipids may completely infuse before the parenteral nutrition solution is completed. If this occurs, discontinue the lipids as you would other "add-on" or **piggyback** solutions and discard the tubing appropriately.

Some facilities mix the lipid emulsion with dextrose and amino acids in one bag to create a total nutrient admixture or "three-in-one" formulation and administer it to the patient over a 24-hour period. A special filter is used with this solution to prevent the lipids from coalescing.

CYCLIC TPN

People receiving long-term parenteral nutrition receive **cyclic TPN.** This means that after the patient has been stabilized on a prescribed solution given continuously over a 24-hour period, the administration may be adjusted to allow it be given over fewer hours. **Cycling**

allows the body to adjust to the infusion of nutrient solutions and avoids sudden changes in blood glucose levels while receiving the prescribed nutrients over 12 to 18 hours rather than over 24 hours. This strategy provides for greater mobility and less restriction for the patient (ASPEN, 2001).

During "cycling," the TPN solution is started at a slow rate at the beginning of the day. When the patient is responding effectively to the initial rate, the rate is gradually changed so that more solution is administered each hour until the patient is receiving the prescribed calories and nutrients over a shorter length of time. This process is called cycling up.

At the end of the infusion, the solution is cycled down before stopping. This means that the rate is slowed gradually, allowing the patient's body to adjust to the dropping blood glucose infusion rate. Blood glucose levels are monitored (using a glucometer and blood from a finger stick) 2 hours after parenteral nutrition is initiated and 30 minutes after its completion. See Figure 51-3 for an example of a cycling form.

DISCONTINUING TPN

When parenteral nutrition is to be discontinued completely, the procedure is similar to starting TPN but reversed. The dosage per hour is gradually decreased before stopping altogether. The person is getting less solution each hour. This is often referred to as "tapering down." Again, the blood glucose is monitored to evaluate the patient's response. After the infusion is terminated, an isotonic glucose solution is often administered to prevent rebound hypoglycemia. When discontinuing TPN, always check the physician's order for the tapering down plan.

GENERAL PROCEDURE FOR ADMINISTERING PARENTERAL NUTRITION

ASSESSMENT

1. Assess the patient who is to receive parenteral nutrition. The following data are essential.
   a. *The patient's diagnosis.* **R:** The diagnosis indicates whether the patient will be on long-term or short-term therapy and indicates any at-risk complications for this patient. For example, is the patient a diabetic and have a need for close blood glucose monitoring?
   b. *The patient's age and medical condition.* **R:** If the patient is an infant, an elderly adult, or in precarious health, the impact of parenteral nutrition

DATE	TIME	PHYSICIAN'S ORDERS	NOTED BY
		TPN CYCLING ORDERS FOR NON-BMT PATIENTS	
12/26/06	1000	(1.) CYCLE SCHEDULE	

(Final goal: _2_ liters at night over _12_ hours)

	DATE	START TIME	BAG#	LITERS	RATE	HOURS
DAY 1	12/26	1900	5	1	110	10
DAY 2	12/27	0500	6	1	110	10
DAY 3	12/27	1900	7	1.5	135	16
DAY 4	12/28	1900	8	1.5	155	14
DAY 5	12/29	1900	9	1.5	185	12

(2.) TAPERING:

Start infusion at 50 ml/hour for 1/2 hour.

End infusion at 50 ml/hour for 1/2 hour.

(3.) Infuse ___500___ ml intravenous Fat Emulsion 10%/20%

every ___day___. Infuse over ___4 - 6___ hours.

Begin when TPN started.

(4.) Heparin Lock catheter when TPN completed.

(5.) DC all sliding scale insulin coverage.

DC previous chemstick orders.

DC urine fractionals.

(6.) Obtain chemsticks each day of Cycle Schedule:

   a. 2 Hours after TPN initiated

   b. 1/2 hour after TPN completed

   c. Notify Dr. ___Norman___ if chemstick results are

   >240 or <60.

7. DC chemsticks when Cycle Schedule is completed if chemstick results are

within normal limits.

DATE ___12/26/06___ RPh/RN SIGNATURE ___Nancy Alkins, RN___

PHYSICIAN SIGNATURE ___N. Norman___

A DRUG EQUIVALENT MAY BE DISPENSED UNLESS CHECKED ☐

SIGNATURE IS REQUIRED FOLLOWING ENTRY OF EACH ORDER

HOSPITAL MEDICAL CENTER

FIGURE 51-3 "Cycling" form used by the physician to prescribe the rate of flow.

therapy on other body systems may be much greater than if the patient is in relatively stable health.

c. *Height and usual weight.* **R:** This information gives baseline data for monitoring the patient's fluid and nutritional status.

d. *Intake and output.* **R:** Intake and output records are important observations for assessing daily nutritional and fluid status and detecting early emergence of complications.

e. *Allergies.* Some patients have allergic reactions to tape or iodine-based solutions commonly used to prepare and maintain the CVC insertion site. Other patients may have allergies to components of the solutions. **R:** Reactions can typically be avoided if known allergies are reported before starting therapy.

f. *Patient's vital signs.* Patients receiving parenteral nutrition have their vital signs measured every 4 hours. **R:** From baseline measures, fluctuations in vital function and possible complications can be detected before they are severe. For example, an elevated temperature may indicate a catheter-related infection.

g. *Knowledge of procedure.* **R:** Awareness of the procedure and side effects may facilitate early detection of problems through patient self-monitoring.

h. *Mental status.* **R:** An alteration in mental status may be an indicator of fluid volume.

2. Assess the patient's unit to determine which items of equipment are in the room and which need to be obtained. **R:** To determine the need for additional equipment before beginning the procedure.

ANALYSIS

3. Critically think through your data, carefully evaluating each aspect and its relation to other data. **R:** This enables you to determine specific problems for this individual in relation to parenteral nutrition.

4. Identify specific problems and modifications of the procedure needed for this individual. **R:** Planning for the individual must take into consideration the individual's problems.

PLANNING

5. Determine individualized patient outcomes in relation to the administration of parenteral nutrition, including the following. **R:** Identification of outcomes guides planning and evaluation.

a. The right *patient* receives the right *parenteral solution* in the right *volume* at the right *time*.

b. The solution is administered at the right *rate*.

c. The patient experiences the desired effects from the solution(s) administered.

d. The patient's blood sugar and vital signs remain stable and the patient experiences no adverse effects from the solution(s) administered.

6. Remove the solution from the refrigerator 1 hour before use to warm it to room temperature and to check the container for correct content of solution, its expiration date, and the solution itself for any cloudiness or particulate material (Fig. 51-4). **R:** Infusion of a cold solution can cause pain, venous spasm, and hypothermia. Checking the content ensures that the patient is receiving the prescribed solution and that it is safe for use. If the solution is cloudy, it may be contaminated and cannot be used. Solutions must be used within 24 hours of preparation.

Safety Alert

Note: If the TPN solution is not available when scheduled to be hung or the solution runs out before the next bag is delivered, hang a container of dextrose 10% in water ($D_{10}W$) until the prescribed solution is available. This prevents sudden hypoglycemia.

HA ORDERS

DATE: ___3-17-06___

Dextrose ___25___ %   Amino Acids ___5___ %
Rate ___1___ L/Day   _____ cc/hr
Volume _____

NaCl _____	mEq/ _30_	Date ord. _____
Na Acetate_____	mEq/ _____	Date ord. _____
K Cl _____	mEq/ _25_	Date ord. _____
K Phos _____	mEq/ _15_	Date ord. _____
K Acetate_____	mEq/ _____	Date ord. _____
Ca Gluc _____	mEq/ _____	Date ord. _____
Mg SO$_4$ _____	mEq/ _8_	Date ord. _____
		Date ord. _____
		Date ord. _____
Reg. Insulin _0_ u/ _____		Date ord. _____

MVI _____10__ ml/Day
Trace Minerals _1_ ml/Day
Vit. K _____10__ mg/wk   *(Sun.)*
Vit. C ___500_____ mg/Day

Lipids __20__ % __500__ cc/Day
Rate: _50_ cc/hr

Maintenance IV rate: _____ cc/hr
Maximum IV rate: _____ cc/hr

FIGURE 51-4 In various settings, a hyperalimentation (HA) form is used by the nurse to check the contents of the parenteral nutrition formula.

7. Obtain the specific type of equipment that is needed (see a through e below). **R:** An **infusion pump** ensures both the right rate and the right amount over time. A pump eliminates changes in flow rate that may occur with a change in activity. The IV filter traps bacteria and particles that can form in the TPN solution tubing. Tubing should be changed every 24 hours because the high glucose content and protein component can promote bacterial growth (O'Grady, et al., 2002). Connections must be secure, but twist-on connections are usually present on the lines used for TPN. Tape may leave sticky residue around the connection and is avoided if possible. Tape the connections if a twist-on connection is not present.

   a. Infusion pump (if not already in the room)
   b. Tubing with filter for infusion pump; use tubing with a 0.22 micron filter for dextrose- and a 1.2 micron filter for lipid-containing admixtures. New tubing is used with each bag of solution or changed after 24 hours.
   c. Alcohol wipe
   d. Clean gloves
   e. Tape for connections, if needed

IMPLEMENTATION

Action	Rationale
8. Wash or disinfect your hands.	To decrease the transfer of microorganisms that could cause infection.
9. Pull off the rubber or plastic cover on the bag or bottle and insert the spike of the tubing into the port.	To pierce the seal and allow the tubing to fill.
10. Prime the tubing with solution, following the directions for the specific infusion pump in use.	To purge air from the system and avoid air embolus.
11. Cover the distal end of the tubing with the sterile cap before carrying it to the bedside.	To maintain asepsis.
12. Identify the patient, using two identifiers.	Verifying the patient's identity helps ensure that you are performing the right skill for the right patient.
13. Explain the procedure and rationale to the patient and family members if present.	Explaining the procedure helps relieve anxiety or misperceptions that the patient may have about a procedure or activity and sets the stage for patient participation.
14. Hang the bag on the IV pole.	To prepare for the infusion.
15. Raise the bed to an appropriate working position based on your height.	To allow you to use correct body mechanics and protect yourself from back injury.
16. Wash or disinfect your hands.	To decrease the transfer of microorganisms that could cause infection.
17. Inspect the site of the central or peripheral line.	To detect signs of inflammation and infection. If these signs are present, contact the prescriber. Usually you will continue to administer TPN while a decision is made regarding treatment.

(continued)

Action	Rationale
18. Administer the parenteral nutrition.	
a. Thread the tubing through the infusion pump according to the manufacturer's directions.	So the pump will work correctly.
b. Put on clean gloves.	To protect yourself from contact with blood and to protect the patient from introduction of microorganisms.
c. For a CVC, clamp the central venous line.	To prevent air from entering the catheter when the patient inhales and intrathoracic pressure drops.
d. Scrub the connection point on the CVC or the correct port on a multi-**lumen** CVC with an alcohol wipe and let dry.	To decrease the potential for microbial contamination of the IV.
e. Attach the administration tubing to the CVC or to the appropriate port in a multi-lumen CVC and twist on the connector that covers the junction of the tubing and the CVC. If no twist-on connector is present, tape the connection in a manner that allows the tape to be removed easily for the next tubing change (Fig. 51-5).	To ensure that the parenteral nutrition is given into an appropriate vein and to prevent accidental dislodging of the tubing, contamination of the solution, and the potential for air embolism.

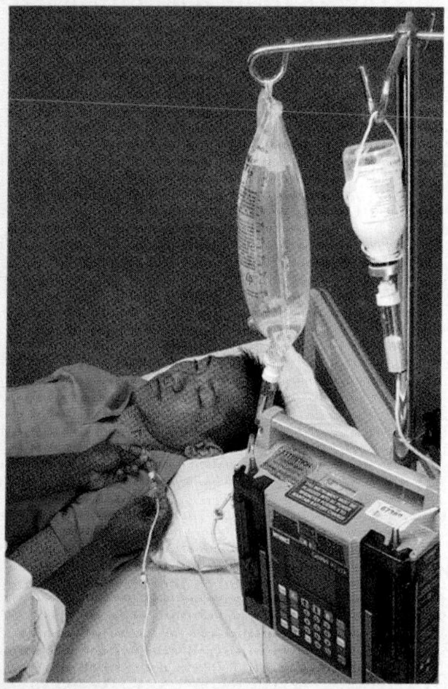

FIGURE 51-5 Connecting the tubing that will deliver the lipids (fat emulsion) to the patient through the central venous site.

Action	Rationale
f. Set the correct rate on the infusion pump. Infuse the initial parenteral nutrition solution gradually at 25 to 50 mL/hour for 30 minutes.	To provide a period of time for the patient to adjust to the higher glucose level.

(continued)

Action	Rationale
19. Monitor the patient's response by assessing vital signs every 10 minutes for 30 minutes. Then, check the blood glucose within 4 hours of beginning the procedure. If no adverse reactions occur, the rate may be adjusted to the prescribed flow rate. If the patient is being cycled up or down, set the rate accordingly.	To detect adverse response(s) quickly. The desired final rate provides for the prescribed nutrients over 24 hours and stabilizes blood glucose levels.

EVALUATION

20. Evaluate using the individualized patient outcomes previously identified, including the following. **R:** Evaluation in relation to desired outcomes is essential for planning future care.
   a. The right *patient* received the right *parenteral solution* in the right *volume* at the right *time*.
   b. The solution was administered at the right *rate*.
   c. The patient experienced the desired effects from the solution(s) administered.
   d. The patient's blood sugar and vital signs remained stable and the patient experienced no adverse effects from the solution(s) administered.

DOCUMENTATION

21. Complete right *documentation*. Document the administration of parenteral nutrition as you would administration of any IV solution. Vital signs and blood glucose levels are usually recorded on flow charts. Record any adverse reactions on the nursing progress notes. **R:** Documentation is a legal record of the patient's care and therapy and communicates nursing activities to other nurses and caregivers.

◼ POTENTIAL ADVERSE OUTCOMES AND RELATED INTERVENTIONS

1. Patient develops hyperglycemia.
Intervention: Limit dextrose concentration to less than 25% if possible. Monitor blood glucose level every 4 to 6 hours. Communicate with the physician regarding the possible need to add a sliding-scale insulin therapy.
2. Patient develops hypoglycemia.
Intervention: Gradually slow the rate of the infusion when discontinuing parenteral nutrition. Assess blood glucose levels.
3. Patient experiences sharp chest pain, dyspnea, decreased breath sounds, and/or cyanosis, indicating pneumothorax or hemothorax.
Intervention: Stop the infusion immediately. Obtain a chest x-ray order from the prescriber. Monitor vital signs and breath sounds. Assist with chest tube placement if necessary.

SPECIFIC PROCEDURE FOR ADMINISTERING FAT EMULSIONS (LIPIDS)

To administer fat emulsions, follow the steps of the General Procedure for Administering Parenteral Nutrition as modified below. The modified steps have been included completely, and the steps of the General Procedure that remain the same are referenced.

Procedure for Administering Lipids

ASSESSMENT

1-2. Follow steps 1 and 2 of the General Procedure: Assess the patient receiving parenteral nutrition for the first time for diagnosis, age, and medical condition, height and usual weight, intake and output, allergies, usual vital signs, knowledge of procedure, and mental status. Assess the need for equipment to be obtained.

ANALYSIS

3-4. Follow steps 3 and 4 of the General Procedure: Think through your data, and identify specific problems and modifications.

PLANNING

5. Determine individualized patient outcomes in relation to fat emulsions, including the following. **R:** Identification of outcomes guides planning and evaluation.
   a. The right *patient* receives the right *fat emulsion solution* in the right *volume* at the right *time*.
   b. The solution is administered at the right *rate*.
   c. The patient experiences the desired effects from the solution(s) administered.
   d. The patient experiences no adverse effects from the solution(s) administered.
6. Obtain the lipid emulsion. Check the label carefully against the order and check the expi-

ration date on the bottle. **R:** To ensure that you are administering the right solution to the right patient.

7. Obtain the specific type of equipment that is needed.

   a. Macrodrip, vented tubing without filter. If a pump is being used, use the type of tubing specific to the pump. **R:** A filter would be obstructed by the lipids and the IV would not flow. A vent is essential to allow the fluid to flow out of the glass bottle.

   b. Needleless connector for IV access

   c. Alcohol wipe to disinfect connection

   d. Clean gloves to protect yourself from contact with body fluids

   e. Tape for connections if needed

IMPLEMENTATION

Action	Rationale
8. Follow step 8 of the General Procedure: Wash or disinfect your hands.	
9. Remove the metal band around the top of the bottle without touching the sterile black cap beneath. Insert the spike of the tubing into the port of the bottle.	Aseptic technique prevents contamination of tubing.
10-17. Follow steps 10 to 17 of the Procedure for Parenteral Nutrition. Prime the tubing, replace the sterile cover over the end of the tubing, identify the patient (two identifiers), explain the procedure, hang the bottle on the IV pole, raise the bed, wash or disinfect your hands, and inspect the IV site.	
18. Administer the lipids.	
a. Thread the tubing through the pump if one is being used.	So the pump will work correctly.
b. Put on clean gloves.	To protect yourself from contact with blood and to protect the patient from introduction of micro-organisms (O'Grady, et al., 2002).
c. Identify the Y-port on the TPN tubing that is below the filter to use for the lipids.	Lipid solutions have an increased viscosity that will obstruct the flow by being trapped in the filter.
d. Scrub the port with an alcohol wipe and allow it to dry.	To decrease the potential for microbial contamination of the IV set-up.
e. Insert the needleless connector and twist it on firmly, or secure the connection with tape (see Fig. 51-5).	To prevent accidental disconnection of lipids and consequent contamination of solution.
f. Set the correct rate on the pump, or using the roller clamp, manually time the lipids. Infuse the initial dose slowly, giving a **test dose**: a 10% solution should begin at 1 mL/minute for 15 to 30 minutes; maximum rate of 80 to	A slow rate allows more time to observe for an ana-phylactic (serious allergic) reaction.

(continued)

Action	Rationale
125 mL/hour or over 4 hours. A 20% solution should begin at 0.5 mL/minute for 15 to 30 minutes; maximum rate of 63 mL/hour or over 8 to 10 hours (McConnell, 2001).	
19. Monitor the patient for adverse responses: assess vital signs and observe for rash or breathing difficulties.	To detect adverse response(s) quickly.

EVALUATION

20. Evaluate using the individualized patient outcomes previously identified, including the following. **R:** Evaluation in relation to desired outcomes is essential for planning future care.
   a. The right *patient* received the right *fat emulsion solution* in the right *volume* at the right *time*.
   b. The solution was administered at the right *rate*.
   c. The patient experienced the desired effects from the solution(s) administered.
   d. The patient experienced no adverse effects from the solution(s) administered.

DOCUMENTATION

21. Document a lipid infusion as you would any IV solution. Record any untoward reactions on the nursing progress notes. **R:** Documentation is a legal record of the patient's care and therapy and communicates nursing activities to other nurses and caregivers.

Acute Care

Should a patient be discharged from the acute care area on total parenteral nutrition either to home or to a long-term facility, instructions and orders are necessary to provide continuity of care. Referrals are made to a home health agency for the homebound patient. Care coordination for the patient discharged to long-term care is needed so that care is consistent with the needs of the patient.

Long-Term Care

Many long-term care facilities accept residents who are receiving parenteral nutrition. In some facilities, the solutions are prepared and delivered by a commercial medical supply company. The general proce-
dure for assessing the resident and administering and monitoring parenteral nutrition must be conscientiously followed to ensure safety. Your responsibility as part of the nursing staff is to be knowledgeable and competent in administering parenteral nutrition to residents. Older adults are at a greater risk for alterations in skin integrity, nutritional imbalances, and fluid and electrolyte imbalances; close monitoring of these residents is essential.

Home Care

A client may need parenteral nutrition for an extended time after discharge. The nurse teaches the procedure to the client and caregiver(s) and gives demonstrations along with written directions. The caregiver demonstrates the procedure within the hospital environment before the client goes home. It is important that the client and the caregiver feel comfortable and confident before the procedure is performed in the home. The solutions are prepared as ordered by the physician, and the caregiver is taught to add vitamins or insulin, if needed, at specific designated times.

The general procedure is the same as that used in the hospital or long-term facility. In urban areas, the solutions and equipment are available from a number of commercial companies. These companies usually make deliveries to the home at least twice weekly. They also are a resource to the family if any difficulties arise after the nurse or nutritionist makes an initial home visit. In suburban and rural areas, the family may have to make special arrangements regarding where and how to obtain the solution and equipment for the procedure.

Home health agencies monitor the client and reinforce the teaching that the caregiver needs to maintain parenteral nutrition in the home, to recognize signs of impending problems such as infection, and to implement emergency interventions.

Ambulatory Care

The nurse in the ambulatory care setting provides an ongoing assessment of the CVC site, monitors intake and output, weight changes, blood glucose levels, and laboratory results. Written daily logs of information should be maintained. A home caregiver should see the nurse in this setting as another resource besides the home care agency for additional instructions and to answer questions as to what signs and symptoms are important to report.

LEARNING TOOLS

DEVELOP YOUR BACKGROUND KNOWLEDGE

1. Review the Learning Outcomes.

2. Read the section on total parenteral nutrition in your assigned text.

3. Look up the Key Terms in the glossary.

4. Review this module and mentally practice the techniques described. Study so that you would be able to teach these skills to another person.

DEVELOP YOUR SKILLS

In the practice setting, select one other student and work in pairs. Alternate so that each has the opportunity to practice with the equipment and perform each of the following procedures. The student who is not participating at a given time can observe and evaluate the performances of the other.

1. Examine the parenteral nutrition and fat emulsion equipment. Identify the following:
   a. simulated orders for parenteral nutrition and fat emulsion
   b. practice parenteral nutrition solution and fat emulsion bottle
   c. an infusion pump
   d. pump or regular tubing for the parenteral nutrition solution and tubing for the fat emulsion bottle

2. After checking the order against the printed label on the bottle or bag, practice setting up the parenteral nutrition solution and fat emulsion bottle, using the appropriate tubing. Insert the tubing into the pump or an existing parenteral nutrition line.

3. Set the flow rate and operate the pump.

4. Practice documenting the parenteral nutrition and lipids on an IV record form.

DEMONSTRATE YOUR SKILLS

In the clinical setting

1. Consult with your instructor regarding the equipment and policies and procedures for administering parenteral nutrition, including lipids, in the agency to which you are assigned.

2. With your instructor's supervision, administer parenteral nutrition and fat emulsions (lipids). Evaluate your performance with the instructor.

3. Make appropriate assessments and take any action needed to prevent complications with parenteral nutrition. Use the Performance Checklist on the CD-ROM in the front of this book as a guide. Evaluate your performance with the instructor.

CRITICAL THINKING EXERCISES

Evaluate each of the following situations and describe how you would respond.

1. The parenteral solution bag you are to hang has a label that indicates that multivitamins have been added, but the solution is clear.

2. The site of the patient's central line is slightly reddened, but the solution flow is not obstructed.

3. The alarm on the pump goes off several times.

4. The lipid bottle arrives on the unit and the solution appears to be separating, so there is an oil solution at the top and white solution at the bottom.

5. After receiving the first container of parenteral nutrition, the patient has a blood glucose level of 205 mg/dL.

SELF-QUIZ
SHORT-ANSWER QUESTIONS

1. List two types of parenteral nutrition.

   a. _____

   b. _____

2. List four areas of assessment that are essential to monitor while a patient is receiving total parenteral nutrition.

   a. _____

   b. _____

   c. _____

   d. _____

3. Why are total parenteral nutrition solutions started at slower rates and gradually increased in speed?

_____

4. Why is an infusion pump always used to infuse the parenteral nutrition solution?

_____

5. Why is peripheral parenteral nutrition usually given for a limited time?

_____

6. Why is a glucose solution greater than 10% dextrose administered through a CVC?

_____

MULTIPLE CHOICE

_____ 7. A common complication of parenteral nutrition is
a. hyperglycemia.
b. weight loss.
c. indigestion.
d. dependent edema.

_____ 8. Lipids may be given along with parenteral nutrition to supply the patient with
a. proteins.
b. carbohydrates.
c. fats.
d. trace minerals.

_____ 9. Total parenteral nutrition would be appropriate to use for which type of patient?
a. One for whom a weight gain of 10% above current body weight is desired
b. A patient with inflammatory bowel disease
c. All elderly patients
d. A patient who is NPO for 48 hours

_____ 10. Lipids are available in what concentration?
a. 35%
b. 20%
c. 5%
d. 50%

_____ 11. Lipids are administered through an IV line below the filter because
a. the lipids do not mix well with the parenteral nutrition solution.
b. the lipids are free of bacteria and particles that do not require filtering.
c. the molecules are too large to pass through the filter and would clog the tubing.
d. filters large enough for use with lipids are not available.

_____ 12. Orders for total parenteral nutrition are reviewed by the physician
a. every 48 hours.
b. every 8 hours.
c. every 12 hours.
d. every 24 hours.

Answers to the Self-Quiz questions appear in the back of the book.

Administering Blood and Blood Components

KEY TERMS

acute hemolytic transfusion
   reaction
allergic transfusion reaction
allogeneic
anaphylactic transfusion reaction
apheresis

autologous transfusion
circulatory overload
compatibility testing
febrile nonhemolytic transfusion
   reaction (FNTR)
fibrinogen
hypothermia

red blood cells (RBCs)
septic transfusion reaction
thrombocytopenia
transfusion-related acute lung
   injury (TRALI)
type and crossmatch
white blood cells (WBCs)

OVERALL OBJECTIVE

▸ To safely administer blood components and to effectively manage reactions that may occur.

LEARNING OBJECTIVES

The student will be able to

1. Assess the patient and family's educational needs, cultural and religious beliefs, and informed consent for transfusion.
2. Assess the patient's physical status in relation to receiving a transfusion.
3. Analyze assessment data to identify the specific individual concerns that are present for the patient related to administering a transfusion.
4. Determine appropriate patient outcomes of the transfusion and recognize the potential for adverse outcomes.
5. Plan the transfusion, including appropriate equipment and supplies.
6. Safely administer the whole blood or blood component.
7. Evaluate the patient's clinical status during the transfusion.
8. Evaluate the effectiveness of the transfusion and the need for additional blood components.
9. Document the transfusion correctly.
10. Document any evidence of possible transfusion reaction.

Blood components may be administered for various reasons, including to improve oxygen-carrying capacity, to prevent or control bleeding due to **thrombocytopenia** (low platelet count) or platelet dysfunction, and to replace clotting factors. Because complications may occur with the administration of blood or blood components, the nurse must understand these complications, initiate a plan of care to prevent them, and intervene appropriately when they occur.

NURSING DIAGNOSES

With transfusion, the patient's nursing diagnoses may be associated with symptoms indicating the need for transfusion of any blood component, symptoms or risks identified during nursing assessment, or adverse effects the patient has experienced with previous transfusions. Common nursing diagnoses pertaining to transfusion include

- Activity Intolerance: weakness related to decreased number of **red blood cells (RBCs)** (anemia) or loss of blood
- Deficient Fluid Volume: related to hemorrhage
- Excess Fluid Volume: related to increase in vascular fluid volume during or following transfusion

- Impaired Comfort: (e.g., chills, fever, or itching) related to transfusion reaction
- Deficient Knowledge: related to transfusion, indications for transfusion, risk of transfusion-transmitted infections, potential adverse outcomes of transfusion
- Risk for Bleeding: related to abnormal levels of clotting factors, thrombocytopenia, or low fibrinogen count (hypofibrinogenemia)
- Risk for Spiritual Distress: related to beliefs about blood transfusion. Some individuals do not accept blood transfusion for religious reasons.
- Anxiety: related to receiving blood transfusion
- Risk for Infection: related to low white blood cell (WBC) count

DELEGATION

The administration of blood and blood components has such a high potential for serious adverse effects that it is never delegated to unlicensed staff. In many facilities, even nursing students never administer blood but may observe the procedure performed by a registered nurse and provide observations and data collection during the transfusion.

BLOOD COLLECTION METHODS

There are three blood donor sources for routine blood collection: unrelated donor (allogeneic), directed donor, and autologous (or self).

UNRELATED DONOR

Most blood transfused to patients is **allogeneic** blood, which is blood donated by unrelated volunteer donors. Through a laboratory process, the blood from each donor is typed (ABO group and Rh type) and tested for a variety of transfusion-transmitted diseases, such as hepatitis B, hepatitis C, human immunodeficiency virus (HIV), human T-cell lymphotropic virus (HTLV), West Nile virus, and syphilis. If any of the tests are positive, the blood is discarded, and the donor is notified.

DIRECTED DONOR

In some cases, blood may be donated by a directed donor (i.e., a donor chosen by the patient). The donor may or may not be related to the patient, but the blood, which must be compatible with the patient's blood, is designated for use by the patient for whom the donation is given. The blood undergoes the same tests as blood from unrelated donors. There is no scientific evidence that blood from directed donors is safer than blood from unrelated donors.

AUTOLOGOUS DONOR

For patients anticipating a future planned surgery, an option may be autologous blood donation, whereby the patient donates his or her own blood in advance of potential need. The units are stored and later infused back to the patient during the perioperative period. As much as possible, an adequate number of units should be collected, to minimize the need for transfusing blood from other donors. It is best when autologous blood is donated as far in advance of surgery as practical, beginning 3 to 5 weeks before surgery, to allow for optimal compensatory red blood cell (RBC) regeneration. The patient may be placed on oral iron supplements to aid in hemoglobin regeneration. Ordinarily, the last donation should occur more than 72 hours before surgery to allow for volume replacement (American Association of Blood Banks [AABB], 2004).

To be eligible for autologous donation, the patient must have a hematocrit value of 33% or greater. The donated whole blood or RBCs are labeled for the patient and stored until ready for use. Unused autologous blood is discarded and never released into the general blood supply.

Although **autologous transfusion** eliminates the risk of infectious disease transmission and may represent the safest possible option for some patients, it is not risk-free. Risks of bacterial contamination, volume overload, and **acute hemolytic transfusion reaction,** resulting from administrating the wrong unit to the wrong patient, are not eliminated. A potential disadvantage of autologous donation is that the patient may experience anemia prior to the scheduled surgery. People for whom receiving blood from others is not acceptable due to religious belief may accept autologous blood.

WHOLE BLOOD AND BLOOD COMPONENTS

When a unit of whole blood is donated, it is most commonly separated into individual components including RBCs, platelets, plasma, and cryoprecipitate. These components are more frequently given to patients than whole blood. Each component can be selectively ordered to treat a patient's specific transfusion need. Individual component therapy better utilizes blood resources because components made from one unit of whole blood can treat multiple patients.

Prior to administering a blood component, you must have specific information about that component, just as you have specific information about medications that are administered. Descriptions, indications, and compatibility requirements of whole blood and other blood components are discussed below (see also Table 52-1).

WHOLE BLOOD

A unit of whole blood is approximately 500 to 570 mL, composed of 450 to 500 mL of blood from a donor and 63 to 70 mL of anticoagulant-preservative solution (Brecher, 2002). It contains no functional platelets or **white blood cells (WBCs).** It is stored in a monitored blood refrigerator between 1° and 6°C until issued to a patient for transfusion.

RED BLOOD CELLS (RBCs)

An RBC unit is prepared by removing most of the plasma from a whole blood unit. One unit of RBCs equals approximately 250 to 400 mL, composed of 160 to 275 mL of RBCs suspended in varying amounts of plasma and anticoagulant-preservative solution (AABB, 2002). It contains no functional platelets or WBCs. It is stored in a monitored blood refrigerator between 1° and 6°C until issued to patients for transfusion.

PLATELETS

Platelets (thrombocytes) are an essential contributor to the clotting process. A platelet concentrate unit is derived from a whole blood unit and consists of platelets suspended in approximately 40 to 70 mL of plasma

table 52-1. **Blood Components**

Composition	Storage	Indications
Whole blood (an entire unit of blood as obtained from the donor plus the anticoagulant-preservative)		
■ 500 to 570 mL (450–500 mL of blood from a donor and 63–70 mL of anticoagulant-preservative solution)	In temperature-monitored blood refrigerator between 1° and 6°C until issue. May be returned to transfusion service for use at a later time, if unit temperature has not exceeded 10°C after being issued; some transfusion services allow for return within 30 minutes.	■ Rarely used; individual blood components are usually given rather than whole blood. ■ Acute, massive blood loss ■ Special needs, such as neonatal exchange transfusion or cardiopulmonary bypass surgery
Red blood cells (the component that remains after most of the plasma is removed from a whole blood unit)		
■ Approximately 250–400 mL composed of 160–275 mL of RBCs suspended in varying amounts of plasma and anticoagulant-preservative solution	In temperature-monitored blood refrigerator between 1° and 6°C until issued to the patient care area. May be returned to transfusion service for use at a later time, if unit temperature has not exceeded 10°C after being issued; some transfusion services allow for return within 30 minutes.	■ Severe bleeding ■ Symptomatic anemia (dyspnea, tachypnea, tachycardia, pallor, and fatigue) ■ Even when symptomatic anemia is not present, most patients require an RBC transfusion when hemoglobin level falls below 6–7 g/dL. ■ For hemoglobin levels between 6 and 10 g/dL, provider must evaluate individual patient's clinical status and risk factors to determine need for RBC transfusion. ■ For hemoglobin levels > 10 g/dL, RBC transfusion is not usually required, but may be required for some patients.
Platelets (cell fragments that contribute to the clotting process, formerly called thrombocytes)		
Whole blood platelet concentrates ■ Suspended in approximately 40–70 mL of plasma ■ Normally, multiple platelet concentrates (4–8 units) are pooled in one bag to equal a therapeutic adult dose. Pediatric dose is based on child's weight. **Platelets obtained by apheresis** ■ Suspended in approximately 200–400 mL of plasma ■ 1 unit is equal to approximately 4–8 units of pooled platelet concentrates.	Room temperature (20°–24°C) in a platelet incubator with continuous gentle agitation until issue. After issue, stored at room temperature; should never be refrigerated	■ To treat bleeding in patients with thrombocytopenia (< 50,000–100,000 platelets/microliter) or abnormal platelet function ■ Given prophylactically to prevent bleeding in patients with severe thrombocytopenia (<10,000–20,000 platelets/microliter); may be given at platelet counts higher than this range to patients undergoing surgery or an invasive procedure
Plasma (fluid portion of the blood)		
■ 1 unit of FFP or thawed plasma contains between 200–250 mL of plasma. ■ Fresh frozen plasma (FFP) has a normal concentration of all clotting factors. ■ Thawed plasma's levels of clotting factor V and factor VIII decline during storage.	FFP is separated from whole blood soon after collection and frozen at −18°C or below. Once thawed for use, FFP may be stored for up to 24 hours, or FFP may be relabeled as thawed plasma and and stored for up to 5 days. Thawed FFP and thawed plasma units are stored in a temperature-monitored blood refrigerator until issue.	■ To replace clotting factors in patients with multiple clotting factor deficiencies (as evidenced by a prolonged PT or aPTT or an elevated INR) and active bleeding ■ As prophylaxis to prevent bleeding in patients with multiple factor deficiencies and in need of surgery or an invasive procedure ■ For rapid reversal of anticoagulation resulting from warfarin (Coumadin) use in a bleeding patient or in a patient requiring emergency surgery ■ To treat thrombotic thrombocytopenia purpura (TTP)
Cryoprecipitate (concentrated source of certain plasma proteins)		
■ Each unit is suspended in approximately 15 mL of plasma. ■ Contains clotting factors including fibrinogen, von Willebrand factor, factor VIII, and factor XIII	Stored frozen (−18°C or below). Once thawed for use, cryoprecipitate is stored at room temperature; it should never be refrigerated.	■ For patients with hypofibrinogenemia (<80–100 mg/dL) and active bleeding ■ For patients with hypofibrinogenemia (<80–100 mg/dL) who are undergoing an invasive procedure
Granulocytes (a type of white blood cell, also called neutrophils)		
■ Large numbers of granulocytes, 20–50 mL of RBCs, and 200–300 mL of plasma and varying numbers of platelets	Stores poorly, viability diminishes rapidly. Once available, should be administered as soon as possible, but may be stored at room temperature (20°–24°C) for up to 24 hours.	■ To treat severe neutropenia (absolute neutrophil count < 500/microliter) in patients with serious bacterial or fungal infections unresponsive to standard medical therapy ■ To treat life-threatening infection in patients with congenital granulocyte dysfunction

(AABB, 2002). It also contains varying numbers of WBCs and a very small amount of residual RBCs. Normally, multiple platelet concentrates (4 to 8 units) are pooled together into one bag to provide a therapeutic dose for adult patients. For pediatric patients, a therapeutic dose is calculated using the patient's weight.

Platelets may be derived from another method of collection called **apheresis.** Apheresis uses a machine to withdraw whole blood from a donor. The machine selectively collects platelets suspended in plasma and returns the RBCs to the donor. This collection method allows a therapeutic adult dose of platelets to be collected from a single donor in one collection. One unit of platelets obtained by apheresis contains approximately 200 to 400 mL. Varying numbers of WBCs and a very small amount of residual RBCs are also contained in each unit. One unit of platelets obtained by apheresis is equal to approximately 4 to 8 units of pooled platelet concentrate units derived from whole blood units. Platelets are stored at room temperature (20° to 24°C) in a platelet incubator that provides continuous gentle agitation until units are issued for transfusion.

PLASMA

Plasma is the fluid portion of the blood and is composed of 91% water, 7% protein, which includes the clotting factors, and 2% carbohydrate. It is free of RBCs, platelets, and WBCs. Fresh frozen plasma (FFP) is plasma that has been separated from whole blood shortly after collection and frozen at −18°C or below. Once thawed and prepared for transfusion, the plasma may be labeled as FFP and stored for up to 24 hours, or the plasma may be labeled as thawed plasma and stored for up to 5 days. Thawed units are stored in a monitored blood refrigerator until issued to patients for transfusion. FFP contains a normal concentration of all the clotting factors; thawed plasma's levels of clotting factor V and factor VIII decline during storage (Brecher, 2002). One unit of FFP or thawed plasma contains approximately 200 to 250 mL of plasma. Clotting factors are indicated by prothrombin time (PT), activated partial thromboplastin time (aPTT), and international normal ratio (INR).

CRYOPRECIPITATE

Cryoprecipitate is a concentrated source of certain plasma proteins prepared from FFP. It contains clotting factors including **fibrinogen,** von Willebrand factor, factor VIII, and factor XIII (AABB, 2002). It contains no RBCs, platelets, or WBCs. Each unit is suspended in approximately 15 mL of plasma. Cryoprecipitate is refrozen after preparation and is stored in a monitored blood freezer (−18°C or below). It is thawed by the transfusion service laboratory before being sent to the patient for transfusion. Cryoprecipitate should remain at room temperature.

GRANULOCYTES (NEUTROPHILS)

A granulocyte unit is usually collected from a single donor using an apheresis machine. This component contains large numbers of granulocytes, variable numbers of lymphocytes, 20 to 50 mL of RBCs, and 200 to 300 mL of plasma (AABB, 2002). It may contain large numbers of platelets up to an amount equivalent to that found in 6 to 10 units of pooled platelets. Depending on the needs of the patient, some blood collection facilities may prepare platelet-poor granulocytes, which contain a small number of platelets. In urgent neonatal situations, granulocytes may be prepared from a unit of fresh whole blood. Transfusion of a granulocyte unit should be started as soon as possible after it is available because granulocytes do not store well, and their viability diminishes rapidly over time. If this is not possible, a unit may be stored at room temperature for up to 24 hours.

COMPATIBILITY TESTING: TYPE AND CROSSMATCH

Before a component containing a significant number of RBCs (i.e., RBCs, whole blood, granulocytes) is issued for a patient, **compatibility testing** is completed. Compatibility testing, done in the transfusion service laboratory, involves a **type and crossmatch** to help ensure that the unit is compatible with the patient, thereby preventing an acute hemolytic transfusion reaction, which can occur when incompatible RBCs are administered. The American Association of Blood Banks' *Technical Manual for Blood Banks* provides a comprehensive explanation of compatibility testing (see Table 52-2 for blood component compatibility) (AABB, 2002).

First, the patient's blood is tested to determine its ABO blood group and Rh type. Of the many different antigens on the surface of an RBC, the most clinically significant are those antigens that determine the ABO group and Rh type.

Four blood groups are in the ABO system of blood typing: A, B, AB, and O (Table 52-3). The blood group is determined by the presence or absence of the A or B antigens on the surface of the RBCs. If only the A antigen is present, the blood is group A; if only the B antigen is present, the blood is group B; if both A and B antigens are present, the blood is group AB; and if neither A nor B antigens are present, the blood is group O. By the age of 3 to 4 months, people naturally develop antibodies to the A or B antigens (anti-A or anti-B) they lack. Therefore, those with group A type blood produce antibodies against the B antigen (anti-B), those with group B produce anti-A, those with group AB produce neither, and those with group O produce both anti-A and anti-B. These antibodies are present in the plasma.

table 52-2. ABO Group and Rh Type Blood Component Compatibility

Patient Blood Type	Compatible Whole Blood	Compatible RBCs	Compatible Granulocytes	Compatible Plasma*
Group O Rh positive	Group O Rh positive Group O Rh negative	Group O Rh positive Group O Rh negative	Group O Rh positive Group O Rh negative	All ABO groups and Rh types are acceptable.
Group O Rh negative	Group O Rh negative	Group O Rh negative	Group O Rh negative	All ABO groups and Rh types are acceptable.
Group A Rh positive	Group A Rh positive Group A Rh negative	Group A Rh positive Group A Rh negative Group O Rh positive Group O Rh negative	Group A Rh positive Group A Rh negative Group O Rh positive[†] Group O Rh negative[†]	Group A Rh positive Group A Rh negative Group AB Rh positive Group AB Rh negative
Group A Rh negative	Group A Rh negative	Group A Rh negative Group O Rh negative	Group A Rh negative Group O Rh negative[†]	Group A Rh positive Group A Rh negative Group AB Rh positive Group AB Rh negative
Group B Rh positive	Group B Rh positive Group B Rh negative	Group B Rh positive Group B Rh negative Group O Rh positive Group O Rh negative	Group B Rh positive Group B Rh negative Group O Rh positive[†] Group O Rh negative[†]	Group B Rh positive Group B Rh negative Group AB Rh positive Group AB Rh negative
Group B Rh negative	Group B Rh negative	Group B Rh negative Group O Rh negative	Group B Rh negative Group O Rh negative[†]	Group B Rh positive Group B Rh negative Group AB Rh positive Group AB Rh negative
Group AB Rh positive	Group AB Rh positive Group AB Rh negative	Group AB Rh positive Group AB Rh negative Group A Rh positive Group A Rh negative Group B Rh positive Group B Rh negative Group O Rh positive Group O Rh negative	Group AB Rh positive Group AB Rh negative Group A Rh positive[†] Group A Rh negative[†] Group B Rh positive[†] Group B Rh negative[†] Group O Rh positive[†] Group O Rh negative[†]	Group AB Rh positive Group AB Rh negative
Group AB Rh negative	Group AB Rh negative	Group AB Rh negative Group A Rh negative Group B Rh negative Group O Rh negative	Group AB Rh negative Group A Rh negative[†] Group B Rh negative[†] Group O Rh negative[†]	Group AB Rh positive Group AB Rh negative

Note: Platelets and cryoprecipitate: Consult facility policy, as practice varies.
*Plasma may be given without regard to Rh type. An Rh-positive or an Rh-negative patient may receive either Rh-positive or Rh-negative plasma.
[†]May require volume reduction; check facility's policy.
Compiled from data in Puget Sound Blood Center. (2005). *Blood components reference manual.* Seattle, WA: Author.

Blood is also classified as either Rh positive or Rh negative. The Rh type is determined by the presence or absence of the D antigen on the surface of the RBCs. If the D antigen is present, the blood is Rh positive; if it is absent, the blood is Rh negative. Unlike people with anti-A and anti-B antibodies, which occur naturally, people who are Rh negative do not develop antibodies against the D antigen (anti-D) they lack unless exposed to Rh-positive RBCs either through pregnancy or transfusion. This is also true in most other cases of antibody development to red cell antigens; there must be exposure to foreign red cell antigens either through transfusion or pregnancy before antibodies are produced.

Basic to safe administration of RBCs and blood components containing a significant number of RBCs is avoiding transfusing antigen to a patient having antibodies against that antigen. Table 52-2 provides information on the compatibility of various blood components based on the patient's blood type. For example, a patient with group A blood must not be given group B or group AB RBCs because the anti-B antibodies in the patient's plasma will react with the B antigens on the surface of the transfused RBCs. This antigen-antibody reaction triggers a series of immune responses, which results in the destruction of the infused RBCs and may cause a serious and possibly fatal acute hemolytic transfusion reaction.

table 52-3. ABO Blood Group System

Blood Group	Antigens on the RBCs	Antibodies in the Plasma
A	A	Anti-B
B	B	Anti-A
AB	A and B	None
O	None	Anti-A and Anti-B

Rh-positive patients can receive either Rh-positive or Rh-negative blood components. Rh-negative patients should receive only Rh-negative RBC-containing components. This includes RBCs, whole blood, granulocytes, and platelets. Although platelet components contain very few RBCs, enough are present potentially to cause anti-D development in an Rh-negative patient. It is important to avoid anti-D formation in patients, especially in women with childbearing potential.

Besides A, B, and D antigens, there are hundreds of other antigens that may be present on the surface of an RBC and to which a person may be sensitized. People may develop RBC antibodies to these RBC antigens through pregnancy or transfusion. An antibody screen and a crossmatch are used to test the patient's plasma for clinically significant RBC antibodies. This antibody screen is performed to select compatible units of RBC–containing blood components.

Compatibility testing is not required for platelet, plasma, or cryoprecipitate transfusion orders. As long as the patient's blood type is known at the transfusion service, it is not necessary to send a blood sample for typing and crossmatching when ordering these components.

EQUIPMENT AND SUPPLIES

Blood components must be administered using equipment and supplies that ensure safe transfusion.

VENOUS ACCESS

Blood components may be administered through either a peripheral or a central venous catheter (CVC). A 19-G or larger catheter is commonly used because it will accommodate variable flow rates. If the patient is an adult with small veins or an infant or young child, a 20- to 25-G catheter may be used. Using a small-lumen catheter will not cause hemolysis of the infusing RBCs, provided high pressure is not used to force the component through the catheter. A small catheter size will limit the rate at which a component can infuse.

ADMINISTRATION SETS AND FILTERS

All blood components including whole blood, RBCs, platelets, plasma, cryoprecipitate, and granulocytes must be infused through a sterile administration set that contains a filter (usually 150 to 260 micron pore size) designed to remove small clots and particulate matter that may accumulate during storage. A standard blood administration set includes tubing, an in-line blood component filter, and a drip chamber. The administration set may be primed with either 0.9% sodium chloride (normal saline) solution or the blood component.

Refer to the manufacturer's guidelines, and follow recommended priming instructions. The filter should be entirely saturated with normal saline solution or the blood component before the infusion starts to be sure the entire filter is utilized.

Most standard blood administration sets can be used to filter 2 to 4 units of blood components before debris accumulates and slows the flow rate. However, because the maximum number of units that can be infused varies with different types of administration sets, always check the manufacturer's guidelines, or follow the facility's policy when determining this maximum number. Filters should not be left hanging for more than 4 hours because of the hazard of bacterial proliferation. Platelets should not be infused through the same administration set that was used to transfuse RBCs because the platelets may become trapped in the filter that contains red cell debris. If it is necessary to transfuse platelets after RBCs, use a new blood component administration set.

A Y-type blood administration set or a straight blood administration set (Fig. 52-1) may be used to infuse blood components. Most commonly, Y sets are used for the infusion of RBCs, whole blood, or granulocytes; either a Y set or a straight set is used for the infusion of platelets, plasma, and cryoprecipitate. A Y set allows the administration set to be easily primed with normal saline solution attached to one infusion spike of the Y tubing. Once primed, the blood component is attached to the second infusion spike. Y sets are preferable when normal saline solution is needed for component dilution or for flushing the line after the transfusion is completed.

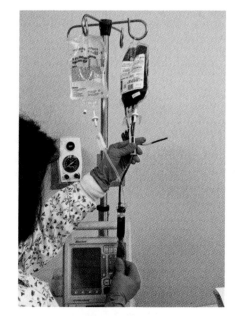

FIGURE 52-1 Y-type blood administration set, which differs from a straight blood administration set by including the set-up for infusing saline solution.

Note: For pediatric patients, a facility may issue blood components in a syringe, or policy may allow for blood components to be withdrawn through a blood administration set into a syringe and administered via a syringe pump.

Some facilities may use specialized filters called leukocyte reduction filters when transfusing whole blood, RBCs, or platelets for specific patients. Because these filters have special priming and use requirements, carefully follow the manufacturer's instructions. Do not flush a leukocyte reduction filter with normal saline solution after the transfusion is completed.

INFUSION PUMPS

Many facilities use infusion pumps to transfuse blood components because they allow the infusion rate to be controlled precisely. As long as the pump is approved by the manufacturer for the transfusion of blood components, its use is acceptable. Because practice varies, it is also necessary to determine and follow the policy regarding pump use at each facility.

COMPATIBLE IV SOLUTIONS

Many facilities have policies stating that the only solution that may be added directly to a blood component or infused through the same tubing with the blood component is normal saline solution. This restriction prevents the addition of incompatible IV solutions such as 5% dextrose in water (D_5W), which can cause RBC hemolysis, and lactated Ringer's solution (and other solutions containing calcium), which can cause clot formation. Other solutions may be added to blood components if they are approved by the Food and Drug Administration (FDA) or if there is documentation showing the addition of the solution is safe and does not harm the blood component (AABB, 2004).

BLOOD WARMERS

Blood warmers are not required for most transfusions. However, they are indicated for several specific clinical situations, primarily for rapid, large-volume transfusions. Transfusing large quantities of cold refrigerated blood components (whole blood, RBCs, FFP, thawed plasma) rapidly can cause **hypothermia** and induce associated physiologic changes, including coagulopathies and cardiac arrhythmias, which may lead to cardiac arrest. Blood warmers are recommended for the following transfusion situations: massive transfusion, infusion rate greater than 50 mL/minute for 30 minutes or more in adults, infusion rate greater than 15 mL/kg/hour in children, and infants receiving exchange or large-volume transfusion (Hrovat, et al., 2002).

There are many different types of blood warmers. Only warmers specifically designed for use with blood components and approved by the FDA or validated by the transfusing facility may be used to warm blood. The manufacturer's guidelines must be followed closely because overheating a blood component can cause RBC hemolysis. Warming platelet, cryoprecipitate, and granulocyte components is not indicated because warming may cause these components to be less effective (Hrovat, et al., 2002).

ADMINISTERING INTRAVENOUS MEDICATIONS

In general, a medication should not be added directly to a blood component or administered through the same tubing with the blood component. Medications may cause clotting, hemolysis, or other changes in the blood. In addition, the blood component may alter the therapeutic effect of the medication. If the IV line being used to administer the blood component must be used to give medications (e.g., when emergency medications must be given and another IV access is not available), stop the transfusion, thoroughly flush the line with normal saline solution before and after medication administration, and then restart the transfusion.

Safety Alert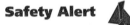

Although not recommended, administering a medication through the same tubing with the blood component may be done if the medication is FDA approved for this use or if there is documentation showing that the addition of the medication is safe and does not harm the blood component.

CONSENT FOR BLOOD TRANSFUSIONS

A transfusion has many risks as well as potential benefits. The patient's primary care provider is responsible for obtaining informed consent from the patient, family, and/or guardian. Consent is considered informed when a discussion has included the nature and character of the transfusion of blood components, the anticipated benefits of transfusion, the recognized potential serious risks and complications, and any available treatment alternatives to transfusion, including no transfusion. In addition, the patient must be given an opportunity to ask questions. Prior to administering a transfusion, the nurse is responsible for checking that informed consent is documented in the patient's record. However, transfusion must not be delayed when a life-threatening emergency exists and time does not allow for informed consent (Brecher, 2002).

GENERAL PROCEDURE FOR ADMINISTERING RBCs AND WHOLE BLOOD

The instructions in the following general procedure include the fundamental nursing actions needed to administer RBCs and whole blood safely. The specific procedures that follow the general procedure provide instructions for administering other blood components and call for the nurse to use many steps of the general procedure and to vary others. Of course, steps of the procedure should always be in accord with your healthcare facility's policies and procedures.

ASSESSMENT

1. Review the prescribed transfusion order. The order includes the specific type of blood component (such as whole blood or RBCs), any required special attributes (e.g., irradiation, leukocyte reduction, CMV negative [tested negative for cytomegalovirus antibodies]), the number of units or volume to be transfused, and the infusion rate if the rate is not a standard protocol. **R:** To verify that the component type is appropriate and that the dose and rate of transfusion are within a safe range for the specific patient.

2. Check for a signed informed consent form for transfusion. If the consent is not present, notify the prescriber. **R:** Documentation of informed consent is required prior to beginning a transfusion, except for emergency lifesaving transfusions. Transfusion must not be delayed when a life-threatening emergency exists and time does not allow for informed consent. Informed consent helps ensure that the patient understands the risks, benefits, and alternatives of transfusion.

3. Review the patient's hematocrit or hemoglobin level that triggered the RBC or whole blood transfusion order. **R:** To determine the laboratory value at which the specific patient has developed symptomatic anemia and verify that the transfusion is indicated.

4. Assess the patient and family's cultural and religious beliefs related to transfusion. **R:** To determine if concerns must be addressed prior to beginning the transfusion.

5. Assess the patient and family's need for education regarding transfusion. **R:** To determine the patient/family knowledge level and allay fears related to transfusion procedure.

6. Assess for history of transfusion reaction. **R:** To determine whether pre-transfusion medications or administration modifications (e.g., decreasing the rate of transfusion) or special attributes (e.g., leuko-

cyte reduction) are required to help prevent transfusion reactions.

7. Obtain the patient's history and physically assess the patient for signs and symptoms of anemia, including dyspnea, tachypnea, tachycardia, dizziness, confusion, pallor, and fatigue. **R:** Signs of symptomatic anemia must be documented to provide baseline data needed to evaluate the effectiveness of transfusion.

8. Perform physical assessment for any current symptoms that are similar to those that may be experienced during a transfusion reaction, including the following: dyspnea, rales, fever, chills, hypertension or hypotension, rash, itching, and nausea/vomiting. **R:** To establish a baseline of symptoms from which to assess changes in the patient's clinical status during and following the transfusion. The changes may indicate an adverse outcome of the transfusion.

9. Assess the patient for cardiac, renal, or pulmonary disease or signs and symptoms of fluid volume excess. **R:** To determine if a slower rate of transfusion is necessary.

10. Assess existing IV access for patency and size; a size 19-G or larger cannula is preferred. Size 20- to 25-G access may be used for infants and other patients with small veins. **R:** To ensure that proper venous access is available before the blood component is requested.

ANALYSIS

11. Critically think through your data, carefully evaluating each aspect and its relation to other data. **R:** To determine specific problems for this individual in relation to the transfusion.

12. Identify specific problems and modifications of the procedure needed for this individual. **R:** Planning for the individual must take into consideration the individual's problems.

PLANNING

13. Determine individualized patient outcomes in relation to this transfusion by considering the following. **R:** Identification of outcomes guides planning and evaluation.
    a. The right *patient* receives the right *blood* component, in the right *amount*, by the right *route*, at the right *time*.
    b. The blood component was administered over the correct length of time.
    c. Decreased or absent signs and symptoms of anemia
    d. Post-transfusion hematocrit and/or hemoglobin (if ordered) levels show an appropriate increase when compared to pre-transfusion test results.

e. Absence of adverse effects related to the transfusion

14. Plan for the approximate start time of the transfusion and for the insertion of an IV access device in advance of that time if necessary. In some settings, an IV nurse must be contacted to start the IV. **R:** To maximize efficiency and ensure that the transfusion can be completed within 4 hours of the component leaving monitored refrigeration or prior to expiration, whichever is sooner.

15. Gather the necessary equipment (e.g., basic equipment for starting an IV infusion, if needed) in addition to the following (see Module 47, Preparing and Maintaining Intravenous Infusions).

   a. Y blood administration set or straight blood administration set (see Fig. 52-1) as appropriate. For pediatric patients, your facility may issue blood components in a syringe; or in the patient care area, blood components may be withdrawn though a blood administration set into a syringe and administered via syringe pump.

   b. A 100 mL or larger bag of normal saline solution for use with a Y blood administration set, if indicated.

   c. An infusion pump to precisely control the rate of the transfusion. *Be sure to select a blood administration set with tubing that is compatible with the infusion pump.*

   d. Blood warmer, if rapid, large-volume transfusion is required to prevent hypothermia, cardiac arrhythmias, or cardiac arrest induced by the rapid, large-volume transfusion of cold blood components. (*Note:* Blood components that are warmed cannot be used at a later date.)

    e. Clean gloves to prevent potential contact with blood components

16. Obtain the RBCs or whole blood from the transfusion service just before beginning the transfusion

---

box 52-1   *Storage and Handling of Refrigerated Blood Components**

1. Whole blood, red blood cells (RBCs), and plasma (post-thawing) are stored only in monitored blood refrigerators (i.e., refrigerator equipped with a temperature monitoring and alarm system).

2. Transfusions must be completed within 4 hours from the time the unit is removed from monitored refrigeration or prior to the expiration date/time whichever is sooner.

3. RBCs, whole blood, or plasma components cannot be returned to the transfusion service's inventory if the unit temperature has exceeded 10°C. To ensure that a unit has not exceeded this maximum temperature, most facilities will only accept a unit back into inventory if it is returned within 30 minutes from the time it was removed from monitored refrigeration.

4. All blood components that are issued and not transfused must be returned to the transfusion service for documentation that the patient did not receive the unit and for proper disposal, if required.

5. Some facilities have monitored blood refrigerators in the patient care areas. When a refrigerated blood component is transferred from the transfusion service for storage in a monitored blood refrigerator on the patient care area, the unit temperature cannot exceed 10°C.

---

*This policy has been established to decrease the risk of bacterial proliferation, which may occur when units are stored out of monitored refrigeration. Adapted from Brecher, M. E. (Ed.). (2002). *AABB technical manual for blood banks* (14th ed.). Bethesda, MD: American Association of Blood Banks.

---

and verify that the dose is correct. **R:** RBCs and whole blood must be stored only in special blood refrigerators that are designated for blood storage and monitored to maintain the correct temperature (Box 52-1).

IMPLEMENTATION

Action	Rationale
17. Wash or disinfect your hands.	To decrease the transfer of microorganisms that could cause infection.
18. Compare the unit and the transfusion tag (Fig. 52-2) to the prescriber's order, including any required special attributes (e.g., irradiation, leukocyte reduction, CMV negative).	To ensure that the correct component has been issued for transfusion.

(continued)

Central 206-292-6525   UDL 206-522-2462

Puget Sound Blood Center
research   medicine   blood & tissue services
921 Terry Ave., Seattle, WA 98104

IF THE UNIT IS TRANSFUSED
RETAIN THIS COPY
AS A PERMANENT PART OF
THE PATIENT'S RECORDS

Bellevue 425-453-4560   Renton 425-656-7900

Issued on: 7/20/05 at   8:38
Inspected by: 4464

Hospital   **LOCAL HOSPITAL**

Last Name   **PATIENT**

First   **SAMPLE**

Middle   **A**

Patient ID Number   **123456**

Component   **LEUKOREDUCED AS5 RBC**

Unit Number   **CB91544**

Expiration Date and Time: 23:59 on 8/17/05

Compatibility Results: **COMPATIBLE**
Do not transfuse after: 23:59 on 7/23/05

Patient Blood Type   **O POSITIVE**

Component Blood Type   **O POSITIVE**

Patient Requirements Per Blood Center Records   IRRADIATED LEUKOREDUCED RBC

Processes Performed on Component   IRRADIATED LEUKOREDUCED RBC

I have verified all of the following:
- ❏ The name and hospital number on the patient's identification band is identical to that on this Transfusion Report.
- ❏ The unit number, ABO/Rh and expiration date/time on the unit label is identical with that on this Transfusion Report.
- ❏ The unit is normal in appearance.

VERIFIED and STARTED BY _____ Date _____ Time _____
VERIFIED BY _____ Date _____ Time _____

Comments:

UNIT RECORD this section is to remain attached to blood bag
Hospital   LOCAL HOSPITAL
Patient Name   PATIENT SAMPLE A
ID Number   123456

Component   LEUKOREDUCED AS5 RBC
Unit Number   CB91544

Lab staff must complete this section if component is returned to the Blood Center. The component has been stored in a monitored device at the temperature range indicated on the component label.
YES _____   **NO** _____   Verified By:

1006956

LAB RECORD   ELEC CROSSMATCH
Hospital   LOCAL HOSPITAL
Patient Name   PATIENT SAMPLE A
ID Number   123456

Component   LEUKOREDUCED AS5 RBC
Unit Number   CB91544
Billed Processes   IRRADIATED LEUKOREDUCED RBC

Puget Sound Blood Center

1006956

FIGURE 52-2 Example of a transfusion tag. (Reprinted with permission from Puget Sound Blood Center.)

Action	Rationale
19. Inspect the blood component bag for leaks or abnormal appearance.	A unit with an abnormal appearance is unacceptable for transfusion because this may indicate compromised quality of the unit (e.g., bacterial proliferation, damage, clots, hemolysis). Such a unit must be returned to the transfusion service; a replacement unit should be obtained.
20. Carefully verify the patient's identification and blood component unit identification with another authorized individual (usually another registered nurse or a physician) at the patient's bedside.	To ensure that the right patient receives the right blood component unit.
a. Ask the patient, family member, or guardian to state the patient's name, if able, and compare with the name on the patient's identification band.	Comparing the stated name to the name on the patient's identification band helps ensure that the correct identification band has been placed on the patient.

b. Identify the patient, using two unique identifiers, with one nurse verifying the identifiers on the patient's identification band, and the other nurse simultaneously verifying the identifiers on the transfusion tag and the prescriber's order. This process usually includes one nurse reading the identifiers from one source while the other nurse checks the information on the other sources.
 	
     (1) State the patient's name and then spell out each letter of the patient's name on the patient's identification band and compare with the transfusion tag and the order.
 	
     (2) Read the patient's medical record number or other unique identifier on the patient's identification band and compare with the transfusion tag and the order.
	Verifying the patient's identity prevents treatment errors and helps ensure that the correct blood component is transfused to the correct patient. Because a transfusion error may have serious or fatal consequences, identification must be verified by two people.

c. Verify that the information on the transfusion tag attached to the blood component matches the information on the unit bag label. One nurse reads the transfusion tag while the other checks the unit bag label. You and the other verifier must document that all of the information is correct and acceptable, either on the transfusion tag attached to the unit or on a form specified by your facility (Fig. 52-3). Verify the following.	Careful checking helps ensure transfusion of the correct unit. Clerical or distribution errors may occur at the transfusion service. For example, a transfusion tag may be attached to the wrong unit, or an expired unit may be issued for transfusion. Because a transfusion error may have serious or fatal consequences, information on the blood unit and the transfusion tag must be verified by two people.

(continued)

Action	Rationale
(1) Unit number **(2)** ABO group and Rh type **(3)** Expiration date **(4)** Expiration time, if documented	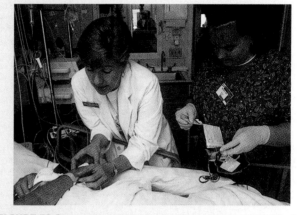 **FIGURE 52-3** Two registered nurses verify the patient's identification and blood component unit identification.
d. Verify that the expiration date and time of the patient's compatibility testing (type and crossmatch) on the transfusion tag attached to the unit has not passed.	Compatibility testing determines whether the patient has developed RBC antibodies. Testing must be performed within 3 days prior to blood transfusion. Verifying that the expiration date and time have not passed helps ensure that a unit is transfused while the compatibility testing is valid.
e. Verify that the ABO/Rh of the blood component is compatible with the patient's ABO/Rh on the transfusion tag attached to the unit.	ABO/Rh compatibility is essential to avoid transfusion reactions.
f. Do not proceed unless all comparisons match exactly and all items are correct and acceptable. Consult with another RN for an additional check, and then contact the transfusion service if any discrepancy exists or if any items are incorrect.	Verifying the patient's identity and identifying the correct blood unit helps ensure that you are administering the correct blood component to the correct patient. A wrong blood component given to a patient is a potentially fatal error and requires precise safeguards.
21. Explain the procedure you are about to perform to the patient/family. The explanation should include **a.** kind of blood component that will be transfused **b.** reason for the transfusion **c.** steps in the procedure, including the need for frequent observation and vital signs **d.** approximate duration of the transfusion **e.** expected outcome	Explaining the procedure helps relieve anxiety or misperceptions that the patient/family may have about transfusion and sets the stage for patient participation.

(continued)

Action	Rationale
f. signs and symptoms of a transfusion reaction and the need to immediately report any changes in the patient's condition during or following the transfusion	
22. Measure and record the patient's blood pressure, temperature, pulse, and respirations before starting the transfusion.	Baseline vital signs allow you to detect changes that may indicate a possible transfusion reaction.
23. Prepare the equipment as follows:	
a. Put on clean gloves.	
b. Select a blood administration set. If using a Y set, proceed to step 23c. If using a straight set, proceed to step 23d. Consult your facility's policy for pediatric transfusion when blood is administered via syringe using a syringe pump.	
c. *Prepare the Y blood administration set:* Follow guidelines on package instructions.	
(1) Close all control clamps on the Y set.	Filling the tubing completely prevents instilling air into the IV.
(2) Insert one spike of the administration set into the port of the normal saline solution and hang the bag on the IV pole.	
(3) Open the clamp closest to the bag of normal saline solution.	
(4) Partially open the clamp on tubing of unused spike apparatus.	
(5) Allow normal saline solution to flow through tubing and fill the filter and tubing of unused spike. Ensure that the filter chamber is completely saturated. Close clamp on tubing of unused spike.	All blood components must be filtered with a blood administration set to remove blood clots or particles that may harm the patient.
(6) Squeeze and release the drip chamber on the normal saline solution until approximately one-quarter full.	

(continued)

Action	Rationale
(7) Remove the sterile cap at the end of the main tubing. Partially open clamp on main tubing line and prime remainder of blood administration set with normal saline solution. Ensure that all air is purged from line; reclamp and recap.	
(8) Gently rock the blood component.	To help resuspend any blood cells that may have settled.
(9) Insert the spike into the blood component port and hang the unit on the IV pole.	
d. *Prepare the straight blood administration set:* Follow guidelines on package instructions.	
(1) Close clamp on the blood administration set.	
(2) Gently rock the blood component.	To help resuspend any blood cells that may have settled.
(3) Insert the spike of the administration set into the blood component port.	
(4) Invert blood component and filter.	
(5) Open clamp and gently squeeze filter until filter is fully saturated with the blood component, and the drip chamber is one-quarter full; reclamp.	
(6) Return blood component and filter to upright position and hang the unit on the IV pole.	
(7) Remove the sterile cap at the end of the tubing and partially open clamp to prime remainder of the blood administration set with the blood component. Ensure that all air is purged from line; reclamp and recap.	
24. Remove the sterile cap from the end of the blood administration set and connect it directly to the hub of the IV catheter. Do not piggyback a blood component into an existing IV line.	Transfusing directly through the hub of the IV catheter helps prevent infusion with incompatible solutions and reduces the possibility of the blood administration set disconnecting from the venous access.

(continued)

Action	Rationale
25. Begin the transfusion. If using a Y set, open the clamp below the blood component. Partially open the clamp on the main tubing, check for patency, and establish appropriate starting rate. Except when urgent transfusion is required, a transfusion should be started slowly. For adults, calculate the flow rate to administer approximately 25 to 30 mL during the first 15 minutes. For pediatric patients, calculate the flow rate to administer approximately 2 mL/kg/hour during the first 15 minutes, not to exceed a rate of 120 mL/hour.	Severe transfusion reactions may occur after a small volume of the blood or blood component has been transfused. A test-dose of the transfusion, initiated at a slow rate, may detect an acute reaction before a larger volume is infused.
26. Stay with the patient, if possible; otherwise, frequently observe the patient during the first 15 minutes of the transfusion.	To detect possible reactions and complications before a large volume has transfused.
27. Monitor vital signs 15 minutes after the start of the transfusion, or sooner if the patient's condition warrants. Compare with baseline measurements.	To monitor for signs of possible transfusion reaction.
28. If the patient is tolerating the transfusion, the infusion rate may be increased to the rate indicated by the medical order, patient's condition, or facility policy. Most RBC and whole blood transfusions are completed within 2 to 3 hours. However, a slower rate of transfusion may be required if the patient is susceptible to fluid volume excess. A faster rate may be required during emergent transfusion. RBC and whole blood transfusions must be completed within 4 hours from the time the unit was removed from temperature-monitored refrigeration or prior to the expiration date/time, whichever is sooner.	The rate should be individualized for each patient.
29. Assess the patient periodically (at least every 20 to 30 minutes) for symptoms of transfusion reaction, patency of the IV, and rate of transfusion.	To detect possible transfusion reactions and ensure appropriate rate of transfusion.
30. If a transfusion reaction occurs, follow the procedure in Box 52-2. See also Table 52-4 and Figure 52-4.	To avoid additional transfusion of a component that is implicated in a possible transfusion reaction, to provide medical care during a possible transfusion reaction, and to facilitate transfusion reaction workup.

(continued)

box 52-2 *Acute Transfusion Reaction Management Guidelines*

For an acute reaction other than a mild allergic reaction (hives [urticaria]), follow all of the steps below. For a mild allergic reaction, omit step 6. Always refer to your facility's policy and provider's orders for specific requirements.

1. Stop the transfusion. Stay with the patient. Ask for help from another nurse, if needed. Measure vital signs. Do not discard the unit, administration set, or any attached IV fluids; keep the entire set intact.
2. Notify the patient's provider and the transfusion service.
3. Maintain IV access, because it may be necessary to give medications and IV fluids for treatment of the reaction. Hang new IV tubing with new normal saline solution to maintain IV access. To avoid infusing any additional amount of the component into the patient, do not flush or use the blood component administration set for IV access.
4. Complete a clerical check to ensure that the correct unit was given to the right patient:
   - Confirm that the patient's name and patient's record number on the unit's transfusion tag agree with the patient's identification band.
   - Confirm that the unit number, ABO group, and Rh type on the unit's transfusion tag agree with the information on the unit bag label.
   - If the clerical check reveals a discrepancy, notify the transfusion service.
5. Treat the symptoms in accord with the provider's order, and closely monitor vital signs and symptoms.
6. Follow your facility's procedure for performing a transfusion reaction workup. Steps may include submitting the following to the transfusion service or laboratory:
   - Blood bag with attached administration set/IV fluids; keep entire set intact.
   - Completed transfusion reaction form (see Fig. 52-4).
   - Post-transfusion blood samples from the patient to check for hemolysis and, when indicated, to perform bacterial blood cultures and other laboratory tests, as prescribed.
   - Fresh urine sample, if the patient's urine is discolored (pink, red, dark).
7. Thoroughly document the reaction and treatment of the reaction.

Adapted from Brecher, M. E. (Ed.). (2002). *AABB technical manual for blood banks.* (14th ed.). Bethesda, MD: American Association of Blood Banks.

table 52-4. Acute Transfusion Reactions

Type of Transfusion Reaction	Cause	Possible Signs and Symptoms	Clinical Management (Treat per prescriber's order)	Prevention
Acute hemolytic transfusion reaction (AHTR)	Usually caused by the transfusion of ABO-incompatible RBCs. Antibodies (anti-A and/or anti-B) in the patient's plasma attach to the corresponding antigens on the incompatible transfused RBCs, resulting in RBC lysis.	Fever, chills, hypotension, nausea, vomiting, tachycardia, dyspnea, lower back pain, anxiety, hemoglobinemia (free hemoglobin in the plasma), red/dark urine (hemoglobinuria—free hemoglobin in the urine), vascular collapse, shock, unexplained bleeding, oliguria, acute renal failure, disseminated intravascular coagulation (DIC)	Stop transfusion immediately (follow steps 1–7 in Box 52-2). Treat symptoms. Treat shock, if present, with IV fluids, vasopressors, or corticosteroids as needed; maintain blood pressure with IV fluids; give diuretics/IV fluids to maintain renal output (monitor urine output); may require dialysis if renal failure occurs; treat for DIC with active bleeding as needed; do not transfuse additional blood components until approved by the transfusion service.	Careful identification of patient and accurate labeling of the compatibility (type and crossmatch) sample when ordering red-cell-containing blood components (whole blood, RBCs, granulocytes) Careful identification of patient and blood component before transfusion
Febrile nonhemolytic transfusion reaction (FNTR)	Antibodies in the patient's plasma directed against WBCs or platelets Biologic response modifiers, including cytokines, that accumulate in the unit during storage	Fever (> 1°C), chills, rigors. Symptoms often occur near the end or after the end of the transfusion.	Stop transfusion immediately (follow steps 1–7 in Box 52-2). Give antipyretics (but avoid aspirin) as needed for fever. Give meperidine as needed for severe chills (rigors).	Consider premedication with an antipyretic (avoid aspirin) 30 to 60 minutes prior to future transfusion; opinions vary on whether premedication is indicated. Repeated reactions warrant use of leukocyte-reduced whole blood, RBCs, and platelets.

(continued)

table 52-4. Acute Transfusion Reactions (Continued)

Type of Transfusion Reaction	Cause	Possible Signs and Symptoms	Clinical Management (Treat per prescriber's order)	Prevention
Mild allergic (urticarial)	Sensitivity to foreign plasma proteins in the transfused component	Localized urticaria (hives), itching, flushing	Stop transfusion immediately (follow steps 1–5 and 7 in Box 52-2). Give antihistamine. If symptoms are mild and subside or resolve, resume transfusion slowly. Complete transfusion as long as symptoms do not worsen or return. Do not restart transfusion if symptoms are moderate to severe or if fever, pulmonary symptoms, or any other symptoms develop.	Premedicate with an antihistamine prior to future transfusions.
Anaphylactic	Severe sensitivity to foreign plasma proteins in the transfused component. Patients with IgA deficiency and IgA antibodies (anti-IgA)	Respiratory distress, stridor, wheezing, chest tightness, bronchospasm, laryngeal edema, hypotension, abdominal cramps, nausea, vomiting, fever absent. Symptoms usually have an immediate onset shortly after the start of the transfusion.	Stop transfusion immediately (follow steps 1–7 in Box 52-2). Administer epinephrine, steroids, antihistamines, and/or provide oxygen support as appropriate.	Premedicate with steroids or an antihistamine prior to future transfusions, infuse slowly, and monitor patient closely. Order washed components (RBCs, platelets) for future transfusions. If available, administer IgA-deficient components for IgA-deficient patients with IgA antibodies. Autologous transfusions may be an option for some patients' transfusion needs.
Transfusion associated circulatory overload (TACO)	Inability of the circulatory system to accommodate an increased vascular fluid volume (increased risk in infants, elderly, and patients with cardiopulmonary disease or renal failure)	Dyspnea, hypertension, tachycardia, headache, cough, rales, restlessness, neck vein distension, pulmonary edema, congestive heart failure	Stop transfusion immediately (follow steps 1–7 in Box 52-2). Place patient upright with feet in a dependent position. Administer diuretics, oxygen, morphine, therapeutic phlebotomy if severe.	Infuse transfusion at a slower rate. Diuretics may be indicated. If clinical condition allows, divide amount of volume transfused over time. For example: request that a unit be divided into two or more aliquots and transfuse over a longer time period, or transfuse one unit of RBCs on one day and the second unit on the following day.
Transfusion-related acute lung injury (TRALI)	Donor leukocyte antibodies from transfused component react with patient's leukocytes. Less common, patient's leukocyte antibodies react with leukocytes in the transfused blood component. May be caused by other mechanisms. Results in microvascular damage in the lungs	Dyspnea, hypoxemia, bilateral pulmonary edema, hypotension, fever, normal pulmonary capillary wedge pressure (noncardiogenic)	Stop transfusion immediately (follow steps 1–7 in Box 52-2). Provide oxygen; intubation is often required; vasopressors as needed	Notify blood center to remove from inventory any co-components made from the same donor; if donor has leukocyte antibody, blood center will determine need to defer donor from future donations. If leukocyte antibody is present in the patient, order leukocyte-reduced components for future transfusions.
Septic transfusion reaction related to bacterial contamination	Bacteria enter the blood component during collection or processing and the bacterially contaminated blood component is transfused. More common in platelets than RBCs or whole blood, rarely implicated in plasma or cryoprecipitate	High fever (> 2°C), chills, rigors, nausea, vomiting, diarrhea, hypotension, shock	Stop transfusion immediately (follow steps 1–7 in Box 52-2). Treat hypotension/shock (IV fluids, vasopressors), broad-spectrum antibiotics after collecting patient blood culture specimens, antipyretics. Send remainder of transfused unit for gram stain and culture and collect patient blood specimens for culture.	Careful inspection of the unit to check for abnormalities before initiating transfusion. Proper storage and handling of blood components. Notify blood center to remove from inventory any co-components made from the same donor; blood center will determine need to defer donor from future donations.

Clinical management information is provided as a general guideline. Treat patient based on prescriber's order.

REPORT OF SUSPECTED TRANSFUSION REACTION

TIME RECEIVED

Puget Sound Blood Center research | medicine | blood & tissue services

CENTRAL	Ph. (206) 292-6525	FAX (206) 343-1780
BELLEVUE	Ph. (425) 453-4560	FAX (425) 453-5095
UDL	Ph. (206) 522-2462	FAX (206) 522-5948
RENTON LAB	Ph. (425) 656-7900	FAX (425) 656-7945

NOTE: TRANSFUSION REACTION EVALUATIONS SHOULD BE TREATED AS AN EMERGENCY AND REPORTED IMMEDIATELY.

Instructions:
- ☐ Stop Transfusion. Do not discard unit or infusion set.
- ☐ Notify patient's MD. If culture of component and patient is ordered, send bag and patient samples to **hospital** laboratory.
- ☐ Maintain IV access
- ☐ Monitor vital signs frequently
- ☐ Perform clerical check*
- ☐ Draw and send one or two anticoagulated (EDTA) specimens as specified by your policy to the **hospital** lab STAT with this form
- ☐ Obtain urine sample. Send red/dark urine to the **hospital** laboratory
- ☐ If transfusion is to be discontinued, send the blood bag, infusion set, and any attached IV fluids with this form to the Puget Sound Blood Center.

*Perform clerical check:
1. Name and hospital ID number on the **Transfusion Report** agree with the **patient's identification band.** ☐ Yes ☐ No
2. The blood bag number and ABO-Rh on the **Transfusion Report** agree with the information on the **blood bag label.** ☐ Yes ☐ No

If no, explain _____

PERSON REPORTING _____

PATIENT'S PHYSICIAN _____

PATIENT'S DIAGNOSIS _____

PHONE RESULTS TO:
(NURSE OR PHYSICIAN NAME) _____

SERVICE OR UNIT & TELEPHONE NUMBER _____

BLOOD PRODUCT
UNIT NUMBER IMPLICATED _____

Component:
- ☐ Red blood cells
- ☐ Fresh frozen plasma
- ☐ Platelets
- ☐ Cryoprecipitate
- ☐ Whole Blood

Amount infused (est.) _____
Pre-medication:
- ☐ Tylenol
- ☐ Benadryl
- ☐ Other_____

Time and Vital Signs:
THE INFORMATION IN RED IS REQUIRED

Start of Transfusion	Time of Reaction
Date/Time:	Date/Time:
BP	BP
P	P
T	T
R	R
O$_2$ Sat _____	O$_2$ Sat _____

Signs and Symptoms (new onset with or after transfusion)
- ☐ Fever
- ☐ Shaking chills
- ☐ Flushing or hives
- ☐ Urticaria
- ☐ Periorbital edema
- ☐ Wheezes
- ☐ Difficulty breathing
- ☐ Persistant severe hypoxia
- ☐ Anaphylaxis
- ☐ Nausea/vomiting
- ☐ Back or chest pain
- ☐ Dark/red urine

Is the patient now back to baseline? ☐ Yes ☐ No

If no, explain _____

Date & Time
Specimen collected _____

Person drawing specimen X _____

Person verifying Patient I.D. X _____

Hospital Laboratory:
Centrifuge of one EDTA tube reveals hemolysis? ☐ Yes ☐ No
Tech Initials _____
Culture of bag sent to hospital laboratory ☐ Yes ☐ No
☐ Routed to the Blood Center

_____
DATE & TIME

Immediately send one EDTA tube, the blood bag, infusion set with attached IV fluids, and this report to the Blood Center.

Note: Name must exactly match name on sample label.

Name on Sample LAST	FIRST	M.I.
Hospital Identification Number		
Hospital/Institution		
Social Security Number	Sex (M/F)	Date of Birth (mm/dd/yr)

99-32007 (7/04)

19-9-026 03

FIGURE 52-4 Form for reporting suspected transfusion reaction. (Reprinted with permission from Puget Sound Blood Center.)

Action	Rationale
31. On completion of the transfusion, put on gloves and perform one of the following:	To maintain or discontinue IV access following transfusion.
a. *To resume infusion from a Y blood administration set:*	
(1) Clamp the blood tubing closest to the blood component bag.	
(2) Partially open the clamp between the normal saline solution and allow solution to flush the blood administration set tubing to transfuse the RBCs or whole blood remaining in the tubing to the patient. Do not perform this step if using a leukocyte reduction filter; a leukocyte reduction filter should never be flushed with normal saline solution after the transfusion is completed.	
(3) Clamp the tubing on the main tubing line and remove it from the catheter hub.	
(4) Insert the tubing of the previous IV infusion into the catheter hub and adjust the flow rate.	
b. *To resume infusion from a straight blood administration set:*	
(1) Clamp the blood tubing and remove it from the catheter hub.	
(2) Immediately connect the tubing to the normal saline solution or the syringe of normal saline solution to the administration set to flush the catheter.	
(3) Flush the catheter with normal saline solution and then remove either the solution tubing or the syringe from the catheter hub.	
(4) Insert the tubing of the previous IV infusion into the catheter hub and adjust the flow rate.	
c. *If the IV infusion is to be discontinued or an IV lock is to be inserted,* follow the instructions in Module 47.	

(continued)

Action	Rationale
32. Monitor vital signs and compare them with baseline measurements and measurements obtained during the transfusion.	To monitor for signs of possible transfusion reaction.
33. Discard the blood component bag and the administration set in a biohazard container, or return to the transfusion services in a biohazard bag as specified by your facility's policy.	To dispose of biohazardous materials properly.
34. Remove gloves, and wash or disinfect your hands.	To decrease the transfer of microorganisms that could cause infection.

EVALUATION

35. Evaluate using the individualized patient outcomes in relation to this transfusion as previously identified. **R:** Evaluation in relation to desired outcomes is essential for planning future care.
   a. The right *patient* received the right *blood component*, in the right *amount*, by the right *route*, at the right *time*.
   b. The blood component was administered over the correct length of time.
   c. Decreased or absent signs and symptoms of anemia
   d. Post-transfusion hematocrit and/or hemoglobin (if ordered) show an appropriate increase when compared to pre-transfusion test results.
   e. Absence of adverse effects related to the transfusion

DOCUMENTATION

36. Complete right *documentation:* Document the procedure and any evidence of a transfusion reaction, including the following. **R:** Documentation is a legal record of the patient's care and therapy and communicates nursing activities to other nurses and caregivers. Documentation of evidence of possible transfusion reaction may be used to prescribe pre-transfusion medications to help prevent reactions in the future and will provide information regarding the care provided while the patient may have been experiencing a transfusion-related adverse effect.
   a. Vital signs obtained prior to, during, and after the transfusion
   b. The name of the component (whole blood or RBCs), unit number, transfusion start and end date/time, and the identification of the transfusionist.
   c. The volume of the transfusion; include the volume as IV intake on the intake and output flow sheet.
   d. Evidence of possible transfusion reaction; if you suspect a transfusion reaction, document interventions instituted and patient outcome.

◼ POTENTIAL ADVERSE OUTCOMES AND INTERVENTIONS

Each transfusion is associated with the potential for adverse outcomes, including acute transfusion reactions and transfusion-transmitted diseases.

1. Acute transfusion reactions: Although the transfusion of blood components is usually safe, each transfusion is associated with the potential for adverse effects. Acute transfusion reactions, their associated signs and symptoms, clinical management and prevention are described in Table 52-4. It is important that the nurse can recognize a potential reaction and intervene immediately.

Intervention: When any signs or symptoms of a potential transfusion reaction occur, immediately stop the transfusion to prevent any additional amount of the component from infusing, and follow your facility's transfusion procedure. Use the steps in Box 52-2 as a guideline. Measures may be instituted to prevent or minimize transfusion reactions, such as administering pre-transfusion medications (e.g., an antihistamine) to prevent a mild **allergic transfusion reaction** or slowing the rate of the transfusion to avoid **circulatory overload.** However, all transfusion reactions cannot be completely eliminated.

2. Transfusion-transmitted diseases: Although improved laboratory testing has decreased the risk of contracting certain infections from transfusion, there is still risk. All types of blood components pose a risk of transmitting diseases from viruses, bacteria, parasites, and other infectious agents. Contracting HIV, hepatitis B, and hepatitis C may be of highest concern to patients because these viruses are generally well-known. However, it is bacteria, not viruses, that are the most common infections transmitted via transfusion. Bacterial contamination of whole blood, RBCs, or platelets can cause life-threatening sepsis. See "Septic transfusion reaction related to bacterial contamination" in Table 52-4 for further information. There have been few case reports of bacterial contamination with plasma or cryoprecipitate because these components are stored in freezers; the very cold temperature does not support bacterial proliferation. Because the risk for contracting viruses, bacterial infections, parasites (e.g. malaria), and other diseases from transfusion can change over time, consult with the transfusion service to obtain the most current risk estimates.

Intervention: Report all symptoms of a potential transfusion-transmitted disease to the provider. All suspected cases of infection also should be reported to your transfusion service and the blood center from which the donation was obtained.

Specific Procedure for Administering Platelets

ASSESSMENT

1-2. Follow steps 1 and 2 of the General Procedure: Review the transfusion order; check for valid consent.

3. Review the patient's platelet count and treatment plan that triggered the platelet transfusion order. **R:** To determine the reason for the platelet transfusion, such as thrombocytopenia, bleeding, or planned surgical procedure, and to verify that the transfusion is indicated.

4-6. Follow steps 4 to 6 of the General Procedure: Assess the patient and family's cultural and religious beliefs and need for education; assess for history of transfusion reaction.

7. Obtain patient's history and physically assess the patient for signs and symptoms of thrombocytopenia including purpura (tiny pin-prick hemorrhages under the skin), ecchymosis (bruising), and bleeding. More serious complications of thrombocytopenia include acute hemorrhage and intracranial bleeding. **R:** These assessments detect signs and symptoms of thrombocytopenia and provide baseline data to evaluate effectiveness of transfusion.

8-9. Follow steps 8 and 9 of the General Procedure: Perform physical assessment in regard to symptoms that are similar to a transfusion reaction to obtain a baseline; assess clinical status for susceptibility to fluid volume excess.

10. Assess existing IV access for patency. Platelets may be transfused through any size catheter. **R:** Patency ensures that proper venous access is available before the blood component is requested from the transfusion service.

ANALYSIS

11-12. Follow steps 11 and 12 of the General Procedure: Think through your data, and identify specific problems and modifications.

PLANNING

13. Determine individualized patient outcomes in relation to the platelet transfusion, considering the following. **R:** Identification of outcomes guides planning and evaluation.
   a. The right *patient* receives the right *platelets*, in the right *amount*, by the right *route*, at the right *time*.
   b. The platelets were administered over the correct length of time.
   c. Appropriate increase in post-transfusion platelet count, if ordered; blood for a post-transfusion platelet count may be drawn 10 to 60 minutes after completion of the platelet transfusion.
   d. No evidence of new bleeding or bruising
   e. Evidence that pre-transfusion bleeding ceased or is reduced
   f. Absence of adverse effects related to the transfusion

14. Plan for the approximate start and end time of the platelet transfusion and for the insertion of an IV access device if necessary. **R:** These determinations maximize efficiency and ensure that the platelets will be administered prior to their expiration date and time.
   a. Determine the expiration date and time of the platelet component. The expiration date and time vary depending on the processing required to prepare the component but are usually within 3 or 4 hours from the time of issue.
   b. Determine the approximate start time of the transfusion to allow for completion of the transfusion prior to the expiration date and time.

15. Follow step 15 of the General Procedure (omitting step d): Gather the necessary equipment. Include basic equipment for starting an IV infusion if needed: appropriate Y type or straight blood administration set, a 100-mL or larger bag of normal saline solution for use with a Y blood administration set if indicated, an infusion pump to precisely control the rate of the transfusion, clean gloves to prevent potential contact with blood components.
   Note: Use of a blood warmer to infuse platelet components is not indicated.

16. Obtain the platelet component from the transfusion service just prior to beginning the transfusion. Platelets are stored at room temperature and must not be refrigerated. **R:** To prevent incorrect storage of platelets in the patient care area.

IMPLEMENTATION

Action	Rationale
17-20. Follow steps 17 to 20 of the General Procedure (omit steps 20d and 20e): Wash or disinfect your hands, compare the blood component to the prescriber's order, inspect blood component bag for leaks or abnormal appearance, verify the patient's identification and blood component unit identification. *Note:* Compatibility testing (cross matching) is not required for platelet components. Criteria for ABO compatibility of platelets varies among facilities. Verify that the ABO/Rh of the platelet component is compatible with the patient's ABO/Rh according to your facility's policy.	
21-27. Follow steps 21 to 27 of the General Procedure: Explain the procedure to the patient/family, measure and record baseline vital signs, prepare the equipment, connect the blood administration tubing to the hub of the IV access, begin the transfusion slowly, observe the patient during the first 15 minutes, and measure vital signs 15 minutes after the start of the transfusion, or sooner if indicated.	
28. If the patient is tolerating the transfusion, the infusion rate may be increased to the rate indicated by the medical order, patient's condition, or facility policy. Most platelet transfusions are completed within 45 to 90 minutes. However, a slower rate of transfusion may be required if the patient is susceptible to fluid volume excess, or a faster rate may be required during emergent transfusion. The transfusion must be completed prior to the expiration date and time.	The rate should be individualized for each patient.
29-34. Follow steps 29 to 34 of the General Procedure: Assess for symptoms of transfusion reaction; provide patient care if a transfusion reaction occurs and perform transfusion reaction workup; discontinue infusion on completion of transfusion; measure post-transfusion vital signs; discard blood component bag and administration set in biohazard container, or return to transfusion service in biohazard bag per policy; remove gloves, and wash or disinfect your hands.	

EVALUATION

35. Follow step 35 of the General Procedure: Evaluate using the individualized patient outcomes in relation to this transfusion as previously identified:
    a. The right *patient* received the right *platelets*, in the right *amount*, by the right *route*, at the right *time*.
    b. The platelets were administered over the correct length of time.
    c. Appropriate increase in post-transfusion platelet count, if ordered
    d. No evidence of new bleeding or bruising
    e. Evidence that pre-transfusion bleeding ceased or is reduced
    f. Absence of adverse effects related to the transfusion

DOCUMENTATION

36. Follow step 36 of the General Procedure: Complete right *documentation*. Document vital signs, name of the component, unit number, transfusion start and end date/time, identification of the transfusionist, volume transfused, and any evidence of possible transfusion reaction.

Specific Procedure for Administering Fresh Frozen Plasma (FFP) or Thawed Plasma

ASSESSMENT

1-2. Follow steps 1 and 2 of the General Procedure: Review the transfusion order; check for valid consent.
3. Review the patient's prothrombin time (PT), activated partial thromboplastin time (aPTT), or international normalized ratio (INR), and treatment plan that triggered the plasma transfusion order. **R:** To determine the reason for the plasma transfusion, such as low levels of clotting factors or planned surgical procedure, and to verify that the transfusion is indicated.
4-6. Follow steps 4 to 6 of the General Procedure: Assess the patient's and family's cultural/religious beliefs and need for education; assess for history of transfusion reaction.
7. Obtain patient's history and physically assess the patient for signs and symptoms of coagulopathy (coagulation abnormalities), including ecchymosis (bruising), oozing or bleeding, and more serious complications, such as hemorrhage and intracranial bleeding. **R:** To detect signs of signs and symptoms of clotting factor deficiencies and

provide baseline data to evaluate effectiveness of transfusion.

8-9. Follow steps 8 and 9 of the General Procedure: Perform physical assessment in regard to symptoms that are similar to a transfusion reaction to obtain a baseline; assess clinical status for susceptibility to fluid volume excess.
10. Assess any existing IV access for patency. Plasma may be transfused through any size catheter. **R:** To ensure that proper venous access is available before you request the unit of plasma from the transfusion service.

ANALYSIS

11-12. Follow steps 11 and 12 of the General Procedure: Think through your data, and identify specific problems and modifications.

PLANNING

13. Determine individualized patient outcomes in relation to this plasma transfusion, considering the following. **R:** Identification of outcomes guides planning and evaluation.
    a. The right *patient* received the right *FFP or TP*, in the right *amount*, by the right *route*, at the right *time*.
    b. The FFP or TP is administered over the correct length of time.
    c. Absence of the signs and symptoms of coagulopathy
    d. Correction of abnormal PT, INR, aPTT, if ordered
    e. Absence of adverse effects related to the transfusion
14. Follow step 14 of the General Procedure: Plan for the approximate start and end time of the plasma transfusion and for the insertion of an IV access if necessary.
15. Follow step 15 of the General Procedure: Gather the necessary equipment. Include basic equipment for starting an IV infusion if needed: appropriate Y type or straight blood administration set; a 100-mL or larger bag of normal saline solution for use with a Y blood administration set if indicated; an infusion pump to precisely control the rate of the transfusion; blood warmer, if rapid, large-volume transfusion is required; and clean gloves to prevent potential contact with blood components.
16. Obtain plasma from the transfusion service just before beginning the transfusion. **R:** Plasma must be stored only in blood refrigerators that are designated for blood storage and monitored to maintain the correct temperature (see Box 52-1).

IMPLEMENTATION

Action	Rationale
17-20. Follow steps 17 to 20 of the General Procedure (omit step 20d): Wash or disinfect your hands, compare the blood component to the prescriber's order, inspect blood component bag for leaks or abnormal appearance, verify the patient's identification and blood component unit identification, verify ABO/Rh of the plasma unit is compatible with patient's ABO/Rh. *Note:* Compatibility testing (crossmatching) is not required for plasma components.	
21-27. Follow steps 21 to 27 of the General Procedure: Explain the procedure to the patient and family; measure and record baseline vital signs; prepare the equipment; connect the blood administration tubing to the hub of the IV access; begin the transfusion slowly; observe the patient during the first 15 minutes; measure vital signs 15 minutes after the start of the transfusion, or sooner if indicated.	
28. If the patient is tolerating the transfusion, the infusion rate may be increased to the rate indicated by the medical order, patient's condition, or facility policy. Most plasma transfusions are completed within 45 to 90 minutes. However, a slower rate of transfusion may be required if the patient is susceptible to fluid volume excess, or a faster rate may be required during emergent transfusion. The transfusion must be completed prior to the expiration date and time.	The rate should be individualized for each patient.
29-34. Follow steps 29 to 34 of the General Procedure: Assess for symptoms of transfusion reaction; provide patient care if a transfusion reaction occurs and perform transfusion reaction workup; discontinue infusion on completion of transfusion; measure post-transfusion vital signs; discard blood component bag and administration set in biohazard container, or return to transfusion service in biohazard bag; remove gloves, and wash or disinfect your hands.	

EVALUATION

35. Follow step 35 of the General Procedure: Evaluate using the individualized patient outcomes in relation to this transfusion as previously identified:
    a. The right *patient* received the right *FFP or TP*, in the right *amount*, by the right *route*, at the right *time*.
    b. The FFP or TP is administered over the correct length of time.
    c. Absence of the signs and symptoms of coagulopathy
    d. Correction of abnormal PT, INR, or aPTT, if ordered
    e. Absence of adverse effects related to the transfusion

DOCUMENTATION

36. Follow step 36 of the General Procedure: Complete right *documentation*. Document vital signs, name of the component, unit number, transfusion start and end date/time, volume transfused, identification of the transfusionist, and any evidence of possible transfusion reaction.

Specific Procedure for Administering Cryoprecipitate

ASSESSMENT

1-2. Follow steps 1 and 2 of the General Procedure: Review the transfusion order; check for valid informed consent.
3. Review the patient's fibrinogen level and treatment plan that triggered the cryoprecipitate transfusion order. **R:** To determine the reason for the cryoprecipitate transfusion, such as hypofibrinogenemia (fibrinogen <80 to 100 mg/dL) and bleeding or hypofibrinogenemia and a planned surgical procedure, and to verify that the transfusion is indicated.
4-6. Follow steps 4 to 6 of the General Procedure: Assess the patient's and family's cultural and religious beliefs and need for education; assess for history of transfusion reaction.
7. Obtain patient's history and physically assess the patient for signs and symptoms of hypofibrinogenemia, including oozing or bleeding and more serious complications, such as hemorrhage and intracranial bleeding. **R:** To help detect signs and symptoms of hypofibrinogenemia and provide baseline data to evaluate effectiveness of transfusion.
8-9. Follow steps 8 and 9 of the General Procedure: Perform physical assessment in regard to symptoms that are similar to a transfusion reaction to obtain a baseline; assess clinical status for susceptibility to fluid volume excess.
10. Assess existing IV access for patency. Cryoprecipitate may be transfused through any size catheter. **R:** To ensure that proper venous access is available before the cryoprecipitate is requested from the transfusion service.

ANALYSIS

11-12. Follow steps 11 and 12 of the General Procedure: Think through your data, and identify specific problems and modifications.

PLANNING

13. Determine individualized patient outcomes in relation to this cryoprecipitate transfusion, considering the following. **R:** Identification of outcomes guides planning and evaluation.
    a. The right *patient* received the right *cryoprecipitate*, in the right *amount*, by the right *route*, at the right *time*.
    b. The cryoprecipitate is administered over the correct length of time.
    c. Appropriate increase in the post-transfusion fibrinogen level, if ordered
    d. No evidence of new bleeding
    e. Evidence that pre-transfusion bleeding has ceased or is reduced
    f. Absence of adverse effects related to the transfusion
14. Plan the approximate start and end time of the cryoprecipitate transfusion and for the insertion of an IV access if necessary. **R:** To maximize efficiency and to ensure that the cryoprecipitate will be administered prior to the expiration date and time and within 4 hours of spiking the unit.
    a. Determine the expiration date and time of the cryoprecipitate. The expiration date and time varies depending on the processing required to prepare the component but is usually within 3 to 6 hours from the time of issue.
    b. Determine the approximate start time of the transfusion to allow for the completion of the transfusion prior to the expiration date and time or within 4 hours of spiking the unit, whichever comes first.
15. Follow step 15 of the General Procedure (omit step d): Gather the necessary equipment. Include basic equipment for starting an IV infusion, if needed: appropriate Y type or straight blood administration set, a 100-mL or larger bag of normal saline solution for use with a Y blood admin-

istration set if indicated, an infusion pump to precisely control the rate of the transfusion, and clean gloves to prevent potential contact with blood components.

Note: Use of a blood warmer to infuse cryoprecipitate is not indicated.

16. Obtain the cryoprecipitate from the transfusion service just prior to beginning the transfusion. Cryoprecipitate is stored at room temperature and must not be refrigerated. **R:** To prevent incorrect storage of cryoprecipitate in the patient care area.

IMPLEMENTATION

Action	Rationale
17-20. Follow steps 17 to 20 of the General Procedure (omit 20d and 20e): Wash or disinfect your hands; compare the blood component to the prescriber's order; inspect blood component bag for leaks or abnormal appearance; verify the patient's identification and blood component unit identification. *Note:* Compatibility testing (crossmatching) is not required for cryoprecipitate. Criteria for ABO compatibility of cryoprecipitate varies among facilities. Verify that the ABO/Rh of the cryoprecipitate is compatible with the patient's ABO/Rh according to facility policy.	
21-27. Follow steps 21 to 27 of the General Procedure: Explain the procedure to the patient and family; measure and document baseline vital signs; prepare the equipment; connect the blood administration tubing to the hub of the IV access; begin the transfusion slowly; observe the patient during the first 15 minutes; measure vital signs 15 minutes after the start of the transfusion, or sooner if indicated.	
28. If the patient is tolerating the transfusion, the rate may be increased to the rate indicated by the medical order, patient's condition, or facility policy. Most cryoprecipitate transfusions are completed within 25 to 35 minutes. However, a slower rate of transfusion may be required if the patient is susceptible to fluid volume excess or a faster rate may be required during emergent transfusion. The transfusion must be completed prior to the expiration date and time or within 4 hours of spiking the cryoprecipitate, whichever comes first.	The rate should be individualized for each patient.

(continued)

Action	Rationale
29-34. Follow steps 29 to 34 of the General Procedure: Assess for symptoms of transfusion reaction; provide patient care if a transfusion reaction occurs and perform transfusion reaction workup; discontinue infusion on completion of transfusion; measure post-transfusion vital signs; discard blood component bag and administration set in biohazard container, or return to transfusion service in biohazard bag per policy; remove gloves, and wash or disinfect your hands.	

EVALUATION

35. Follow step 35 of the General Procedure: Evaluate using the individualized patient outcomes in relation to this transfusion as previously identified:

a. The right *patient* received the right *cryoprecipitate*, in the right *amount*, by the right *route*, at the right *time*.

b. The cryoprecipitate is administered over the correct length of time.

c. Appropriate increase in the post-transfusion fibrinogen level, if ordered

d. No evidence of new bleeding

e. Evidence that pre-transfusion bleeding has ceased or is reduced

f. Absence of adverse effects related to the transfusion

DOCUMENTATION

36. Follow step 36 of the General Procedure: Complete right *documentation:* Document vital signs, name of the component, unit number, transfusion start and end date/time, identification of the transfusionist, volume transfused, and any evidence of possible transfusion reaction.

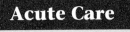

Acute Care

Transfusions in the acute care setting may be given emergently or as a routine treatment. Transfusing a blood component during an emergency does not diminish the need to carefully complete the pre-administration check to verify that the correct blood component is being transfused to the correct patient. Clerical errors are the most common cause of fatal hemolytic transfusion reactions. Drawing a type and crossmatch blood specimen from one patient and labeling it with another patient's unique identifiers

(e.g., drawing blood from Joseph Smith and labeling it with John Smith's name and patient record number) and failing to properly verify patient identity immediately prior to transfusion (e.g., giving John Smith's blood to Joseph Smith) are two of the most frequent types of clerical errors leading to transfusion-related deaths.

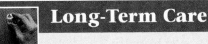

Long-Term Care

Residents in long-term care facilities occasionally receive blood components. The care facility must have a written policy and procedure for transfusion. An employee of the facility is often required to pick up the blood component from the blood center, verifying that the resident's name and identification attached to the unit matches the intended recipient. The nurse administering the blood component must be competent with regard to the transfusion policies and procedures to ensure safe administration.

Elderly residents, especially those with diminished cardiac reserve or chronic anemia, are susceptible to fluid volume excess or congestive heart failure, which may be exacerbated if the blood component is infused too rapidly. Misinformation regarding transfusion may produce a heightened sense of anxiety about the procedure. Actively listen and give clear, calm, supportive explanations to allay any fear that may be expressed.

Home Care

The administration of blood in the home can have serious consequences because the availability of medical intervention, equipment, and medications to treat serious transfusion reactions may be limited. In addition, reimbursement for home transfusions is not always available. Informed consent for transfusion should be obtained from individuals receiving blood components in the home. The benefits and additional risks of home transfusion as well as the alternative of in-hospital or outpatient transfusion should be included in the discussion. Home care administration of blood components has merits in that it avoids having very ill and weak individuals who are receiving care in the home transported to and from an acute care setting for this procedure. Only specially trained and competent licensed professionals can administer blood components. Some blood centers will not release blood components to an agency unless they are reassured that the agency administering the component has adequate procedures and trained transfusionists.

Ambulatory Care

Not all individuals requiring transfusion are hospitalized; many receive transfusion in an ambulatory care setting. For example, individuals with cancer needing transfusion following chemotherapy or individuals with chronic anemia may require transfusion that may be performed on an outpatient basis. Billing practices of the facility and the availability of reimbursement should be evaluated prior to scheduling a transfusion. Individuals receiving transfusion in the ambulatory care setting should be monitored following the transfusion and prior to leaving the facility. They should be provided written instructions of the signs and symptoms that require follow-up with a healthcare provider.

LEARNING TOOLS

DEVELOP YOUR BACKGROUND KNOWLEDGE

1. Review the Learning Outcomes.

2. Review the section on blood transfusion in this module and in your assigned text.

3. Look up the Key Terms in the glossary.

4. Mentally practice the techniques described in this module. Study so that you would be able to teach these skills to another person.

5. Read the clinical policy and procedure for transfusions at your facility.

6. Read the clinical policy and procedure for obtaining informed consent for transfusion at your facility, if available.

DEVELOP YOUR SKILLS

In the practice setting, practice the following skills. You may partner with another student or your instructor.

1. Examine the blood administration equipment. Identify each of the following:
   a. Y-type blood administration set
   b. straight blood administration set
   c. blood administration set for use with infusion pump
   d. infusion pump
   e. forms for recording blood administration

2. Read the directions on the package regarding how to set up the blood administration set you will be using.

3. Set up a blood administration set as though you were going to administer a blood component. Use normal saline in place of a blood component. Use a Y set with an additional bag of normal saline or a straight set per policy at your facility.

4. Regulate the drip rate for an adult transfusion so that 30 mL of the blood component are delivered for the first 15 minutes of the transfusion.

5. If infusing by gravity, refer to the package of the blood administration set to determine the drops per milliliter delivered by the drip chamber.

6. If using an infusion pump, set the appropriate rate on the pump.

7. Assume that the first 15 minutes of the transfusion were well tolerated. Regulate the drip rate so that 320 mL of the blood component will be delivered over 2 hours.

8. Demonstrate what you would do if it were necessary to stop the transfusion because of a suspected transfusion reaction.

9. Practice documenting the following.
   a. The administration of 1 unit of RBCs with a volume of 350 mL: the transfusion was started at 13:00 (1:00 p.m.) and completed at 15:00 (3:00 p.m.); document as appropriate to your facility.
   b. The recipient of the blood experiences a mild allergic transfusion reaction (hives and itching localized to the upper chest and face). Simulate appropriate nursing history and physical assessment; indicate required nursing interventions; document as appropriate to your facility.

DEMONSTRATE YOUR SKILLS

In the clinical setting

1. Identify the rationale for the administration of a blood component to a specific patient.

2. Read the transfusion tag attached to a blood component and determine
   a. ABO group and Rh type of the patient.
   b. ABO group and Rh type of the blood component.
   c. unit number.
   d. expiration date and time of the unit and, for RBC–containing units (i.e., whole blood, RBCs, and granulocytes), the expiration date and time of the compatibility testing (type and crossmatch).

3. Read the label on the blood component and determine
   a. ABO group and Rh type of the blood component.
   b. unit number of the blood component.
   c. expiration date and time of the blood component.

4. Consult with your instructor regarding the opportunity to set up and administer a blood component to an adult or pediatric patient or to observe a transfusion. Evaluate your performance with the instructor.

CRITICAL THINKING EXERCISES

1. You started a transfusion of RBCs 10 minutes ago. The patient reports feeling anxious and is experiencing nausea and chills. Plan your immediate nursing actions and assessments, giving the rationale for each. Also describe your interaction with the patient.

2. You are caring for an adolescent patient with leukemia for whom 2 units of pooled platelet concentrates have been ordered prior to surgery. Her platelet count is 15,000/microliter, and she weighs 60 kg. Where would you find the information to determine whether this would be an appropriate dose? If the source indicates this is not an appropriate dose, what would be your next action? Describe how you would proceed with the platelet transfusion, beginning with obtaining the platelets from the facility's transfusion service. Compare the steps in administering platelets with those for transfusing RBCs. Explain why certain steps are different.

SELF-QUIZ

SHORT-ANSWER QUESTIONS

1. Name the four blood groups in the ABO system.
   a. _____
   b. _____
   c. _____
   d. _____

2. List four types of acute transfusion reactions.
   a. _____
   b. _____
   c. _____
   d. _____

3. List four signs and symptoms of an acute hemolytic transfusion reaction.
   a. _____
   b. _____
   c. _____
   d. _____

4. List the primary indications for the transfusion of RBCs
   _____

5. List two indications for the transfusion of platelets.
   a. _____
   b. _____

6. List the primary indication for the transfusion of cryoprecipitate.
   _____

7. List the first action you would take in the event a patient was experiencing a suspected acute hemolytic transfusion reaction.
   _____

MULTIPLE CHOICE

_____ 8. An individual with group O blood naturally produces which antibody or antibodies?
   a. Anti-A but not anti-B
   b. Anti-B but not anti-A
   c. Anti-A and anti-B
   d. No ABO antibodies

_____ 9. An individual with group AB blood has what ABO antibody circulating in the plasma?
   a. Anti-A
   b. Anti-B
   c. Anti-D
   d. No ABO antibody

_____ 10. Which blood components should never be refrigerated?
   a. Platelets only
   b. Platelets, cryoprecipitate, and granulocytes
   c. RBCs and whole blood only
   d. RBCs, whole blood, and FFP that has been thawed

_____ 11. Fresh frozen plasma contains clotting factors. What laboratory tests are used to determine if a patient has low levels of clotting factors?
   a. Hemoglobin
   b. Hematocrit
   c. Platelet count
   d. Prothrombin time (PT), activated partial thromboplastin time (aPTT), and international normal ratio (INR)

_____ 12. RBCs may be indicated for a patient with which of the following?
   a. Platelet dysfunction
   b. Low level of clotting factors
   c. Abnormal PT and aPTT
   d. Symptomatic anemia

_____ 13. When beginning a transfusion, the nurse
   a. transfuses the blood component slowly for the first 15 minutes to test the effect on the patient and observe for signs and symptoms of a potential transfusion reaction.
   b. transfuses the first 100 mL quickly over 1 minute to test the effect on the patient.
   c. transfuses half of the blood component unit as fast as possible to identify any potential adverse transfusion reaction.
   d. transfuses the entire blood component unit as fast as possible to prevent an adverse transfusion reaction.

_____ 14. If the patient identification information on the transfusion tag attached to the blood component does not match the corresponding information on the patient's identification band,
   a. do not transfuse; contact the transfusion service.
   b. begin the transfusion and then notify the transfusion service of the discrepancy.
   c. discard the unit.
   d. ask the patient to accept the transfusion with a discrepancy in patient identification information.

_____ 15. A routine transfusion of 1 RBC unit for an adult is usually completed within
   a. 6 hours.
   b. 4 to 6 hours.
   c. 1½ to 2 hours (up to 4 hours).
   d. 30 minutes.

Answers to the Self-Quiz questions appear in the back of the book.

MODULE 53

Administering Epidural Medications

KEY TERMS

analgesic	neurotoxic
anesthetic	opioid
dura	paraparesis
epidural	particulate
narcotic	pruritus

OVERALL OBJECTIVE

▸ To prepare and administer medications safely, using the epidural route.

LEARNING OUTCOMES

The student will be able to

1. Assess the patient effectively with regard to the medication ordered and the use of the epidural route of administration.
2. Analyze assessment data to determine special problems or concerns that must be addressed to successfully administer the medication ordered by the epidural route.
3. Determine appropriate patient outcomes for the medication(s) administered and recognize the potential for adverse outcomes.
4. Plan appropriate strategies to ensure that the patient receives the medication ordered by the epidural route.
5. Administer medications safely and accurately, using the epidural route.
6. Evaluate the patient's response to the medication(s) administered.
7. Document the medication administered, including the epidural site and the patient's response according to facility policies.

The technology associated with providing pain relief is constantly expanding. One aspect of this technology is the administration of opioids and **anesthetic** agents through an **epidural** catheter. To provide effective care and optimum pain relief, nurses caring for patients with epidural catheters must understand the location of the catheter, how the system works, and the specific actions of the medications instilled.

NURSING DIAGNOSES

■ Acute Pain is the nursing diagnosis most often associated with patients receiving an epidural analgesic; for example, patients who have had surgery. The nursing diagnosis of acute pain specifies pain of 6 months duration or less; some individuals have what might be termed "long-term acute pain." This is the patient who has had intractable or severe long-term pain associated with cancer or other life-threatening conditions.

DELEGATION

Administration of epidural medications is not delegated to assistive personnel. They may be asked to observe for and report specific effects (both desired and adverse) of medications the nurse has administered. However, the nurse is always responsible for evaluating the effect(s) of all medications administered.

WHAT IS AN EPIDURAL CATHETER?

Epidural catheters are silicone catheters that are used to administer a medication into the epidural or subarachnoid space. The catheter usually is placed in surgery by a physician (most commonly an anesthesiologist). The internal end of the catheter may be in the epidural space in the lumbar region or in the thoracic region based on the anatomic location of the pain. The higher on the spine that the catheter is placed, the more vigilant the nurse must be in regard to respiratory effects.

When the epidural catheter is used to deliver medications for long-term control of chronic pain such as cancer pain, it may be sutured in place and tunneled through the subcutaneous tissue to an exit site on the abdomen (Fig. 53-1).

When the catheter is intended for short-term use (such as postoperatively), it may not be sutured in place. The temporary catheter exits on the back, under the insertion site dressing. To protect the catheter, an extension tubing is commonly attached and secured with wide adhesive tape along the spine to the shoulder where the port at the end of the catheter is accessible.

The catheter is the same type used to administer regional anesthetic for childbirth and some types of surgery. In some instances, a low-dose anesthetic agent, such as bupivacaine (Marcaine) is infused continuously into an epidural catheter to provide pain relief. When regional anesthetic agents are used in an epidural catheter, many states require that they be administered by an anesthesiologist or nurse anesthetist because of the risk of serious complications. The nurse who does administer low-dose anesthetic agents must have special education

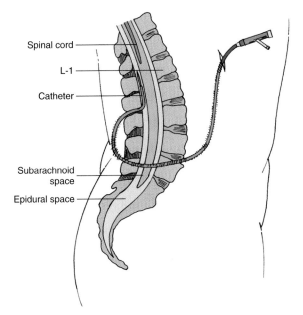

Spinal cord

L-1

Catheter

Subarachnoid
space

Epidural space

FIGURE 53-1 Tunneled epidural catheter for long-term use.

to be able to respond immediately to the complications that may occur.

This module discusses the administration of **opioid (narcotic) analgesics** by direct injection or infusion into an epidural catheter. Although potential problems are associated with the use of opioids in this manner, they are not as serious as those from the use of anesthetic agents. Therefore, opioids such as morphine, hydromorphone, and fentanyl are commonly administered by registered nurses using the epidural route. Some facilities require that nurses attend special in-service education classes and be certified in the use of epidural catheters before assuming this responsibility.

Many facilities have a special form on which the physician's orders for epidural medications and care are written. Use of these forms ensures that complete orders are written clearly. Computerized order entry systems also provide templates to facilitate complete orders. Such forms usually include medication, dose, and method of administration. Scheduled assessment may be included in the orders. Additionally, the form includes specific orders for treating the various complications outlined later in this module. In other facilities, the orders are less detailed and there are standardized protocols in place for assessment and management of epidural catheters.

ADVANTAGES OF EPIDURAL NARCOTIC ADMINISTRATION

The major advantage of epidural administration of opioids is that a lower total daily dose is needed to maintain adequate pain relief. Additionally, much of the drug

dose attaches to receptors in the spinal cord before reaching the central nervous system. This action allows the person to be more alert, more mobile, and have fewer central nervous system effects while remaining pain-free. Opioids given epidurally also have a more prolonged effect than those administered through other routes, such as the oral route. Administered orally, medications must first be absorbed in the gastrointestinal tract and then transported through the liver. In the liver, some breakdown occurs before the drug gets to the central nervous system (the "first pass" effect). Administered epidurally, medications bypass the GI tract. Respiratory depression is less common with epidural administration than with intravenous (IV) administration, as are other side effects of opioids, such as nausea, constipation, and dizziness. Epidural medications can be given by intermittent or continuous infusion.

CARE OF THE EPIDURAL CATHETER EXIT SITE

The temporary epidural catheter is covered with a surgical dressing after insertion, and this dressing is not usually changed. If a dressing change is necessary, follow the directions for sterile dressing change. The care of the exit site for the permanent epidural catheter is usually identical to the care of the exit site of a surgically implanted central venous catheter. The catheter has been tunneled under the skin to provide a barrier to infection ascending along the exterior of the catheter. Be sure to follow the procedure outlined for your facility, or follow the general procedure for central venous catheter (CVC) site care outlined in Module 49, Caring for Central Venous Catheters.

ADMINISTERING A MEDICATION THROUGH AN EPIDURAL CATHETER

Epidural narcotics can be injected intermittently into the epidural catheter. The medication gradually diffuses across the **dura** to contact opiate receptors in the spinal cord. Because of this gradual diffusion, the injections are only needed every 8 to 12 hours. The amount used is often small, but because it is concentrated where the receptors are located, pain relief is maintained.

Any medication or solution administered epidurally must be free of preservatives because the preservatives used to prevent bacterial growth in common injectable medications are toxic to the nervous system (**neurotoxic).** Dilute solutions of the active medication are used to facilitate the gradual absorption of the drug.

PROCEDURE FOR ADMINISTERING EPIDURAL MEDICATIONS BY INTERMITTENT INJECTION

To carry out this procedure, follow the steps of the General Procedure for Administering Oral Medications (Module 44) as modified below. The modified steps are included completely and references are made to the steps of the General Procedure that remain the same.

ASSESSMENT

1. Follow step 1 of the General Procedure: Review the medication record.
2. Examine the medication administration record (MAR) for accuracy and completeness as prescribed by your facility. When checking the medication order, verify that the epidural route is to be used, and determine the location of the epidural catheter and whether it is temporary or permanent. **R:** To promote accuracy and completeness of medication administration.

3-4. Follow steps 3 and 4 of the General Procedure: Review medication information with special attention to how the medication acts by the epidural route, and assess the patient's abilities, especially the ability to change position.

5. Assess the patient (see a to e below). **R:** To ensure that adverse effects are identified before additional medication is administered and that additional medication is not given to a patient who is not stable.
   a. Pain level using a standard scale (e.g., 0 to 10, with 0 being no pain and 10 being the greatest pain)
   b. Respiratory rate
   c. Blood pressure and pulse rate
   d. Ability to move lower extremities
   e. Sedation level

ANALYSIS

6-7. Follow steps 6 and 7 of the General Procedure: Critically think through your data, carefully evaluating each aspect and its relation to other data, and identify specific problems and modifications of the procedure needed for this individual.

PLANNING

8. Follow step 8 of the General Procedure: Determine individualized patient outcomes in relation to the particular epidural medication(s) prescribed for the patient, including the following.
   a. The right *patient* receives the right *medication* in the right *dose* by the *epidural route* at the right *time*, and at the right *rate*.
   b. The patient experiences desired level of pain relief.
   c. The patient experiences no adverse effects from the medication (Table 53-1).
9. Obtain the supplies needed.
   a. A 10- or 12-mL syringe with a 20-G needle or needleless safety connector to administer the diluted preservative-free narcotic. In addition, you will need a small syringe if the narcotic comes in an undiluted form and must be drawn and measured before dilution. **R:** The syringe must be the correct size to measure the pain medication accurately and a second larger syringe is needed for diluting the medication.
   b. A filter needle. **R:** This may be used to draw the medication to make sure that no **particulate** matter is in the drug solution.
   c. A needleless connector for administering the medication. **R:** Needleless devices prevent needle-stick injuries.

   d. Povidone-iodine wipes to use in preparing the medication and in giving the injection. **R:** As an antiseptic solution, povidone-iodine is more acceptable than alcohol, which is neurotoxic and causes pain. Therefore, it is not used when preparing medications for epidural administration or on the injection port of an epidural catheter.
   e. Sterile 2- × 2-inch gauze squares. **R:** Gauze squares are used to wipe off the povidone-iodine from the cap before administering the medication. Povidone-iodine leaves a sticky residue.
   f. Clean gloves to protect you from contact with body fluids

IMPLEMENTATION

Action	Rationale
10. Wash or disinfect your hands.	To decrease the transfer of microorganisms that could cause infection.
11-14. Follow steps 11 to 14 of the General Procedure: Access the official MAR and	

(continued)

table 53-1. Sample Assessment Protocol: Patients With New Epidural Catheters

Objective Data	Scale and Action	Frequency
Pulse Respiration (R)	Note any drop. R less than 10—Obtain O$_2$ saturation/pulse oximetry. R less than 8—Give naloxone 0.4 mg IV stat; obtain O$_2$ saturation/pulse oximetry; notify physician.	Monitor relevant data Every 30 min × 2 Then every 1 h × 2 Then every 4 h × 24 h Then every 8 h
Blood pressure	Note any drop. Notify physician if systolic pressure falls below 100.	
Sedation	*Scale:* 3 = Awake and responding 2 = Sleeping but responds to normal voice 1 = Sleeping but responds to loud voice/movement 0 = Sedated, does not respond *Action:* Level 1—Obtain O$_2$ saturation/pulse oximetry; call physician. Level 0—Give naloxone 0.4 mg IV stat; obtain O$_2$ saturation/pulse oximetry; call physician stat; obtain arterial blood gas (ABGs) level stat.	
Mental state	Light-headed Confused: Notify physician.	
Pain	0–10, with 0 as no pain and 10 as the highest possible pain.	
Pruritus	Present Absent	
Muscle strength and control	Note extremities checked. Weak versus normal strength	

Skin sensation	*Sensation scale*
	   N = Normal
	   T = Tingling
	   Nb = Numbness
	   A = Absent
	Anatomic location
	S1–S5: Ankle/foot
	L1–L5: Groin/pelvis/thigh
	T1–T12: Umbilicus
	T1–T4: Nipple level
	C1–C5: Hand	

Postural blood pressure	Note excessive postural drop. Patient ambulates with assistance.	Begin this assessment before first ambulation and continue every 8 h until stable.
Urinary output	Compare with intake.	Every 8 h

Action	Rationale
read the name of the medication to be given; access the epidural medication, check the label on the medication and compare the medication label to the MAR before picking it up (first check); and pick up the medication and check the label again (second check).	
15. Prepare the epidural medication.	
a. Verify that the medication available is labeled "preservative free." Use a prediluted preservative-free narcotic solution (such as Duramorph) or a preservative-free narcotic (such as morphine, fentanyl, or hydromorphone	Preservatives used in standard multiple-dose vials may be toxic to nervous tissue. Some facilities do allow narcotics with preservatives to be used in long-term epidural catheters as long as they are diluted with preservative-free saline solution. Be sure you follow the policy in your facility. *(continued)*

Action	Rationale
labeled as preservative-free) and preservative-free 0.9% sodium chloride (normal saline) solution for diluting the narcotic.	
b. Complete all required documentation regarding a controlled substance before proceeding.	Medications given by the epidural route for pain management are controlled substances.
c. Calculate the volume of medication needed.	Most medication orders are written in terms of milligrams of the drug. You will need to read the label to determine how many milligrams are found in each milliliter to calculate how many milliliters you are to give.
d. Draw the medication in one of the following ways.	
(1) *For a prediluted narcotic:*	
(a) Draw the dilute medication into the large syringe using a standard needle or filter needle.	
(b) Change to a needleless connector or safety needle for administration.	
(2) *For an undiluted narcotic:*	
(a) Draw the medication into the small syringe using a standard needle or a filter needle and recap the needle. If a filter needle was used at this time, change to a standard needle.	The medication can be accurately measured in the small syringe. The standard needle can be capped because it is still sterile and not a hazard to staff.
(b) Draw 10 mL of preservative-free saline solution into the large syringe and then pull back to allow enough space for the narcotic.	A large volume of fluid permits the narcotic to contact the optimum number of receptors. The large syringe can measure the large amount of saline solution accurately, and the space in the syringe will allow you to mix the medication with the solution.
(c) Cap the needle, remove the needle from the large syringe, and discard it in the sharps container.	The needle can be capped because it is still sterile and not a hazard to staff. Removing the needle should only be done with the needle covered to prevent accidental needle stick. You will be replacing the needle, so you do not need to keep it.
(d) Hold the needle carefully while you insert the needle from the small syringe into the tip of the large syringe. Inject	This mixes the medications in the same syringe and results in a dilute solution.

(continued)

Action	Rationale
the narcotic into the saline in the large syringe.	
(e) Replace the needle on the large syringe with a safety needle, or attach a needleless connector if a needleless system is in use at your facility.	To prevent needle-stick injury.
(f) Gently rotate the syringe.	To mix the narcotic and saline solution.
e. Recheck the medication record, the label on the medication container, and your syringe.	For the third check.
16-20. Follow steps 16 to 20 of the General Procedure: Prepare any additional medications to be given at this time, check each medication label against the MAR once again, obtain the patient identification to be taken to the patient's bedside. Identify the patient (two identifiers) and explain how the medication will be administered.	
21. Administer the medication into the epidural port as follows.	
a. Make sure there is adequate lighting, and position the patient for access to the injection port, raising the bed if needed.	To enable you to see the injection port and work without back strain.
b. Put on clean gloves.	To protect yourself from contact with body fluid.
c. Identify the epidural catheter injection port. (Two nurses may need to do this. Follow the procedure in your facility.)	To be sure that the correct port is being used. Many facilities require that this be double-checked because of the serious consequences of erroneously using an IV line of some kind.
d. Clean the injection cap on the epidural catheter with a povidone-iodine wipe.	To remove microorganisms and decrease the potential for infection.
e. Dry the injection cap with the sterile 2- × 2-inch gauze square.	Povidone-iodine may form a sticky residue if left on the cap.
f. Insert the needle or needleless connector into the cap.	To access the epidural catheter.
g. Aspirate. If blood returns, or if more than 1 mL of clear fluid is aspirated, do not give the medication; remove the syringe and report to the physician.	If blood returns, the catheter may have eroded into a blood vessel. Clear fluid may indicate that the catheter has eroded into the subarachnoid space.

(continued)

Action	Rationale
h. Inject the medication steadily. If you cannot inject the medication, check the tubing for kinks. If you still cannot inject, withdraw the syringe and report it to the physician.	You are injecting the medication into the epidural space, where it will be used gradually. It is not like an IV medication, which goes immediately into the circulation. If the patient indicates discomfort, slow the injection. It may be difficult to instill medication because the catheter is small and long. The catheter may become occluded and need to be replaced.
i. Remove the needle and syringe from the catheter. Confirm that the cap of the catheter is secured in place. It should connect with a twist lock connector. In some facilities, the cap is taped in place for extra security.	The catheter must remain sealed by the cap. Securing the cap prevents it from falling off.
22. Follow step 22 of the General Procedure: Leave the patient in a comfortable position and lower the bed if it was raised.	
23. Follow step 23 of the General Procedure: Discard the syringe and needle in the closest sharps container without replacing the needle guard.	
24. Follow step 24 of the General Procedure: Remove gloves, and wash or disinfect your hands.	

EVALUATION

25. Evaluate using the individualized patient outcomes previously identified:
   a. The right *patient* received the right *medication* in the right *dose* by the *epidural route,* at the right *time,* and at the right *rate.*
   b. The patient experienced desired level of pain relief (use same pain scale as before medication administration).
   c. The patient experienced no adverse effects from the medication (see Table 53-1). **R:** Evaluation in relation to desired outcomes is essential for planning future care.

DOCUMENTATION

26-27. Follow steps 26 and 27 of the General Procedure. Complete right *documentation.* Document the name of the medication, the dose, time, route, and your signature on the correct patient's record. Also record assessment data, such as the pain level assessed on a consistent scale; respiratory rate, pulse rate, and blood pressure; and observations for potential adverse responses, such as **pruritus** and hypotension. These assessments are completed at regularly scheduled intervals, such as every hour initially then gradually moving to every 2 hours and every 4 hours as pain relief and patient's response are stabilized. A special flow sheet may be used for documenting pain management and any identified adverse effects (Fig. 53-2).

POTENTIAL ADVERSE OUTCOMES AND RELATED INTERVENTIONS

1. Urinary Retention: related to disturbed innervation of the bladder caused by the narcotic's effect on spinal receptors.
Intervention: Measure urinary intake and output and palpate the bladder for distention. The nurse may need to consult with the physician regarding catheterization.

2. Risk for Injury: related to administering IV medications or solutions into an epidural catheter.
Intervention: Because the epidural catheter looks like an IV catheter, a special safety concern is clearly identifying these two lines and not confusing them. Medications

ANALGESIA MONITORING RECORD

Date	5-22-06											
Time		1000	1200	14	16	18	20					
Resp. Rate		24	22	20	22	18	20					
Pain Scale • Appropriate box												
5-Excruciating												
4-Horrible												
3-Distressing		*	*									
2-Discomforting				*	*							
1-Mild						*	*					
0-None												
Sedation Scale												
SL-Sleeping/Not assessed 1-Alert 3-Rousable, drowsy frequently 2-Drowsy, occas. somnulent, hard to arouse		1	1	1	1	1	1					
Side Effects/Other Monitoring												
List if present: N-Nausea R-Respiratory Depression P-Pruris O-Other (write in) U-Urinary retention		∅	∅	∅	∅	∅	∅					
Numbness Level (local anesthetic/See reverse)		N/A										
Motor Function (only for local anesthetics) Y-Able to move knees U-Unable		N/A										
Analgesics and/or Local Anesthetics												
Type	morphine sulfate											
Rate	1 ml/hour											
1–Cont. infusion		✓	✓	✓	✓	✓	✓					
☐IV ☒ Epi ☐ SQ												
New syringe/Bag hung (✓)												
Volume hung (cc)		50										
2-PCA Dose volume (ml)												
☐IV ☐ Epi Lockout time (min)												
4 hr. limit												
3–New syringe hung (✓)												
4–Other Medications given (✓) (see M.A.R. for details)												
5–Total Narcotics infused per 8 hrs				4 mg								

Init	Signature	Init	Signature
WW	W.Wentzel RN		

Roberts, Jeffrey M. Age 67
000-00-0000
Dr. McCarty

ADDRESSOGRAPH

FIGURE 53-2 Flow sheet for monitoring pain managed by drugs supplied by epidural catheter.

intended for IV use may be neurotoxic, and the dosage of narcotic given epidurally may be life-threatening when given by direct IV push. In some facilities, a brightly colored label specifying "epidural catheter" is placed on the epidural line next to the injection port. In other facilities, the policy is that two nurses verify the epidural line immediately before giving any medication. Both of these safeguards may be used. As a safety measure, a large, very legible label may be placed on the line next to any port (if there are several ports on the line, use a label for each port). Some facilities specify that an administration tubing without ports must be used for epidural lines. This helps to prevent administration into the wrong port. Also, as a student, you should always have a registered nurse identify the line with you. In all cases, follow the hospital policy. In many facilities, students do not administer medications by the epidural route, although they may assist the registered nurse in this task.

3. Acute head pain: related to leakage of cerebrospinal fluid from the site around the catheter.
Intervention: Notify the physician when new head pain occurs. A variety of medical interventions may be used to treat this complication.

4. Risk for infection if cerebrospinal fluid leaks around the catheter. This creates a pathway for micro-

organisms to travel into the wound and cause an infection.
Intervention: Monitor temperature and inspect the catheter site. Change the cap on the tubing at regular intervals, depending on the frequency of use, to prevent leakage from repeated puncture. Check your facility's policy for the frequency of changing the cap on the tubing. Report any indication of infection to the physician immediately.

5. Impaired skin integrity: related to a skin rash. Pruritus that is sometimes accompanied by a rash is a fairly common adverse response to epidural narcotics.
Intervention: For some individuals, it is only mildly annoying and may be alleviated by lotion on the skin. For others, it is extremely uncomfortable, necessitating administration of a narcotic antagonist. As the narcotic antagonist relieves the pruritus, it also diminishes the pain relief. Therefore, the narcotic antagonist may be given in small increments to attempt relief of the pruritus without loss of pain control. If that is unsuccessful, another drug or method of pain management is necessary.

6. Ineffective breathing pattern progressing to respiratory depression with respiratory rate below 8 per

minute. Although one of the advantages of epidural narcotic administration is less-frequent respiratory depression than with other methods of narcotic drug administration, breathing problems related to respiratory depression still can occur. It is more likely to occur if the patient is lying flat while an infusion is given because the medication ascends along the dura. Breathing problems also may occur if there is a large absorption into the vascular system from the epidural site.

Intervention: When the first dose of medication is given, pay particular attention to respiratory assessment and prepare for immediate intervention. An emergency cart with a self-inflating rebreathing (Ambu) bag should be available for emergency treatment. The physician may order a narcotic antagonist such as naloxone if the patient's respiratory rate drops to less than 8 breaths per minute.

7. Reversible **paraparesis** (weakness of the lower extremities) may occur because of the effect of the medication on the motor nerves from the lower extremities. This may occur if a medication with a preservative or one not intended for epidural use is injected into the catheter, causing an adverse response of nervous system tissue.

Intervention: Discontinue the medication and notify the physician. Fortunately, this complication is usually reversible if the medication causing the problem is discontinued and the tissue is given an opportunity to recover.

8. Hypotension may occur because of the narcotic's action on receptor sites that control vascular responses.

Intervention: Special attention to safety is necessary because hypotension may cause dizziness. Have the patient call for assistance before getting out of bed. Help the patient to exercise the legs before getting up and then to move slowly. A narcotic antagonist is ordered only if the blood pressure drop is precipitous because it would also reverse the pain relief.

9. Neural irritation, characterized by abnormal sensations in the lower extremities that may include tingling and numbness, may be related to particulate matter in the medication solution.

Intervention: Place a 0.22-micron filter on the epidural catheter to make sure that no particulate matter, which might cause local irritation, is injected into the catheter.

PROCEDURE FOR ADMINISTERING EPIDURAL MEDICATIONS BY CONTINUOUS INFUSION

For patients with long-term pain, such as those with major trauma, a complicated recovery, or cancer, continuous infusion of an epidural narcotic may be used for pain management. The continuous infusion is set up using an IV pump that is volume controlled to provide the precise control of the dosage that is needed. Review Module 48 for information on setting up IV pumps. Follow the Procedure for Administering Epidural Medications (above) with the modifications described below.

ASSESSMENT

1. Follow step 1 of the General Procedure: Review the medication record medications to be given.
2. Examine the medication administration record (MAR) for accuracy and completeness as prescribed by your facility. When checking the medication order, verify that the epidural route is to be used, the location of the epidural catheter, and whether it is temporary or permanent. **R:** The epidural route requires special safeguards and must be carefully differentiated from the more common IV route. Teaching will differ based on whether the catheter is temporary or permanent.

3-5. Follow steps 3 to 5 of the General Procedure: Review medication information with special attention to how the medication acts by the epidural route; assess for pain level, blood pressure and pulse rate, ability to move extremities, and sedation level.

ANALYSIS

6-7. Follow steps 6 and 7 of the General Procedure: Critically think through your data, carefully evaluating each aspect and its relation to other data, and identify specific problems and modifications of the procedure needed for this individual.

PLANNING

8. Follow step 8 of the General Procedure: Determine individualized patient outcomes in relation to the particular epidural medication(s) prescribed:
   a. The right *patient* receives the right *medication* in the right *dose* by the *epidural route* at the right *time,* and at the right *rate.*
   b. The patient experiences the desired level of pain relief.
   c. The patient experiences no adverse effects from the medication (see Table 53-1).
9. Obtain the supplies needed, which may include the following. **R:** Planning ahead allows you to proceed more safely and effectively and to give the injection accurately.

 a. Volume-controlled IV pump: After obtaining the pump, determine how you will set the pump to deliver the correct rate of infusion. **R:** Setting the pump accurately is essential for safety. You will usually need to calculate a flow rate (in milliliters of solution per hour) to deliver the ordered milligrams of drug hourly.

Some pharmacies print this information on the label, but others do not because it is confusing if the dose changes while the same IV bag is in use. In some facilities, policy requires that two nurses verify the dose calculation for an epidural medication. As a student, you should always have your instructor or another registered nurse double-check your calculation for safety.

Note: A patient-controlled analgesia pump that has a mechanism for administering a basal rate as well as intermittent patient-actuated doses also may be used for continuous infusion of epidural narcotics. **R:** These pumps have many safeguards in their operation that provide additional protection to the patient.

b. Special pump tubing. **R:** Accuracy depends on specialized tubing.

c. Appropriate in-line filter if one is not already on the epidural catheter. **R:** The filter ensures particulate-free medication.

d. Safety needle or needleless connector. **R:** Safety devices prevent needle-stick injuries.

e. Povidone-iodine swabs for cleaning the epidural catheter port. **R:** As an antiseptic, povidone-iodine is preferred over alcohol, which is neurotoxic and causes pain; therefore, alcohol is not used when preparing medications for epidural administration nor is it used on the injection port of an epidural catheter.

f. Sterile 2- × 2-inch gauze squares. **R:** Gauze wipes are used to remove the povidone-iodine from the cap before administering the medication. The povidone-iodine leaves a sticky residue.

g. Tape and labels indicating "epidural line" for safety

IMPLEMENTATION

Action	Rationale
10-14. Follow steps 10 to 14 of the General Procedure: Wash your hands; access the official MAR and read the name of the medication to be given; access the epidural medication IV bag; check the label on the medication and compare the medication label to the MAR before picking it up (first check); and pick up the medication and check the label again (second check). Verify that the medication dispensed is labeled "preservative-free" or the label specifies "for epidural use."	
15. Prepare the epidural medication.	
a. Attach the pump tubing to the medication container, set up the pump, and attach the filter and safety needle or needleless connector to the line.	The pump ensures stable drug delivery. The filter prevents particulate matter from entering the epidural space. The safety devices prevent inadvertent needle sticks.
b. Place an "epidural" label on the tubing.	The label helps all staff accurately identify the tubing.
c. Recheck the MAR and the infusion bag label (third check) and calculate the hourly flow rate.	To be sure that the medication is delivered at the correct rate.
16-20. Follow steps 16 to 20 of the General Procedure: Prepare any additional medications to be given at this time, check	

(continued)

Action	Rationale
each medication label with the MAR once again, plan for the patient identification to be taken to the patient's bedside, identify the patient (two identifiers), and explain how the medication will be administered.	
21. Administer the epidural medication only if assessment reveals that the patient's condition is stable. Proceed as follows:	
a. Make sure there is adequate lighting, and position the patient for access to the injection port. Raise the bed if needed.	To enable you to see the injection port and work without back strain.
b. Put on clean gloves.	To protect yourself from contact with body fluid.
c. Identify the epidural catheter injection port. (Two nurses may need to do this.)	To make sure that the correct port is being used. Many facilities require that this be double-checked because of the serious consequences of erroneously using the wrong line.
d. Clean the injection cap on the epidural catheter with a povidone-iodine swab.	To remove microorganisms and decrease potential for infection.
e. Dry the injection cap with the sterile 2- × 2-inch gauze square.	Povidone-iodine may form a sticky residue if left on the cap.
f. Attach the infusion set to the epidural catheter by inserting the needle or needleless connector into the injection cap. Tape the connection, or use the built-in system connector to secure the two lines.	To access the epidural catheter and to make sure that the line stays intact.
g. Turn on the pump and set it according to the manufacturer's directions to deliver the prescribed dose per hour.	To ensure ongoing accurate dosage.
22. Follow step 22 of the General Procedure: Leave the patient in a comfortable position and lower the bed if it was raised.	
23. Discard povidone-iodine wipes and syringes into the sharps container.	To protect others from injury.
24. Follow step 24 of the General Procedure: Remove your gloves, and wash or disinfect your hands.	

EVALUATION

25. Evaluate using the individualized patient outcomes previously identified:

    a. The right *patient* received the right *medication* in the right *dose* by the *epidural route* at the right *time,* and over the correct length of time.

    b. The patient experienced the desired level of pain relief (use same pain scale as before medication administration).

    c. The patient experienced no adverse effects from the medication (see Table 53-1). **R:** Evaluation in relation to desired outcomes is essential for planning future care.

DOCUMENTATION

26-27. Follow steps 26 and 27 of the General Procedure. Document the name of the medication, the dose, time, route, and your signature on the correct patient's record. Also record assessment data, such as the pain level assessed on a consistent scale; respiratory rate, pulse rate, and blood pressure; and observations for potential adverse responses, such as pruritus and hypotension. These assessments are completed at regularly scheduled intervals such as every hour initially, then gradually moving to every 2 hours and every 4 hours as pain relief and patient's response are stabilized. A special flow sheet may be used for documenting pain management and any identified adverse effects (see Fig. 53-2).

Acute Care

Patients with a variety of surgeries may be managed postoperatively with epidural pain medication. This method of pain management often provides excellent pain relief without drowsiness or other adverse effects. The patient can turn, move, and rapidly return to functioning.

Long-Term Care

Residents with permanent epidural catheters in place may be transferred from acute care to long-term care facilities for convalescence or terminal care. In the past, this was rare; therefore, nurses in these settings may be inexperienced in the use of epidural catheters. The acute care staff may arrange for learning materials and educational opportunities to support the long-term care nursing staff in providing quality care to the resident with an epidural catheter. This type of cooperative planning for effective care management is increasingly common. Procedures in long-term care will be the same as in acute care.

Home Care

Both intermittent and continuous epidural narcotics are used in the home setting to provide pain management to individuals with terminal or intractable pain. Permanent epidural catheters are usually placed while the individual is hospitalized, and response to the medications can be carefully monitored. The client and family caregivers must be instructed in the techniques of epidural medication administration before the client is discharged for home care. Some agencies provide excellent written and illustrated materials to support home care, including specific directions, drawings, and a place for record keeping. In addition, family caregivers will need to learn how to care for the catheter exit site. After initial teaching in the hospital, a home care nurse is needed for ongoing assessment and support for the client and family.

LEARNING TOOLS

DEVELOP YOUR BACKGROUND KNOWLEDGE

1. Review the Learning Outcomes.

2. Read the section on epidural analgesia in your assigned text.

3. Look up the Key Terms in the glossary.

4. Review this module and mentally practice the techniques described. Study so that you would be able to teach these skills to another person.

DEVELOP YOUR SKILLS

In the practice setting, select another student and work in pairs.

1. Changing so that each has the opportunity to play the role of the patient, perform each of the procedures below. Any student who is not participating at a given time can observe and evaluate the performances of the others.

    a. Prepare and administer an epidural medication by injection.

    b. Prepare and administer an epidural medication by infusion.

2. When you feel confident in your skill, ask your instructor to check your performance.

DEMONSTRATE YOUR SKILLS

In the clinical setting

1. Consult with your instructor regarding the opportunity to participate in caring for a patient with an epidural catheter in place. Use the Performance Checklist on the CD-ROM in the front of this book as a guide.

2. Evaluate your performance with the instructor.

CRITICAL THINKING EXERCISES

1. Katherine Stover has returned from surgery with a temporary epidural catheter in place. You are planning for her care. She has stated that she is not having any pain, but her back is itching and she would like some lotion rubbed on it. As you make your plans for care, identify what assessment will be most important. Summarize the concerns you might have for her.

2. Jonathan Baker has been diagnosed as being terminally ill with metastatic cancer that has spread to his spine. He was admitted for placement of an epidural catheter for pain control. He will be going home with his son. His son and daughter-in-law plan to care for him with the help of hospice nurses. Evaluate Mr. Baker's immediate and long-term care needs; then formulate the plans you will make. Identify a variety of resources to assist this family.

SELF-QUIZ

SHORT-ANSWER QUESTIONS

1. Give two reasons that epidural narcotics may be used instead of oral narcotics.

   a. _____

   b. _____

2. Identify two safety precautions related to the administration of epidural narcotics.

   a. _____

   b. _____

3. How does the exit site care differ for a temporary and a permanent epidural catheter?

   _____

4. List four adverse responses to epidural narcotics.

   a. _____

   b. _____

   c. _____

   d. _____

5. What action would be taken if the patient experiences respiratory depression from an epidural narcotic?

   _____

6. What action is commonly taken if the patient experiences pruritus from an epidural narcotic?

   _____

7. What assessment should the nurse make to determine whether there is any neural irritation in the patient with an epidural catheter?

   _____

8. Giving a narcotic antagonist to relieve pruritus has what effect on pain control?

   _____

MULTIPLE CHOICE

_____ 9. Advantages of epidural administration of opioids include which of these? (Choose all that apply.)
   a. A lower total dose is needed to maintain adequate pain relief.
   b. Respiratory depression is less common.
   c. Much of the drug dose attaches to receptors in the spinal cord before reaching the central nervous system.
   d. The effect is less prolonged.

_____ 10. Any medication or solution administered epidurally must meet which of these criteria?
   a. It must be sterile.
   b. It must contain preservatives to prevent infection.
   c. It must not be diluted.
   d. All of these.

_____ 11. Adverse effects from epidural medications include which of these? (Choose all that apply.)
   a. Increase in pulse rate
   b. Drop in blood pressure
   c. Pruritis
   d. Confusion

Answers to the Self-Quiz questions appear in the back of the book.

REFERENCES AND SUGGESTED RESOURCES: UNIT 9

Alexander, M., & Corrigan, A. (Eds.). (2004). *Core curriculum for infusion nursing.* (3rd ed.). Philadelphia: Lippincott Williams & Wilkins.

American Association of Blood Banks (AABB). (2004). *Standards for blood banks and transfusion services.* (22nd ed.). Bethesda, MD: Author.

American Association of Blood Banks (AABB), America's Blood Centers & American Red Cross. (2002). *Circular of information for the use of human blood and blood components.* Bethesda, MD: Author.

ASPEN Board of Directors. (2001). Guidelines for the use of parenteral and enteral nutrition in adult and pediatric patients. *Journal of Parenteral & Enteral Nutrition, 26*(1S).

Brecher, M. E. (Ed.). (2002). *AABB technical manual for blood banks.* (14th ed.). Bethesda, MD: American Association of Blood Banks.

Bunce, M. (2003). Central lines. *RN, 66*(12), 29–32.

Centers for Disease Control and Prevention. (2002). Guideline for the prevention of intravascular-catheter-related infections. *Morbidity and Mortality Weekly Report, 51* (No. RR-10), 1–29.

Centers for Disease Control and Prevention. (1988). Update: Universal precautions for prevention of transmission of human immunodeficiency virus, hepatitis B virus, and other bloodborne pathogens in healthcare settings. *Morbidity and Mortality Weekly Report, 37,* 1–7.

Centers for Disease Control and Prevention. (1987). Recommendations for prevention of HIV transmission in healthcare settings. *Morbidity and Mortality Weekly Report*(Suppl. 36), 25–185.

Chaiyakunapruk, N., Veenstra, D. L., Lipsky, B. A., et al. (2002). Chlorhexidine compared with povidone-iodine solution for vascular catheter-site care: A meta-analysis. *Annals of Internal Medicine, 136*(11), 792–801.

Chan, H. S. C. (2001). Effects of injection duration on site-pain intensity and bruising associated with subcutaneous heparin. *Journal of Advance Nursing, 35*(6), 882–992.

Fahs, P. S., & Kinney, M. R. (1991). The abdomen, thigh, and arm as sites for subcutaneous heparin injections. *Nursing Research, 40*(4), 204–207.

Frey, A. (2003). Drawing blood samples from vascular access devices: Evidence-based practice. *Journal of Infusion Nursing, 26*(5), 285–293.

Hankins, J., Lonsway, R. A. W., Hedrick, C., et al. (Eds.). (2001). *The infusion nurses society: Infusion therapy in clinical practice* (2nd ed.). Philadelphia: W. B. Saunders.

Hrovat, T. M., Passwater, M., & Palmer, R. N. (Contributors). (2002). *Guidelines for the use of blood warming devices.* Bethesda, MD: American Association of Blood Banks.

Institute of Medicine—I.O.M. (2000). *To err is human: Building a safer health system.* National Academies Press. (Online). Available at http://books.nap.edu/openbook/0309068371/html/index.html.

Intravenous Nurses Society. (2000). Infusion nursing standards. *Journal of Intravenous Nursing, 23*(65), 1–88.

Joint Commission on Accreditation of Healthcare Organizations. (2004). *Accreditation manual for hospitals.* Chicago: Author.

Joint Commission for the Accreditation of Healthcare Organizations. (2004). Prohibited abbreviations. (Online). Available at www.jcaho.org. Retrieved Aug. 15, 2004.

Joint Commission on Accreditation of Healthcare Organizations. (2004). National patient safety goals 2005. Questions about goal # 3 (Online). Available at http://www.jcaho.org/accredited+organizations/patient+safety/05+npsg/05_npsg_faqs.htm. Retrieved June 29, 2005.

McConnell, E. A. (2001). Clinical do's and don'ts: Administering total parenteral nutrition. *Nursing2001, 31*(7), 17.

National Institute for Occupational Safety and Health (NIOSH). (1999). *NIOSH alert: Preventing needlestick injuries in healthcare settings.* DHHS (NIOSH) Publication No. 2000–108. (Online). Available at www.cdc.gov/niosh/2000-108.html. Retrieved Sept. 10, 2004.

O'Grady, N. P., Alexander, M., Patchen-Dellinger, E., et al. (2002). Guidelines for the prevention of intravascular catheter-related infections. *MMWR,* (Aug. 9) 51 (RR10), 1–26. (Online). Available at http://www.cdc.gov/mmwr/preview/mmwrhtml/rr5110a1.htm.

Occupational Safety and Health Administration (OSHA). (2001). Needlestick Safety and Prevention Act, Pub. L., No. 106–430. (Online). Available at www.osha.gov. Retrieved November 2, 2005.

Pellowe, C. M., Pratt, R. J., Harper, P., et al. (2003). Infection control: Prevention of healthcare-associated infection in primary and community care. Section 5. Central Venous Catheterization. *Journal of Hospital Infection Control, 55* (Suppl. 2), 1–127.

Pugent Sound Blood Center. (2005). *Blood components reference manual.* Seattle, WA: Author.

Shelton, P., & Rosenthal, K. (2004). Sharps injury prevention: Select a safer needle. *Nursing Management, 35*(6), 25–31.

Singapore Ministry of Health. (2002). *Prevention of infections related to peripheral IV devices.* Singapore: Singapore Ministry of Health.

Smeltzer, S., & Bare, B. (2003). *Brunner and Suddarth's textbook of medical-surgical nursing,* (10th ed.). Philadelphia: Lippincott Williams & Wilkins.

South Western Staffordshire Primary Care Trust. (2005). *Clinical guidelines district nursing and intermediate care.* (Online). Accessed at http://www.sws-pct.nhs.uk/policies/Clinical/DNICT03.pdf.

Ward, J. (2003). Nutrition support to patients undergoing gastrointestinal surgery. *Nutrition Journal, 2*(1), 18.

Weinstein, S. M. (1997). *Plumer's principles & practice of intravenous therapy* (6th ed.). Philadelphia: Lippincott Williams & Wilkins.

Zeraatkari, K., Karimi, M., Shahrzad, M. K., et al. (2005). Comparison of heparin subcutaneous injection in thigh, arm, & abdomen. *Canadian Journal of Anesthesia, 52,* A60.

Answers to Self-Quiz Questions

MODULE 1 AN APPROACH TO NURSING SKILLS
SHORT-ANSWER QUESTIONS

1. a. Right to self-determination/consent
    b. Right to information upon which to base decisions
    c. Right to privacy/confidentiality
    d. Right to safe care
    e. Right to personal dignity
    f. Right to individualized care
    g. Right to assistance toward independence
    h. Right to criticize and obtain changes in care

2. Any one of the following: calling patient by preferred name, helping person to be physically clean and attractive, always pulling drapes and closing doors for privacy

3. a. The right task
    b. The right circumstances
    c. The right person
    d. The right direction/communication
    e. The right supervision/evaluation

4. a. Assessment
    b. Analysis/Nursing Diagnosis
    c. Planning
    d. Implementation
    e. Evaluation

5. Gathering data, analyzing data, and identifying the problems present

6. Organized, purposeful, disciplined thinking, focused on deciding what to believe or do

7. By conceptualizing nursing process as a cyclical in nature, with every component interacting with every other component, and with critical thinking at the center

8. a. Correct technique
    b. Organization
    c. Dexterity
    d. Speed

9. Past practice and sound deductive reasoning from known facts

10. To identify the outcomes of nursing action

11. Imagine yourself performing the actions in the procedure while "feeling" and "seeing" yourself doing the movements and skills described.

MODULE 2 DOCUMENTATION
SHORT-ANSWER QUESTIONS

1. a. Source oriented
    b. Problem oriented

2. Any two of the following: narrative, SOAP, APIE, DARP

3. To clearly communicate information and to avoid the appearance of bias

4. Underline "States upset over upcoming surgery."

5. Draw a line through the 225 mL and write "Wrong amount" above it. Add "175 mL urine" at the end.

6. The facility

7. Patients have a right to the information contained in the record. Usually there is a procedure to follow in the facility.

MULTIPLE CHOICE

8. b

9. c

10. a

MODULE 3 BASIC BODY MECHANICS
TRUE/FALSE

1. T
2. T
3. F
4. F
5. T
6. F

SHORT-ANSWER QUESTIONS

7. These muscles may become tired or injury to the back may occur.

8. It is easier to move an object on a level surface than to move it up a slanted surface against the force of gravity.

9. Enlarging the base of support in the direction of the force to be applied increases the amount of force that can be applied.

10. It takes less energy to hold an object close to the body than at a distance from the body; it is also easier to move an object that is close.

MODULE 4 BASIC INFECTION CONTROL
SHORT-ANSWER QUESTIONS

1. To avoid creating air currents that will transfer microorganisms

2. To avoid contaminating your hair with what might be on your hands and to avoid getting what might be on your hair on your clean hands

3. Microorganisms move by gravity.

4. To provide a barrier between your clean hand and the contaminated faucet handle

5. To protect the mucous membranes of the eyes, mouth, and nose from potential contact with contaminated substances

6. To prevent potential needle-stick injuries with contaminated objects

7. To prevent your hands from becoming grossly contaminated with pathogens

8. To protect the mucous membranes of the eyes, mouth, and nose from potential contact with contaminated substances

9. To reduce the number of microorganisms on the hands and thus prevent their spread

10. To minimize environmental contact with the contaminated surface of the gloves

11. Visible soil must be washed from hands with soap and water because microorganisms may be protected from contact with a disinfectant by the material on the hands.

MULTIPLE CHOICE

12. a, b, c, and d

13. a, b, and d

14. a, b, c, and d

15. a, c, and d

16. d

17. c

18. d

MODULE 5 SAFETY IN THE HEALTHCARE ENVIRONMENT
SHORT-ANSWER QUESTIONS

1. a. The facility is complex and unfamiliar.
   b. Patients are more vulnerable.
   c. Equipment may be hazardous

2. Any five of the following: good body mechanics; walking, not running; keeping to the right in hallways; turning corners and opening doors carefully; using stretchers properly; using brakes on beds, wheelchairs, and stretchers; using elevators correctly

3. Any three of the following: bed in low position; bed alarm in place; adequate lighting in room; no clutter in the room

4. Use three-pronged plugs, check for frayed cords, use only approved appliances

5. Any three of the following: falls, contractures, pressure sores, dehydration, chronic constipation, functional incontinence, loss of bone mass and muscle tone, loss of ability to move around independently

6. Make appropriate assessments, and plan for a safe environment.

7. Most maintain a strict nonsmoking policy for patients, visitors, and staff. Patients who insist on smoking may be escorted to an outdoor area.

8. a. Be familiar with code procedure.
   b. Remove patients from immediate vicinity of fire.
   c. Initiate code.
   d. Return to unit if you did not call code.
   e. Never use elevators.
   f. Return patients to rooms, and close doors.
   g. Calm patients.
   h. Follow directions of person in charge.
   i. Stand in hallway.
   j. Evacuate according to procedure if necessary.
   k. Remain calm.
   l. Wait for directions at all-clear signal.

9. To be knowledgeable, report as designated, and perform skills as predetermined by plans

MULTIPLE CHOICE

10. c

11. a, b

12. a, b, c, d

MODULE 6 MOVING THE PATIENT IN BED AND POSITIONING
SHORT-ANSWER QUESTIONS

1. So as not to be working against the gravitational pull

2. a. Promotes physical progress
   b. Adds to the patient's self-esteem

3. Dislocation of the shoulder

4. The patient's trunk

5. a. For the patient's comfort and safety
   b. To make sure there is no undue pressure on parts

6. a. To prevent pressure ulcers
   b. To prevent joint contractures
   c. to improve muscle tone and circulation

7. Trochanter roll

8. Flexed forward

9. a. Feet in space between mattress and footboard
   b. Roll placed under ankles

10. Develop a teaching plan, and teach the proper method of moving and positioning residents or affected family members.

MULTIPLE CHOICE

11. b
12. b
13. c

MODULE 7 PROVIDING HYGIENE
SHORT-ANSWER QUESTIONS

1. A bath blanket provides warmth and is more absorbent than a sheet.

2. Prevents fine scratches on the surface of the glasses caused by dust particles.

3. The a.m. care includes using the toilet, bedpan, or commode; washing face and hands; and brushing the teeth—preparing for breakfast.

4. The p.m. care includes using the toilet, bedpan, or commode; washing face and hands; brushing the teeth; backrub and possibly a fresh gown and clean pillowcase—preparing for sleep.

5. Equipment for shampoo includes pitcher for water, a trough with a receptacle to receive shampoo water, plastic sheet, towels, shampoo, conditioner (optional), hair dryer.

6. Wipe off the hearing aid with dry tissue, turn off the battery, place in a container in the bedside drawer until the patient returns.

MULTIPLE CHOICE

7. c
8. c
9. d
10. b
11. c

MODULE 8 ASSISTING WITH ELIMINATION AND PERINEAL CARE
SHORT-ANSWER QUESTIONS

1. a. Observe infection control measures.
   b. Be aware that the procedure of assisting with elimination and perineal care can be embarrassing and create uncomfortable feelings.
   c. When assisting a patient with elimination, approximate the normal position as closely as possible.

2. a. Raise buttocks and slide bedpan in place.
   b. Rolling patient onto bedpan

3. a. Postpartum patient or patient who has had perineal surgery
   b. Patient with an indwelling catheter
   c. Patient who is incontinent

4. a. Postpartum or surgical patient: Remove dressing or pads, place a waterproof pad under patient, and position on a bedpan. Pour tepid tap water or the solution used in your facility over the perineum. Rinse with clear water. Using cotton balls, gauze, or wipes, wipe from anterior to posterior. Clean gently. Use extra gauze square or cotton balls, but use each only one time, and then discard into waste bag. Replace any pads or dressings. Remove bedpan and discard the contents.
   b. Patient with catheter: Wash the perineal area thoroughly with soap and water. Clean around the entire insertion site. Rinse and dry.
   c. Patient who is incontinent: Place a waterproof pad under the patient; wash the perineum, using warm water and mild soap. Gently separate the labia of the female patient as you clean. Clean with washcloth from front to back. Use different sections of the washcloth for each stroke. For the male, begin with the penile head and move downward along the shaft. Retract the foreskin for the uncircumcised patient to clean. Be sure to replace the foreskin when cleaning is completed. Rinse and dry.

5. To prevent contamination of the vaginal area from the anal area.

6. The nurse is coming into contact with body fluids and substances, such as mucous membranes. Cross-contamination from another patient is a possibility.

MULTIPLE CHOICE

7. d
8. c
9. b
10. b
11. c
12. c

MODULE 9 BEDMAKING AND THERAPEUTIC BEDS

SHORT-ANSWER QUESTIONS

1. a. Patient is safe.
    b. Patient is comfortable.

2. Method is more time efficient and less fatiguing to the nurse

3. Keep side rails up on the side of the patient

4. May decrease the effectiveness of the mattress in preventing pressure relief

5. The bed may become firm by pressing a button or switch that turns off the motor.

MULTIPLE CHOICE

6. b
7. d
8. a
9. b
10. c
11. b
12. c

MODULE 10 ASSISTING PATIENTS WITH EATING

SHORT-ANSWER QUESTIONS

1. (In any order)
    a. Environment
    b. Emotions
    c. Physical disability
    d. Dentures

2. (In any order)
    a. Hot or cold temperature foods
    b. Cooked vegetables, ground meat
    c. Pureed fruits, pudding
    d. Thickened liquids

3. (In any order)
    a. Water, tea, coffee, or soda
    b. Tough, stringy, hard, or dry foods
    c. Sticky foods
    d. Neutral temperature foods

MULTIPLE CHOICE

4. c
5. b
6. a

TRUE/FALSE

7. F
8. F
9. T
10. F

MODULE 11 ASSESSING TEMPERATURE, PULSE, AND RESPIRATION

SHORT-ANSWER QUESTIONS

1. 98.6°F or 36°C

2. Any four of the following: age, infection, environmental temperature, exercise, emotional status, or metabolism

3. a. Radial
    b. Carotid
    c. Femoral

4. 60 to 100

5. 12 to 20

6. a. Infection
    b. Pain
    c. Exercise
    d. Fever

MULTIPLE CHOICE

7. d
8. c
9. b
10. d
11. c
12. b

MODULE 12 MEASURING BLOOD PRESSURE

SHORT-ANSWER QUESTIONS

1. 140/80/70

2. Low-pitched sounds are heard more easily with the bell.

3. The period without sounds between when the first faint Korotkoff sounds are heard and when clear, sharp Korotkoff sounds are heard at a lower level when the cuff pressure is reduced.

4. By pumping the hand bulb on the blood pressure cuff to a point 30 mm of mercury beyond the point at which you last felt a pulse.

5. The blood pressure reading will be too high.

6. a. You may not hear a beat at the actual high pressure and, therefore, miss the systolic pressure.
   b. You may also erroneously note the diastolic as lower than it is.

MULTIPLE CHOICE

7. a, c, d

8. a

9. b

10. a

11. a

12. b

MODULE 13 MONITORING INTAKE AND OUTPUT

SHORT-ANSWER QUESTIONS

1. Sweat

2. Increased urine output

3. a. Infants
   b. Elderly

4. Daily weights reflect the patient's overall state of fluid balance

5. a. Urine
   b. Vomit
   c. Diarrhea stool

6. Confusion

MULTIPLE CHOICE

7. a

8. c

9. b

10. a

11. a

12. d

MODULE 14 NURSING PHYSICAL ASSESSMENT

SHORT-ANSWER QUESTIONS

1. Any five of the following: color, odor, size, shape, symmetry, movement

2. a. What is being done
   b. Why is it being done
   c. What can the patient do to assist in the process

3. a. Size
   b. Shape
   c. Equality

4. Head elevated to 45 degrees or greater

5. Breasts are sensitive during menses.

6. It can change bowel sounds.

7. Bronchial obstruction, chronic lung disease, or shallow breathing

8. Pneumonia caused by consolidation

9. If the sound occurs in relationship to the heartbeat rather than respiration, then it is a pericardial friction rub and not pleural.

10. Mitral valve area at the 5th intercostal space just inside the midclavicular line

11. a. Consultation with healthcare team members
    b. Review of records and reports
    c. Review of literature
    d. Interview
    e. Observation

MULTIPLE CHOICE

12. d

13. a

14. b

15. c

MODULE 15 COLLECTING SPECIMENS AND PERFORMING COMMON LABORATORY TESTS

SHORT-ANSWER QUESTIONS

1. Assess the patient for signs or symptoms of problems that would relate to abnormality. Notify the physician as appropriate. Depending on the

test, physician notification may be delayed. All results, normal or abnormal, should be documented according to facility policy.

2. There may be a "quick-reference" guide on the unit that would provide necessary information. For any questions, or if a quick guide is not available, refer to the facility's Policy/Procedure Manual.

3. a. Getting the right amount of specimen
   b. In the right container
   c. From the right patient
   d. Tested in the right way

4. Whenever there is any possibility of contact with blood or body fluids

5. All specimens should be placed in the appropriate container with a tightly fitting lid. They should be placed in a biohazard plastic bag, according to facility policy.

TRUE/FALSE

6. T

7. F

8. F

9. F

10. F

MODULE 16 ADMISSION, TRANSFER, AND DISCHARGE
SHORT-ANSWER QUESTIONS

1. A discharge planner

2. Any one of the following: elevated temperature, new or unusual pain, change in a wound

3. To enable them to carry out effective care at home

4. To identify problems that must be addressed immediately

MULTIPLE CHOICE

5. b

6. b, c, d

7. b

8. c

9. a, b, c, d

10. d

11. a, c, d

12. a, b, c, d

13. b, d

MODULE 17 ASSISTING WITH DIAGNOSTIC AND THERAPEUTIC PROCEDURES
SHORT-ANSWER QUESTIONS

1. a. Meeting the physical and psychological needs of the patient
   b. Gathering necessary equipment and assisting the physician

2. Because bleeding at the site could be excessive if the patient is taking anticoagulants.

3. a. Privacy
   b. Set up and clean a surface for equipment.
   c. Obtain appropriate equipment.
   d. Maintain sterile field if necessary.

MULTIPLE CHOICE

4. c

5. a

6. c, d

7. b, c

MODULE 18 TRANSFER
SHORT-ANSWER QUESTIONS

1. Any two of the following: They give the patient a sense of security; they prevent slipping; they prevent foot injury; they protect against contaminated floors.

2. Ease the patient back onto bed or chair of origin or gently to the floor. Protect the patient's head.

3. Chair must be placed on left side, extra support may be needed, right leg must be braced with nurse's leg or knee while pivoting.

4. To provide a firm handhold and support for the nurse when transferring the patient

5. a. Bed to chair: one-person minimal assist
   b. Bed to chair: two-person maximal assist

6. To prevent a blood pressure drop (orthostatic hypotension) or dizziness

7. When moving the supine patient between bed and stretcher

MULTIPLE CHOICE

8. b

9. b

10. d

MODULE 19 AMBULATION: SIMPLE ASSISTED AND USING CANE, WALKER, OR CRUTCHES

SHORT-ANSWER QUESTIONS

1. Any four of the following: maintain muscle tone, restore muscle tone, stimulate respiratory system, stimulate circulatory system, improve psychological well-being, facilitate elimination

2. Falls

3. They give better support, are less likely to slip, and usually stay on better.

4. A transfer and ambulation belt, a cane, a walker, or crutches

5. Crutches should extend from the floor, about 6 inches out from the foot, to the side of the chest 2 inches under the axilla.

6. Four-point gait

7. Push up from arms of the chair (or the bed).

8. Opposite the weak leg

9. Hold both in one hand.

10. Three-point gait

11. Crutches, weak leg, strong leg

12. Any three of the following: stairs, narrow doors, rugs, furniture placement, inadequate lighting.

MULTIPLE CHOICE

8. b

9. b

10. c

MODULE 20 IMPLEMENTING RANGE-OF-MOTION EXERCISES

SHORT-ANSWER QUESTIONS

1. a. To maintain joint mobility
   b. To prevent lengthy rehabilitation

2. a. When increasing the level of energy expended or the level of circulation is potentially hazardous
   b. When joints are swollen or inflamed or there is injury near the joint

3. Flexors

4. Elbow, knee, and ankle; the joint moves in one plane to extend outward to 180° and to flex to an acute angle.

5. Thumb; flexion, extension, abduction, adduction, and opposition

6. Gliding

7. Active

8. Supination

9. Abduction

MULTIPLE CHOICE

10. d

11. b

12. c

MODULE 21 CARING FOR PATIENTS WITH CASTS AND BRACES

SHORT-ANSWER QUESTIONS

1. a. Plaster of Paris
   b. Synthetic materials, including thermoplastic and fiberglass

2. a. Hard
   b. Inexpensive

3. a. Lightweight
   b. Not damaged by water

4. Preexisting skin breakdown or infection may require treatment and follow up.

5. a. Folded down stockinette
   b. Petaling

6. a. Motion
   b. Sensation
   c. Pain

7. a. Cotton padding
   b. Plastic
   c. Metal

8. The weight and confinement of the brace may disturb balance.

MULTIPLE CHOICE

9. d

10. b

11. b

12. c

13. b

MODULE 22 CARING FOR THE PATIENT IN TRACTION OR WITH AN EXTERNAL FIXATION DEVICE

SHORT-ANSWER QUESTIONS

1. Any two of the following: Bucks, Bryant's, Russell's, Pelvic, Cervical halter

2. Sterile saline, cotton-tip applicators, half-strength hydrogen peroxide, topical antibiotic

3. a. Footboard or footrest
   b. Plantar-flexion and dorsiflexion exercises

4. a. Constipation
   b. Anorexia
   c. Skin breakdown
   d. Urinary stasis

MATCHING

5. (1) b, d
   (2) b, a
   (3) a, b, f
   (4) a, b
   (5) b, g
   (6) b, c, h
   (7) b

MULTIPLE CHOICE

6. d

7. c

MODULE 23 ISOLATION PROCEDURES

SHORT-ANSWER QUESTIONS

1. a. To protect the patient
   b. To protect the environment and others in that environment

2. Droplet Precautions

3. Standard Precautions are sufficient for this patient.

4. Any three of the following: private room, sign on door, leave stand outside door for equipment, laundry hamper inside room, wastebasket lined with plastic, thermometer, and blood pressure equipment

5. No special precautions are used.

6. Thoroughly wash your hands.

7. To protect the patient from infection

MULTIPLE CHOICE

8. b

9. d

10. d

11. b

MODULE 24 BASIC STERILE TECHNIQUE: STERILE FIELD AND STERILE GLOVES

SHORT-ANSWER QUESTIONS

1. A disinfectant is a process or liquid that kills microorganisms other than spores, whereas

sterilization is the complete elimination of microorganisms including spores.

2. Sterile conscience is a moral mandate to monitor and correct one's behavior in the absence of others.

3. Liquid or moisture promotes the bacteria spread through a process of wicking, which may cause objects to become contaminated.

4. Fungicide

5. Acrylic nails have been shown to harbor microorganisms, especially yeast and fungi.

MULTIPLE CHOICE

6. d

7. d

8. b

9. c

10. b

11. a

MODULE 25 SURGICAL ASEPSIS: SCRUBBING, GOWNING, AND CLOSED GLOVING

SHORT-ANSWER QUESTIONS

1. Any three of the following: mask, eyewear, gown, gloves, shoe cover. All protect the wearer from contact with blood or body fluids.

2. 2 to 6 minutes

3. Subungual area/nail beds

4. Hands clasped together above the waist in front. This prevents the hands from inadvertently touching a nonsterile surface.

MULTIPLE CHOICE

5. c

6. b

7. c

MODULE 26 ADMINISTERING ENEMAS

SHORT-ANSWER QUESTIONS

1. Any three of the following: return flow, premixed, medicated, cleansing

2. a. Patient response (pain, cramping)
   b. Characteristics of stool
   c. Change in baseline vital signs
   d. Patient's ability to use toilet

3. a. Oil retention
   b. Medicated

4. 7 to 10 cm

5. 500 to 1,000 mL.

6. a. In preparation for a diagnostic test
b. For relief of constipation

MULTIPLE CHOICE

7. c

8. b

9. a

10. c

MODULE 27 ASSISTING THE PATIENT WHO REQUIRES URINARY CATHETERIZATION

SHORT-ANSWER QUESTIONS

1. a. Anxiety
b. Infection risk
c. Pain

2. Nurse failed to allow patient to verbalize concerns

3. a. Normal to experience urgency and frequency
b. May feel minimal amount of burning
c. Encourage intake of fluids
d. Measure output for next 24 hours

4. Any two of the following: patient response, patient's ability to void, intake and output

5. Any two of the following: to maintain patent tubing, to instill medication into the bladder, to remove clots

MULTIPLE CHOICE

6. b

7. c

8. c

9. c

10. a, b, c, e

11. a

12. c

13. d

MODULE 28 CARING FOR THE PATIENT WITH AN OSTOMY

SHORT-ANSWER QUESTIONS

1. An opening from the ileum (small intestine) onto the abdominal wall

2. The drainage is liquid and contains digestive enzymes, which increases the potential for skin breakdown.

3. Red and smooth mucous membrane surface without ulceration

4. A portion of the ileum is dissected and folded back on itself to form a structure for urine storage similar to the bladder. An advantage is that the patient performs self-catheterization and does not wear an appliance.

5. Seated on a toilet or commode

6. Approximately 1,000 mL

7. Approximately 15 minutes

8. Approximately 30 minutes after the patient gets up from the toilet

9. Because of the potential for urinary tract infection

10. a. Health teaching
b. Referring patient and family to community resources

MULTIPLE CHOICE

11. b

12. a

13. d

14. a

MODULE 29 INSERTING AND MAINTAINING A NASOGASTRIC TUBE

SHORT-ANSWER QUESTIONS

1. Any three of the following: enteral nutrition, administering medications, irrigating the stomach, gastric suction

2. To avoid damaging the mucosa on insertion

3. Prevention of nausea and gagging

MULTIPLE CHOICE

4. c

5. a

6. c

7. c

8. b

MODULE 30 ADMINISTERING TUBE FEEDINGS

SHORT-ANSWER QUESTIONS

1. After each feeding and before and after medication administration; to provide fluids required by the patient or ordered by the physician.

2. Test the secretions for glucose content. Secretions containing formula will have a high glucose content.

3. Check the policy manual or the physician's orders. You may need to withhold the feeding.

4. Sudden change in consistency of diet.

5. Instilling a pancreatic enzyme solution to digest and dissolve the obstruction.

MULTIPLE CHOICE

6. a

7. c

8. b

9. b

10. a

11. c

12. a

MODULE 31 ADMINISTERING OXYGEN
SHORT-ANSWER QUESTIONS

1. a. Nasal cannula or prongs
   b. Nasal catheter
   c. Transtracheal catheter
   d. Mask

MULTIPLE CHOICE

2. c

3. b

4. d

5. b

6. b

7. a, b, c, d

8. d

MODULE 32 RESPIRATORY CARE PROCEDURES
SHORT-ANSWER QUESTIONS

1. To promote expansion of alveoli and expectoration of secretions

2. 2:1

3. To use the force of gravity to help drain pulmonary secretions

4. a. Head elevated and then
   b. Lean to the right

   c. Lean to the left
   d. Leaning forward 30 to 45 degrees
   e. Leaning backward 30 to 45 degrees
   f. Lying on the abdomen, back, and sides while horizontal

5. a. Head slightly down (30 to 45 degrees) and then
   b. Supine
   c. Right side but halfway to back
   d. Right side lying
   e. Prone

6. To help loosen pulmonary secretions

7. To encourage the patient to breathe deeply

MULTIPLE CHOICE

8. a

9. a

10. d

MODULE 33 ORAL AND NASOPHARYNGEAL SUCTIONING
SHORT-ANSWER QUESTIONS

1. a. To keep the patient calm
   b. To facilitate compliance

2. To prevent the transfer of microorganisms to the patient's respiratory tract

3. A closed system helps to maintain sterility.

4. Place the unconscious patient in the lateral position, facing toward you.

5. a. To promote drainage of secretions
   b. To prevent aspiration

6. 15 seconds

7. Three

MULTIPLE CHOICE

8. a

9. a

10. d

MODULE 34 TRACHEOSTOMY CARE AND SUCTIONING
MULTIPLE CHOICE

1. a, c, d

2. b

3. a

4. d

5. a

6. d

MODULE 35 CARING FOR PATIENTS WITH CHEST DRAINAGE
SHORT-ANSWER QUESTIONS

1. a. To remove air
   b. To remove fluid
   c. To restore the normal negative intrapleural pressure

2. Air in the pleural space

3. Anteriorly through the second intercostal space, because air rises

4. a. Promotes drainage because of gravity
   b. Prevents backflow of bottle contents into pleural space

5. Controls amount of suction applied to the chest tube

6. a. Airtight system except for vent in waterseal bottle
   b. Vent open
   c. Waterseal in operation

7. Tension pneumothorax

8. To confirm that the lung has reexpanded

MULTIPLE CHOICE

9. b, c

10. c

11. a

12. b

MODULE 36 EMERGENCY RESUSCITATION PROCEDURES
SHORT-ANSWER QUESTIONS

1. Shake the person and say loudly, "Are you all right?"

2. Because the most common cause of arrest in the pediatric age group is primary respiratory arrest or an obstructed airway, the procedure is to assess the patient and provide approximately 1 minute of rescue support before activating Emergency Medical Services.

3. Flat, with the neck straight

4. Locate the trachea and slide your fingers toward yourself to the hollow beside it.

5. By placing your thumb on the outside of the infant's upper arm and pressing gently with your index and middle fingers on the inside of the upper arm

6. 1½ inches above the xiphoid process

7. Clutching the neck in the area of the larynx between the thumb and index finger

8. In the midline, below the xiphoid process of the sternum but above the navel

9. Only in the unconscious patient to attempt to grasp a foreign body and remove it

MULTIPLE CHOICE

10. a, b, c, d

11. a, b

MODULE 37 APPLYING BANDAGES AND BINDERS
SHORT-ANSWER QUESTIONS

1. a. To provide support
   b. To protect wounds
   c. To protect and hold underlying dressings

2. a. Circular
   b. Spiral
   c. Reverse spiral
   d. Figure-eight
   e. Recurrent fold

3. A joint

4. Distal to proximal

5. To promote venous return and prevent deep vein thrombosis and pulmonary embolism

6. Severe arterial disease of the lower extremities

7. a. To hold layer dressings in place
   b. For support

8. Any two of the following: stretch net bandages are easy to wash, provide air circulation, and are comfortable for the patient.

9. Safety pins have hard, sharp surfaces and cause tissue damage if the patient rests on them.

MULTIPLE CHOICE

10. d

11. c

MODULE 38 APPLYING HEAT AND COLD
SHORT-ANSWER QUESTIONS

1. Any three of the following: the very young and the elderly are more susceptible to negative effects of heat and cold therapies; a sensation of warmth or coolness dissipates in short time; the maximum length of time a heat or cold treatment should be left in place is 20 minutes; injuries are more likely to occur when you apply moist heat or cold; the length of time the body is exposed to heat or cold, as well as the size of the skin area being treated, affects the ability of the body to tolerate the treatment.

2. a. The specific treatment applied
    b. The length of time left in place
    c. The patient's response.

MULTIPLE CHOICE

3. a
4. c
5. c
6. b
7. c
8. b
9. b

MODULE 39 ADMINISTERING EAR AND EYE IRRIGATIONS
SHORT-ANSWER QUESTIONS

1. a. Cleaning
    b. Instilling medications

2. Eye

3. Ear

4. a. Excessively high temperature
    b. Excessive pressure
    c. Incorrect solution concentration

5. One of the following: When the tympanic membrane is not intact, or when there is an organic foreign body present

6. To prevent the spread of microorganisms from one eye to the other

7. When any splashing might occur

MULTIPLE CHOICE

8. d
9. b
10. c

MODULE 40 PROVIDING WOUND CARE
SHORT-ANSWER QUESTIONS

1. Three of the following: protection, absorption, application of pressure, maintain a moist surface

2. a. To appropriate technique
    b. To observe and describe the wound
    c. To use appropriate dressing materials

3. a. Amount
    b. Color
    c. Consistency
    d. Odor

4. Any three of the following: edges approximated, smooth contour, minimal inflammation, minimal edema

5. Nonadherent

6. Paper tape

7. To protect the skin from large amounts of drainage

8. This action prevents spreading microorganisms from one site to another.

9. To debride the wound

MULTIPLE CHOICE

10. a, b, c
11. d
12. a
13. c

MODULE 41 PROVIDING PREOPERATIVE CARE
SHORT-ANSWER QUESTIONS

1. a. To establish a baseline
    b. To detect elevated temperature that may signal infection

2. a. Drug allergies
    b. Food allergies
    c. Latex allergy and skin (contact) allergies

3. a. To provide progress reports regarding the patient
    b. To consult in an emergency situation

MULTIPLE CHOICE

4. b
5. d
6. a
7. c

MODULE 42 PROVIDING POSTOPERATIVE CARE
SHORT-ANSWER QUESTIONS

1. Any four of the following: blood pressure (BP) cuff, IV pole, thermometer, oximeter, oxygen, suction

2. Any six of the following: pulse, BP, temperature, pulse oximetry value, skin color, level of consciousness, dressing status, respiratory rate and rhythm

3. a. Color
b. Clarity
c. Amount

4. a. Early ambulation
b. Coughing and deep breathing
c. Frequent position changes

5. a. Notify surgeon immediately.
b. Elevate patient's legs.
c. Do not leave patient alone.

MULTIPLE CHOICE

6. d

7. a

8. d

9. b

MODULE 43 PROVIDING POSTMORTEM CARE
SHORT-ANSWER QUESTIONS

1. Any three of the following: rigor mortis, livor mortis, skin indentation, algor mortis

2. To prevent discoloration and indentation of the underlying hand if folded over the chest

3. a. IVs
b. Nasogastric tubes
c. Urinary catheters
d. Oxygen equipment

4. Any two of the following: straighten the unit, soften the lights, provide chairs

5. Any two of the following: make sure the family knows they can see and hold the infant; wrap the infant in a receiving blanket, and carry as you would a living baby; provide a nursery crib if the family is not comfortable holding the baby; offer the family the opportunity to be alone.

6. The realization of offering an extension of life to another

7. Viability and usefulness of tissues

8. Any three of the following: persons who die suddenly when in apparent good health and without medical attendance within 36 hours preceding death; circumstances indicate death caused entirely or in part by unnatural or unlawful means; suspicious circumstances; unknown or obscure causes; deaths caused by any violence whatsoever, whether the primary cause or any contributory factors in the death; contagious disease; bodies that are not claimed; premature and stillborn infants

9. An examination of the body after death

10. a. To determine cause of death
b. To gather scientific knowledge
c. To add to statistical data

MULTIPLE CHOICE

11. c

12. c, d

13. b

MODULE 44 ADMINISTERING ORAL MEDICATIONS
SHORT-ANSWER QUESTIONS

1. a. Right drug
b. Right dose
c. Right route
d. Right patient
e. Right time
f. Right documentation

2. (1) As it is taken out of the storage site; (2) after it is in hand; (3) before a stock bottle is replaced or when all unit doses are obtained or before a unit dose is administered

3. a. Name, birthdate, or patient number on identification band
b. Patient states any of these same items

MULTIPLE CHOICE

4. d

5. b

6. a

7. c

8. c

9. b

10. b

11. a

12. a

13. d

14. c

15. b

MODULE 45 ADMINISTERING MEDICATIONS BY ALTERNATIVE ROUTES

SHORT-ANSWER QUESTIONS

1. Because of the danger of aspiration pneumonia with oil-based solutions

2. Ethmoidal and sphenoidal sinuses

3. Any three of the following: to protect, to soften, to soothe, to relieve itching

4. a. Dorsal recumbent position with knees flexed
   b. Sims' position

5. Beyond the internal sphincter

6. To help the patient relax

7. By taking a deep breath and fully exhaling, then by inhaling when the puff is activated, and continuing to breathe in around the mouthpiece

MULTIPLE CHOICE

8. a

9. c

10. b

MODULE 46 ADMINISTERING MEDICATIONS BY INJECTION

SHORT-ANSWER QUESTIONS

1. a. Glass
   b. Disposable plastic
   c. Prefilled
   d. Cartridge

2. There are 100 units of insulin in 1 mL.

3. a. Length
   b. Gauge

4. a. Vials
   b. Ampules

5. Vial

6. Any three of the following: almost complete absorption, more rapid absorption, gastric disturbances do not affect the medication, patient does not have to be conscious or rational

7. 25-G, ½-inch needle

8. a. Upper arms
   b. Anterior aspect of thighs
   c. Lower abdominal wall

9. Intramuscular route

10. 1½-inch needle

11. a. Greater trochanter
    b. Crest of the ilium
    c. Anterior superior iliac spine

12. Any three of the following: no large nerves or blood vessels, cleaner, less fatty, several positions can be used, better for small children because gluteus medius muscle not well developed until after a child walks

13. a. Small muscle, so not capable of absorbing large amounts of medication
    b. Danger of injury to the radial nerve

14. To see whether the needle has penetrated a blood vessel

MULTIPLE CHOICE

15. a

16. a, d

MODULE 47 PREPARING AND MAINTAINING INTRAVENOUS INFUSIONS

SHORT-ANSWER QUESTIONS

1. A controlled-volume set such as Peditrol, Soluset, and Volutrol or a microdrip set

2. A secondary infusion set that connects into the primary set

3. A bottle must have room air enter in order to empty. This may allow contaminants into the fluid. The bag collapses to empty so that no contaminated air enters.

4. Replace the IV bag immediately.

5. a. Hang the second bag at a height greater than the primary bag.
   b. Clamp the primary bag's tubing and closely monitor until the secondary bag is completed; then unclamp the primary bag and allow it to continue infusing.

6. a. Infuse at 31 drops per minute.
   b. Infuse at 24 drops per minute.
   c. Infuse at 33 drops per minute.
   d. Infuse at 33 drops per minute.

7. IV bag or bottle every 24 hours; infusion set every 72 hours (or less)

8. The drip rate regulates the time over which the infusion is given; too much fluid over a short period of time will simply be excreted or will cause fluid volume overload; too little fluid may not meet the body's needs for fluid.

9. a. Apply pressure over the IV site for several minutes after removing the IV catheter
   b. Apply pressure just medial to the IV site for several minutes after removing the IV catheter.

10. a. IV infiltrated
    b. IV tubing kinked
    c. IV bag or bottle is hanging too low.
    d. Compression above the IV site by a tourniquet or BP cuff
    e. Particulate matter or clotted blood in the IV catheter or tubing

11. a. Warmth at the site
    b. Redness at the site
    c. Edema at the site
    d. Tenderness at the site

12. a. Edema at the site
    b. Coolness at the site
    c. Blanching of the site
    d. Tenderness at the site
    e. Slowing of the IV rate

13. a. Note location.
    b. Note IV device (type and size).
    c. Note dressing—is it clean and occlusive?
    d. Note date of insertion.
    e. Note appearance of site.
    f. Note if fluids are infusing and, if so, is rate correct?

MULTIPLE CHOICE

14. a, b, c

15. a, b, c

16. a, c, d

17. a, b, c

18. a, b

19. a

MODULE 48 ADMINISTERING INTRAVENOUS MEDICATIONS
SHORT-ANSWER QUESTIONS

1. Drug reference information should be reviewed. Always inject according to manufacturer's guidelines, but if none are given, a general rule may be that no syringe-held bolus should be given faster than 1 mL per minute.

2. Medication added to containers should be agitated because the medication could be trapped in the injection port, or it may separate and float either to the top or bottom of the bag depending on its viscosity.

3. a. Alter or negate the effects of the drug(s)
   b. Cause the patient to experience adverse reactions

4. a. Review the package insert information provided with the medication
   b. Review a drug reference for current information. Pharmacists can often provide information and current updates on medications.

5. To provide venous access without having to utilize continuously infusing fluids or medications to keep the vein patent

6. Syringe infusion pumps must have the syringe properly positioned in the pump to accurately dispense the medication.

7. To maintain a patent venous access so that blood does not flow back into the lock and clot, causing the IV to become nonfunctioning

8. They usually contain 50 to 100 mL.

MULTIPLE CHOICE

9. d

10. b, c

MODULE 49 CARING FOR PATIENTS WITH CENTRAL VENOUS CATHETERS
SHORT-ANSWER QUESTIONS

1. a. To permit the infusion of solutions that would be too irritating to peripheral veins
   b. When peripheral veins have been used extensively or are otherwise unsuitable for intravenous lines

2. a. Infection
   b. Air embolism

3. a. To allow for assessment of the entry site
   b. To thoroughly cleanse the area and remove debris
   c. To replace potentially contaminated dressings with sterile ones

4. To provide a chemical and mechanical barrier to microbes

5. Because it might easily be mistaken for a peripheral IV. This could have serious consequences.

6. The Hickman catheter has an internal diameter of 1.6 mm and can be used for drawing blood and administering nutrients, fluids, and medications. The Broviac catheter has an internal diameter of 1.0 mm and cannot be used for drawing blood but can be used for all infusions.

7. Repeated punctures of the cap with needles large enough to draw blood will damage the cap, leading to leakage.

8. To prevent air from entering and causing an air embolism

9. A noncoring needle (sometimes called a Huber needle)

MULTIPLE CHOICE

10. b, c, d

11. d

12. c

MODULE 50 INITIATING INTRAVENOUS THERAPY

SHORT-ANSWER QUESTIONS

1. a. May imply serious illness
   b. Pain
   c. Immobility

2. Any two of the following: to maintain daily fluid requirements, to replace past losses, to provide a large amount of fluid rapidly, to provide medication

3. Scalp; less chance of dislocation because there is less movement in that area

4. a. Applying a tourniquet or blood pressure cuff
   b. Hand pumping
   c. Placing arm in dependent position
   d. Applying warm, moist heat

5. Chlorhexidine gluconate

6. Use a back-and-forth movement with friction for 30 seconds

7. a. Date
   b. Time
   c. Type of device
   d. Catheter gauge
   e. Initials

8. a. The need for fluids is absent, but the need for IV access remains.
   b. The need for IV access is intermittent.

MULTIPLE CHOICE

9. c

10. a, b, c, d

MODULE 51 ADMINISTERING PARENTERAL NUTRITION

SHORT-ANSWER QUESTIONS

1. a. Total parenteral nutrition
   b. Partial parenteral nutrition

2. a. Intake and output
   b. Daily weight
   c. Blood glucose monitoring
   d. Vital signs

3. To allow the body to physiologically adapt to the increased dextrose concentrations

4. An infusion pump monitors and regulates precise fluid volumes.

5. Frequent incidence of phlebitis with higher dextrose concentrations

6. Due to the concentration of the parenteral nutrition solutions, they must be delivered to a large blood volume for rapid dilution.

MULTIPLE CHOICE

7. a

8. c

9. b

10. b

11. c

12. d

MODULE 52 ADMINISTERING BLOOD AND BLOOD COMPONENTS

SHORT-ANSWER QUESTIONS

1. a. A
   b. B
   c. AB
   d. O

2. Any four of the following are acceptable: acute hemolytic transfusion reaction, febrile nonhemolytic transfusion reaction, mild allergic (urticarial) transfusion reaction, anaphylactic transfusion reaction, circulatory overload, transfusion-related acute lung injury (TRALI), septic transfusion reaction related to bacterial contamination

3. Any four of the following symptoms are acceptable: fever, chills, hypotension, nausea, vomiting, tachycardia dyspnea, lower back pain, anxiety (sense of impending doom), hemoglobinemia (free hemoglobin in the plasma), red/dark urine (hemoglobinuria—free hemoglobin in the urine), vascular collapse, shock, unexplained bleeding, oliguria, acute renal failure, disseminated intravascular coagulation (DIC)

4. Symptomatic anemia

5. Any two of the following indications are acceptable: prevent bleeding in patients with severe thrombocytopenia, treat bleeding in patients with abnormal platelet function, treat bleeding in patients with thrombocytopenia

6. Bleeding due to hypofibrinogenemia

7. Stop the transfusion

MULTIPLE CHOICE

8. c
9. d
10. b
11. d
12. d
13. a
14. a
15. c

MODULE 53 ADMINISTERING EPIDURAL MEDICATIONS

SHORT-ANSWER QUESTIONS

1. a. To decrease the side effects and allow the patient to be more alert
   b. To allow lower doses of narcotics to be used

2. a. Identification of the catheter
   b. Observation for adverse reactions

3. A permanent catheter is dressed in the same way as an indwelling central intravenous catheter. A temporary catheter has an occlusive dressing that is not changed until the catheter is removed.

4. Any four of the following: respiratory depression, urinary retention, hypotension, pruritus, reversible paraparesis

5. Administer the ordered narcotic antagonist.

6. An antihistamine is given. If that is not successful, a narcotic antagonist is given in small incremental doses.

7. Patient reports abnormal sensations in the lower extremities that may include tingling and numbness.

8. It diminishes the pain relief.

MULTIPLE CHOICE

9. a, b, c
10. a
11. b, c, d

Standard Precautions

The following guidelines were developed to prevent the transmission of infection during patient care for all patients, regardless of known or unknown infectious status.

Hand Washing/Hand Hygiene

- Wash hands/perform hand hygiene after touching blood, body fluids, secretions, excretions, and contaminated items, whether or not gloves are worn.
- Wash hands/perform hand hygiene immediately after gloves are removed, between patient contacts, and when otherwise indicated to avoid transfer of microorganisms to other patients or environments.
- Wash hands/perform hand hygiene between tasks and procedures on the same patient to prevent cross-contamination of different body sites.
- Use a plain (nonantimicrobial) soap or alcohol-based hand rub for routine hand washing.
- Use an antimicrobial agent or waterless antiseptic agent for specific circumstances (control of outbreaks or hyper-endemic infections). (See Contact Precautions.)

Gloves

- Wear clean, nonsterile gloves when touching blood, body fluids, secretions, excretions, and contaminated items.
- Put on clean gloves just before touching mucous membranes and nonintact skin.
- Change gloves between tasks and procedures on the same patient after contact with materials that may contain a high concentration of microorganisms.
- Remove gloves promptly after use, before touching non-contaminated items and environmental surfaces, and before going to another patient.
- Wash hands/perform hand hygiene immediately after removing gloves.

Mask, Eye Protection, Face Shield

- Wear a mask and eye protection or a face shield to protect mucous membranes of the eyes, nose, and mouth during procedures and patient care activities that are likely to generate splashes or sprays of blood, body fluids, secretions, or excretions.

Gown

- Wear a clean, nonsterile gown to protect skin and prevent soiling of clothing during procedures and patient care activities that are likely to generate splashes or sprays of blood, body fluids, secretions, or excretions.

- Select a gown that is appropriate for the activity and amount of fluid likely to be encountered.
- Remove a soiled gown as promptly as possible and wash hands/perform hand hygiene to prevent the transfer of microorganisms to other patients or environments.

Patient Care Equipment

- Handle used patient care equipment soiled with blood, body fluids, secretions, and excretions in a manner that prevents skin and mucous membrane exposures, contamination of clothing, and transfer of microorganisms to other patients and environments.
- Ensure that reusable equipment is not used for the care of another patient until it has been cleaned and reprocessed appropriately.
- Ensure that single-use items are discarded properly.

Environmental Control

- Ensure that the hospital has adequate procedures for the routine care, cleaning, and disinfection of environmental surfaces, beds, bed rails, bedside equipment, and other frequently touched surfaces.
- Ensure that procedures are being followed.

Linen

- Handle, transport, and process used linen soiled with blood, body fluids, secretions, and excretions in a manner that prevents skin and mucous membrane exposures and contamination of clothing and that avoids transfer of microorganisms to other patients and environments.

Occupational Health and Bloodborne Pathogens

- Take care to prevent injuries when using needles, scalpels, and other sharp instruments or devices:
  When handling sharp instruments after procedures
  When cleaning used instruments
  When disposing of used needles
- Never recap used needles or otherwise manipulate them by using both hands or use any technique that involves directing the point of the needle toward any part of the body.
- Use either a one-handed scoop technique or a mechanical device designed for holding the needle sheath.
- Do not remove used needles from disposable syringes by hand and do not bend, break, otherwise manipulate used needles by hand.

(continued)

- Place used disposable syringes and needles, scalpel blades, and other sharp items in appropriate puncture-resistant containers as close as practical to the area in which the items were used.
- Place reusable syringes and needles in a puncture-resistant container for transport to the reprocessing area.
- Use mouthpieces, resuscitation bags, or other ventilation devices as an alternative to mouth-to-mouth resuscitation methods in areas where the need for resuscitation is predictable.

Patient Placement

- Place a patient who contaminates the environment or who does not or cannot be expected to assist in maintaining appropriate hygiene or environmental control in a private room.
- If a private room is not available, consult with infection control professionals regarding patient placement or other alternatives.

Adapted from (1996) Guideline for isolation precautions in hospitals. *Infection Control and Hospital Epidemiology, 17,* 53–80 and (2002). Guideline for hand hygiene in health-care settings. *Morbidity and Mortality Weekly Report, 51*(RR-16), 1–45.

Glossary

A

abdominal breathing—respirations in which the abdominal muscles and diaphragm are active; the abdomen moves out on inspiration and in on expiration; also called diaphragmatic breathing

abduction—the act of drawing away from the median line or center of the body

accommodation—the adaptation or adjustment of the lens of the eye to permit the retina to focus on images or objects at different distances

acetone—a colorless volatile solvent; commonly used as a synonym of ketone body; see ketone bodies

acid—a substance that ionizes in solution to free the hydrogen ion; turns litmus paper pink

acuity—the degree of seriousness of a person's illness

acute care—healthcare provided for a person who has a current problem that is expected to resolve within a limited time period

acute hemolytic transfusion reaction—the breakdown of red blood cells causing a systemic reaction by the body, most commonly the result of transfusing ABO–incompatible red blood cells

additive—a substance that is added to a medication or intravenous solution

adduction—the act of drawing toward the median line or center of the body

adherent—property of a material allowing it to stick to some other object or surface

adhesions—scar tissue that attaches surfaces within the body that are normally separate from one another

adhesive—sticky, adherent

ADLs—activities of daily living

advance directive—a legal document in which an individual makes known his or her wishes with regard to healthcare, especially with regard to the use of extraordinary measures at the end of life

adventitious sounds—abnormal sounds, as in the lungs

advocate—a person who speaks on behalf of another

aeration—exchanging oxygen and carbon dioxide between the blood and inspired air in the lungs

afebrile—without fever

affected—involved, such as the part of the body involved with pain or disease

agility—the state of being nimble or of moving with ease

AIDS (acquired immunodeficiency syndrome)—a viral disease of the immune system causing decreased immune function that can be transmitted through the blood and certain body substances of infected persons

Airborne Precautions—isolation precautions used for patients known or suspected to have serious illnesses in which infectious agents are transferred on droplet nuclei or dust particles that may remain suspended in the air and that spread easily on air currents

air embolism—a bubble of air moving within the circulatory system

air embolus—see air embolism

airway—the passageway by which air circulates in and out of the lungs; a device used, generally when a patient is not fully alert to prevent the tongue from slipping back and occluding the throat and air passages

alcohol-based hand rub—hand hygiene product that may be used for hand antisepsis throughout surgical procedures

algor mortis—the gradual decrease in body temperature that occurs as circulation slows and stops after death

alignment—arrangement of position in a straight line; used to refer to body parts being positioned so that they are in correct relationship with no twisting

alimentary—pertaining to nutritive material or to the digestive tract

alkaline—having characteristics of a base; neutralizes an acid

allergic transfusion reaction—reaction to a blood transfusion in which the recipient experiences an antibody reaction to allergens in the donor's blood, characterized by hives and itching, flushing, anxiety, breathing problems, and other discomfort

allergy—an abnormal body hypersensitivity to a specific antigen that is ordinarily harmless

allogeneic—pertaining to someone other than self

alternating pressure mattress—a plastic mattress attached to a motor that alternately inflates and deflates the tubular sections of the mattress so that the pressure against any one section of the patient's body changes constantly. It is placed over the regular mattress on the bed.

alveoli—air sacs of the lungs, at the termination of a bronchiole

AMA—against medical advice

ambient—surrounding; encircling; used to describe the normal air found in a room as ambient air

Ambu bag—a device composed of a face mask and a large bag made of a flexible material that is used to force air into the lungs using positive pressure

ambulate—to walk from place to place

ambulatory surgery—surgery during which a patient is admitted and discharged within a 24-hour period

amino acids—organic compounds containing both an amino (nitrogen) group and a carboxylic acid (carbohydrate-related) group that is the basic component of the protein molecule

amniotic—fluid within the uterus that surrounds the fetus

amoeba—any of various protozoans of the genus Amoeba and related genera, occurring in water, soil, and as internal animal parasites, characteristically having an indefinite, changeable form and moving by means of pseudopodia

ampule—a small, sealed, sterile glass container that usually holds a parenteral medication

analgesic—any substance that relieves pain

anal sphincter—the two ringlike muscles that close the anal orifice. One is called the external anal sphincter; the other, the internal anal sphincter. The actions of both sphincters control the evacuation of feces.

analysis—the process of critically examining data for patterns and cues to identify nursing diagnoses, collaborative problems, potential problems, and areas of strength or growth; the second phase of the nursing process

anaphylactic transfusion reaction—an immediate, life-threatening allergic reaction to allergens in a blood component; commonly causes respiratory distress and vascular collapse

anastomose—see anastomosis

anastomosis—surgical connection of two tubular organs

anatomic position—a body position in which body parts are in correct relation to one another and in which correct function is possible

aneroid manometer—an air-pressure gauge that indicates blood pressure by a pointer on a dial

anesthesia—the total or partial loss of sensation

anesthesiologist—a physician with special training in the science and skill of administering anesthetic agents

anesthetics—agents that affect nerve function; general anesthetics induce complete lack of consciousness and all sensation and motion; local or regional anesthetics induce a loss of sensation and motion in an area served by the nerves affected

anesthetist—a nonphysician who is skilled in administering anesthetic agents

anorectal—referring to the distal portion of the digestive tract, including the entire anal canal and the distal 2 centimeters of the rectum

anorexia—loss of appetite

anoxia—a pathologic deficiency of oxygen

antecubital space—a depression in the contour of the inner aspect of the elbow; also called antecubital fossa

anticoagulant—any substance that suppresses or counteracts coagulation, especially of the blood

antiembolism stockings—elastic compression stockings applied to lower extremities to promote venous return, also called compression stockings, support stockings, or TEDs

antiemetic—an agent used to prevent vomiting

antimicrobial—capable of destroying or suppressing the growth of microorganisms; agent that reduces bacterial counts

antineoplastic—an agent that inhibits the growth of abnormal cell tissues or neoplasms

antipyretic—a medication that lowers body temperature

antiseptic—agent with antimicrobial actions; any substance that halts the growth of microorganisms, not necessarily by killing them

apex—the narrow or cone-shaped portion of an organ; in the heart, the point located in the area of the midclavicular line near the fifth left intercostal space; in the lung, the narrower, more pointed, upper end

apheresis—obtaining blood components from a donor by withdrawing blood, circulating it through a machine that selectively collects the desired component, and then returning the remaining portion of the blood to the donor

apical—pertaining to the apex

apical pulse—the heartbeat heard through a stethoscope held over the apex of the heart

APIE charting—a problem-oriented style of documenting; A: assessment data regarding any problem, P: problems identified, I: interventions, and E: evaluation

apnea—absence of respiration

appliance—any device worn by a person to facilitate the meeting of basic needs; for example, any device worn to contain drainage from a stoma

approximated—touching; e.g., wound edges that are touching

armboard—a firm, flat, padded device that is used to straighten the arm and/or hand to keep an infusing intravenous line in place

arrhythmia—any irregularity in the force or rhythm of the heartbeat; also called dysrhythmia

ascending colon—the portion of the colon on the right side of the abdomen that extends from the junction of the small and large intestine to the first major flexion near the liver

ascites—an abnormal accumulation of serous fluid in the abdominal cavity

ascitic fluid—see ascites

aseptic—preventing contamination by microorganisms; see also surgical asepsis

asepto syringe—a medical instrument that is used to aspirate and instill a fluid. The tip is graduated in size so that it fits into tubings of various sizes; the rounded bulb is used to create suction to fill the barrel and pressure to expel the fluid.

asphyxiation—suffocation

aspirate—to inhale foreign matter into the lungs; also to draw fluid into a container by suction, see also aspiration

aspiration—inhalation of fluid or an object; also removal of gases or fluids by suction

aspiration pneumonia—pneumonia caused by aspirating foreign material, such as gastric contents into the lungs

assessment—the process of gathering data; the first step in the nursing process

asymmetry—inequality or difference in form or function on opposite sides of the body

atelectasis—alveolar collapse resulting in impaired gas exchange

auricle—the external part of the ear; the pinna

auscultation—listening with a stethoscope to the sounds produced by the body

auscultatory gap—during the measurement of blood pressure, a period when the Korotkoff sounds heard initially over the brachial artery disappear and then resume at a lower level as the pressure is reduced

autoclave—a device that establishes special conditions for sterilization by steam under high pressure

autologous transfusion—a blood transfusion of the person's own blood that was donated previously or recovered and processed during a surgical procedure

automated external defibrillator—a battery-operated, electronic device that can be attached to a nonresponsive person's chest to sense cardiac rhythm and administer a defibrillating shock automatically

autopsy—an examination of the body after death to determine the cause of death and to further scientific investigation

axilla—armpit; axillae (pl)

B

bacteria—single-celled plantlike microorganisms that can cause disease

ball-and-socket joint—a joint in which a ball-shaped end of a bone rests in a socketlike cavity; examples are the shoulder and hip

barrel—in a syringe, the cylinder that holds the fluid

barrier—anything that acts to obstruct or prevent passage; a boundary or limit

base—the broad or wide end of an organ; in the heart, the area located at the second left and right intercostal spaces at the sternal borders; in the lungs, the wide lower end

base of support—that which makes up the foundation of an object or person and supports the weight

bedboard—a thin board, often hinged for easy use and storage, that is placed underneath a mattress to provide a firmer sleeping surface

bed cradle—an archlike device (like an inverted cradle) designed to keep bed linens off the feet and lower legs of patients, particularly those with edema, leg ulcers, burns, or surgical wounds on the lower extremities

bedpan—a metal or plastic receptacle for the elimination needs of bedridden persons

bell—on the stethoscope, the cone-shaped head that is most often used for listening to heart sounds

bevel—on a needle, the slanting end that contains the opening

bifurcation—the point at which a structure divides or separates into two parts or branches

bilirubin—a yellowish pigment that is derived from the destruction of hemoglobin

binder—a type of bandage, worn snugly around the trunk or body part to provide support

biopsy—procedure by which a tissue specimen is removed for laboratory analysis

bivalving—the process of using a cast saw to cut a cast in half lengthwise when the cast causes skin problems or undue pressure. The two parts of the cast are then held together by an elastic bandage when the patient is moving.

bladder scan—ultrasonic test procedure that measures the volume of urine being retained in the bladder

bloodborne—referring to those microorganisms that are transported by blood and specific body fluids such as semen, vaginal secretions, and spinal fluid

body language—conveying thoughts or meanings through the posturing or positioning of the body

body mechanics—the analysis of the action of forces on the body parts during activity

Body Substance Precautions—a set of behaviors designed to prevent the transmission of micro-organisms that are transported by any body substance such as urine, saliva, and feces; a term largely replaced by the use of Standard Precautions

body substances—fluids and moist matter created by the body, such as feces, urine, nasal secretions, vomit, blood, and sputum

bolus—a measured amount of medication delivered at one time, usually into a vein or intravenous device

bone marrow—soft material that fills the cavities of bones and contains blood forming cells

bounding pulse—a body pulse that strikes the fingers with excessive strength

bowel impaction—hardened, dry feces in the rectum that the person is unable to pass

brachial artery—an artery that supplies blood to the shoulder, arm, forearm, and hand

bradycardia—an abnormally slow heartbeat, usually defined as below 60 beats/minute

bradypnea—respirations that are regular in rhythm but slower than normal in rate (usually below 12 respirations/minute in the adult). Bradypnea may be normal during sleep.

breathing—inhaling and exhaling air

bronchi—the branches of the trachea that lead directly to the lungs

bronchial—pertaining to or affecting one or more bronchi; see bronchi

bronchioles—the fine, thin-walled, tubular branches of a bronchus

bronchoscopy—a diagnostic and therapeutic procedure performed by a physician to observe the bronchial structures; insertion of a bronchoscope through the patient's mouth down into the bronchus to visualize abnormalities and remove secretions

Broviac catheter—a single-lumen intravenous catheter with an internal diameter of 1.0 mm designed to be surgically implanted into a large central vein

bruit—an abnormal sound that results from circulatory turbulence

buccal—pertaining to the cheeks or oral cavity

butterfly—a type of tape that is used to secure two wound edges together; a device that is used to start intravenous infusions; named for its plastic "wings," which are used to secure the device in place

button—a small, round, plastic device that is used to plug a tracheostomy opening

C

cachexia—extreme wasting of the body

cane—a rehabilitative device used as an aid in walking

cannula—a tube that is inserted into a bodily cavity to drain fluid or to insert medication; a tubing used to deliver oxygen to the nostrils; an intravenous access device

canthus—the corner at either side of the eye that is formed by the meeting of the upper and lower eyelids. The inner canthus is the corner next to the nose; the outer canthus is the corner to the outside of the face.

capnogram—a graphic readout of carbon dioxide throughout the ventilation cycle

capnography—a mechanism that measures carbon dioxide in expired air

capsule—a soluble gelatinous sheath that encases a dose of oral medication

carbon dioxide—colorless, odorless gas formed during metabolic processes and expelled in normal breathing

cardiac arrest—cessation of heart action

cardiac output—the amount of blood pumped by the heart in a minute; the volume pumped in each stroke times the number of beats per minute. In the normal resting adult, it is usually 2.5 to 3.6 L/minute.

cardiac sphincter—a circular muscle between the esophagus and the stomach that opens at the approach of food; the food then moves into the stomach as a result of peristalsis

caries—decayed matter of bone or tooth

cariogenic—that which contributes to the formation of dental caries

carotid artery—either of the two major arteries in the neck that carry blood to the head

carotid pulse—the wave of blood that is palpable as it passes through the carotid artery

cast padding—a "waffled" padding, consisting of soft, thin cotton layers between two outer layers of closely woven cotton, used to provide cushioning between the patient's skin and a cast

catheter—a slender flexible tube of metal, rubber, or plastic that is inserted into a body channel or cavity to distend or maintain an opening; often used to drain or to instill fluids

catheterization—see catheterize

catheterize—insertion of a catheter to drain or instill fluid

catheter-tip syringe—any syringe that has a smooth, funnel-type tip to allow it to fit tightly into any type of tubing

caustic—able to burn, corrode, dissolve, or otherwise eat away by chemical action

cauterize—a technique that uses high heat to coagulate protein, thereby sealing blood vessels or cutting through tissue

cecostomy—a surgically devised opening directly from the cecum to the abdominal wall

Celsius—a temperature scale, devised by Anders Celsius, that registers the freezing point of water at 0°C and the boiling point at 100°C under normal atmospheric pressure; also called centigrade

center of gravity—a point in an object or person at which gravitational pull functions as if the entire weight of the object or person were at that single point

centigrade—see Celsius

central venous catheter (CVC)—an intravenous catheter inserted into a central vein, such as the subclavian or the internal jugular vein, to deliver therapeutic drugs or fluids to the central circulation

cephalic vein—a large superficial vein of the upper arm

cerebrospinal fluid (CSF)—the serum-like fluid that bathes the lateral ventricles of the brain and the cavity of the spinal cord

cerumen—a yellowish waxy secretion of the external ear; earwax

cervical collar—a device worn around the neck that prevents flexion, extension, and rotation of the cervical spine and supports the head; may be constructed of foam rubber or rigid plastic

cervical traction—traction applied to the cervical spine by the use of weights attached by ropes to either skull tongs or a chin harness

chart—the official, legal record of healthcare

charting by exception—a documentation method that may use a flow chart to reduce time spent writing; normal findings may be indicated on the chart by a symbol, such as a checkmark, and only abnormal findings are described

Cheyne-Stokes respirations—a cyclic pattern of respirations that gradually increase in depth followed by respirations that gradually decrease in depth, with a short period of apnea between cycles

chronic wound—a wound, such as an ulcer resulting from poor circulation, that fails to exhibit healing and persists over a long time

circadian rhythm—the approximately 24-hour cyclic pattern of rest and activity in humans

circular bandage—a bandage wrapped in circular fashion, overlapping several times to encircle an affected body part

circulation—movement of blood, lymph, and other fluids throughout the body

circulatory overload—a situation in which the volume of fluid circulating in the body is more than the heart can handle adequately; overload can develop if a large amount of blood or fluid is infused in a short period

circumcise—to surgically remove the prepuce (foreskin) of the penis

circumduction—a circular movement of the eye or of a body part such as the head

citrated blood—blood that is prevented from coagulating by the presence of citrate-phosphate-dextrose or acid-citrate-dextrose

claustrophobia—a pathologic fear of confined places

Clinitron bed—a special bed with a mattress filled with ceramic beads that move constantly when air is blown through them, thereby eliminating continuous pressure on any one body point and minimizing shear during movement while decreasing pain

clockwise—the direction in which the hands of a clock move

closed suctioning—a type of sterile suctioning system that is connected to the patient continuously and is changed every 24 to 72 hours

clove hitch—a knot that consists of two turns, with the second held under the first

CMS (circulation, motion, and sensation)—abbreviation that denotes the focus of a neurovascular assessment of an extremity

collaborative problem—a patient's problem that the nurse must assess for, identify when present, and report to the physician for treatment

colonoscopy—visual examination of the colon with a flexible fiberoptic instrument called a colonoscope; may include obtaining tissue samples for analysis

colostomy—a surgically devised opening directly from the large intestine to the abdominal wall

comatose—unconscious

combustion—process whereby burning occurs

commode—a portable toileting device that resembles a chair on wheels and a seat that lifts to reveal a recessed pan or container for the collection of urine and feces

common vehicle transmission—term used to denote the mode by which diseases are transmitted by food or water

communication—the process by which information is shared from one person or group or one cell to another

compartment syndrome—a pathologic condition that occurs when there is increased tissue pressure within a limited space (e.g., muscle compartment). It is caused by the progressive development of arterial and nerve compression and reduced blood supply.

compatibility testing—testing performed to select compatible red blood cell–containing components (e.g., whole blood, red blood cells, granulocytes); testing includes determination of ABO group and Rh type, antibody screen, and crossmatch

compatible—capable of integrating and/or agreeing with; not causing complications

complete blood count (CBC)—measurement that establishes the values of a variety of components of the blood, usually including red blood cell count, white blood cell count, hemoglobin, and hematocrit

compression-only CPR—delivery of chest compressions without rescue breathing for the person who has suffered cardiopulmonary arrest

compression stockings—stockings designed to provide compression to the lower extremities and thus aid venous return, also called anti-embolic stockings, support stockings or TEDs

compromised host—a person with a suppressed immune system, who is therefore less capable of self-protection against pathogens

computerized order entry (COE)—an electronic method for physician orders to be input directly into the computer by the physician

computerized record—a mechanism for documenting data regarding a patient through the use of a computer file

concentration of solution—the amount of a specified substance in a unit amount of another substance; may be expressed as a percentage (20% solution), or as a ratio (1:1000), or as a weight in a fluid amount (100 mg/L)

concurrent—happening at the same time or place

condyloid joint—a joint in which a knuckle-shaped end of a bone rests in an oval depression; examples are the wrist, fingers (excluding the thumb), and toes

confidentiality—the right to have personal matters kept private

conjunctival sac—the saclike inner fold of membrane on the lower eyelid

consensual reaction—when both pupils move and focus together

consent—to make a personal decision regarding any healthcare

consolidation—the process of becoming solid or the condition of being solid; used to describe the lung as it fills with exudate in pneumonia

constriction—a feeling of pressure or tightness

Contact Precautions—isolation precautions used when the infectious agent can be spread by contact with the patient's skin or by surfaces within the room

contaminate—to introduce microorganisms to an object or person

contaminated—having been in contact with microorganisms

contamination—presence of potentially pathogenic microorganisms

continent urinary reservoir (CUR)—a surgical procedure in which a portion of the ileum is used to create a bladderlike structure for the collection of urine; a "nipple" valve on the skin surface allows intermittent self-catheterization

continuous bladder irrigation (CBI)—a method that uses continuous flow of an irrigant to maintain patency of a urinary catheter

contracture—a shortening of a muscle that causes distortion or deformity of a joint

contraindicate—to indicate the inadvisability of an action—for example, in treatment

convergence—two objects moving toward one another; e.g., when both pupils follow a point as it moves closer to the nose and both move medially (toward the nose)

coroner—a public officer whose primary function is to investigate by inquest any death thought to result from other than natural causes

cough reflex—an involuntary nerve response that causes a cough

counterbalance—using your weight and the patient's weight as a balance to assist in lifting or moving

counterclockwise—opposite of clockwise; see clockwise

countertraction—exerting pull in opposition to a traction system

crackles—a sound similar to hair strands being rubbed together that is heard upon auscultation of the lungs and indicates moisture in small airways

cradle—see bed cradle

cranium—the portion of the skull that encloses the brain

critical care—healthcare provided for acute, life-threatening illness

critical thinking—organized, purposeful, disciplined thinking focused on deciding what to believe or do; both an attitude and an approach to ideas and decisions

crutch—a staff or support that is used as an aid in walking; usually has a crosspiece that fits under the armpit and often used in pairs

culture—the growing of microorganisms in a nutrient medium

culture and sensitivity (C&S)—a laboratory test in which a swab or smear of specimen tissue is placed in a nutrient medium to allow microorganisms to grow. If microorganisms do grow, the culture is then tested with various antibiotics to determine whether the microorganisms are sensitive to the effects of these antibiotics. If the antibiotic destroys the microorganism, the microorganism is considered sensitive to the antibiotic. If the microorganism is not destroyed, it is considered to be resistant.

cyanotic—the presence of a bluish discoloration of the skin due to oxygen deficiency

cycling—occurring in a pattern of regular repeated events; usually refers to total parenteral nutrition or tube feeding schedules in which the daily intake is provided during a set number of hours followed by a number of hours without feeding

cytology—study of cells; a laboratory test in which cells are examined microscopically

D

dangling—rising in bed from a supine position to a sitting position and allowing the legs to dangle over the side of the bed to prevent dizziness (orthostatic hypotension) upon transfer to a standing position, or a chair, or the like

DARP charting—documentation in progress notes, which is keyed to emphasize **d**ata, **a**ction, **r**esponse, and **p**lan

data—information, especially material that is organized for analysis or used as a basis for decision-making

dead-air space—the portion of the airway in which gas exchange does not take place

debride—to remove dead or necrotic tissue from the surface of a wound

deceased—complete cessation of respiration, heartbeat, and blood pressure; dead

decubitus ulcer—a lesion of superficial tissue caused by pressure that interferes with blood supply, specifically one caused by remaining in a decubitus (lying) position for prolonged time; also called a pressure ulcer

defecation—the act of expelling bowel contents

defibrillation—stopping irregular contractions of the heart and restoring normal rhythm by means of drugs or electric shock

dehiscence—unintentional wound edge separation; the splitting or bursting open of a wound, usually of the abdomen

dependent edema—see edema

depilatory—chemical hair removal agent

dermatologic—pertaining to the skin

descending colon—the portion of the colon on the left side of the abdomen that extends from the major flexion at the spleen to the point where the colon again flexes into the sigmoid portion

descending colostomy—a colostomy performed on a portion of the descending colon

dexterity—skill in the use of the hands

dextrose—a simple sugar found in animal and plant tissue; also called glucose

dialysis cannula—a surgically inserted tube that provides access to the circulatory system for hemodialysis

diaphoresis—perspiration, especially copious or medically induced perspiration

diaphragm—a muscular membranous partition that separates the abdominal and thoracic cavities and that functions in respiration; on a stethoscope, the flat, drumlike head that is used most often for listening to lung and bowel sounds

diarrhea—pathologically excessive evacuation of watery feces

diastole—the normal rhythmically recurring relaxation and dilatation of the heart cavities during which the cavities are filled with blood

diastolic blood pressure—the lowest pressure reached in the arteries during the heart's resting phase, identified by the cessation of Korotkoff sounds

digestion—process by which food is converted into substances that can be absorbed by the gastrointestinal system

digital—pertaining to a finger; e.g., a digital examination is one carried out with a finger

dignity—inherent worth; worthy of respect

dilation—the condition of being enlarged or stretched

diluent—a substance that is used to dilute or dissolve

discharge planner—the professional who takes primary responsibility for planning for referrals for home healthcare or nursing home placement and assists with locating resources for care

disinfect—to clean or rid of pathogenic organisms

disinfectant—agent (or process) that destroys, neutralizes, or inhibits the growth of pathogenic microorganisms other than spores

disinfection—see disinfectant

displacement—the act whereby a substance is replaced by another either in weight or in volume

distal—in anatomy, located far from the origin or line of attachment

distention—bloat and turgidity from pressure within; usually refers to the stomach, bowel, or bladder; may also refer to the dilated blood vessel when filled with blood

diuresis—the increased production and output of urine

diuretic—a drug that increases the production and output of urine

diversion—re-routing, deviation; in regard to controlled substances, indicates use for other than the intended recipient

donor—one who donates blood, tissue, or an organ for use in a transfusion or transplant

dorsal recumbent position—a position in which the person lies on the back with knees bent

dorsalis pedis—an artery located on the top of the foot, used for palpating the pedal pulse

dorsiflexion—bending or moving a part toward the dorsum or back

dose—a specified quantity of a therapeutic agent, prescribed to be taken at one time or at stated intervals

double-barrel colostomy—a colostomy in which there are two openings—one that leads to the proximal colon and one that leads to the distal colon

double T-binder—a binder with two tails that is used to hold a dressing in place on the perineum of a male patient so that the testicles are not restricted

droplet nuclei—microscopic particles (5 microns or less) that become airborne when surrounded by moisture and that may carry infectious agents to be dispersed widely by air currents

Droplet Precautions—isolation precautions used when infectious agents are transferred on large particle droplets (which tend to settle out of the air rapidly)

droplets—moist particles spread into the air when an individual coughs, sneezes, or even talks or from equipment for suctioning. They may carry infectious agents. Droplets are large, quickly settle out of the air, and are different from droplet nuclei.

dullness—in reference to percussion, not sharp or intense

dura—the outermost of the three membranes covering the spinal cord and brain

dysphagia—difficulty in swallowing

dyspnea—difficulty in breathing

E

edema—an excessive accumulation of serous fluid in the tissues. Dependent edema is fluid that has accumulated in the lower areas of the body due to gravity; periorbital edema is fluid that has accumulated in the soft tissue around the eyes; and pretibial edema is fluid that has accumulated over the tibia.

effluent—a substance that flows out; general term used to refer to any of the different substances that may flow out of the various types of ostomies

egg crate mattress—a foam mattress that has rounded projections and indentations resembling an egg crate; used to diminish pressure on tissues

elastic bandage—bandage constructed of a heavy, stretchable material; usually applied to an extremity, providing pressure

electroencephalogram (EEG)—a record or tracing of brain waves; product of electroencephalography

electroencephalography—see electroencephalogram

electrolyte—substance that dissociates into ions in solution; in the body, electrolytes are critically important chemicals

elemental feeding—nutrients for use in tube feeding that can be absorbed without the need for further digestion

embolus—a moving particle in the bloodstream

emulsify—to combine two solutions that do not normally mix into one liquid, resulting in a suspension of globules

endoscopy—procedure for visualizing the interior of a bodily canal or a hollow organ such as the colon, bladder, or stomach

endotracheal tube—a rubber or plastic tube that is placed in the trachea to keep the airway open

enema—solution that is instilled directly into the rectum and large intestine to dilate and irritate the intestinal mucosa, increasing peristalsis and promoting evacuation of feces and flatus

enteral—within the gastrointestinal tract

enteral feedings—nutrients given by way of a tube passed into the gastrointestinal tract, through the nose, or directly into the stomach or jejunum

enteric—referring to the small intestine

enterostomal therapist—a person, often a nurse, with specialized preparation in the care of individuals with ostomies and skin management problems

epidural—outside of the dura mater that covers the brain and spinal cord

epigastrium—the upper middle region of the abdomen

epithelial—related to the cellular surface of the skin or mucous membrane

epithelialization—the process by which the body creates epithelial tissue for wound healing

ergonomics—the science of fitting a task to a person's anatomic and physiologic characteristics in order to enhance efficiency and well-being

erythrocyte—red blood cell

esophagus—the portion of the gastrointestinal tract that extends from the pharynx, through the chest, to the stomach

estimated blood loss (EBL)—an estimate of blood lost during surgery; data of importance to nurses in the postanesthesia care unit

ethical—pertaining to or dealing with principles of right and wrong

ethical rights—rights that the healthcare community recognizes as important to the patient's well-being but that may not be included in actual laws

ethmoid sinus—the open cavity in the ethmoid bone that lies between the eyes and forms part of the nasal cavity

ethnic—characteristic of a religious, racial, national, or cultural group

eupnea—normal, unlabored respirations

eustachian tube—narrow opening that connects the middle ear to the pharynx that serves to equalize pressure on either side of the tympanic membrane

evaluation—the process of determining the outcomes of a course of action

eversion—turned in an outward direction

evisceration—internal organ protrusion after dehiscence occurs

exception—something that does not conform to normal rules or situations

excoriate—to chafe or wear off the skin

excoriation—breakdown of the outer surface of the skin characterized by redness, inflammation, and abrasion

excretion—the process of eliminating waste matter, such as feces, urine, or sweat

exhalation—breathing out

expectorate—to eject from the mouth; spit

expiration—exhalation; also death

explosive—pertaining to a sudden, rapid, violent release of energy

extension—the act of straightening a joint

external disaster—a disaster occurring in the community that may affect the medical facility

external fixation device—a system of pins and wires passing through bone and connected to a rigid external metal frame consisting of circular rings with interconnecting rods that hold fractured bone in place

external rotation—moving a body part outward on an axis

extravasation—movement of intravenous fluid out of the vascular system; often used to refer to the inadvertent administration of a vesicant medication into the tissues

exudate—fluid drainage from cells

F

face shield—a barrier that protects the face from splashed fluids

Fahrenheit—a temperature scale that registers the freezing point of water at 32°F and the boiling point at 212°F under normal atmospheric pressure

fanfold—to fold or gather in accordion fashion; for example, the top linen of a bed toward the bottom or one side

fat emulsions—a form of fats in which the particles are finely disbursed so as to form a smooth fluid; sometimes referred to as lipids

febrile—having an elevated body temperature

febrile nonhemolytic transfusion reaction—reaction that occurs when the recipient is sensitive to white blood cells or plasma proteins in the transfused blood component; primarily manifested by fever and chills

feces—waste matter excreted from the bowels

femoral artery—either of the two large arteries that carry blood to the lower abdomen, the pelvis, and the lower extremities, femoral pulse is counted at the groin over a femoral artery

fenestrated tracheostomy tube—a tracheostomy tube that allows air to pass through the larynx, allowing the individual to talk while the tracheostomy tube is in place

fever—abnormally high body temperature

fiberglass cast—a "light" cast, made of fiberglass, that is impermeable to water

fibrin—an insoluble protein essential to clotting of blood

fibrinogen—a protein found in the plasma of the blood that is converted into fibrin, which is essential to the blood clotting process

figure-eight bandage—a bandage that is wrapped around a body part in a figure-eight configuration

finger stick—a lancing method used to obtain a drop of blood for testing by piercing the tip of the finger

first intention healing—uncomplicated wound healing that occurs when tissue is constructed between two wound surfaces that touch; see primary intention healing

fixation—holding an object in a fixed position. Used to refer to holding broken bones in a correctly aligned position for healing

flaccid—lacking firmness; soft and limp; flabby

flashback—blood return in the hub or tubing that indicates the IV catheter is in the vein

flatness—in percussion, a short high-pitched sound without resonance or vibration

flatus—gas generated in the stomach or intestines and expelled through the anus

flexion—bending of a joint

flow chart—see flow sheet

flowmeter—a mechanical device that monitors the flow of oxygen or other gases or liquids

flow sheet—also called flow chart; a schematic representation of a sequence of operations or events

fluid balance—a state in which the fluid intake and output are approximately equivalent

fluid overload—a situation in which there is more fluid in the circulatory system than it can handle; also called circulatory overload

focus charting—style of charting in which narrative notes are organized by entering an area of concern such as a body system or need and the entering data, actions, and evaluation related to that area

Foley catheter—a rubber urethral catheter with an inflatable balloon at its end; when inflated, the balloon holds the catheter in place

footboard—a board or small raised platform against which the feet of a patient in bed are supported or rested

footdrop—the abnormal permanent plantar flexion of the foot that results from paralysis or injury to the flexor muscles

footrest—a canvas sling or padded bar at the distal end of a leg cast used to support the foot; the small platforms attached to a wheelchair that support the feet

foreign-body airway obstruction (FBAO)— airway occluded by a foreign body, such as meat or a bone; may be life-threatening

foreskin—the loose fold of skin that covers the glans of the penis; the prepuce

Fowler's position—a position in which the patient is in bed on his or her back with the head elevated approximately 60 degrees (also called mid-Fowler's position). Traditionally, knees were also elevated, but this is seldom done today. The degree of elevation of the head can vary: in semi-Fowler's position (low Fowler's position), the head is at a 30-degree angle from the horizontal; in high Fowler's position, the head is as close to 90 degrees as possible.

fracture pan—a container of metal or plastic with a lower edge, or lip, than a conventional bedpan; used for purposes of elimination by bedridden patients, especially those with a fractured hip or in a cast

friction—the rubbing of one object or surface against another

full weight-bearing (FWB)—act of bearing full weight on a body part, such as the leg or legs

funeral director—a licensed person who is responsible for a body from the time of death until ultimate disposition; see mortician

funeral home—a place where the deceased are prepared for burial or cremation; see mortuary

G

gag reflex—a reflex action that results in gagging or vomiting when the pharynx is stimulated

gait—a way of moving on foot; a particular fashion of walking or running

gait (transfer) belt—a strong, webbing belt with a safety release buckle used to provide support for a patient during transfer and ambulation; sometimes called a transfer and ambulation belt or simply a transfer belt

gastric gavage—introducing a feeding by tube into the stomach

gastric secretions—enzymes produced by the glands of the lining of the stomach that digest certain components in food. Examples are hydrochloric acid and pepsin

gastric sump tube (Salem)—a gastric intubation tube having two lumens; one is used to apply suction, and the second is used to provide an air vent to limit the level of suction that can be applied

gastrostomy—a surgical opening into the stomach; usually for feeding by tube

gatched bed—a hospital bed that can be bent and raised at the knee area

gauge—a measurement of the diameter of a cylinder, used to indicate the size of a needle; a large number indicates a smaller diameter

gauze bandage—a bandage of a soft, meshlike material. This type of bandage is usually used to wrap a part of the body; the material may or may not be stretchable.

gavage—feeding by means of a tube

generic name—in reference to drugs, the name assigned to a chemical compound by the federal Food and Drug Administration; example of a drug known by its generic name is aspirin

genital area—the body area that contains the external reproductive organs

genitalia—external male or female reproductive organs

girth—the distance around a body part, usually referring to the abdomen

gliding joint—a joint in which a bone glides over the surface of another. The foot and vertebrae of the spine have gliding joints.

glucose—a dextrose sugar

gluteal settings—an isometric exercise that involves contraction of the gluteal muscles where there is little or no movement. The desired benefit for the immobile person is increased venous blood flow. On a long-term basis, the exercise may contribute to increased muscle mass, tone, and strength.

goggles—a barrier device to protect the eyes from splashed fluids

gooseneck lamp—an adjustable lamp with a slender flexible shaft

granulation—the process by which new tissue forms on the surface of a wound

graphic record—refers to a graph, such as one used to refer to the record of temperature, pulse, and respiration

gravida—a pregnant woman; used with numerals to designate the number of pregnancies a woman has had regardless of outcome

gravity—the force exerted by the earth on any object, tending to pull the object toward the center of the earth

green cast—a cast that is still damp or not thoroughly hardened

Groshong catheter—a central venous catheter that is inserted surgically and emerges from a subcutaneous tunnel on the chest; characterized by a special tip that eliminates the need for heparin to maintain patency of the catheter

guaiac—a natural resin that is used as a reagent to test for blood in specimens, often used to refer to any test for occult blood in a specimen

guarding—muscle rigidity that may occur because the patient is nervous or ticklish, or it may indicate an acute inflammatory process

gurgles—a bubbling sound of moisture in large airways heard upon auscultation of the lungs

H

hairline fracture—a simple fracture of a bone that is not displaced; shows on x-ray films as a "hairline" image

healing ridge—ridge that is visible about 4 days after surgery or an injury; the body molds the ridge into a flatter scar as healing progresses

Health Insurance Portability and Accountability Act (HIPAA)—federal legislation that contains requirements for protecting the privacy of individual protected health information

healthcare system—all the individuals, organizations, and agencies that provide health services and health financing considered as a whole

health status—a person's level of ability in meeting his or her own needs

Heimlich maneuver—an emergency procedure (also called subdiaphragmatic abdominal thrusts) devised for relieving foreign body airway obstruction

Hematest—a brand name for a product that is used to detect blood in fecal specimens; commonly used to refer to the test itself

hematuria—blood in the urine

hemodilution—the dilution of blood by other fluids; done purposefully before surgery when a patient's blood is donated and then replaced with intravenous fluids. The donated blood is returned to the patient during or after the surgical procedure as replacement for the diluted blood lost during surgery.

hemolytic reaction—a reaction in which red blood cells are broken down as a result of incompatibility of the donor's red blood cells and the recipient's red blood cells

hemophilia—a hereditary, plasma-coagulation disorder principally affecting males but transmitted by females and characterized by excessive, sometimes spontaneous bleeding

hemophiliac—a person who suffers from hemophilia

hemopneumothorax—presence of blood and air in the pleural space

hemorrhage—excessive bleeding

hemostasis—prevention or limiting of bleeding

hemothorax—presence of blood in the pleural space

heparin lock—a device filled with heparinized saline anticoagulant solution, used to provide ready access to a vein, making an infusing IV line unnecessary; also called IV lock

heparinoid—any of several compounds closely related to heparin given for similar indication but less likely to cause some adverse effects

hepatitis—inflammation of the liver, caused by infectious or toxic agents, characterized by jaundice and usually accompanied by fever and other systemic manifestations

Hickman catheter—an intravenous catheter with an internal lumen diameter of 1.6 mm designed to be surgically implanted into a large central vein. Both single- and multiple-lumen models are available.

hinge joint—a joint in which the convex end of one bone rests on the concave surface of another; examples are the elbow, knee, and ankle

HIPAA—Health Insurance Portability and Accountability Act; an act of the federal government that provides standards for ensuring patient privacy in regard to healthcare

Homans' sign—pain in the dorsal calf when the foot is firmly flexed; may be indicative of thrombophlebitis

homeostasis—the tendency of all living tissue to restore and maintain itself in a condition of balance or equilibrium

horizontal—parallel to or in the plane of the horizon

hub—on a needle, the portion that attaches to a syringe or tubing

humerus—the long bone of the upper part of the arm, extending from the shoulder to the elbow

humidifier—an apparatus that increases the humidity in a room; device that moisturizes air

hydraulic—moved or operated by a fluid, especially water under pressure

hydrogen peroxide—a colorless, strongly oxidizing liquid made of hydrogen and oxygen

hydrometer—instrument used to determine specific gravity

hyperalimentation—nutrition provided outside of the alimentary tract; another term for parenteral nutrition; the introduction of nutrients into a large vein

hypercalcemia—an excessive amount of calcium in the serum; greater than 10.5 mg/dL

hyperextension—extension of the joint beyond the straight position

hyperglycemia—an excessive amount of glucose in the blood; greater than 120 mg/100 mL

hyperkalemia—an excessive amount of potassium in the blood; greater than 5 mEq/L

hypertonic—having a higher osmotic pressure than body fluid, causes fluid to shift from the compartment of lower osmotic pressure to the compartment of higher osmotic pressure

hyperventilation—abnormally fast or deep respiration in which excessive quantities of air are taken in and excessive carbon dioxide is expelled, causing buzzing in the ears, tingling of the extremities, and sometimes fainting

hypocalcemia—a deficit in calcium in the blood, less than 4.5 mEq/L

hypostatic pneumonia—pneumonia caused by lack of movement

hypothermia—a condition in which body temperature is lower than that necessary for body processes to function adequately

hypotonic—having a lower osmotic pressure than body fluid, causes fluid to shift from the compartment of lower osmotic pressure to the compartment of higher osmotic pressure

hypoventilation—abnormally slow or shallow respirations that result in inadequate air movement and thus inadequate oxygenation

hypovolemic shock—a state of shock that is caused by an abnormally low volume of body plasma

hypoxemia—inadequate oxygenation of the blood

hypoxia—an oxygen deficiency of body tissues

I

ileobladder—see ileoconduit

ileoconduit—a type of urinary diversion, a surgically constructed pathway for urinary drainage in which a segment of ileum is detached from the rest of the bowel, the ureters are attached to this ileal segment, and one end of the segment is closed while the other opens onto the abdomen in a single stoma; also called ileobladder and ileoloop

ileoloop—see ileoconduit

ileostomy—a surgically devised opening from the ileum to the abdominal wall, the drainage of which is liquid and contains some digestive enzymes

iliac crest—the highest portion of the broad rim of the hip bone

immunosuppression—the suppression of the body's natural immune system by drugs or disease

impaction—compressed material in a confined space; for example, hardened feces in the bowel

implementation—the carrying out of a plan of action; the fourth step of the nursing process

implied consent—agreement to a procedure or program that is implied by a persons previous actions or statements

increased intracranial pressure—a state of higher than normal pressure within the cranium

incubate—to provide conditions for growth; to warm to promote development and reproduction of microorganisms

induration—swelling, hardening

indwelling catheter—a catheter that remains in place over a long time

inferior vena cava—the large vein that returns blood to the heart from the lower body

infiltration—leaking of fluid from an intravenous line into the tissue surrounding the vein

inflammation—localized heat, redness, swelling, and pain as a result of irritation, injury, or infection

inflatable cuff—a plastic balloonlike device, such as the one around a tracheostomy tube that, when filled with air, expands, creating a closed system through the tracheostomy tube and into the lungs

informed consent—consent given when a person has sufficient information to make a decision with an adequate understanding of both the benefits and potential adverse consequences

Infus-a-port—trade name of a surgically inserted, subcutaneous central venous access port for delivery of fluids and medication

infused—introduced into the body through a vein

infuser—a device used to provide multiple subcutaneous injections; consists of a needle or catheter that is placed into the subcutaneous tissue and is connected to a small port attached to the skin into which the injection can be given

infusion—solution introduced into a blood vessel; commonly, a vein

infusion pump—a mechanical device used to control the rate and volume of fluids administered parenterally

ingested—see ingestion

ingestion—intake of food, liquids, or other substances by swallowing

inpatient—a person who has been admitted to an acute care facility

inspection—a careful, critical visual examination

inspiration—the act of breathing in; inhalation

instill—to pour in drop by drop; commonly used to indicate very slow fluid introduction

instillation—the process of pouring in drop by drop; commonly used to indicate a slow process of introducing fluid

integument—skin

intensive care unit (ICU)—an area of a hospital set aside for the care of the critically ill

intercostal space—the space between the ribs

interdigital—between the fingers (digits)

intermittent—stopping and starting at intervals

intermittent infusion adapter—a device used to convert a regular intravenous needle into a IV lock; see heparin lock

internal disaster—a disaster occurring within the medical facility

internal rotation—moving a body part inward on an axis

intracranial pressure—the pressure maintained within the enclosed skull or cranium. When pressure is greater than normal, the term increased intracranial pressure is used.

intradermal—injected into the skin layers

intramuscular (IM)—injected into the muscle tissue

intraoperative—occurring during the surgery; inside the operating room

intravenous—placed into a vein; often used to refer to the fluid being given directly into a vein

intubation—the placement of a tube into an organ or passage; often used to refer to placing an endotracheal tube into the trachea

invasive—any procedure that involves the insertion or placement of a device through the skin or into a body orifice or cavity

inversion—turning in an inward direction

irrigant—fluid used for irrigation

irrigate—to wash out with water or a medicated solution

isolation—a set of actions taken so that organisms cannot be readily transferred from a person with an infection to another person

isometric exercises—contracting and relaxing the muscles voluntarily without obvious movement of the part

isotonic—having the same osmolarity or osmolality as another fluid; fluids isotonic with the blood do not cause the movement of fluids from one body compartment to another

isotope—a radioactive substance used for diagnosis and treatment

IV cannula—a general term referring to all types of percutaneous devices used for vascular access, including small steel needles (as found on butterfly and scalp vein devices) and plastic catheters

IV lock—a device filled with normal saline or heparinized solution used to provide vascular access; also called heparin lock

J

JCAHO—Joint Commission for the Accreditation of Healthcare Organizations; a voluntary organization that acts as the primary accrediting body for acute care hospitals. JCAHO also accredits home care agencies and long-term care facilities.

jejunum—the second portion of the small intestine that extends from the duodenum to the ileum

K

ketone bodies—substances synthesized by the liver as a step in the metabolism of fats; may be present in abnormal amounts in disorders such as uncontrolled diabetes mellitus

Korotkoff's sounds—the characteristic sounds, produced by the pressure of blood entering the artery during systole, that are heard on auscultation of an artery after it has been occluded

Kussmaul's respirations—deep rapid respirations, often seen in states of acidosis or renal failure

kyphosis—an exaggerated posterior curvature of the thoracic spine; produces a "humped" back

L

labia—the lips or folds of tissue that surround the female perineum

lactase—an enzyme secreted by the intestine and necessary for the digestion of lactose (sugar found in milk)

laminar airflow hood—a device that provides a controlled flow of microorganism-free air layers within a hood; used to create an environment for the sterile preparation of medications

lancet—a small, sharp device for piercing the tissue

laparotomy—a surgical incision into any part of the abdominal wall

lateral—toward the side; away from the midline of the body

lather—a light foam that is formed by soap or detergent agitated in water

lavage—washing, especially of a hollow organ (stomach or lower bowel) by repeated injections of water

left lateral position—lying on the left side with the top leg placed forward for balance

legal rights—rights that are supported by law and upholdable in court

legibility—capable of being read or deciphered

lesion—a wound or injury in which tissue is damaged

Levin's tube—a slender rubber or plastic tube that is usually used for decompression or naso-gastric feedings; also called nasogastric tube

lingula—the projection from the lower portion of the upper lobe of the left lung

liniment—a medicinal fluid that is applied to the skin by rubbing

lipids—fats; term used to indicate the fat emulsion given as part of total parenteral nutrition

liter—the metric equivalent of 1.0567 quarts, equal to 1,000 milliliters

lithotomy position—a position in which a person lies on the back with legs flexed and spread apart

litmus paper—white paper that is impregnated with litmus and is used as an acid-base indicator

liver biopsy—excision of liver tissue for micro-scopic examination

livor mortis—skin discoloration that occurs after blood circulation stops due to the release of hemoglobin from the red blood cells that are breaking down

LOB (loss of balance)—abbreviation used to expedite documentation related to activity; indicator of the presence or absence of loss of balance during standing, transfer, or ambulation

lobes—subdivisions of the lungs that are bounded by fissures and connective tissue

local—of or affecting a limited part of the body; not systemic

logrolling—turning a patient so that the entire body turns at one time with no twisting

loss of balance—see LOB

Luer-Lok—a brand name that is commonly used to refer to a type of syringe tip that fastens securely to a needle by a twisting action

lumbar puncture (LP)—also called spinal tap; the insertion of a needle into the spinal canal for purposes of withdrawing spinal fluid or instilling contrast media

lumbosacral—pertaining to the lumbar and sacral regions of the spinal column

lumen—the inner, open space of a needle, tube, or vessel

lung—spongy, saclike respiratory organs

M

maceration—skin area softened by prolonged contact with moisture, followed by deterioration

macrodrip—intravenous infusion administration set that delivers 10 to 20 drops/mL

macular—a skin rash consisting of separate, circular flat reddened spots

malleable—capable of being shaped or formed

malnutrition—a condition in which a person has less than the body's requirements of essential nutrients

manometer—an instrument that measures the pressure of liquids and gases

MAR—see medication administration record

meatus—the opening of the urethra onto the surface of the body

medial—toward the midline of the body

mediastinal shift—movement of the heart and great vessels toward one side of the chest due to intrathoracic pressure in the opposite side of the chest

mediastinal tube—a chest drainage tube used to drain secretions from a surgical wound in the mediastinum

mediastinum—an area in the center of the chest that contains the heart, great vessels, trachea, esophagus, thymus gland, and lymph nodes

medical asepsis—clean technique used to reduce the number of microorganisms; the technique designed to prevent the spread of microorganisms from one person (or area) to another

medical examiner—a public official, usually a forensic pathologist, whose function it is to investigate deaths that result from traumatic causes (homicide, suicide, accident) and sudden natural deaths in the absence of medical attention

medication administration—the process of giving medications to an individual or group

medication administration record (MAR)—record that identifies, lists, and documents the medications administered to a patient

meniscus—the curved upper surface of a liquid column

mental practice—a technique of reviewing a manual activity in the mind while "feeling" and "seeing" oneself performing each step correctly

metabolism—the complex of physical and chem-ical processes concerned with the disposition of the nutrients absorbed into the blood following digestion

methicillin-resistant *staphylococcus aureus* (MRSA)—a strain of a common microorganism that does not respond to treatment with the antibiotic methicillin. MRSA is a serious nosocomial infection spread through simple contact.

microdrip—intravenous infusion administration set that delivers 60 gtt/mL

microorganisms—animals or plants of microscopic size, especially viruses, bacteria, fungi, or protozoans

midclavicular line—an imaginary line running vertically through the midway point of the clavicle or collarbone

midline catheter—catheter inserted into a large upper arm vein to deliver solutions that do not require the large blood flow of the central veins; can be used for 2 to 4 weeks

military time—a system for noting time in which time is recorded as part of a 24-hour cycle, beginning at midnight. Hours before 10:00 a.m. are noted with a zero before the hour; minutes after the hour are noted immediately after the numbers for the hour. For example, 15 minutes after 1:00 a.m. would be recorded as 0115; the hours after noon are numbered 13, 14, and so on, so 15 minutes after 1:00 p.m. would be 1315.

minibottle—a small container for intravenous infusion solutions

Minimum Data Set (MDS)—a standardized data collection form that is required in nursing homes by federal government regulations

mini–IV bag—small plastic bags containing intravenous medications in 50 to 100 mL of fluid

mitered corner—a method of folding a sheet or blanket to achieve a smooth angled covering over the corner of the mattress

morgue—a place in a healthcare facility where the bodies of deceased patients are temporarily held pending release to a mortician, coroner (medical examiner), or other authorized person

mortician—a funeral director and embalmer who is responsible for the care and disposition of a deceased person

mortuary—a place where a deceased person is prepared for burial or cremation

MRSA (See methicillin-resistant *staphylococcus aureus*)

mucous—description pertaining to mucus (adjective)

mucus—the viscous suspension of mucin, water, cells, and inorganic salts that is secreted as a protective lubricant coating by glands in the mucous membranes (noun)

N

narcotic—drug derived from opium or opiumlike compounds (opioids) with potent analgesic and sedative effects and with the potential for dependence, tolerance, and addiction

nares—the openings in the nasal cavities; the nostrils

narrative charting—the traditional style of recording data on a patient's record in a time-sequenced storylike form

nasal mucosa—the mucous membrane lining of the nose

nasal speculum—an instrument used to dilate the nostrils for purposes of inspecting or treating the nasal passages

nasogastric tube—a long slender rubber or plastic tube that is introduced through the nose and esophagus into the stomach for purposes of feeding or aspiration

nasopharynx—the part of the pharynx immediately behind the nasal cavity and above the soft palate

nasotracheal tube—a tube that is inserted through a patient's nose into the trachea to maintain an open airway

nebulizer—a device that converts a liquid into a fine spray

necrosis—the death of living tissue

needle—the part of a drug or fluid delivery device that pierces the skin

needleless system—a method of access to IV tubing that does not utilize sharp instruments for puncture

net binder—a tube made of netlike material that is used to secure dressings to the body

neurosensory—sensory function that is innervated by the nervous system, relating to seeing, hearing, smelling, tasting, and feeling

neurotoxic—damaging to neural tissue

neurovascular status—neurologic (motor and sensory components) and circulatory functioning of a body part

next-of-kin—the closest relative of a person

noncoring needle—a needle constructed so that it cuts a slit in a rubber stopper or diaphragm and does not cut out a cylindrical core

nonvolumetric—refers to a kind of IV infusion pump designed to deliver solution at a constant *rate* (not volume) over a specified period

normal flora—usual microorganisms that inhabit the body and may serve as part of the body's natural defense mechanisms

normal saline—a solution of sodium chloride with the same osmolality or tonicity as body fluid, 0.9% saline

nosocomial—acquired in a healthcare institution

NPO—nothing by mouth; nothing to eat or drink, from the Latin *non per os*

nursing diagnosis—the intellectual processes of sorting and classifying data collected, recognizing patterns and discrepancies, comparing these with norms, and identifying patient responses to health problems that are amenable to nursing intervention; also the end statement of the nursing analysis, which includes a statement of the problem and its etiology

nursing history—the initial data gathered through interview by the nurse

nursing process—a thoughtful, deliberate use of a problem-solving approach to nursing

nystagmus—involuntary (vertical or horizontal) rapid, rhythmic movement of the eyeball

O

objective—based on observable phenomena

objective data—data that can be seen or measured

obturator—any device that closes the opening in a channel, such as a tracheostomy tube

occiput—the posterior, inferior portion of the cranium

occult—hidden

ocular—of or pertaining to the eye

ointment—one of the numerous, highly viscous or semisolid substances that are used on the skin as a cosmetic, an emollient, or a medicament; an unguent; a salve

ombudsman—an official designated to act as an advocate for a member of the public in disputes with a healthcare agency

open suctioning—the traditional method of suctioning, where a new suction catheter is opened and used each time the patient needs suctioning

ophthalmic—of or pertaining to the eye or eyes; ocular

ophthalmoscope—an instrument that consists of a light and a disk with an opening through which the interior of the eye is examined

opioid—drug derived from opium or opiumlike compounds, with potent analgesic and sedative effects, and with the potential for dependence, tolerance, and addiction; a narcotic

opposition—positioned opposite one another; for example, the thumb to the fingers

organ/tissue donation—a donation of organs and/or tissues for transplantation through a personal pre-death bequest or through the bequest of the family after death

organization—systematic approach to technical skills

oronasal—the area between the mouth and the nose

oropharynx—the part of the pharynx between the soft palate and the upper edge of the epiglottis

orthopnea—a state in which a person has difficulty breathing in the recumbent position and is relieved by sitting upright or standing

orthopneic—see orthopnea

orthostatic hypotension—a sudden drop in blood pressure that is caused by a change in position, from lying to sitting or standing; may cause dizziness, fainting, and falling; also called postural hypotension

osmolarity—refers to the number of osmotically active particles in a unit of fluid

ostomate—a person who has an ostomy

ostomy—a surgically constructed opening from a body organ to the exterior of the body

otic—of or pertaining to the ear

otoscope—an instrument for inspecting the ears, consisting of a light and a cone

out of bed (OOB)—refers to movement from lying in bed to sitting or standing to maintain and restore muscle tone, stimulate respiration and circulation, and improve elimination

outpatient—a patient who comes to the hospital, clinic, or dispensary for diagnosis and/or treatment but does not remain for ongoing care

ova—the female reproductive cells of animals; eggs

oximetry—see pulse oximetry

oxygenation—treating, combining, or infusing with oxygen

oxygen saturation—a measurement of the oxygen content of the blood compared with the oxygen capacity of the blood expressed as a percentage; calculated by dividing the oxygen content by the oxygen capacity

P

packed red blood cells—components of blood that make up the blood product remaining after most of the plasma is removed from whole blood

palpation—examining or exploring by touch

para—prefix used with numerals to designate the number of pregnancies a woman has had in which a viable fetus (over 20 weeks' gestation or 500 g weight) is produced

paracentesis—the insertion of a trocar into the abdominal cavity for the removal of excess fluid

paralysis—loss or impairment of the ability to move or have sensation in a bodily part as a result of injury to or disease of its nerve supply

paralytic ileus—bowel inactivity and paralysis resulting in abdominal distension and acute obstruction

paraparesis—A weakness or partial paralysis of the lower extremities

parasites—any organisms that grow, feed, and are sheltered on or in a host organism while contributing nothing to the host's survival

parenteral—administered into the body in a manner other than through the digestive (enteral) tract; for example, through intramuscular or intravenous injection

parenteral fluid—fluid given directly into tissues or blood vessels

parietal pleura—the serous membrane that lines the walls of the thoracic cavity

Parkinson's position—supine position with the patient's head tilted back hanging over the edge of the bed and tilted to one side, to facilitate the administration of nose drops

partial weight-bearing—see PWB

particulate matter—material made up of particles, often airborne or undissolved in a liquid

password—a code that provides an individual with access to data or computerized files

patellar tendon—a continuation of the quadriceps tendon that leads from the patella to the tibia

patent—open; unobstructed

pathogen—any agents, especially microorganisms, such as bacteria or funguses, that cause disease

pathogenic organism—a microorganism that causes disease

pathologist—a physician who specializes in pathology

pathology—the study of structural and functional changes caused by a disease process

pectoralis muscles—four muscles of the chest

pedal pulse—a pulse wave that can be palpated over the arteries of the feet

penis—external male reproductive and urinary organ

Penrose drain—a flat, soft, latex tubing; used to provide drainage from a surgical wound, or to act as a tourniquet

percussion—a process of striking a finger held against the body surface with a fingertip of the opposite hand and listening to the resulting sound as part of assessment; also the striking of a hand on the chest wall to produce a vibration or shock that loosens secretions retained in the lungs

percutaneous—refers to any device or substance that enters the body through the skin

percutaneous endoscopic gastrostomy (PEG)—the insertion of a "mushroom" catheter through the abdominal wall into the stomach, using an endoscope to ensure correct placement within the stomach

percutaneous introducer—a special device used to insert a tracheostomy at the patient's bedside

perineum—the portion of the body in the pelvic area that is occupied by urogenital passages and the rectum

perioperative—the time around surgery; includes immediate preoperative, intraoperative, and postoperative periods

periorbital edema—edema around the eyes or the orbits

peripherally inserted central catheter (PICC)—intravenous catheter that is inserted into a peripheral vein and threaded into the vessel until the tip reaches a central vein

periphery—the outermost part or region, away from the center of the body

peristalsis—wavelike muscular contractions that propel contained matter along the alimentary canal

personal protective equipment (PPE)—equipment or clothing used by healthcare personnel to protect themselves from direct exposure to patient blood or body fluid. Types of PPE include gloves, gowns, protective eyewear, head coverings, foot coverings, and face shields and masks.

petaling—forming adhesive or moleskin "petals" by cutting strips into pointed or rounded ends and tucking around the rough edges of a cast in such a way that the skin is protected

pH—a measure of the acidity or alkalinity of a solution; 7.0 is neutral, numbers below that indicate an acid solution, and numbers above it indicate an alkaline solution, in a range of 1 to 14

pharynx—the section of the digestive tract that extends from the nasal cavities to the larynx, there becoming continuous with the esophagus; functions as a passageway for both food and air

PHI—protected health information; information about the patient that relates to his or her health problems or healthcare

phlebitis—inflammation of a vein

physical practice—performing the movements for a skill to develop proficiency

piggyback—an intravenous infusion setup in which a second container is attached to the tubing of the primary container through a short tubing apparatus

pinna—the flaring portion of the external ear that aids in the reception of sound waves; the auricle

pinwheel—a wheel-like instrument with sharp points that is used to test peripheral sensation of the body

pitting edema—type of edema seen when fingertips pressed into the tissue leave a depression behind; rated on a scale of 1+ to 4+

pivotal joint—a joint in which the axis or protuberance rests in the atlas or cavity of another; the neck is an example of a pivotal joint

planning—the second step in the nursing process, in which information is reviewed and synthesized to form goals and a plan of action

plantar flexion—bending the foot so that the toes point downward

plasma—the liquid portion of the blood after red and white blood cells and platelets are removed

plaster of Paris—cast material made of calcium sulfate, which, when combined with water, forms gypsum, producing a light but rigid and durable structure

platelets—small, disk-shaped cell fragments in the blood that adhere to any damaged surface and begin the clotting process; also called thrombocytes

pleural friction rub—sound caused by the rubbing together of inflamed and roughened pleural surfaces

pleural space—a potential space formed by the visceral and parietal pleura and containing only enough lubricating fluid to allow the two surfaces to slide smoothly over each other during inhalation and exhalation

pleural tube—a chest drainage tube used to drain secretions from the pleural space

plunger—in a syringe, the pistonlike rod that expels the fluid from the barrel

pneumonitis—acute inflammation of the lung

pneumothorax—accumulation of air or gas in the pleural cavity; occurs as a result of disease or injury or sometimes is induced to collapse the lung in the treatment of tuberculosis or other lung diseases

popliteal artery—the major artery that extends from the femoral artery down behind the knee

popliteal space—the hollow area behind the knee joint

Port-a-cath—trade name of a surgically inserted subcutaneous central venous access port

positive nitrogen balance—a condition in which the amount of nitrogen taken into the body is greater than the amount excreted

postanesthesia care unit (PACU)—a nursing unit where patients are cared for as they emerge from anesthesia immediately following surgery; formerly termed recovery room (see also postanesthesia recovery room)

postanesthesia recovery room (PARR)—area of the hospital set aside for the care of the immediate postoperative patient; also called recovery room (RR) or postanesthesia care unit (PACU)

post-exposure prophylaxis (PEP)—refers to providing medical treatment to an individual after known exposure to a serious communicable disease, before disease develops

postmortem examination—see autopsy

postoperative bed—also called the surgical bed or anesthetic bed; bed made so that a patient can be transferred after surgery from stretcher to bed with a minimum of motion and discomfort, then easily and quickly covered with bed linens, including a blanket, to prevent chilling

postural drainage—using positioning and the force of gravity to help drain lung secretions

postural hypotension—a sudden drop in blood pressure that is caused by a change in position, from lying to sitting or standing; may cause dizziness, fainting, and falling; also called orthostatic hypotension

prefilled cartridge—disposable glass container with an attached needle that fits into a holder for injection; contains a single dose of medication

preformed water—the water content of ingested foods

pressure ulcer—erosion of the skin and potentially the underlying tissue, commonly over bony prominences, caused by excessive pressure; sometimes called a decubitus ulcer

pretibial edema—fluid accumulated in the tissue over the tibia

primary intention healing—uncomplicated wound healing that occurs when tissue is constructed between two wound surfaces that touch; see also first intention healing

prism glasses—eyeglasses that direct the vision upward and then horizontally so that a patient in the supine position can see television or read books

privacy—the right to have matters of a personal nature not shared with anyone who does not have a need to know them

problem-oriented medical record (POR or POMR)—a system of keeping medical records organized according to the patient's problems

proctoscopy—procedure by which a physician uses a hollow lighted instrument called a proctoscope to examine and treat the rectum and lower part of the sigmoid colon

Proetz position—the patient is supine with a pillow or other support under the shoulders so that the head tilts straight back to facilitate the administration of nose drops

profuse—plentiful, overflowing, copious

pronation—turning the palm or inner surface of the hand or forearm downward

prone position—a position in which the patient lies on the abdomen with the head turned to one side

prongs—sharp or pointed projections; a device that delivers oxygen at the nostrils

prophylactic—acting to defend against or to prevent something, especially disease

protected health information—see PHI

protein—an organic compound that contains amino acids as its basic structural unit

protocol—a formal process for addressing a particular situation

protuberance—an area of the body that protrudes above the usual surface, such as a distended abdomen or enlargement over a joint

proximal—near the center part of the body or a point of attachment, or origin

pruritus—itching

psi—pounds per square inch; a measure of pressure that is applied against an object

ptosis—paralytic drooping of the upper eyelid caused by nerve failure

pulley—a grooved wheel that allows free movement of a rope

pulmonary embolus—obstruction of the pulmonary artery or one of its branches by an embolus

pulse deficit—the difference in rate between apical and radial pulses

pulse oximetry—a procedure for measuring the oxygen saturation of the blood by measuring the reflectance of light transmitted through a translucent part of the skin such as the ear lobe or fingertip by hemoglobin; also called oximetry

pulse pressure—the difference between systolic and diastolic blood pressure readings

pureed—pulverized and strained, as in food

purulent—containing or secreting pus

PWB (partial weight bearing)—an abbreviation used to expedite documentation related to activity; used when the patient can bear only partial weight on the affected lower extremity

pyloric valve—the valve between the stomach and the duodenum

pyrexia—fever

Q

quad cane—a cane with a four-legged base for stability

quadriceps setting—an isometric exercise that involves contraction of the quadricep muscles where there is little or no movement. Potential benefits are increased venous blood flow; on a long-term basis increased muscle mass, tone, and strength occur.

quadriplegia—paralysis of all four extremities

R

radial—body area on the thumb side of the forearm at the wrist

radial artery—the artery that descends from the brachial artery along the radius of the arm; most common and convenient site for measuring pulse rate of an adult

radial deviation—bending the hand on the wrist in the direction of the thumb (toward the radius bone)

radiolucent—a surface through which x-rays can be taken

rales—abnormal or pathologic respiratory sounds heard on auscultation; also called crackles

reagent—a substance that is used in a chemical reaction to detect, measure, examine, or produce other substances

rebound tenderness—the pain or discomfort that is experienced when pressure is quickly withdrawn from an area

recipient—person receiving something, such as blood, tissue, or an organ as a transfusion or transplant

reconstituted—characterized by mixing a powder with a liquid to become a solution; used to describe a powdered medication prepared for injection

record—documentation of care provided; legal document

recovery room (RR)—an area of a hospital set aside for the care of the immediate postoperative patient; also called postanesthesia care unit (PACU)

recumbent—lying down position

recurrent fold bandage—a bandage that is wrapped in such a way that it recurs, or folds over, on itself

red blood cells (RBCs)—blood cells that carry oxygen; also called erythrocytes

reduction—in relationship to a fracture, the process of placing the fractured ends in alignment so that bone healing can occur

referral—a specific plan for directing a patient or client to other healthcare resources

reflectance—infrared technology used to measure the temperature; used in tympanic thermometers

reflex contraction—an involuntary response of muscle contraction

reflex hammer—a small rubber-headed hammer that is used to test body reflexes; also called a percussion hammer

reflux—the return of fluid substance backward through a valve that is not working correctly. For example, esophageal reflux refers to stomach contents moving into the esophagus; ureteral reflux refers to urine moving from the bladder into the ureters.

regurgitate—to vomit

regurgitation—see regurgitate

renal calculi—kidney stones

repetitive strain injury—also called repetitive stress injury; injury resulting from repetitive motion over time; an example is carpal tunnel syndrome

repose—condition of rest, calm, and tranquility

reservoir—a container used to hold a fluid for continuous administration, such as in tube feeding

resonance—in percussion, a vibrating sound that is produced in the normal chest

respect—regard for the intrinsic worth of a person

respirator—a mechanical apparatus that administers artificial respiration; a ventilator

respiratory arrest—the sudden cessation of breathing

respite—an interval of rest or relief

resuscitate—to revive or restore to life

retention catheter—see indwelling catheter

retraction—an abnormal pulling in of soft tissue of the chest on inspiration; commonly seen in the supraclavicular, intercostal, and substernal areas

reverse spiral bandage—a bandage that is applied, usually on a limb, in a circular fashion with a reverse fold

rhonchi—coarse rattling sounds that are produced by secretions in the bronchial tubes; also called gurgles

rhythm—pattern of motion or activity; in reference to the heart, pattern of pulsations

right atrium—the chamber on the right side of the heart that receives unoxygenated blood from the body

rigor mortis—muscle stiffening after death

roll bandage—bandaging material that has been rolled to provide for easier application; commonly used to refer to rolls of gauze

rotation—a circular movement around a fixed axis

Roto-Rest bed—an electrically operated special bed that turns side to side continuously. Cervical, thoracic, and rectal areas can be cared for through posterior hatches.

route—in reference to medication, a path of administration

rubber-shod hemostat—the presence of rubber tubing over the tips of hemostats or Kelly clamps to make them less traumatic to tissue or less likely to damage a tube on which the clamp is placed

S

saddle joint—a joint, such as the thumb, in which two bones rest together in convex-concave position

saliva—the secretion of the salivary gland, which contains mucus and digestive enzymes

salvaged blood transfusion—a transfusion using blood that is recovered and processed during a surgical procedure in order to be reinfused into the patient

sanction—authoritative permission or approval; conversely, specific disapproval by a formal group

sanguineous—containing blood as in sanguineous drainage

SBA (standby assist)—an abbreviation used to expedite documentation related to activity; used when the patient needs someone present during activity (especially transfer and ambulation) for assessment and possible assistance even if that individual usually does not need to provide actual support

scab—the hardened crust over a wound formed by dried exudates

scalpel—a sharp surgical knife

sclerosed—development of connective tissue or scarring; sclerosis of a blood vessel occludes the vessel

scoliosis—an abnormal lateral curvature of the spine

secondary intention healing—healing that occurs through granulation beginning at the base of the wound, also called second intention healing

secretions—substances that are exuded from cells or blood

segment—a subdivision of a lobe of the lung

self-care—the ability to manage one's own life in such a way as to meet one's own needs

self-determination—the right to make personal decisions

semi-Fowler's position—a supine position with the head raised 12 to 18 inches; see also Fowler's position

sensory deprivation—a lower level of sensory input than that required by an individual for optimum functioning

septicemia—an infection in which the pathogens are circulating in the bloodstream

septic transfusion reaction—systemic infection caused by the transfusion of a bacterially contaminated blood component with signs and symptoms that may include high fever (>20° Celsius), chills, rigors, nausea, vomiting, diarrhea, hypotension, or shock

sequential compression device—an electronic device used to provide intermittent compression over the lower leg and/or thigh to promote venous return and prevent deep vein thrombosis and pulmonary embolism; amounts of pressure may be adjusted on an attached control unit

serosanguineous—containing serum and blood as in serosanguineous drainage

serous—containing, secreting, or resembling serum

serum hepatitis—a form of hepatitis caused by a virus transmitted primarily by blood and body fluids; also called hepatitis B

shaft—on a needle, the long narrow stem

shear—a situation in which there are two parallel forces, each acting in a different direction. For example, when a patient is sitting up in bed, friction causes skin to adhere to bedding and exerts a force on the skin holding it in place, and body weight causes underlying tissue to move downward in a parallel but opposite direction to the force of the friction.

shearing force—the sum of the two parallel forces acting in opposite directions

shock—a state of insufficient blood supply to vital tissue as a result of a massive physiologic reaction to bodily illness or trauma, usually characterized by marked loss of blood pressure and the depression of vital processes; caused by hemorrhage, infection, trauma, and the like

shroud—a cloth used to wrap a dead body

side-lying position—a position in which the patient is on the side with the head supported on a low pillow

sigmoid flexure—the distal portion of the colon, which appears as an S-shaped curve preceding the rectum

sigmoidoscopy—procedure in which a physician uses a tubular instrument with a light, called a sigmoidoscope, for inspection and treatment of the sigmoid colon

silicone—a flexible material used in the manufacture of tubes and prosthetic devices

Sims' position—a side-lying position with the top leg flexed forward

singultus—hiccup

six rights—systematic checks and careful procedures implemented to promote safe medication administration; check for the right *drug,* right *dose,* right *route,* right *time,* right *patient,* and right *documentation*

skin barrier—an agent to protect the skin from the discharge of urine or feces

skull tongs—device inserted into each side of patient's cranium as an attachment for the application of traction

skull tongs traction—see skull tongs

sling—commercially produced or homemade fabric device used to rest or immobilize the arm in a right-angle position

slough—necrotic or dead tissue that is separated from the living tissue in a wound

smegma—a thick whitish substance, composed of epithelial cells and mucus, which is found around external genitalia

Snellen chart—a chart printed with black letters in gradually decreasing sizes, used in testing vision

SOAP—an acronym for a format used to record progress notes in relation to an identified problem consisting of **s**ubjective data, **o**bjective data, **a**ssessment (analysis), **p**lan

sordes—accumulation of dried secretions and bacteria in the mouth caused by not eating, mouth-breathing, and inadequate oral hygiene

speaking valve—a valve that can be placed over a cuffed tracheostomy tube to allow the patient to speak

specific gravity—a measurement of the concentration of urine; overhydration leads to a low specific-gravity figure; dehydration results in a high figure

sphenoid sinus—the open area in the center of the sphenoid bone that lies at the base of the brain

sphincter—a circular muscle that controls an internal or external orifice

sphygmomanometer—an instrument that measures blood pressure in the arteries

spiral bandage—a bandage that is applied, usually on a limb, in a circular ascending fashion

splinting—holding the incisional area firmly; minimizing movement to decrease pain. Splinting can be accomplished by spreading the hands and holding them firmly over the incision, or the patient can hold the incision with his or her own hands, or a pillow can be held firmly over the incision area to splint it.

spore—an asexual, usually single-celled reproductive organism that is characteristic of non-flowering plants, such as fungi, mosses, and ferns; a microorganism in a dormant or resting state that is especially resistant to destruction

spreader bar—a bar that extends across a traction frame to allow traction pull to be aligned as needed

sputum—expectorated matter that contains secretions from the lower respiratory tract

stab wound—a small intentional wound made with a scalpel in order to introduce a trocar, tube, or drain

staging—a system of describing the characteristics of a tissue or lesion, such as a tumor or a pressure ulcer, using numbered categories; standardized pressure ulcer staging is provided by using the National Pressure Ulcer Advisory Panel's classification system

Standard Precautions—CDC guidelines for preventing transmission of microorganisms; includes protecting the self from contact with any moist body substance, including feces, urine, nasal secretions, vomitus, and sputum; includes all of the measures that are a part of Universal Precautions

stereotype—a presumed form or pattern that is attributed to a group and generalized to an individual

sterile—absence of microorganisms

sterile conscience—a moral mandate to monitor and correct one's behavior in the absence of others

sterile technique—a method of functioning that is designed to maintain the sterility of sterile objects

sterilization—complete elimination of micro-organisms

sterilize—to render sterile; see also sterile

sternum—a long, flat bone that forms the midventral support of most of the ribs; the breastbone

stertorous—refers to respiration characterized by a heavy snoring sound

stethoscope—an instrument that is used for listening to sounds produced in the body; also see bell and diaphragm

stock supply—medications kept in a general supply to be dispensed to individual patients

stockinette—a soft, stretchy, ribbed material that comes in a tube shape of different circumfer-ences. When pulled over a body part, it provides a smooth surface and protection from the inner surface of a cast.

stoma—the opening on the skin of any surgically constructed passage from a body organ to the exterior of the body

stomatitis—an inflammation of the oral mucosa

stopcock—a valve that regulates a flow of liquid through a tube

straight abdominal binder—a large cloth that is placed snugly around the lower part of the trunk to give support or to secure a dressing

straight catheter—a plain catheter without a bulb or balloon on its end

stylet—a thin metal wire or probe that fits inside a catheter or tube, making it more rigid and easier to insert

subclavian vein—a vein of the upper body that lies under the clavicle

subcutaneous (SC)—pertaining to tissue beneath the layers of the skin

subcutaneous catheter port—a wholly implanted device for access to a central vein consisting of a flexible intravenous line and a rounded metal reservoir with a rubber diaphragm, which is entered through a skin puncture with a special needle; see Port-a-Cath

subcutaneous emphysema—air trapped in the subcutaneous tissue that "crackles" when palpated

subdural—immediately under the dura mater that covers the brain and spinal cord

subjective—personal; in assessment, refers to information from the patient's viewpoint

subjective data—see subjective

sublingual—beneath the tongue

subungual—under a fingernail or toenail

suction—withdrawing (gas or fluids) through the use of negative pressure

superior vena cava—the large vein that returns blood to the heart from the upper body and head

supination—turning or placing the hand and forearm so that the palm is upward

supine position—position in which the person lies flat on the back

supporting muscles—the broad muscles of the body (back, abdomen, and legs) that facilitate effective body mechanics

suppository—a solid medication that is designed to melt in a body cavity other than the mouth

suppurating—see suppuration

suppuration—the formation or discharge of pus

suprasternal notch—the notched bone forma-tion that occurs at the uppermost end of the sternum

surgical asepsis—technique designed to main-tain the sterility of previously sterilized items and to prevent the introduction of any micro-organisms into the body

surgical bed—see postoperative bed

suspension—a relatively coarse, noncolloidal dispersion of solid particles in a liquid

sutures—the thread, gut, or wire used to stitch tissues

symmetry—the equal configuration of opposite sides

symphysis pubis—the area at the front center of the pelvis, where the pubic bones from either side fuse into one bone

symptoms—perceptions of illness reported by the individual experiencing them

synovial fluid—a secretion of the synovial sac surrounding a joint; a clear fluid that acts as a lubricating agent for the movement of the joint

syringe—a medical instrument that is used to aspirate and inject fluids

syrup—a concentrated solution of sugar in water; a medicinal syrup has a drug added to the solution

systemic—of or pertaining to, or affecting, the entire body

systole—the rhythmic contraction of the heart, especially of the ventricles, by which blood is driven through the aorta and pulmonary artery after each dilation, or diastole

systolic blood pressure—the highest pressure reached in the arteries, created by the contraction of the ventricles of the heart

T

tablet—a small, flat pellet of medication that is taken orally

tachycardia—an abnormally rapid heartbeat, usually defined as more than 100 beats/minute, in the adult

tachypnea—very rapid respirations

taut—pulled or drawn tight

T-binder—a binder with a single tail that is used to hold a dressing in place on the perineum of a female patient

technical competence—skill in the performance of tasks

technical proficiency—see technical competence

TEDs—a brand name that is commonly used as a synonym for compression or antiembolism stockings; see antiembolism stockings

temporal artery—one of the two three-branched arteries that lie at the temple of the head

tension pneumothorax—a situation in which air gets trapped in the pleural space leading to buildup of pressure, which collapses the lung and causes mediastinal shift

tepid—lukewarm

test dose—a small amount of any substance that is given in order to assess for adverse reactions before regular administration is begun

testes—the bilateral external male genitalia that produce semen

thermistor—a resistor made of semiconductors that has resistance that varies rapidly and predictably with temperature; able to measure extremely small temperature changes

thoracentesis—the insertion of a chest tube into the pleural space of the chest for the removal of abnormal fluid or air

thoracotomy—a surgical incision into the chest wall

thready pulse—a weak, faint pulse

three checks—a safety measure used to ensure procuring of correct drug. The label is checked (1) before picking up the medication, (2) while holding it in the hand, and (3) after returning the container to its storage place.

three-way catheter—a catheter that can be connected to irrigant by one channel and to drainage by another

thrombocytopenia—fewer than normal number of platelets

thrombophlebitis—inflammation of a vein resulting from a thrombus (blood clot)

thrombus—clot formed in a blood vessel

thyroid gland—a two-lobed endocrine gland that is located in front of and on either side of the trachea

tidaling—fluctuation of the water level in the long tube in the waterseal bottle of a chest drainage system

tidal volume—the volume of air moved in or out during a normal breath

toe pleat—a method of folding top bed linen to provide extra room for the feet

tolerance—in activity, the capacity to endure

Toomey syringe—a large-barreled syringe with a graduated tip that fits into tubing

topical—applied or pertaining to a local part of the body

torsion—the act or condition of being twisted or turned; the stress caused when one end of an object is twisted in one direction and the other end is held motionless or twisted in the opposite direction

torso—the trunk of the human body

tortuous—having or marked by repeated turns or bends; winding; twisting

tourniquet—any device that is used to stop temporarily the flow of blood through a large artery in a limb

trachea—a thin-walled tube of cartilaginous and membranous tissue that descends from the larynx to the bronchi, carrying air to the lungs

tracheal ring—the proximal, cartilaginous ringlike structure that surrounds the trachea

tracheostomy—a surgically devised opening into the trachea from the surface of the neck

traction—a pulling force applied to bones; usually used to reduce bone fractures

trade (brand) name—name given to a generic drug by the manufacturer of the drug; an example of a trade name is Tylenol (acetaminophen is the generic drug); see generic name

transdermal—in reference to medication; topical administration route by which some medications are absorbed from the skin to provide systemic effects

transfer belt—see gait (transfer) belt

transfer needle—a double-ended needle used to transfer medication from the medication container to the fluid container prior to intravenous administration

transfusion related acute lung injury (TRALI)—a reaction that occurs when the blood component contains leukocyte antibodies that react with the patient's leukocytes, causing damage to the pulmonary microvasculature. Possible signs and symptoms include dyspnea, hypoxemia, bilateral pulmonary edema, hypotension and fever.

Transmission-Based Precautions—a system for establishing isolation precautions for the patient with an infection; based on the way the particular infection is transmitted

transtracheal—across the trachea; in reference to catheters that deliver oxygen directly into the trachea. A transtracheal catheter is a small-diameter plastic tube with several openings near the tip; it is surgically inserted into the trachea to deliver oxygen with reasonable safety and economy.

transverse colon—the portion of the colon across the top of the abdomen from the hepatic flexure to the splenic flexure

transverse colostomy—a colostomy performed on a portion of the transverse colon

trapeze—a short, horizontal bar suspended from a frame over the top of a bed; a trapeze is used by the patient to facilitate moving in bed and transferring

tremor—an involuntary trembling motion of the body

Trendelenburg's position—position in which the head is lower than the feet, with the body on an inclined plane

triage—a process that prioritizes patients according to their condition so that the most expedient and appropriate treatment can be given to a large number of patients

trocar—a small, sharp, pointed metal rod used as an instrument to enter a body cavity

trochanter—the bony processes below the head of the femur; often used to refer to the greater trochanter, which is on the lateral aspect of the femur

trochanter roll—a cylindrical roll made from a sheet, bath towel, or pad that is placed firmly beside the hip to stabilize the hip joint and prevent the leg from rotating outward

tube feeding—the process of providing nutrients through a tube directly into the gastrointestinal tract for the person who is unable to eat a regular diet; liquid formula of nutrients instilled through a tube for the patient who is unable to eat a regular diet

tuning fork—a small two-pronged instrument that, when struck, produces a sound of fixed pitch; used to test auditory acuity

tunneling—extension of undermining; tunneling occurs when a wound opens into deeper tissue; see undermining

turgor—normal tissue fullness in relationship to superficial body fluids

twist support—a strong plaster bar between two casted extremities or between a casted extremity and the body cast, formed by twisting a wetted plaster roll during the application of a cast

tympanic—referring to the drumlike covering of the middle ear or to drumlike sounds heard on auscultation

tympanic membrane—the thin, semi-transparent, oval-shaped membrane that separates the middle ear from the inner ear; also called eardrum

tympany—in percussion, a low-pitched, drumlike sound

type and crossmatch—a laboratory process carried out prior to transfusion to avoid hemolytic transfusion reaction; the process is used to identify whether the donor's and the recipient's blood are compatible. First, the blood group (A, B, AB, or O) and Rh type is determined. Next, testing is performed to determine if the recipient has antibodies that may interact with the donor's red blood cells.

U

ulnar deviation—bending the hand on the wrist in the direction of the ulna, toward the fifth, or small finger

umbilicus—navel, belly button

undermining—process characterized by extension of an open wound under the wound edges

unit dose—a system of dispensing drugs in which each dose is packaged and labeled individually

Universal Precautions—a set of behaviors designed to prevent the transmission of blood-borne microorganisms by being used on all patients at all times

ureterostomy—a surgically devised opening in which a ureter is brought out to drain directly through a stoma onto the abdomen

urethra—the tubular structure leading from the bladder to the surface of the body

urethral meatus—the opening of the urethra onto the surface of the body through which urine is passed

urinal—a receptacle for urine that is used by bedridden patients

urinalysis—the chemical analysis of urine, which commonly includes color, clarity, pH, specific gravity, and checks for glucose, red blood cells, casts, and white blood cells

urination—the act of excreting urine

urine refractometer—a microscope-like instrument that refracts a beam of light through a drop of urine to give a reading of specific gravity; may be used by nurses on the patient care unit

urinometer—an instrument that is used to determine the specific gravity of urine using the principle of displacement

uvula—the small, conical fleshy mass of tissue that is suspended from the center of the soft palate above the back of the tongue

V

vagina—the passage leading from the external genital orifice to the uterus in female mammals

vaginal—pertaining to the vagina

vaginal speculum—an instrument that is used to dilate the vagina for purposes of inspecting or treating the vaginal passages or to obtain a specimen for a diagnostic test

vancomycin-resistant *staphylococcus aureus* (VRSA)—a strain of a common microorganism that is resistant to the antibiotic vancomycin. This organism is responsible for serious nosocomial infections that can be spread through simple contact.

vasoconstriction—a decrease in the lumen of blood vessels created by contraction of smooth muscle in the vessel wall

vasodilation—an increase in the lumen of blood vessels created by the relaxation of smooth muscle in the vessel wall

vectorborne transmission—the method by which diseases are transmitted via an intermediate host, such as a mosquito

venipuncture—the puncture of a vein; for example, in drawing blood or administering intravenous fluids and medication

venous—of or pertaining to a vein or veins

venous pressure—the pressure of blood in the veins; often measured in the superior vena cava. This measurement, called central venous pressure (CVP) is normally between 4 and 10 cm water.

venous thrombosis—formation of a blood clot inside a vein

ventilator—a mechanical device used to assist the patient to breathe, but patient must have an artificial airway in place, such as an endotracheal, nasotracheal, or tracheostomy tube

ventricular fibrillation—a cardiac arrhythmia characterized by rapid contractions of the ventricular muscle fibers without coordinated ventricular contraction; frequent cause of cardiac arrest

vesicant—any agent that can cause blistering or necrosis of tissue

vial—a small glass container that is sealed with a rubber stopper; may be used for single or multiple doses of a parenteral medication

vibration—a rapid, rhythmic to-and-fro motion used on the chest to loosen secretions

visceral pleura—the serous membrane that covers the outside walls of the lungs

viscosity—the degree of resistance to flow; thickness

vital signs—blood pressure, respiratory rate, pulse rate, and temperature

void—to empty any body cavity; most commonly the emptying of urine from the bladder through the urethra; to urinate

volumetric—refers to infusion pumps; i.e., devices that deliver a specific desired *volume* over a specified period

VRSA (See vancomycin-resistant *staphylococcus aureus*)

vulva—the external female genitalia, includes the labia majora, the labia minora, the clitoris, and the vestibule of the vagina

W

walker—a rehabilitative device used for support while standing or walking

walking heel—a metal or plastic implant embedded in the heel of a plaster or fiberglass leg cast to facilitate walking

waterbed—a special water-filled mattress used to distribute pressure evenly over the body

waterseal drainage—chest drainage system that allows air to escape through a vent but prevents air from traveling back into the pleural space

WBT (weight bear as tolerated)—an abbreviation used to expedite documentation related to activity; used when the patient is permitted to bear as much weight as is comfortable on the affected lower extremity

weight-bearing—the ability of the body to bear weight; the side on which the weight of the body can be placed while standing; for example, partial weight-bearing indicates that an individual cannot stand solely on the affected limb and must have other means of support

wheal—a small acute swelling on the skin; may be caused by intradermal injections or by insect bites and allergies

wheezes—hoarse whistling sounds, produced by breathing, that are considered abnormal

whiplash—injury of the neck or cervical spine due to a sudden whiplike motion of the body

whole blood—blood drawn from a living human being, which contains all blood components and is prepared for use in transfusion

white blood cells (WBCs)—leukocytes, the infection-fighting blood cells

windowing—the procedure of cutting an opening in a cast to allow for observation, care of the skin underneath, and relief of pressure

XYZ

xiphoid process—the lower tip of the sternum at the level of the seventh rib

Yankauer suction-tip catheter—a special catheter tip designed for oral suctioning

Z-track—a method for injecting medications that are particularly irritating or which stain the tissues; injection method that prevents medication from leaking out through the needle track

Index

Page numbers followed by b indicate box; those followed by f indicate figure; those followed by t indicate table.

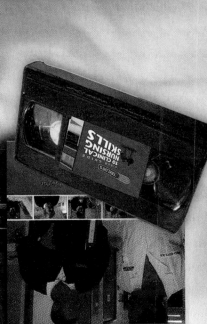